COMPREHENSIVE MATERNITY NURSING

PERINATAL AND WOMEN'S HEALTH

SECOND EDITION

Martha Ann Auvenshine, R.N., Ed.D
Professor/Chairman
Department of Nursing
California State University, Hayward, CA

Martha Gunther Enriquez, R.N., N.N.P., M.S.N.
Executive Director
Women and Infant Services
Alta Bates-Herrick Hospital, Berkeley, CA

JONES AND BARTLETT PUBLISHERS
Boston   Portola Valley

This book is dedicated to my parents, Corinne Clark and Ewell H. Auvenshine, on the occasion of their 60th wedding anniversary. They have instilled within me a love for God and family, respect for learning and an optimistic view of living for which I will always be grateful.

M.A.A.

To my husband, Tony M. Enriquez, for his love, patience, understanding, support, and encouragement. And to my children, Marco, Kayla, and Nicolas for sharing their lives with me.

M.G.E.

© 1990 by Jones and Bartlett Publishers, Inc.
All rights reserved. No part of this book may be reproduced, stored in a retrieval system, or transcribed, in any form or by any means—electronic, mechanical, photocopying, recording, or otherwise—without the prior written permission of the publisher.

Editorial, sales, and customer service offices:
Jones and Bartlett, etc
20 Park Plaza
Boston, MA 02116.

Printed in the United States of America
10 9 8 7 6 5 4 3 2 1

Library of Congress Cataloging-in-Publication Data
Comprehensive Maternity Nursing: Perinatal and Women's Health, Second Edition
    Includes bibliographies and index.
    1. Obstetrical nursing.   2. Perinatology.
I. Auvenshine, Martha Ann.   II. Enriquez, Martha Gunther.
RG951.M325   1989   610.73'678   88-28472

Production: *Editing, Design & Production, Inc.*
Text Design: *Mina Greenstein*
Cover Design: *Rafael Millán*
Illustrations: *Karl Nicholason*
Photography: *Jeff Weissman*

Additional credits appear on page 1024.

The selection and dosage of drugs presented in this book are in accord with standards accepted at the time of publication. The authors and publisher have made every effort to provide accurate information. However, research, clinical practice, and government regulations often change the accepted standard in this field. Before administering any drug, the reader is advised to check the manufacturer's product information sheet for the most up-to-date recommendations on dosage, precautions, and contraindications. This is especially important in the case of drugs that are new or seldom used.

ISBN 0-086720-421-4

Contributors

Linda Larssen Avery, RPT, ACCE
Physical Therapist
Alta Bates-Herrick Hospital
Private Practice
Berkeley and Oakland, California
Chapter 22

Christine Berman, MPH, RD
Nutrition Consultant
Private Practice
Kentfield, California
Chapter 28

Stephanie Berman, MSW, LCSW
Chief, Pediatric/Perinatal Social Services
Department of Patient and Family Services
Mount Zion Hospital and Medical Center
San Francisco, California
Chapter 35

Mary Anne Blum, RN, MSN
Assistant Professor
College of Nursing
The State University of New Jersey, Rutgers
Doctoral Candidate
Adelphi University
Chapter 31

Barbara F. Blumenthal, MA, MPH, RD
Program Specialist
Alameda County Health Care Services
Oakland, California
Chapter 12

Elizabeth O. Bridston, ED.D, MSN, RN
Assistant Professor
Bemidji State University
Bemidji, Minnesota
Chapters 43 and 44

Carolyn Spence Cagle, PH.D., RN
Associate Professor
Harris College of Nursing
Texas Christian University
Fort Worth, Texas
Chapters 13 and 42

M. Therese (Terri) Casey, MSN, ARNP
Patient Care Manager, NewLife Center/Gyn
St. Francis Hospital and Medical Center
Topeka, Kansas
Chapter 6

Penny S. Cass, PH.D., RN
Undergraduate Program Director and
  Assistant Professor of Nursing
Oakland University
Rochester, Michigan
Chapter 17

Bonita Cross, RN, MSN
Director of Associate Degree Nursing Program
Holmes Junior College
Grenada, Mississippi
Chapter 30

Marsha D. M. Fowler, PH.D., RN
Associate Professor, School of Nursing
 and Graduate School of Theology
Azusa Pacific University
Azusa, California
   Chapter 7

Elaine Gebhardt, RN, MAN, MPH, PH.D.
Nurse Researcher
Irving Healthcare System
Irving, Texas
Lead Teacher in Maternity Nursing
The University of Texas at Arlington
School of Nursing
Arlington, Texas
   Chapter 37

Pamela Gill, RN, MSN
Perinatal Clinical Specialist
Children's Hospital of San Francisco
Assistant Clinical Professor
Department of Family Health Care Nursing
University of California, San Francisco
San Francisco, California
   Chapter 10

Barbara Goddard
Associate Professor, Childbearing Nursing
College of Nursing
South Dakota State University
Brookings, South Dakota
   Chapter 15

Theresa Kraince Gorman, RN, MS
Lecturer
California State University, Hayward
Hayward, California
   Chapter 3

Carolyn A. Grubb-Phillips, RNC, PH.D.
Associate Professor
University of Texas
School of Nursing at Galveston
Galveston, Texas
   Chapter 11

Harriet A. Harrell, RN, NNP, BSN
Assistant Director of Neonatal Nurse
 Practitioners
University Medical Center
University Physicians, Inc.
Arizona Health Sciences Center
University of Arizona
Tucson, Arizona
   Chapter 33

Carol Harte, MSW
Perinatal Social Worker
Alta Bates-Herrick Hospital
Berkeley, California
   Chapter 38

Sandra C. Hesterly, RN, MS
Associate Director, Nursing Services
Alta Bates-Herrick Hospital
Berkeley, California
   Chapter 8

Linda Welsch Jensen, RN, MN
Assistant Professor
Kearney State College
Kearney, Nebraska
   Chapters 1 and 19

Janet Kirksey, RN, BSN
Co-Founder, Coordinator
S.A.N.D.
(Support After Neonatal Death)
Alta Bates-Herrick Hospital
Berkeley, California
   Chapter 36

Megan Kirshbaum, PH.D.
Executive Director
Through the Looking Glass
Berkeley, California
   Chapter 39

Joanne McManus Kuller, RN, MSN
Neonatal Clinical Nurse Specialist
Alta Bates-Herrick Hospital
Berkeley, California
Assistant Clinical Professor
Department of Family Health Care Nursing
University of California, San Francisco
San Francisco, California
   Chapters 25, 26 and 27

Patricia P. Kyzar, BSN, MSN
Assistant Professor
University of North Alabama
School of Nursing
Florence, Alabama
   Chapter 2

Linda Lefrak-Okikawa, RN, NNP, MS
Neonatal Clinical Nurse Specialist
Oakland Children's Hospital
Oakland, California
   Chapter 32

Carol Mikusa L'Esperance, RN, MSN, IBCLC
Breastfeeding Consultant, Assistant Professor of Nursing
Presbyterian Hospital and University of New Mexico
Albuquerque, New Mexico
Chapter 21

Donna Lee Loper, RN, MS, CNS
Nursery Clinical Coordinator
San Francisco General Hospital
San Francisco, California
Chapter 9

Carolyn Houska Lund, RN, MS
Neonatal Clinical Nurse Specialist
Oakland Children's Hospital
Oakland, California
Chapter 32

Patricia Zirkel Lund, ED.D, RN
Assistant Professor
School of Nursing
Columbia University
New York, New York
Chapter 4

Janet M. Mayorga, PH.D., RN
NAACOG Certified OB/Gyn Nurse Practitioner
Director of Nursing Services
HCA Sun Valley Regional Hospital
El Paso, Texas
Chapters 5 and 40

Eunice C. Messler, BA, MN, ED.D.
Professor and Assistant Dean, Undergraduate Program
School of Nursing
East Carolina University
Greenville, North Carolina
Chapters 16 and 18

Mary E. Müller, MS, RN
Doctoral Candidate
University of California
San Francisco, California
Chapter 20

Katherine Marcia Nelson, RN, MS
Perinatal Clinical Specialist
Alta Bates-Herrick Hospital
Berkeley, California
Chapter 41

Gaile Ellington-Rinne, MED, MA
Disabled Parent Educator, Disability Right Consultant and Clinical Dependency Treatment Specialist, and Psychotherapist
Berkeley, California
Chapter 39

Marsha Keiko Sato, RN, MN
Assistant Professor
Department of Nursing
Mount St. Mary's College
Los Angeles, California
Chapter 23

Linda Seppanen, RN, PH.D.
Health Systems Consultant
Productive Systems
Route One, Box 12B
Winona, MN
Chapter 24

Joyce Thies Smyrski, RN, BSN, MSN
Education Consultant
North Carolina Board of Nursing
Raleigh, North Carolina
Chapter 14

Mary Edna Stevens, RN, MS
Associate Professor
California State University, Hayward
Hayward, California
Chapter 3

Catherine Rose Tobin, RN, MS
Nursing Director, Neonatal Services
Alta Bates-Herrick Hospital
Berkeley, California
Chapter 34

ACKNOWLEDGMENTS

Without the assistance of others this book would not have been revised. Our special recognition is extended first of all to those nurse colleagues who chose to contribute their time and effort through the revision of the manuscript. They were committed to the long-range effects that this content would have on the care of the client and family. They did this work unselfishly and without any monetary rewards. We also extend thanks to our families and friends who have provided encouragement, support and assistance.

There are individuals whose tireless efforts and professional encouragement we want to recognize by name:

Barbara McSorley, Administrative Secretary, Alta Bates-Herrick Hospital, Berkeley, California

Susan Cobb, Secretary, Department of Nursing, California State University, Hayward

Kay Kammerer, Librarian, Alta Bates-Herrick Hospital

Michelle Miller, Senior Nursing Student, California State University, Hayward

Elizabeth Bridston, R.N., Ed.D., Bemidji, Minnesota

Foreword

At this time in the history of prenatal care, it is a heroic task to take on the work of writing a textbook on maternity nursing. In contrast to the recent past when the rules and regulations appeared written in stone and were in large part related to the principles of good hygiene, practice today is finally under critical evaluation both by the practitioner and the consumer.

A significant stimulus for close review and study of maternity practices began in England in the 1970s when the British Government established the National Perinatal Epidemiology Unit at Oxford with Dr. Ian Chalmers as director. At its initiation, the president of the Royal College of Obstetricians and Gynecologists wrote "Obstetricians have to examine critically and objectively their present practices with a view to excluding features which are superfluous, wasteful, doubtful, useful, and sometimes harmful." Next year the National Perinatal Unit will publish a landmark critical review of all randomized trials related to the care of infants and their mothers from 1945 to 1985. This will allow those working in the field to evaluate and review the effectiveness of all their present procedures and practices.

Brigette Jordan, in her book entitled *Birth in Four Cultures*, has, in my opinion, produced the best explanation of why our maternity practices became so rigid and lacking in experimental support when she noted that "Any way of doing birth consists of beliefs and practices which are mutually dependent and internally consistent. The work of maintaining consistency and the systems operation is accomplished by a continuous process of justification which draws on standards from the local definition of birth." These procedures . . . are part of the system rather than grounded in independent objective standards. She notes that "This is not a flaw peculiar to birthing, but is characteristic of evaluations from the inside out where the judged provide the criteria for the judging." She also notes that "there is nothing wrong in this as long as everyone realizes that they are system specific and that they are not, however, elevated to scientific criteria." The extensive evaluations now underway are questioning our system specific criteria. This major review of our present maternity care practices is examining whether practices, that in some cases have been part of our care for the past fifty years, have any efficacy.

Appropriately, in this era of evaluation of care practice, this book is organized with two overlapping approaches. First the reader is introduced to maternity nursing as a specialty moving from historical developments to planning and implementation of change in the future. Simultaneously the reader is exposed, not only to changes within the specialty as they relate to society and family, but also to changes that relate to the individual patient during each period of pregnancy.

This new edition is expanded with revisions in every chapter and special emphasis on women's health and perinatal nursing. There is a new chapter on perinatal infections focusing on sexually transmitted diseases as they relate to women's health care issues as well as chapters on resuscitation of the high risk newborn, maternal and neonatal transports, and strategies for mobilizing families in perinatal crises. A major goal of this valuable book is to prepare the learner for any problems encountered during the perinatal period.

The unique focus of the book is that it is centered around the theory of change. Each unit focuses on change as it relates to maternity nursing, women's health, and perinatal care with complete chapters on the parent with physical disabilities, the father's role, adolescent pregnancy, substance abuse, perinatal loss, and alternative birthing.

The detailed nursing care plans provided in this book along with the rationale for each procedure along with detailed references are especially helpful in understanding the essentials of maternity care.

Appropriately, the authors approach both the medical and behavioral needs of the mother, father, and infant. They explore in detail the problems in both hospital and home care. Extensive care outlines are presented for many procedures and special problems, and the authors share their many years of practical experience covering a wide range of situations from minor to major clinical problems. Fortunately, the authors describe the management of each of the clinical situations in sufficient detail to simplify even complicated problems and procedures. I encourage the reader to inspect carefully even small details of each diagram since they can have a major impact on care.

The value of collaboration across many disciplines is beautifully illustrated throughout this book as the many subspecialties including anatomy, ethics, behavior, psychology, pharmacology, physiology, and genetics are interwoven by the authors into practical maternity nursing. The authors have performed a real contribution by including the disabled parent (the mother who is deaf or blind, or with a spinal cord injury). The book is rich in interesting areas including the role of society in changing care practices. The book also examines new areas of prenatal care including ultrasonography and amniocentesis, and evaluates the "technology" of childbirth, as well as how normal parents develop a close attachment to their healthy or sick infants.

The authors are to be commended for their creative work in preparing this special book. I hope they will accept the challenge to revise this valuable textbook in the light of the major ongoing, critical evaluation of all our maternity care practices.

MARSHALL H. KLAUS, M.D.
Director of Academic Affairs
Children's Hospital Oakland
Adjunct Professor of Pediatrics
University of California San Francisco

Preface

The first edition of this text was designed to provide a base of knowledge to allow safe practices in maternity nursing with a focus on family-centered care. The second edition continues this trend and emphasizes women's health and perinatal nursing.

Perinatal nursing is the practice of professional nursing in response to the need to achieve the goal of reproductive health. It includes the care of the patient/client from the period preceding childbirth through the first four weeks of neonatal life. Perinatal nursing includes the events of the reproductive experience to the end of the postpartum period, as well as the interrelationship of the experience of childbearing on the newborn. Throughout the period of pregnancy from the first four weeks of intrauterine life, the conditions and diseases that affect the fetus and newborn are studied, along with resulting nursing care and treatment.

In the area of women's health, there is a comprehensive chapter on contraception including male and female anatomy and physiology, types of birth control, practical information on various birth control methods for the patient, and types of abortions. There is also a new chapter on perinatal infections which focuses on sexually transmitted diseases as they relate to women's health care issues. The book includes a unit on the high risk mother, infant, and family. This unit has new chapters on resuscitation of the high risk newborn, maternal and neonatal transports, and strategies for mobilizing families in perinatal crises.

The goals of perinatal nursing set forth in this text are: 1. utilization of an extensive knowledge base; 2. early detection and prevention of reproductive failure; 3. improved collaboration between patient, family, and health care teams; and, 4. expansion of research efforts by nurses.

The unique focus of this book is that it is centers around the theory of change. Each unit focuses on change as it relates to maternity nursing, women's health, and perinatal care. The nurse's understanding of the change process is vital to the development of an awareness of human behavior. The perinatal nurse encounters many facets of change. Within the social system the nurse must recognize changes that affect the family structure, roles, and value systems. There are constant changes in legislation that govern the practice of perinatal nursing. While change is slow, it is constant and dynamic, ever present. The reader is given a definition of change and then is moved from historical developments within maternity nursing to planning and implementing change within the nursing specialty. Changes within society are explored as they affect the perinatal client and family.

Other features of this new text include chapters on the parent with physical disabilities, the father's role, adolescent pregnancy, substance abuse, perinatal loss, alternative birthing, and perinatal infections. Each chapter contains specific behavioral objectives to guide learning. It is our intention to provide a resource for both nursing students and nurses specializing in perinatal nursing.

Contents

Contributors, v
Foreword, ix
Preface, xi

UNIT ONE

CHANGE IN PERINATAL NURSING TODAY

1 *Change Defined* 3

Behavioral Objectives 3
Definitions of Change and Related Terms 4
  *Planned Change, 5 • Change by Drift, 6
  • Participants in the Change Process, 6*

Change Theorists, Theories, and Process of Change 7
A Change Model for Nurses 9
  *Level I: Unfreezing—Assessment and Diagnosis, 9
  • Level II: Moving, 13 • Level III: Refreezing, 16*

Successful Change 17
  *Driving Forces, 17 • Restraining Forces, 17
  • Implementation, 17 • Adoption and Internalization, 17*

Failure to Change 18
Change in the Family 18
Summary 19

2 *Historical Developments in Maternity Nursing* 22

Behavioral Objectives 22
Definitions 23

Women's Roles in Society and Childbearing 24
Early History to Nineteenth Century 24
  *Ancient Civilization, 24 • Ancient Greece, 26
  • Christianity, 27 • The Middle Ages, 27 • The
  Renaissance, 27 • The Eighteenth Century, 29*

The Nineteenth Century 29
  *Early Nursing Education in the United States, 30
  • Changes to Prevent Puerperal Sepsis, 30 • The
  Beginning of Modern Nursing, 31*

Into the Twentieth Century 33
  *Margaret Sanger, 33 • Midwifery in the United
  States in the Early Twentieth Century, 34*

Changes in the Recent Past 36
  *Governmental and Voluntary Agencies, 36 • New
  Knowledge, Methods, and Techniques, 38 • Changes
  in Nursing Education, 38 • The Consumer
  Movement and Childbirth Education, 39 • The
  Women's Movement, 41 • Effecting Legislative
  Changes, 41 • Change Agents in the Recent Past, 42*

Birth Rate 42
  *Maternal Mortality Rates, 43 • Infant Mortality
  Rates, 44 • Perinatal Mortality, 45*

Effecting Change in the Future 45
Summary 47

3 Changes Related to Women's Health: Issues of Contraception 50

Behavioral Objectives 50
Anatomy and Physiology 51
Historical Perspective 51
Factors Influencing Contraceptive Use 52
Consideration in Choosing a Contraceptive Method 54
Effectiveness, 54 • Safety/Risks, 54 • Future Contraceptive Plans, 55

Barrier Methods of Contraception 55
Diaphragm, 56 • Cervical Cap, 57 • Condom, 58 • Spermicides, 59 • Contraceptive Sponge, 61 • Oral Contraceptive Pills, 63 • Intrauterine Device (IUD), 65

Sterilization 67
Female Sterilization, 68 • Male Sterilization, 68

Fertility Awareness Methods 70
Calendar Method, 70 • The Temperature Method, 70 • The Ovulation Method, 70 • Safety and Effectiveness, 70 • Sexual Effects, 71

Other Methods of Contraception 71
Lactation, 71 • Abstinence, 71 • Coitus Interruptus, 72 • Postcoital Methods 1: Abortion, 72 • Postcoital Methods 2: "Morning After" Pill, 73 • Douching, 73

Future Trends in Contraception 74
The Nursing Process and Contraception 74
Assessment, 74 • Nursing Diagnosis, 75 • Planning, 75 • Implementation, 75 • Evaluation, 76

Summary 76

4 Change in Family Roles 79

Behavioral Objectives 79
Definitions 81
Evolution of the Family 84
Evolution of Parenting 84
Factors Influencing Family Roles 88
Allocation of Power and Decision Making, 88 • Value Placed on Education, 88 • Locus of Control, 88 • Time Orientation, 88 • Perception of Roles, 89 • Socioeconomic Status, 89

Family Developmental Levels and Tasks 89
Stage 1: Establishment Phase, 89 • Stage 2: Expectant Family and Childbearing Phases, 89 • Stage 3: The Family with a Preschooler, 91 • Stage 4: The Family with a Schoolage Child, 91 • Stage 5: The Family with a Teenager, 91 • Stage 6: The Family as a Launching Center, 91 • Stage 7: The Family in the Middle Years, 91 • Stage 8: The Aging Family, 92 • Aldous's Family Development Stages, 92 • Using Knowledge About Family Development, 92

The Nurse and the Family—Assessments, Interventions, and Strategies 92
Levels of Functioning, 92

Problems with Changing Roles 93
Summary 96

5 Change in Society: Roles and Expectations 98

Behavioral Objectives 98
Change in Society: Past and Present 99
Alternative Family Lifestyles 100
Single-Parent Families, 100 • Adoption, 101 • Homosexual Parents, 102

Scientific and Technologic Advances: Alternative Parenting 103
Artificial Insemination, 103 • In Vitro Fertilization, 104 • Low Ovum Transfer, 105 • Surrogate Mothers, 105 • Oocyte Donation, 106 • Sex Selection, 106 • Genetic Engineering, 107

Summary 108

6 Cultural Aspects of Childbearing 110

Behavioral Objectives 110
Culture 111
How Individuals Experience Culture 112
Culture's Role in Childbearing 112
Society's Expectations for Behavior 113
Family Planning, 113 • Pregnancy, 114 • Prenatal Management, 114 • Intrapartal Management, 114 • Postpartal Management, 115 • Management of the Newborn, 115 • Guidelines for Nurses, 115 • Components of a Cultural System, 115 • The Kay-Galenic Framework, 115 • The Newton Framework, 122 • Nursing's Role, 123

Summary 124

7 Ethics and Perinatal Nursing 129

Behavioral Objectives 129
Ethics: Some Basic Concepts 130
Ethics and Law, 130 • Obligation and Moral Character, 131

Bioethics and Nursing 131
Tools for Decision Making: Principles and Rules in Bioethics 134
Justice, 134 • Autonomy, 136 • Nonmaleficence, 140 • Beneficence, 142

Summary 143

8 Legal Issues in Perinatal Nursing 145
  Behavioral Objectives 145
  Historical Background and the Framework of Law 146
  Nurse Practice Acts 147
  Expanded Roles in Perinatal Nursing 148
   Clinical Nurse Specialists, 148 • Nurse Practitioners, 149 • Nurse-Midwives, 149
  The Rights of Patients 150
   Trends in Patients' Rights, 150 • Communication About Patients, 150

  Current Legal Controversies in Perinatal Nursing 152
   A Fetal "Right to Life" Amendment, 152 • The Rights of Defective Newborns, 152
  AIDS 153
  Surrogacy 153
  Summary 154

UNIT TWO

CHANGE: THE PRENATAL PERIOD

9 Physiologic Changes in the Fetus 159
  Behavioral Objectives 159
  Ovarian and Endometrial Cycles 160
   Follicular Development and Ovulation, 160 • Corpus Luteum, 161 • Endometrial Cycle and Changes in Cervical Mucosa, 162 • Menstruation, 163
  Gametogenesis 163
   Spermatogenesis, 163 • Oogenesis, 164
  Fertilization 165
  Implantation 170
  The Decidua 170
  Placental Development 170
  The Umbilical Cord 174
  Embryonic Development 174
  Fetal Development 177
   Weeks 9–12, 177 • Weeks 13–16, 178 • Weeks 17–20, 178 • Weeks 21–24, 179 • Weeks 25–28, 179 • Weeks 29–32, 180 • Weeks 33–36, 180 • Weeks 37–40, 180
  Organ System Development and Function 181
   Placental Function, 181 • Fetal Nervous System, 182 • Fetal Circulatory System, 184 • Fetal Renal System, 187 • Fetal Gastrointestinal System, 189
  Summary 192

10 Physiologic Changes in the Maternal System 194
  Behavioral Objectives 194
  Signs and Symptoms of Pregnancy 195
   Presumptive Signs and Symptoms of Pregnancy, 195 • Probable Signs of Pregnancy, 196 • Positive Signs of Pregnancy, 198 • Estimation of Gestational Age, 198

  Effects of placental hormones 199
   Human Chorionic Gonadotropin, 199 • Human Placental Lactogen, 199 • Estrogen, 199 • Progesterone, 199
  Changes in the Reproductive System 200
   Uterus, 200 • Cervix, 200 • Vagina, 201 • Breasts, 202 • Perineum, 203
  Changes in the Cardiovascular System, 203
   Heart, 203 • Changes in Blood Pressure and Volume, 203
  Changes in the Respiratory System 203
  Changes in the Renal System 205
  Changes in the Digestive System 206
   Stomach, Esophagus, and Intestine, 206 • Mouth and Teeth, 206 • Liver, 206
  Changes in the Musculoskeletal System 206
  Changes in Skin and Associated Structures 206
   Pigmentation, 207 • Hair, 207 • Connective Tissue, 207 • Blood Vessels of the Skin, 207
  Metabolic Changes 207
   Weight Gain, 207 • Protein Metabolism, 207 • Carbohydrate Metabolism, 207 • Fat Metabolism, 208 • Mineral Metabolism, 208 • Water Metabolism, 208
  Changes in the Endocrine System 208
   Pituitary Gland, 208 • Thyroid Gland, 209 • Parathyroid Gland, 209 • Adrenal Glands, 209 • Pancreas, 209
  Changes in the Immunologic System 209
  Minor Discomforts of Pregnancy 210
  Summary 210

11 Psychologic and Emotional Changes of Pregnancy: Mother and Family 218

Behavioral Objectives 218
The Concept of a Developmental Crisis 219
Pregnancy as a Developmental Crisis 220
Psychologic Changes of Pregnancy for the Woman 222
The First Trimester, 222 • The Second Trimester, 223 • The Third Trimester, 224

Development of Maternal Identity 227
The Process of Maternal Role Taking 228
Mimicry, 228 • Role Play, 228 • Fantasy, 228 • Introjection-Projection-Rejection/Acceptance (IPR/A), 228 • Grief Work, 229

Maternal Tasks 229
Seeking Safe Passage for Self and Baby, 229 • Securing Acceptance, 230 • Learning to Give of Self, 231 • Binding-in to the Unknown Baby, 232

The Father's Experience 233
The Sibling's Experience 237
The Grandparents' Experience 239
The Nurse's Role 240
Summary 241

12 Maternal Nutrition 243

Behavioral Objectives 243
Historical Perspectives 244
The Importance of Nutrition in Pregnancy 244
Nutritional Needs 246
Energy, 247 • Protein, 247 • Iron, 248 • Calcium, Phosphorus, and Magnesium, 248 • Zinc and Iodine, 249 • Fat-Soluble Vitamins, 249 • Water-Soluble Vitamins, 249 • Supplementation, 250

Nutritional Assessment 250
The Health Care Team, 250 • Nutritional Risk Factors, 250 • The Client Interview and Nutritional History, 251 • Assessment Tools, 254 • Daily Food Guide, 254 • Biochemical Tests, 255 • Anthropometric Assessment, 256 • Weight Gain and Control, 256 • Weight Control During Lactation and Postpartum, 259

Nutritional Risk Factors of Pregnancy 260
Teenage Pregnancies, 260 • Spacing of Pregnancies, 261 • Low Income, 261 • Weight Control, 261 • Smoking, Alcohol, and Drugs, 261 • Pica, 261

Influences on Eating Behavior: Promoting Optimal Nutrition 261
Ethnic Influences, 261 • Cultural Influences, 262 • Common Discomforts During Pregnancy, 264

Beyond Pregnancy and Lactation 265
Summary 265

13 Prenatal Diagnosis and Fetal Well-Being 267

Behavioral Objectives 267
Sonography 268
Definitions and Indications, 268 • Procedure and Interpretation, 268 • Nursing Roles, 269

CAT Scan 270
Definitions and Indications, 270 • Procedure and Interpretation, 270 • Nursing Roles, 270

X-Rays (radiography) 270
Definitions and Indications, 270 • Procedure and Interpretation, 271 • Nursing Roles, 271

Amniocentesis 271
Definitions and Indications, 271 • Assessment of Fetal Maturity, 278 • Procedure and Interpretation, 278 • Nursing Roles: Genetic Counseling, 279

Fetal Monitoring 282
Definitions and Indications, 282 • Procedure and Interpretation, 282 • Nonstress Test, 282 • Contraction Stress Test/Oxytocin Challenge Test (CST/OCT), 289 • Nursing Roles, 289

Fetal Biophysical Profile 291
Placental Hormones and Enzymes 292
Definitions and Indications, 292 • Procedure and Interpretations, 294 • Nursing Roles, 295

Fetoscopy 295
Definitions and Indications, 295 • Procedure and Interpretation, 296 • Nursing Roles, 297

Placental Grading 297
Definitions and Indications, 297 • Procedure and Interpretation, 298 • Nursing Roles, 298

Chorionic Villus Sampling 298
Definitions and Indications, 298 • Procedure and Interpretation, 298 • Nursing Roles, 299

Percutaneous Umbilical Blood Sampling (PUBS) 299
Definitions and Indications, 299 • Procedure and Interpretation, 300 • Nursing Roles, 300

Summary 300

14 Methods of Childbirth Preparation 303

Behavioral Objectives 303
History of Prenatal Education 304
Prior to the Second World War, 304 • Following the Second World War, 304 • The Influence of Dick-Read, 304 • The Influence of Lamaze, 305 • The Influence of Bradley, 305 • The Influence of Kitzinger, 305 • Cesarean Birth Classes, 306 • Hypnosis and Yoga, 306

Childbirth Classes 306
The Bradley Method, 306 • The Lamaze Method, 308

Key Elements of Prenatal Education 310
 Timing and Location, 310 • Target, 310 • Structure, 310 • Economics, 311 • Types of Classes, 311 • Assessment of Learning Needs, 311 • Teaching Strategies, 312 • Content, 312 • Father's Needs, 313

Summary 313

15 The Role of the Nurse in the Prenatal Period 315

Behavioral Objectives 315
Preconceptual Counseling 316
Nursing Assessment of the Pregnant Patient 317
 Health History, 317 • General Health Assessment, 319 • Assessment of the Breasts, 322 • Assessment of the Abdomen, 323 • Pelvic Examination, 328

Psychosocial/Emotional Assessement, 329
Maintenance and Promotion of Health for the Pregnant Patient 330
 Continuing Prenatal Education, 332 • Development of Relationships, 332

Anticipatory Guidance 334
Summary 334

UNIT THREE

CHANGE: THE INTRAPARTAL PERIOD

16 The Labor Process: Change in the Mother and Fetus 339

Behavioral Objectives 339
Theories of Labor Onset 340
Biophysical Changes in the Mother During Labor 340
 Uterus, 340 • Uterine Contractions, 342 • Other Changes in Maternal Systems, 344

Fetal Attributes 344
Pelvic Characteristics 347
Premonitory Signs of Labor 350
Stages of Labor 351
 First Stage of Labor, 351 • Second Stage of Labor, 353 • Third Stage of Labor, 353 • Fourth Stage of Labor, 356

Duration of Labor 356
Summary 359

17 The Nurse's Role During the Intrapartal Period 361

Behavioral Objectives 361
Labor and Delivery as Stressors 362
The Nurse's Role in Assessment 362
 Nursing Assessment of the Fetal Heart Rate: Periodic Auscultation, 362 • Nursing Assessment of Uterine Contractions, 363 • Electronic Fetal Monitoring, 363 • Evaluation of Interactions of Significant Others, 365 • Emotional and Psychologic Considerations, 366 • The Use of Touch, 373

The Nurse's Role in Examinations 373
 General Role, 373 • Assessment of the Uterus, 373 • Rectal and Vaginal Examinations, 373

Technology 373
 Care of the Patient as Opposed to Care of the Machine, 374 • Special Patient Considerations, 374

Assessment of Fetal Distress 374
 Assessment of Uterine Contraction Tracings, 375 • Periodic Fetal Scalp Blood Sampling, 376

Summary 378

18 Comfort Management During Labor and Delivery 379

Behavioral Objectives 379
Research on Pain Mechanisms 380
Factors Influencing Pain in Labor 381
 Cultural Influences, 381 • Past Experience, 382 • Psychologic Factors, 382

Measurement of Pain 382
Pain in Labor 384
 First and Second Stages, 384 • Physiologic Effects of Pain in Labor, 384

Role of the Nurse in Pain Assessment 385
Approaches to Relieving Pain in Labor 387
Pharmacologic Approaches 387
 Effects of Drugs on the Fetus, 388 • Systemic Medications, 388 • Regional Anesthesia, 390 • Inhalation Analgesics, Inhalation Anesthesia, and General Anesthesia, 395 • Sensory Modulation Approaches, 396

Psychologic Approaches 396
Summary 398

19 Care of the Newborn Immediately Following Birth 399

Behavioral Objectives 399
Preventing Asphyxia 400
Initial Assessment: The Apgar Score 402
Hypothermia 405
   Thermal Control in the Infant, 405 • Maintaining a Neutral Thermal Environment, 407

Hypoglycemia 409
Hypercarbia 409
Hypotension 409
Blood Tests 409

Preventing Infection 410
   Cord Care, 410 • Preventing Eye Infection, 410

Preventing Hypoprothrombinemia 412
Examining for Congenital Anomalies 412
Facilitation of Attachment 413
   Hugs, Holding, and Bonding, 413 • Cultural Customs and Individual Preferences, 415

Spiritual Care 415
Identification 415
Charting 416
Certificates 418
Summary 418

UNIT FOUR
CHANGE: THE POSTPARTAL PERIOD

20 Maternal Physiologic Adaptation 423

Behavioral Objectives 423
The Reproductive System 424
   Involution, 424 • The Progressive Process, 426

The Cardiovascular System 426
   The Coagulation and Fibrinolytic Systems, 426 • Vital Signs, 427

The Endocrine System 427
The Gastrointestinal System 428
The Renal System 428
The Musculoskeletal System 428
The Immune System 428
   Blood-Type Incompatibilities, 428 • Rubella, 429

Other Changes 429
Return to the Steady State 430
   "Afterpains," 430 • Body Image, 430 • Rest and Ambulation, 430 • Disequilibrium, 431 • Hypothermic Reactions, 431

Problems and Special Considerations 431
   Spinal Headache, 431 • Morphine Epidurals, 432 • Episiotomies and Lacerations, 432 • Hemorrhoids, 433 • Hematomas, 433 • Bladder Trauma and Urine Retention, 433

Summary 434

21 Breastfeeding: Physiology and Management 436

Behavioral Objectives 436
History and Trends 437
   History, 437 • Trends, 437

Anatomy and Physiology of the Breast 438
   Anatomy of the Breast, 439 • Physiology of Lactation, 440

Nursing Management of Successful Breastfeeding 441
   Support Needs, 441

Encouraging Demand Feeding 445
   Information Needs, 447

Breastfeeding Problems 451
   Engorgement, 451 • Sore Nipples, 452 • Difficult Attachment, 452 • Slow Weight Gain, 453 • Colicky Baby, 453 • Mastitis, 453

Adapting Breastfeeding to Special Situations 454
   Mother-Infant Separation, 454 • Breastfeeding Twins, 459 • Infant With a Cleft Lip or Palate, 459 • Cesarean Birth, 460 • Induced Lactation and Relactation, 460 • Drugs and Breastfeeding, 461

Summary 461

22 Postpartum Exercises 465

Behavioral Objectives 465
Early Postpartum Restoration: Day 1 466
   Initial Comfort Measures, 466 • Pelvic Floor (Kegel) Exercises, 466 • Positions of Comfort, 467 • Basic Diaphragmatic Breathing Exercise, 468 • Pelvic Realignment Exercise, 468 • Lower Extremity Exercises, 469 • Body Mechanics: First Transfers, Posture, and Early Ambulation, 470 • Relaxation, 471 • Massage, 472

Postpartum Restoration: Day 2 472
   Comfort Measures, 473 • Position of Comfort, 473 • Body Mechanics: Caring for the Infant, 474 • Abdominal Exercises, 475 • Head Lift, 476 • Cervical and Thoracic Exercises, 476 • Visualizations, 477

Postpartum Restoration: Day 3 478
Progressive Abdominal Exercises, 478 • Low Back Exercises, 480

Postcesarean Section Restoration 480
Comfort Measures and Body Mechanics, 481 • Postsurgical Exercises: Day 1, 482 • Beginning Restoration Exercises: Days 2 through 4, 483 • Progressive Restoration Exercises: Day 5, 483 • Relaxation, 483

Discharge Planning 483
Summary 485

23 The Nurse's Role in the Postpartum Period 486

Behavioral Objectives 486
Physical Assessment 487
Vital Signs, 487 • Lungs, 487 • Breasts, 487 • Abdomen, 487 • Suprapubic Area, 488 • Vaginal and Perineal Area, 489 • Back, 490 • Lower Extremities, 490 • Other Considerations, 490

Assessment of Mothering Behaviors 491
Phases of Maternal Behavior, 492 • Maternicity, 493 • Mother-Infant Bond, 494

Role Transition to Motherhood 496
The Process of Transition, 496 • Factors Influencing Transition, 497 • Supportive Interventions, 497

Early Hospital Discharge 499
Summary 500

24 Parent Education: Teaching/Learning 501

Behavioral Objectives 501
The Role of the Nurse in Education During Postpartum 502
Learning Theories 503
Behavioristic Theories, 503 • Gestalt or Cognitive-Field Theories, 505 • Theories as Guides for Teaching—Learning Principles, 507

Influences on Learning 508
Psychologic Factors, 508 • Environmental Factors, 509 • Organizational Factors, 510

Teaching—Learning Transactions 510
Postpartum Curriculum 510
Defining Objectives, 511 • Analyzing the Task, 512 • Determining Entering Behaviors, 513 • Developing an Individual Plan, 517 • Selecting Materials and Techniques, 518 • Teaching, 521

Special Teaching Considerations 521
Multiple Births, 521 • Premature Births, 521 • Evaluating, 521 • Documenting, 524

Summary 527

UNIT FIVE

CHANGE: THE NEONATAL PERIOD

25 Extrauterine Life Adaptation 531

Behavioral Objectives 531
Intrauterine Life 532
Pulmonary Function, 532 • Fetal Circulation, 533

Pulmonary Extrauterine Life Adaptation 533
First Breath, 533 • Mechanical, Sensory, and Chemical Factors as Negative Stressors, 536 • Establishment of Rhythmic Respirations, 537

Circulatory Extrauterine Life Adaptation 538
Cord Clamping, 538

Adaptation of Other Systems 539
Thermoregulation, 539 • Endocrine System, 540 • Metabolic Changes, 541 • Gastrointestinal System, 541 • Hepatic System, 542

Periods of Reactivity 542
First Period of Reactivity, 542 • Sleep Period, 544 • Second Period of Reactivity, 544

Transitional Period After Birth 544
Summary 544

26 Assessment of the Normal Newborn 546

Behavioral Objectives 546
The Importance of Assessment 547
Classification of Newborn Infants 547
Birth Weight, 547 • Gestational Assessment, 548 • Estimation of Gestational Age, 548

Physical Assessment 549
Factors that Influence Examination, 549 • Equipment, 551 • Symmetry, 551 • General Appearance of the Newborn, 551 • Systematic Evaluation of the Newborn, 551 • Skin, 551 • Head, 555 • Neck, 558 • Chest, 559, • Abdomen, 559 • Genitals, 560 • Extremities, 561 • Spine, 562 • Buttocks, 562 • Rectum, 562

Neurologic Assessment 563
Posture, 563 • Muscle Tone, 567 • Reflexes, 567

Behavioral Assessment 570
Brazelton Neonatal Behavioral Assessment Scale, 571 • Sleep/Wake Cycle, 574 • Assessment of Sensory Status, 575 • Examination at Discharge, 576

Summary 576

27 Care of the Normal Newborn 579

Behavioral Objectives 579
Routine Care of the Normal Newborn 579
Safety of the Newborn, 580 • Prevention of Infection, 581

Concepts for Care for the Newborn 590
Admission/Transitional/Observation Nursery, 590 • Central Nursery, 590 • Rooming-In, 591 • General Infant Care Routines, 594

Summary 597

28 Infant Nutrition 599

Behavioral Objectives 599
Infant Growth and Development Needs 600
Physical Growth, 600 • Assessment of Growth, 600 • Mental and Psychosocial Growth, 601

Nutritional Requirements 601
Energy Needs, 601 • Carbohydrates, 602 • Protein, 602 • Fats, 602 • Water, 602 • Minerals, 602 • Vitamins, 603 • Recommended Dietary Allowances, 604 • Assessment of Nutritional Status, 605 • Infant Feeding, 605 • Physiological Considerations, 608

Psychosocial Needs 608
Support of Successful Feeding, 608 • Breastfeeding, 609 • Formula Feeding, 610 • Solid Food Additions, 613

Small, Underdeveloped Infants 614
Physical Characteristics, 614 • Food and Feeding, 615

Infant Nutritional Therapy Needs 617
Planning Nutritional Care, 618 • Special Infant Needs, 618 • Gastrointestinal Problems, 619 • Conditions Requiring Special Formulas, 619

Summary 621

29 Infant Attachment and Stimulation 623

Behavioral Objectives 623
Maternal Behavior in Animals 624
Human Maternal Attachment Behavior 625
Development of the Attachment Process, 625 • Parent-Infant Attachment Behaviors, 627 • Infant Attachment and the Premature Infant, 629

The Importance of Infant Stimulation 630
Sensorimotor Intelligence, 630 • Reciprocity, 631

Maternal Actions and Their Effects on Infants 632
Tactile Stimulation, 632 • Auditory Stimulation, 632 • Stimulation of Preterm Infant, 633

Infant Characteristics Affecting Relationships 634
Appearance, 634 • Visual Responses, 634 • Olfactory Abilities, 634 • Gustatory Responses, 634 • Physiologic State and Responsiveness, 635 • Smiling, 635 • Crying, 636

The Nurse's Role 636
Education of Parents, 636 • Implementation of a Stimulation Program, 637

Summary 638

UNIT SIX

HIGH RISK MOTHER, INFANT AND FAMILY

30 Problems During Pregnancy 643

Behavioral Objectives 643
Hypertensive States in Pregnancy 644
Risks to Mother and Infant, 644 • Medical Intervention, 645

Premature Labor 647
Risks to Mother and Infant, 649 • Medical Intervention, 649

Diabetes Mellitus 649
Risks to Mother and Infant, 650 • Medical Intervention, 650

Infections 652
Risks to Mother and Fetus, 654 • Medical Intervention, 654

Postpartal Infection 657
Etiology/Diagnosis, 658 • Incidence, 658 • Pathophysiology/Clinical Aspects, 658

Hemorrhagic Disorders 660
Risks to Mother and Infant, 662 • Medical Intervention, 662

Postpartal Hemorrhage 665
Etiology/Diagnosis, 665 • Incidence, 666 • Pathophysiology/Clinical Aspects, 666

Pulmonary Embolism: Thromboembolic Disease 669
Incidence/Diagnosis, 670 • Pathophysiology/Clinical Aspects, 670 • Findings, 671 • Management, 674 • Amniotic Fluid Embolus, 675

Summary 675

31 Problems During the Intrapartal Period 679

Behavioral Objectives 679
Cesarean Section 680
Indications, 681 • Description of Procedure, 681 • Possible Complications, 685

Induction of Labor 691
Indications, 691 • Description of Procedure, 691 • Possible Complications, 694

Dystocia 695
Causes of Dystocia, 695 • Risks to Infant, 695 • Medical Intervention, 696

Fetal Distress 701
Risk to Infant, 702 • Medical Interventions, 704

Hemorrhagic Disorders 704
Risks to Mother and Infant, 707 • Medical Intervention, 707

Summary 707

32 The High-Risk Newborn 710

Behavioral Objectives 710
The Premature Infant 711
Physical Characteristics, 711 • Physiological Characteristics, 712

The Small-For-Gestational-Age Infant 722
Etiology, 728 • Physical Characteristics, 729 • Physiologic Characteristics, 729

The Postmature Infant 734
Physical Characteristics, 734 • Physiological Characteristics, 734

Summary 739

33 Resuscitation of the High-Risk Newborn 740

Behavioral Objectives 740
Physiologic Differences of the Newborn 741
Identifying Infants at Risk 741
Prepartum (Maternal), 742 • Intrapartum, 742 • Postpartum, 742

Preparation for Resuscitative Interventions 742
Criteria for Resuscitation 743
Resuscitation Techniques 745
ABCs of Neonatal Resuscitation 745
A. Assessment/Airway/Agitation, 745 • B. Breathing, 745 • C. Cardiac/Circulation, 746 • D. Drugs, 747 • E. Environment, 747

Procedures Needed in Neonatal Resuscitation 748
Bag and Mask Ventilation, 748 • Endotracheal Intubation, 749 • Cardiac Compressions, 752 • Peripheral Venous Access, 753

Summary 754

34 Maternal and Neonatal Transport 756

Behavioral Objectives 756
Concept of Transport 757
The Transport System 757
Neonatal Transport, 757 • Maternal Transport, 758 • Organization, 759 • Communication, 760 • The Team, 760 • Equipment, 761 • Administrative Aspects, 764 • Medicolegal Aspects, 766

The Transport Process 767
Outreach, 767 • The Referral Call, 767 • Before Team Departs Receiving Hospital, 767 • Care After the Team Arrives at Referral Hospital, 773 • Documentation, 776 • Before Departure from Referral Hospital, 776 • Management en route, 777 • Transition of Care at the Perinatal Center, 777

Modes of Transport 778
Ground Ambulance, 778 • Fixed-Wing Aircraft, 778 • Helicopter, 778

Return Transports 779
Summary 779

35 Care of the High-Risk Family: Strategies for Mobilizing Families in Perinatal Crisis 781

Behavioral Objectives 781
The High-Risk Family 782
Case Presentation 1, 783 • Case Presentation 2, 784

Needs of the High-Risk Family 785
Preparing the Antepartum Family for the Birth of a Preterm Infant, 785 • Family Meetings, 786 • Telephone Communication, 787 • Changes in Status, 787

Supporting the Family 787
Counseling Suggestions, 788 • Referrals for Long-Term Support, 789 • Preparation for Discharge, 789

Summary 790

36 Perinatal Loss 791

Behavioral Objectives 791
Coping with Loss 792
Individual Reactions, 792 • Siblings' Reactions, 792 • Grandparents' Reactions, 792

Physiology of Perinatal Loss 792
Miscarriage/First Trimester Loss, 792 • Abortion, 793 • Antepartum Fetal Death, 793 • Genetic Abortion, 793 • Stillbirth, 793 • Neonatal Death, 794

The Psychology of Perinatal Loss 794
First Trimester, 794 • Second Trimester, 794 • Third

Trimester, 794 • Neonatal Death, 794 • Genetic Abortion, 794 • Subsequent Pregnancies, 795 • Nursing Intervention, 796 • The Health Care Team, 796 • Providing Information, 796 • Self-Help Organizations, 796 • Grief Responses, 799 • Practical Information, 800

Summary   800

UNIT SEVEN

CHANGE AND VARIATIONS

37 The Father's Role   805

Behavioral Objectives   805
The Meaning of Pregnancy for Fathers   806
The Father's Participation in Labor and Birth   807
Benefits of Father Participation to the Mother   808
  Emotional Support, 808 • The Gatekeeper Function, 809 • Pain Control, 809 • The Father's Influence on Mother-Infant Bonding, 810

Benefits of Father Participation to the Father   810
Benefits of Father Participation to the Infant   811
  Engrossment, 812 • Illness and Death of the Newborn, 814

Preparation of Fathers,   814
  Culture, 814 • Attitudes of Nurses, 815

Guidelines for Father Participation   817
Summary   818

38 Adolescent Pregnancy   821

Behavioral Objectives   821
Statistics   823
Issues Involved in the Increase in Adolescent Pregnancy   823
  Sex Education and the Adolescent, 823 • Contraception and the Adolescent, 825

The Stage of Adolescence in Relation to Adolescent Pregnancy   826
The Pregnant Adolescent   826
  Psychologic Characteristics and Risk Factors, 826 • Physical Characteristics and Medical Risks, 827

The Adolescent Patient in the Antepartum Period   828
  Early Intervention: Making Choices and Assessing Needs, 828 • Continuation of Education, 830 • Prenatal Care, 831 • Involving the Adolescent Father, 833

The Adolescent Patient During Labor and Delivery   834

The Adolescent in the Postpartum Period   836
  The Hospital Stay, 836 • Follow-Up Needs and Assessment, 836

Resources and Referrals   838
New Approaches and Programs   841
Summary   842

39 The Parent with a Physical Disability   844

Behavioral Objectives   844
The Deaf Parent   846
  The Heterogeneity of Deaf Culture, 847 • The Role of Planning, 848 • Focusing on One Cultural Issue: Will the Baby be Deaf, 850

The Blind Parent   851
  Identifying the Visually Disabled Person, 851 • The Attitudinal Problem, 851 • The Effect of Blindness on a Pregnant Woman, 851 • The Effect of the Childbearing Process on Blindness, 852 • Care and Treatment Issues, 853 • Techniques to Enrich and Improve Obstetric Care for the Blind Parent, 854

The Parent with a Spinal Cord Injury   855
  Issues in Maternal and Infant Well-being, 855 • Experience of Premature Labor, 858 • Autonomic Dysreflexia or Hyperreflexia, 858 • Delivery, 859 • Outcome: The Baby, 859

The Parent with Multiple Sclerosis   862
  The Genetic Issue, 862 • MS and Pregnancy Research, 862 • Information and its Communication, 863 • The Role of Planning, 863 • Social and Emotional Considerations When Plans Go Awry, 864

Parenting Issues   865
  Parenting Anxieties, 865 • Planning, 866 • Parenting Strategies, 867

Summary   868

40 Substance Abuse   872

Behavioral Objects   872
Definitions of Drug Terms   873
Characteristics of Drug Abusers   873

Drug Abuse During Pregnancy 874
Fetal Effects of Maternal Substance Use and Abuse 875
Chemical Teratogenesis, 875 • Alcohol, 875 • Marijuana, 884 • Narcotics, 885 • Caffeine, 886 • Cigarette Smoking, 887 • Prescribed and Over-the-Counter Medications, 888

Summary 889

41 *Sexually Transmitted Diseases: Impact on Perinatal Infections* 891

Behavioral Objectives 891

Gonorrhea 892
Epidemiology and Incidence, 892 • Maternal Issues, 893 • Newborn Issues, 893

Syphilis 893
Epidemiology and Incidence, 893 • Maternal Issues, 893 • Treatment, 895 • Newborn Issues, 895 • Nursing Issues, 895

Chlamydia 896
Epidemiology and Transmission, 896 • Maternal Issues, 896 • Newborn Issues, 897 • Screening, 897 • Nursing Issues, 897

Cytomegalovirus 897
Epidemiology and Transmission, 898 • Maternal Issues, 898 • Newborn Issues, 898

Human Papilloma Virus 898
Epidemiology and Transmission, 899 • Maternal Issues, 899 • Newborn Issues, 899 • Nursing Issues, 900

Herpes Simplex Virus 900
Epidemiology and Transmission, 900 • Maternal Issues, 900 • Newborn Issues, 901 • Treatment and Prevention, 902 • Maternal Issues, 902 • Newborn Issues, 903 • Nursing Issues, 903

Hepatitis B 903
Epidemiology and Transmission, 904 • Maternal Issues, 904 • Newborn Issues, 905 • Prevention, 905

Human Immunodeficiency Virus 906
Epidemiology and Transmission, 906 • Maternal Issues, 907 • Newborn Issues, 908 • Nursing Issues, 909

Summary 909

UNIT EIGHT

IMPLEMENTING CHANGE

42 *Alternative Birthing Methods* 915

Behavioral Objectives 915
Historical Overview of Childbearing Beliefs 916
Family-Centered Maternity Care 917
Current Practices, 917 • Improvements in Family-Centered Maternity Care, 918 • The Role of the Nurse-Midwife, 920 • Family-Centered Maternity Care in Hospitals, 920

Home Birth 920
Advantages of Home Birth, 920 • Disadvantages of Home Birth, 922 • A Back-Up System for Home Birth, 923 • The Nurse-Midwife's Role in Home Birth, 923

Out-of-Hospital Birthing Centers 924
Advantages of Out-of-Hospital Birthing Centers, 924 • Disadvantages of Out-of-Hospital Birthing Centers, 925 • Childbearing Centers, 925

In-Hospital Birthing Centers 925
Advantages of In-Hospital Birthing Centers, 925 • Disadvantages of In-Hospital Birthing Centers, 927 • Preparation for Use of a Birthing Center, 928

Leboyer Birth 929
Vaginal Birth after Cesarean Birth 930
Other Alternative Birthing Concepts 931
Maternal Position in Labor, 931 • Maternal Positions for Delivery, 931

Summary 932

43 *Caring in Perinatal Nursing* 935

Behavioral Objectives 935
Caring and Nursing Education 936
Historical Perspective 936
The Paternalistic Focus, 936 • Science and Technology, 937 • Nursing as an Art and a Science, 938 • Caring as Human Sensitivity, 939 • The Nurse's View of the Patient, 940 • The Patient's Responsibility for Self-Care, 940 • The Patient's Compliance to Medical Regimen, 941

The Nurse as a Professional 941
Accountability, 941 • Advocacy, 942

Summary 944

44 Research for Change 946
   Behavioral Objectives 946
   The Research Process and Perinatal Nursing 947
      Types of Research, 947 • Investigative Methods, 948 • Applicability of Investigative Methods to Perinatal Nursing Research, 950

   The Research Process and the Change Process 951
   Nurse Research in the Perinatal Field 952
   Summary 953

APPENDIXES

APPENDIX A	*The Florence Nightingale Pledge*	959
APPENDIX B	*Standards for Obstetric, Gynecologic, and Neonatal Nursing*	960
APPENDIX C	*Standards of Maternal-Child Health Nursing Practice*	961
APPENDIX D	*A Patient's Bill of Rights*	963
APPENDIX E	*The Pregnant Patient's Bill of Rights and Responsibilities*	965
APPENDIX F	*Resources for Prenatal Educators*	968
APPENDIX G	*Resource Organizations Concerned with Parent or Infant Needs*	969
APPENDIX H	*The Development of Family-Centered Maternity/Newborn Care in Hospitals*	970
APPENDIX I	*Organizations for Alternative Birthing*	974
APPENDIX J	*Resources for Parents with Disabilities*	976
APPENDIX K	*Instructions for Use of Contraceptives*	978
APPENDIX L	*Audiovisuals on Pregnancy, Childbirth and Parenting*	989
APPENDIX M	*Infections Representing Potentially Serious Threats During Pregnancy*	990
APPENDIX N	*Perinatal HIV Guidelines*	993
APPENDIX O	*Testing for HIV-Clinical Diagnosis*	996
APPENDIX P	*Preparation for Neonatal Transport*	998

INDEX 1003

CREDITS 1024

Comprehensive

Maternity

Nursing

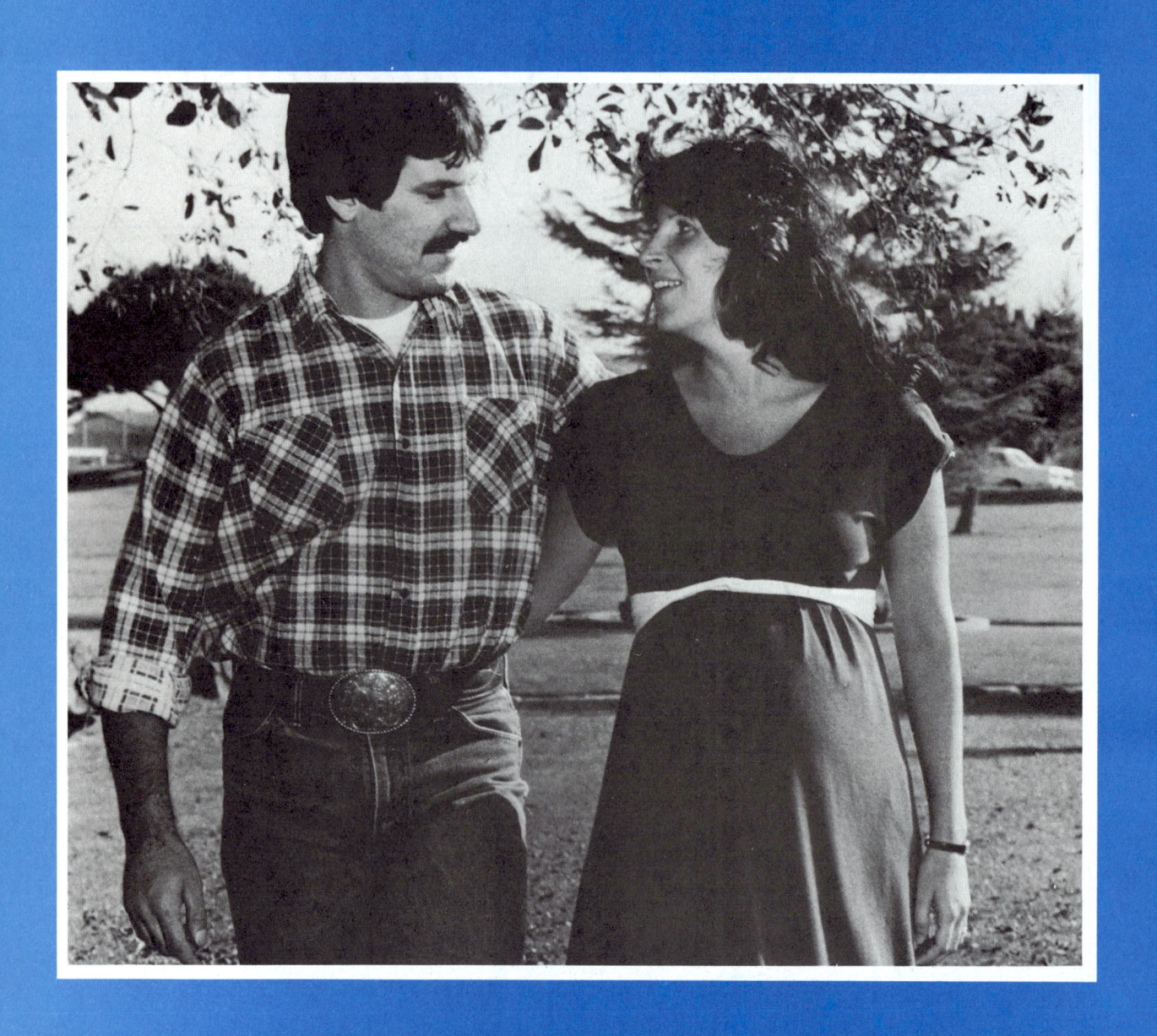

UNIT ONE

CHANGE IN PERINATAL NURSING TODAY

1

Change Defined

BEHAVIORAL OBJECTIVES

Upon completion of this chapter, the reader should be able to:

- Discuss why nursing knowledge includes the thorough study and application of the change process.

- Define and differentiate the terms equilibrium (steady state), change, change agent, and target system.

- Discuss a model for change that incorporates the nursing process.

- Describe an assessment of the setting for change, including status quo, motivators for change, and resistors to change.

- Discuss roles the nurse plays in the change process.

- Describe strategies nurses can use to implement change, giving examples of change projects in which nurses have participated.

- Discuss the need for research of the change process.

To change has been defined as to make different the form, nature, content, future cause of something; to transform or correct; to become altered or modified (*Random House College Dictionary*, 1982).

Nurses are constantly being affected by change and are effecting change, even though they may not consciously choose to be part of the process. Changes occur continuously in the health care system as new technology and consumer education demand an increase in health care options. Some of the changes that have occurred within the last few decades in the maternity care system include birthing chairs, birthing beds, birthing rooms, birthing centers, spouses, siblings, and other supportive companions (daula) attending the birth, labor and delivery postpartum recovery rooms (LDPR), Lamaze childbirth classes, rooming in, fetal monitoring, neonatal intensive care centers, *in vitro* fertilization, and intrauterine surgery. Increased medical technology has made observation of the fetus by ultrasound, amniocentesis, and fetal monitoring commonplace, increasing the possibility of salvaging more infants (see Chapter 13).

With all these advances in technology, it is still questionable whether health care or the quality of the health of all people has improved. Few health care systems match the ideal and contain all the recommended optimal levels of access, comprehensiveness, continuity, coordination, and accountability (Andreapoulos, 1974). Consumers are dissatisfied with the depersonalization and fragmentation of care in maternity nursing, as evidenced by movements toward home birth and other forms of health care at home (Rushmer, 1975). Health care has become a competitive business (Young, 1982).

Childbirth is always a time of change and adaptation for the client and her family. These changes in the physical, emotional, social, and developmental needs of the family can become chaotic, even precipitate a crisis. The maternity client's needs have undergone rapid change—in part because of an increase in single parenting, mobility of the population, and modern-day economic and social pressure.

Nurses' roles have changed with increasing use of technology, expanding drug discovery, and proliferation of knowledge in the medical and behavioral sciences. The technology of monitoring is replacing personal observation, computers are replacing charts, and a battery of inhalation therapists, physical therapists, occupational therapists, and other health care personnel may be replacing nurses! Care has become fragmented and more costly, but not necessarily better (Rushmer, 1975). The professional nurse must assume a more independent role that will potentiate change for the health system and its clients.

There is a great need for the nurse to become an effective change agent rather than a victim of change. In maternity nursing the nurse must become sensitive to ways in which change will result in improvement in the health care of the client and the family. The nurse can become an agent for change by actively intervening to create a desire for change. If the nurse is satisfied with the situation as it exists, he or she will hardly be interested in changing, because the change agent must begin by disturbing the established order of things. A reversal in perceived role from *victim*, or one caught in a situation, to *agent of change*, one in charge of moving a situation, must occur. The nurse must be a professional who is skilled in both the theory and the practice of planned change. The nurse must be able to use a systematic and deliberate system to collaborate and to coordinate activities to bring about alterations in clients, nursing, and the health care delivery system (Michigan State University College of Nursing, 1980). Efforts at planning social change have been widely used since 1950, but only within the last decade have theories of social change been applied to the health care industry (Blum, 1974).

This chapter defines equilibrium, steady state, change by drift, and planned change and describes several models and strategies the nurse can use to bring about planned change.

DEFINITIONS OF CHANGE AND RELATED TERMS

Equilibrium has been defined as a relatively balanced state between simultaneously driving and restraining forces, naturally maintained by adaptive responses that promote healthful survival. A steady state in the organism or system is maintained by coordinated physiologic processes or feedback mechanisms. Various sensing, feedback, and control mechanisms function to effect and maintain this steady state, which depends in a sense on every part of the body always knowing what all parts are doing (Urdang and Swallow, 1983). It is commonly known that *steady state* is the continuing "identity" of a system—where equilibrium implies open and static systems.

Concepts used to describe change include:

Any present state is a dynamic equilibrium of simultaneously operating driving and restraining forces (Lewin, 1951).

Homeostatic or reactive change occurs in response to an outside stimulus of some kind and is directed toward reestablishing balance between the system and its environment. Change is defined as any planned or unplanned alteration in the status quo in an organism, situation, or process (Lippitt, Watson, and Westley, 1958).

Reformulation of a social structure involves disequilibrium and the occurrence of a new equilibrium (Etzioni, 1964).

Change and continuity are two halves. Continuity includes the traditions and status quo patterns of behavior. Change implies the development of a new level of adaptation (Spradley, 1980).

Planned Change

The first step in conceptualizing the role of the nurse as change agent is to select a definition of change. Several questions may help with the definition:

1. Are all modifications and fluctuations within the environment to be defined as change?
2. What differentiates change from chaos?
3. Can change occur only in planned, controlled situations, or can it be an unplanned disruption of the established process?
4. Is change progressive or viewed with suspicion and dread?
5. How is homeostasis related to change?
6. Is homeostasis or change the more desirable state?

The following definitions of planned change have been summarized by social scientists:

Change is an alteration in the structure and function of a social system (Rogers, 1962).

Change is the method that employs social technology to help solve problems of society (Bennis, Benne, and Chin, 1969).

Change is the induction of new patterns of action, belief, and attitudes among substantial segments of a population (Schein, 1969).

Change is an innovation through discovery or invention, diffusion, or alteration (Lenski, 1970).

Planned change is the result of a conscious, deliberate, and collaborative effort intended to improve the operation of a system and to facilitate acceptance of the improvement by involved parties (Havelock, 1973).

Developmental social change is change within an existing social system, adding to it or improving it rather than replacing some of its key elements (Gerlach and Hine, 1973).

Social change is a quantitative process that occurs through time (Hamblin, Jacobsen, and Miller, 1973).

Change is viewed as differentiation, reintegration, and adaptation (Smith, 1973).

Change is the conscious, deliberate, and collaborative effort to improve the operations of a system, whether it be self-system, social system, or cultural system through the utilization of scientific knowledge (Bennis et al., 1976).

Change is relearning on the part of an individual or group in response to newly perceived requirements of a given situation requiring action and resulting in a change in the structure or functioning of social systems (Zaltman and Duncan, 1977).

Recently, definitions of the change process have been adapted to nursing. Some of these definitions are found in the nursing literature:

Change as a process is deliberate and collaborative, involving a change agent (the health provider) and a target system (the client) (Brooten, Hayman, and Naylor, 1978).

The change process can be defined as a process of leadership and accountability, a means of adaptation and problem solving—alteration by choice and deliberation as distinctly differing from change by indoctrination, coercion, natural growth and accident (Douglass and Bevis, 1979).

Change is an alteration in the behavior of an individual or group of individuals as a result of their redefining a situation; it is the creation of something different (Sumner and Philips, 1981).

Change is any significant departure from the status quo. It is the process of moving within, between, and among systems at three levels, which include (Gillies, 1982):

First-level change—alteration occurs in the change agent, the nurse.

Second-level change—altered behavior in the change agent effects behavioral change in the target system, those individuals with whom the nurse has direct contact.

Third-level change—complex alteration of forces affects the entire system, involving client and health care setting.

Synthesizing from the writings of social scientists and nurses, change can be described as a process that is either planned or unplanned.

Planned change is defined as a deliberate effort to improve the client system, which is composed of four subsystems: the individual personality, the group, the organization, and the community. The help of an outside agent is engaged to make this improvement. Problem solving is a major thrust of planned change (Lippitt, Watson, and Westley, 1958). *However, in nursing we would define change as planned change, a process of deliberate and collaborative action between the nurse and the client resulting in alterations in the behavior of both, within the health care setting.*

Change by Drift

Change cannot always be planned, but even many sudden uncontrollable changes such as earthquakes, tornadoes, or major injury accidents can be better managed if there is a plan. Change by drift, on the other hand, occurs by happenstance, and the system is only cognizant that change has occurred in retrospect (Reinkemeyer, 1970).

Nursing has too often allowed profession and environment to change by drift. This option may be chosen consciously, but usually such change has occurred without nurses even noticing. Change by drift is marked by passivity and a failure to think through consequences and set goals. The pattern is one of reacting rather than leading and acting. Nurses have two alternatives: to utilize models to aid in the implementation of planned change, or to let change occur spontaneously without attempting to control the process or the outcome. Not all change can be planned, but a plan can often be used to control spontaneous changes that occur (Brooten, Hayman, and Naylor, 1978).

Participants in the Change Process

Within the planned change process there are two main participants: *a professional helper* (change agent) and a *help-needing system* (client, target) involved in a (usually) voluntary relationship focused on the solving of a current or potential problem via use of scientific knowledge. This relationship is conceived by both parties as being temporary, collaborative, deliberate, and equal in power (Green, 1983).

Change Agent
The *change agent* is any individual or group operating to change the status quo in the target (client)

TABLE 1–1. Insider and Outsider as Change Agents

Insider as Change Agent

Advantages
1. Knowledgeable about the system.
2. Speaks the language.
3. Understand the norms.
4. Identifies with the system's needs and aspirations.
5. Is a familiar figure.

Disadvantages
1. May lack perspective and not see the whole.
2. May not have special skills or knowledge relevant to the change.
3. May not have an adequate power base.
4. May not have independence of movement, time.
5. May have to live down past failures.

Outsider as Change Agent

Advantages
1. Starts fresh.
2. Has perspective.
3. Independent of power structure.
4. Is expected to bring in new ideas and aid the system.

Disadvantages
1. Is a stranger.
2. May have different cultural habits, language.
3. May not understand the group norms and concerns.
4. May not care enough about the system to preserve essential parts.

SOURCE: Olson (1979).

---

system so that a relearning of roles is involved (Zaltman and Duncan, 1977). A change agent has been described as a professional who influences innovative decision making in a direction seen as desirable by a change agency (Rogers and Shoemaker, 1971). The change is seen as an external agency trying to communicate the need for change in the target system. Change agents have been described as helping professionals who have roles that involve the stimulation, guidance, and stabilization of change in organizations. The change agent is one employed by the client (target) system (Jones, 1969). Lippitt, Watson, and Westley (1958) describe a change agent as a person outside of the system, but Bennis (1976) and Olson (1979) assert that this person can be part of the system. Olson has identified advantages and disadvantages of the change agent's being part of the system or being an external consultant, some of which are included in Table 1–1.

A change agent has been defined as a professional who relies on a systematic body of knowledge to guide the change process. The change agent should be able to help plan as well as to accomplish change. An effective change agent will actively involve all persons concerned with the situation (Brooten, Hayman, and Naylor, 1978).

In summary, a change agent is a person or group that assesses the client's interactions with the health care system, diagnoses the problem, and collaborates to bring about alterations within the system to improve the client's health care. The terms *nurse* and *change agent* should be used interchangeably.

Target System

The *target system* is that which the change agent attempts to alter. The target system may be an individual, a group of people, an agency, an organization, or a social institution (Brooten, Hayman, and Naylor, 1978). The term target system in this chapter will be used to describe the client with which the nurse is seeking to facilitate the change, whether it be an individual, a family, other nurses, health care personnel, or an entire health care system (Fig. 1–1).

CHANGE THEORISTS, THEORIES, AND PROCESS OF CHANGE

Most writing about the change process has been in social science fields; however, in recent years several nurses have written about the use of the change process in many areas of nursing (see Table 1–2).

Kurt Lewin (1890–1947) was a social scientist who used a systematic theory to analyze causal relationships and to build scientific constructs. Prior to his work, most social science was based on speculative systems. Lewin formulated a general theory of change that he used to study diverse situations of planned change such as psychotherapy, childrearing, industrial management, race relations, and community development.

Lewin (1951) theorized that there are three basic steps in the change process: (1) unfreezing, (2) moving, and (3) refreezing. He described *unfreez-*

Planned Change
Who and Where

The Change Agent	The Change Relationship	The Client	The Change Process
also known as the professsional helper, the consultant	also known as the Consultative Relationship, the Therapeutic Relationship, the Helping Relationship	also known as the changee or the help-needing system	also known as Problem solving process Nursing process Caring process
Examples: nurses at all levels teachers ministers consultants therapists social workers group leaders		**Examples:** individuals families small groups organizations committees staffs companies faculties	

FIGURE 1–1. Components of planned change.
SOURCE: Adapted from Green, C.P. 1983. Teaching strategies for the process of planned change. *The Journal of Continuing Education in Nursing:* 14(6) p. 17.

TABLE 1-2. The Elements of Change

Lewin (1951)	Lippitt, Watson, and Westley (1958)	Rogers (1962)	Havelock (1973)	Bailey and Claus (1975)	Brooten, Hayman, and Naylor (1978)
Unfreezing	Development of a felt need for change Establishment of a change relationship	Awareness Interest	Building a relationship Diagnosing the problem Acquiring the relevant resources	Defining overall needs, purposes, goals Defining problem	Assessment: a. Interest b. Motivation c. Environment
Moving	Clarification or diagnosis of the client's problem Examination of alternatives, routes, and goals: establishing goals and intentions of action Transformation of intentions into actual change efforts	Evaluation Trial	Choosing the solution Gaining acceptance	Specifying constraints, capabilities, resources, claimant groups Specifying approach Stating behavioral objectives Listing alternative options Analyzing options Choosing approach	Planning a. Support group b. Goals c. Resistance to change and power groups d. Developing strategies Implementation
Refreezing	Generalization and stabilization of change Achieving a terminal relationship	Adoption or rejection	Stabilization and self-renewal	Controlling and implementing decisions Evaluating effectiveness of action	Evaluation Stabilization

ing as the stage in which the motivation for change is created. There are three ways individuals in the target system can become aware of the need for change (unfreezing):

1. Lack of confirmation—inability of system to meet expectations.
2. Guilt anxiety—uncomfortable feeling about action or lack of action.
3. Psychologic safety—former obstacle to change has been removed.

Moving is the planning and initiation of change. *Refreezing* is the stage in which change is integrated and stabilized. For change to be permanent there must be internalization of the change into the target's value system (Lewin, 1951).

Lewin uses concepts of mathematical force fields to explain the forces of the change process. The present state, or status quo, is defined as a dynamic equilibrium of simultaneously driving and restraining forces. Lewin's premise is that increasing the driving forces and decreasing the restraining forces makes change possible. Thus, unfreezing occurs when the status quo is interrupted, and moving occurs when driving forces are increased and restraining forces are decreased (Fig. 1-2).

Lewin's theory has been modified many times, but all its modifications seem to include the concept of planned change. These elements in the planned change process have been identified as (1) building a relationship, (2) diagnosing the problem, (3) acquiring relevant resources, (4) choosing the solution, (5) gaining acceptance, and (6) stabilization and self-renewal. Theories of change can be divided into two major categories or models:

1. *Social interaction model:* begins when the potential receiver becomes aware of the innovation and becomes psychologically and behaviorally involved, showing interest, seeking

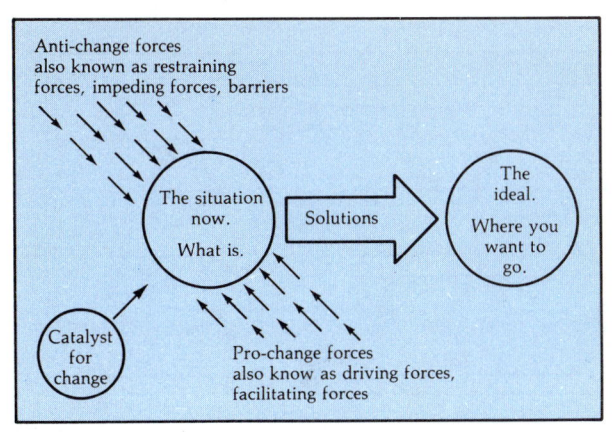

FIGURE 1–2. The forces of change.
SOURCE: Green (1983)

information, evaluating, and participating in trial and adoption.

2. *Problem-solver model:* focuses on the effort of a target system to solve its own particular problem. One example is the Claus-Bailey nursing decision-making systems model, which was developed as an instructional tool for teaching graduate nursing students to become better problem solvers, decision makers, and change agents (Bailey and Claus, 1975). This model can be utilized for change by delineating the nursing actions relevant to each of Lewin's three basic steps of the change process as follows:

Unfreezing: (1) define overall needs, purposes, and goals; (2) define the problem.
Moving: (3) specify constraints, capabilities, resources, and claimant groups; (4) specify approach to the problem solution; (5) state behavioral objectives; (6) list alternative solutions; (7) analyze options; (8) choose plan; (9) control and implement decisions.
Refreezing: (10) evaluate effectiveness of action.

A problem-solving model for change that is similar to that used in the nursing process was described in 1978 by Brooten, Hayman, and Naylor. They specify that the *assessment phase* must include a thorough and accurate assessment of the interest, the motivation, and the environment for change. During the *planning phase* the support group is formed and involved in formulating short-term and long-term goals and in choosing strategies for the *implementation* and *evaluation* phases. Sources of power and sources of resistance to the process are identified and considered in the planning. After implementation is begun, periodic evaluation is recommended. The process ends with stabilization into a dynamic equilibrium that always leaves room for innovation and improvement.

Figure 1–3 is a model of the change process. The change model used for this chapter is an adaptation of the nursing process model by Brooten but also includes some facets of other models previously discussed (Table 1–3).

A CHANGE MODEL FOR NURSES

Level I: Unfreezing—Assessment and Diagnosis

Tasks of the first assessment level include (1) building a therapeutic relationship, (2) assessing the status quo, (3) determining what will motivate the target system, and (4) identifying barriers to change.

BUILDING A THERAPEUTIC RELATIONSHIP Establishing a rapport, a feeling of trust, and open communication is the first step of the change process, whether the client system is a person seeking health care, an institution, a community, or a policy-making government committee. There is almost always some suspicion aroused when a newcomer arrives in a group, particularly if that newcomer rushes in with plans to change the situation. Because the present structure or procedures have been established and maintained with what might be considered great amounts of vested interest, any threat to upset the status quo may be viewed with alarm and therefore not welcomed. Early attempts to bring about change tend to stimulate the use of defense mechanisms. When resistance occurs, a comprehensive assessment of the target system is rendered almost impossible. The process of change cannot be accomplished in isolation. It must enlist the participation of the target system from the beginning. For example, if the target system is a maternity client who has been a heavy smoker for many years, a quick lecture about the harmful effects of smoking will probably not be effective. Using clear communication and giving consideration to the client's ideas, opinions, and feelings will lead to the develop-

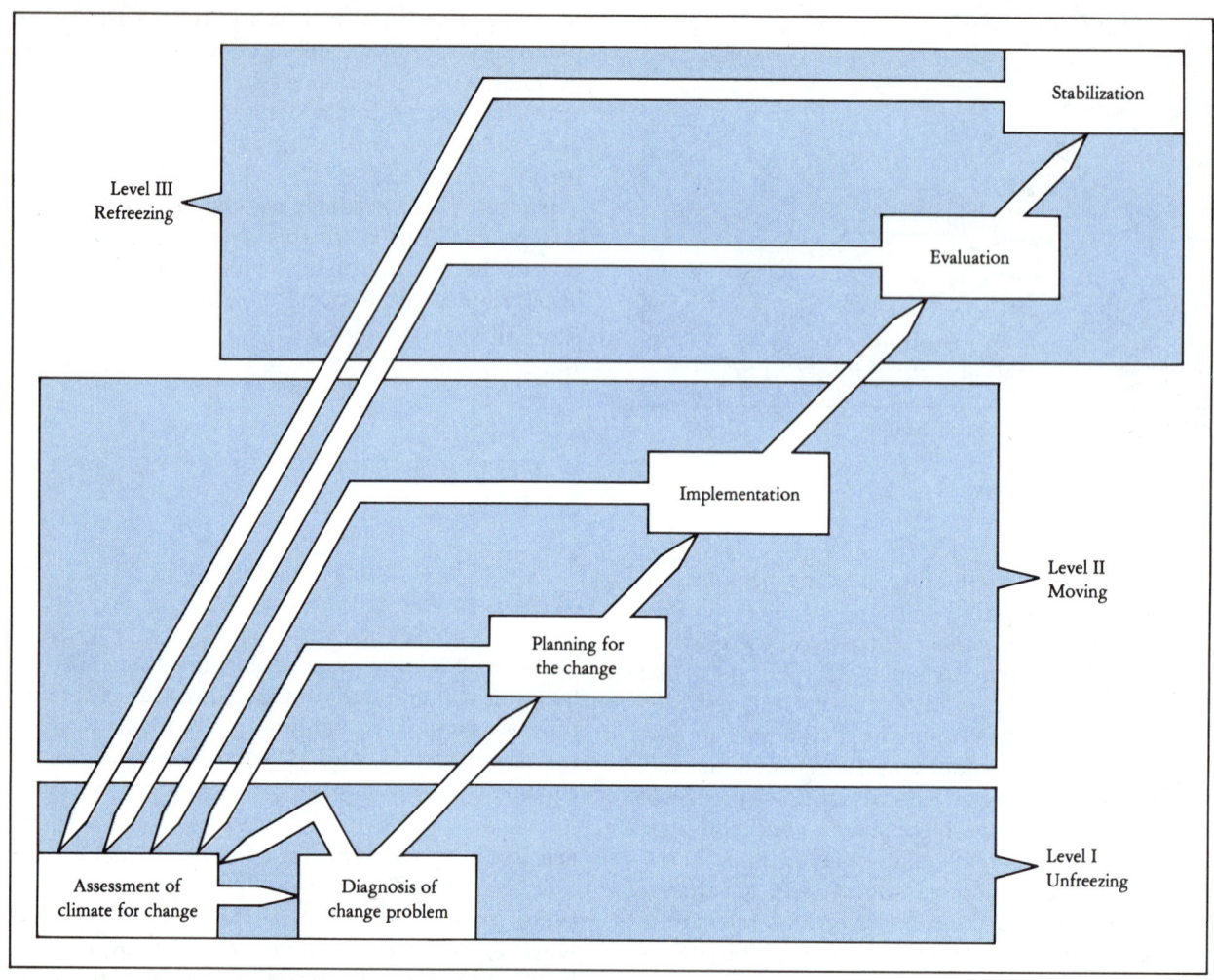

FIGURE 1–3. The nursing process as related to steps in the change process. At any time there may be a movement back toward the original state that called for a change.

ment of trust, and will facilitate effective problem solving (Douglass and Bevis, 1979).

Building personal relationships with co-workers and other persons in the health care system is also important for the nurse. Learning to share the perspectives and feelings of others while developing a knowledge of culturally delicate areas will help to build rapport and to develop a sense of trust. The nurse as change agent should develop empathic understanding for co-workers as well as clients. Credibility builds trust. A solid core of technical knowledge along with the ability to perform basic nursing skills is important in maximizing credibility among health care professionals. Licensing credentials and a demonstration of competence are important in gaining the respect of the client. Although the nurse may immediately see many aspects of the health care system that he or she would like to change, the first priority should be to build confidence in his or her nursing care. The nurse must demonstrate competence in the ability to provide effective, safe nursing care to clients. As the nurse demonstrates confidence and ability to give competent nursing care, he or she may assume the role of change agent.

Joining professional organizations and other organizations in the community will help the nurse become acquainted with a broad range of persons, some of whom may be helpful in the implementation of change. These affiliations may also be helpful in gathering information about community resources and available alternatives to the status quo.

The nurse as change agent should be aware of

TABLE 1-3. Nursing Process for Change

Phase	Action
Unfreezing	Assess climate for change and diagnose the problem a. Build relationship b. Assess status quo c. Assess motivators d. Assess resistors
Moving	Plan for change and implement a. Negotiate goals b. Establish objectives and assign roles c. Analyze resources d. Select approach e. Determine strategy
Refreezing	Evaluate—adopt or revise Stabilize or terminate relationship

current changes occurring within the community, state, nation, and world and their effect on the health care system.

ASSESSING THE STATUS QUO Once a therapeutic relationship is established, the status quo, or the current situation, should be assessed. This situation could include a state of wellness, illness, equilibrium, or chaos. The client or target system may be in a state of illness and need a change in order to return to a steady state. A change such as childbirth occurring and the client system may need to reach a new level of equilibrium before an accurate or conclusive assessment can be performed. If the target system is an individual person or a family, a holistic assessment should be obtained. This includes data collection in the areas of physical, psychosocial, cultural, behavioral, emotional, intellectual, and spiritual functioning. When the target system is co-workers, assessment of mental abilities, knowledge, and educational preparation may be necessary in order to define deficits and to determine the need for additional training. When the target system is a health care agency, similar categories can be used for assessment. Physical environment, space, and accessibility are important if the change agent is considering the establishment of new facilities or services. The environment may need rearrangement, repainting, or even rebuilding for client comfort or convenience. Availability of funding may need to be considered, particularly if new facilities or services are to be provided.

Table 1-4 lists characteristics of static and future-oriented target systems identified by Lippitt (1973). These characteristics can be assessed in the organizational target system and usually include a mixture of the characteristics in Table 1-4.

Assessment should begin with initial interviews and orientation (Fig. 1-4). During interviews there should be a clear exchange of expectations between the nurse and the client/target system. The nurse should determine who is responsible for decision making in the target system. Identifying the persons who have power, both formally and informally, will give the nurse insight into the best method for initiating change. The nurse should be alert to any opportunity to become an active part of the health care system. Becoming involved with policy making—for example, being a member of committees for audit and quality control—frequently entails extra work, and such groups usually welcome volunteers. By becoming involved in the work of a committee, the nurse can begin to influence the health care system through active participation.

DETERMINING WHAT WILL MOTIVATE THE TARGET SYSTEM Motivation of the target system for change means that there is a willingness to work to accomplish identified change goals. When working with a client, the nurse should remember that an individual's desire to continue to live a useful life is often the key to recovery or rehabilitation. Internal motivation is derived from a hierarchy of needs. The basic physiologic needs such as air, food, water, and sleep must be met before the higher ones of safety and security, love and belonging, self-esteem, and self-actualization can be addressed. Any of these needs can become motivators for change (Maslow, 1970).

Maslow's theory can be applied to individuals, groups, and institutions. For example, a large hospital did not have many services available to the night shift. The new vice-president for nursing implemented a night cafeteria cart, thereby providing a meal service. The night security force was increased, which helped to meet the workers' safety and security needs. Administration made weekly night rounds to visit with employees and listen to their concerns, thus meeting some belonging and self-esteem needs. The staff became much more supportive of the administrators' efforts for change and the improvement of nursing care.

TABLE 1–4. Characteristics of Static and Future-oriented Organizations

Paramater	Static Organizations	Future-Oriented Organizations
Structure	Rigid: permanent committees, reverence for constitution and bylaws, tradition Hierarchical: chain of command Role definitions narrow Property bound and restricted	Flexible: temporary task force, readiness to change constitution and bylaws, departure from tradition Linking: functional collaboration Role definitions broad Property mobile and regional
Atmosphere	Internally competitive Task centered, reserved Cold, formal, aloof	Goal oriented People oriented, caring Warm, informal, intimate
Management and philosophy	Controlling: coercive power Cautious, low risk Errors: to be prevented Emphasis on personnel selection Self-sufficient: closed system concerning resources Emphasis on conserving resources. Low tolerance for ambiguity	Releasing: supportive power Experimental, high risk Errors: to be learned from Emphasis on personnel development Interdependent: open system concerning resources Emphasis on developing and using resources. High tolerance for ambiguity
Decision making and policy making	High participation at top, low at bottom Clear distinction between policy making and execution Decision making by legal mechanisms Decisions treated as final	Relevant participation by all those affected Collaborative policy making and execution Decision making by problem solving Decisions treated as hypotheses to be tested
Communication	Restricted flow, constipated One way—downward Feelings repressed or hidden	Open flow: easy access Two way—upward and downward Feelings expressed

SOURCE: Lippitt (1973).

A discussion of motivation is essential to the topic of change. Motivation focuses on two sets of factors—extrinsic and intrinsic. *Extrinsic* factors include company policy, administration, supervision, work conditions, and salary. *Intrinsic* factors are achievement, recognition, the work itself, self-growth, and interpersonal relationships (Herzberg, 1968). When considering motivation for change, the mission, goals, and purposes of the target system should be examined. For example, if a woman is pregnant and her goal is to have a healthy baby, she will be motivated to improve nutrition.

The discrepancy between what one does, wants, or expects and what is obtained is often a powerful motivator (Brooten, Hayman, and Naylor, 1978). The climate for change often becomes more favorable as the discrepancy becomes greater. The place to begin change is at those points where some stress exists. Stress may give rise to dissatisfaction with the status quo and thus become the motivator for change (Bennis et al., 1969). For motivation to be sustained, individuals must feel that they have some control over the situation and that the change will help solve the problem (Zaltman and Duncan, 1977). Motivating or driving forces must be strong in order to overcome restraining or resisting forces.

IDENTIFYING BARRIERS TO CHANGE Resistance to change can be analyzed according to the same holistic assessment used for analyzing the status quo. *Resistance* has been defined as any conduct

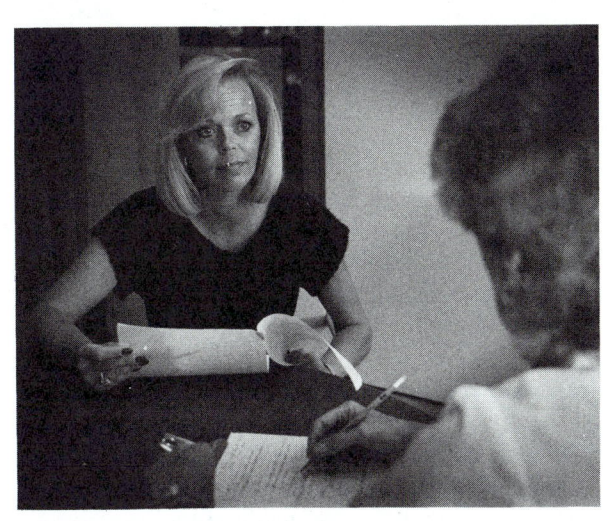

FIGURE 1–4. Assessment begins with the initial interview.

that serves to maintain the status quo in the face of pressure to alter it (Zaltman and Duncan, 1977).

If resistance to change is to be assessed, certain barriers or resisting forces must be identified. These are:

1. *Physical and economic barriers.* Inadequate facilities and inadequate funding are factors to be considered when working with clients. Teaching a mother how to prepare a formula by sterilizing bottles will be ineffective if there is no money to buy the bottles or powdered formula.
2. *Cultural and social barriers.* The traditions, customs, and values of an ethnic or religious group are cultural barriers. If a certain ethnic group values large families, group members may distrust a nurse who is stressing the use of birth control methods. The economic and health conditions of an area may create a barrier to change. Some cultures require high birth rates so that there will be enough children to help the family earn a living. Resistance to change may occur if the change agent is from another cultural or ethnic group.

    Change may be seen as a threat to the established norm. Resistance may be met from homogeneous groups. For example, teenagers may be unwilling to use birth control methods unless others in their group have attended family planning clinics.

    The strength of resistance to change is proportional to the emotional and economic investment in the status quo. For example, changes in leadership of a nursing unit may cause the nursing staff to feel threatened. If the new head nurse immediately seeks to change some procedures that the staff worked hard to develop, the red flags of resistance will rally. Resistance occurs more frequently when the system has been stable and the personnel are satisfied with current conditions.

    Some people see advances in technology as threatening. Rather than seize the opportunity that a computer can give to improve care, many nurses may be reluctant to learn the new technology necessary for its efficient, effective use.
3. *Psychologic barriers.* Some of the most powerful restraining forces are psychologic barriers. Habit is a restraining force. When an obstetrician has used the delivery table for years, he or she is reluctant to change to a birthing chair, because the old method is familiar and comfortable. The fear of failure is a strong force.

    Dependence and superego needs often cause resistance. Children tend to incorporate the values, attitudes, and beliefs of those who care for them. Outbursts of rebellion frequently occur during adolescence, but the typical adult has been found to agree with his parents on language, religion, education, politics, and childrearing (Watson, 1966).

Resistance to change is natural and not always bad. Attempts to change some parts of a structure may make the building collapse. It is vital to assess all aspects of a problem setting carefully before initiating change (Gillies, 1982).

Level II: Moving

Planning for Change
When a need for change has been identified, the moving phase (the actual change) occurs. This phase is one in which the nurse as change agent seeks the involvement of others in the health care system. Reasons for involving others are as follows: (1) involvement tends to decrease resistance, (2) responsibility should be shared by more than a few, and (3) group work tends to be more effective in problem solving for better health care.

NEGOTIATING GOALS   In determining change goals, the change agent should consider the nature and scope of the change, the target of the change, and the key people who will initially help to accomplish the change.

The formal goals of the health care system are usually stated in written form. There are also informal, unwritten goals of the employees. Both types of goals must be considered before the initiation of any change. Group dynamics and previously established interpersonal relationships may be utilized as the nurse helps the target system to determine its mutual goals for health care. The nurse will want to involve consumers in goal planning. The free exchange of ideas by health care personnel and consumers regarding goals and subgoals allows the establishment of specific, legitimate goals and establishes a common base for the beginning of the change process.

ESTABLISHING OUTCOME OBJECTIVES AND ASSIGNING ROLES Outcome objectives should be specifically stated and measurable so that signs of success can be noted and reinforced. Both short-term and long-term goals should be formulated. Critical objectives should be distinguished from noncritical ones for better task accomplishment. This process of distinguishing objectives helps to resolve disputes, clarify points of confusion, and aid evaluation.

Again, the participation of the target system is essential for accomplishing explicit and definitive task analysis (Douglass and Bevis, 1979). Formation and assignment of task groups according to the task, the time limitations, and the capabilities of the participants enables each member to contribute optimally. Organizing participants around tasks decreases the power focus and increases the goal orientation of the work groups.

Assignment of roles is one of the most critical parts of the change process. The target system should select who will act as the change agent for implementation. The change agent should have administrative capabilities, so that the change process can be managed effectively. The nurse must consider objectively the limits of his or her own resources and decide how best to facilitate the change, as a leader or as a catalyst. The nurse will want to keep actively involved in planning the change.

The following is an example of objectives set in a change project. The project was undertaken in a community hospital by a nursing instructor and an assistant nursing administrator to improve maternal and child health services to the benefit of both the consumer and the nursing student. There were five objectives:

1. To initiate family bonding in the delivery room for all patients.
2. To help the parents acquire parenting skills by having the infant at the mother's bedside for as long as she desires.
3. To prepare maternity nurses who will care for both the mother and infant so that job satisfaction is increased.
4. To initiate a continuing education program for maternity nurses so that they can better meet the physical, psychologic, and educational needs of the parents.
5. To provide a model of professional nursing for students to give them better opportunities to learn the nursing process in a maternal–child health setting.

The following strategies were chosen:

1. A survey of consumers was to be carried out to assess satisfaction with the services of the maternity unit.
2. A continuing education program was to be developed, to include classes on "Your Sexuality" and "Family-Centered Maternity Care".
3. A survey of staff nurses was to be conducted to measure job satisfaction. This survey would be repeated at 6- to 12-month intervals to determine whether the objectives of the change had been met.

This was an excellent opportunity for nursing service and nursing education to collaborate on a change project to improve the care of the client (Mizner and Barraro, 1979).

ANALYZING RESOURCES A thorough analysis of the capabilities and limitations of the change agent, the health care system, and interest groups affected by the decision for change must be made before change strategies are selected. Factors to be analyzed include time, financial support, equipment, facilities, interaction and assistance within the organization, manpower, outside assistance, and the environment.

Careful attention should be given to identifying special interest groups that might enhance the change, whether they are part of the formal organization or the informal organization.

In the process of goal negotiation in a

nurse–client relationship, the nurse must spend a considerable amount of time talking with the family about its health situation. Often the family's first expression of the nature of the problem is not the underlying issue of concern. If the work is to be successful, family members must also be involved in the problem. Family members may have conflicting goals that make compromise necessary before any progress can occur in the change process.

SELECTING AN APPROACH Formulating several alternative approaches to achieving a goal enables the group to select the alternative most nearly in keeping with group needs. This process of formulating alternative solutions is referred to as brainstorming, and it can be effective if innovative ideas are compatible with the resources identified.

Change agents should be sensitive to the needs and perspectives of the target system in designing solutions for change situations.

Determining Strategy

Approaches to change may be classified as facilitative, re-educative, persuasive, and power strategies.

FACILITATIVE STRATEGIES Facilitative strategies furnish important financial, social, or other resources that will enable the change to take place. A problem may arise if only limited resources are available. Many nursing strategies are facilitative in that the change agent assists the target system in making the change. Facilitative strategies are appropriate when the target system is committed to the change and the change agent's only function is to make the change easier. Simply furnishing services may not produce change if the target system is not committed.

REEDUCATIVE STRATEGIES Reeducative strategies are feasible when there is plenty of time so that they may be used in advance of the innovation itself. Childbirth classes that prepare the couple to help themselves cope with the changes during and after childbirth is one example. Reeducative strategies are more effective if they are also participative.

PERSUASIVE STRATEGIES Persuasive strategies tend to create change by reasoning, urging, and inducement. Advertisement is a common form of a persuasive strategy that may reflect facts accurately or may be false. Persuasive strategies can be necessary if the target system has a felt need but cannot choose a solution. For example, the nurse can present the alternatives for infant feeding to a patient but should not use persuasion for one method over another, such as breast over bottle feeding. Lottery tickets were suggested to improve attendance in a nutrition class, but were not implemented because the practice was considered unethical.

POWER STRATEGIES Power strategies involve the use of authority, coercion, or manipulation to obtain the target system's compliance. Although this may be immediately effective in obtaining change, the target system may not internalize the change and may later neglect parts of it or even sabotage the change. Use of power or coercion implies that the target system is externally motivated and tends to conflict with a broader objective in change: to encourage self-care and internal motivation (Zaltman and Duncan, 1977).

OVERCOMING RESISTANCE While designing the change strategies, the health care professional should consider how to overcome the resistance to the change. Resistance has some value in that it can force the leadership to clarify the purpose and goals of the change. Before or during this level of moving, the resistance should be identified and an attempt should be made to understand the leadership's perception. The change agent should avoid interpreting the resistance as a personal challenge. Defensive attitudes, censorship, control, or punishment could result. Usually being open to feelings and actively including resistors in the plans will lessen resistive efforts.

Implementation of Change

During implementation, five management functions must be accomplished: planning, organizing, staffing, leading, and controlling (Bailey and Claus, 1975). Timing is important; change should not be rushed. Explicit rewards or recognition of individual or group achievement reinforces changing behavior and promotes continuing efforts toward the realization of goals. Implementation must be carefully coordinated, and leaders should be open to feedback from personnel and clients. The individuals in the system need to feel that they are contributing to the improvement of health care.

The target system's cooperation with the change agent can be maximized if individuals within the target system perceive that the change agent is helping them gain more influence in the change process. Allowing frequent feedback and providing external rewards will help increase the enthusiasm for change.

The change agent should expect an initial period in which change efforts will not be rewarded by quick change. The change agent should be prepared to operate under stressful conditions without becoming defensive when confronted by the target system as it deals with the anxiety and frustration sometimes associated with the change. The nurse needs to show persistence and patience in maintaining good interpersonal relationships with the target system and practicing the art of compromise and tact.

Here are some tactics, suggested by Gillies (1982), that may be helpful in implementing change:

1. Try to create differences of opinion and dialogue by stirring up the situation.
2. Discover the discrepancy between the reality of the change and how it is perceived.
3. Introduce major ideas slowly in informal, one-to-one contacts with employees during coffee or lunch breaks.
4. Link the objectives of a proposed change to personal goals of key employees and groups.
5. Start with those individuals most receptive to the proposal.
6. Strive for some early successes; these heighten employee motivation.
7. Analyze change from the adversary's point of view.
8. Persistently and repeatedly enunciate the plans in clear and simple language.
9. Persuade any clique opposing the change to change sides and work for it.
10. Divide any clique of powerful antagonists.
11. Stay only slightly ahead of the targets, report the steps taken, and explain the next steps.
12. Help employees develop new problem-solving and human relations skills.
13. Entice each worker into some overt behavioral commitment to the change.
14. Learn the art of compromise.
15. Use positive reinforcement.
16. Provide additional skill training and psychologic support for middle management.
17. Build a psychologic support system for change agents.
18. Utilize news media and consumer support.

The setting should be considered carefully when the change agent selects which of these tactics to use. If used inappropriately they may retard rather than facilitate the implementation of planned change.

Level III: Refreezing

Evaluation

An evaluation process should be undertaken from the first steps of the change. It should include frequent feedback from the target system. Evaluation provides a method of assessing the effects of change and points out areas where it may be necessary to restructure or modify the plan.

Here are some guidelines for effective evaluation, adapted from Bailey and Claus (1975):

1. Evaluation should be planned in advance so that it is not done haphazardly.
2. Evaluation should be conducted in terms of objectives and goals that were set during the planning stage.
3. Evaluation should be objective, based upon uniform and agreed-upon standards and procedures.
4. Evaluation should be verifiable; its results must be reliable and subject to replication.
5. Evaluation should be a participative, cooperative effort involving all who were involved in the change, either as actors or individuals who were affected by it.
6. Evaluation should be specific, pinpointing strengths and weaknesses, achievements and deficiencies.
7. Evaluation should be both quantitative and qualitative.
8. Evaluation should be feasible in time, work, and cost.
9. Evaluation should result in useful information rather than information that merely satisfies curiosity.

There are several different paths that adoption of a change can take. If the change is accepted, it may be adopted and continued as is, or it may be further revised and refined before institutionalization. The change may be rejected, but later adopted, or the change may be completely rejected. Sometimes the change may be accepted in policy, but if not accepted by the people performing the procedure, it may be performed inconsistently and eventually rejected (Rogers, 1962).

Stabilization

The change must involve the target system in the change process from the stages of initial assessment through implementation and evaluation. Internalization of the change by the target system results in refreezing. A system of external sanction and reward can be established for a period of time, but unless the change is internalized into the habits and value system of the client system, it will not be permanent. If the target system changes because of fear, pressure, coercion, or a desire to please the nurse, the change will probably be only temporary.

SUCCESSFUL CHANGE

Here is an outline of a successful change project—the acquisition of a birthing chair (see Fig. 1–5). This project was reported by Jensen (1982).

Driving Forces

1. The factory was nearby (identification with area).
2. Consumers were asking for a birthing chair.
3. Some physicians were friends of a physician who helped develop the chair.

Restraining Forces

1. The cost was $5000, and there was no money in the budget because a new delivery table had been bought the previous year.
2. Some physicians were against the change.
3. There was some nursing staff resistance.

Implementation

1. The nursing staff used some work time to tour the factory and see the chair being made.
2. Some smaller changes were implemented (remodeling the delivery area, change to 10-hour shifts) that built the credibility of the change agent and the relationship between change agent and target system.
3. The fund drive started with the director's donation.
4. Community organizations were involved in fund raising.

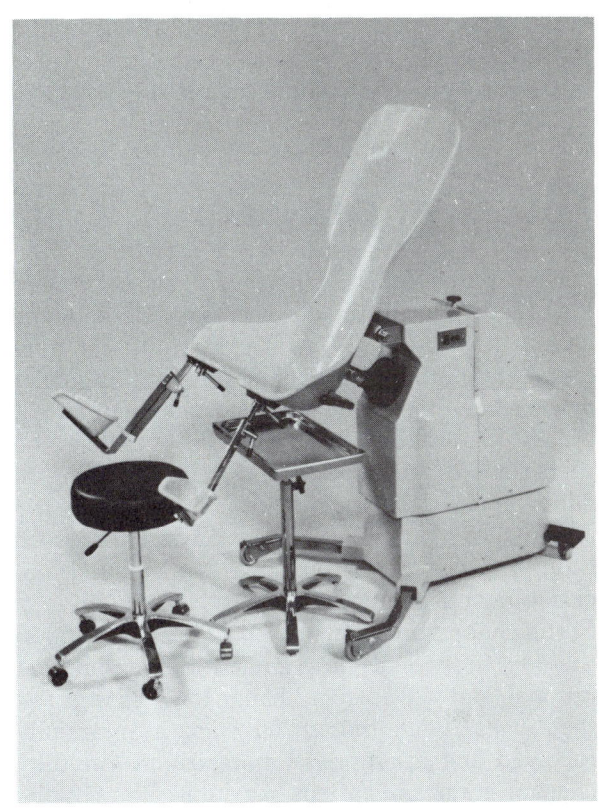

FIGURE 1–5. A modern birthing chair.
SOURCE: Courtesy of Century Manufacturing Company.

5. Staff members were involved as speakers and by participating in publicity photos.
6. A nursing research proposal was made for data to be gathered at another hospital with a birthing chair and at the hospital without a chair.
7. The salesman offered the birthing chair free of charge for a trial period.
8. The local news media announced the arrival of the birthing chair and described its advantages.
9. The staff offered clients the option of using the chair. Clients asked to use the chair.
10. Physicians were allowed to discuss the changes needed with the salesman and to order a custom-made birthing chair.
11. The fund-raising drive was successful, and the birthing chair was purchased.

Adoption and Internalization

The birthing chair was originally used for almost all deliveries (unless two births occurred at the same time or the patient desired an alternative).

Now, some 5 years later, the hospital has built a birthing center and is adjusting to the use of birthing rooms. The birthing chair is now used less frequently.

FAILURE TO CHANGE

Several pitfalls of the change process have been identified. Sometimes the necessary steps of the change process are not carried out carefully enough. Another hospital bought a birthing chair at the same time as the study hospital mentioned, but it has seldom been utilized, because the physicians did not like it and were unwilling to adapt their delivery methods to discover the advantages found by other physicians. Even though the chair was purchased, it is stored in a closet most of the time.

The change process is based on the assumption that all individuals are guided by reason, are rational, and will accept a change that will improve their lives. Even though all steps are carefully followed and appropriate strategies are carefully chosen, some individuals may never accept the change. For example, even with education and ready availability, many families may resist the adoption of family planning methods.

Other reasons for the failure of the change process may include poor definition of change goals or problems. Sometimes symptoms of the problem may be mistaken for causes, and so the change efforts may be misdirected. There may have been a failure to consider the social and physical context of the situation. When there is ineffective use of resources, frustration increases and the change process may not succeed. This has happened in some federally funded programs (Zaltman and Duncan, 1977).

CHANGE IN THE FAMILY

Almost daily the role of the nurse can be described as "facilitating family change." As families participate in the birthing process there are many difficult changes to which they must adjust, e.g. there are role changes, such as becoming a mother, father, brother, sister, grandmother, or grandfather. Economic changes occur as the family adjusts to providing for the needs of another member. Changes in the physical environment are also necessary to allow for the additional bed and other equipment associated with an infant. New tasks of parenting and physical care such as bathing, diapering, and feeding must be learned. The

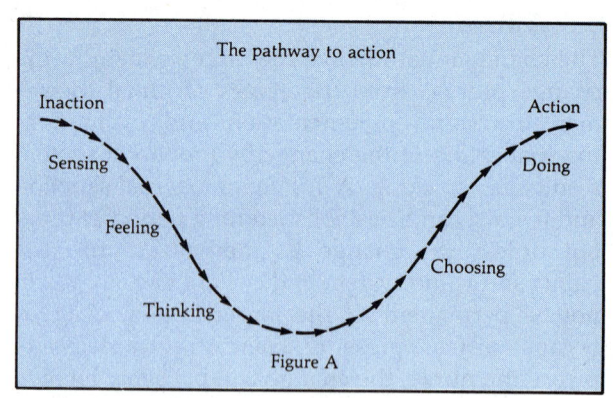

FIGURE 1-6. The pathway to action.
SOURCE: Welter (1985).

mother experiences many physical, hormonal, and metabolic changes during pregnancy and puerperium, and both parents experience developmental, emotional, and psychological changes during pregnancy, childbirth, and parenthood. Even if the pregnancy has been desired and planned, there will be times when these changes will meet resistance.

The attitude and the interactions of the nurse can facilitate the change process for these clients. Individual assessment of the client's motivations and obstacles to change is very important. Clients in developmental changes frequently need time to express their feelings. They may be too preoccupied with the changes in their lifestyles, emotions, and relationships to prioritize the health teaching they are receiving. The pathway to action begins with a sensing and clarification of feelings and thinking, before a client can move forward to choosing and doing (Fig. 1-6).

Some changes I need to make in my own life	The obstacles to making these changes	Some ways I could be more helpful in reducing the resistance of others to change

FIGURE 1-7. A format for clients.
SOURCE: Welter (1985).

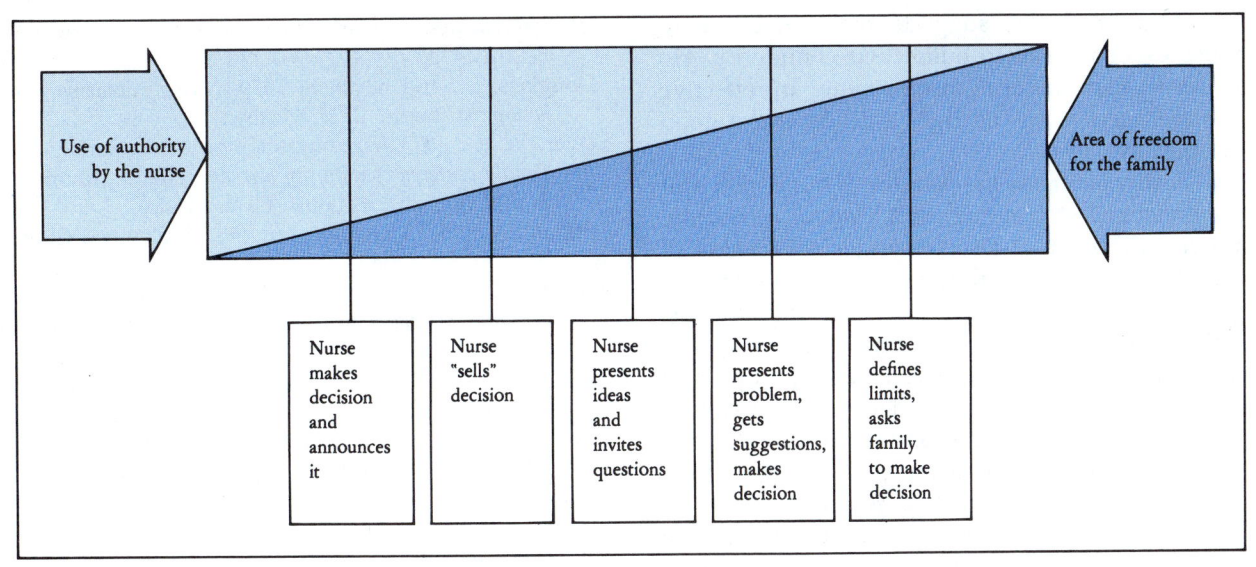

FIGURE 1–8. Continuum of leadership behavior adapted for nurses.
SOURCE: Dyer (1973).

A nursing diagnosis which can be utilized with many family clients is: "Family coping: potential for growth." Interventions such as teaching clients about the normal growth and development of children, communication skills, stress management skills, and other anticipatory guidance may facilitate the change process. Unique strengths should be identified and affirmed. The nurse change agent may help clients to identify obstacles to change and alternatives to overcome these resistors. Clients can learn to utilize the change process in solving their own problems. Figure 1–7 illustrates a format that can easily be taught to clients.

When a nurse is working within a family, the degree of responsibility each actor assumes depends on three kinds of forces:

1. *Forces in the nurse.* The degree to which the nurse will assume the authority or give more to the family will depend on personal feelings of security in giving authority to others, confidence in the family, the nurse's own training and experience, and his or her own value system of what is felt to be appropriate.
2. *Forces in the family system.* The amount of freedom that the family assumes depends on their readiness for freedom of action, their past experience and skill, their level of knowledge, and their understanding of the situation.
3. *Forces in the situation.* In addition to the nurse and the family, certain situational factors must be considered: the health situation, the time pressures, and the demands from one's superiors.

These forces must be taken into account as the nurse decides what degree of authority is appropriate and what degree the family should assume. To meet the goal of finally leaving the family in a state of autonomy, ready to handle its own health problems, the nurse should try to move in the direction of more and more authority and freedom for them (Dyer, 1973). Figure 1–8 shows how authority may be divided between the nurse and the family.

SUMMARY

Nurses may play a variety of roles in the change process, depending on their education, experience, capabilities, and status in the organization. They may be involved in any or all of the phases of the change process, working with individuals, families, or other nurses. A nurse may serve as a facilitator, data gatherer, motivator, supporter, idea supplier, resistor, protector, catalyst, integrator, climate creator, consultant, role model, or change agent.

The three most common excuses nurses give for staying silent when they think something needs to be changed are referred to as the three P's: *perfection, procrastination,* and *paralysis.* The perfection excuse uses the rationalization that the "perfect" time for suggesting the change has never happened yet. The procrastination excuse similarly always puts off the change until tomorrow, which never comes. In paralysis the nurse has made a decision to quit trying, perhaps because of past change failures. She or he has decided not to do anything outside the narrowest limits of the job. Paulson (1981) suggests that nurses using these excuses need to build their confidence. He believes that anyone can become an effective change agent with the right attitude and a good support system.

Whether acting as the director of nursing, a unit supervisor, a staff nurse, or a student nurse, the nurse can effect or affect change. Awareness of changes occurring in the world, the government, the health care industry, and the community is important for any change agent. Nurses should keep active contacts with consumer groups and ask for their ideas and preferences. They should continuously evaluate care and study their individual units for needed changes. Reading professional magazines describing recent innovations and research helps keep nurses alert to alternative kinds of care. Nurses need to add to the body of nursing knowledge by carrying out more research on the use of the change process with clients and organizations.

Nothing in life is quite so certain as change. We hope that the change agents of the future will be those educated, skilled nurses who care about other people and who will take control of the mechanistic health care system to effect change toward a more humanistic, comprehensive health care for all clients.

REFERENCES

Taking charge of change in hospital. *J. Nursing.* March:540–543.

Health care politics. Chicago: University of Chicago Press.

1973. *Standards of care for nursing practice.* Kansas City: Association.

Andreapoulos, S. 1974. *Primary care: Where medicine fails.* New York: John Wiley & Sons.

1979. Change, conflict, continuing education, competency. *Supervisor Nurse.* April:26–35.

Smith, A.; Smith, M.; and Snider, M., eds. 1979. *McGraw-Hill nursing dictionary.* New York: McGraw-Hill.

Bailey, J., and Claus, K. 1975. *Decision making in nursing.* St. Louis: C. V. Mosby.

Bennis, W.; Benne, D.; and Chin, R. 1969. *The planning of change.* 2nd ed. New York: Holt, Rinehart, & Winston.

Bennis, W.; Benne, D.; Chin, R.; and Corey, K. 1976. *The planning of change.* 3rd ed. New York: Holt, Rinehart, & Winston.

Blum, H. 1974. *Planning for health.* New York: Human Sciences Press.

Brooten, D.; Hayman, L.; and Naylor, M. 1978. *Leadership for change.* Philadelphia: J. B. Lippincott.

Clinical research: Instrument for change. *J. Nurs. Admin.* 8(12):27–32.

Douglass, L., and Bevis, E. 1979. *Nursing leadership in action.* St. Louis: C. V. Mosby.

Dyer, W. G. 1973. Planning change in the family. In *Family centered community nursing,* eds. A. Reinhart and M. Quinn. St. Louis: C. V. Mosby.

Etzioni, A. 1964. *Modern organizatins.* Englewood Cliffs, N.J.: Prentice-Hall.

Gerlach, L. P., and Hine, V. H. 1973. *Lifeway leap: The dynamics of change in America.* Minneapolis: University of Minnesota Press.

Gillies, D. 1982. *Nursing management.* Philadelphia: W. B. Saunders.

Green, C. P. 1983. Teaching strategies for the process of planned change. *J. Cont. Educ. Nurs.* 14(6):

Hamblin, R. L.; Jacobsen, R. B.; and Miller, J. L. 1973. *A mathematical theory of social change.* New York: John Wiley & Sons.

Havelock, R. 1973. *The change agent's guide to innovations in education.* Englewood Cliffs, N.J.: Educational Technology.

Herzberg, F. 1968. One more time: How do you motivate employees? *Harvard Business Review.* 46(1):53–62.

Jensen, L., 1982. *A comparative study of primiparous women delivering in a birthing chair and on a delivery table.* Unpublished master's thesis, Wichita State University.

Jones, G. N. 1969. *Planned organizational change: A study in Change Dynamics.* New York: Praeger.

Kramer, M. 1974. *Reality shock.* St. Louis: C. V. Mosby.

Lenski, G. E. 1970. *Human societies.* New York: McGraw-Hill.

Lewin, K. 1951. *Field theory in social science.* New York: Harper & Row.

Lippitt, G. I. 1973. Hospital organization in the post-industrial society. *Hosp. Prog.* 54:55–64.

Lippitt, R.; Watson, J.; and Westley, B. 1958. *The dynamics of planned change.* New York: Harcourt, Brace.

Maslow, A. 1970. *Motivation and personality.* New York: Harper & Row.

Michigan State University College of Nursing. 1980. *Role characteristics of the graduate–FNC graduate program.* Graduate handbook. Unpublished.

Mizer, H. E., and Barraro, A. 1979. Change for nursing service and education. *Nurs. Clin. N. Amer.* 14(2):337–345.

Olson, E. 1979. Strategies and techniques for the nurse change agent. *Nurs. Clin. N. Amer.* 14(2):323–386.

Paulson, T. 1981. Yes, you can change the system. *Nursing Life.* Sept./Oct.:26–31.

Reinkemeyer, G. 1970. Nursing's need: A commitment to an ideology of change. *Nurs. Forum.* 9:341–355.

Rogers, E. 1962. *Diffusion of innovations.* New York: Free Press.

Rogers, E. M., and Shoemaker, F. L. 1971. *Communication of innovations: A cross-cultural approach.* New York: Free Press.

Rushmer, R. 1975. *Humanizing health care: Alternative futures for medicine.* Cambridge, Mass.: MIT Press.

Schein, Edgar H. 1969. The mechanisms of change. In *The planning of change*, 2nd ed., eds. W. G. Bennis, K. D. Benne, and R. Chin. New York: Holt, Rinehart, & Winston.

Smith, A. D. 1973. *The concept of social change.* London: Routledge & Kegan Paul.

Spradley, B. 1980. Managing change creatively. *J. Nurs. Admin.* 10(5):32–37

Sumner, P. E., and Philips, C. R. 1981. *Birthing rooms: Concept and reality.* St. Louis; C. V. Mosby.

Urdang, L., and Swallow, H., eds. 1983. *Mosby's medical and nursing dictionary*, 3rd ed. St. Louis; C. V. Mosby.

Watson, G. 1966. *Concepts for social change.* Cooperative project for educational development series, vol. 1. Washington, D.C.: National Training Laboratories.

Welter, P. 1985 *Connecting with a friend.* Wheaton, Ill.: Tyndale, pp. 68, 72.

Young, D. 1982. *Changing childbirth.* Rochester: Childbirth Graphics.

Zaltman, G., and Duncan, R. 1977. *Strategies for planned change.* New York: John Wiley & Son.

2
Historical Developments in Maternity Nursing

BEHAVIORAL OBJECTIVES

Upon completion of this chapter, the reader should be able to:

- Identify major events in the history of maternity nursing.

- Discuss the changes in statistical data in the development of maternity nursing.

- Compare the actions of historical and present change agents to components of change theory discussed in Chapter 1.

- Compare the profession of maternity nursing today with nursing in previous periods in history.

- State contributions that can be made in the future by practioners of maternity nursing.

To evaluate the present status of maternity nursing and to plan for future changes, we must know about past changes. Throughout history, many of the needs of childbearing families have not been met by the health care system. Today, maternity nurses are effecting many changes in care to meet expressed and implied needs of consumers. Changes are occurring so rapidly that the overall effect could be termed revolutionary. New knowledge and new techniques are continually being discovered. Even with the many improvements in care to childbearing families, those families and maternity nurses are continually identifying problems that require future changes. This dynamic state of change makes maternity nursing exciting and stimulating but, at the same time, anxiety-producing and demanding.

Studying the history of childbearing leads today's maternity nurses to an appreciation of the current status of maternity nursing. This study enables learners to develop an appreciation of the difficulties overcome in the past, the significance and value of change agents and their contributions to families, and the many positive accomplishments of the profession they aspire to.

DEFINITIONS

Definitions of maternity nursing have changed as nursing has changed. Archeologic discoveries and the earliest written historical records tell us that there have always been nursing roles in all societies. The term *nurse* usually meant someone who provided nurture and caring for infants, children, families, and the physically ill. The role of nurse was usually assumed by a woman. Younger women were usually taught nursing by older women in their families or communities.

The term *midwife* has usually referred to a woman who provides primary care for childbearing women, including delivering their infants. In some instances, husbands, male family members, or other men provided care. Physicians sometimes attended parturient women, especially those with complications in childbirth. In this role, physicians were sometimes called *male midwives*.

One of the main reasons why women usually cared for other women was the common, strict distinction between men and women in societies. Women and their health problems were usually considered beneath the dignity of legitimate physicians. In addition, there were some societies in which people believed that it was immoral for physicians or male midwives to provide health care for women.

Physicians gradually became primary health care providers for women during the period between the Renaissance and the twentieth century. As the profession of medicine evolved during this time, some physicians began to specialize in the medical care of childbearing women. This specialty was called *obstetrics*, and the physicians who practiced it were called *obstetricians*. In the twentieth century obstetrics gradually moved from care in the home to care in the hospitals. Nurses who provided care in obstetric departments of hospitals were called *obstetric nurses*. Obstetrics was defined as "the science and the art of human reproduction" (Bookmiller and Bowen, 1954). The word comes from the French *obstetrix* for *midwife*, and means literally "to stand before." The definition has expanded during the early twentieth century to include health care during the prenatal, intrapartal, and postpartal periods.

As recently as the mid-twentieth century, widely used nursing textbooks defined obstetrics but not obstetric nursing. The reason for this was that *obstetric nursing* was theoretically dependent on obstetrics for its structure and practice, particularly in hospitals, where the majority of maternity nurses worked. Private duty nurses and visiting nurses (later called public health nurses) of the later nineteenth and early twentieth centuries worked more independently than hospital nurses; however, obstetric nursing at that time was based on the medical model of obstetrics. Obstetric nurses assessed childbearing women and infants and planned, implemented, and evaluated their care during the prenatal, intrapartal, postpartal, and neonatal periods.

Legally, nurses practiced in roles that were primarily dependent on physicians for direction. In actuality, they functioned interdependently and independently, depending on the situation. When physicians were present, especially in hospitals and clinics, nurses were usually dependent on the physicians for direction. When physicians were not present, nurses were required to function independently. For instance, if the physician was absent for deliveries, obstetric nurses delivered babies, although this was not legally sanctioned by nurse practice acts. Nurses were expected by physicians and health care agencies, especially hospitals, to be more independent at night than during the day. They were also expected to act more independently in hospitals and clinics that lacked medical interns and residents. These situations still exist today.

Nurses continually faced the dilemma of providing the health care that clients needed while at the same time practicing within legal boundaries. Obstetric nurses recognized that the maternity care system was not meeting many of the expressed needs of consumers. They also realized that there were many ways, within legal limits, that nurses could help these clients. Gradually, nurses began to change the base of practice from the obstetric medical model to a client-centered model of care. As a result, the term *maternity nursing* has evolved. Maternity nursing is the subsystem of health care in which the nurse collaborates with the expectant family and others to help them prevent or adapt to problems that may arise during the prenatal, intrapartal, postpartal, neonatal, and interpartal periods of childbearing. The nurse assesses, plans with the family and others, implements nursing measures, and evaluates whether those measures are meeting the goals that were set by the nurse and family members.

Beginning courses in maternity nursing enable students to begin to function in the professional maternity nursing role. Graduate level courses teach beginning professional nurse practioners to specialize for roles as *advanced registered nurse practitioners* (ARNP). ARNP roles include those of nurse practitioners, clinical nurse specialists, and nurse-midwives. So that nurses in these roles can meet the needs of consumers, the nursing profession has made efforts to expand legal limits through revisions in many states' nurse practice acts. These efforts have been successful, although some compromises have been required because of those who have been resistant to the expansion of the nurse's role.

WOMEN'S ROLES IN SOCIETY AND CHILDBEARING

Women's roles in Western European society have affected both childbearing and nursing. Although some individual women were influential and powerful, until about 100 to 150 years ago, most women had little control over their own lives. Few received any formal education, and those who did certainly were far less educated than men of the same period. Women usually belonged, literally, to their fathers or male relatives until marriage. Then they belonged to their husbands. Women could seldom own property. When they did, it usually became the property of their husbands at the time of marriage. In civilized societies, fathers usually chose husbands for their daughters. Sometimes leaders of tribes or governments chose husbands. Because of this, married couples usually had social, religious, economic, and physical similarities. If childbearing couples were congruent physically, there was less likelihood of difficulty in childbirth due to fetopelvic disproportion. In many cases, childbirth was a natural, uncomplicated process. However, if complications arose, mothers often suffered prolonged and exhausting pain, bled profusely, had convulsions, developed sepsis, and died. Women had many pregnancies during their childbearing years and miscarriages were common. Even when they delivered healthy infants, they often had to suffer the loss of their children to infections and other causes.

Much of the suffering of women resulted from their status in society. They were considered expendable except as childbearers. The status of women in society has directly affected the importance of nursing, because nurses have nearly always been women. Even today only a small percentage of nurses are men. Early histories of health care were recorded by men because they were the ones in society who could write. Women discovered natural cures that were handed down orally from woman to woman (Stevenson, 1981). Men were the ones who were taught to read and write, so they recorded their own views and achievements. They discussed nurses as ignorant peasant-midwives and medieval witches.

EARLY HISTORY TO NINETEENTH CENTURY

Ancient Civilization

Because of the status of women in society, little is recorded about childbirth in very early history. However, since the customs of primitive tribes change slowly, studies of health practices of primitive cultures may provide insight into prehistoric and ancient cultures (Graham, 1951; Bullough and Bullough, 1978). Various authors have described many different customs related to childbirth (Figs. 2–1—2–4). In some primitive tribes mothers assumed kneeling, squatting, or sitting positions for delivery of their newborns. Newborn infants were often bathed with either cold or warm water and treated with applications of various substances—grease, sand, or red or black dye (Graham, 1951; Bullough and Bullough, 1978). In some primitive cultures fathers participated in both labor and delivery. Sometimes wives sat on their husband's lap and reclined against him, with the husband's legs spread on either side. Both husband and midwife applied pressure on the contracting uterus. In many other cultures, husbands were excluded from participation in childbirth because of fears, superstition, customs, or taboos (Graham, 1951).

Women were often treated with cruel and painful methods, particularly when they developed complications in childbirth. The ancients believed

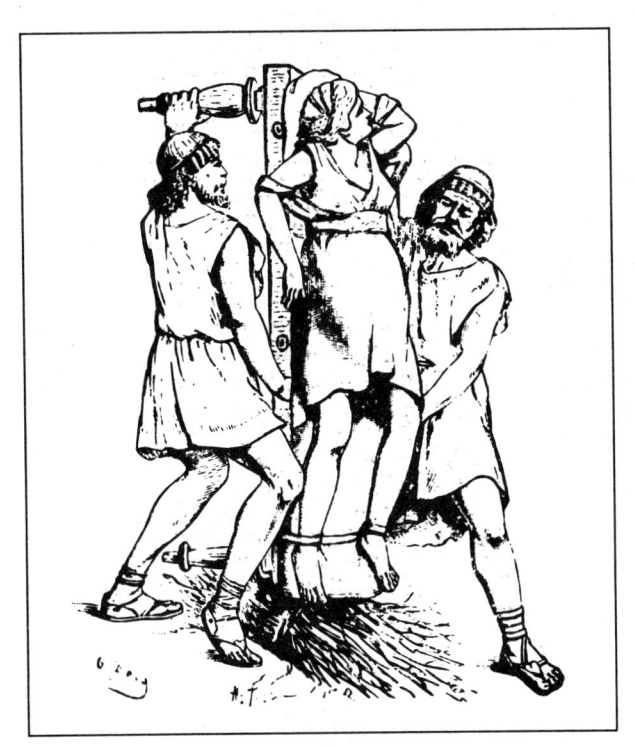

Historical Developments in Maternity Nursing 25

FIGURE 2–1. Childbirth in antiquity. The pregnant woman was tied to a table and moved up and down to speed labor.
SOURCE: The Bettmann Archive, Inc.

that unborn babies actively initiated labor and moved themselves out of their mothers' bodies. In some cultures mothers were vigorously shaken, held upside down, or both to speed the birth. Sometimes wild horses were released to charge at women about to deliver, turning aside immediately before trampling them. This torture was supposed to frighten the woman into delivery or scare the child out of the woman's body. In other

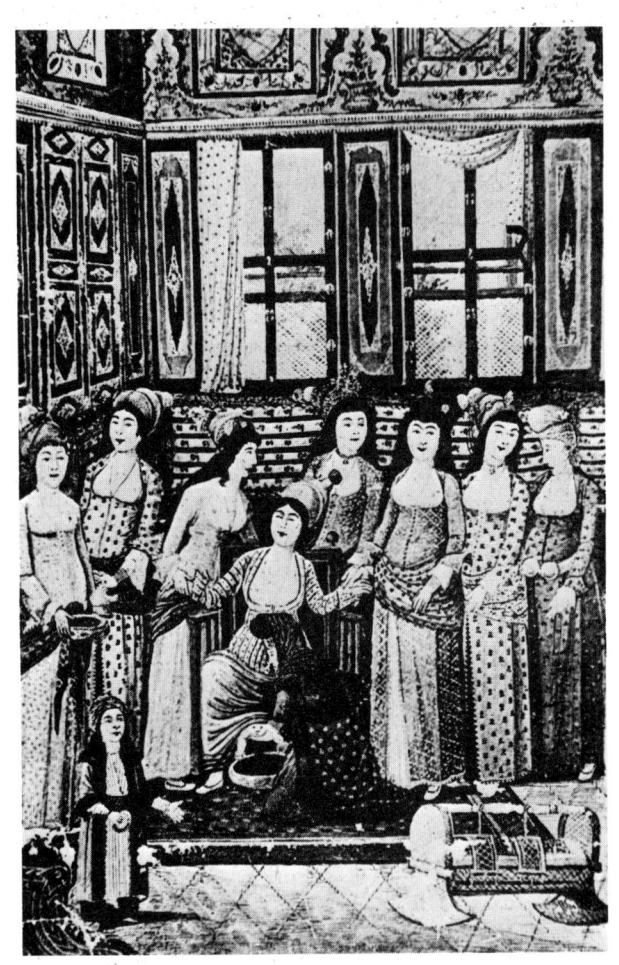

FIGURE 2–2. Childbirth in a Turkish home. Note the birthing stool.
SOURCE: The Bettman Archive, Inc.

instances, food was used to coax the baby into the extrauterine world. In some groups mothers either bit into or ate part of the placenta after its delivery.

Findley (1939) concludes that primitive people

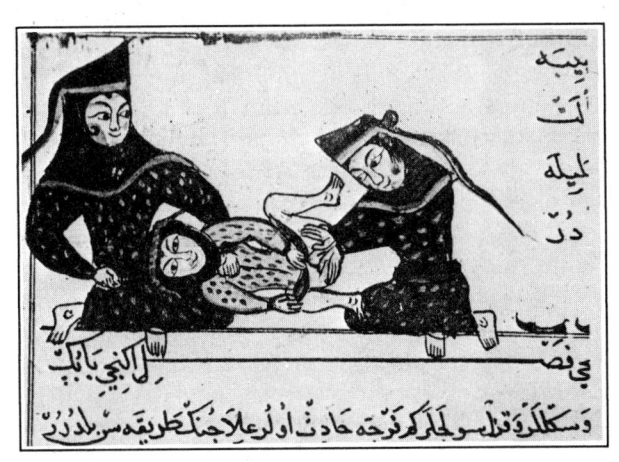

FIGURE 2–3. Turkish female physician assisting with birth, 1466.
SOURCE: The Bettmann Archive, Inc.

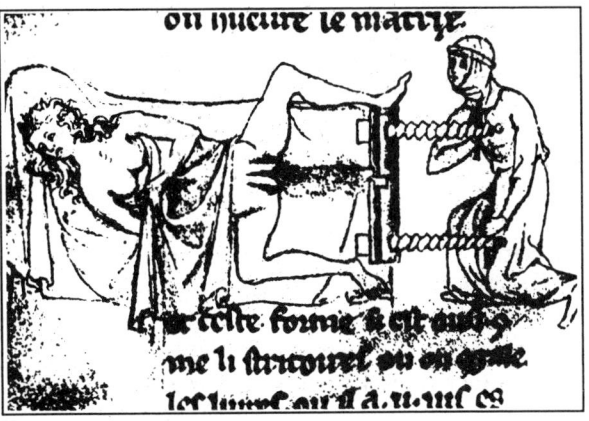

FIGURE 2–4. Vaginal examination using vaginal dilator as described by Arabs.
SOURCE: Bettmann Archive, Inc.

were unable to "conceive of logical sequences," and because of this, they lived in mystery and fear. In many societies roles in medicine and religion were mixed. Priests were also medicine men.

Records of early civilization in the Bible offer examples of women who acted as nurses for infants and children. The importance of women midwives in the management of childbirth is discussed (Gen. 35:17; Exod. 1:15–21). Birthing stools are mentioned. The Song of Solomon refers to giving birth under an apple tree. This may have been common (Graham, 1951). Commands to bathe after coitus and to avoid intercourse with menstruating or parturient women reflect the attitudes toward sex hygiene in the Mosaic period (Findley, 1939). Mosaic law includes public health laws that have relevance today. Bathing, diet, contagious diseases, and circumcision are discussed. Some of these practices were similar to those in Egypt, Persia, and other countries in the Middle East.

Graham (1951) states that the Egyptian papyri are the oldest medical records. One of these, the Ebers papyrus, a perfectly preserved roll of papyrus that dates from 1550 B.C., was found in an Egyptian tomb in 1872. It discusses childbirth, abortion, and various diseases of women, including breast problems. Interventions such as douches of dates in milk, dates in hog's bile, garlic and horn of a cow, bile of a cow, and cassia and oil are mentioned. The belief that the sex of the unborn infant could be predicted by observing the color of the pregnant woman's face is discussed. The papyrus also discusses a milk and semen mixture prescribed for various ailments by a goddess who was called the first woman doctor in history.

Maternity care providers were categorized, even in very early cultures. Egyptian maternity care providers were referred to as ordinary midwives and physician midwives. In China and Japan only midwives were permitted to care for women. In India there were "womenhelpers" (Findley, 1939). In many early civilizations, physicians assisted only with difficult births.

In many cultures, particularly those that were Mohammedan and Oriental, some type of "circumcision" was performed on girls. Usually the clitoris and labia minora were removed to prevent promiscuity and the enjoyment of sex (Graham, 1951).

In early Irish childbirth practices, women delivered the mother while she knelt on a feather mattress and leaned against a chair in front of her. After the delivery, the mattress was burned to prevent the spread of infection. The mother and newborn were kept together, and the mother was usually allowed out of bed by the third day and resumed chores by the fifth day (Dolan, 1973).

Ancient Greece

In ancient Greece midwives were called "naval cutters" (Findley, 1939). Aristotle spoke of their wisdom and intelligence. Some were of the high social orders and were intelligent and skillful. For example, the mother of Socrates and the wife of Pericles were midwives.

Agnodice the Athenian, who lived in ancient Greece, was an early change agent. She became concerned about the "chaste and noble women of Athens" who were being maltreated by "man-wives." These physicians were attempting to have restraining laws passed that would allow them a monopoly on the practice of midwifery. Because of her concern for childbearing women, Agnodice went to Alexandria to study midwifery. She return to Greece, put on men's clothing, and proceeded to practice her profession in Athens. She was brought to court, and there she revealed that she was a woman. She was acquitted after women of high social rank defended her to the court. After her victory, the city of Athens licensed midwives to practice midwifery and to treat diseases of women (Findley, 1939).

The Greek culture was significantly advanced beyond previous cultures. Greek medicine was more similar to modern medicine than was any other medical practice in history. Hippocrates (460–379 B.C.) was recognized as the greatest physician of his day. He is accepted as the father of medicine. Many medical books of this period are attributed to this Greek physician (Bullough and Bullough, 1978). His writing has few childbirth references, although one woman's puerperal sepsis is discussed. Bullough and Bullough (1978) indicate that very little is recorded about nursing because it was implemented by women, who were kept distinctly separate from men. During this period, physicians, who were usually men, rarely attended at births. They usually assisted only with very difficult deliveries. If mothers could not deliver babies vaginally, physicians had to destroy the babies and cut them out piece-meal. Midwifery and gynecology were not as advanced as other areas of medicine (Graham, 1951).

Soranus (A.D. 98–138) has been called the father of obstetrics. He was born in Ephesus, studied in

Alexandria, and practiced in Rome during the times of Trajan and Hadrian (Graham, 1951). He was the first to write about podalic version, a procedure largely forgotten during the next 1300 years. He wrote about pregnancy, the birthing chair, and abortion. He taught midwives to use warm hands with trimmed, smooth nails. He urged discretion. He wanted women to be taught to examine themselves and to use rancid oil, honey, cedar oil, thin strips of lint, and pessaries for contraception. He advocated supporting the perineum with a linen pad when the head was advancing during delivery to prevent tearing. There may have been obstetricians of the caliber of Soranus in the next 1400 years, but if there were, everything they wrote or did is lost. He taught rational midwifery and child care that was based on knowledge and divorced from the superstition that had been prevalent for centuries (Graham, 1951).

Galen (A.D. 130–200) was another Greek physician who practiced in Rome. In brilliance and influence he surpassed even Hippocrates but lacked his depth, selflessness, and serenity (Graham, 1951). He wrote over 300 books, some of which contain scattered references to midwifery and gynecology. He was arrogant, uncompromising, and impatient. He made enemies of his colleagues, and turned to the laity for support. He was "fiercely combatted in his own time by his envious colleagues"; however, physicians for centuries considered him infallible (Findley, 1939). These Greek physicians had probably never dissected women's bodies, but their descriptions of anatomy are remarkably accurate for their day. After Galen, most of the civilized world's medicine began to decline into superstition, numerology, mysticism, astrology, and sheer ignorance.

Christianity

The spreading influence of Christianity led to the promotion of feelings of compassion for those in need of health care. Christ's teachings promoted elevation of the status of women, and some Christians followed those teachings. Although this tenet of Christianity was ignored in many instances, Christiantity did foster the development of nursing as an occupation. The New Testament mentions several instances of women who functioned in nursing roles. Phoebe, a deaconess, is described as "a succourer of many" and of Paul himself (Rom. 16:1–2). Widows are cited as relieving the afflicted (1 Tim. 5:9–10). Early Christian religious orders provided organized nursing services for centuries.

Historical literature mentions few organized groups of nurses until 660, when a small number of volunteers became the Sisters of Hotel Dieu. Stewart (1962) calls this the oldest order of nuns devoted to nursing alone.

The Middle Ages

During the Middle Ages, only the Arabian physicians practiced medicine according to some of the scientific methods used by earlier physicians. The Moslem world erected magnificent hospitals during the eighth to the tenth centuries (Griffin and Griffin, 1973).

In most of the "civilized world" filth and diseases, particularly syphilis and bubonic plague, were widespread. Bettman (1956) indicates that women in the Middle Ages were in great danger of puerperal sepsis and sheer butchery. The status of women remained low. In addition, they were considered to be "sisters of Eve" and represented "sin incarnate." It was thought that they deserved to suffer, especially in childbirth, because Gen. 3:16 states that Eve should bring forth children in sorrow.

Beginning around the twelfth or thirteenth century, crusaders to the Holy Land brought chastity girdles back to Europe. These were metal devices that encircled women's hips. They had openings with protruding metal teeth over the areas of the vulva and anus. They were kept locked. These devices, used for several hundred years, are displayed in museums today (Findley, 1939).

Nursing has always been affected by military campaigns and military health care. During the Middle Ages there were three male military nursing orders—the Knights of St. John, the Teutonic Knights, and the Knights of St. Lazarus. There were also corresponding orders of women who cared for women in their special hospitals (Griffin and Griffin, 1973).

The Renaissance

The Renaissance brought many advances in most areas of life; however, the most backward field of medicine during this period was obstetrics. In 1522, one male physician, a Dr. Theutt of Hamburg, wanted to study the process of birth. Men were not allowed in the lying-in chambers, so he dressed as a woman to observe a woman's labor and delivery. He was discovered and burned at the stake (Graham, 1951). In this same period some authorities believed what whipping the mother in labor might upset her so that the baby would be born. Physicians were sometimes called by midwives to assist with extremely difficult deliveries. Those physicians were called *male midwives*.

Leonardo da Vinci (1452–1519) dissected bodies in Rome to learn how to portray accurately the human body in art. For centuries dissection of dead bodies had been forbidden. Da Vinci was the first to show an accurate drawing of the uterus (see Fig. 2–5). Arantius, an Italian of the same period, described the gravid uterus and its contents at different periods of pregnancy (Bookmiller and Bowen, 1954).

In 1500 a Swiss sow-gelder, Jacob Nufer, performed a successful cesarean section upon his wife, who lived for years afterward (Graham, 1951). For centuries before, cesarean section had usually been performed as a last resort and usually on a dead woman. (At one time, it was though that the term *cesarean section* was so named because Julius Caesar had been delivered in that manner. This idea has been discounted by some historians). William P. Dewees (1768–1841), a professor of obstetrics at the University of Pennsylvania, believed that the procedure on a living mother was known to the ancient Jews. Other historians agree that the Talmud refers to this surgical procedure.

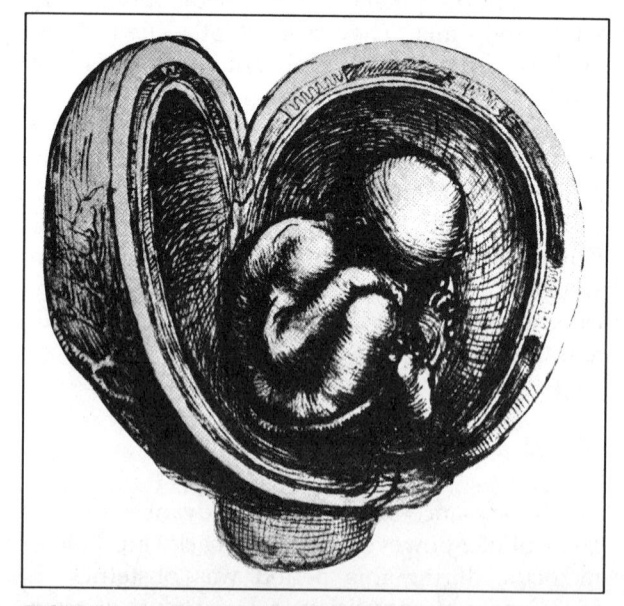

FIGURE 2–5. Fetus *in utero* from a drawing by Leonardo da Vinci.
SOURCE: The Bettmann Archive, Inc.

However, it was performed rarely on living women until the introduction of surgical aseptic techniques.

Until the fifteenth century, when printed medical books were introduced, the majority of the older medical documents were unused. In 1513 Eucharius Roesslin published *Rosegarden of pregnant women and midwives,* which was used as an obstetric textbook for 200 years. It was merely a review of previous documents. Thomas Raynalde plagiarized it and renamed it the *Byrth of mankind* in 1545. It "had some sensible suggestions" but "effected no immediate reforms" (Bettmann, 1954, p. 107). In 1595 Scipione Mercurio reported a cesarean section on a living mother in his midwifery handbook. *LcCommare O Reccoglitrice,* published in Venice in 1596 by G. B. Ciotti, describes the technique of cesarean section.

William Harvey (1578–1657), a brilliant student of great Italian teachers, discovered the circulation of the blood and also wrote about the physiology of childbirth. He has often been called the father of modern medicine because he is credited with establishing the principle of the physiologic experiment (Griffin and Griffin, 1973).

Ambroise Pare (1510–1590), a French barber-surgeon, is credited as having rediscovered podalic version. In 1668 Francois Mauriceau, a famous French obstetrician, published a treatise on midwifery that was advanced for its time. Most of these famous obstetricians taught midwives. Louise Bourgeois (1563–1637), a well-known French midwife of this period, advocated the use of podalic version.

In the late sixteenth century a school for midwives was established at Hotel Dieu in Paris. This school was recognized for improving the character of midwives. Hospitals in this period were used only by poor, destitute parturient women.

Although the Hindus and the Greeks used implements to deliver stillborns and the Arabs used some obstetric forceps, credit is generally given to the Chamberlens for inventing modern obstetric forceps. William Chamberlen was a Huguenot who escaped persecution in France and went to England in 1569. He had two sons and a grandson, all named Peter, who were obstetricians. The Chamberlens are given credit for inventing the forceps (Findley, 1939). Some of the Chamberlens taught midwives and even championed their rights. These physicians were usually opposed by the College of Physicians for their work with midwives, for being mercenary, and for gaining fame because of the secret of their *instru-*

ments of iron, which they guarded for five generations (Findley, 1939).

In 1620 the physician Fuller and his wife, a highly esteemed midwife, came to Massachusetts on the *Mayflower*. Anne Hutchinson was another early midwife in America. She went to Boston in 1634, but when she was banished for noncompliance with the religious beliefs of this community, she went to Rhode Island. When she served as midwife to a friend who had an anencephalic infant, Hutchinson was accused of being a witch, and she moved again. She was later killed in an Indian raid.

Prominent lay people have had significant influence on changes effected in historical times. In 1663, Mlle. La Valliere, mistress of Louis XIV of France, was attended by a physician (male midwife), Le Sieur Boucher. Louis hid and watched La Valliere's labor and delivery. Later, in 1682, Jules Clement delivered the French Dauphine. These and similar events in other countries led to people in lower social groups following the examples of the nobility. It gradually began to be accepted for men to be present and to serve as attendants during childbirth.

The Eighteenth Century

In England William Smellie (1697–1763) introduced new types of forceps and wrote an important book on midwifery that has recently been reprinted (Smellie, 1974; Fig. 2–6). This book discussed rules for using forceps as well as for measuring to differentiate between contracted and normal pelves (Bookmiller and Bowen, 1954). It contains incorrect information, and lacks the scientific rationale on which contemporary practice is based, but it discusses many concepts that are relevant today.

Midwives have been licensed or regulated throughout history. Bookmiller and Bowen (1954) cite an eighteenth-century New York City ordinance that required midwives to take an oath including the promise to help any woman in labor, whether rich or poor; to identify the true mother and father of the newborn; to prevent the newborn's being murdered or hurt; to consult with other midwives as the need arose; to avoid giving medicine to produce abortion; to avoid concealing the birth of bastards; and to be of good behavior.

William Shippen, a prominent U.S. physician who had studied with Smellie in England, initiated a midwifery course in Philadelphia in 1762. He was later a professor of anatomy, surgery, and midwifery at the University of Pennsylvania.

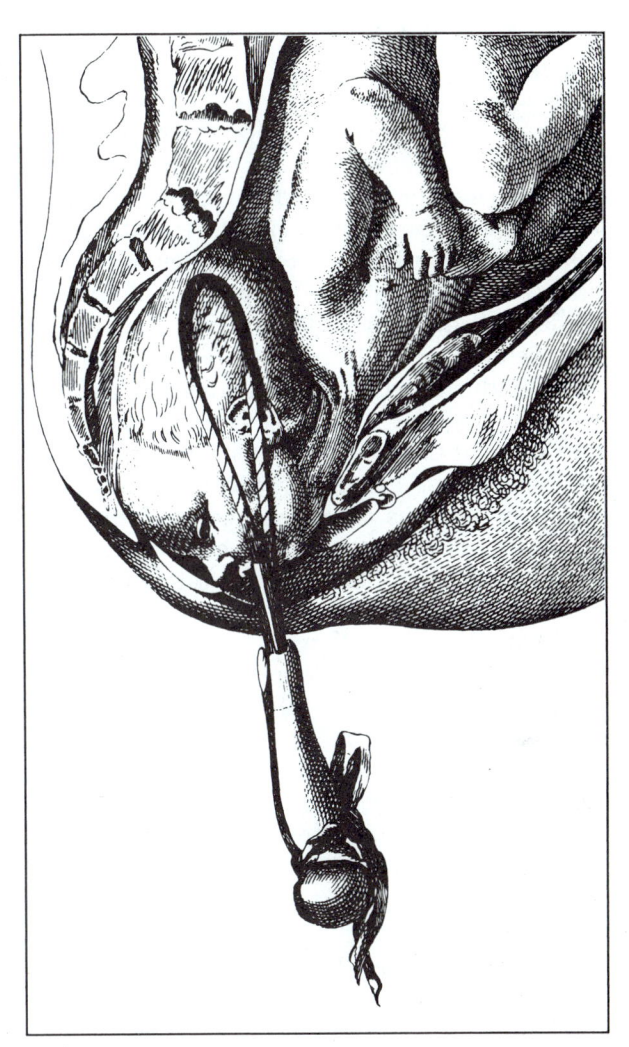

FIGURE 2–6. Forceps bound with leather strips applied to child. After treatise on midwifery by Smellie (1974).
SOURCE: The Bettman Archive, Inc.

THE NINETEENTH CENTURY

An English physician, Sir James Y. Simpson (1811–1870), has received credit for first using anesthesia in childbirth. He used chloroform, although this was strongly opposed by clergymen who believed women should suffer pain in childbirth. Simpson's work influenced Dr. John Snow, who used chloroform for Queen Victoria while she was giving birth to her seventh child (McGrellis, 1976). The queen was so beloved and admired by her subjects that this event was largely responsible for initiating widespread use of anesthesia in childbirth.

Early Nursing Education in the United States

Nursing education in the United States was influenced by Elizabeth Blackwell, the first woman to graduate from a U.S. medical school. Blackwell had been refused admission at several medical schools because she was a woman. Bendiner (1980) relates that she had to be accepted by all 129 male students at the Geneva (New York) Medical College before she could enroll as a student there. After graduation from medical school in 1849, she went to England and then to France to study midwifery at La Maternité, which was recognized as the greatest European school of midwifery. However, she was prevented from studying there because she was blinded in one eye by a gonococcal infection she contracted while caring for someone with gonorrhea.

Blackwell and a colleague, Marie Zakrzewska, helped found the New York Infirmary for Women in 1857. They also worked together to establish educational opportunities for nurses and, in 1872, were involved in the establishment of the first recognized school of nursing in the United States at the New England Hospital for Women and Children (De Young, 1972). Blackwell was a friend of Florence Nightingale (Dolar, 1973; Bullough and Bullough, 1978).

Early nursing education was also influenced by the religious orders that had included organized nursing groups and also some lay orders. A lay order of nurses called the Sisters of Charity had been organized by St. Vincent de Paul in 1633 in France, but it became the "most widespread and best beloved of all nursing orders" of the period (Stewart, 1962).

In the United States Elizabeth Bayley Seton was the director of the Sisters of Charity of St. Joseph, established in Maryland in 1809. Other Catholic sisterhoods in the United States established hospitals with schools of nursing. These hospitals and schools have made many positive contributions to maternity care by fostering high standards of nursing and implementing policies that promote family-centered care. For example, the hospitals operated by Catholic religious orders were among the first to have rooming-in in obstetric departments of hospitals

In 1826 a Protestant group of deaconesses was organized under the direction of Pastor Theodor Fliedner and his wife, Friederike. They opened a hospital and home for deaconesses at Kaiserwerth on the Rhine in Germany. Friederike wrote "the first work on nurses' training ever written by a woman" (Goodnow, 1948). After Friederike died in 1842, Pastor Fliedner married Caroline Bertheau, who had been in charge of nursing at a hospital in Hamburg. The work at Kaiserswerth grew until there were 1600 deaconesses, 32 deaconess houses, and 400 fields of work, including both England and Pennsylvania. Both deaconesses and nurses in religious orders worked long, grueling hours for room and board; they were given no salary. The influence of these organizations contributed to the policies and practices of early hospital schools in the United States. Many of those schools, from the late nineteenth century to the mid-twentieth century, provided room, board, and education (called training) in return for assigned and supervised nursing work. There were varying ratios of class time to clinical work; students were generally exploited until accreditation by the National League for Nursing Education began to be sought by these and other schools of nursing.

Changes to Prevent Puerperal Sepsis

One of the most significant changes in the history of maternity care was the institution of proper handwashing to prevent the spread of puerperal fever. Puerperal fever was mentioned in the writing of both Hippocrates and Galen (Pritchard and MacDonald, 1976). However, epidemics of the disease were first reported at the beginning of the sixteenth century. This was the period when the first obstetric hospital wards (called lying-in wards) were opened. Even then, most women still had babies at home. Only the very poor and outcast went to the hospitals. Many of the childbearing women in hospitals were unmarried or were prostitutes. In these early obstetric hospital wards, where midwives usually delivered the women, many of the patients died from puerperal fever. There was little scientific knowledge of infectious disease, particularly of its cause. Two men were primarily responsible for determining the cause of puerperal fever.

Oliver Wendell Holmes

Oliver Wendell Holmes (1809–1894) was a physician, teacher, writer, and professor of anatomy at Harvard Medical School. He was an interesting, humorous speaker and a good writer. In 1840 he heard a medical report of the death of a colleague after performing an autopsy on a woman whose cause of death was puerperal fever (Bookmiller and Bowen, 1954). There had been scattered reports in the eighteenth century of the infectious nature of this killer of childbearing women, but they were largely ignored. In 1843 Holmes published *The contagiousness of puerperal fever,* in which he demonstrated that this disease was spread by physicians who went from patient to patient without cleansing their hands. He was criticized by his peers, especially the obstetricians of the day. One objected because it seemed to him preposterous that gentlemen could carry infection on their hands. In spite of criticism, Holmes reprinted his work with additions in 1855. He taught medicine for nearly half a century, and he tried to obtain admission for women to Harvard Medical School. His persistence, scholarly writing, and use of effective communication skills and interpersonal relations enabled him to effect the significant change of handwashing between examinations of parturient women.

Ignaz Phillip Semmelweis

Ignaz Phillip Semmelweis (1818–1865), a Hungarian physician who was a contemporary of Holmes, is considered a heroic but tragic change agent by many historians. Semmelweis studied in Budapest and then graduated from medical school in Vienna in 1844. In that year he began work at the Vienna Lying-in Hospital, where students of both medicine and midwifery studied.

Medical students and physicians, including Semmelweis, dissected and studied cadavers. Medical students were taught in the First Obstetric Clinic (ward). They examined and delivered women there. Midwifery students were taught in the Second Obstetric Clinic. Childbearing women pleaded to go to the second clinic because so many women died in the first clinic, where the mortality rate was three times the rate in the second clinic. When Kalletschka, a friend and colleague of Semmelweis, died of puerperal sepsis after cutting a finger during an autopsy, Semmelweis became determined to investigate the disease thoroughly. There had been concern in the medical group about the high mortality rates, but they were attributed to various factors other than infection. After extensive data collection and analysis, Semmelweis concluded that physicians and medical students were spreading disease by going directly from dissecting cadavers to examining parturient women. He required that everyone wash their hands in a chloride of lime solution between patients. There was a dramatic drop in mortality rates, particularly in the first clinic. The mortality rate dropped from 12.4 to 1.27 percent in two months (Bettmann, 1954). Kalisch and Kalisch (1978) report that the mortality rate dropped over 90 percent between 1846 and 1848. Graham (1954) states that it fell from 11.4 to 3.8 percent in a year, and that in the following year it was only 1.27 percent. The rate for the midwives in the second year was 1.33 percent.

Even so, Semmelweis was vehemently opposed by his colleagues. He called another physician a murderer and a Nero, as well as blaming his superior for the terrible conditions in the wards. Persecuted by his colleagues, he left Vienna in 1858 and went to Budapest, where he faced similar experiences (Bettmann, 1954).

Semmelweis published *The aetiology, concept and prophylaxis of childbirth fever* in 1861. It was ridiculed in Europe and America for years afterward (Kalisch and Kalisch, 1978). Graham (1954) states that Semmelweis was a poor writer. This, coupled with his poor interpersonal relations, hampered the acceptance of his work. He died in an insane asylum of an infection that was probably septicemia.

Changes leading to the prevention of puerperal fever were influenced further by the work of Louis Pasteur (1822–1895) and Sir Joseph Lister (1827–1912), who worked to prove the germ theory and to promote antiseptic techniques in the care of wounds.

The Beginning of Modern Nursing

Florence Nightingale (1820–1910), the founder of modern nursing, influenced all of nursing, including maternity care. Nightingale, an extraordinary person, was famous and honored in her own lifetime for the contributions she made to society.

Nightingale was born in Florence, Italy, to wealthy upper-class English parents. Although most girls of her day were not formally educated, she was taught Greek, Latin, French, German, Italian, philosophy, and history by her father. A governess taught her music and drawing (Bullough and Bullough, 1969). Wealthy and deeply religious, she grew up protected, because women were thought to be weak and vulnerable.

Because of her Christian beliefs, she was concerned about those who were ill and needed care, and she was particularly interested in the state of hospital care of the ill and injured. At this time the status of nursing as an occupation was very low. In *Martin Chuzzlewit,* Charles Dickens described despicable characteristics of nurses of that day. This widely read author created the characters Sairey Gamp and Betsy Prig, who were ignorant, lazy, dirty, uncaring, selfish nurses. This view of nurses, prevalent in the United States as well as England, was changed, in part, because of the influence of Florence Nightingale and her work.

Nightingale believed that nurses needed to provide more than compassion, sympathy, tenderness, and kindness. She realized that she and others would need *knowledge* to become effective in the care of the sick and the prevention of illness. She studied literature about hospitals and the care of the sick.

In addition, she went to Kaiserswerth and to the Sisters of Charity in Paris to study their methods. Despite strong family opposition to all her efforts to become a nurse, she came back to England and took over the superintendency of a hospital there.

This background prepared her to go to the Crimea with her own group of nurses. Nightingale's friend, Secretary of War Sidney Herbert, asked her to improve the hospital conditions for the wounded and sick British soldiers in the Crimean War. Thousands of British soldiers had been dying because of the filth, vermin, rodents, and lack of care in the military hospital wards.

Nightingale and her nurses literally transformed the wards, but not without opposition. Nightingale was responsible for her nurses, but all the nurses were responsible to the military medical officers, who were opposed to their work, especially at first (Palmer, 1983). She encouraged good public relations with the officers. The nurses proceeded cautiously, kept records of their achievements, and finally won recognition for back-breaking work and compassionate and knowledgeable care.

Although she worked within the system, Nightingale maintained high standards. She introduced cleanliness in the wards, proper cooking of food, and clean bedding. She obtained clothing and even medical supplies for patients and organized a "lying-in hospital" for wives of the soldiers. She was responsible for lowering the mortality rate in the military hospital from 60 percent to about 1 percent (Kalisch and Kalisch, 1978). After returning from the Crimea to England, Nightingale used her considerable influence with the public and government authorities to quietly work for reforms in the army and in hospitals as well as in nursing.

Kalisch and Kalisch (1983) relate a story that exemplifies her response to those with whom she disagreed. When she heard that a physician who had fought her work in the Crimea had been awarded the K.C.B. (Knight Commander of the Order of the Bath), she wrote to her influential friend Sieney Herbert, referring to the physician as the Knight of the Crimean Burial Grounds. She has been portrayed in a film as having made that statement directly to the physician; however, she did not use such tactics. During those times even women of influence had to use manipulative skill in effecting changes in a world dominated by men.

She also used writing to effect change. In 1858 she wrote *Notes on matters affecting the health, efficiency, and hospital administration* of the British Army, which influenced leaders of government and the military to reform many of the injustices suffered by British soldiers. During that same year she wrote *Notes on hospitals*. In 1859 she wrote *Notes on nursing*, which served for years as a standard textbook on nursing (Kalisch and Kalisch, 1978). Palmer (1983) lists a bibliography of her work.

The people of England were so grateful for her service that they rewarded her with the Nightingale fund, which she used to start a nursing school at St. Thomas' Hospital in 1860. The school's admission standards and training program were very strict. She also helped found a school for the first public health nurses (called visiting or district nurses).

In addition, Nightingale emphasized the need for nurse-midwifery education (Graham, 1951). In 1871 she published a "monumental statistical report on the subject of obstetrical mortality" (Palmer, 1983).

Nightingale received many honors from her countrymen, from political leaders, and from Queen Victoria. Her work was influential in effecting changes in other countries as well as in the British empire. "Nightingale nurses" from schools she established went to other countries, including the United States, to introduce their methods. This led to vastly improved nursing education and practice (Stewart, 1962).

Nightingale's admonitions are relevant today. She advised proceeding carefully and slowly, trying out changes, and maintaining flexibility (Palmer, 1983). Historical accounts of her life offer the reader examples of changes that have had immeasurable influence on the status of women and nursing today. Accounts of her work have continued to serve as direction for implementation of change.

Nightingale was a strong supporter of the International Red Cross, founded by the Swiss humanitarian Henri Dunant in 1864. Clara Barton, an American Civil War nurse, aroused American interest in the Red Cross. She was an early leader of the American Red Cross (ARC), which was organized in 1881. The ARC later recruited, taught, and certified registered nurses to teach expectant couples about pregnancy, childbirth, and baby care, providing an early influence in the childbirth education movement.

INTO THE TWENTIETH CENTURY

Margaret Sanger

Margaret Sanger (1883–1966) was another nursing change agent whose life serves as a role model for those desiring to make improvements in maternity health care delivery. A citizen of the United States, she was the public health nurse (visiting nurse) who opened the first birth control clinic in America in 1916 in Brooklyn, New York. She was an educated, dedicated, courageous, altruistic humanitarian who displayed effective public relations, initiative, and persistence.

Historical sources differ on the date of her birth but agree that she was the sixth of eleven children. Early in her life she nursed her mother, who died of tuberculosis at the age of 48. Sanger was very much aware that her mother died at a much younger age than her father, who lived to be 80.

Her mother's illness motivated her to become a physician; however, she could not afford medical education. *Who's who of American women,* vol. I (1958) states that Margaret Sanger attended Claverack College in Hudson, New York, and graduated from the Nurses Training School of White Plains Hospital. She also studied at the School of Manhattan Eye and Ear Hospital. She married William Sanger, a prosperous architect, in 1900. They had two sons and a daughter.

Sanger's work as a public health nurse brought her into contact with childbearing families who had more children than they could properly feed or clothe. Among those families, maternal and infant mortality rates were particularly appalling. Mothers literally begged for information that would help them prevent additional births (Sanger, 1938). The turning point in Sanger's life was her experience with the 28-year-old mother of three who aborted herself and then died 3 months later after another self-abortion (Kalisch and Kalisch, 1978).

Margaret Sanger studied the problems of the poverty-stricken with whom she worked. She identified their problem and millions of others like them as that of too many births due to ignorance of contraception. In order to begin to find solutions to the problem, she studied independently in libraries in the United States. She concluded that there was no information on contraception available in this country.

Because of the deficit of information in the United States, she visited France and learned about methods the French had used for generations to prevent large families (Sanger, 1938). After returning to the United States she published periodicals and other literature about limiting births. In 1914 she started *Woman Rebel,* a periodical. Such publications were forbidden by the Comstock Law, which classified birth control information as obscene and pornographic and also prohibited contraception and abortion. In her literature she coined the phrase *birth control.* She also enlisted the help of her family and others, particularly wealthy, influential people who were also concerned about this problem.

When she sent her literature through the mails, the U.S. Justice Department indicted her on nine counts of violation of the Comstock Law. She realized she could go to the penitentiary for 45 years. When the agents came to arrest her, she spent 3 hours telling them "the tragic stories of conscript of motherhood" (Sanger, 1938). They agreed with her that the Comstock Law should not exist.

Sanger realized that she was not prepared to defend her case in court. After writing a letter of explanation to the judge of her case, she left her family and went to Canada to prepare her defense. She later went to England and then to the Netherlands, where birth control was accepted and the maternal mortality rate was one-third that in the United States. She traveled in other European countries gathering information about birth control. Soon after she returned to the United States (in 1915) her daughter died of pneumonia. *Who's who of American women* (1958) states that eminent friends of the birth control movement used influence with President Wilson to have the case against Sanger dropped. According to Kennedy (1970), her husband was arrested in 1915 and went to jail for a time.

In 1916, Sanger and her sister, Ethel Byrne, who was also a nurse, as well as Fania Mindell, opened a birth control clinic and were arrested after approximately 1 week of operation. In court, she challenged the law that forbade the dissemination of birth control information. The judge sentenced her to 30 days in the workhouse, and Sanger served that sentence. She continued her work as a teacher, held conferences, and founded organizations concerned with birth control. One organization was the National Birth Control League (Sanger, 1938). She was arrested several other times.

Even though her family was supportive, her work eventually took its toll on her family life, and she was divorced in 1920. In 1922 she married Noah H. Slee, a wealthy patron of the birth control movement.

In 1928 she founded the National Committee on Federal Legislation for Birth Control, which later became the Planned Parenthood Federation of America. In addition to *Women Rebel*, she also published the *Birth Control Review*. She wrote ten books which were published between 1916 and 1931. Her autobiography was published in 1938.

From 1910 to 1930 there was a decline of 38 percent in the birth rate in women between the ages of 15 and 44 (Kalisch and Kalisch, 1978). Gerson (1970) attributes to Sanger the major milestone of the New York Academy of Medicine's 1931 resolution to support birth control. The American Medical Association announced support in 1937. Lader and Meltzer (1969) indicate that Sanger spoke to a House committee in the U.S. Congress in 1932 as an authority on birth control. She was honored for her work with an honorary L.L.D. from Smith College in 1949, and in 1952 she founded the International Planned Parenthood Federation.

Margaret Sanger devoted her life to the work of the birth control movement. After effecting changes in the United States, she traveled widely in other parts of the world, including Russia. She worked for birth control in those countries also, particularly in India. Her determination and her diligence in pursuing her goals, as well as her use of effective strategies for effecting changes, made her one of the most admired figures of this century. She is one of 21 nurses in the Nursing Hall of Fame established by the American Nurses' Association in 1976.

Midwifery in the United States in the Early Twentieth Century

During the nineteenth century, affluent European families continued to follow the lead of nobility in many civilized countries by having physicians come into their homes to deliver children. The less affluent and the poor still relied on midwives, even into the early twentieth century. This was also true in the United States.

Because of public concern over maternal and infant mortality rates, government, especially the federal government, organized programs to save lives of mothers and infants. Nurses were active in both the assessment of needs and the planning of these programs. They recognized that scientific advances made in the health care system were inaccessible to lay midwives. In addition, there were no standards against which their work could be measured and no licensure to indicate their competence to the family consumers of their care. These lay midwives received much of the blame for the status of maternity care in the United States. At that time obstetrics was not necessarily a part of medical education, there was no prenatal care, and adequate hospital facilities for complications in childbirth were lacking (Varney, 1980). Sanger (1938) wrote that "few people wanted to enter hospitals; they were afraid they might be 'practiced' upon, and consented to go only in desperate emergencies. Sentiment was especially vehement in the matter of having babies." Women preferred their own bedrooms for their deliveries. Dolan (1973) states that there were many women who delivered without a physician and that a quarter of those were delivered by untrained women, especially in rural and underserved areas. A survey in New York City indicated that untrained people delivered 40 percent of the infants and that there were 3000 of those attendants in the city (Bullough and Bullough, 1978). Although some nurses were taught midwifery, the movement was not as successful in the United States as it was in many other areas of the world. Elsewhere, nurse-midwives provided care for those without maternity complications and referred clients with complications to physicians. Nurse-midwifery was one of the first of the expanded roles of nursing. However, it evolved slowly because of the opposition of organized medicine, which promoted physicians' dominance over the entire area of maternity care.

One movement toward change in the status of maternity care was for a federal Children's Bureau. A nurse, Lillian Wald (1867–1940), has been given credit for suggesting this bureau. She also is a member of the Nursing Hall of Fame (American Nurses' Association, 1983). The first legislative effort to create the bureau failed in 1906, but President Theodore Roosevelt convened the First White House Conference on Children in 1910. This was a group of professionals and lay people who recommended the bureau, and in 1912 the Children's Bureau became a reality. This bureau conducted a study that indicated that infant mortality rates were approximately 124 per 1000 live births. Data analysis led to the conclusion that there was a close correlation between such high rates and poor maternal health. Studies of maternal mortality were used as rationale for initiating prenatal, intrapartal, and postpartal care.

Another effort by the federal government to effect changes for better maternity care was the passage of the Sheppard-Towner Act in 1921. This act ensured that public health nurses would train lay midwives but would not practice. The phasing out of lay midwives was encouraged and lay midwifery became illegal in many states (Bullough and Bullough, 1977). Nurse-midwives had been expected to practice among the poor and in rural areas where there were few physicians (Bullough and Bullough, 1977; Dolan, 1973). When they also practiced in other areas, the opposition of organized medicine effected the repeal of the Sheppard-Towner Act in 1929.

Because of studies in New York City that indicated maternity care was inadequate, maternity centers were organized in 1917. A central organization, the Maternity Center Association (MCA), was established in 1918. The MCA has promoted educational programs in New York City and other areas of the United States and has provided teaching aids for such programs.

Although research studies have shown that there was a need for better maternity care, either there were too few physicians to provide that care or consumers did not seek their care. Several schools for lay midwives were organized, but they operated only until the 1930s, when medical schools began to teach obstetrics and it became an established specialty (Varney, 1980).

Goodnow (1948) states that Europe and England gave excellent training in midwifery. In Europe most studied midwifery only; however, in England, most studied nursing first. At that time (1948), practically all registered nurses were also registered midwives. Some of those nurse-midwives came to the United States. Nurse-midwives "had never quite been accepted by American physicians or by nursing itself" (Bullough and Bullough, 1969, p. 213). Nurses were taught in hospitals that their role was to support and help physicians.

One of the leading American change agents who helped expand the role of nurse-midwife was Mary Breckinridge (1881–1965). (Fig. 2–7). She was from a prominent American family: her grandfather was vice-president of the United States, and her father was the U.S. Ambassador to Russia. Her autobiography, *Wide neighborhoods* (1952), dis-

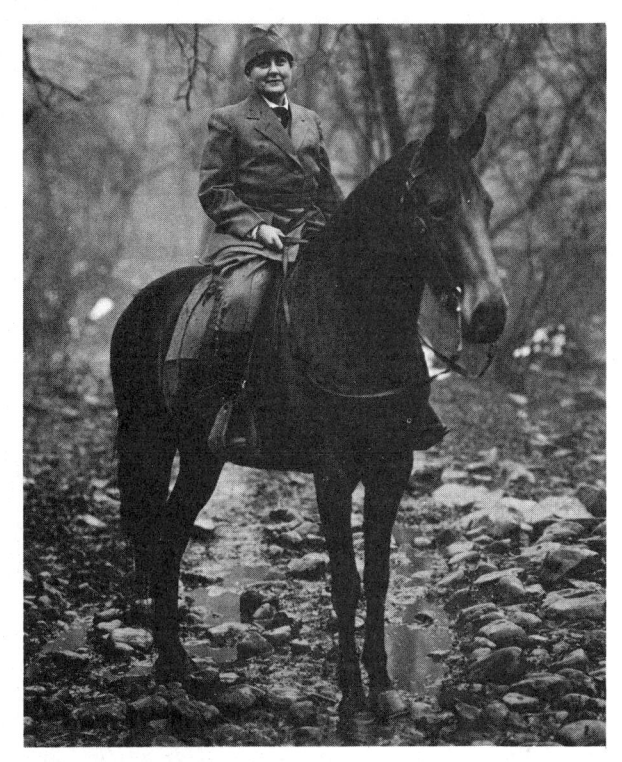

FIGURE 2–7. Mary Breckinridge.
SOURCE: Reproduced with permission from the Frontier Nursing Service, Hyden, Kentucky.

cusses the delivery of her young brother in Russia by a midwife, an early influence on her life's work.

The loss of her first husband, small son, and infant daughter probably influenced her to attend New York's St. Luke's Hospital, where she graduated from nursing school. She was very interested in the high maternal and infant mortality rates in the United States. After studying statistical data, she concluded that in the United States there were more women lost in childbirth than in wars. She assessed the health needs of the mountain people in her native state of Kentucky and decided that there was an urgent need there for improved and comprehensive maternity care.

She was so motivated by the needs of childbearing families that she went to England to study nurse-midwifery. She also visited Scotland. Some of the nurse-midwives she met came back to Kentucky with her. As a group, they began to initiate plans and interventions to improve maternity care in that area. All of the nurse-midwives were certified from the Central Midwives' Board in either Scotland or England. They established the Frontier Nursing Service in 1925.

These nurse-midwives established the first rural health center of the service in Hyden, Kentucky. Kalisch and Kalisch (1978) state that they established eight districts of 78 square miles each. *Granny midwives*, ignorant and superstitious women, delivered babies in the areas. By building a log cabin inhabited by two nurse-midwives in each district, the nursing service made itself accessible to the people in the area. The country was hilly and without proper roads. The nurses traveled to homes on horseback or in jeeps if people could not come to the cabins. The charges for health care were $1 a year and $5 for complete maternity care. Breckinridge contributed her own money to support the service and used her influence to obtain other funds. Clients with medical problems were referred to physicians.

All of the 16 nurse-midwives on the staff of the Frontier Nursing Service became charter members of the American Association of Nurse-Midwives, a Kentucky association they organized in 1928 (Breckinridge, 1952). They kept careful records of their clients. Their maternal and infant death rates were very low compared to the overall U.S. rates. In 1932, a Dr. Dublin wrote that if their services were available to women in the United States generally, 10,000 mothers' lives and 30,000 infants' lives would be saved. Breckinridge (1952) also reported that children of their childbearing families even had higher intelligence scores at 4 years of age than the norm. This was undoubtedly due to the prenatal health care, including nutritional teaching, provided by the nurses. Breckinridge's inclusion in the Nursing Hall of Fame is a tribute to her life's work in organizing and administering the Frontier Nursing Service, which served as a model to illustrate the contributions this expanded role in nursing made in improving maternity care in the United States and other parts of the world.

Both the Frontier Nursing Service and the Maternity Center Association developed nurse-midwifery educational programs. The first program in the United States was the Lobenstein Midwifery School, which began in 1931. This school was a result of the efforts of the Association for the Promotion and Standardization of Midwifery, which was incorporated in early 1931 by the medical board of the Maternity Center Association. Ralph Waldo Lobenstein, M.D., and Mary Breckinridge were charter members of the board. Varney (1980, p. 18) states that "Lobenstein worked tirelessly to bring about the establishment of nurse-midwifery services and education until his death in 1931."

The first school became known as the Maternity Center Association School of Nurse-Midwifery in 1934. Then the Maternity Center Association and the Lobenstein Midwifery Clinic merged. The clinic provided prenatal care, and nurse-midwives and physicians provided intrapartal and postpartal care in families' homes unless complications required hospitalization. These services made 7099 deliveries between 1932 and 1958, with 6116 occurring in the homes of the childbearing women. The MCA mortality rate was 0.9 compared to 10.4 for the same district as a whole, and 1.2 for a leading hospital in New York City.

The Maternity Center Association school and its graduates have been involved in the organization of all schools of nurse-midwifery in the United States with the exception of the Frontier Graduate School of Midwifery, which was begun by the Frontier Nursing Service in 1939. Today there are several schools across the United States.

Most of the early graduates of these schools did not practice clinical nurse-midwifery because of the need for their services in public health agencies at local, state, and federal levels, in hospitals, and in schools of nursing as teachers, administrators, consultants, and researchers (Varney, 1980). In the past decade many state legislatures have changed nurse practice acts to allow nurse-midwives to practice.

CHANGES IN THE RECENT PAST

Changes in maternity nursing have occurred rapidly during the recent past. Factors influencing these changes have been the growth of governmental and voluntary health services; new knowledge, methods, and techniques; the expansion of undergraduate and graduate education in colleges and universities, which led to expanded roles for nurses; the consumer movement, which fostered participation of families in childbirth education and in maternity care; the women's movement, which promoted assertiveness of women in gaining control of their own lives; and the increased effectiveness and unity of nurses in effecting legislative changes in nurse practice acts to allow legal expansion of nursing roles.

Governmental and Voluntary Agencies

Early in this century the federal government initiated programs to improve maternal and child health. Gradually the government's involvement in maternal and child health programs grew, in spite of opposition from groups who feared socialized medicine. These programs have been vastly expanded during the recent past. Some of the more significant actions of the federal government that have brought about better maternity care are the following:

1909–1979 White House conferences regarding children have been held every 10 years.

1912 The Children's Bureau was formed and was initially concerned with reducing the high maternal and infant mortality in the United States. Aims included the improvement of maternal and infant care and the development of standards of care for mothers and children. The Children's Bureau has also included programs for aid to dependent children, child welfare, crippled children's services, genetics, family planning, adolescent pregnancy, and regionalization of perinatal care (Gold, 1983).

1921 The Sheppard-Towner Act was passed. It was repealed in 1929.

1935 The Social Security Act was passed. It has been amended many times.

1948 The World Health Organization became an official agency of the United Nations.

1953 The Department of Health, Education, and Welfare (DHEW) was founded.

1965 Medicare and Medicaid were provided under amendment to the Social Security Act.

1972 The states were required to implement Medicaid.

1972 The Women, Infants, and Children (WIC) Program was initiated to provide nutritional supplements to pregnant and lactating women, and to infants and young children at risk because of inadequate income and nutrition.

1975 Title XX, an amendment to the Social Security Act, provided funds for family planning.

1980 DHEW became the Department of Health and Human Services (DHHS) and the Department of Education.

One branch of the DHHS, the Public Health Service (PHS), has many programs for disease prevention and health promotion. It collects and analyzes statistical data regarding citizens' health status, and then plans goals and interventions for maternal and infant health. The Office of Disease Prevention and Health Promotion of the Public Health Service has programs specifically designed to motivate citizens to strive for and maintain "wellness." The emphasis is on "wellness" and sickness and teaches citizens what we can all do to "help ourselves to health" (U.S. Department of Health and Human Services, 1982, p. iii).

There are many similar educational and motivational programs that promote preventive and promotional health practices for children, adolescents, and adults. The DHHS publication *Prevention 82* (1982) discussed the various organizations within the bureaucratic framework of DHHS and illustrated how the agencies utilize large amounts of federal tax monies to develop educational materials, programs, and curricula to provide preventive health service to families. Many other publications have also detailed reports of the activities of DHHS. Reference rooms of most university libraries contain many of these U.S. government documents that contain data about maternity care programs and statistics. (Refer to these documents for further information about maternal and infant programs.)

There are several programs in which governmental and voluntary agencies cooperate to improve the health of mothers and infants. One such program is the National Health Promotion Network, whose goal is to conduct sound health promotion programs. The Office of Disease Prevention and Health Promotion, a DHHS agency, cooperates with the following voluntary agencies: The National Coalition of Hispanic Mental Health and Human Services Organization, the National Urban League, the National Board of the Young Men's Christian Association, and the American National Red Cross. These voluntary agencies have large networks of community volunteers, including maternity nurses.

Another example of governmental and voluntary cooperation to improve maternal and infant health is that of the Healthy Mothers/Healthy Babies' public information program that was begun in 1981. This program aims to provide information on healthy behavior to low-income pregnant women and women planning pregnancies. The Public Health Service cooperates in this effort with approximately 40 other agencies. Some of the organizations and agencies cooperating with the Public Health Service are the American Nurses' Association, the American College of Obstetricians and Gynecologists, the American Academy of

Pediatrics, the March of Dimes, Birth Defects Foundation, the National Parent-Teachers Association, and the U.S. Department of Agriculture.

It is important for nurses to participate in planning and utilizing governmental and voluntary services. Many maternity nurses are actively involved in these organizations. All nurses need to know about these organizations in order to encourage consumer use of the services provided by the organizations and to contribute nursing knowledge and expertise in the planning and implementation of these services.

New Knowledge, Methods, and Techniques

Some of the more significant recent advances which have improved nursing practice are:

1940   The Rh system of antigens was discovered.

1951   Dame Kate Campbell reported the relationship between oxygen and retrolental fibroplasia.

1952   Virginia Apgar, M.D., proposed her method of initial screening of the newborn.

1958   Phototherapy was initiated for treatment of hyperbilirubinemia.

1963   Rho Gam was first reported in the U.S.

early 1970s   Lung maturity studies were initiated.

late 1970s   Rubella vaccine was routinely given to postpartal women.

Other recent advances include the introduction of monitoring of the fetus and uterine contractions, and the medical and nursing specialties of neonatology and perinatology. These specialties led to intensive care facilities for high-risk pregnant women and new born infants. The intensive care facilities were located in large medical teaching hospitals. These facilities provided care that saved the lives of high-risk newborns that would have previously been lost. The concept of regionalization was conceived in the late 1960s and early 1970s to maximize accessibility to these high-risk centers. Regionalization is implemented by designating hospital nurseries as one of three levels, depending on the health care providers and facilities available in each hospital. Level I, the primary level, includes smaller and less sophisticated hospitals, which usually provide maternal and infant care for uncomplicated courses of childbirth. Level II includes hospitals located in more densely populated areas that go beyond emergency and uncomplicated care to include care for most high-risk patients. In order to avoid costly and unnecessary duplication, these hospitals transport patients with complicated, high-risk problems to the tertiary level, or Level III, hospitals. The regional program is ideally coordinated from this level. Regionalization allows distribution and access to all patients, fosters communication among health professionals, contributes to the establishment of standards of care, and provides continuing educational programs. Level III units conduct research that has improved care for high-risk maternity clients (Hawkins, 1980). The neonatal intensive care nurseries are located in Level III units. Therefore, the needs of the family and measures to insure family support are of primary importance in planning nursing care.

The *test-tube baby* is another recent advance in medical science. Edwards and Steptoe in 1980 documented the contributions of nurses to the work that led to the birth of the first test-tube baby, Louise Joy Brown, in England on July 25, 1978. As with most significant changes, a great deal of controversy arose over this development. Clergy widely discussed the ethical and moral questions regarding *in vitro* fertilization. News media presented the sensational aspects of such a departure from centuries of natural conception. Study and research were continued, and there have been other healthy babies born after *in vitro* fertilization. On January 8, 1980, Virginia health authorities announced that, for the first time, a United States birth clinic would use the Edwards–Steptoe method of conception. Since then there have been other babies born in the United States by using this method. It has given hope to thousands of couples who would not otherwise be able to have children (see Chapter 5).

Changes in Nursing Education

An additional factor that influenced changes in the maternity care system was the movement of basic nursing education from hospital schools of nursing to colleges and universities. In the early 1900s most nurses worked outside of hospitals because nursing students provided most of the nursing service in hospitals. When educational standards were raised, hospitals began to close their nursing schools, because they became too expensive to operate when students were no longer utilized for nursing service.

As hospital schools decreased in number, colleges and universities began to open schools of nursing with money from private and governmental sources. These programs sought a faculty with advanced degrees. Nursing faculties in the 1950s had received most of their graduate degrees in education (Bullough and Bullough, 1978); however, master's and doctoral degree programs in nursing have rapidly increased in number since that time, as have the numbers of nurses with master's and doctoral degrees in nursing.

Many universities opened programs for advanced registered nurse practitioners. These included nurse practitioner programs; nurse-midwife programs—with and without master's degrees; and clinical nurse specialist programs granting master's degrees. Presently, nurses may further specialize and conduct extensive research at the doctoral level. Nurses in these expanded roles have effected many changes that have promoted family-centered maternity care.

The Consumer Movement and Childbirth Education

The consumer movement of the past 20 to 30 years has encouraged childbearing families to assertively voice their concerns about maternity health care. Families want to be active participants in childbearing. They also want some control over this developmental crisis in their lives. These concerns have led to cooperation between consumers and maternity health care providers in making many changes in the delivery of maternity care. One of the cooperative efforts was the initiation and expansion of childbirth education programs throughout the United States.

The childbirth education movement has itself provided stimuli for many changes in the delivery of maternity care. As has already been mentioned, until the twentieth century, most deliveries in the United States occurred at home. As obstetrics and gynecology became an established medical specialty and physicians gained dominance in the care of childbearing women, deliveries began to occur more commonly in hospitals. In 1900, 90 percent of deliveries in the United States occurred in the home. By 1950, 90 percent of American women had babies delivered by physicians in hospitals (Gilgoff, 1978).

One of the obstetric medical practices that paralleled the trend toward hospitalization was the use of anesthesia for delivery. Other practices associated with maternity care in hospitals were partial separation of the mother from her newborn baby and complete separation of other family members from the baby during postpartum hospitalization. Mothers were heavily sedated and given amnesic drugs in labor. They were given anesthesia and placed in lithotomy positions for delivery. Because of anesthesia, more forceps deliveries were performed. All these practices sometimes resulted in complications. Many women accepted anesthesia because they feared childbirth. Such fears were promoted by discussions of complications and death during childbearing in literature and movies. Margaret Mitchell's *Gone with the Wind* is an example of a widely read and viewed book and movie that depicted death due to childbearing

Families also accepted the rigid rules "to prevent infection" imposed by hospitals. Mothers were not allowed food or any oral liquids during labor because anesthesia was planned. They routinely had the entire genital area shaved and were given enemas upon admission to labor rooms. They were put to bed and kept on their back "to hasten labor"; and, because of sedation and analgesia, parturient women were strapped on to delivery tables with arms and legs restrained completely. Episiotomies became routine, including "extra sutures to make women like virgins once more" so that husbands' sexual pleasures would be enhanced. All of these practices led to controversies among health professionals as well as consumers.

Even though clients of the maternity health care system tolerated some of these practices, there was growing dissatisfaction with the emphasis on "unnatural" as opposed to "natural" methods of childbirth. From the beginning of the trend toward hospitalization and primary care by physicians until the present, there has been increasing use of invasive and unnatural scientific and technologic innovations for parturient women. There have been differing opinions among health care providers regarding the advisability of all these practices. Use of fetal and uterine monitoring has become routine in many institutions. Cesarean delivery rates approximate 25 percent in some areas. Consumers have voiced grave concerns about these pathologic approaches to childbirth.

Other authors, many of whom were mothers, criticized hospital maternity care (Wessel, 1973; Sousa, 1976; Gilgoff, 1978). T. Berry Brazelton (1961, 1971), a well-known pediatrician and author, warned professionals and consumers about drugs given to the mother in labor and delivery, and their effects on the baby.

During the 1960s there were publications about the phenomenon of maternal–infant attachment and bonding. One of the earliest researchers in this field was John Bowlby (1965). He wrote a report, *Maternal care and mental health*, in 1951 for the World Health Organization (WHO), that collated expert opinions on the subject. In 1962 Mary Salter Ainsworth reported work to WHO that was included with Bowlby's work in a publication entitled *Child care and the growth of love* (1965), which was abridged and edited by Margery Fry. This book, published for the general public, discussed maternal deprivation and the concept of attachment between mother and child.

Klaus and Kennell (1976) discussed the research that led them to conclude that there is a *sensitive period* during which conditions are optimal for maternal–infant attachment. Their illustrations and rationale provided "one of the most important influences on the medical establishment's decision to return control of childbirth to parents" (Lamb and Hall, 1982). Authorities disagree as to whether or not Klaus and Kennell's conclusions are true; however, their reports provided impetus for change toward family-centered maternity care (see Chapter 29).

All of the literature about natural childbirth and bonding has stimulated interest among the general public in promoting prenatal education for childbearing couples. Mothers who had already given birth collaborated with nurses and others to teach classes that provided couples with knowledge and techniques for participating in labor and delivery processes that were as natural as possible.

Many nurses have established independent private practices in childbirth education. In collaboration with consumers and with other maternity health care providers, they have identified problems, planned strategies for change, implemented interventions, and evaluated those interventions. They have continued to provide liaison between consumers and providers of maternity health care.

Consumers and childbirth educators have been involved in the formation of several organizations to promote family-centered care. Two organizations for childbirth educations are the International Childbirth Education Association (ICEA) and the American Society for Psychoprophylaxis in Obstetrics (ASPO). Both organizations provide educational programs and certification for childbirth educators.

During the mid-twentieth century few maternity health care providers encouraged breastfeeding. Sometimes they actively discouraged it. Along with the movement toward natural childbirth came the movement toward breastfeeding. In 1956 breastfeeding mothers organized the La Leche League, an organization that provides encouragement through meetings between experienced and inexperienced breastfeeding mothers. It also publishes information for mothers and health care professionals who work with mothers who breastfeed (see Chapter 21).

In the past few years, many health care providers have encouraged breastfeeding. Until the 1600s women traditionally fed infants by breast for varying periods of time. There are some recorded instances of mothers who did not breastfeed their infants, but the vast majority of babies were nourished this way. Sometimes mothers had their infants fed by other lactating women called "wet nurses." Babies were seldom artificially fed. About the time of the Industrial Revolution, some mothers began to feed their infants animal milk and liquid foods instead of human milk. Even until the 1920s and 1930s few women fed infants artificially because of high morbidity and mortality rates among infants who were not breastfed. With advances of science that allowed safe artificial feeding, the numbers of mothers who used this method increased.

In many Third World countries pharmaceutical companies succeeded in their advertising depicting healthy babies who had been formula-fed. Formula-feeding caused increased mortality and poverty in these countries because of unhygienic practices and the need to spend disproportionate amounts of already low incomes on these formulae (Riordan and Countryman, 1980). The World Health Organization became involved in reversing this trend.

In the United States since the 1960s increasing numbers of mothers have breastfed. Mothers most likely to breastfeed are those who are better educated, live in suburbs rather than inner cities, have been educated about childbirth, belong to the La Leche League, and are interested in natural ways of living (Riordan and Countryman, 1980).

Childbirth educators, particularly those who were nurses, have effected profound changes in maternity health care. When these educators encouraged consumers to assertively voice their concerns and expectations to health care providers, many of the previously discussed maternity care practices of hospitals were modified. One important change is the decrease in the use of analgesia and anesthesia during childbirth, resulting in a decrease in respiratory depressions of neonates.

Many other changes have occurred to promote family-centered maternity care. Fathers or significant others who have attended childbirth education classes have been allowed to remain with mothers during labor and delivery to coach them and actively participate in the childbearing experience. These fathers or significant others were also allowed to help care for newborns in mothers' rooms on partpartum wards. Parents were allowed to visit sick newborns in nurseries. Many of the hospital rules that separated families had existed for years in order to promote asepsis and prevent infection. Each time changes were made to allow more participation of family members in care during hospitalization, these rules had to be modified. These changes always required consideration of consumers' wishes as well as continued protection of hospital clients from infection. Consumers, childbirth educators, and professional health care providers have collaborated successfully to effect these desired changes.

The Women's Movement

The women's movement has also had a profound influence on maternity care. Many changes have occurred in nursing because of changes in women's roles and status in society. The primary reason that nursing was subservient to medicine for years was that nurses were nearly always women and physicians were usually men. Women in the workplace have traditionally been given lower status and lower-paid jobs, often receiving lower pay that men for the same jobs. Women are "struggling to cope with the challenges of being a minority and a largely powerless group, they are questioning attitudes, feelings, and behavior that they formerly took for granted" (Lytle, 1977). Women from the 1960s to the present have made strides toward attaining greater independence and recognition in society. Women now have many more opportunities in traditionally male areas of work. Much larger percentages of students in medicine, law, engineering, and other professions are women.

Women continue to hold leadership positions in government. Sandra Day O'Connor was appointed as the first woman Justice of the Supreme Court of the United States in 1981. Also, in 1981, Jeane Kirkpatrick was appointed the permanent representative from the United States to the United Nations. In 1982 Faye G. Abdellah was promoted to deputy surgeon general of the U.S. Public Health Service. She was "the first nurse, and the first woman, to hold that post with the 184-year-old Public Health Service" ("News," April 1982). Margaret Heckler, a former U.S. Congresswoman from Massachusetts, was appointed Secretary of the Department of Health and Human Services in 1983. This agency had more than 145,000 workers and a budget of $276 million. During the same year, Elizabeth Dole was appointed Secretary of Housing and Urban Development.

More women were also serving in national, state, and local offices in 1983. In 1971 there had been 15 women in Congress, 362 women in state legislatures, and 7 mayors of cities with a population over 30,000. By 1983 there were 24 in Congress, 992 in state legislatures, and 76 mayors. At the National Women's Political Caucus in 1983, national presidential candidates indicated they believed women would strongly influence the next presidential election (O'Reilly, 1983). And, in fact, Geraldine Ferraro became the first woman vice-presidential candidate on a major party ticket in 1984.

Effecting Legislative Changes

The success of the women's movement has encouraged nurses to strive for more independence and recognition in the health care system. Nurses' roles are expanding, and nurses are working toward true professionalization of their vocation. Many are striving to develop independent practices as well as collaborative relationships with other professionals, particularly physicians. Nursing literature documents the success of these efforts (Huntington and Shores, 1983); however, there have been continuing reports of the efforts of the medical profession to prevent changes that allow nurses these opportunities. Nurses have successfully worked together during the recent past to effect legislative changes in nurse practice acts that allowed more expanded roles, and these successes have been reported in nursing journals. There were about 30 registered nurses serving as state legislators in 1983, and the Nurses' Coalition for Action in Politics (NCAP) reported 83 percent success among the political candidates it endorsed ("News," 1983a).

Change Agents in the Recent Past

In the recent past nurse change agents have tried to effect change through the courts. One of them was a male nurse in Little Rock, Arkansas, who was denied the opportunity to work in his requested area of labor and delivery in the obstetric department of a hospital. In 1983 only 2 percent of nurses were men. Men had previously faced discrimination from those inside and outside the nursing system. They were expected to practice only in certain areas of nursing, and obstetric or maternity nursing was not one of them. Until the civil rights and women's movements, many male nursing students did not receive the same educational experiences as female students. In the 1950s it was common for male students to spend most of their obstetric clinical classes in the newborn nursery rather than in the prenatal clinic, labor and delivery, or postpartum. This has gradually changed so that both male and female students have opportunities for clinical experiences in all areas of maternity nursing.

It has been very unusual for male nurses to practice in maternity care. In some institutions men were barred from this health care system. The male nurse mentioned previously resigned from the hospital that had denied his request to work in labor and delivery. He then sued the hospital charging discrimination based on sex. His suit was dismissed by the United States District Court. He appealed, but the Appeals Court ruled that the question was moot since he was no longer at the hospital (Regan, 1982).

Two other change agents in the recent past are Susan Sizemore and Victoria Henderson. These two nurse-midwives established a private practice in Nashville, Tennessee, in partnership with an obstetrician, Darrel Martin, who provided supervision to the self-employed nurses. Hospitals in Nashville denied them admitting privileges for their practice. Then the State Volunteer Mutual Insurance Company (SVMIC), which was owned by physicians, canceled Martin's malpractice insurance later the same year (1980). The two nurse-midwives, the physician, and former clients of the nurse-midwives filed a multimillion-dollar antitrust action against the insurance firm, the three hospitals, and five physicians ("News," 1982b). The suit, filed in a federal district court, charged the defendants with violating Sections 1 and 2 of the Sherman Antitrust Act, which restricts attempts to monopolize and to conspire to restrain trade. The nurse-midwives received a great deal of support from lay people in the Nashville area. They also received publicity locally and in national nursing literature. Their courageous action gained community and national support for the practice of nurse-midwifery and illustrated the need for more unity among nurses in effecting changes.

The assertive stance by the nurse-midwives and the physician influenced the Federal Trade Commission to review the case. Although the insurance company canceled Martin's malpractice insurance, it continued to insure physicians who *employed* nurse-midwives. In 1983 the Federal Trade Commission threatened legal action against SVMIC for violating antitrust laws. The commission said that the firm limited competition in three ways: "by preventing physicians and nurse-midwives from collaborating; by denying consumers choice of services; and by blocking the growth of nurse-midwifery" ("News," 1983d). These change agents utilized some of the same strategies that earlier nursing change agents used. All of them provide role models for the future.

BIRTH RATE

Local, state, and federal agencies, particularly the health agencies, collect statistical data on childbearing. These statistics provide information for the assessment of maternity care. Birth rates, maternal mortality rates, infant mortality rates, and perinatal mortality rates are a few of the kinds of statistics that are collected. *Birth rate* is defined as the number of births per 1000 people in the population. In 1915 there were only ten states that registered births, but by 1935 all states had mandatory birth registration (Varney, 1980).

Birth rates fluctuate in response to historical events. Figure 2–8 shows the reported changes in birth rates in the U.S. from 1920 to 1984. There was a decline in birth rates during the late 1920s and the 1930s due to the severe economic depression of that time. After the end of the Second World War, there was a surge in birth rates, called the "baby boom." Figure 2–8 also shows an increase during the late 1950s and early 1960s, at which time there was economic prosperity in the U.S. The birth rates began to decline as the women's movement encouraged women to find jobs outside the home; however, as the "baby boomers" had children, the birth rates rose.

The first-birth rates for women in their 30s began to rise during the 1970s as recorded by the National Center for Health Statistics (NCHS,

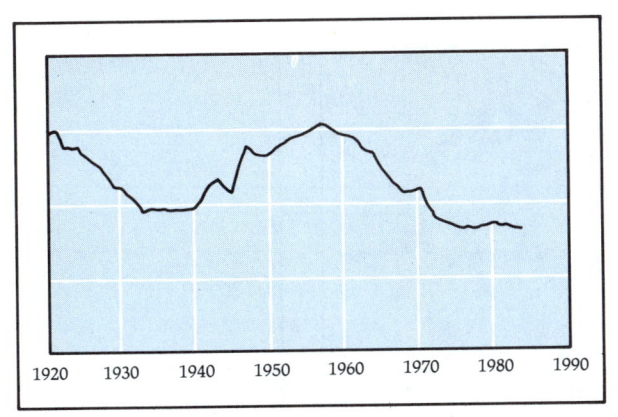

FIGURE 2–8. Changes in birth rates in the United States, 1920–1984.
SOURCE: DHHS (1982).

TABLE 2–1. Rank orders of causes of maternal deaths.

1949	1977
1. Toxemias	1. Sepsis
2. Sepsis and abortions	2. Hemorrhage
3. Hemorrhage	3. Toxemias
4. Ectopic pregnancy	4. Ectopic pregnancy

SOURCE: Adapted from Federal Security Agency (1951) and Pratt (1982).

1986b). On the other hand, the birth rates in 1984 for "teenagers 15–19 years dropped to the lowest levels observed in the U.S. since 1940, and for women 20–24 years, to the lowest levels ever observed" (NCHS, 1986b, p. 1).

The birth rate in the U.S. was 15.5 in 1983 and 1984. Provisional data from 1985 indicate that the rate was 15.7 (NCHS, 1986c). During the 12 months ending April, 1987, the birth rate was 15.4 (NCHS, 1987b).

Maternal Mortality Rates

Maternal mortality rates are now defined as the numbers of deaths from complications of pregnancy, childbearing, and the puerperium per 100,000 live births. Figure 2–9 shows changes in maternal mortality rates from 1915 to 1950. There was an increase during the First World War, followed by a decrease between 1920 and 1925. Figure 2–9 also illustrates an increase during the Great Depression. After 1930, there was a remarkable decline in maternal mortality rates. Pratt (1982) states that in 1930 the U.S. maternal mortality rate was almost 700 per 100,000 live births, but by 1940 the rate was reduced to 376. By 1950 the rate was 83.3 per 100,000 live births.

The main causes of maternal deaths in the U.S. have changed since 1949. Table 2–1 lists the rank order of causes of maternal deaths in 1949 and the rank order of causes of maternal deaths in 1977.

Toxemias of pregnancy, which had been the major cause of maternal deaths in 1949, was relegated to third place, and sepsis became the leading cause of death in 1977. Abortion was not listed by Pratt (1982) as a cause in 1977, due probably to the 1973 Roe v. Wade U.S. Supreme Court decision to allow women legal abortions.

Table 2–2 lists data from the U.S. vital statistics system regarding maternal mortality. The table illustrates the disparity between white and black maternal mortality rates which still exists today, even though the rates have fallen significantly since 1950.

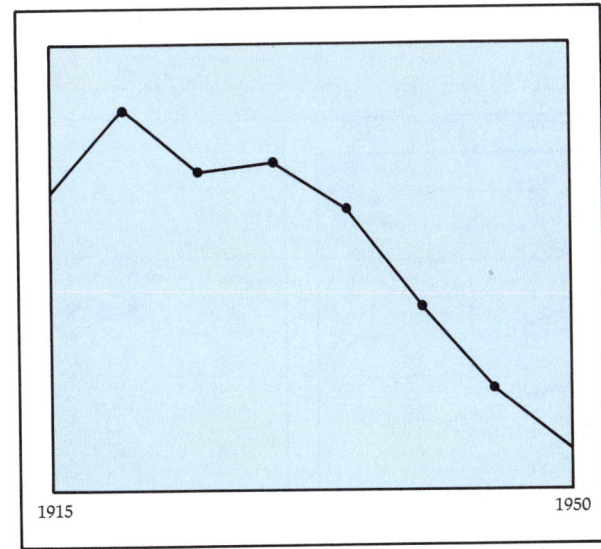

FIGURE 2–9. Changes in maternal mortality rates, 1915–1950, in 5-year intervals.
SOURCE: DHHS (1982).

TABLE 2–2. Maternal mortality rates (all ages, crude).

	1960	1970	1979	1980	1981
White	26.0	14.4	6.4	6.7	6.3
Black	103.6	59.8	25.1	21.5	20.4
Total	37.1	21.5	9.6	9.2	8.5

SOURCE: NCHS (1984).

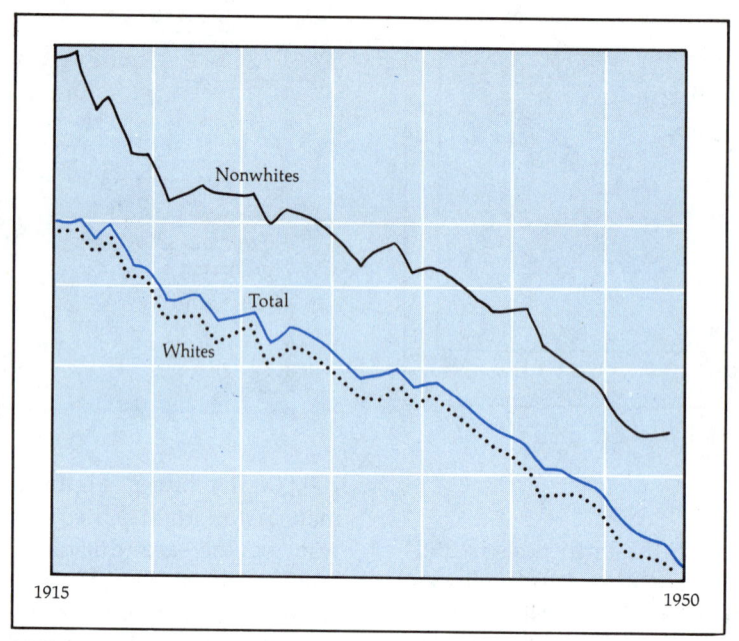

FIGURE 2–10. Infant mortality rates by race, 1915–1949, in 5-year intervals.
SOURCE: Federal Security Agency (1952).

Infant Mortality Rates

The *infant mortality rate* is defined as those deaths during the first year of life per 1000 live births. Infant deaths decreased from approximately 100 per 1000 live births in 1900 to about 29.2 in 1950 (Pratt, 1982). Figure 2–10 shows a sharp decline in infant mortality rates from 1915 to 1950 in both white and black infants, whereas Fig. 2–11 shows white and black infant death rates from 1950 to 1981. Even though all the rates have declined by large percentages, there has continued to be great disparity in the rates of white and black infant mortality. The NCHS (1984, p. 12) states that "a large portion of the difference . . . can be attributed to a higher incidence of low birth weight among black infants." Even though the survival of infants of low birth weight in the U.S. has improved, weight has been a major factor in the deaths of infants.

There has been a slower decline during the very recent past in infant death rates, although rates are

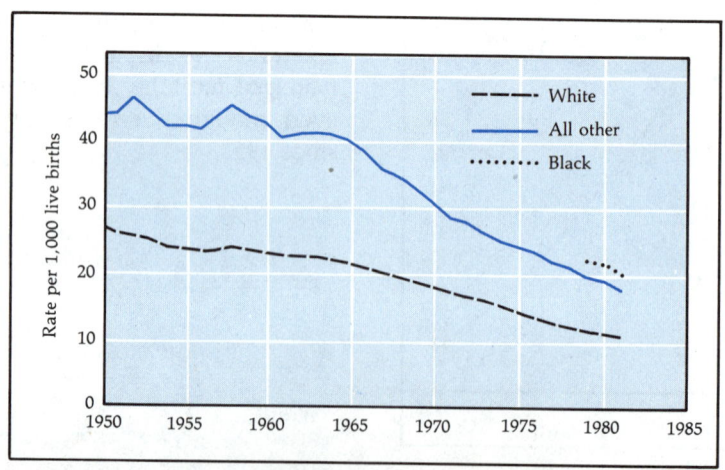

FIGURE 2–11. Infant mortality rates by race, 1950–1981.
SOURCE: NCHS (1968a).

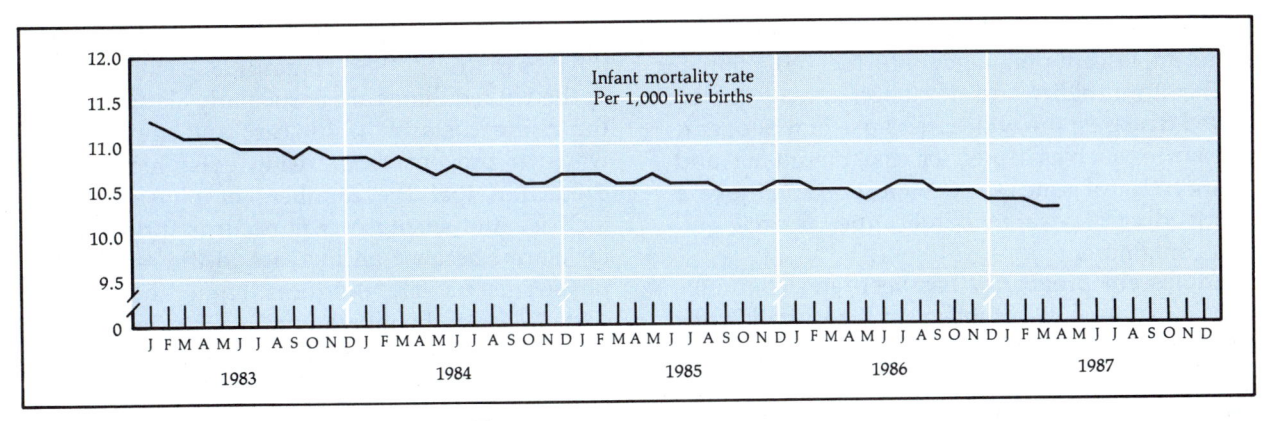

FIGURE 2–12. Infant mortality rates, 1983–1987.
SOURCE: NCHS (1987b).

still declining each year. The steady decline during 1983 to April, 1987, is illustrated in Fig. 2–12: provisional data from NCHS show that the rate has fallen from 10.8 in 1984 to 10.6 in 1985 (NCHS, 1986c).

Perinatal Mortality

Perinatal mortality, broadly defined, refers to all spontaneous fetal deaths occurring after 20 weeks of pregnancy, and neonatal deaths (birth up to 28 days of age). The term has been used since the late 1940s because researchers knew that large number of fetuses and infants were lost immediately before and after delivery (NCHS, 1986a). After 1979, NCHS published data with three definitions within the period broadly defined above. However, in a 1986 report, the NCHS used the definition of perinatal mortality to denote fetal deaths of 28 weeks or more gestation and neonatal deaths of less than 7 days, because almost 75 percent of all perinatal deaths occur in this period, and the definition is generally used for international comparisons. The perinatal rate was defined as "the number of perinatal deaths per 1,000 live births and fetal deaths" (NCHS, 1986a, p. 3) of 28 weeks or more gestation. Even though NCHS publishes both perinatal and infant mortality rates, the news media still usually refer to infant death rates when discussing maternity statistics. Between 1950 and 1981 the perinatal rate dropped from 32.5 to 12.6 (NCHS, 1986a).

In 1981 there was disparity between white and non-white live births weighing 2500 grams or less. Six percent of white and 11 percent of non-white live births were of low birth-weight. Black women accounted for 82 percent of births in the non-white statistics. The NCHS (1986a) stated that infants of low birth-weight comprised approximately 75 percent of all neonatal deaths.

EFFECTING CHANGE IN THE FUTURE

Even though many radical changes have occurred in maternity nursing care in the past, many problems remain for the nursing profession to address in the future. One of these problems is that families are still dissatisfied with maternity services, particularly hospital services. This dissatisfaction leads to families searching for alternatives to hospital care. One alternative has been for families to have babies in their own homes (White, 1983). Gilgoff (1978) states that 15 percent of all births in California are in clients' homes. There are some physicians and nurse-midwives who attend deliveries in the clients' homes, but this practice is opposed by most organized medical groups.

Another alternative was pioneered by Ruth Watson Lubic, a nurse-midwife who is the general director of the Maternity Center Association (MCA) in New York City. Lubic is a change agent whose work led to the establishment of a prototype birthing center at the MCA in 1975. Nurse-midwives provide most of the care, and the cost at this center is about half that estimated by Blue Cross/Blue Shield for the average hospital costs of normal childbirth. There have been over 100 other birthing centers established since the one at MCA (Lubic, 1983). Others are in the planning stages. The National Association of Childbearing Centers was established in 1983 to set standards for and to gather data about these centers.

Other problems that have been identified include: adolescent pregnancy; a further reduction in perinatal morbidity and mortality; sexually transmitted diseases; the widespread use of teratogenic substances such as drugs, tobacco, marijuana, and alcohol; ethical issues such as abortion and the care and feeding of severely handicapped infants; and cost containment.

Adolescent pregnancy has been and continues to be a major health problem. In the United States approximately 1 million teenagers become pregnant each year. Because of this, the DHHS created the Office of Adolescent Pregnancy Programs (OAPP) in 1978. This office was created with bipartisan congressional support to help establish networks of community-based services for adolescents—those who wish to avoid pregnancy as well as those already pregnant or already parents (DHHS, 1982). Nurses can provide knowledge and expertise in planning and implementing the many changes needed to reduce this enormous health care problem (see Chapter 35).

Other changes must be made to reduce perinatal morbidity and mortality. Perinatal morbidity involves conditions and the diseases that may seriously impair infants' future social and economic lives. The primary aim of WHO is "the attainment by all citizens of the world by the year 2000 of a level of health that will permit them to lead a socially and economically productive life" (DHHS, 1982).

The United States has fallen behind the other industrialized nations of the world in reducing infant mortality. Hughes et al. (1986) state that the United States has dropped from sixth in the 1950–1955 ranking of nations to a tie for last place in the 1980–1985 ranking by the United Nations Children's Fund (UNICEF). The national objective of the DHHS is to have no more than nine infant deaths for each 1000 live births by 1990 (DHHS, 1982). It is unlikely that this goal will be met.

Although there have been dramatic decreases in maternal and infant mortality, there are still significant differences in these rates among whites and blacks. Black women in 1980 were three times as likely as white women to suffer maternal mortality. In 1980 the black infant mortality rate was almost twice that for white infants (NCHS, 1983). By studying data related to these statistics from the perinatal period, nurses can prepare themselves to participate in making changes to lower them.

Nurses can also effect changes that will lower costs for maternity care. Cost containment will require the efforts of both the private and public sectors. Health care costs approached 10 percent of the U.S. Gross National Product (GNP) in 1983 ("News in Brief," 1982; Hager, 1983). Corporations in the United States are particularly alarmed about the rising costs of health care and are studying ways to prevent them rising even higher. The prediction that the numbers of physicians will increase and surpluses will occur is further cause for alarm, because an increase in the numbers of physicians usually produces higher health care costs. Most of the inflation in health care costs has been due to increases in hospital costs. Maternity nurses can effect changes that will decrease these costs in the future by providing such alternatives as birthing centers, home health care, and education about preventive measures and self-care.

In order to effect successfully desired changes in the future, nurses must work with each other and with other groups of health care providers. There are several collaborative organizations for nurses. The American Nurses' Association (ANA), the professional nursing organization, has a Council on Maternal and Child Health Nursing.

Sexually transmitted diseases are a serious problem at the present time and will probably remain so in the future. Acquired immunodeficiency syndrome (AIDS) is a fatal sexually transmitted disease which is causing devastation in our society. The human immunodeficiency virus (HIV) is the cause of AIDS and has infected between 1 and 2 million Americans (Fauci, 1987). Maternity nurses are vitally concerned about preventing the spread of the disease because maternity patients and their families may harbor the virus (see Chapters 5 and 42). Research is continually being conducted regarding the dangers to health care professionals who care for patients with the HIV.

The widespread use of alcohol, drugs, and other teratogens is a monumental problem for families in the childbearing cycle. Maternity nurses must educate themselves about this problem and work to effect changes to decrease the use of harmful substances.

Ethical issues such as abortion and the care of handicapped infants are continually being discussed in the news media. Today, there are groups with various aims which are working continually to influence the legislation and policies of the federal and state governments which will promote each group's values and beliefs. As members of society, nurses should clarify their own values and be able to participate in these processes of change which will effect better care for childbearing families.

The Nurses' Association of the American College of Obstetricians and Gynecologists (NAA-

COG) is a specialty organization for maternity and gynecologic nurses. This group was organized in 1969. Both NAACOG and ANA set standards, provide credentials through certification, and provide continuing education for maternity nurses. Nurses who participate in their meetings have the opportunity to work with other nurses in an organized, united way that is much more likely to accomplish changes than nurses working individually. Leaphart (1983), Mallison (1983), and other nursing leaders advocate unity in nursing through the National Federation for Specialty Nursing Organizations (NFSNO), which first met in the early 1970s. This organization includes 27 nursing organizations plus ANA. Nursing can have a powerful voice in health care if nurses are united.

In the future nurses will need to collaborate more closely with other health care providers. In the past, in many instances, individual physicians have been mentors and advocates for nurses and, in some instances, have worked with them as colleagues. However, even though individual physicians have worked for the advancement of nursing, medical organizations have usually opposed legislative changes that would allow more independence and an expansion of nursing roles. Nurses should strive for more cooperation and collaboration between nurses and all other groups of health care providers, particularly physicians. Nurses need to convey to other providers what nursing involves, what nurses can do, and what service nurses can provide for clients that no other practitioners are providing. Nurses want to practice nursing, not medicine. This should be made clear to physicians so that role expansion and independence are less threatening to them.

The process of collaboration could be enhanced by nurses' becoming more powerful. A primary source of power is knowledge. Nursing research has generated knowledge which is used to provide better services to childbearing families. Maternity nurses must continue to add to the unique body of nursing science by conducting research which generates and tests nursing knowledge (see Chapter 45). Nurses can also become more powerful and effect positive changes for maternity patients through the political process.

Many desired changes will be effected through legislation. Serevino (1982) states that "one in 44 registered women voters is a nurse." This means that nurses have power in sheer numbers that could be used in the future to make legislative changes allowing more independence and recognition for nurses in meeting needs of consumers. Eunice Cole, the ANA president, has stressed that "the nation's 1.6 million registered nurses are a growing political force that must be reckoned with wherever women's rights or health-promoting measures are at issue" ("News in Brief," 1982).

Change agents need power to bring about changes. Nurses can gain power through unity, collaboration, research, and working in the political system.

SUMMARY

The study of the evolution of maternity care from the earliest recorded history through the present provides direction for future changes. In the past the maternity care system changed because the society it served changed. Historical developments affected both the practice and the practitioners of maternity care for childbearing women and their families. Changes were made because change agents responded to the needs of consumers of health care.

Each individual who practices maternity nursing can effect changes in his or her society by supporting and helping families during the changes required of them by childbearing. When families cope successfully with childbearing, they are better able to begin childrearing. Successful childrearing strengthens societies that compose the nation and ultimately the world. Collectively, maternity nurses can make an enormous difference in the health and well-being of families.

REFERENCES

ANA requests nominations for Nursing Hall of Fame. 1983. *Amer. Nurse.* 15(8):16.

Bendiner, E. 1980. Elizabeth Blackwell: Heresy with intelligence. *Hospital Practice.* 15(6):109–128.

Bettmann, O. L. 1956. *A pictorial history of medicine.* Springfield, Ill.: Charles C. Thomas.

Bookmiller, M. M., and Bowen, G. L. 1954. *Textbook of obstetrics and obstetric nursing.* 2nd ed. Philadelphia: Saunders.

Bowlby, J. 1965. *Child care and the growth of love.* 2nd ed. England: Penguin Books.

Brazelton, T. B. 1961. Effect of maternal medication on the neonate and his behavior. *J. Pediatrics.* 58:513–518.

Breckinridge, M. 1952. *Wide neighborhoods.* New York: Harper & Row.

Bullough, B., and Bullough, V. 1977. Introduction and overview. In *Expanding horizons for nurses,* eds. B. Bullough and V. Bullough. New York: Springer-Verlag.

Bullough, B., and Bullough, V. L. 1978. *The care of the sick: The emergence of modern nursing.* New York: Prodist.

Bullough, V. L., and Bullough, B. 1969. *The emergence of modern nursing.* 2nd ed. Ontario: Collier-Macmillan.

Department of Health and Human Services. 1982. *Prevention 82.* DHHS (PHS) Publication No. 82-50157.

De Young, L. 1972. *The foundations of nursing.* St. Louis: C. V. Mosby.

Dolan, J. A. 1973. *Nursing in society: A historical perspective.* 13th ed. Philadelphia: Saunders.

Fauci, A. S. 1987. Nurses play a critical role in care of AIDS patients. *Amer. Nurse* 19(7):17.

Federal Security Agency. 1952. *Vital statistics* 26(17).

Findley, P. 1939. *Priests of Lucina.* Boston: Little, Brown.

Gerson, N. B. 1970. *The crusader.* Boston: Little, Brown.

Gilgoff, A. 1978. *Home birth.* New York: Coward, McCann and Geoghegan.

Goodnow, M. 1948. *Nursing history.* 8th ed. Philadelphia: Saunders.

Graham, H. 1951. *Eternal Eve.* Garden City, N.Y.: Doubleday.

Griffin, G. J., and Griffin, J. K. 1973. *History and trends of professional nursing.* St. Louis: C. V. Mosby.

Hager, M. 1983. 290 billion a year and growing. *Consumers Digest.* 22(4):10–12.

Hawkins, M. M. 1980. Nursing and regionalization of perinatal services. *J. Obstet. Gynecol. Neonatal Nurs.* 9:215–217.

Hughes, D.; Johnson, K.; Rosenbaum, S.; Simons, J.; and Butler, E. 1986. *The health of American's children: The maternal and child health data book.* Washington, D.C.: Children's Defense Fund.

Huntington, J. A., and Shores, L. 1983. From conflict to collaboration. *Am. J. Nurs.* 83:1184–1186.

Kalisch, B. J., and Kalisch, P. A. 1983. Heroine out of focus: Media images of Florence Nightingale. *Nurs. Health Care.* 4:270–278.

Kalisch, P. A., and Kalisch, B. J. 1978. *The advance of American nursing.* Boston: Little, Brown.

Kennedy, D. M. 1970. *Birth control in America: The career of Margaret Sanger.* New Haven, Conn.: Yale University Press.

Klaus, M. H., and Kennell, J. H. 1976. *Maternal–infant bonding.* St. Louis: C. V. Mosby.

Korones, S. B. 1983. To be or not to be: Who decides for the newborn? *Childbirth Educator.* 2(3):42–45.

Lader, L., and Meltzer, M. 1969. *Margaret Sanger: Pioneer of birth control.* New York: Thomas Y. Crowell.

Lamb, M. E., and Hall, E. 1982. Bonding: The emphasis on early contact needs to be reexamined before it backfires. *Childbirth Educator.* 2(1):19–23.

Leaphart, E. 1983, Editorial. *J. Obstet. Gynecol. Neonatal Nurs.* 12:151.

The legal side. 1983. *Am. J. Nurs.* 83:1202–1203.

Lewis, E. P. 1983. For the nurse writer's bookshelf. *Am. J. Nurs.* 82:1116–1118.

Lubic, R. W. 1983. Where to give birth: Birthing center. *Childbirth Educator.* 2(4):26–38.

Lytle, N. A., ed. 1977. *Nursing of women in the age of liberation.* Dubuque, Iowa: William C. Brown.

Mallison, M. B. 1983. Editorial: Gadfly to the profession. *Am. J. Nurs.* 83:1141.

McGrellis, N. M. 1976. Labor and delivery 120 years ago. *J. Obstet. Gynecol. Neonatal Nurs.* 5(3):56–58.

National Center for Health Statistics. 1983. Advance report of final mortality statistics, 1980. *Monthly Vital Statistics Report.* 32(4), Supplement. U.S. Department of Health and Human Services: Public Health Service.

National Center for Health Statistics. 1984. *Health United States* 1984. DHHS Pub. No. (PHS) 85–1232. Hyattsville, MD: Public Health Service.

National Center for Health Statistics. (1986a). Perinatal mortality in the United States: 1950–81. *Monthly Vital Statistics Report.* 34(12), Supplement. DHHS Pub. No. (PHS) 86–1120. Hyattsville, MD: Public Health Service.

National Center for Health Statistics. (1986b). Advance report of final natality statistics 1984. *Monthly Vital Statistics Report.* 35(4), Supplement. DHHS Pub. No. (PHS) 86–1120. Hyattsville, MD: Public Health Service.

National Center for Health Statistics. (1986c). Annual summary of births, marriages, divorces, and deaths, United States 1985. *Monthly Vital Statistics Report.* 34(13). DHHS Pub. No. (PHS) 86–1120. Hyattsville, MD: Public Health Service.

National Center for Health Statistics. (1987a). Births, marriages, divorces, and deaths for November 1986. *Monthly Vital Statistics Report.* 35(11). DHHS Pub. No. (PHS) 87–1120. Hyattsville, MD: Public Health Service.

News. 1982a. *Am. J. Nurs.* April. 82:519, 527.

News, 1982b. *Am. J. Nurs.* June. 82:914.

News, 1983a. *Am. J. Nurs.* January. 83:7.

News. 1983b. *Am. J. Nurs.* March. 83:345.

News. 1983c. *Am. J. Nurs.* June. 83:858.

News. 1983d. *Am. J. Nurs.* August. 83:1119, 1123.

News in Brief. 1982. *Am. J. Nurs.* September. 82:1336.

News in Brief. 1983. *Am. J. Nurs.* July. 83:988.

O'Reilly, J. 1983. Getting a gender message. *Time.* July 25:12–13.

Palmer, I. S. 1983. From whence we came. In *The nursing profession: A time to speak,* ed. N. L. Chaska. New York: McGraw-Hill.

Pratt, M. W. 1982. The demography of maternal and child health. In *Maternal and child health practices: Problems, resources, and methods of delivery,* eds. H. M. Wallace, E. M. Gold, and A. C. Oglesby. New York: John Wiley & Sons.

Pritchard, J. A., and MacDonald, P. C. 1976. *Williams Obstetrics.* 15th ed. New York: Appleton-Century-Crofts.

Regan, W. A. 1982. Sex discrimination charges: Male nurses. *The Regan Report on Nursing Law.* 23(3):2.

Riordan, J. R., and Countryman, B. A. 1980. Basics of breastfeeding—Part I: Infant feeding patterns past and present. *J. Obstet. Gynecol. Neonatal Nurs.* 9:207–210.

Ryan, J. 1983. Editorial: Groups affirm nursing's stances; let's move ahead. *Amer. Nurse.* 15(7):4.

Sanger, M. 1938. *Margaret Sanger: An autobiography.* New York: W. W. Norton.

Serevino, J. 1982. Editorial. *J. Obstet. Gynecol. Neonatal Nurs.* 11:208.

Smellie, W. 1974. *A treatise on the theory and practice of midwifery.* Facsimile printing of the 1st ed. New York: Cassell and Collier Macmillan and Robert E. Krueger.

Sousa, M. 1976. *Childbirth at home.* Englewood Cliffs, N.J.: Prentice-Hall.

Stevenson, J. S. 1981. The nursing profession: From the past into the future. *National Forum.* 61(4):9–10.

Stewart, I. M., and Austin, A. L. 1962. *A history of nursing.* 5th ed. New York: Putnam's.

Varney, H. 1980. *Nurse-midwifery.* Boston: Blackwell.

Wessel H. 1973. *Natural childbirth and the family.* New York: Harper & Row.

White, W. G. 1983. Part II: Out of hospital: Home birth. *Childbirth Educator.* 2(4):33–36.

Who's who of American women. 1958. Chicago: Marquis.

3

Changes Related to Women's Health: Issues of Contraception

BEHAVIORAL OBJECTIVES

Upon completion of this chapter, the reader should be able to:

- Discuss the difference in the availability of contraceptives over the past three decades.

- Identify factors influencing the female partner's use of contraception.

- Identify factors influencing the male partner's use of contraception.

- Discuss general areas of consideration which will influence contraceptive behavior.

- Discuss the significance of the proposed assessment guide for use with clients regarding contraception.

- Identify a possible intervention for the chronic noncontraceptor.

- Discuss the value of combination barrier methods of contraception with examples.

- Discuss a method of contraception which reduces the risk of sexually transmitted diseases

The realistic possibility of a woman having control over her fertility is one of the main reasons for the expanding, and improving, role of women today. Still, contraception is a long way from being a simple matter. Many women are not effective users of contraception and find themselves pregnant. On average, a woman aged between 13 and 45 has approximately 32 or more fertile years in her lifetime (DHEW, 1985). That is at least 380 monthly cycles or 380 chances to get pregnant or not to get pregnant, as she chooses. Many women who are pregnant do not wish for another child in the near future. Thus pregnancy often becomes a great motivator for change, an unfreezer (see Chapter 1). There is then a natural window for evaluation, teaching, and the possible improvement of contraceptive practice. If this is effectively acted upon by the nurse it can lead to a higher level of wellness for the client and her partner because of fertility management. To be able to do this, the nurse must be well prepared with information about the factors influencing contraceptive behavior and specific knowledge of each available method for contraception. This chapter will give that information. Instructions for the use of each method are included in Appendix K. They are designed specifically for use in client teaching.

ANATOMY AND PHYSIOLOGY

In considering contraception, it is assumed the reader is knowledgeable about basic anatomy and physiology. Three illustrations indicating male and female reproductive anatomy are presented in conjunction with a diagram of physiology of the menstrual cycle (see Figs. 3–1, 3–2, and 3–3).

HISTORICAL PERSPECTIVE

The results of a recent survey of 7000 women show that less than 50 percent between the ages of 15 and 44 used contraception the first time they had sexual intercourse. Almost 25 percent of the women did not use contraception for at least a year after becoming sexually active, but 95 percent did report using contraception at some time. The report also found that younger women who had more recently become sexually active were much more likely to be using contraception from the beginning (Collomb, 1987).

This last finding gives encouragement that contraception and knowledge about it may be coming "out of the closet." As recently as the 1960s, people had to inquire surreptitiously of friends how to go about getting a diaphragm, and would often have to travel great distances to secure one. There were actually federal, state, and local laws severely restricting access to contraception information. These effectively prohibited public health nurses from discussing contraception.

Into this environment of the 1960s burst "the pill" and the reproductive revolution. The repressive laws have been repealed, contraceptives are now widely available in every community, and nurses are encouraged to promote contraception.

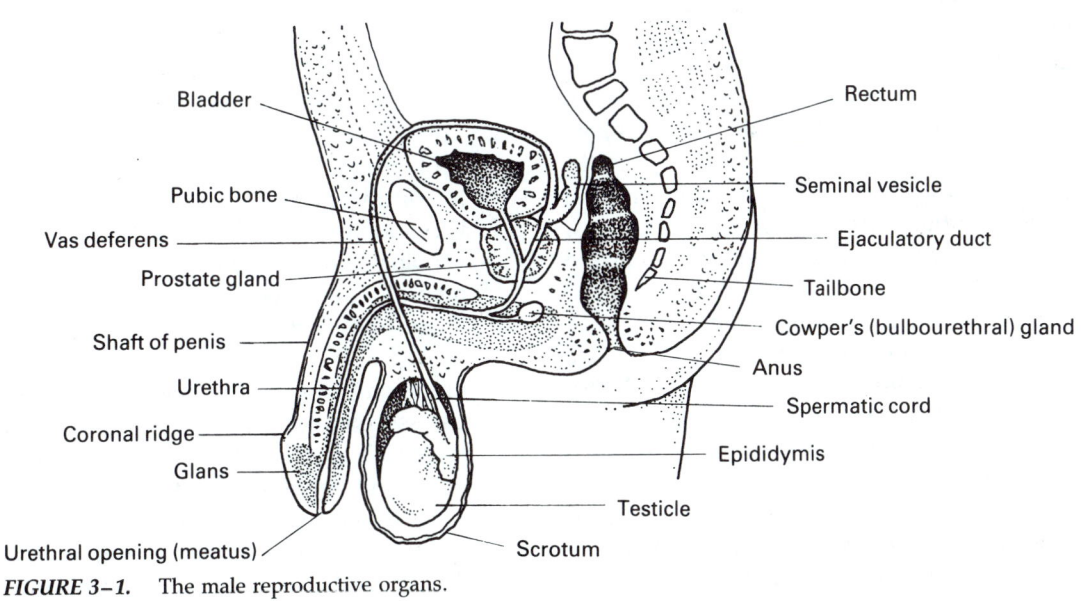

FIGURE 3–1. The male reproductive organs.
SOURCE: Nass and Fisher (1988).

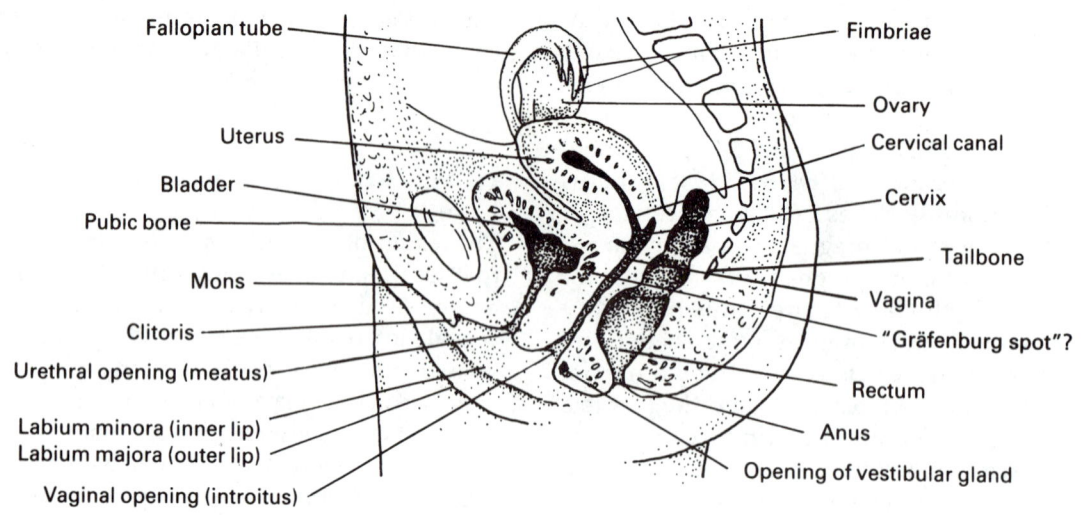

FIGURE 3-2. The internal female reproductive system (side view).
SOURCE: Nass and Fisher (1988).

Still, dissemination and application of contraceptive knowledge has been very slow in the United States. It is estimated that 1.1 million teenagers under 18 will still get pregnant in 1988 (Children's Defense Fund, 1987).

FACTORS INFLUENCING CONTRACEPTIVE USE

There are many reasons why people do not use contraception, even though they do not want to become pregnant. A common reason is inadequate knowledge. One survey has shown that about half of sexually active teenage females, aged 15–19, thought they could not become pregnant (Henshaw and O'Reilly, 1983). A survey of urban mothers showed that only one-third knew when during the menstrual cycle a woman is most likely to become pregnant (Presser, 1977).

There are many social, religious, and cultural factors which affect the use of contraceptives. Those factors tend to be quite different for married than for single women. Also, a modern orientation may emphasize such things as career activities, whereas a more traditional one will emphasize childbearing and home activities (Miller, 1986). Resistance to contraceptive use may also be influenced by one's attitudes about virility and reproduction, or beliefs among certain ethnic groups that widespread contraception is a means to promote genocide (Mazurkewicz, 1983). The behavior of friends and family, social norms (school, church), and ideas and values expressed through the mass media all exert an influence (Miller, 1986). The health care provider's manner of interacting with the client may also affect contraceptive use.

Aside from the many factors influencing "ordinary" contraceptive decisions, there is also the problem of the chronic noncontraceptor. The degree to which the nurse is able to learn the person's feelings and attitudes about contraception can make the difference in whether counseling is effective or not. Some of the factors which may contribute to contraceptives not being used include:

1. Irresponsibility, not in the classic sense, but in the sense of being unable to respond to one's fertility.
2. Low or non-existent self-esteem, a particular problem with very young women. The inability to contracept may reinforce this.
3. Questionable comprehension, a particular problem with learning disabled people, the mentally retarded, the poorly educated, and those unable to read. The approaches have to be tailored so that the person can actually understand the contraceptive instructions.
4. Unassertive behavior, often related to low self-esteem, but which can be rooted in the continuous, subtle messages for women not to be aggressive. A contraceptive response (or nonresponse) may be a retreat into unassertiveness.
5. Anger, with the refusal to contracept and the

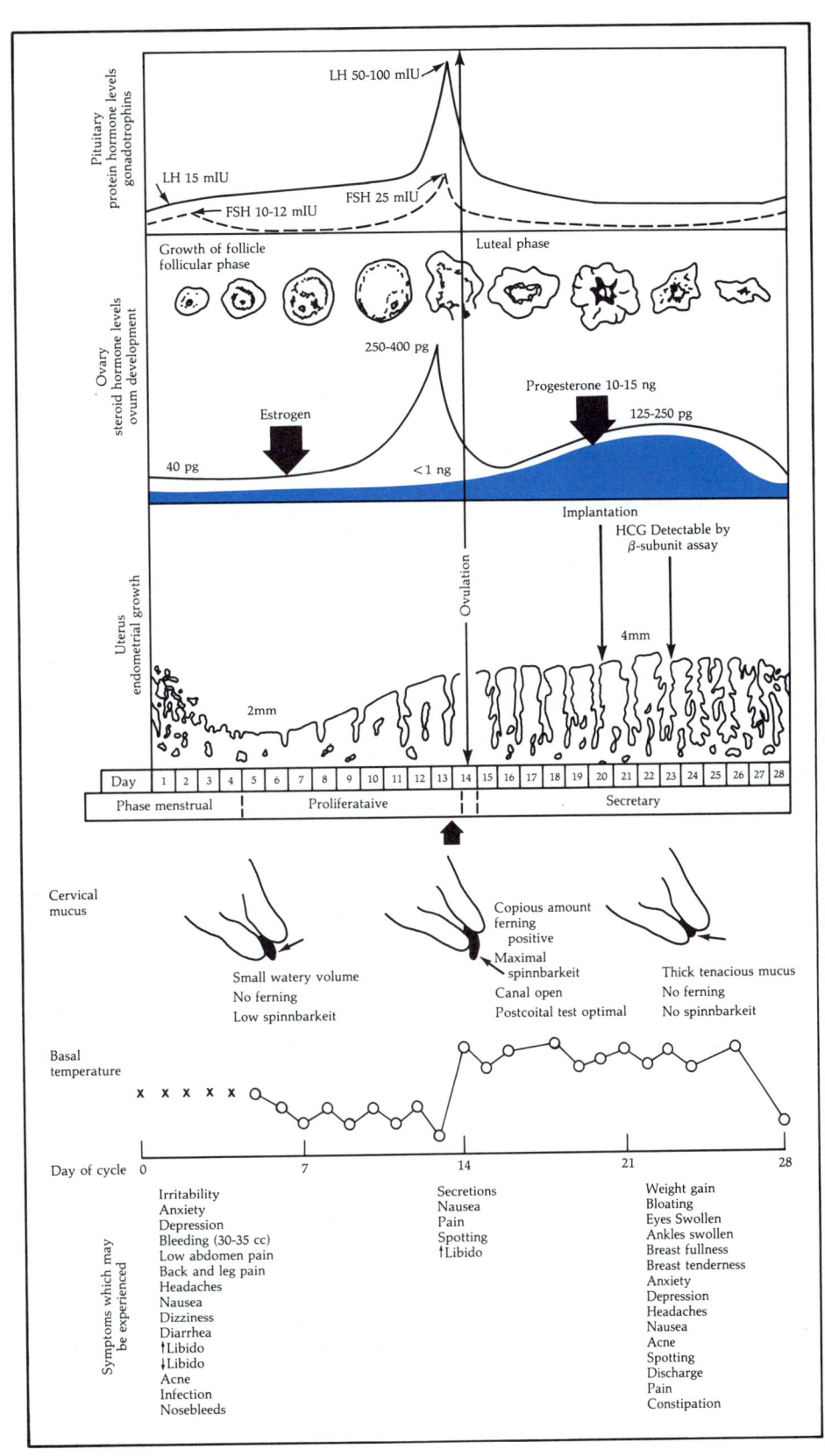

FIGURE 3–3. A diagram of menstrual physiology.
SOURCE: Hatcher et al. (1984).

possible resulting pregnancy becoming a punishment for the object of the young woman's anger, which may be a parent, a sexual partner, or even herself.
6. Unconscious desire to be pregnant to test one's fertility.
7. Sexuality conflicts or denial of sexuality, with the avoidance of contraception being a way of denying that one is a sexual being.
8. Risk-taking behavior, particularly in those with risk-taking lifestyles.
9. Ambivalence about the method of choice and, therefore, the method will not be used effectively. If the young woman is afraid that the pill causes cancer despite the evidence, she will probably not take it effectively. Or, if she is not confident about the diaphragm's effectiveness, she will probably not use it consistently (Collomb, 1987).

There are four general areas of consideration that influence the choice and use of contraception:

1. Motivation to avoid conception.
2. Risk of conception with the perceived risk possibly being even more important than the actual risk.
3. A set of attitudes and beliefs of both partners that govern contraceptive preferences and the adoption of specific methods.
4. Interaction that takes place between each user and the method (Miller, 1986).

CONSIDERATIONS IN CHOOSING A CONTRACEPTIVE METHOD

In choosing a contraceptive method, three major considerations are:

1. *Effectiveness:* how well will a method work for a specific person (and will she have an abortion if the method fails)?
2. *Safety:* do the risks of a specific method outweigh the benefits for the couple?
3. *Future reproductive plans:* will the person want children in the future?

Effectiveness

The comparison of failure rates of contraceptive methods is often a beginning point for discussion in choosing a method. As a person realizes the inherent differences in effectiveness of the methods, there develops a more focused need to consider different options in a given situation. Table 3–1 compares these rates.

Safety/Risks

All contraceptives have risks which may be categorized as:

1. *Dangers of the method itself:* death, hysterectomy, infection, loss of fertility, pain or nuisance side-effects.
2. *Potential risks in terms of inconvenience:* intercourse less pleasant, too great an expense, partner dissatisfaction, embarrassment.
3. *Risks associated with failure and pregnancy:* danger to the woman, degree of disruption of life.
4. *Noncontraceptive benefits:* therapeutic effects of oral contraceptives or protective effects of methods against STDs (Hatcher et al., 1986).

Putting voluntary risks into perspective in comparison to contraceptive risks, as in Table 3–2, helps to understand the problem. However, even

TABLE 3–1.	Contraceptive Method Failure Rates
Method	Failure Rate: Typical Users (%)
Tubal ligation	0.04
Vasectomy	0.15
Injectable progestin	0.25
Combined birth control pills	2.0
Progestin-only pills	2.5
IUD	5.0
Condom	10.0
Diaphragm (with spermicide)	19.0
Sponge (with spermicide)	10–20
Cervical cap	13.0
Foams, creams, jellies, and vaginal suppositories	18.0
Coitus interruptus	23.0
Fertility awareness technique (Basal body temperature, mucous method, calendar, and "rhythm")	24.0
Douche	40.0
Chance (no method of birth control)	90.0

SOURCE: Adapted from Hatcher et al. (1984).

TABLE 3-2. Putting Voluntary Risks Into Perspective

Risk	Chance of Death in a Year
Smoking	1 in 200
Motorcycling	1 in 1000
Automobile driving	1 in 6000
Playing football	1 in 25,000
Using tampons (toxic shock)	1 in 350,000
Having sexual intercourse (PID)	1 in 50,000
Preventing pregnancy:	
Oral contraception: nonsmoker	1 in 63,000
Oral contraception: smoker	1 in 16,000
Using IUDs	1 in 100,000
Using barrier methods	None
Using natural methods	None
Undergoing sterilization	
Laparoscopic tubal ligation	1 in 20,000
Vasectomy	None
Deciding about pregnancy:	
Continuing pregnancy	1 in 10,000
Terminating pregnancy:	
Illegal abortion	1 in 3000
Legal abortion:	
Before 9 weeks	1 in 400,000
After 16 weeks	1 in 10,000

SOURCE: Adapted from Hatcher et al. (1984).

if the odds of a complication are one in a million, to the one person who gets that complication, it is 100 percent reality.

Attention to contraindications in choosing a method can help to greatly reduce the degree of risk for a given person and a given method. Contraindications can be ranked on three levels:

1. *Absolute contraindications:* the method must not be used. For example, a person with PID must not use an IUD.
2. *Strong relative contraindications:* strongly advise not to use the method. For example, a person over 30 who smokes should not use oral contraceptive pills.
3. *Other relative contraindications:* method may be used if there is adequate clinical monitoring for early signs of trouble. For example, a

family history of hypertension in prospective pill users.

Future Contraceptive Plans

If the client plans to have any children in the future, then the choice of method should protect fertility. Some examples of this principle are:

1. Sterilization should be considered permanent in spite of the number of surgical reversals which are attempted.
2. The risk of infection makes the IUD a poor choice for a woman who wants more children.
3. The oral contraceptive pill may be the ideal contraceptive for the young, non-smoking woman who wants to be sexually active for a long period of time before bearing children.

BARRIER METHODS OF CONTRACEPTION

In the discussion of barrier methods of contraception, keep in mind that there are two general types, mechanical barriers and chemical barriers. The most common chemical barrier is nonoxynol-9. It is enjoying increasing popularity because of its germicidal properties which make it helpful in preventing some STDs. Though each barrier method can be used alone, the effectiveness rate is not great. If two methods, one mechanical and one chemical, are used together correctly and consistently, the resulting effectiveness rate is extremely high. Common examples of these combinations are condoms and foam, diaphragm and cream, or the one condom now available in the United States, Ramses-Extra, which is coated with spermicide.

Success with all nonpermanent contraceptives appears to be greater for patients who do not desire any future pregnancies compared with those who are uncertain or who plan pregnancy in the future. The effectiveness of barrier methods is influenced by a variety of factors, such as frequency of intercourse, inherent fertility of the couple, risk-taking habits and attitudes, motivation to prevent pregnancy, inherent effectiveness of the barrier method being used, specific method characteristics that enhance or interfere with proper use, clinical and educational approaches used to educate each user properly, and the ability of the user to use the method correctly (Hatcher et al., 1986).

Diaphragm

How it Works/How it is Obtained

In the form of a round, shallow dome of thin rubber stretched over a flexible ring, the diaphragm acts as a mechanical barrier. It covers the cervix, making it difficult for sperm to enter and travel up to the uterus (see Fig. 3–4). In addition, spermicide is placed in the cup of the diaphragm because the blocking mechanism is not very reliable by itself. Diaphragms come in different sizes and they must be fitted by trained health personnel. A set of graduated flexible rings is used to determine the correct fit depending on the size and shape of the vagina and the size and position of the cervix. After the fitting, the woman must have adequate opportunity to learn how to place and remove the diaphragm by herself. One study has shown that effectiveness can be greatly improved if the woman returns in 1 week with the diaphragm in place, so that the position and fit can be checked for accuracy (Hatcher et al., 1986).

Use, Safety, and Effectiveness

The diaphragm has a lower rate of effectiveness than either birth control pills or IUDs. Failure rates for the diaphragm are reported to be between 2 and 19 pregnancies per 100 women using the device for 1 year (Hatcher et al., 1986). There are both "user" and "method" failures. The woman's memory and motivation are important influences on effectiveness because this method requires consistent and correct use. Other problems relating to effectiveness are the diaphragm slipping out of position due to improper insertion or a poor fit. Also, even a well-fitted and properly inserted diaphragm can become dislodged during intercourse because sexual excitation may cause expansion of the vagina and movement of the uterus. This is a particular problem when the woman is on top of the man or if the penis is removed and reinserted into the vagina during plateau levels of arousal (Masters, Johnson, and Kolodny, 1988).

The diaphragm is a very safe contraceptive because it has no effect on body processes or later fertility, though toxic shock syndrome has been reported in relation to its use. The danger signs of toxic shock syndrome are fever above 101°F, diarrhea, vomiting, muscle aches and/or a sunburn-like rash (see Hatcher et al., 1986, for a

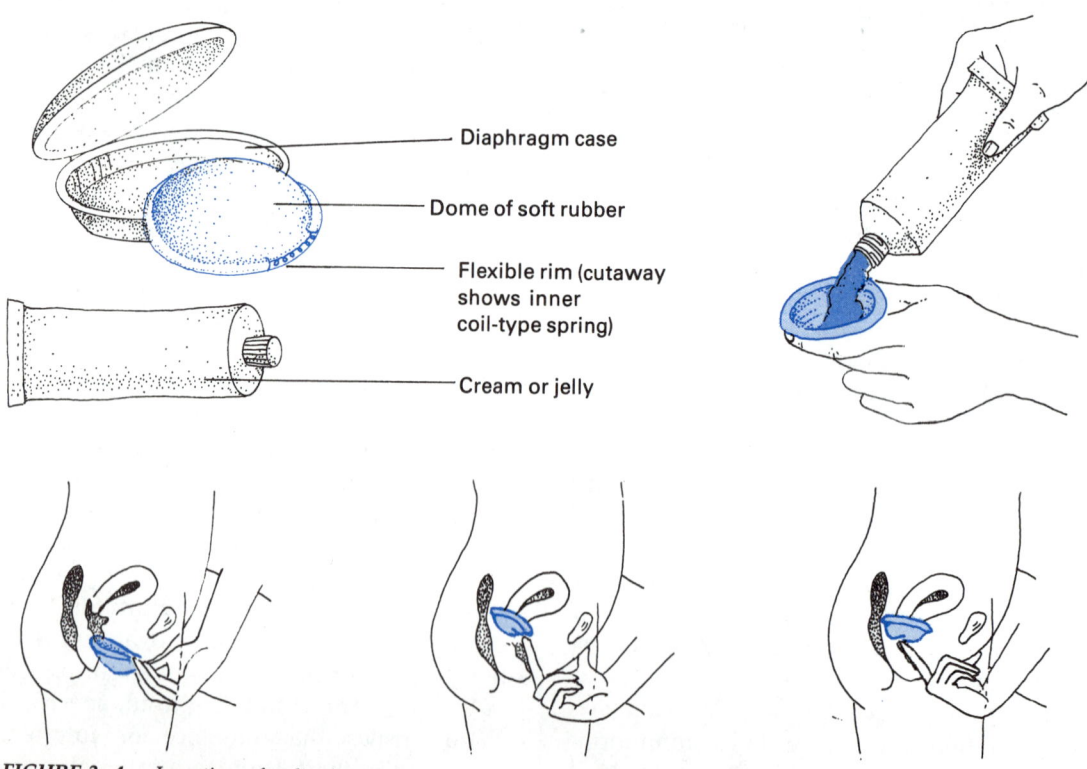

FIGURE 3–4. Insertion of a diaphragm.
SOURCE: Nass, Libby, and Fisher (1987).

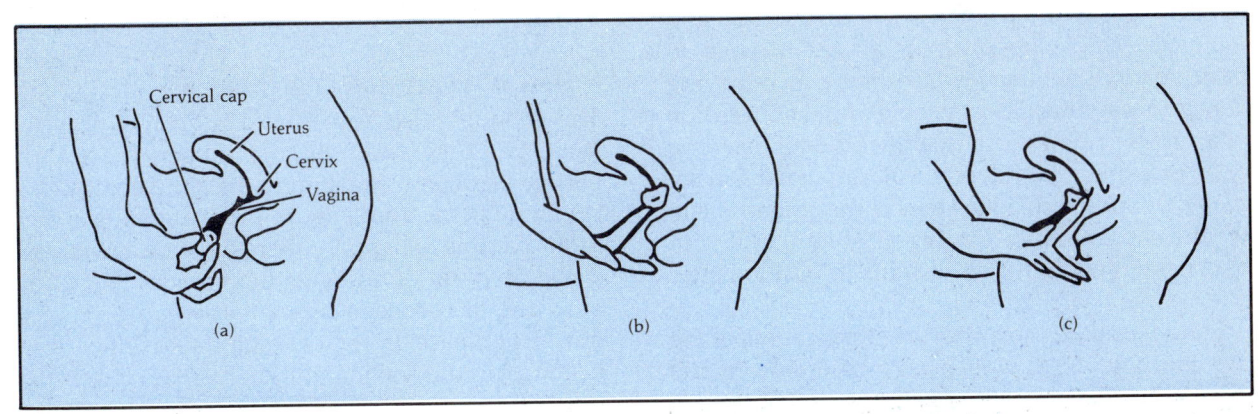

FIGURE 3–5. Insertion of a cervical cap.
SOURCE: Adapted from Hatcher et al. (1986).

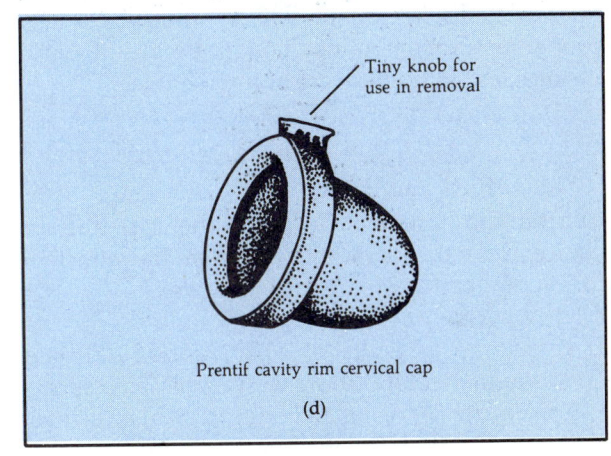

detailed discussion of diaphragm side-effects and contraindications).

Sexual Effects

The primary sexual effect of the diaphragm is interference with sexual arousal due to the time taken to insert the diaphragm if it has not been put in place in advance (Masters, Johnson, and Kolodny, 1988). However, insertion can be incorporated as part of sex play. Either partner may find diaphragm use unaesthetic. The use of spermicides can make diaphragm insertion very slippery and awkward, especially when first learning to use one. An oversized diaphragm may cause pain for one or both partners at the time of intercourse. Some men state that diaphragm use causes intercourse to feel different (Masters, Johnson, and Kolodny, 1988). Partners may find the taste or smell of the spermicide unpleasant if they engage in oral sex.

Cervical Cap

How it Works/How it is Obtained

The cervical cap is like a large thimble made of rubber. It fits tightly over the cervix where it is held in place by suction (see Fig. 3–5). It is a barrier method of contraception similar to the diaphragm. The cervical cap may be an effective means of contraception by itself without cream or jelly. However, particularly at or near the time of ovulation, it is suggested that a spermicide is used with the cap (CSUH Student Health Center, 1983).

The cap has been used extensively in other countries for many years. In the United States, it was not approved by the Food and Drug Administration (FDA) until 1988. Until then the cap was available from a limited number of places participating in FDA studies. It appears that FDA approval in May, 1988 will lead to much wider availability and popularity of the cap.

Use, Safety, and Effectiveness

The cap has been approved for use by women with normal pap smears. A repeat pap smear should be carried out in 3 months. If there is any abnormality, the person should stop using the cap. The soft rubber caps which are currently available are not suitable for prolonged vaginal retention in most women. This is because of problems with a strong odor after 36–48 hours in the vagina, and because of the theoretical risk of toxic shock syndrome. Manufacturers' recommendations which accompany the cap suggest the use of spermicide inside the cap (to fill one-third of the cup). They specify time rules for insertion and removal (Hatcher et al., 1986).

Possibly the most important factor influencing

effectiveness is the woman's skill of insertion and removal. Ample opportunity for the woman to have supervised practice inserting and removing her cap is essential. Most people find that insertion of a cap is somewhat more difficult than insertion of a diaphragm, and removal can be distinctly tricky. A common suggestion is that each person try the cap first during a period of low fertility in her cycle to verify that it remains in position after intercourse (Hatcher et al., 1986).

Studies to date show that the effectiveness of the cap is about 85%, which is comparable to the diaphragm (Hatcher et al., 1986). Many failures are due to faulty technique (no spermicide or improper instruction on insertion) or because the cap is not used with every act of intercourse.

Side-effects and Safety

Contraindications which make the cap a poor choice for women or may prevent the effective fitting of a cap at a particular time are:

1. Infections: a history of Toxic Shock Syndrome or vaginal colonization with *Staphylococcus aureus*, acute cervicitis, pelvic or vaginal infection.
2. Allergy to rubber (latex) or spermicide.
3. Lack of medical personnel qualified to fit the cap or an inability of the client or partner to learn the correct technique.
4. Anatomical abnormalities, or normal variations of the cervix or vagina that preclude satisfactory fit. An extremely shallow or extremely long cervix, severe cervical laceration, or a vaginal septum are some anatomical problems that may make cap fitting impossible.
5. Abnormal pap smear, or undiagnosed vaginal or cervical lesions.
6. Cervical biopsy or cryosurgery within the past 6 weeks.
7. Full-term delivery within the past 6 weeks (Hatcher et al., 1986).

Sexual Effects

The sexual effects of the cervical cap are similar to those of the diaphragm. The male partner may experience pain or lack of sensation due to the firmness and placement of the cap. Partners may find the taste or smell of the spermicide unpleasant if they engage in oral sex. As yet, no research data documents the role the cap may play in the presentation of STDs, but it is thought that it will be at least as effective as the diaphragm.

Condom

How it Works/How it is Obtained

The condom, also known as a rubber or prophylactic, is a thin sheath of latex rubber. It acts as a barrier because it fits snugly over the erect penis keeping sperm from entering the vagina (see Fig. 3–6). For this to happen, there must be a reservoir at the tip of the condom (either because it is made with one or because space is left when putting it on). This space is for collecting the semen and keeping it from leaking into the vagina. This is the only effective non-surgical contraceptive method for males. There are no health risks associated with condoms.

Condoms do not require a prescription. They are inexpensive but they are not reusable. They are available to anyone and can be purchased in drugstores, supermarkets, family planning clinics, and men's rooms in restaurants, bars, and gas stations. Condoms come in many different styles: lubricated, colored, flavored, ribbed to provide more stimulation for the female and, recently, coated with spermicide as well as lubricant. Infrequently, latex condoms may cause genital irritation, necessitating the use of condoms made of tissue from lamb intestine (Masters, Johnson, and Kolodny, 1988).

A "female condom" is expected to be on the market in the United States by the end of 1988. It will be a disposable, latex device which fits loosely inside the vagina and covers the perineum. This is designed to provide more protection against sexually transmitted diseases than traditional condoms can do because it should effectively prevent any contact with body secretions for the men and the women. Because the device does not fit closely against the penis, it can be made much thicker for safety without reducing male sensitivity (Robertson, 1988). Female sensitivity seems questionable. These devices are already in use in Europe where they are called fem-shield or vaginal shield.

Safety and Effectiveness

The condom can be a very reliable method of contraception if used properly and consistently. The theoretical failure rate is 2 pregnancies per 100 couples using condoms for a year (Hatcher et al., 1986). Effectiveness almost equals that of oral contraceptive pills when condoms are used routinely in combination with a vaginal spermicide. However, studies have shown that couples using the condom as their only method of contraception risk an overall failure rate of 10–20 pregnancies per

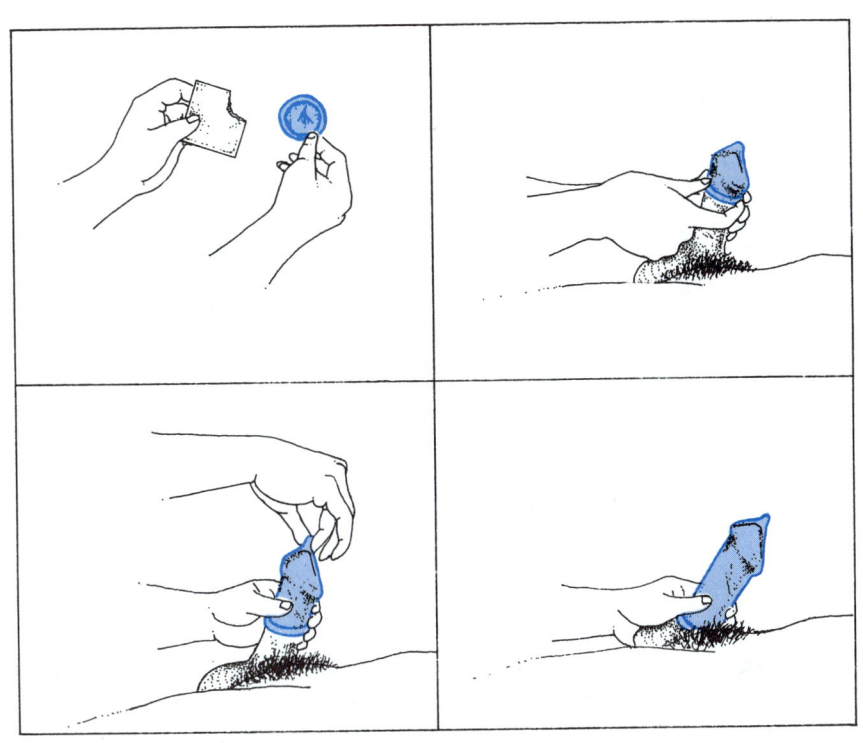

FIGURE 3-6. Application of a condom.
SOURCE: Nass, Libby, and Fisher (1987).

100 couple years (Masters, Johnson, and Kolodny, 1988). Obviously this method requires effort, motivation, and knowledge to prevent unwanted pregnancies.

One aspect of the safety of condoms is their contribution in disease prevention: they may prevent cancer of the cervix, and they can provide considerable protection against some sexually transmitted diseases. However, some precautions must be taken to insure protection. The penis must be protected at all times during foreplay which includes genital sex play. Condoms must be undamaged prior to use, must be correctly applied before and correctly removed after intercourse, and must remain undamaged after use (Dirubbo, 1987).

Sexual Effects

There are several sexual advantages to using condoms. Clearly, the male participates in and shares responsibility for contraception which can be very pleasing to the female. When vaginal lubrication is a problem, use of lubricated condoms can be helpful. Postcoital secretions for the woman can be greatly reduced or eliminated (if this is seen as a problem). Men who have difficulty controlling ejaculation may find the condom beneficial (Masters, Johnson, and Kolodny, 1988).

The sexual disadvantages of condom use include interrupted spontaneity, although application can be incorporated into foreplay. A common complaint is a decreased sensation of the penis when wearing a condom. For men who have problems with erection, the condom is probably a poor contraceptive choice: it calls attention to the degree of erection and may increase "performance anxiety" (Masters, Johnson, and Kolodny, 1988). Men may even be unable to maintain an erection while putting on the condom. Also, to reduce the chance of spillage of semen into the vagina, the penis must be removed from the vagina soon after ejaculation, even though this does interfere with the intimate mood (Masters, Johnson, and Kolodny, 1988).

Spermicides

How they Work/How they are Obtained

Spermicides are vaginal chemical contraceptives and are effective in two ways: the chemical ingredient kills sperm, and the material containing this chemical also acts as a mechanical barrier blocking the entrance to the cervix. In order for these effects to occur, the spermicide must be placed properly in the vagina (see Figs. 3-7 and 3-8). Spermicides come in several forms: foams (some with prefilled

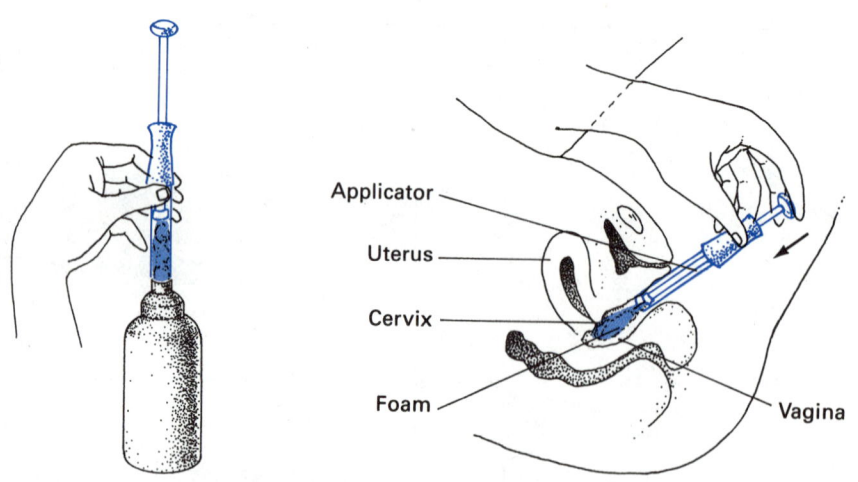

FIGURE 3–7. Insertion of contraceptive foam.
SOURCE: Nass, Libby, and Fisher (1987).

applicators which may be especially convenient for women with physical disabilities), jellies, creams, and tablets or suppositories. There are such individual differences in the many products on the market that the manufacturers' insert in each package must be consulted regarding use and effectiveness. Because spermicides do not require a prescription, they are readily available in drugstores or family planning clinics.

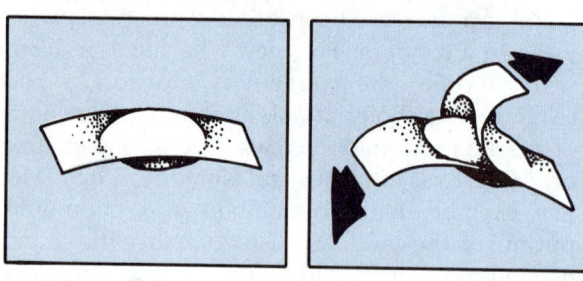

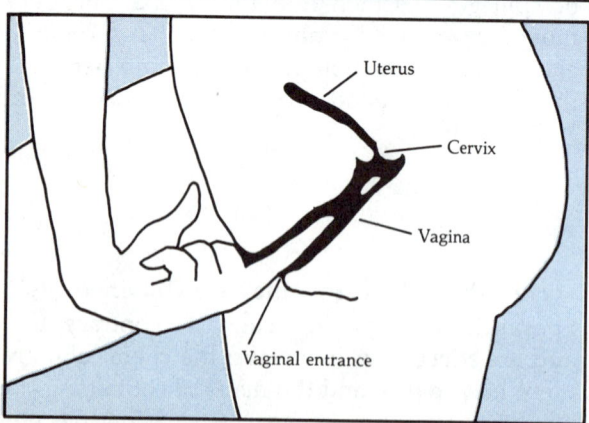

FIGURE 3–8. Insertion of a vaginal suppository.
SOURCE: Planned Parenthood/Alameda-San Francisco (1983).

Safety and Effectiveness

As with the condom, spermicidal products must be used correctly and routinely to be effective. Several studies report failure rates of less than 5 pregnancies per 100 couples using these methods for a period of 1 year (Masters, Johnson, and Kolodny, 1988). However, the failure rates during actual use are approximately 15 pregnancies per 100 couple years due to inconsistent and incorrect use of spermicides.

Some specific problems which contribute to failures using this method include incorrect insertion of the spermicide into the vagina, having intercourse more than once without inserting more spermicide, disregarding the time limits for effectiveness, using outdated products (expiration dates are on the labels), or using an almost empty container so there is not enough foam to adequately fill the applicator. This last problem is easily solved by having a backup can available.

Creams and jellies should be used only with another method of birth control such as a diaphragm or condom. In general, foam and suppositories are considered much more effective. Foam is an especially versatile method and may be used alone as a contraceptive or in combination with condoms as a backup method, for added lubrication, or as protection against sexually transmitted diseases. As a contraceptive, foam may be used during the first month of oral contraceptive use or while waiting to begin the first pack of pills (Hatcher et al., 1986). Foam is an excellent choice when a couple have decided to start a family but want to wait several months after stopping the pills. Diaphragm users may want to insert foam before having intercourse a second time (Hatcher et al., 1986). Foam is an all-purpose backup method to have at home. IUD users may use it during the first months or as a midcycle method to increase the effectiveness of an IUD, condom, or fertility awareness methods (Hatcher et al., 1986). If a couple is using condoms and one should accidentally break, foam can be used as an emergency backup method.

Though they are safely absorbed by the body, spermicides can cause burning or irritation of the vagina or penis—this occurs in about 1 in 20 people. It can often be alleviated by switching to a different product (Masters, Johnson, and Kolodny, 1988).

Possible spermicide toxicity engendered intense public debate with the publication in 1981 of controversial research findings reporting a possible link between spermicide use near the time of conception and the occurrence of fetal abnormalities. Subsequent researchers have found there are no adverse fetal effects related to spermicide use.

There is increasing evidence that spermicides provide some protection against sexually transmitted diseases such as gonorrhea (Cates, Weisner, and Curran, 1982). They also seem to help in preventing pelvic inflammatory disease (Masters, Johnson, and Kolodny, 1988).

Sexual Effects

The use of spermicides can interfere with spontaneity, but this can be compensated for by including their use as part of foreplay. It takes 20–30 minutes for the suppositories or tablets to dissolve, so they cannot be used if the couple is in a hurry. Spermicides may interfere with oral sex because of their unpleasant taste, and they are often considered messy and to provide too much lubrication (Masters, Johnson, and Kolodny, 1988).

Contraceptive Sponge

How it Works/How it is Obtained

The contraceptive sponge, marketed under the brand name "Today," is a 2-inch by 1-inch, round, polyurethane sponge permeated with the commonly used spermicide nonoxynol 9. This sponge is to be inserted into the vagina so that the concave side (which looks like a dimple) will fit over the cervix (see Fig. 3–9). Because the sponge comes in one size only and is not anchored in place in any way, there is a real possibility that it can become dislodged during intercourse. The sponge is effective for three reasons: it contains spermicide; it is a mechanical barrier partially preventing sperm from entering the cervix; and it is thought to trap and absorb sperm. After moistening the sponge with about two tablespoons of water and squeezing it gently until foam appears (which indicates the spermicide is activated), the sponge should be inserted in the vagina. This can be done either moments before intercourse or up to 18 hours before. This is considered a very convenient contraceptive because of this time factor and because:

1. It is considered easier to insert than a diaphragm though there can be problems with removal.
2. It is effective for up to 24 hours without any need of reapplication of spermicide regardless of how many times the user has intercourse.
3. There is no need to clean up any mess as the sponge is disposable. It can only be used once and it is not messy or drippy like some spermicides.
4. It is ordorless, tasteless, and unobtrusive (Masters, Johnson, and Kolodny, 1988).

This sponge was approved by the Food and Drug Administration in April, 1983. It is readily available in drugstores and family planning clinics. It does not require a prescription or fitting by trained health care personnel. Detailed instructions come in each box and must be studied well before use.

Safety and Effectiveness

Effectiveness of the sponge is almost equal to that of the diaphragm. The user failure rate is approximately 17 per 100 woman years (Grimes, 1986). These failures are attributed to poor user motivation and incorrect use of the sponge (Masters, Johnson, and Kolodny, 1988), e.g. the sponge is often removed too soon after intercourse. If the sponge is used in combination with a condom, the effectiveness rate is significantly improved (Masters, Johnson, and Kolodny, 1988).

One study has shown that those who have already been pregnant are twice as likely to become pregnant using the sponge as are nulliparous (never pregnant) users (Hatcher et al., 1986). Because the sponge comes in one size only, it is apparently too small for these women. On the other hand, this difference could be related to the inherent fertility or intercourse frequency of these women (Hatcher et al., 1986).

The sponge can cause mild irritation of the

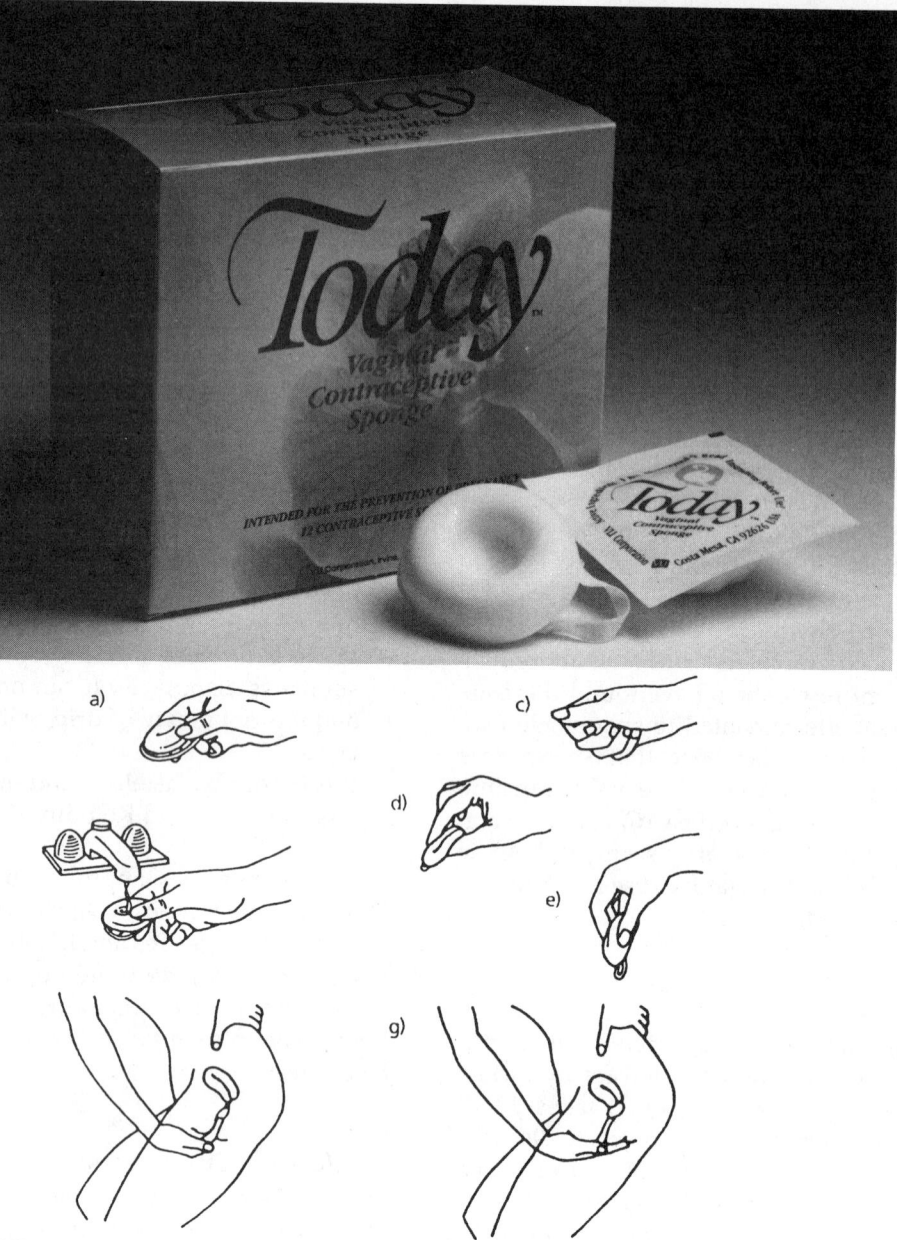

FIGURE 3–9. The contraceptive sponge.
SOURCE: Masters, Johnson, and Kolodny (1988).

vagina or penis in 3–5 percent of users. This is usually related to the spermicide.

Because the sponge is so new, not enough data has been gathered to fully assess its safety. However, there have been rare occurrences of toxic shock syndrome (10 per 100,000 users per year, similar to the 5–10 cases per 100,000 users of tampons). For this reason, the sponge should not be left in for more than 24 hours (Hatcher et al., 1986). Also, there may be as yet unidentified risks associated with the much stronger dose of nonoxynol-9 (1 g) compared to one application of other spermicide products (60–100 mg). Any adverse systemic effects have not been reported (Hatcher et al., 1986).

Sexual Effects

Because of convenience, the sponge does not interfere with spontaneity. The most important feature is the fact that the sponge can be left in for up to 18 hours before intercourse without the need for repeated applications of spermicide for multiple acts of intercourse. Usually couples do not feel the sponge during intercourse (Masters, Johnson, and Kolodny, 1988). Being odorless and tasteless, it does not interfere with oral sex. Some women have found that the sponge absorbed excessive vaginal secretions and caused vaginal dryness. Still other women reported absorption of secretions and ejaculate as a desirable effect of sponge use (Hatcher et al., 1986).

Oral Contraceptive Pills

How they Work/How they are Obtained

Oral contraceptive pills (OCPs) are synthetic hormones which act on the pituitary to block the normal cyclic output of FSH and LH, which prevents ovulation (see Fig. 3–3 for a diagram of basic physiology). In addition, OCPs contain a synthetic progesterone hormone, progestogen, which inhibits the development of the lining of the uterus, making implantation difficult. Progestogen also thickens the cervical mucous, thus decreasing the chance that sperm can get through.

There are two types of OCP. The combination pill contains both a synthetic estrogen and progesterone. These pills are taken daily beginning 4 days after a period begins (fifth day of the menstrual cycle) until the pack is empty. The combined pills come in low-, medium-, and high-dose ranges. For example, a woman who experiences a contraceptive failure on a mid-range dose may be a candidate for a higher-dose OCP. If one pill in the cycle is missed, two should be taken on the next day. If more than one is missed, it is likely that the pill will not be effective and another form of contraception must be used until the fifth day of the next cycle (Hatcher et al., 1986).

The newer minipill is distinctly different from the combined pill. The minipill contains progestogen only and in smaller doses. These pills can be very helpful for those experiencing estrogen-excess side-effects from the combined pill (Hatcher et al., 1986). The minipill is taken every day of the cycle even during menstruation. Ideally, because pregnancy rates are the highest during the first 6 months of minipill use, a second method of contraception should be used as a backup during this time. However, this should not be pushed strongly if it will interfere with the woman's use of the minipill. Some women use a backup method during midcycle for the duration of minipill use to improve effectiveness (Hatcher et al., 1986).

Both types of pill are available by prescription only. Minimally, a brief history and physical examination, including a pelvic examination, are necessary before the pills are prescribed. Thereafter, a yearly visit to the health care provider is required, making this an expensive method for some women.

Oral contraceptives may reduce the body's ability to use food nutrients. An oral contraceptive pill user should be sure to include foods containing folic acid, Vitamin B_2 (riboflavin), Vitamin B_6, and Vitamin C in her diet (Washoe County Health Department, 1985; see Table 3–3).

Hatcher et al. (1986) discuss some pertinent concerns when prescribing pills for young teenagers. For example, it is ideal if the teenager has 6–12 regular periods before starting the pills, but, if the teenager is already having intercourse, the medical and social risks of pregnancy probably outweigh the risks of taking oral contraceptives. This is true

TABLE 3–3. Nutrition and Family Planning: Oral Contraceptives

If you notice	*The Pill may cause*	*What foods can help*
Nervous tension, moodiness	A drop in Vitamin B_6 in the blood	Foods high in Vitamin B_6: meat, fish, poultry, whole grain breads and cereals
Fatigue	Increased body need for folic acid—this could lead to *anemia*	Foods high in folic acid: dark, green, leafy vegetables, citrus fruit, liver
Weight gain, bloating, breast tenderness	Salt and water retention (an estrogen effect)	Reduce your salt intake. See your health care provider if symptoms persist. Cut down on high-calorie foods to avoid weight gain
Lighter periods	Less blood loss; less iron loss means more iron retained by the body	This is beneficial. Change in diet not usually necessary unless iron blood levels are low

SOURCE: Washoe County Health Department (1985).

even if she has not started having menstrual periods. For premenarchal teens, height limitation due to premature closure of the epiphyses is not a problem when taking estrogen in the current low-dose pill. And epiphyseal closure is significantly advanced in menstruating teenagers (Hatcher et al., 1984). All minor side-effects such as nausea or spotting should be taken seriously in teenagers, for they are much more likely to discontinue pill use because of such problems (Hatcher et al., 1984).

Effectiveness

Only sterilization has a higher effectiveness rate than oral contraceptive pills. Theoretically, statistics indicate that only one pregnancy will occur among 200 women using the combined pill for 1 year (Hatcher et al., 1986). User negligence accounts for the actual failure rate of 2–3 pregnancies per 100 women using combined pills annually (Ory, Forrest, and Lincoln, 1983). The minipill, however, is less effective than the combined pill. In fact, failure rates are similar to those of the IUD, with perfect use of the method resulting in 1–2 pregnancies per 100 women annually. Women commonly forget to take a pill resulting in actual use rates of 5–10 pregnancies per 100 women annually (Masters, Johnson, and Kolodny, 1988).

The pill's effectiveness can be lowered somewhat in combination with certain prescription drugs. The medications listed in Table 3–4 may alter the body's breakdown of estrogen in the pill, thereby making it less effective.

Side-effects and Safety

Oral contraceptive pills have probably been studied more intensively than any medication in history. They have been in common use since the 1960s. The evidence shows greater health benefits than risks for many users, particularly for young, nonsmokers. The safety of OCP use is greatly improved when those whose histories indicate known contraindications are factored out of the study sample (Masters, Johnson, and Kolodny, 1988).

Some benefits of taking the pill include: protection against ovarian and uterine lining cancer and ovarian cysts; for many women, a reduced menstrual flow, more regular cycles and less menstrual cramping; premenstrual tension may be reduced; pelvic inflammatory disease is only half as common (Centers for Disease Control, 1983; Mishell, 1982; Senayake and Kramer, 1980).

TABLE 3–4. Adverse Oral Contraceptive Drug Interactions

Interacting Drugs	Adverse Effects
Anticoagulants, oral	Decreased anticoagulant effect
Barbiturates	Decreased contraceptive effect
Carbamazepine	Decreased contraceptive effect
Guanethidine	Decreased guanethidine effect
Hypoglycemics, oral	Decreased hypoglycemia
Phenytoin	Decreased contraceptive effect
Primidone	Decreased contraceptive effect
Rifampin	Decreased contraceptive effect
Tetracyclines	Decreased contraceptive effect
Troleandomycin	Jaundice
Tuberculin Skin Test	Depressed sensitivity

When taking any of these medications:
1. Additional methods of contraception may be necessary.
2. Breakthrough bleeding may indicate diminished contraceptive effect.

ADAPTED FROM: Hatcher et al. (1984).

Bothersome, but usually not serious, side-effects mimic those of pregnancy such as headache, vision problems, nausea, breast tenderness, edema, skin rashes, and constipation. Also associated with OCP use can be weight gain or loss, increased vaginal secretions, and increased susceptibility to vaginal infections (Masters, Johnson, and Kolodny, 1988). (For a detailed discussion of pill side effects as they change or stay constant over time, see Hatcher et al., 1986.) OCPs create a marked progesterone influence in the vagina causing a decrease in vaginal acidity. This allows the *Candida* pathogens to grow, leading to a close relationship between OCP use and a higher incidence of candidiasis. Candidiasis can be recognized by its curd-like, pasty discharge, pain on wiping or voiding, vulvar itching or burning, and dyspareunia (Robertson, 1987).

Less common but more troublesome side-effects caused by the pill include high blood pressure, diabetes, migraine headaches and/or eye problems, disturbance in liver function and rarely jaundice or liver tumors, possible birth defects if taken during pregnancy, a possible link with depression and, most seriously, disorders of the circulatory system. The disorders include thrombophlebitis, pulmonary embolus, heart attack, and stroke. About 1 in 27,000 using the pill annually dies from these cardiovascular complications (Ory, Rosenfeld, and Landman, 1980).

All these risks are dramatically increased for women who smoke and for those over the age of 35. The combination of these two contraindications and OCP use is particularly dangerous.

It is the estrogen in combined pills which is thought to be associated with certain cardiovascular diseases. Since minipills are progestogen-only pills, they are theoretically safer than combined pills. However, studies proving this have not been carried out (Hatcher et al., 1986).

This has been a brief discussion of the side-effects and contraindications of OCPs. For detailed information on these topics, see Hatcher et al. (1986) and Dickerson (1983). Another useful source of information is the package insert accompanying each packet of pills.

Certainly when comparing the safety risks of OCPs to other methods, the statistics do not favor OCP use. However, safety is a relative matter when balancing the marked effectiveness of OCP use in preventing pregnancy versus the risk of certain health problems. For example, the mortality rates during pregnancy and childbirth in underdeveloped countries are much higher than those of the highly advanced health care system in the United States. In this instance, the benefits of pill use significantly outweigh the risks even for those women over 35 (Masters, Johnson, and Kolodny, 1988). Safety issues associated with OCP use can also be put into perspective by comparing them with the risks of everyday living (see Table 3–2).

Sexual Effects

Spontaneity and intimacy may be more easily achieved with OCP use because there is no interruption of sexual activity. However, sexual response to use of the pill is a highly individual matter. In general, responses can be categorized as either biological or psychological (Masters, Johnson, and Kolodny, 1988). For example, if a woman gets a yeast infection which is typically associated with OCP use, she will be likely to curtail sexual activity. If OCPs decrease or eliminate premenstrual and menstrual cramps, then it is possible the woman will feel less fatigued and more sexually responsive. Psychological attitudes can also enhance or hinder a woman's sexual response and function. For example, a woman using OCPs may feel liberated from the fear of pregnancy allowing her to relax and enjoy her sexual responsiveness. Conversely, guilt brought on by conflicts with religious beliefs or a desire for children may inhibit sexual interest and enjoyment. Overall, most women currently using OCPs report no change from previous sexual patterns (Masters, Johnson, and Kolodny, 1988).

Intrauterine Device (IUD)

How it Works/How it is Obtained

The IUD or intrauterine device is made of plastic and comes in various sizes and shapes (see Fig. 3–10). It is inserted through the vagina and cervix into the uterus where it remains in place until removal by the physician or another health care provider. IUDs act by interfering with or preventing implantation of the fertilized egg in the lining of the uterus. This is thought to occur in several ways: mechanical action of the IUD may dislodge the fertilized egg; a local inflammatory reaction may irritate the uterine lining preventing implantation; hormonal production may alter the development of the uterine lining inhibiting implantation; and antibodies that destroy sperm may be increased (Belcastro, 1986).

IUDs come in two forms, medicated or nonmedicated. The medicated IUD such as the Progestasert-T, contains a synthetic form of the hormone, progesterone, which is slowly released into the uterus. Medicated copper IUDs release copper into the uterus where it is believed to slow down hormone production necessary for implantation (Belcastro, 1986).

Currently, the Progestasert-T and the Copper T 380A are the only IUDs available in the United States. Although the FDA continues to approve the sale and insertion of IUDs, the manufacturers of IUDs have voluntarily removed their products from the market due to liability issues (Klitsch, 1988).

Placement of the IUD in the uterus must be done by a trained health care professional. The woman must be examined to rule out pregnancy since insertion in the presence of an existing undetermined pregnancy can cause abortion. For this reason, insertion is usually performed during, or shortly following, a menstrual period (Hatcher et al., 1986). Evaluation for gonorrhea, *Chlamydia*, and other pelvic infections is also done prior to

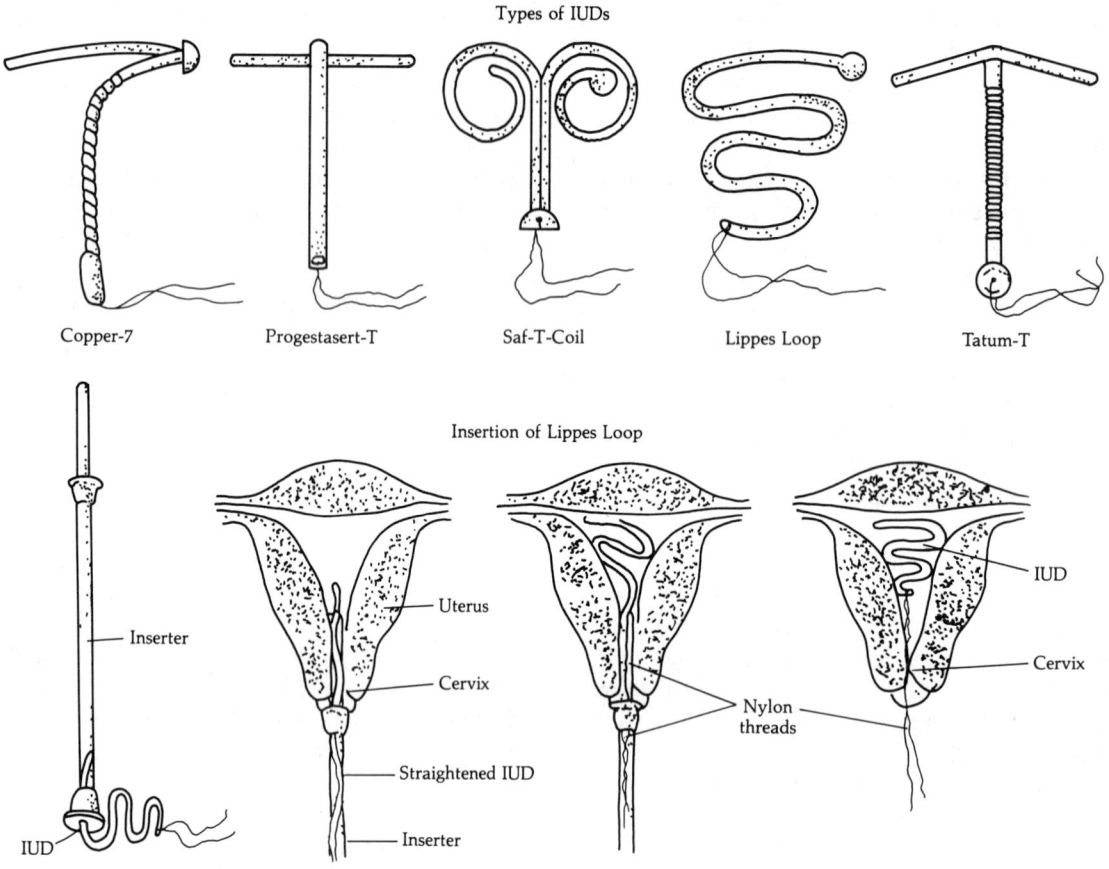

FIGURE 3–10. Types of IUD and insertion of a Lippes loop.
SOURCE: Nass, Libby, and Fisher (1987).

IUD insertion to prevent dissemination of bacteria into the uterus or Fallopian tubes.

Safety and Effectiveness
The failure rate among 100 women using the IUD for 1 year ranges between one and six pregnancies. Differences in effectiveness rates are affected by the size and shape of the IUD, the presence of medication, and patient variables such as age, parity, and frequency of intercourse (Hatcher et al., 1986). Failures are commonly attributed to undetected expulsion of the IUD which accounts for about one-third of the pregnancies among IUD users. Expulsion occurs more frequently in nulliparous women and during menstruation. Women using IUDs without copper or progesterone are twice as likely to expel the IUD (Piotrow, Rinehart, and Schmidt, 1979).

The most serious safety risk associated with IUD use is perforation of the uterus. This usually happens at the time of insertion and occurs at the rate of about 1 per 1000 insertions (Masters, Johnson, and Kolodny, 1988). There may be no immediate symptoms, although sudden pain and loss of blood commonly occurs requiring abdominal surgery to remove the IUD. Breastfeeding significantly increases the risk of perforation (Merz, 1983).

IUD insertion should cause only fleeting discomfort. However, some health care providers recommend taking 2–3 aspirin tablets or prostaglandin inhibitors (Advil, Nuprin) before insertion. These medicines block the release of prostaglandins, thereby decreasing uterine cramping. To check for proper placement of the IUD, the woman must be shown how to feel for the plastic threads coming through the cervix and partially extending into the vagina. The lengthening of the string or an inability to locate the string means the woman should return for a checkup.

Side-effects/Safety
The most common side-effects of the IUD are uterine bleeding and painful cramps which lessen

considerably after the first 3 months of IUD use. However, these problems severely affect about 10–15 percent of women necessitating removal of the IUD (Hatcher et al., 1986). Most women notice an increase in the length and amount of menstrual flow along with some spotting between periods. However, women using the Progestasert-T have reported a decrease in menstrual flow (ALZA, 1987). Iron deficiency anemia has been associated with increased blood loss.

Recent studies support the conclusion that the IUD is a relatively low-risk method when used by a fully informed, monogamous woman (Hutchings et al., 1985). Women for whom oral contraceptive pills are medically contraindicated may find this method more suitable. It may be ideal for those women who forget to take pills or are physically unable to use barrier methods.

The risk of pelvic infection is four times greater in women using the IUD and does not decrease with continued use. The IUD tail is thought to be an excellent reservoir for infections which are spread by travelling up the string to the ovaries and Fallopian tubes causing pelvic inflammatory disease (PID). PID is usually a sexually transmitted disease caused by infection with gonorrhea, *chlamydia*, or other bacteria. The chances of getting PID increase significantly with more than one sexual partner. PID can lead to permanent blockage of the tubes and sterility. For this reason, another method of contraception is recommended for women intending to become pregnant in the future.

Some women become pregnant while using the IUD. If the IUD remains in place during pregnancy, the risk of spontaneous abortion is about 50 percent. Removal of the IUD after conception occurs results in a 30-percent chance of spontaneous abortion. There is some concern that medicated IUDs such as the Progestasert-T may cause birth defects, although this relationship has not been established (ALZA, 1987). Unlike most other contraceptives, the IUD does not prevent ectopic pregnancy which, if undetected, can seriously compromise the health of the mother (see Chapter 14). Studies indicate there is a 5-percent chance of pregnancy developing outside the uterus. This risk is more pronounced in women using the Progestasert-T as compared to the copper-releasing IUDs (ALZA, 1987).

The IUD is contraindicated for women who are pregnant or have a history of ectopic pregnancy, currently have a pelvic infection, or have an increased risk of getting PID. Any woman with hematologic or immunosuppressive disorders, or abnormalities of the pelvic organs or heart valves should not use the IUD. Limited access to health care services also prohibits IUD use since many complications require immediate treatment. Any woman who is concerned about her future fertility should not use the IUD.

For a detailed discussion of side-effects and contraindications of the IUD, see Hatcher et al. (1986).

Sexual Effects

The IUD is highly effective in preventing pregnancy and requires no precoital planning. The IUD may cause painful intercourse for either the man or woman. Some men complain of penile sensitivity or irritation from contact with the IUD string in the vagina (Masters, Johnson, and Kolodny, 1988). Some women experience pain, usually because of improper placement of the IUD or the presence of pelvic infection. Ten percent of users report decreased sexual interest when painful cramps or bleeding are present, and a small number of users find that intense uterine contractions with orgasm lessen sexual enjoyment (Masters, Johnson, and Kolodny, 1988).

STERILIZATION

Other than abstinence, sterilization affords the highest degree of contraceptive protection. The popularity of both male and female sterilization is increasing. One recent estimate indicates that about 25 percent of American married couples will use sterilization within 2 years after the birth of their last wanted child, and that more than 50 percent will undergo sterilization within 10 years after their last child (Westhoff and McCarthy, 1979). Though these procedures are safe, effective, and permanent, their permanence can become a drawback if there is a change in feeling or circumstances. There is ever-increasing success with attempts at microsurgical reversal of sterilizations, but the results are still so questionable that sterilization should be considered a permanent procedure.

Each state has different regulations outlining requirements for consent for sterilization. Commonly, when public funds are used to pay for the procedure, the consent form must be signed 30 days in advance. This becomes important when a pregnant client desires to be sterilized at the time of delivery (Hatcher et al., 1986).

Female Sterilization

How it Works

Female sterilization operations block the Fallopian tubes, which prevents the union of sperm and egg (see Fig. 3–11). Though the operation is commonly called tubal ligation (tying the tubes), that is rarely done alone today. Other methods that cut, clip, or block the tubes are much more effective. Using a laparoscope, the tubes are cut and cauterized. Only a 1-inch incision is required. No scar is visible if it is done through the umbilicus. The procedure can be carried out during a laparotomy for some other reason or because of technical difficulties. Hysterectomy also has the effect of sterilization. However, it is not commonly done for that reason alone (Hatcher et al., 1986).

Effectiveness

Failures occur at the rate of 3–4 pregnancies per 100,000 tubal sterilizations. The failures occur if the procedure is performed without adequate pregnancy testing and the woman is already pregnant. There are virtually no side-effects to tubal sterilization other than those occurring in the first few days after surgery and these relate to the surgery itself, such as bleeding and infection (Masters, Johnson, and Kolodny, 1988).

Sexual Effects

There is no physical reason to have sexual difficulties after tubal sterilization. There is neither a change in hormones, since the ovaries are intact, nor in sexual anatomy. Some women show increased sexual interest because they no longer fear pregnancy. A few may encounter problems if they were pushed into the sterilization by a husband or for health or economic reasons: this may lead to a decreased interest in sex. There may also be problems with lowered responsiveness if a person feels "incomplete" or "less than a woman." This can be related to a religious background in which sex is considered unnatural or sinful if it is separated from its reproductive potential (Masters, Johnson, and Kolodny, 1988).

Male Sterilization

How it Works/How it is Obtained

Vasectomy is the surgical cutting and tying of each vas deferens (the tube which carries the sperm) in the scrotum (see Figure 3–12). This blocks the passage of sperm from the testes to the upper part of the vas deferens. It does not stop sperm production which accumulates in the epididymis. In this mass of tubes at the back of each testis, phagocytes engulf and destroy the sperm. At the time of the operation, some sperm are already above where the vasectomy is done. Therefore, it usually takes about a dozen ejaculations (often this may take as long as 6–8 weeks depending on frequency of intercourse) after the operation before the ejaculate is free of sperm and the man is considered sterile. The couple should use other

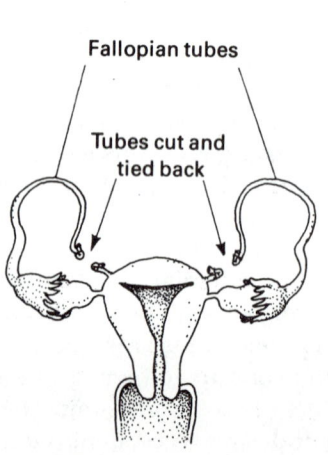

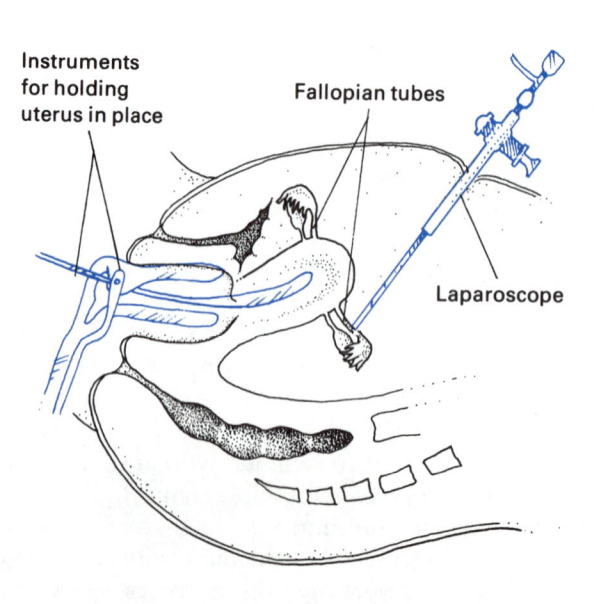

FIGURE 3–11. Female sterilization.
SOURCE: Nass, Libby, and Fisher (1987).

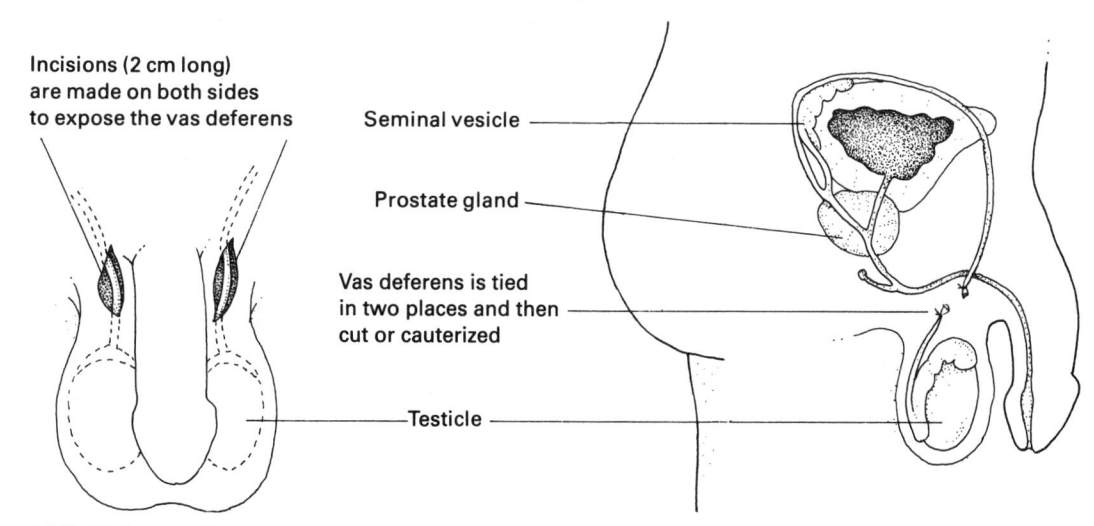

FIGURE 3-12. Vasectomy.
SOURCE: Nass, Libby, and Fisher (1987).

methods of contraception until two consecutive semen exams show no sperm are present. One of the problems in getting a man to agree to vasectomy is his reluctance to complete this necessary followup. The reality of producing the semen sample for inspection can be too embarrassing. Men should be reassured that the amount and consistency of the ejaculate is practically unchanged, since under 5 percent of seminal fluid comes from the testis and epididymis (Masters, Johnson, and Kolodny, 1988). There is no change in the man's ability to get an erection and vasectomy does not affect hormone production. There are no long-term health risks created by a vasectomy. Although about one-half to two-thirds of men will develop antibodies to sperm following vasectomy, there is no current evidence to support pathologic complications arising from this condition (Hatcher et al., 1986).

Vasectomy is a simple surgical procedure requiring only about 15–20 minutes. It is usually done under local anesthesia in a physician's office or clinic. Though the man can go home immediately, it is wise to avoid strenuous physical activity for approximately 2 days. Minor swelling, pain, and temporary skin discoloration occur in about 50 percent of the men (Wortman, 1975). Ice packs and a well-fitted scrotal supporter can reduce discomfort. The rate of medical complications such as bleeding and infection is less than 5 percent (Wortman, 1975).

Effectiveness

The failure rate for vasectomy is 0.15 percent, making it the safest and easiest type of surgical contraception (Hatcher et al., 1986). Most failures can be attributed to reanastomosis of the cut ends of the vas deferens (they grow back together), a poor surgical technique, or failure to completely clear the ejaculate of sperm before having intercourse (Wortman, 1975).

Reversing vasectomies has had mixed success and requires special training. Clinical success (fertility) ranges between 18% and 60%. Successful reanastomosis depends on several factors including the type of initial surgical procedure and the length of time since it was done. In China there is active research underway using a compound (SHUG device) which may be injected into the vas deferens for occlusion but does not cause scarring. It is hoped that it can be removed later to reverse the vasectomy (Hatcher et al., 1986).

Sexual Effects

Because the worry about becoming pregnant or using contraceptives has been removed, people generally find that sex is more spontaneous and fun after a vasectomy. Less than 1 man in 20 reports decreased sexual pleasure after a vasectomy. Close to 50 percent claim increased pleasure and about 25 percent report an increase in frequency of intercourse. There may be some discord or sexual dysfunction if the man expects special recognition or gratitude in return for having the surgery or if the woman resents not being able to have more children or, in the case of remarriage, if the new couple wants children. Men who have a history of sexual problems may be poor candidates for a vasectomy. They may be more prone to developing psychological impotence or other difficulties after the surgery (Masters, Johnson, and Kolodny, 1988).

FERTILITY AWARENESS METHODS

Periodic abstinence from intercourse during times of the menstrual cycle when fertility is most likely is the basis of the fertility awareness methods of contraception, i.e. 5 days before ovulation allowing for sperm life and 3 days after ovulation allowing time for the egg to die after being released. The aim of the methods is to identify the approach of ovulation, the time of its occurrence, and the fertile days after the event. These methods are acceptable for couples with religious concerns about contraception. These methods may be used as an adjunct to other means of contraception. They are also an effective program for teaching teenagers their own reproductive physiology.

Calendar Method

The calendar or rhythm method is used to calculate a woman's fertile period (days where intercourse will not lead to pregnancy) based on the lengths of previous cycles. Ovulation should occur approximately 14 days (±2 days) before the start of the next menstrual period.

To calculate the fertile period, a record must be kept of the length of each menstrual cycle for 6–8 months. The first day of the fertile period is calculated by subtracting 18 from the length of the shortest cycle. The end of the fertile period is found by subtracting 11 from the number of days in the longest cycle. If a woman's shortest cycle is 27 days and her longest is 33 days during her "record keeping" time, she must abstain from intercourse beginning on cycle day 9 (27−18=9) and continue abstention until day 22 (33−11=22). The fertile days would be days 9–22, 13 days when intercourse would not be permitted (Hatcher et al., 1986).

The Temperature Method

Using a basal body thermometer, the woman records her temperature daily for 3–4 months. Right before ovulation, the basal body temperature (BBT) drops slightly and then rises noticeably 24–72 hours later. Protected intercourse should begin on the first day of the menstrual cycle and continue for 3 days after the rise in temperature is detected (Hatcher et al., 1986). Unprotected intercourse should be avoided if no temperature rise is detected in a full menstrual cycle (Hatcher et al., 1986).

The Ovulation Method

The ovulation or Billings method is based on changes which occur in the consistency and appearance of cervical mucous just before ovulation. A woman's fertile period can be determined by observing these changes. During ovulation, cervical mucous becomes thin and clear with a stretchy consistency much like raw egg white. When the mucous has returned to a yellow viscous color, usually 4 days after clear mucous begins, intercourse is considered safe. The cervix also becomes more difficult to feel in the vagina because it tends to soften in texture and pull up towards the vagina during ovulation. Dilatation of the cervical os also occurs at this time. It is important not to confuse other mucous-like substances such as lubricants and spermicides with midcycle secretions (Hatcher et al., 1986).

Safety and Effectiveness

A history of irregular periods or irregular intervals between menses, anovulatory cycles, and irregular temperature charts make this a difficult approach to use (Hatcher et al., 1986). Stress or an irregular lifestyle contributes to these problems. Therefore, these methods are generally not appropriate for mothers of young children, women with high stress jobs, or women who are ill or travel. Women who douche cannot use the mucous method because they cannot observe changes in the mucous since it is washed away. Unwillingness to part with sexual spontaneity and unwillingness or an inability to keep careful records are possible relative contraindications. An advantage of this system is there are few, if any, absolute contraindications to these methods (Hatcher et al., 1986).

The effectiveness of these methods individually is very poor. Using them in combination does enhance effectiveness. The calendar method is the least reliable with failure rates of approximately 15–45 per 100 woman years (Ross and Pietrow, 1974). Unless the woman's cycle is very regular, long periods of abstinence from intercourse will be required. Difficulty in interpretation makes the temperature methods inaccurate. The BBT chart does not indicate ovulation in about 20 percent of ovulatory cycles (Bauman, 1981). Many woman probably have difficulty noting the cyclic changes in their cervical mucous. Women who have a vaginal infection (which may itself create a discharge) usually cannot use this method. In a 1981 study of 725 women, an overall failure rate of 22.3 per 100 woman years was noted (WHO, 1981).

Risk-taking during the fertile phase is suspected by WHO researchers as the cause of more accidental pregnancies than difficulty interpreting BBT and mucous patterns. They concluded that it is still not possible to estimate accurately the length of the fertile life span of spermatozoa within the female reproductive tract. If sperm survive in the female tract 5 or more days, unprotected intercourse in the preovulatory phase would be difficult to justify (Hatcher et al., 1986).

The data that suggest that fertilization of an overripe ovum is associated with an increased incidence of fetal wastage and birth defects are not convincing one way or the other. If there is an increased risk of abnormal offspring when failures occur, it is very low (Hatcher et al., 1986).

Sexual Effects

Major sexual difficulties are usually not associated with the use of fertility awareness contraceptive methods. The need for abstinence creates unusual pressures to have intercourse on "safe" days, regardless of whether the couple feel like it or not, which can create problems as can the fear of pregnancy (Masters, Johnson, and Kolodny, 1988). To prevent frustration from long periods of abstinence, the couple may be counseled on other lovemaking techniques (Hatcher et al., 1986). In addition, some couples may use a barrier method of contraception to allow intercourse on the unsafe days. Fertility awareness methods tend to promote greater communication, cooperation, and awareness of reproductive anatomy and physiology between partners.

OTHER METHODS OF CONTRACEPTION

Lactation

How it Works

The same hormone that stimulates milk production, prolactin, also decreases the level of luteinizing hormone necessary for maintaining the menstrual cycle. Lactation does not postpone menstruation indefinitely. This postpartum amenorrhea can last for 2–3 months in nonbreastfeeding women and for 4–24 months in those who are breastfeeding. Hatcher et al. (1986) state that "the longer a woman breast-feeds, the more likely it is that menstruation will return while she continues to breastfeed. The more frequently an infant suckles, the longer will the return of menses be delayed." A reduction from full breastfeeding to partial breastfeeding as other foods are added to the baby's diet may cause the menstrual cycle to resume (Hatcher et al., 1986).

Use and Effectiveness

Breastfeeding as generally practiced in the United States is not a reliable method of contraception. Only when breastfeeding is practiced on demand, around the clock, can it be considered a contraceptive. Women living in more developed nations find it particularly difficult to adhere to such rigorous feeding patterns (Hatcher et al., 1986). Statistics reveal that nearly 80 percent of breastfeeding women will ovulate before they have their first period and possibly as early as 2 months after delivery. A total of 3–7 percent of breastfeeding women will become pregnant before they have their first menstrual period (Hatcher et al., 1986).

Contraception during Breastfeeding

When choosing a contraceptive method to use during breastfeeding, one that will not interfere with establishing the milk supply in the immediate postpartum period should be chosen. Contraceptives begun at the time of the 6-week postpartum checkup are less likely to interfere with breastfeeding since lactation is firmly established by then. The methods which do not interfere with lactation are spermicides, barrier methods, IUDs (medicated or not), tubal ligation, and abstinence (Hatcher et al., 1986).

The studies are contradictory regarding the effect of the minipill on lactation. However, if a hormonal contraceptive is desired, the progestin-only minipill is recommended (Hatcher et al., 1986). It can be started immediately postpartum or at the 6-week checkup. In addition, a policy statement has been issued by the American Academy of Pediatrics approving the use of combined pills in lactating women once effective lactation is well established. Two studies reported in Hatcher et al. (1986) show that there is little or no effect on the infant from exposure to oral contraceptives. The transfer did not seem to exceed the physiologic effect that would occur once the woman resumed ovulation.

Abstinence

Abstinence, i.e. refraining from sexual intercourse, remains a commonly chosen option in the United States and in other areas of the world, despite the increase in pressure from society to participate in sexual activity. Historically, this has probably been the most important method of curtailing human fertility. Other than sterilization, it is the only absolute means of contraception for a fertile person. It can be used when intercourse is medically unwise.

It is important to distinguish between those who are not having sexual intercourse of their own volition from those whose abstinence is dysfunctional or forced upon them. Though the latter may require help, the former deserve respect, encouragement, and support. Even those choosing abstinence should at least have the knowledge of easily available methods of contraception should their decision change. This is particularly true for couples who are choosing noncoital forms of sexual intimacy. Intimate sex without intercourse exists as a contraceptive option in many cultures (Hatcher et al., 1986).

Coitus Interruptus

The withdrawal method (coitus interruptus) is an age-old method of conception control. The couple may have intercourse until ejaculation is imminent but then the penis must be withdrawn from the vagina. Ejaculation must occur away from the vagina and female external genitalia. There are some advantages in that it requires no devices or chemicals and has no cost and no medical side-effects. However, an overwhelming disadvantage is its actual failure rate of 23 pregnancies per 100 women per year (Hatcher et al., 1986).

Drops of pre-ejaculatory fluid can escape at any time prior to ejaculation. Any drop can contain millions of sperm. Multiple orgasms within a short span of time increases the likelihood of escape of this fluid with subsequent contraception failure. This method demands a great degree of self-control at a time when the natural feeling is to achieve deeper penetration. This interruption of the sexual response cycle can lead to markedly diminished pleasure for the couple as well as increased potential for contraceptive failure (Hatcher et al., 1986).

Postcoital Methods 1: Abortion

Abortion is defined as the spontaneous or induced expulsion of the products of conception before the fetus is legally viable. Viability is currently legally defined as between 20 and 28 weeks of gestation and between 500 and 1000 g of weight. There are many different types or classifications of abortion but for the purposes of contraception, a voluntary interrupted pregnancy (VIP) is usually the term given to abortion by surgical or medical methods.

Abortions have been performed for many centuries. It was discussed by Plato and Aristotle. But it was not until a United States Supreme Court decision (*Roe* vs. *Wade*) in January, 1973, that it became a legal right for women in America to choose whether or not to have an abortion (Hatcher et al., 1986).

The times at which abortions are carried out and the type of procedure appropriate to the period are as follows:

1. *First trimester abortion:* carried out during the first 3 months of pregnancy with gestational age determined from the onset of the last menstrual period (LMP). The most common method is vacuum aspiration of the uterine contents, which requires only 3–5 minutes. It is usually carried out under local anesthesia on an outpatient basis. The woman can leave the setting in 1–4 hours.
2. *Second trimester abortion:* carried out between 14 and 24 weeks of gestation. Several methods are used in this period. Dilation and evacuation (D&E) involves dilating the cervix and removing the contents by vacuum aspiration. This can be carried out under general anesthesia or a paracervical block. Dilation and curettage (D&C) involves dilating the cervix and scraping the uterine lining, and usually requires general anesthesia. A hysterotomy, the surgical opening of the uterus through the abdomen, can be carried out under general anesthesia. Chemical abortions stimulate contractions of the uterus causing expulsion of the contents. Three primary medicines used are prostaglandins, hypertonic saline, or hypertonic urea. Chemical abortions take many hours, involve physical and emotional discomfort during contractions, and require vaginal delivery of a dead fetus (Hatcher et al., 1986).
3. *Menstrual extraction:* carried out without positive diagnosis of pregnancy. The uterine contents are vacuum aspirated. With the increased sensitivity of current pregnancy tests, this is rarely, if ever, needed.

Adjunctive techniques may be used to reduce discomfort or facilitate completion of the abortion.

Laminaria, a small stick of compressed seaweed, is inserted in the cervix to speed dilatation of the cervical os. It does require an extra visit to the doctor or clinic for insertion about 24 hours before the abortion. Intravenous oxytocin is commonly used with the D&C method and with other second-trimester methods to facilitate uterine contractions (Hatcher et al., 1986).

Danger signs to watch for after an abortion include a fever of 100.4°F or greater taken orally; abdominal pain or severe cramps; heavy bleeding that lasts longer than 3 weeks; abdominal tenderness that intensifies with walking, coughing or pressure; foul-smelling vaginal discharges; medication reaction resulting in a rash, hives, or asthma; and menses failing to resume within 6 weeks (Hatcher et al., 1986).

Though some people still believe that such things as eating certain foods and vigorous exercise will lead to abortion, this is not true. Inserting objects into the uterus such as wire coat hangers or knitting needles to induce abortion is very dangerous and can lead to fatal infections or bleeding (Masters, Johnson, and Kolodny, 1988).

Safety

Deaths from a legal abortion in the United States occur at a rate of approximately 1 per 100,000 procedures performed on healthy women with no history of medical problems (Lebolt, Grimes, and Cates, 1982). Today, abortion is safer than childbirth. Approximately 20 deaths per 100,000 pregnancies occur as compared to only 4 deaths per 100,000 induced abortions (Grimes and Cates, 1980).

Abortions carried out during the first trimester are simplest and safest. After this, complications such as bleeding, infection, and perforation of the uterus are more common.

Studies on long-term post-abortion complications are contradictory. At this time there is no clear evidence that one early abortion carries any risk to future pregnancies. Some early studies have shown that women who have had two or more abortions may have a greater risk of premature deliveries or miscarriages in future pregnancies. More recent studies of abortions using smaller instruments have shown no increased risk (Planned Parenthood, 1982).

Psychological Aspects of Abortion

For most women, the emotional benefits outweigh the psychological risks (Nadelson, 1978). Psychiatric referrals occur in less than 3 women in every 100,000 who have had an abortion (David, 1978). For many women, having an abortion is based on a good evaluation of the realities of her situation and culminates in feelings of relief. Even then, short-lived feelings of guilt, sadness, and loss are common. Pre-abortion and post-abortion counseling should be offered in conjunction with this procedure.

Another aspect of the abortion experience is the male's reaction. Men may initially try to approach the decision in an abstract, intellectual way (Shostak, McLouth, and Seng, 1984). Later they find themselves having to deal with feelings of hurt, guilt, or anger. Few abortion centers offer counseling for the men: some counselors choose to focus only on the woman. Others say that the men seem disinterested in the service. As conception control moves toward shared responsibility by both partners, the question of the man's reaction will warrant recognition in relation to abortion as well as other methods.

This has been a brief overview of the subject of abortion. For detailed information, see Hatcher et al. (1986).

Postcoital Methods 2: "Morning After" Pill

Both birth control technology and human behavior are imperfect. This leads to the use of postcoital contraception. Some of the methods used are "morning after" pills, "morning after" IUD insertion, or menstrual extraction. Pills may be either high-dose estrogens or progestins which should be taken within 24 hours of coitus. There is also a pill, marketed in the United States as Ovral, which can be used up to 3 days after intercourse, but preferably within 12–24 hours (Hatcher et al., 1986).

Douching

Douching is not a reliable contraceptive method. Sperm enter the cervical os as soon as 15 seconds after ejaculation. The failure rate is greater than 40 percent. This is true even if spermicide is used in the solution. It is unnecessary to douche after intercourse but, if a woman wishes to do so, any douching should be delayed 6–8 hours after intercourse if a vaginal spermicide has been used (Hatcher et al., 1986).

FUTURE TRENDS IN CONTRACEPTION

Considerable research efforts directed towards the control of female and male fertility will continue to provide new contraceptive alternatives. In the female, long-acting forms of contraceptive hormones released from vaginal rings, injectable microcapsules, or biodegradable rods are being studied. Currently, the most advanced such device is the Norplant System. It contains a set of six small capsules filled with levonorgestrel that are injected subcutaneously in the upper arm and supply contraceptive protection for 5–7 years (Population Council, 1983). Other research has focused on producing hypothalamus blocking agents which prevent pituitary release of LH and FSH, thereby disrupting initiation of ovulation. An antipregnancy vaccine is being studied as well as a self-administered pill, liquid, or vaginal tampon that would induce menstrual flow at the expected time of menstruation.

Tubal occlusion is a sterilization procedure performed by injecting liquid silicone rubber that solidifies and forms a plug. Supposedly, the plug can be removed to reverse the sterilization effect, although research is proving doubtful in this regard (Hatcher et al., 1986).

New directions in male contraception are aimed at developing a male birth control pill. Various combinations of estrogen, progesterone, and testosterone have been tried but have either proved to have incomplete effects on blocking spermatogenesis or caused a profound drop in sexual interest in males. An oral antifertility compound, Gossypol, is currently being used in China. Gossypol is a phenol compound made from cottonseed oil which acts on sperm metabolism to immobilize or kill sperm cells. Side-effects such as dizziness, fatigue, dry mouth and, rarely, a decreased libido, have been reported. A protein substance made in the testes, inhibin, signals the hypothalamus and pituitary gland to control production of FSH. Now a synthetic form of inhibin has been developed which suppresses sperm production without affecting sexual function.

THE NURSING PROCESS AND CONTRACEPTION

Assessment

With an antepartum client, the question of contraception should be raised in the second trimester. This will allow time for investigation and education for those who need to make a new or initial decision about contraception. At a minimum, the subject should be discussed again in the immediate postpartum period to see if plans continue as before. It should be raised again at the time of the 6-week postpartum checkup to see that arrangements are working smoothly.

In obtaining the database from clients, the nurse needs to be clearly aware of the factors influencing contraception decisions and practices. Both the cognitive and emotional factors have been discussed in detail in this chapter. It is also wise to remember that contraception is a two partner issue. For adequate assessment, the database needs to include information from both partners' perspective. Just as surely as the female does, the male may have conflicting feelings about pregnancy and contraception himself. In addition, his feelings may be in conflict with hers. One study has shown that appreciable differences in the partners' values occurred in 25 percent of cases. At the same time, one spouse's perception of the other's values was incorrect 50 percent of the time (Miller, 1986).

Also, remember that the database interview will be influenced by the sexual attitudes, knowledge, and experience of both the client and the nurse. This is in addition to the more obvious influence of the contraceptive attitudes, knowledge, and experience of both partners. A caregiver must be well-prepared in advance of the interview so that one's knowledge, nonjudgmental attitudes and skills will enable the client to explore the necessary questions and answers. A caregiver must avoid imposing personal values by understanding and accepting his or her own sexuality so the values of others can be accepted nonjudgmentally. The caregiver is not required to agree with the values of the client but rather to respect the right of the patient to have and act on a personal belief system (Swanson and Forrest, 1984).

In structuring an interview which will focus on sexuality and contraception, it is especially important to provide for privacy and avoid interruptions. It is also important to carefully adjust one's language to terms which can be understood by the client. To do this, ask the client what names he/she uses for the functions or the parts of the anatomy being discussed, and clarify what the client means by street terms used. If the interviewer is uncomfortable with the street terms being used, or if the terms are not appropriate, the interviewer can use both terms. For example: going down or oral sex; pulling out in time or withdrawal (Swanson and Forrest, 1984).

The specific questions to elicit a contraceptive history from a perinatal client as adapted from Swanson and Forrest (1984) are:

1. Is this a planned or unplanned pregnancy? If the answer is "unplanned," it may be appropriate to explore her feelings about this further before moving into the contraception question.
2. Were you using contraception before the pregnancy? If so: What kind? Did it work? How did you use it? What education did you have about it? How did you like it? How did your partner like it? How did it affect your sex life? Is there anything you would like to change about your method? If not: Why not?

If appropriate, continue with:

3. How important is contraception to you and your partner?
4. What are the wishes of both partners about future pregnancies? (This question is of special significance to the single woman and the career woman.)
5. Are there religious or cultural problems with contraception?
6. Have you become pregnant in the past using contraception? What type? Why?
7. Have you had any diseases which would interfere with contraception (includes both physical disabilities, chronic diseases, and STDs)?
8. Menstrual history: Do you miss periods? Cycle vary in length? Problem with cramping? Any bleeding between periods? Any premenstrual problems?
9. Do you have any questions about contraception?

Nursing Diagnosis

Certainly the choice of a nursing diagnosis applied to contraception will be based on each individual client's situation. There may be more than one diagnosis for each client, depending on the problems identified by the nurse. The diagnosis is generally made after analyzing the database. It becomes the basis for developing a personalized care plan. The diagnosis may change over time based on the nurse's continuing evaluation of the patient's response to care. The following diagnoses (Kim, McFarland, and McLane, 1987) are listed as possibly applicable to contraction concerns:

- Anxiety
- Comfort, altered: pain
- Coping, ineffective family: compromised
- Coping, family: potential for growth
- Coping, ineffective individual
- Family processes, altered
- Fear
- Growth and development: altered (this diagnosis may be especially appropriate for the mentally retarded or developmentally delayed client)
- Health maintenance, altered
- Infection, potential for
- Knowledge deficit (specify)
- Noncompliance (specify)
- Powerlessness
- Self-concept, disturbance in: body image
- Self-concept, disturbance in: self-esteem
- Sexual dysfunction

Planning

There are primarily two types of plans which will be formulated. One is assistance in decision making about a contraceptive method, and the other is a teaching plan to correct a knowledge deficit about contraception in general or about a specific method (one in use or one just chosen). In assisting the client to select a method of contraception, the information contained in the database must be compared to the use and effectiveness information and contraindications for each method. This should lead to the closest match between the client's requirements and future life plans compared to a method's advantages and constraints. In this decision-making process it should be remembered that men basically remain the dominant decision makers in many homes and most societies: "Male permission and agreement can be crucial even when the method is anatomically female-directed" (Swanson and Forrest, 1984).

Implementation

For those plans leading to choosing a method of contraception, the nurse's role in implementation is one of referral to a provider if medical intervention is required. If not, the nurse should provide information about places where "over-the-counter" contraceptives are available at the cheapest prices. Some suggested providers of contraceptives are:

- Planned Parenthood
- School or university health clinics

- Community clinics
- Private medical doctor

For those plans leading to education about a contraceptive method, remember to include both partners whenever possible. Particularly if it is an over-the-counter method include ample opportunities for a return demonstration. In this instance, the nurse will probably be the only health care provider doing teaching. Examples of this are: have the woman use the equipment for instilling foam, actually filling, emptying and cleaning it; be certain she can locate the vagina anatomically; condoms can be applied to a banana, practicing the correct procedure; the person must be taught to fully understand the danger signals of the method, if there are any—this is most important with the pill and IUD. For the pill users, be sure to include a discussion of possible drug interactions and diminished effectiveness (see Table 3–4). If a developmental or physical disability prevents a client from using an appropriate contraceptive method, then a partner or someone else may be taught.

In intervening with the chronic noncontraceptor, when the underlying attitudes promoting noncontraception have been identified, counseling can be adjusted appropriately. Be careful to avoid "rescuing" the person or starting to make the decisions for her. The basis for the behavior is not wanting to take responsibility for her own actions. If she wants to blame something (the method) or someone else (the partner), have her list her options and explain to you why she follows that line of reasoning. Try to help her see that she can be in control of one area of her life if she uses contraception effectively. Ask her what she wants to do and how she plans to go about it. Keep reapproaching these questions until you get an answer. Explain options but do not make her decision. Remember the person has freedom of choice and has made a decision not to contracept. The nurse's role is to help the person make a new decision (Collomb, 1987). While many can be reached with support, understanding, and assertive counseling, not everyone wishes help or can change. A person with minimal education and an unstable lifestyle possibly cannot use nonpermanent contraception effectively. The nurse may have to let go, although that can be very hard for health professionals to do.

Evaluation

It is important that the chosen method of contraception works well to prevent pregnancy, the ultimate evaluation. To promote this, and to determine if the nursing diagnoses have been corrected, it is important that follow-up be carried out not only initially but after the method has been used for some time (usually 1–2 months depending on the frequency of intercourse). With methods requiring medical intervention, the client should be sure that a follow-up appointment is arranged to check the fit or placement of the device. The nurse can evaluate the effectiveness of the teaching plan using as appropriate the following questions adapted from a questionnaire in Hatcher et al. (1984):

- Have you been pleased with this method of contraception? Why?
- Have you had any problems using this method?
- Does your partner like the method? Why?
- Is your partner opposed to this method?
- Are you afraid of using this method?
- Would you rather not use this method?
- Have you had trouble remembering to use this method?
- Have you had trouble using this method carefully?
- Do you have unanswered questions about the method?
- Does this method make menstrual periods longer or more painful?
- Does this method cost more than you can afford?
- Does this method ever cause serious problems?
- Do you object to this method because of religious beliefs?
- Are you using this method without your partner's knowledge?
- Has using this method embarrassed you or your partner?
- Are you enjoying intercourse more because of this method? Enjoying it less?
- Does this method interrupt lovemaking?
- Has anyone (including a nurse or doctor) ever told you not to use this method?

If these questions are turning up more problem areas than anticipated in the planning phase, it may be necessary to reinvestigate the congruence between the method and the client's needs. It may be that another method needs to be tried.

SUMMARY

Since the 1960s brought "the pill" and the sexual revolution, contraception and information about it have become readily available in the United States.

However, there is still a great lag in the dissemination and application of this knowledge. Pregnancy can be a time of "unfreezing" and the motivation to improve contraception is generally increased. Effective application of the nursing process in these situations can promote appropriate contraceptive choices and increase self-care knowledge. This will lead to a higher level of wellness through fertility management.

Factors affecting contraceptive practices in four general areas of concern have been discussed. These include:

1. The motivation to avoid conception.
2. The perceived and the actual risk of conception.
3. The contraceptive-related attitudes and beliefs of both partners.
4. The interaction that takes place between the user and the method.

This chapter has included a specific discussion of each method of contraception available in the United States. Each discussion includes information on use, effectiveness, safety, and contraindications. Instructions for the use of these methods, designed for use in client teaching, are included in Appendix K.

Guidance for the application of the nursing process to the client has been presented. This includes an assessment guide, discussion of possible intervention with the chronic noncontraceptor, and an evaluation format.

REFERENCES

Alameda County Health Care Services Agency (ACHCSA). 1984. *Intra Uterine Device*. Oakland, Calif.: Division of Community and Data Services.

ALZA Corporation. 1987. *Progestasert: Intrauterine progesterone contraceptive system*. Palo Alto, Calif.: ALZA Corporation.

Bauman, J. E. 1981. Basal body temperature: Unreliable method of ovulation detection. *Fertility and Sterility*. 36:729.

Belcastro, P. 1986. *The birth control book*. Boston, MA: Jones and Bartlett.

California State University, Hayward (CSUH). 1983. *Cervical cap*. Hayward, Calif.: CSUH Student Health Center.

Cates, W., Jr.; Weisner, P. J.; and Curran, J. W. 1982. Sex and spermicides: Preventing unintended pregnancy and infection. *J. Amer. Med. Assoc.* 248:1636–1637.

Centers for Disease Control. 1983. Oral contraceptive use and the risk of ovarian cancer. *J. Amer. Med. Assoc.* 249:1596–1599.

Children's Defense Fund. 1987. Flier.

Collomb, K. 1987. Understand patient feelings, attitudes to counsel chronic noncontraceptors. In *Contraceptive technology update*, ed. E. M. Robertson. 8(8):99–100.

David, H. P. 1978. Abortion: A continuing debate. *Family Planning Perspectives*. 10:313–316.

Department of Health, Education, and Welfare. 1985. DHEW Pub. No. (HSA) 75-16011. Rockville, Md.: Bureau of Community Health Services.

Dickerson, J. 1983. The pill: A closer look. *Am. J. Nurs.* 83(10):1392–1398.

Dirubbo, N. E. 1987. The condom barrier. *Am. J. Nurs.* 87(10):1306–1309.

Fraser, L. 1988. Pill Politics. *Mother Jones*, p. 42.

Grimes, D. 1986. Reversible contraception for the 1980's. *J. Amer. Med. Assoc.* 255:69–75.

Grimes, D. A., and Cates, W., Jr. (1980). Abortions: Methods and Complications. In *Human reproduction: conception and contraception*, ed. E. S. Hafez, pp. 796–813. Hagerstown, Md: Harper & Row.

Hatcher, R. A.; Guest, F.; Stewart, F.; Stewart, G. K.; Trussell, J.; Cerel, S.; and Cates, W., eds. 1984. *Contraceptive technology, 1984–1985*. 12th ed. New York: Irvington.

Hatcher, R. A.; Guest, F.; Stewart, F.; Stewart, G. K.; Trussell, J.; Cerel, S.; and Cates, W., eds. 1986. *Contraceptive technology, 1986–1987*. 13th ed. New York: Irvington.

Henshaw, S. K., and O'Reilly, K. 1983. Characteristics of abortion patients in the United States, 1979 and 1980. *Family Planning Perspectives*. 15(1):5–15.

Hutchings, J.; Bensson, P.; Perkin, G.; and Sodsrstrom, R. 1985. The IUD after 20 years: A review. *Family Planning Perspectives*. 17(6):244–253.

Jick, H., et al. 1978. Vaginal spermicides and gonorrhea. *J. Amer. Med. Assoc.* 248:1619–1621.

Kim, M. J.; McFarland, G. K.; and McLane, A. M. 1987. *Nursing diagnosis*. 2nd ed. St. Louis: C. V. Mosby.

Lebolt, S. A.; Grimes, D. A.; and Cates, W., Jr. 1982. Mortality from abortion and childbirth. *J. Amer. Med. Assoc.* 248:188–191.

Masters, W. H.; Johnson, V. E.; and Kolodny, R. C. 1988. *Human sexuality*. 3rd ed. Glenview, Ill.: Scott, Foresman and Company.

Mazurkewicz, M. J. 1983. Inability to control reproduction. In *Community health care and the nursing process*, ed. M. J. Fromer, St. Louis: C. V. Mosby.

Merz, B. 1983. Greater IUD perforation risk, lactation linked. *J. Amer. Med. Assoc.* 249:3152.

Miller, W. B. 1986. Why some women fail to use their contraceptive method: A psychological investigation. *Family Planning Perspectives*. 18(1):27–32.

Mishell, D. R., Jr. 1982. Noncontraceptive health benefits of oral steroidal contraceptives. *Am. J. Obstet. and Gynecol.* 142: 809–816.

Nadelson, C. C. 1978. The emotional impact of abortion. In *The woman patient*, eds. M. T. Notman and C. C. Nadelson, Vol. 1, pp. 173–179. New York: Plenum Press.

Nass, G. D., and Fisher, M. P. 1988. *Sexuality today*. Boston, MA: Jones and Bartlett.

Ory, H. W.; Rosenfield, A.: and Landman, L. C. 1980. The pill at 20: An assessment. *Family Planning Perspectives.* 12:278–283.

Ory, H. W.; Forrest, J. D.; and Lincoln, R. 1983. *Making choices and evaluating the health risks and benefits of birth control methods.* New York: The Alan Guttmacher Institute.

Pietrow, P. T.; Rinehart, W.; and Schmidt, J. C. 1979. IUD's: An update of safety, effectiveness, and research. *Population Reports.* Ser. B(3).

Planned Parenthood/Alameda-San Francisco. 1982. *Early abortion by vacuum aspiration.* San Francisco: Planned Parenthood.

Planned Parenthood/Alameda-San Francisco. 1983. *Information on contraceptive vaginal suppositories.* San Francisco: Planned Parenthood.

Planned Parenthood/Alameda-San Francisco. 1986. *Information on contraceptive diaphragm and cream/jelly.* San Francisco: Planned Parenthood.

Planned Parenthood/Napa. 1986. *Condom.* Napa County: Planned Parenthood.

Presser, H. B. 1977. Guessing and misinformation among urban mothers. *Family Planning Perspectives.* 9:11–15.

Reed, T. 1983. Hysteroscopic sterilization: Silicone elastic plugs. *Clin. Obstet. Gynecol.* 26(29):313–320.

Robertson, E. M., ed. 1987. OC user's recurrent candidiasis may require multiple treatment strategies. *Contraceptive Technology Update.* 8(1):9.

Rosenfield, A. 1982. The pill: An evaluation of recent studies. *Johns Hopkins Med. J.* 150:177–180.

Ross, C., and Pietrow, P. T. 1974. Birth control without contraceptives. *Population Reports.* Ser. I(1).

Senanayake, P., and Kramer, D. G. 1980. Contraception and the etiology of PID: New perspectives. Paper presented at the International Symposium on Pelvic Inflammatory Disease, Atlanta, 1–3 April.

Sex Education For Disabled People. 1986. *Information on the condom.* Oakland, Calif.: Sex Education For Disabled People.

Shostak, A.; McLouth, G.; and Seng, L. 1984. *Men and abortions. Lessons, losses, and love.* New York: Praeger.

Swanson, J. M., and Forrest, K. A. 1984. *Men's reproductive health.* New York: Springer.

Washoe County Health Department. *Nutrition and family planning: Oral contraceptives.* Reno, Nevada: Washoe County Health Department.

Westhoff, C. F., and McCarthy, J. 1979. Sterilization in the United States. *Family Planning Perspectives.* 11:147–152.

World Health Organization. 1981. A prospective multicenter trial of the ovulation method of natural family planning II: The effectiveness phase. *Fertility and Sterility.* 36:591–598.

Wortmann, J. 1975. Vasectomy: What are the problems? *Population Reports.* Ser. H(4).

4
Change in Family Roles

BEHAVIORAL OBJECTIVES

Upon completion of this chapter, the reader should be able to:

- Define traditional family roles.

- Define the following:
    Nuclear family.
    Extended family.
  Single-parent family.
    Blended family.
    Family of origin.
  Communal family.

- Describe the purposes the family serves for the individual family member, the family unit, society, and the health care provider.

- Use Duvall's theory to assess the developmental level of the family.

- Determine the types of nursing interventions needed by the family.

- Identify the family's influences on the health status of its members.

The family has long been the basic unit of society and is the institution with the most pervasive effects on its members. The family is the unit that serves as a buffer between the individual and society. When the family unit functions well, some of the effects of society are neutralized, reducing the stress on its individual members. The family provides a setting in which its members can relax, be loved and accepted, and be themselves. Ideally, in the family, the sense of belonging can be met for each individual member.

The family interprets the aspects of society for its members, while continuing to provide new members for that society and to prepare them for their roles.

Within the family, each member has the same basic physical, safety, and belonging needs; yet the family as a unit must balance all the needs of its members—parents, young children, adolescents, and the elderly. The family is also the individual's primary group—the one group with concern for all aspects of each member's life. Each member, however, may belong to several groups in society—a school, a church, an employment setting, a political party, social clubs, or hobby groups (see Fig. 4–1). While membership and activity in these groups may be important to the individual and to facets of his or her growth and development, no single group can meet each member's needs in all areas: physical, social, learning and thought, and inner competencies. Thus, the family is crucial to the development of a strong, integrated self in each of its members; and a strong, healthy sense of self is considered essential to the development of mentally healthy individuals (Gardner, 1980).

In a family unit, any change, either positive or negative, that affects one or more family members

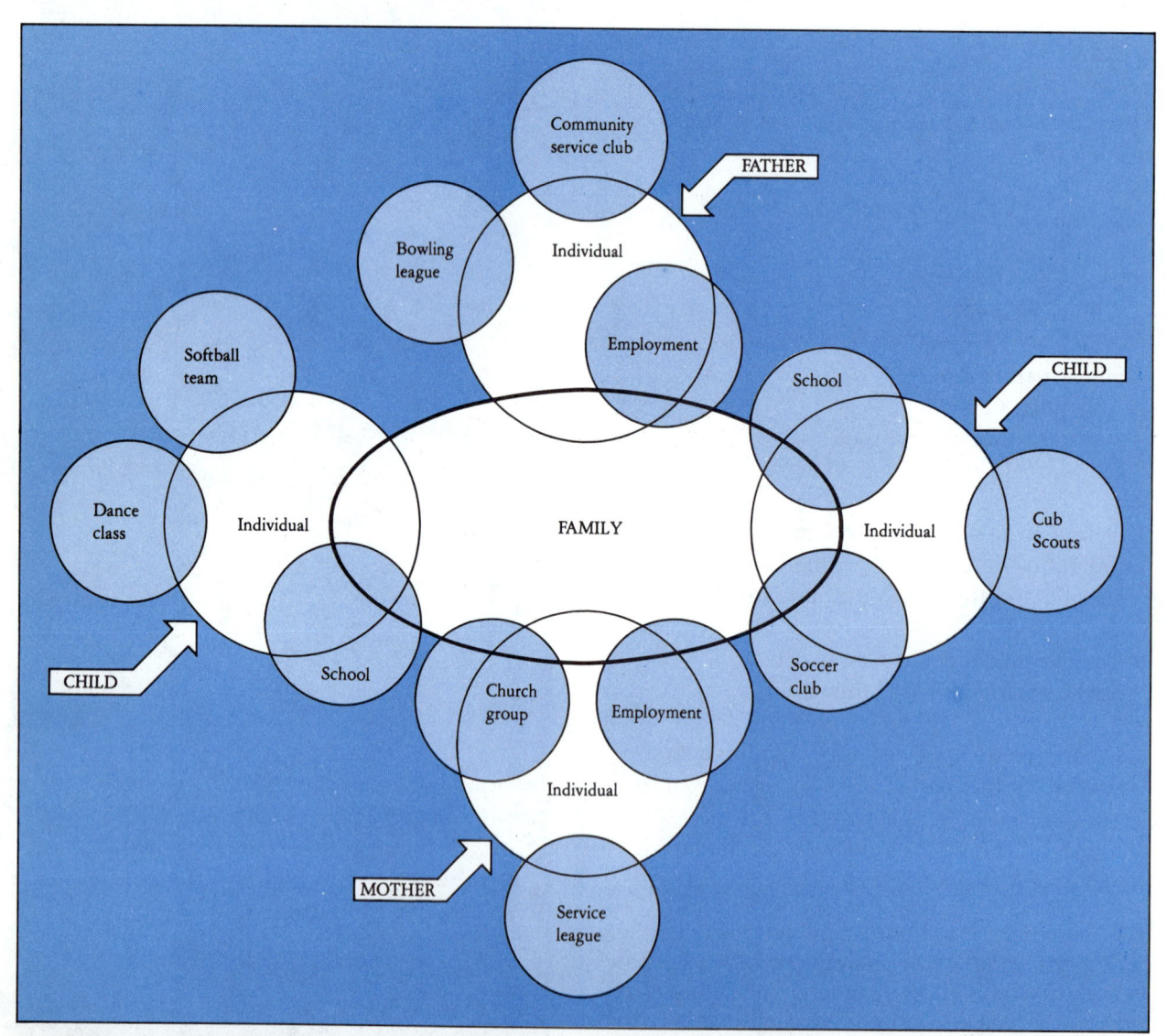

FIGURE 4–1. The family, its members, and its associations.

affects the entire family unit. The healthy, viable family, the "buffer," changes in reaction to stimuli from its environment. This ability to change is a necessary part of any open system and allows for adaptation, and ultimately for survival. The family that cannot, or does not, adapt to change may suffer conflict and eventual disintegration.

The health status and health practices of family members are strongly influenced by family values and beliefs (Friedman, 1981). The young woman pregnant for the first time and seeking prenatal care brings her own value system as well as that of her parents, her siblings, and her mate. These influences may affect her timing in seeking health care, the types of services she desires, her interest in prepared childbirth classes, how she chooses to feed her infant, and the parenting style she will adopt.

A careful nursing assessment of family health practices and values helps the nurse plan interventions with the family to raise their level of wellness. Health practices related to lifestyle affect the entire family. Positive factors adopted by a family during the pregnancy period (such as cessation of cigarette smoking or limiting intake of caffeine and alcohol) may be continued after pregnancy, thus improving the family's health status.

In assessing the entire family, the nurse may identify health problems or risk factors. The nurse may be able to work with family members on these problems or refer them to appropriate sources for care and treatment. When problems in individuals or their relatives are identified early, it may be possible to prevent progression of the problems or their occurrence in new family members.

DEFINITIONS

There is no single definitions for the term *family* in our rapidly changing society. In the 1960s the family was defined traditionally as a group of people having the following characteristics (Burgess, Loche, and Thomas, 1963):

1. Joined together by bonds of marriage, blood, or adoption.
2. Living together in a single household.
3. Interacting and communicating with each other in reciprocal family social roles.
4. Sharing a common culture.

There are many emerging family forms that do not meet these criteria. Horton (1977) described the family as a special kind of social system of two or more interdependent persons who remain united over time and serve as the mediators between the needs of the group's members and the forces, demands, and obligations of society. Several general family types are:

1. *Nuclear family.* The family of marriage, parenthood, or procreation, consisting of husband, wife, and child(ren), either natural, adopted, or both.
2. *Extended family.* The nuclear family plus the relatives of either or both spouses, all living together.
3. *Family of origin.* The family unit into which an individual is born.
4. *Reconstituted or blended family.* A family unit consisting of a widowed or divorced adult, his or her children, and a new mate; a parent, stepparent, children, and stepchildren all living together.
5. *Single-parent (family).* A family consisting of a single (never-married, divorced, or widowed) adult and his or her natural or adopted children.
6. *Communal family.* Households of adults and their children, living in a common geographic area, working together in a common way to achieve the group's goals and ideals.

The spectrum of family forms is summarized in Table 4–1.

Although the form or structural characteristics may vary, families serve common purposes in society. Sussman (1973) has identified five tasks and functions common to all families:

1. Socialization of children.
2. Development of competence of family members to cope with the demands of the organizations within which they must function.
3. Utilization of organizations.
4. Provision of an environment for the development of identities and affectional responses.
5. Creation of satisfaction and a mentally healthy environment conducive to the well-being of the family.

Even when family structures or forms are similar, no two families are identical. Each family has its own strengths and coping patterns. Therefore, each family must be assessed separately, to deter-

TABLE 4–1. Family Forms

Traditional Family Forms

1. Nuclear family—husband, wife, and children living in same household
2. Nuclear dyad—husband and wife alone: childless, or no children living at home
   a. Single career
   b. Dual career
      i. Wife's career continuous
      ii. Wife's career interrupted
3. Single-parent family—one head, as a consequence of divorce, abandonment, or separation (with financial aid rarely coming from the second parent), and usually preschool or school-age children
   a. Career
   b. Noncareer
4. Single adult living alone
5. Three-generation family—may characterize any variant of family forms 1, 2, or 3 living in a common household
6. Middle-aged or elderly couple—husband as provider, wife at home (children have left for college, career, or marriage)
7. Kin network—nuclear households or unmarried members living in close geographic proximity and operating within a reciprocal system of exchange of goods and services
8. "Second career" family—the wife enters the work force when the children are in school or have left the parental home

Nontraditional Family Forms

1. Communal family
   a. Household of more than one monogamous couple with children, sharing common facilities, resources, and experiences; socialization of the child is a group activity.
   b. Household of adults and offspring—a "group marriage", where all individuals are "married" to each other and all are parents to the children; there is usually a charismatic leader
2. Unmarried parent and child family—usually mother and child, where marriage is not desired or possible
3. Unmarried couple and child family—usually a common-law type of marriage with the child their biologic issue or informally adopted
4. Cohabiting couple—unmarried couple living together
5. Homosexual union—persons of same sex living together as "marital partners"

SOURCE: Sussman (1973).

---

mine its needs, and its ability to meet health challenges (Fig. 4–2). Spradley (1985) identifies five family universals:

1. Every family is a small social system.
2. Every family has its own culture and rules.
3. Every family has structure.
4. Every family has certain basic functions.
5. Every family moves through stages in its lifecycle.

When assessing a family, the nurse looks at the family's structural characteristics and at its ability to perform tasks and functions. Otto (1963) proposes the following criteria as useful in determining family strengths:

1. The ability to provide for the physical, emotional, and spiritual needs of individual members.
2. Sensitivity to the needs of individual members.
3. Subjective communication of thoughts and feelings.
4. Support, security, and encouragement.
5. Initiation and maintenance of growth-producing relationships and experiences within and outside of the family.
6. The capacity to maintain and create constructive and responsible community relationships.
7. The ability to grow with and through children.
8. Flexibility in assuming family roles.
9. The ability of self-help and acceptance of help when appropriate.
10. The capacity for mutual respect for the individuality of family members.
11. The ability to use a crisis experience as a means of growth.
12. Concern for family unity, loyalty, and interfamily cooperation.

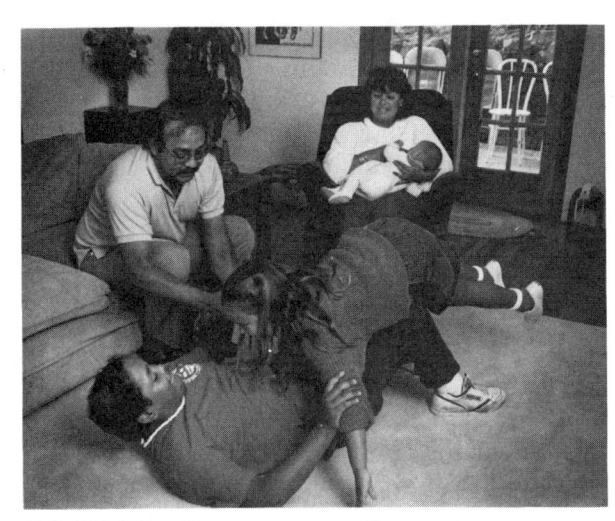

FIGURE 4–2. The nurse assesses the family's structural characteristics.

While the family may take on a variety of forms, some of these forms may not include children. Spradley (1985) has identified family tasks and functions similar to those of Otto and Sussman, but does not specifically mention children. Thus, her criteria may be more universally applied. They are as follows:

1. *Affection:* establishment of a climate of affection; promotion of sexuality and sexual fulfillment; addition of new members.
2. *Security:* maintenance of physical requirements; acceptance of individual members.
3. *Identity:* maintenance of motivation; self-image and role development; social placement.
4. *Affiliation:* development of communication patterns; establishment of durable bonds.
5. *Socialization:* internalization of culture (values and behavior); guidance for internal and external relationships; release of members.
6. *Controls:* maintenance of social control; division of labor; allocation and utilization of resources.

Family functions are best accomplished through flexibility and sharing of tasks and roles, rather than through rigid assignment to a particular individual according to sex or position in the family (Fig. 4–3). The family that is able to share tasks increases its ability to adapt to changes and stressors. A flexible family tends to be more

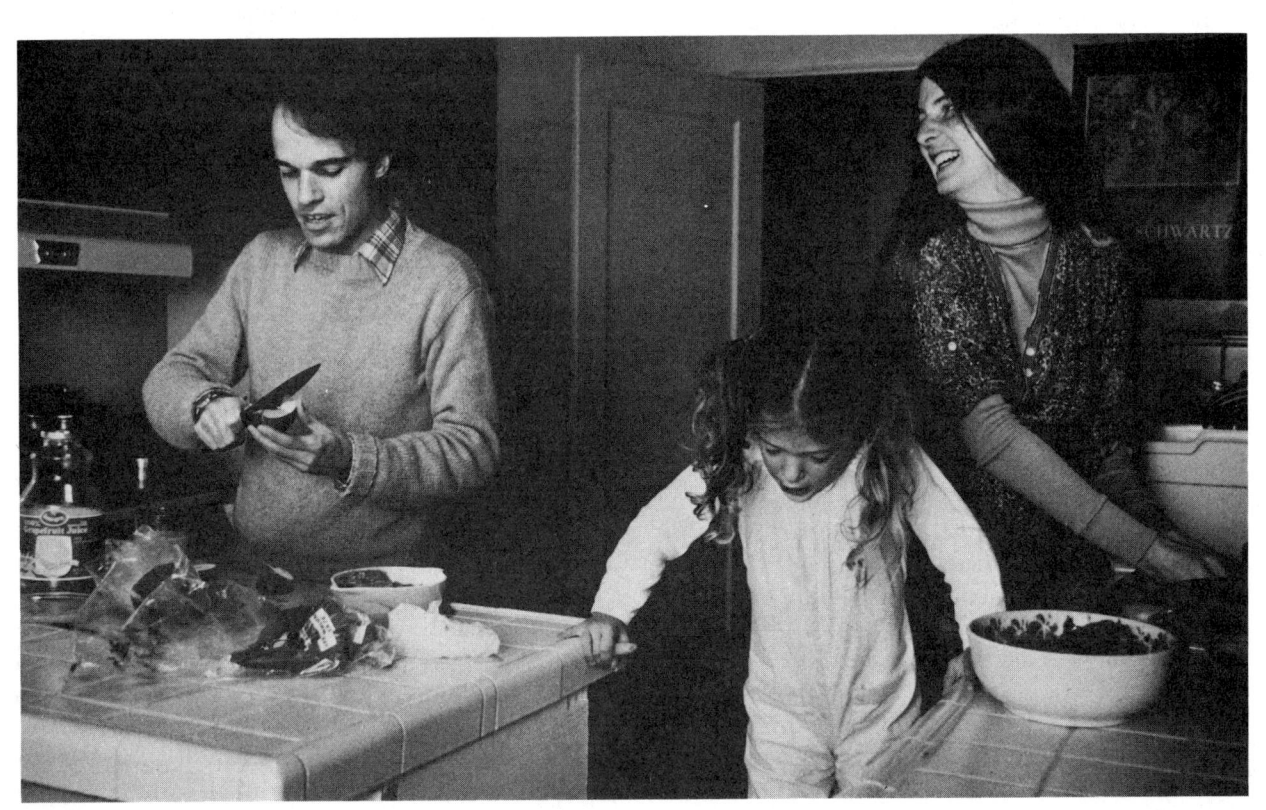

FIGURE 4–3. The sharing of roles increases a family's adaptation to the changes required by pregnancy.

mature and will probably be less likely to react chaotically to the crises of daily life.

Roles are the appointed or understood parts people play in daily life, as defined by their family. In more traditional families, specific roles may be assigned to or expected of each individual. The father-husband role may be assumed by the male, who is also the primary breadwinner, handyman, decision maker and disciplinarian. The mother-wife may be the cook, caretaker of the children, gardener, and seamstress. These are *performance*, or *instrumental, roles*.

There are also *emotional*, or *expressive, roles*, such as protector, nurturer, rebel, leader, and clown. These may be adopted by or assigned to a man, woman, or child, providing family members with guidelines for how to act toward each other and ways to interact with the larger society. Simply stated, roles are prescribed behaviors in a situation (Murray and Zentner, 1985).

In the nuclear family, each individual may have several roles. When an individual who usually fulfills a particular role function suddenly becomes ill or leaves the household, this role must be taken over by another individual. In the case of a prolonged hospitalization of a woman with a high-risk pregnancy, for example, the father-husband may either have to take on more of her instrumental and expressive roles or seek additional help by hiring an extra person or calling on other family members such as grandparents for help. Inability or unwillingness to reallocate the absent mother's roles and functions leaves other family members with unmet physical and emotional needs.

In traditional family patterns where the husband-father works and the wife-mother is a full-time homemaker, definitive role assignments are common. As more women work outside the home, whether for personal satisfaction or out of economic necessity, families are having to adjust to shared role assignments and shared parenting. In 1960, 43 percent of households had only one working spouse. By 1990 it is estimated that 86 percent of households will have more than one wage earner. Only about 7 percent of American families fit the "traditional" profile of working father, homemaker mother, and two children (Nasibitt, 1982).

A sharing of roles between husband-father and wife-mother is becoming more prevalent, as families seek to prevent overloading one adult. With 60 percent of mothers with children under the age of 14 in the labor force (Wallis, 1987), there is a sharing of roles not only in earning income, but in housekeeping and parenting as well. Readjustment of roles and reassignment of tasks may be necessary at the time of a child's birth, when the added task of parenthood begins, and again when the second parent resumes employment (Schuster and Ashburn, 1986). As the wage gap between men and women narrows (see Table 4–2), and more and more women enter more highly paid professions, families may find it sensible for the wife-mother to resume full-time employment as soon as possible after the birth of a child, and have the husband-father assume a larger share of the household and child care responsibilities.

EVOLUTION OF THE FAMILY

Table 4–3 is a historical depiction of the changing family in middle-class North America. Stages I through III describe the family from the agricultural age to the modern age. Stage IV projects future trends. A family today may fit into any of these categories, depending on its socioeconomic status, family characteristics and values, culture, and locale. However, families are beginning to demonstrate more characteristics specific to the informational society. Implications for the future involve the use of home computer systems for education, shopping, electronic mail, communication using modems, and recreation. The home may again become the main base of operation.

EVOLUTION OF PARENTING

Attitudes toward children and parenting have changed markedly as civilization has advanced. Couples initially had no control over their procreative abilities, so childbearing and childrearing were the inevitable consequences of their sexuality. In medieval times, parents showed few attachment behaviors and made little emotional investment in the newborn. Children of that period are not represented in works of literature or art (Tuchman, 1978), which may be indicative of the value of children in that period. Children were cared for by their mothers until the age of 7. After that, boys would be schooled by their fathers for their appropriate role in life—farmer, squire, warrior. Girls were schooled by women for a life of homemaking, servitude, nobility, or the nunnery,

TABLE 4–2. The Wage Gap (figures for full-time workers in selected occupations)

	Women as percent of all workers 1979	1986	Earnings ratio, female to male 1979	1986
Accountants and auditors	34	45	0.60	0.72
Computer programmers	28	40	0.80	0.81
Computer systems analysts	20	30	0.79	0.83
Lawyers	10	15	0.55	0.63
Managers and administrators	22	29	0.51	0.61
Sales of business services	28	34	0.58	0.79
Teachers, elementary school	61	82	0.82	0.95

SOURCE: Pear (1987).

depending on the family's station in life (Tuchman, 1978).

As times began to change, agricultural societies valued children for their economic worth. The wealthy man, the landowner, had many sons who could help him in the fields.

In the early twentieth century health care improved: fewer babies died, child labor laws were enacted, and children became an economic liability, as they contributed less and made increased financial demands on the family for food, clothing, and shelter. While there was increasing personal and emotional investment in children, parents began to desire birth control. The National Birth Control League was founded in 1917, becoming the International Planned Parenthood Federation in 1952, with its goal stated as "every child a wanted child" (Speert, 1980).

With advancing technology, birth control became a choice for many. Today parents have more control over the spacing and number of children in the family.

More couples are giving careful thought to the decision to have children. Many couples choose to postpone childbearing until they feel more secure in their marriage, more financially solvent, and more established professionally. Some postpone having children and then realize that they will be happier without children.

Couples who decide to become parents may have one or more of the following reasons for having a child:

1. Assertion of adulthood.
2. Assertion of sexuality.
3. Fulfillment of cultural expectations.
4. Outlet for personal creativity.
5. Means for self-actualization.
6. Acceptance by peer group.
7. Desire to nurture.
8. Security for later life.
9. Link to immortality.
10. Social status.

Parenthood makes tremendous demands upon the couple. If undertaken at a time when the couple is not secure with its own relationship, it may increase stress. Babies do not respect the needs of parents, in that they are dependent and demanding. If a child prevents other members of a family from reaching their personal goals, resentment may develop and interfere with the family dynamics (Schuster and Ashburn, 1980). The quality of the relationship among members is considered to be the most essential ingredient of healthy family functioning (Lewis, 1979).

Couples need a period of time to adjust to living together, independently of parents, prior to childrearing. They need time to develop ways of handling their money, values, living patterns, and

TABLE 4–3. Historical Stages of Family Living

Family Stage	Purpose	Goal	Motivation	Structure/Roles	Orientation	Societal Expectations
I. Pre-industrial (agricultural)	Economic unit of production	Self-sufficiency	Survival	Closed system; patriarchal structure; dictatorial governance; rigidly defined roles; childrearing = 54% of married life	Children seen as economic necessities, assets, possessions; treated as miniature adults with early indoctrination into adult responsibilities and strong lines between right and wrong	Economic security; protection; religious training; recreation; education; reproduction; health care
II. Industrial (traditional)	Consumptive unit; leisure oriented	Success, domesticity	Quality of living; accumulation of goods	Emerging open system; less patriarchal, but husband still head of household and final authority; autocratic governance; clearly defined roles but not rigid	Children seen as an economic liability after enactment of child labor laws; early assumption of adult role—contribution to family income by 16 or 18	Reproduction; religious training; class- and status-conferring; privacy; identity-conferring
III. Post-industrial (modern)	Consumptive unit; leisure oriented	Self-actualization of members and independence; enhancing potentials of members	Quality of living	Open symmetrical system; shared egalitarian structure; democratic governance; dedifferentiation of roles—flexible and negotiable, depending on who is available and the situation; childrearing = 18% of married life	Children seen as an economic liability had by choice, viewed as persons in their own right; late assumption of adult role, average at 21–22 years; obligation to family is to develop own potentials	Provision of physical needs; fulfillment of emotional and love needs; nurturing—preparing child's personality for modern world; companionship
IV. Informational society (future)	Consumptive unit; leisure oriented	Self-actualization of the individual; enhancing individual potential	Quality of living; accumulation of goods	Shared roles, shared parenting; childbearing shifted to later years—in the 30's; serial marriages, blended families; clearer roles for step-parents	Self-help groups; children economic liability, with costs shared by parents; obligation is to self and one's own children	Independence, autonomy, personal growth and development; greater isolation and less societal interaction in day-to-day life as computer brings outside information, educational programs, and goods into the home

SOURCE: Stages I through III: Tackett and Hunsberger (1981); Stage IV: Naisbitt (1982).

goals. This phase of their relationship is referred to as the *establishment phase*.

Following the establishment phase, the couple enter the *parenthood phase*. Becoming parents will change their lives. It is a turning point with lifelong, irrevocable consequences. Friedman (1957) has described four stages of parenthood:

1. *Anticipatory.* This is the period of pregnancy. The couple discuss how they will have the baby, care for it, raise it, and name it. As they leave this stage, they may realize they will never again be just "a couple".
2. *Honeymoon.* This is a period of initial adjustment to and attachment with the baby. Parents adjust to their new roles and the demands of the baby. They may experience loss of sleep as well as loss of personal freedom.
3. *Plateau.* This is a long period of parental development paralleling childhood. The parents have active roles as mother and father of the growing child, who gradually begins to interact with the larger community.
4. *Disengagement.* During this period the parent–child–family relationship terminates, usually at the time of the child's marriage or when he or she leaves home permanently. Parents are usually relieved of their major childrearing tasks and are free to restructure their lives.

Parenting can be a source of joy, frustration, or a combination of both. One survey (Landers, 1976) revealed that 70 percent of parents say they would not have children if they could relive their lives. Reasons given for this response were:

1. Concerns about world tensions and overpopulation.
2. Interference caused by children in the marital relationship, i.e., financial, emotional, and personal costs.
3. Failure of the children to meet parental expectations.
4. Rejection of parents by the children in later life.

Even Shakespeare's *King Lear* (1605 or 1606) said:

How sharper than a serpent's tooth it is
To have a thankless child.

Several questions may be asked about the responses in Landers (1976) survey. Were the parents' expectations realistic? What was their style of parenting? Did they discuss problems and formulate family goals with their children? The health care facilitator should address these questions to gain insight that will assist parents to engage in active problem solving.

Many changes in parenting behavior have occurred. Half of American women today return to work before their child's first birthday (Wallis, 1987). As a result, there is a tremendous demand for day-care facilities. In 1986, 9 million children were cared for by someone other than their mother (Wallis, 1987). Yet day-care remains hard to find, costly, and not always of high quality. It is not unusual for people to sign up on waiting lists months before the anticipated need for the care. The United States is the only Western industrialized country to not guarantee a working mother the right to a leave of absence after she has a child (Hewlett, 1986). In January, 1987, the United States Supreme Court ruled that states may require businesses to provide maternity leaves with job security; however, only 40 per cent of working women receive this protection through their employers (Wallis, 1987).

The United States also lags behind most industrialized countries, and much of the world, in its support of child care systems. We have neither national maternity, national family, nor national child-care policies. This may reflect respect for the "traditional" motherhood role, but these ideals are not the reality of the late 1980s. More than 100 countries have national policies; many European countries have extensive child care systems which are subsidized and regulated by the government and they also have liberal maternity leave policies, with pay (Hewlett, 1986; Wallis, 1987).

Some American businesses are taking a lead by providing on-site child-care facilities—with sliding-scale fees. These facilities are open at hours that are compatible with the parents' work schedules; parents often take their children for lunch (Wiesler and Thornton, 1983). Wallis (1987) reported that businesses making this investment have found it has paid off in reduced absenteeism and turnover among employees. Some hospitals have converted underutilized beds in their pediatric units to "Sick Bay" facilities, where parents may bring ill children for care while he or she goes to work. Employers are beginning to pay for these benefits. More public schools and community groups are recognizing and responding to the needs for supervised before- and after-school programs for the school age child.

Changes in the ways our children are cared for

have been generating concerns among parents, teachers, psychologists, and sociologists. With fewer people living in extended family situations, and with relatives often far away, this may be the first generation of children reared by strangers. Early separation of parent and infant also affects the parent, often unexpectedly. Harvard pediatrician T. Berry Brazelton has been quoted as saying: "Many parents return to the work place grieving" (Wallis, 1987). The long-term effects of these changes in family life need to be researched.

FACTORS INFLUENCING FAMILY ROLES

Cultural and socioeconomic factors have an impact on family roles. Culture is defined as the ideas, values, and behaviors shared by a group of people—the collection of ways of doing, feeling, and thinking, transmitted from generation to generation by and through the family (Spradley, 1985). Social class affects a family's values, attitudes, and lifestyle, and in combination with cultural background, it provides the family with guidelines for living.

Change occurs slowly in most societal groups, because change implies letting go of or leaving some of the familiar in order to accept the challenge of the new. When families have more demands placed upon them, during times of stress, for example, they may revert to the security of familiar cultural patterns. These patterns provide comfort, solace, and support.

Assessment of the family should include evaluation of (1) allocation of power and decision making, (2) the value placed on education, (3) locus of control, (4) time orientation, (5) perception of roles, and (6) socioeconomic status.

Allocation of Power and Decision Making

The nurse must know the family constellation. Is it an extended, nuclear, or single-parent family? Even if the family is a nuclear one, culture may dictate consultation with older family members on issues related to health care. The family may demonstrate equality in the marital relationship with a division of labor, or all decision making may be delegated to one partner. Will the male partner take an active and supportive role in childbirth preparation, the birth itself, and parenting? Such participation may result in conflict with many values of the dominant culture. For example, is a man who wishes to coach his partner through a labor and delivery scorned by his parents? Is he considered less manly if they both participate in parenting?

Value Placed on Education

The nurse should assess the significance to the couple of education during the childbearing experience. Are the couple ready to learn, or do they prefer to rely upon the assistance of family members? The Indian woman whose child will be cared for by her mother-in-law and nursemaids may see little relevance in baby-care classes, while the nuclear couple having their first child, away from supportive family members, may be eager for classes, readings, and information. Those individuals who do not relate positively to education because of negative past experiences or those with limited reading and verbal skills may feel very uncomfortable about childbirth preparation "classes".

Locus of Control

It is important to assess the family's locus of control. Does their belief system include an *internal* locus of control, a belief that they have some control over events in their lives? For example, if the family's approach is fatalistic and they believe that they have no control over their future (*external* locus of control), the nurse may have difficulty in helping them recognize the value of prenatal care, including classes for childbirth preparation and parenting.

Time Orientation

The nurse should assess the family's time orientation. Is their primary orientation to the past, allowing important events from the past to guide their lives? Some families are present oriented and pay little attention to the past, focusing only vaguely on the future. If a family is future oriented, they may believe that they can improve or change their lives and that planning will affect future events. Middle-class Americans tend to be future oriented. A family's time orientation is an important clue to the likelihood that they will accept preventive health care measures. A present-oriented family may take a passive, day-to-day, crisis-oriented approach to health and illness. When a family is future oriented and has an internal locus of control, its members are more receptive and responsive to prevention, planning, and health teaching (Murray and Zentner, 1985).

Perception of Roles

Careful assessment of the values and beliefs of a family in relation to perception of roles is important. Today's families of childbearing age are likely to have been exposed to a changing value system and may be in the process of choosing a lifestyle that will best develop their personal philosophy of life.

Socioeconomic Status

Differences in socioeconomic strata are not sharply defined. While a family's economic status may be assessed objectively, their economic standing may not always correlate with their views. For example, a high school physical education teacher's economic status may be below that of a blue-collar worker, yet he may pursue golf, a sport often enjoyed by the upper middle class. A family's socioeconomic status also undergoes changes resulting from job layoffs, rising costs of health care, unexpected crises, and surging inflation. How the family perceives their socioeconomic status is important to the nurse in planning nursing care.

FAMILY DEVELOPMENTAL LEVELS AND TASKS

Families, as open systems, undergo continuous change. Eight stages have been defined in the family life cycle. Each stage has a corresponding developmental task. These developmental tasks have been referred to as growth responsibilities (Duvall, 1971). Failure to achieve a certain developmental task leads to unhappiness in the family, disapproval by society, and difficulty with later developmental tasks. The eight stages in the family life-cycle, their relative time duration, and the family group developmental tasks associated with them have been adapted from Duvall (1977) and Spradley (1985) (see Fig. 4–4).

Stage 1: Establishment Phase

At this stage the newly established couple have no children. Developmental tasks of this phase include:

1. Establishing a home base in a place to call their own.
2. Establishing mutually satisfactory systems for getting and spending money.
3. Establishing mutually acceptable patterns of who does what and who is accountable to whom.
4. Establishing a continuity of mutually satisfactory sexual relationships.
5. Establishing systems of intellectual and emotional communication.
6. Establishing workable relationships with relatives.
7. Establishing ways of interacting with friends, associates, and community organizations.
8. Facing the possibility of children and planning for their coming.
9. Establishing a workable philosophy of life as a couple.

Stage 2: Expectant Family and Childbearing Phases

Stage 2 extends from the oldest child's birth until the child is 2½ years old. The developmental tasks of the expectant family phase include:

1. Arranging for the physical care of the expected baby.
2. Developing new patterns for getting and spending income.
3. Redetermining who does what and where authority rests.
4. Adapting patterns of sexual relationships to pregnancy.
5. Expanding communication systems for present and anticipated emotional needs.
6. Reorienting relationships with relatives.
7. Adapting relationships and activities with friends, with associates, and in the community to the realities of pregnancy.
8. Acquiring knowledge about and planning for the specifics of pregnancy, childbirth, and parenthood.
9. Maintaining morale and a workable philosophy of life.

CHANGE IN PERINATAL NURSING TODAY

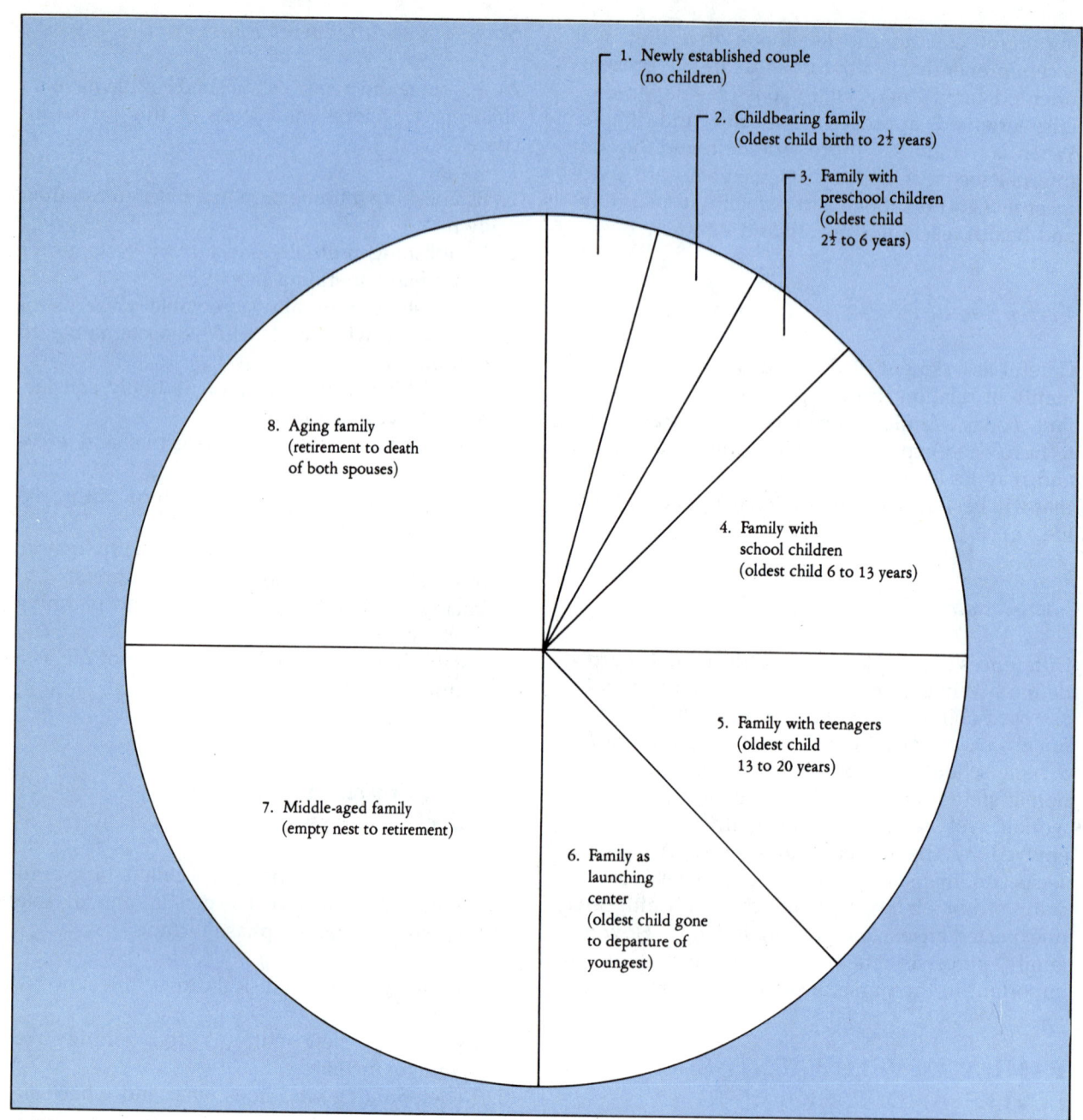

FIGURE 4–4. Eight stages of the nuclear family life-cycle.
SOURCES: Duvall (1971) and Spradley (1985).

1. Newly established couple (no children)
2. Childbearing family (oldest child birth to 2½ years)
3. Family with preschool children (oldest child 2½ to 6 years)
4. Family with school children (oldest child 6 to 13 years)
5. Family with teenagers (oldest child 13 to 20 years)
6. Family as launching center (oldest child gone to departure of youngest)
7. Middle-aged family (empty nest to retirement)
8. Aging family (retirement to death of both spouses)

The developmental tasks of the childbearing phase are:

1. Adapting housing arrangements for the life of the child (referred to as child-proofing the home).
2. Meeting the costs of family living.
3. Reworking patterns of responsibility and accountability.
4. Reestablishing mutually satisfying sexual relationships.
5. Refining intellectual and emotional communication systems for childbearing and childrearing.
6. Reestablishing working relationships with relatives.
7. Fitting into community life as a young family.
8. Planning for additional children in the family.
9. Reworking a suitable philosophy of life as a family.

Stage 3: The Family with a Preschooler

At this stage the family's oldest child is 2½ to 6 years old. Developmental tasks of families with preschool children are:

1. Supplying adequate space, facilities, and equipment for the expanding family.
2. Meeting predictable and unexpected costs of family life with small children.
3. Sharing responsibilities within the expanded family and between members of the growing family.
4. Maintaining mutually satisfying sexual relationships and planning for future children.
5. Creating and maintaining effective communication systems within the family.
6. Cultivating the full potential of relationships with relatives within the extended family.
7. Tapping resources, serving needs, and enjoying contacts outside the family.
8. Facing dilemmas and reworking philosophies of life in ever-changing challenges.

Stage 4: The Family with a School-age Child

During this phase the family's oldest child is 6–13 years old. The developmental tasks to be accomplished are:

1. Providing for children's activities and parents' privacy.
2. Staying financially solvent.
3. Cooperating to get things done.
4. Continuing to satisfy each other as marriage partners.
5. Effectively utilizing family communication systems.
6. Feeling close to relatives in the larger family.
7. Tying in with life outside the family.
8. Testing and retesting family philosophies of life.

Stage 5: The Family with a Teenager

During Stage 5 the oldest child is 13–19 years old. Developmental tasks of the family with a teenager include:

1. Providing facilities for widely differing needs.
2. Working out family money matters.
3. Sharing the tasks and responsibilities of family living.
4. Putting the marriage relationship into focus.
5. Keeping communications systems open.
6. Maintaining contact with the extended family.
7. Growing into the world as a family and as individuals.
8. Reworking and maintaining a philosophy of life.

Stage 6: The Family as a Launching Center

This stage, also known as the contracting family stage, begins as the oldest child leaves home. Developmental tasks of this stage are:

1. Rearranging physical facilities and resources.
2. Dealing with the costs that launching-center families encounter.
3. Reallocating responsibilities among grown and growing children.
4. Coming to terms as husband and wife.
5. Maintaining open systems of communication within the family and between the family and others.
6. Widening the family circle through release of young adult children and recruiting of new members by marriage.
7. Reconciling conflicting loyalties and philosophies of life.

Stage 7: The Family in the Middle Years

Stage 7 begins when the last child has left home. Developmental tasks of this period are:

1. Maintaining a pleasant and comfortable home.
2. Assuring security for the later years.
3. Carrying out household responsibilities.
4. Drawing closer together as a couple.
5. Maintaining contact with grown children's families.
6. Keeping in touch with brothers' and sisters' families and with aging parents.
7. Participating in community life beyond the family.
8. Reaffirming the values of life that have real meaning.

Stage 8: The Aging Family

Stage 8, the final stage of the family, extends from the time of retirement until the second spouse dies. Developmental tasks of the aging family are:

1. Finding a satisfying home for the later years.
2. Adjusting to retirement income.
3. Establishing comfortable household routines.
4. Nurturing each other as husband and wife.
5. Facing bereavement and widowhood.
6. Maintaining contact with children and grandchildren.
7. Caring for elderly relatives.
8. Keeping an interest in people outside the family.
9. Finding meaning in life.

Aldous's Family Development Stages

Aldous (1978) identifies six stages of family development for divorced women who do not remarry:

Stage 1. Women establishing a single-parent family.
Stage 2. Women instituting or reinstituting their work-life career.
Stage 3. Women with adolescents.
Stage 4. Women with young adults.
Stage 5. Women in the middle years.
Stage 6. The retirement of women from work or parental responsibilities.

According to Aldous, widowed women who do not remarry go through similar stages. For women who do remarry, family development tends to follow nuclear family stages.

Using Knowledge About Family Development

Knowledge of the family life-cycle and developmental tasks as identified and described by Duvall, Spradley, and Aldous can assist the nurse in working with individuals and their families. The nurse can use the structure of the family and age of its members to assess the family as being at a particular level. For example, the family with children may be at level that coincides with the age of the oldest child. The nurse can then determine whether developmental tasks prior to that level have been met and whether tasks at the current placement level are being met. These developmental tasks can be discussed with family members as they explore their ever-changing family and can be useful in providing anticipatory guidance for future changes. These developmental tasks can also be useful in helping a family understand why the care and raising of second and subsequent children differ from care and raising of the first. The family itself may be at a more advanced level, and children born into the same family are never exactly alike (Duvall, 1971). Knowledge of family development may also explain why couples who begin childbearing after only a minimal period of time in the establishment phase, with its tasks unmet, many have difficulty meeting the tasks of the childbearing and preschool periods. Such individuals and couples may experience dissatisfaction and unhappiness and may even seek release from the relationship.

THE NURSE AND THE FAMILY—ASSESSMENTS, INTERVENTIONS, AND STRATEGIES

Levels of Functioning

With the current emphasis on family-centered nursing care, the nurse must be able to determine the individual family's needs in order to provide appropriate care. The family's level of functioning should be assessed. Tapia (1972) has identified five levels of functioning and their corresponding characteristics: (1) infancy, (2) childhood, (3) adolescence, (4) adulthood, and (5) maturity.

Level I: Infancy, or Chaotic Families
Families at this level of functioning:

1. Live from day to day without an orientation to the future.
2. Demonstrate distrust of outsiders, with inability to utilize community resources and service.
3. Are hostile or show resistance to offers of help.
4. Are weak parents, showing immaturity and confusion of roles within the family.
5. Function at a survival level.

Level II: Childhood Families

Families at this level, while still somewhat alienated from the community:

1. Have greater ability to trust, and thus have hope for a better way of life.
2. Have parents who, despite some confusion and distortion of roles, are willing to work together to benefit the family unit.
3. Are more able to meet basic survival needs.
4. Are unable to change or to accept change.

Level III: Adolescent Families

Families at the adolescent level:

1. Are normal but have more than the usual number of conflicts and problems.
2. Are more able to meet survival and physical needs, but emotional conflicts cause confusion for children and others.
3. Are characterized by having one parent who is more mature than the other.
4. Are able to look for some solutions to problems; are more future oriented.

Level IV: Adult Families

Families at the adult level of development:

1. Are normal, stable, healthy, and happy and have fewer than the usual number of conflicts or problems.
2. Are able to handle most problems as they arise.
3. Are able to meet physical and emotional needs of family members.
4. May have problems related to growth and developmental tasks.
5. Are willing and able to seek outside assistance to resolve problems.

Table 4–4 summarizes, by family level, the family's ability to meet four basic tasks (Tapia, 1986).

The Nurse's Role

The nurse is viewed differently by each family according to its level of functioning (Tapia, 1972). These views range from "good mother" to expert and partner. A continuum of nursing skills is needed for each level as the nurse works with the family (see Fig. 4–5). Nursing activities range from building a trust relationship at the infancy level to more complex skills as expert, resource person, and provider of anticipatory guidance at the adult level. The mature, independent family no longer requires nursing intervention (Tapia, 1972).

The nurse working with an expectant teenage couple may assess their level of functioning as that of Level II, childhood family. The couple may find it difficult to trust health care workers and may see the nurse as a mother or father figure. The nurse must be fair, setting limits, providing information, and permitting guided, realistic decision making by the couple so that a trust relationship can develop.

A neonatal nurse may assess an experienced family who have cared for previous full-term babies comfortably as being at Level III, the adolescent family, as they learn how to care for their 35-week gestation newborn with a cleft palate. Nursing interventions would include teaching them specific skills for feeding the infant, referring them to appropriate community resources such as support groups, providing anticipatory guidance related to the child's expected growth and development patterns, and helping them to understand the long-term treatment necessary for their child.

PROBLEMS WITH CHANGING ROLES

Change has occurred at a faster pace than many social systems and individuals can comfortably tolerate. With the rapid change in family roles have come problems.

The most obvious problems are intercultural and intergenerational conflicts as people leave the family of origin to formulate their own family units. Lifestyle choices may conflict with long-held values of parents and extended families and may, at times, even conflict with the individual's own belief system. Although an individual may think, or claim, that he or she is free of the tenets of a traditional ethnic or religious upbringing, a man may find, for example, that he is still a cultural Jew in that he wants to have a ritual circumcision for a newborn son.

There may be a lack of support for variant lifestyles from the extended family, support that individuals may not cherish in day-to-day situations but that they miss at crucial life passages, such as childbirth, marriage, or the death of a loved one. Even if extended family members want

TABLE 4–4. *Ability of Families to Meet Basic Family Tasks*

Four Basic Tasks	Family Level				
	I	II	III	IV	V
1 Survival Security	Bare —	Minimal Some	Adequate Adequate	Good Good	Excellent Reasonable
2 Social Emotional	Unclear —	Rigid —	Clear Limited	Good Good	Excellent Excellent
3 Sexuality Training	— —	Barely —	Rigid Limited	Adequate Good	Excellent Excellent
4 Support Growth	— —	— —	Rarely —	Adequate Adequate	Excellent Excellent

SOURCE: Tapia (1986).

to be supportive, they may not know how to give support in circumstances that may be quite alien to their own lifestyles.

Nurses encounter more and more clients without husbands—the unmarried teenager, the unmarried older woman, the woman whose husband has left her, or the couple where one is not yet free to marry because dissolution of a previous marriage is not complete. These women are in need of support in the form of prenatal education, coaching through labor and delivery, praise for their accomplishment in childbirth and their role change to motherhood, and teaching regarding childcare.

Nurses frequently encounter expectant mothers or couples who have not met some of the developmental tasks of Duvall's establishment phase. These individuals are often teenagers experiencing unplanned pregnancies and who are at a higher risk medically and socially. They have not had time to complete their separation from their parents or to establish themselves as individuals and couples. They are likely to experience more role stress and strain and more difficulties in marital adjustment (Friedman, 1981).

Another growing group nurses encounter today is the long-married, career-oriented, older couple experiencing their first pregnancy. Although these pregnancies are usually carefully planned, they carry with them an increased medical risk to mother and child and profound lifestyle changes that the couple, used to their freedom, may find difficult to accept. These achievement-oriented individuals may be unable to accept anything less than a "perfect child" and may overinvest in all aspects of the child's life, resulting in the "superbaby" complex (Langway et al., 1983).

They may also experience the strains of life in a dual-career family. The older couple may each have a career, which Tapia (1986) defined as employment that requires a high degree of commitment and has a continuous developmental character, as opposed to a job. These couples may have invested many years in achieving a certain level of accomplishment in their careers. With parenthood comes a new set of demands, in addition to the existing ones of domestic chores and time for family leisure activities and interactions. Will the couple need outside domestic help? Can they afford it? Can they accept having a child or children, and have someone else be the person with whom the child interacts for the majority of the day?

Can the couple who are used to having freedom to pursue personal and career goals adapt to accommodate the needs of a child? Like many other couples, the older couple may not live near

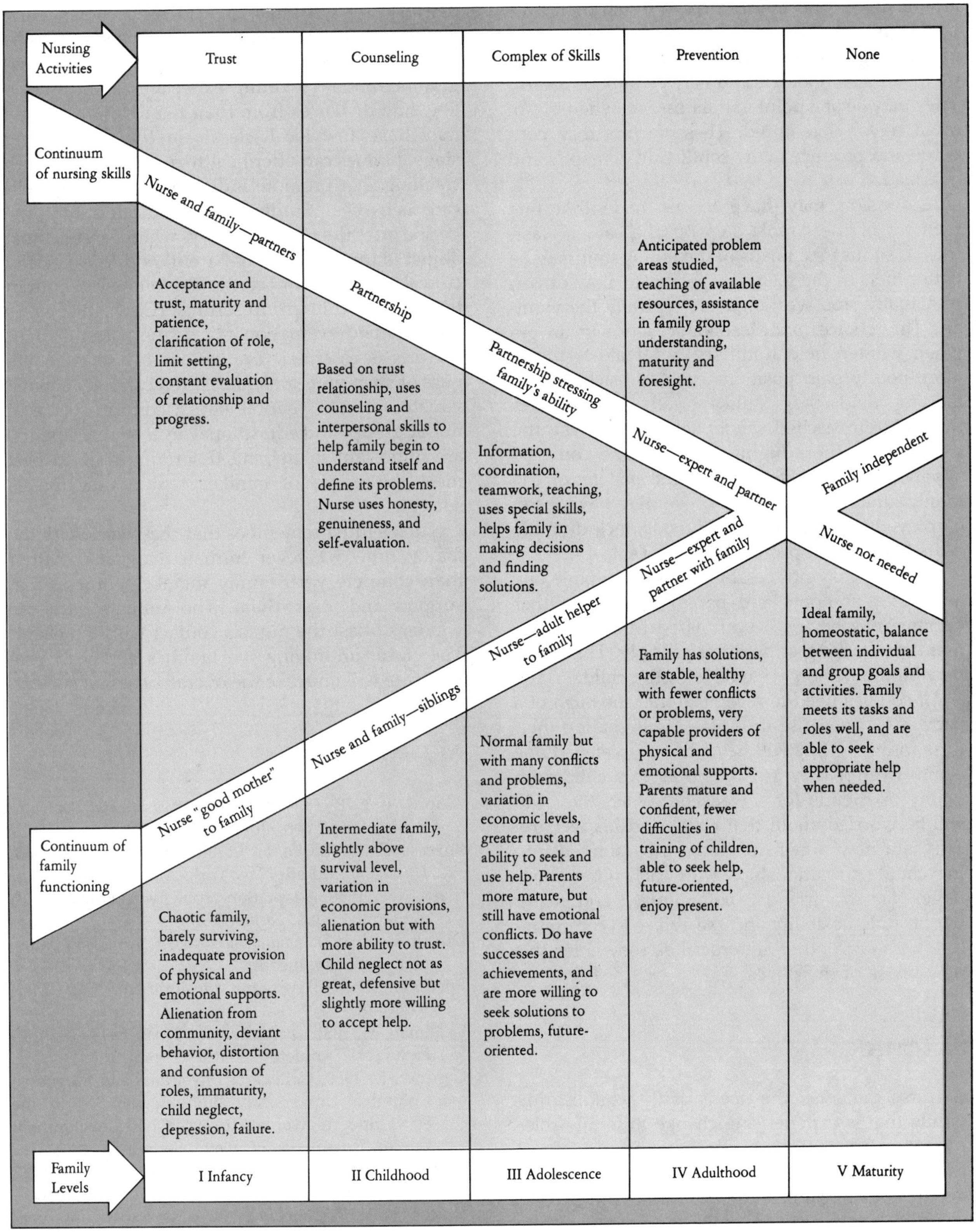

Change in Family Roles 95

Nursing Activities →	Trust	Counseling	Complex of Skills	Prevention	None
Continuum of nursing skills	*Nurse and family—partners*	*Partnership*	*Partnership stressing family's ability*	*Nurse—expert and partner*	*Family independent*
	Acceptance and trust, maturity and patience, clarification of role, limit setting, constant evaluation of relationship and progress.	Based on trust relationship, uses counseling and interpersonal skills to help family begin to understand itself and define its problems. Nurse uses honesty, genuineness, and self-evaluation.	Information, coordination, teamwork, teaching, uses special skills, helps family in making decisions and finding solutions.	Anticipated problem areas studied, teaching of available resources, assistance in family group understanding, maturity and foresight.	*Nurse not needed*
	Nurse "good mother" to family	*Nurse and family—siblings*	*Nurse—adult helper to family*	*Nurse—expert and partner with family*	
Continuum of family functioning	Chaotic family, barely surviving, inadequate provision of physical and emotional supports. Alienation from community, deviant behavior, distortion and confusion of roles, immaturity, child neglect, depression, failure.	Intermediate family, slightly above survival level, variation in economic provisions, alienation but with more ability to trust. Child neglect not as great, defensive but slightly more willing to accept help.	Normal family but with many conflicts and problems, variation in economic levels, greater trust and ability to seek and use help. Parents more mature, but still have emotional conflicts. Do have successes and achievements, and are more willing to seek solutions to problems, future-oriented.	Family has solutions, are stable, healthy with fewer conflicts or problems, very capable providers of physical and emotional supports. Parents mature and confident, fewer difficulties in training of children, able to seek help, future-oriented, enjoy present.	Ideal family, homeostatic, balance between individual and group goals and activities. Family meets its tasks and roles well, and are able to seek appropriate help when needed.
Family Levels →	I Infancy	II Childhood	III Adolescence	IV Adulthood	V Maturity

FIGURE 4–5. A model for family nursing.
SOURCE: Tapia (1972).

any relatives. Those who have invested their time heavily in career pursuits may not have a network of nonwork friends who can assist them. Their own parents are older, and may be in poor health. They may be at a point in their careers when out-of town travel is required. These factors may converge and produce many conflicting demands and overload.

A decision may have to be made that one member of the couple step off the career "fast-track", so that the needs of the family unit may be better met. In the past, the person to slow down, or actually stop working, was typically the woman. This choice made economic sense in an era when women held traditionally female-oriented, more poorly paid positions such as teaching and nursing, fields they could typically re-enter after the children reached school age. In this way the career of the more highly paid husband could be advanced, for the total economic benefit of the family unit. More recently, women have been employed in a wide variety of fields, including the more highly paid professions (see Table 4–2).

A couple may not be able to afford to have one adult stay at home and parent full-time. Other options may be tried, such as part-time employment, or working at home, if possible. The father may be the person at home with the child.

All couples need to recognize that the birth of a baby, especially the first baby, will change their lives forever. They will never be completely alone again. Even if they are able to leave a child with family or friends for a weekend away, they will still be worried about that child, and his welfare. This is a new dimension to be incorporated into the couple's relationships with each other, their larger family, friends, community, and work world. Role flexibility and the ability to communicate with each other are crucial as they enter this new phase of their lives.

SUMMARY

A nurse can meet the needs of the childbearing family that is experiencing change in family roles by acting as a teacher, resource person, direct caretaker, referral source, researcher, or change agent. With consumer support, nurses can encourage hospitals to provide family-centered maternity care options, including paternal as well as newborn rooming-in and early hospital discharge with nurse follow-up in the home.

Primary nursing is an essential component to family-centered care, for it is in this nursing care delivery system that the nurse becomes truly familiar with the family and its needs. This is especially important in our society of high geographic mobility. Young expectant families often live long distances from their family of origin and may have few local friends in the childbearing stage. Nurses can offer health guidance and health teaching that promote individual and family self-care activities. Studies have indicated that the period after the birth of a baby, when parents must adjust to the demands of parenthood, is especially critical and worthy of continued follow-up, both in the home and in group settings (Clark, 1966).

Continued evaluation of existing parent–infant services is essential. Evaluations of the effectiveness of such programs, measured carefully against variables of age, marital status, culture, socioeconomic group, and educational level of participants, are important in helping determine how to best meet the needs of families within our diverse society.

Nurses must remember that they work *with* the family unit, whatever form it may take. Rather than compete with family members, nurses can support and teach them. The family's influence will far outlast the nurse's contact with the client. Therefore, improving the family's ability to provide care will improve the overall health of society.

REFERENCES

Aldous, J. 1978. *Family careers: Developmental change in families.* New York: John Wiley & Sons.

Burgess, E. W.; Locke, H. J.; and Thomas, M. M. 1963. *The family.* 3rd ed. New York: American Book.

Clark, A. L. 1966. Adaptation problems and the expanding family. *Nurs. Forum.* 5:98.

Duvall, E. M. 1971. *Family development.* 4th ed. Philadelphia: J. B. Lippincott.

Friedman, D. 1957. Parent development. *Calif. Med.* 86:25–28.

Friedman, M. 1981. *Family nursing: Theory and assessment.* New York: Appleton-Century-Crofts.

Gardner, R. 1980. College of Physicians and Surgeons, Columbia University. "Building families in the 80's." Speech given at Parson's Child Development Center, Russell Sage College, September 18.

Hewlett, S. A. 1986. *A lesser life: The myth of women's liberation in America.* New York: William Morrow.

Horton, R. 1977. Conceptual basis for nursing interventions with human systems: Families. In *Distributive nursing practice: A systems approach to community health,* eds. J. E. Hall and B. R. Weaver. Philadelphia: J. B. Lippincott.

Landers, A. 1976. If you had to do it over again, would you have children? *Good Housekeeping.* 182(6):100.

Langway, L.: Jackson, T. A.; Zabarsky, M.; Shirley, D.; and Whitmore, J. 1983. Bringing up superbaby. *Newsweek*. March 28:62–68.

Lewis, J. M. 1979. *How's your family?* New York: Brunner/Magee.

Murray, R. B., and Zentner, J. P. 1985. *Nursing concepts for health promotion*. 2nd ed. Englewood Cliffs, N.J.: Prentice Hall.

Naisbitt, J. 1982. *Megatrends*. New York: Warner Books.

Otto, H. A. 1963. Criteria for assessing family strength. *Family Process*. 2:329–338.

Pear, R. 1987. Women reduce lag in earnings but disparities with men remain. *New York Times*, September 4.

Schuster, C. S., and Ashburn, S. S. 1980. *The process of human development—A holistic approach*. Boston: Little, Brown.

Schuster, C. S., and Ashburn, S. S. 1986. *The process of human development*. 2nd ed. Boston: Little, Brown.

Shakespeare, W. 1605 or 1606. *King Lear*.

Speert, H. 1980. *Obstetrics and gynecology in America—A history*. Baltimore: Waverly Press.

Spradley, B. W. 1985. *Community health nursing: Concepts and practice*. 2nd ed. Boston: Little, Brown.

Sussman, M. B. 1973. Family systems in the 1970s: Analysis, policies, and programs. In *Family health care*, eds. D. P. Hymovich and M. U. Barnard. New York: McGraw-Hill.

Tachett, J. J. M., and Hunsberger, M. 1981. *Family centered care of children and adolescents*. Philadelphia: W. B. Saunders.

Tapia, J. A. 1972. The nursing process in family health. *Nurs. Outlook*. 20(4):267–270.

Tapia, J. A. 1986. Fractionalization of the family unit. In *The process of human development*, eds C. S. Schuster and S. S. Ashburn. Boston: Little, Brown.

Tuchman, B. W. 1978. *A distant mirror: The calamitous 14th century*. New York: Alfred A. Knopf.

Wallis, C. 1987. The child-care dilemma. *Time*, June 22.

Wiessler, D., and Thornton, J. 1983. Who'll watch the kids? Working parents' worry. *U.S. News & World Report*. 94(25):67.

5

Change in Society: Roles and Expectations

BEHAVIORAL OBJECTIVES

Upon completion of this chapter, the reader should be able to:

- Identify changes in societal expectations affecting the childbearing years.

- Describe alternative lifestyles and their impact on childbearing and childrearing practices.

- Discuss *in vitro* fertilization, artificial insemination, sex selection, and genetic engineering and their effects on societal expectations and childbearing practices.

- Describe the role of the maternity nurse in dealing with clients who choose alternative lifestyles.

- Define the meaning of nonjudgmental support and give examples of specific communication techniques.

- Clarify personal beliefs and values associated with changes in societal expectations during the childbearing years.

Attitudes, values, and lifestyles in today's society have undergone unparalleled change. There are nearly as many divorces and broken families as marriages. Premarital and extramarital sex have become the norm. Lifestyles have changed radically (Harris, 1981). There are more women in the work force than ever before. Very few children born today will have a home situation in which their mother's main occupation is that of homemaker. There has been a dramatic increase in the number of homosexuals who publicly express their sexual preferences. There are homosexual marriages and homosexuals who become parents. There are test-tube babies and surrogate mothers as well as more babies born to adolescent parents than ever before. The number of single-parent households has increased drastically over the past two decades.

In addition to changes in societal values and expectations, there have been numerous scientific and technologic advances in maternity care, which have made more services available to the childbearing population.

Far reaching changes have taken place in our reproductive capabilities. Huxley's (1956) vision of the future in *Brave New World* seems much closer to reality. Huxley envisioned the abolition of parenthood and the family which would be sanctioned by society as it attempted to improve natural reproduction (Elias and Annas, 1986).

This chapter focuses on alternative lifestyles, the status of women, and family size. Some of the recent scientific and technologic advances in the area of *in vitro* fertilization, artificial insemination, and sex selection are also discussed.

CHANGE IN SOCIETY: PAST AND PRESENT

Middle-class, Anglo-American society is changing so rapidly today that people are not expected to complete their lives in the same kind of world they were born into. In order to survive in times of rapid social change, families need to discover new ways of living in a modern society. In the twentieth century social change has occurred more rapidly than ever before, and families are confronted with many new conditions, problems, and challenges.

Socioeconomic specialists identify four great transitions in history that have affected the human race. The first transition occurred 10,000 years ago when families moved from hunting and food gathering and settled in farming villages. The second transition occurred 5000 years later with the growth of cities. The emergence of a world based on scientific technology was the third transition, and the fourth, known as the "crisis of closure" on the spaceship earth, is now in progress and has caused society to acknowledge that resources are finite. Today's fourth transition has brought about numerous changes in technology, moral principles, attitudes and beliefs, and political systems (Duvall, 1977).

Learning to utilize our own human resources through ingenuity, adaptability, and education is one of today's challenges. In the past, family members spent most of their time together working and playing. They lived according to rigid societal moral rules. Now, the family is more dispersed in work and play, more individualized than family-centered. The social changes that have evolved in this century have forced families to change patterns of living that existed for hundreds of years. Numerous changes in family structure and functions have occurred, with far-reaching implications for society.

The following social trends have been identified as having had a profound impact on the family:

1. A decrease in the size of the family. This has resulted in fewer brothers and sisters to participate in peer socialization. This decrease did not result from increased childlessness or from an increase in families with only one child. It is the result of a decline in families of five or more children. Childlessness remains at approximately 8–10 percent of marriages and one-child families remain at 10 percent.
2. A decline in marriage rates. This decline is most pronounced among late adolescents and those in their early 20s. The decline in marriage rate is accompanied by an increase in unwed motherhood among teenagers.
3. A marked increase in the divorce rate and the rate of remarriage.
4. An increase in the numbers of households made up of single adults, aged adults, unrelated adults, newly married adults, and single parents and their children. In part, this increase reflects a distaste for three-generation households in America that is of long duration.
5. A considerable improvement in the status of women in and out of the family setting. This has resulted in increased education and career opportunities, choice of residence, and control of property (Yinger and Cutler, 1978).

There have been notable changes in the age at which the average American family begins childbearing. Childbearing age is often influenced by culture and socio-economic status. The ideal age for childbearing is a significant question for health care professionals to consider. At one time it was thought that childbearing should begin in the early

20s and end in the 30s. Now, it ranges from pregnancies in early adolescents to women starting their families after age 35.

Teenagers who become pregnant are at greater physical and emotional risk than women in their 20s and early 30s. Women who are aged 35 and over are also subject to some increased health problems. Recently, the number of adolescent girls bearing a child has increased to over 1 million annually. There is also an increase in the number of women over 30 who are having babies. Many young women of childbearing age have delayed marriage and pregnancy in order to pursue a career. There is evidence that with adequate care throughout pregnancy and delivery, both these groups of women are able to deliver healthy babies. In addition, many maternal complications that might arise can be avoided or successfully treated with appropriate care during pregnancy.

There is no perfect age for becoming parents, but there are problems on each extreme of the age continuum (Horowitz, Hughes, and Perdue, 1982). The parenting decision should be based on the couple's ability to balance their needs as parents with the responsibilities of parenting. The available resources and options should also be considered.

ALTERNATIVE FAMILY LIFESTYLES

Single-parent Families

The single-parent family is the most frequent variation of the normative two-parent family structure. It is estimated that over 6 million single parents live in the United States. The vast majority (85 percent) of single-parent households are headed by women (Horowitz, Hughes, and Perdue, 1982).

There are several reasons for the increased number of single-parent households. One major cause is the large number of unmarried adolescent women who become pregnant each year. Over the past several years more than 1 million babies have been born each year to single girls between 12 and 18 years of age. Single-parent households may also result from single parents being allowed to adopt babies. Death, divorce, and separation are responsible for changing some families into single-parent households. An increasing number of fathers are being granted custody of children as a result of death or divorce proceedings and thus are becoming single parents (Horowitz, Hughes, and Perdue, 1982).

Having a single parent affects the health and emotional stability of family members. The children may have lower self-esteem than those of traditional two-parent families. There is often a lack of financial resources in the single-parent household, especially those headed by women, since women in the work force are often paid less than their male counterparts.

Although the majority of single-parent households are headed by women, a small but growing number are headed by men. Single fathers may have difficulty adjusting to the role of parenting alone, but many are very successful. Single-parent fathers may even have a distinct advantage over females in the area of finances because they tend to have larger incomes and greater financial resources.

In single-parent families adequate support systems may be lacking. With only one parent to carry out childrearing responsibilities, there is a need to pay for services that are not supplied by the other parent. If there is a lack of money for these services, the family may become disorganized or disturbed.

Many single parents feel lonely because meaningful adult relationships are limited or lacking. They are often isolated, and life becomes a boring routine of work and childrearing. Often, they experience guilt feelings about their lack of success in maintaining a marriage. Managing the family often becomes extremely difficult for single parents (Horowitz, Hughes, and Perdue, 1982).

Horowitz, Hughes, and Perdue (1982) have pointed out that the health care delivery system typically causes anxiety and concern for single parents and their children in these ways.

1. The family is treated with the approaches appropriate for two-parent families.
2. The problems the family is experiencing are believed to be the result of some deviance from the two-parent norm. Interventions focus on transforming the family into a nondeviant nuclear family.
3. The family is often forgotten or ignored. Problems may be treated as though they do not exist or are considered hopeless or unimportant.

Single parents have difficulty maintaining a balance between the parenting role and the adult role. The health care professional may help the single parent to develop an adequate adjustment in these areas. Accurate assessment of the family's situation is essential. Referral to available community agencies may provide the needed assistance. Self-help groups may help single parents form new relationships and may provide moral support in dealing with problems.

The children of divorced parents may experience feelings of insecurity and guilt. They sometimes believe they are responsible for the separation of their parents. These children need to be encouraged to express their feelings and to develop open communication patterns. They must be reassured that they are loved and were not the reason for the divorce.

When dealing with single-parent families nurses may feel frustrated because they cannot change the reality of the family situation. The caring nurse can offer much needed support to the single parent by listening to their story and helping them understand and work through their feelings regarding parenting and running a household alone. Developing support groups for single parents may also be beneficial.

The maternity nurse may be called upon to provide emotional and physical support for the pregnant young woman who is single because she has not been married or who has become single during pregnancy as a result of divorce, separation, or death. When this situation occurs, the normal psychologic and emotional changes that occur during a pregnancy are complicated by additional psychologic stress. It is important for the nurse to be supportive. The goal is to help the pregnant woman deal with the problems confronting her and to explore the support systems available, such as family members or community agencies. It is essential that the pregnant single woman receive appropriate health care during her pregnancy and delivery in order to maintain her own health and ensure the birth of a healthy baby.

Adoption

Adoption is an alternative to biologic parenting of a child. Adoption may be chosen by couples who (1) are infertile and unable to bear a child, (2) prefer adoption as an alternative to childbirth, or (3) have a serious genetic problem or other health-related reason for not bearing a child. In recent years adoption has also become an option for single individuals who wish to become parents. Adoptions may be handled by an agency, a physician, or a lawyer.

Adoptive parents are referred to as "social" parents (Horowitz, Hughes, and Perdue, 1982). They do not go through the gestation period that the biologic parents do. The adoptive mother does not experience the physiologic changes associated with bearing a child. The gradual changes that occur during pregnancy can assist the biologic parents to adjust emotionally and socially to the birth of their child. Because of the shortage of babies now available for adoption, the adoptive couple may have waited months or years for an available baby. The waiting period is often much longer than the normal 9-month gestation cycle of pregnancy. Liberalized abortion laws, increased use of contraception, and a high percentage of unmarried mothers choosing to keep their babies have contributed to the shortage of babies available for adoption. The limited number of available babies has led couples desiring a child to adopt from racial and ethnic backgrounds different from their own. It also has encouraged some couples to adopt older or handicapped children.

In the past, adoption agencies adhered to rigid requirements regarding prospective parents' age, race, marital status, and religious affiliation. They were very precise in an attempt to match babies and parents. These criteria are no longer an acceptable means of determining the ability to parent. Such practices eliminate many qualified individuals. Changes in these criteria have opened adoption to single men and women and older couples.

Adoptive parents must face the issue of telling their child about his or her adopted status. There is lack of agreement as to the ideal time for telling the child. Some authorities recommend that parents should not feel forced to tell a child about the adoption until the child is mature enough to deal with the information. However, others suggest that a simple explanation should be made by the time the child is 5. When telling a child about being adopted, the developmental level of the child is probably more important than chronological age (Horowitz, Hughes, and Perdue, 1982).

The nurse can assist adoptive parents in dealing with their feelings about adoption. It is important to realize that adoptive parents and their children sometimes require more support than biologic families. The health care delivery system is often actively involved during the adoptive process but then tends to overlook the later needs of these families for support in developing normal family relations.

Homosexual Parents

During the past decade the gay liberation movement has gained considerable attention in the United States. Homosexual men and women have "come out of the closet" and have begun to seek equal recognition.

There are many varieties of homosexual expressions, and the reasons underlying individuals' sexual orientations are quite diverse. Gay men and women who hide their sexual preference from those in the "straight" world avoid many of the social consequences of homosexuality, such as being denied custody of children. Hiding one's sexual identity is perceived by some to cause tremendous emotional pressures and, therefore, many gays have chosen to become more open about their homosexuality.

One of the most controversial areas related to the issue of homosexuality is the desire on the part of some homosexual men and lesbian women to become parents. Although homosexuality itself may not prevent an individual from being a successful parent, there are numerous social difficulties and stigmas that can complicate the situation (Horowitz, Hughes, and Perdue, 1982).

There has been considerable concern expressed regarding the potential dangers for children living in homosexual families and being exposed to sexually transmitted diseases and Acquired Immune Deficiency Syndrome (AIDS) (Rubenstein et al., 1983). This area is still controversial due to limited understanding and the unavailability of a cure or vaccine to prevent the disease. It is known that AIDS is spread by sexual intercourse, infected needles, blood contamination, pregnant mothers, and breastfeeding. However, AIDS is not known to be spread by casual contact and research maintains that even with continued close contact, people who live and work with AIDS patients do not get the disease unless they are exposed by one of the previously mentioned methods (Harris County Medical Society and Houston Academy of Medicine, 1987).

In some areas lesbian mothers have been granted custody of their biologic children in divorce proceedings. Since society views mothers as necessary for childrearing, lesbian mothers have a much greater chance of being granted child custody than homosexual fathers. Few gay fathers have custody of their children, and many have difficulty being granted visitation rights (Horowitz, Hughes, and Perdue, 1982).

Research has indicated that sexual orientation alone is not a reason to prohibit satisfactory parenting. It has been recommended that the approach to "homosexual" custody in divorce cases be determined on the basis of which parent can facilitate maximum growth and development of the child rather than using sexual orientation only. Children in homosexual homes have not been found to demonstrate greater social or emotional maladjustment than those raised in heterosexual single-parent homes with live-in lovers.

At the 1980 American Medical Association (AMA) annual meeting, the House of Delegates voted to study the health care needs of homosexuals. There have been charges that this group is underserved by the health care delivery system. It has been estimated that 5–10 percent of the population has a homosexual orientation and, therefore, the majority of health care providers will come in contact with these individuals at some time or another (AMA, 1982).

Since it is often difficult for members of the health team to be objective when caring for homosexuals, it is important to identify one's own values and ethical beliefs about homosexuality. Homosexuals who are parents need support. Although the health care provider may not agree with the homosexual lifestyle, individualized care should be provided. Homosexual and "straight" parents have similar concerns about parenting. Homosexual parents may also have additional concerns regarding social rejection of their children because of the stigma still associated with homosexuality.

The AMA House of Delegates recommended the following (AMA, 1982):

1. Educate physicians on current research in homosexuality and in taking an adequate sexual history. This should begin in medical school and should be included in continuing education programs.
2. Encourage the development of educational programs for homosexuals to acquaint them with the diseases for which they are at increased risk.
3. Provide physicians with better knowledge of the clinics and health care providers who are willing to become involved in improving the health care of the homosexual population.

Recognition of sexual orientation will enhance the health care provider's ability to provide optimal care to the homosexual patient. There must be a cooperative effort between all health care providers as well as the homosexual community to ensure that this group receives appropriate health care.

SCIENTIFIC AND TECHNOLOGIC ADVANCES: ALTERNATIVE PARENTING

A number of scientific and technologic advances over the past two decades have affected childbearing practices. Such practices as artificial insemination and *in vitro* fertilization have provided help to couples who were previously unable to bear children. These advances pose a number of legal, moral, and ethical questions for the health care professional (see Chapters 6 and 7).

Artificial Insemination

Artificial insemination is a process by which semen is introduced into the female genital tract by mechanical means other than coitus. This procedure is used when a woman is fertile and for some reason it is impossible for her to become impregnated by her mate. In recent years, with the advent of women's liberation, the possibility of artificial insemination for unmarried women has also been discussed.

Two major forms of artificial insemination exist: *artificial insemination homologous* (AIH), which is fertilization using the husband's sperm, and *artificial insemination donor* (AID), which is accomplished by implanting sperm from an anonymous third-party donor into the genital tract of a woman at the time of ovulation. It is used when the father is sterile and infrequently when the couple desires to eliminate some genetic trait carried by the male, such as Rh incompatibility. The need for homologous insemination may occur in the face of physical problems in the father such as ejaculatory difficulties or low sperm count. A study of homologous artificial insemination and oligospermia (low sperm count) revealed a very poor success rate. In 83 inseminations by AIH over a 5-year period, only an 8.3-percent rate of pregnancy occurred (Pakalnis and Makoroto, 1977). *Artificial insemination husband donor* (AIHD) is insemination using a pooled specimen composed of both husband and donor semen. This method is used infrequently in cases of low sperm count in the husband. Generally, this method is chosen to give hope to the couple that the husband's sperm may have fertilized the ovum. Sperm may be collected fresh for immediate use or frozen and stored in sperm banks for later insemination.

According to Glanville Williams (1974), AIH was first performed by John Hunter in London about 1785. AID in humans has been recognized as a treatment for male infertility for over 60 years. It is estimated that by 1964 between 10,000 and 250,000 people in the United States had been born as a result of artificial insemination (Perkins, 1976). Artificial insemination in animals goes back to the second century and is mentioned in Arabian sources in the fourteenth century.

Donor artificial insemination was apparently first performed in 1890 under the greatest secrecy (Goldenberg and White, 1976).

The pregnancy rate using fresh donor semen has been estimated to be from 40 to 50 percent (Fitzgerald, 1975) to as high as 77 percent (Stickler, Keller, and Warren, 1975). The mean conception time is three treatment cycles. The success rate using frozen semen is somewhat less.

To date, performance of AIH has not presented any legal or moral problems. However, many legal, moral, and social questions are raised by AID. Proponents of AID believe that if it is compatible with the couple's and the doctor's beliefs, donor artificial insemination is a completely ethical, moral, and acceptable form of medical therapy. Among reasons given for donor insemination are the increased shortage of babies available for adoption, the desire of the mother to experience pregnancy and pass her characteristics on to the baby, and the husband's wish to share the pregnancy and childbirth with his wife.

It is necessary to specify the legal rights and responsibilities of all parties involved in AID. This includes the prospective mother, her husband, the donor, his wife, and the child born as a result of the insemination process. The majority of states have no formal statutes on the books regarding AID.

Some experts charge that the policy of accepting sperm donors based on a medical history alone may lead to the transmission of genetic disease. Even chromosomal analyses can detect only abnormalities present in the donor and not all the genetic possibilities he may foster (Dunston, 1975). Horne (1976) suggests that the incidence of the transmission of diseases such as gonorrhea and mycoplasm infections is larger than has previously been reported. The practice of paying donors for semen is also controversial. In studies of blood donor programs in which donors were paid, it has been found that there is strong inducement to conceal infections such hepatitis, malaria, and syphilis, and this might also be the case among paid donors for artificial insemination.

When the changing attitudes of society about the rights of people to know their genetic backgrounds, difficulty may arise as a result of protection of the donor's identity. Many doctors do not keep records of the donor's identity. They have a file only on the inseminated mother (Fitzgerald, 1975).

The issue of artificial insemination is far-reaching, and it will probably be at least 25 years before any definite decisions can be made on the positive or negative aspects of AID. Success or failure of treatment should not be measured solely on whether a baby is born but on the long-range sociologic and psychologic effects on the couple and on the child resulting from the process.

The role of the nurse working with a couple desiring to have a child by means of artificial insemination is one of support person, counselor, and educator. The nurse may also be called upon to assist with the actual procedure of artificial insemination. Being aware of the differences between AIH and AID and of the various legal, moral, and ethical issues that may be of concern to couples will enable the nurse to take a supportive, informed approach.

In Vitro *Fertilization*

In 1978 Louise Brown was born in England. She was the first baby born as the result of a procedure known as *in vitro fertilization*. Her birth resulted from many years of research and experimentation by Robert Edwards and Patrick Steptoe. *In vitro* fertilization is one answer for infertile couples who desire a child. Since the first "test-tube" baby was born, centers for *in vitro* fertilization have been established in various locations throughout the United States.

In vitro fertilization offers hope for many infertile couples. It is used with women whose fallopian tubes are obstructed or have been removed. It may also be beneficial for men who have oligospermia, because fertilization *in vitro* requires only 50,000 to 500,000 sperm, whereas *in vivo* fertilization requires a sperm count above 20,000,000/ml. Couples with infertility related to antisperm antibodies, absence of cervical mucus due to destruction of glands, use of diethylstilbestrol (DES) during pregnancy by the woman's mother, or severe cervical dysplasia may also benefit from *in vitro* fertilization (Garner, 1983).

In vitro fertilization involves harvesting a mature oocyte from an ovarian follicle through laparoscopy. The natural menstrual cycle has been used to retrieve an oocyte and human chorionic gonadotropin (HCG) has been administered in conjunction with the natural cycle (Garcia, 1985). Ovulation may be stimulated by the use of ovulation-inducing agents such as clomiphene citrate or human menopausal gonadotropin. These medications produce superovulation in women who ovulate normally, and it is therefore possible to obtain more than one mature oocyte to optimize the chances of conception (Garner, 1983).

The patient is carefully monitored by ultrasonography to follow ovarian follicular development. HCG is administered when follicular development is optimal for obtaining a mature oocyte. When it is determined that ovulation will occur, a laparoscopy is performed in order to remove the oocyte (Garner, 1983).

The oocyte is incubated in a culture medium at 37°C for 8–24 hours. The time of incubation depends on the maturity of the oocyte. About 2 hours before the insemination, a semen specimen is obtained by masturbation. The semen undergoes a special procedure to obtain the 50,000 to 500,000 motile sperm needed for fertilization. The sperm are placed in a Petri dish with an oocyte and placed in the incubator for 12 hours. The oocyte is transferred to a growth medium and returned to the incubator for 28–32 hours. If the oocyte is fertilized, two polar bodies and two pronuclei will appear. About 40 hours after insemination the embryo should undergo cell division. The embryo consists of two or four cells when it is transferred into the uterine cavity. The patient is placed in the knee–chest position if the uterus is antiverted and in lithotomy position if the uterus is retroflexed. The embryo is transferred to the uterus by means of a Teflon catheter. The patient receives progesterone during the early luteal phase because normal corpus luteum function might have been disrupted during follicle aspiration. Couples are advised to refrain from intercourse for 3 days. A pregnancy test is performed 11 days after fertilization. The success rate of embryo transfers is only about 15–20 percent (Garner, 1983).

The nurse must be aware of the couple's anxiety regarding their desire for a pregnancy. They are in a very difficult emotional state. They have usually chosen *in vitro* fertilization as a last resort to infertility. The nurse should assume the role of providing the couple with support and counseling as well as information regarding the procedure. Once pregnancy occurs, the obstetric care is the same as for any pregnant woman, although the couple may suffer from increased anxiety and concern regarding the well-being of their baby. There has been no evidence that *in vitro* fertilization results in a higher number of birth defects than normally conceived pregnancies (Garner, 1983).

Not all ova fertilized outside the womb actually survive to birth, and some have charged that those who do not believe life begins at conception may be careless about such fertilized ova in the pursuit of a successful pregnancy (Ryan, 1983).

Since the first *in vitro* fertilized baby was born, numerous changes and improvements to different aspects of the process have taken place. The success rate is improving and *in vitro* fertilization has become a new therapeutic approach for treating infertility. It is not recommended that *in vitro* fertilization be used as a substitute for other procedures, but rather as a last resort when other methods have failed (Garcia, 1985).

Being aware of his or her own feelings regarding the issue of *in vitro* fertilization will enable the nurse to assume a more effective role when working with these couples.

In vitro fertilization techniques are still being refined and the next decade will see further advances as we continue to improve our understanding of human reproduction.

Low Ovum Transfer

Low ovum transport has been studied as an alternative to *in vitro* fertilization or reconstructive infertility surgery. One of the main reasons for *in vitro* fertilization is to overcome failure of tubal transport of the ovum and spermatozoa. In low ovum transport the oocyte is aspirated from the dominant follicle immediately prior to the expected ovulation and is injected into the lumen of the fallopian tube 1–2 cm above the uterotubal junction. This procedure circumvents the tubal blockage and permits *in vivo* fertilization to take place (Kreitman and Hodgen, 1980).

Low ovum tubal transfer in humans may be able to overcome various forms of irreparable tubal dysfunction to achieve an *in vivo* pregnancy. It is believed low ovum transfer would avert the numerous biologic and ethical problems associated with *in vitro* fertilization.

The health care professional should be aware that low ovum transfer is being investigated as a potential alternative for infertile couples desiring a child. In the future, couples who are candidates may prefer this option over *in vitro* fertilization.

Surrogate Mothers

A *surrogate mother* is a woman who agrees to bear a child for a couple if the male is fertile and the female is infertile. The word *surrogate* may be defined as substitute. The term surrogate mother no longer refers only to one who provides nurturing for a child after birth; it also refers to one who assumes a substitute pregnancy.

The notion of surrogate mothering is quite controversial. The process includes finding a woman who has proven to be fertile and who is willing to be inseminated artificially by the husband whose wife is infertile. The surrogate mother must agree to bear the child and give complete custody to the biologic father. The surrogate mother may receive a fee from the biologic father for delivery of a healthy baby (Franks, 1981).

Numerous legal and ethical questions are associated with surrogate mothering. Recent court rulings have declared that the biologic father has legal rights to the child regardless of the marital status of each parent, provided that the paternal parentage can be reasonably proven (Franks, 1981).

Analogues have been made between today's surrogate motherhood practices and the biblical story of Abraham having a child by Hagar, the handmaiden of Sarah. Opponents of this view believe that in this case Hagar was not a surrogate at all, but an extension of the family unit, even though it was a polygamous union (Krimmael, 1983).

A psychologic study of women who signed up to become surrogate mothers revealed that they had relatively normal personalities. Most wished to become surrogate mothers for a mixture of financial and altruistic reasons. The study did not include any follow-up research on the women after pregnancy, but most indicated that they had given considerable thought to signing over the baby to the biologic father. They viewed this in much the same way as does an unwed mother placing her baby for adoption (Franks, 1981).

Britain has made it a criminal offense for third parties to profit from surrogacy but voluntary surrogacy remains lawful (Brahams, 1987). Germany and France have also established commissions to debate the issue of surrogacy (Palca, 1987). In the United States, commercial surrogate parenting arrangements continue to be a lucrative business, although much controversy surrounds the issue.

The legality of surrogate contracts and whether this constitutes baby selling have been addressed (Cohen, 1984). What happens when a surrogate mother changes her mind? She is, after all, the natural mother of the child. Who has the legal right to the baby? The natural father and his wife based on the surrogate contract or the natural mother?

The New Jersey Supreme Court overturned the lower court ruling in *Stern* vs *Whitehead*, which has been referred to as the "Baby M" case. They ruled that paying a woman to have a baby amounts to illegal baby selling. The maternal rights of the biological mother were returned although the child will remain in the custody of the biological father and his wife. In the decision, the court ruled that the surrogate contract violated New Jersey adoption laws because of the payment. This is the first State Supreme Court ruling regarding a broken surrogate contract (*El Paso Times*, 1988).

Agreeing that "babies should not be exchanged for money", the California State Assembly passed legislation on May 23, 1988, to outlaw contracts under which women are paid to bear children for infertile couples.

The Bill would invalidate any contract in which a woman agreed before she became pregnant to accept payment to bear a child for another couple. The measure would also make it a felony for anyone to assist in the arrangement of a surrogate contract and a misdemeanor for those who advertise for women willing to participate in the arrangement (*San Francisco Chronicle*, 1988).

The health care provider should be aware of the implications surrounding surrogate motherhood and should be prepared to provide support and counsel to all parties involved: the barren wife, the fertile husband, and the surrogate mother. It is also important that the nurse be aware of the legal status of surrogate motherhood as it evolves. Alternatives to this procedure should be discussed before this course of action is taken.

Oocyte Donation

Recently, donation of eggs by a fertile woman to an infertile woman has been reported. The oocyte is removed from the fertile woman by laparoscopy, as in *in vitro* fertilization. The egg is then fertilized *in vitro* by the infertile woman's husband's sperm. If a pregnancy occurs, the embryo is placed into the uterus of the infertile woman who wishes to bear a child. The process of egg donation might be considered similar to AID. Like donor sperm, oocytes may also be frozen. Egg donors generally remain anonymous.

Reasons for using egg donation include severe pelvic disorders preventing egg recovery, risk of genetic disease, ovarian dysgenesis (malformation), failure of ovarian stimulation, and absence of ovaries (Steptoe and Edwards, 1983; Sherman and Annas, 1986).

Sex Selection

Theoretically, there are two methods of choosing the sex of a baby. One is sex preselection before conception, and the other is selective termination of pregnancy if the baby is determined not to be the desired sex. In *sex preselection*, attempts are made to allow only X-bearing or Y-bearing sperm to approach the ovum. Sex selection may be used not only to assure that the child is the desired sex but also as a means of eliminating sex-linked genetic diseases.

Sex preselection has had poor results in the past. Among the methods that have been tried are:

1. *Shettles sex selection technique*

    Preselection of a daughter:

    a. Intercourse should take place 3 days before the estimated day of ovulation without orgasm.
    b. No previous abstinence required, but no intercourse should take place after the prescribed day until an elevated temperature has taken place.
    c. A mild acidic vaginal douche (1 tablespoon of vinegar to 600 ml of water) should be administered before intercourse.

    Preselection of a son:

    a. Intercourse should take place as close to the estimated day of ovulation as possible with orgasm.
    b. Abstinence should be practiced for 5 days before intercourse.
    c. A mild alkaline vaginal douche (1 tablespoon of bicarbonate of soda to 600 ml of water) should be administered prior to intercourse (Simcork, 1985).

2. *Artificial insemination with treated semen.* Attempts to separate X- and Y-bearing sperm have had limited success. The X-bearing sperm is said to be heavier than the Y-bearing sperm. Methods that attempt to separate sperm on the basis of head size, surface charge, or swimming ability have also been ineffective.

A method known as albumin separation has shown some success. In this technique the ejaculate is diluted with equal parts of Tyrode's solution. The diluted specimen is divided into 0.5-ml quantities of washed sperm. The washed sperm are then layered over a 7.5-percent salt-poor human serum albumin medium for 1 hour in a 8 × 75 mm glass column. The sperm layer is then removed by pipette, and the albumin is centrifuged at 2800–3200 rpm for 10 minutes. The sperm are resuspended in the Tyrode's solution and layered over a two-layer column (12.5 percent at the top and 20 percent at the bottom) of human serum albumin. The sperm layer is removed and after a further 30 minutes the 12.5-percent layer is removed. The 20-percent human serum albumin is centrifuged for 10 minutes and the sperm dish is resuspended in 0.25-ml Tyrode's solution, which is finally inseminated high into the cervix. The success rate reported using this three-step, three-layer method is approximately 75 percent male babies. It is noteworthy that women treated with clomid (a nonsteroid compound used to induce labor in anovulatory women) deliver a higher proportion of females in spite of being inseminated with separated sperm (Beernink and Ericsson, 1982).

Techniques such as fluorescence cell sorting are being developed that can identify the sex of a baby as early as 47 days after conception. It has been speculated that some day a pregnant woman may be able to learn the sex of her baby by testing a small amount of blood from a self-administered finger prick (Feil et al., 1984).

An immunological method has also been tried in laboratory mice. In this procedure the female is immunized against proteins (H–Y antigens existing only in male cells and Y-bearing spermatazoa). Vaccination with cells containing these proteins will provoke female antibodies against Y-bearing spermatazoa. Results of studies indicate a slight increase in the number of females born in the vaccinated group. This technique could be used only to preselect girls (Hewitt, 1987).

Dietary methods of sex selection have also been tried, with both parents' dietary intake of certain minerals being studied. The dietary method of sex preselection is based on the dietary ratio of sodium and potassium to calcium and magnesium for a short time prior to conception. A ratio greater than 4 appears to favor boys, while a ratio between 2.8 and 4.0 favors girls (Hewitt, 1987). This method has been said to be 80 percent effective.

Although highly controversial, selective termination of pregnancy as a means of sex selection is almost totally accurate. However, finding out the sex of the fetus requires amniocentesis, which involves certain risks. It cannot be performed before the 15th week of pregnancy. Measuring the testosterone level of the amniotic fluid extracted by amniocentesis is not always accurate. In order to determine the sex of a baby accurately, chromosome studies are needed, and these generally require 2–3 weeks of cell culture for results. With this time lapse, the pregnancy is already near the second trimester, and even proponents of abortion would question the advisability of terminating a normal pregnancy at this stage for reasons of sex selection.

Although it may not be unreasonable to want a child of a particular sex, some experts charge that widespread sex selection could introduce a gross disturbance of the human population structure with adverse social effects. According to one study of 53 women found to be carrying male babies, only one chose abortion, whereas of 47 women carrying girls, 29 chose abortion (Jones, 1977). In China, 100 cases of fetal sex were examined. The sex was wrongly predicted in 6, another 4 ended in spontaneous abortion, and 30 pregnancies were voluntarily terminated, 29 of them girls. Thus, society's preference for males could lead to an imbalance in the population if sex selection were used indiscriminately ("Choosing baby's sex", 1980).

In the future, choosing the sex of a baby by preselection may be available to all. Nurses need to be aware of the scientific advances being made in this area so that they will be able to act as a resource for couples seeking information about sex selection.

Genetic Engineering

Genetic engineering is any artificial process that alters the genetic make-up of an organism or its offspring. It is a process whereby specific genes can be added to or removed from an organism. Recently, experiments to determine how genes work in human beings and other organisms have increased scientific understanding about gene function. This research could be beneficial in developing new ways of treating genetic diseases and other illnesses.

Cloning is the reproduction in a laboratory of an entire organism from a single cell. Although the use of cloning to mass produce human beings still remains within the realm of science fiction, scientists believe that this could become possible. Scientists have already cloned frogs successfully. The process begins with removing the nucleus of a frog egg, which contains the genetic material, and replacing it with the nucleus from one of the millions of cells from an adult frog. The egg with the transplanted nucleus develops into a frog with a set of genes identical to those of the donor. A single frog chosen for certain qualities could parent millions of cloned copies (Ausbel, Beckwith, and Janssen, 1974).

As yet, researchers have not cloned mammals successfully. However, some experts believe that the progress being made in the area of *in vitro* fertilization is a step toward the cloning of human beings. It has been suggested that the technology of *in vitro* fertilization could also be used to replace genetically defective embryos. Scientists have developed ways of removing the nuclei from mammalian cells and then fusing the cells into hybrids that then contain genetic information from both parent cells. Although these investigations are still in the early experimental stages, there is a distinct possibility that a human being could be born as the result of clonal reproduction. It has been predicted that if such technology continues in the nondirected manner that it has so far, a clonal human being could be born within 20–50 years (Ausbel, Beckwith, and Janssen, 1974).

The most dangerous aspects of genetic engineering are its potential misuses. Theoretically, it may become possible to mass produce identical human beings with the traits desired by laboratory administrators.

Of course, some aspects of genetic engineering might be very beneficial to society. Scientists have already transferred the gene for insulin into bacteria, and the altered bacteria have produced insulin. Using such a technique it may be possible to engineer bacteria that could produce human hormones, antibodies, and other proteins. In agriculture, genetic engineering might lead to the development of high-yield crops and livestock, which could help to expand the world's food supply.

According to Anderson (1986) many of the fears regarding genetic engineering or gene therapy are unfounded. He believes we are nowhere near developing master races or Frankenstein monsters, although he does agree that we should be concerned about possible misuses in the future. The best way to prevent the possible misuse of genetic engineering is through a well-informed public.

Gene therapy does have the potential for reducing the suffering and death caused by genetic diseases. At present, whether gene therapy should be initiated before or after birth, is under investigation. It is possible that a number of diseases, especially those involving the nervous system, could be reversed through prenatal gene therapy (Anderson, 1986).

Many geneticists and health care professionals believe the use of these new techniques should be limited to the eradication of serious genetic defects and diseases. Others believe genetic engineering should be used to reduce the world's population (Ausbel, Beckwith, and Janssen, 1974).

SUMMARY

Society is changing rapidly, and this has affected maternity nursing today. The nurse should be aware of changes in societal expectations during the childbearing years and of the implications for nursing and childbearing families of such practices as homosexual parenting, single-parent families, adoption, surrogate mothers, *in vitro* fertilization, artificial insemination, sex selection, and genetic engineering.

REFERENCES

American Medical Association. 1982. Health care needs of a homosexual population. *JAMA*. Council Report, August 13.

Anderson, W. 1986. Prospects for human gene therapy in the born and unborn patient. *Clin. Obstet. Gynecol.* 29(3):586–594.

Ausbel, F.; Beckwith, J.; and Janssen, K. 1974. The politics of genetic engineering: Who decides who's defective? *Psych. Today.* June:30–43.

Beernink, F. J., and Ericsson, R. J. 1982. Male sex preselection through sperm isolation. *Fertility and Sterility.* 38(4):493–495.

Choosing baby's sex. 1980. *Brit. Med. J.* Feb.:272–273.

Cohen, B. 1984. Surrogate mothers: Whose baby is it? *Am. J. Law Med.* 10(3):243–285.

Dunston, G. R. 1975. Ethical aspects of donor insemination. *J. Med. Ethics.* April 41–44.

Duvall, E. M. 1977. *Marriage and family development.* Philadelphia: J. B. Lippincott.

El Paso Times. 1988. February 4.

Feil, R. N.; Largey, G. P.; and Miller, M. 1984. Attitudes toward abortion as a means of sex selection. *Am. J. Psych.* 116:269–272.

Fitzgerald, J. 1975. *Right and birth by artificial insemination.* Richmond, VA: Commonwealth University Press.

Franks, D. D. 1981. Psychiatric evaluation of women in a surrogate mother program. *Am. J. Psych.* 138(10): 1378–1379.

Garcia, J. E. 1985. *In vitro* fertilization. *Obstet. Gynecol. Ann.* 14:45–72.

Garner, C. H. 1983. *In vitro* fertilization and embryo transfer. *J. Obstet. Gynecol. Neonatal Nurs.* 12(2): 75–78.

Goldenberg, R., and White, R. 1976. Artificial insemination. *Connecticut Med. J.* 40(3).

Gomel, V. 1983. An odyssey through the oviduct. *Fertility and Sterility.* 39(2):144–156.

Harris, M. 1981. *America now.* New York: Simon and Schuster.

Herman, E., and Annas, G. J. 1986. Social policy considerations in noncoital reproduction. *JAMA.* 255(1):62–68.

Hewitt, J. 1987. Preconceptional sex selection. 12(3):149, 151–152, 154–155.

Horne, H. 1976. Editorial. *New Engl. J. Med.* October. Horowitz, A.; Hughes, C. B.; and Perdue, B. J. 1982. *Parenting reassessed: A nursing perspective.* Englewood Cliffs, N.J.: Prentice-Hall.

Huxley, A. 1956. *Brave new world.* New York: Modern Library.

Jones, G. 1977. Experts argue blueprints of life at UTEP symposium on genetics. *El Paso Times.* September 21.

Kreitman, O., and Hodgen, G. D. 1980. Low tubal ovum transfer: An alternative to *in vitro* fertilization. *Fertility and Sterility.* 34(4):375–378.

Krimmael, H. T. 1983. The case against surrogate parenting. *The Hastings Center Report.* October: 36–39.

Pakalnis, L., and Makoroto, J. 1977. Reproduction and the test-tube baby. *Canadian Nurse.* February: 34–38.

Palca, J. 1987. US courts and legislatures face implications of surrogacy. *Nature.* 325:184.

Peckins, D. 1976. Artificial insemination and the law. *J. Legal Med.* 4(7):17–22.

Rubenstein, A., et al. 1983. Acquired immune deficiency with reserved T4/T8 ratios in infants born to promiscuous drug addicted mothers. *JAMA.* 249:2350–2352.

Ryan, Father K. 1983. What would you like to know about the Church? *Catholic Digest.* January:100–103.

San Francisco Chronicle. 1988. May 24.

Simcork, B. W. 1985. Sons and daughters—A sex preselection study. *Med. J. Australia.* 142:541–542.

Steptoe, P., and Edwards, R. 1983. Pregnancy in an infertile patient after transfer of an embryo fertilized *in vitro. Brit. Med. J.* 286:1351.

Strickler, R.; Keller, D. W.; and Warren, J. C. 1975. Artificial insemination with fresh donor semen. *New Engl. J. Med.* October:135–138.

Williams, G. 1974. *The sanctity of life and the criminal law.* New York: Alfred A. Knopf.

Yinger, J. M., and Cutler, S. J. 1978. *Major social issues.* New York: Free Press.

6

Cultural Aspects of Childbearing

BEHAVIORAL OBJECTIVES

Upon completion of this chapter, the reader should be able to:

- Describe the characteristics common to the formation and function of all cultures.

- Describe aspects of an individual's life that are culture-dependent.

- Describe areas of variations that occur within and between cultures.

- Discuss the relationship of an individual's culture to her definition of the birth experience.

- Discuss elements of society's expectations for behavior related to pregnancy, birth, the postpartum period, and care of the newborn.

- Determine at least one framework within which the nurse can effectively identify an individual's cultural orientation.

- Discuss the general considerations of nursing or caring for persons of any culture that is different from the caregiver's own.

- Apply the Kay-Galenic or Newton framework to a family of the reader's choice.

- Describe the nurse's role when working with families from diverse cultures.

Culture is the essence of our being. It is the element in our lives that assists us as unique individuals to adapt to membership in our life group. The act of brushing our teeth, the foods we prefer, the language we speak, and the religion we practice are all dictated by our cultural patterning. *Cultural patterning* refers to the process of an individual's orientation to and adoption of the beliefs and practices of a specific group.

An individual's perceptions of illness and health and the behaviors associated with these states are culturally influenced. All societies have certain sets of accepted explanations of birth, illness, and death, with approved practices for the treatment and alleviation of symptoms for each. Because cultural belief systems influence an individual's recognition of illness and selection of health care providers and practices, assessment of cultural beliefs and behaviors is important for the health care professional with a holistic approach to health care. Faced with the demands of providing health care to people from all economic levels, to culturally diverse communities, and to mobile populations, nurses must determine ways to assess cultural patterning and to provide effective care for those persons whose cultural orientations may differ from their own.

In this chapter, emphasis is placed on cultural characteristics that can be assessed for any given group and on the use of this knowledge once it has been obtained. The information presented in this chapter will assist the reader in developing an awareness of the influence of culture on health practices (most specifically during the childbearing period) and in developing the ability to provide individualized health care.

CULTURE

Culture can be defined as "the totality of all the learned and transmitted behaviors of a particular group" (Leininger, 1970). It has also been defined as the socially transmitted system of idealized ways in knowledge, practice, and beliefs along with the artifacts that knowledge and practice produce and maintain as they change in time (Vernon, 1972). Our culture is how we live with ourselves and our birth group as the result of cultural patterning.

There are certain defining characteristics common to the formation and function of all cultures:

1. *All culture is manufactured.* Humans themselves create it. Wherever people settle, they develop patterns for organizing their behavior, relating to others, utilizing natural resources, and creating a meaningful life; culture functions rather like a security blanket (Johnston, 1980).
2. *Culture is learned.* It is not transmitted biologically or genetically but rather through human inteaction. Verbally, it is transmitted through language; nonverbally, it is transmitted through behavior.
3. *Culture is the common property of the group.* It is shared by all group members. No individual knows all of the definitions in his or her group. Children are not taught the entire range of potential human behavior but rather a limited number of behavioral patterns that are appropriate to that group (Johnston, 1980).
4. *Culture is cumulative.* The term *culture* is derived from the Latin word meaning "to grow". Although each group has numerous standardized definitions that it transmits to all new members, each member adds new definitions to these standards throughout his or her lifetime (Rackovsky, 1980).
5. *Culture is constantly changing.* No cultural belief or practice remains static. Changes are usually relatively slow and occur over long periods of time, but they may also occur almost overnight. In general, an observable behavior does not change without a similar change in the belief underlying the behavior.
6. *Culture involves emotional behavior as well as physical behavior.* Beliefs and attitudes underlie behaviors and practices. Culture is so much a part of a person that it becomes a way of thinking and feeling. It decides the person's sense of right and wrong and his or her purpose in life (Rackovsky, 1980).
7. *Culture is integrated and systematized.* Various definitions, beliefs, and practices are interrelated in a logical and reasonable manner. No belief, practice, or custom can function or exist without affecting all the individual's other beliefs and practices (Vernon, 1972).

Until recent years, nursing theory and practice have been presented and performed as if all patients are white, Christian, and of European ancestry (Ruiz, 1981). There has been little acknowledgment or concern by the nursing profession for the relationship between patients' cultural beliefs and their behavior in the health care system. The prevailing philosophy has been that to provide equal care to patients, all patients should be given the same care. Studies in the fields of anthropology, psychology, and sociology, however, give evidence to nursing that patients are done a great disservice when their cultural background is ignored.

Scientific research examines human behavior in an attempt to understand the beliefs and attitudes underlying health customs and practices. By studying these beliefs and attitudes, researchers can arrive at explanations for the cultural solutions to physical problems devised by groups or societies. Such studies attempt to account for similarities and differences in customs of societies and to compare their solutions to problems with those of modern medicine (Kay, 1982).

Comparative studies in the realm of childbearing (Newton, 1970) have effectively identified the relationship of environmental changes to the birthing process by linking findings from the fields of anthropology and psychology. This practice of joining scientific fields, especially nursing and anthropology, can assist the nurse in predicting human motivations and action patterns (Leininger, 1980). There is always a need for research in all scientific fields to effectively broaden the body of knowledge concerning the biopsychosocial event of childbirth (Jordan, 1980).

HOW INDIVIDUALS EXPERIENCE CULTURE

All individuals experience culture as the result of attitudes and behaviors learned through cultural patterning. People's perceptions of their surroundings, their experiences, and their interactions are directly influenced by their expectations of what these will be. Expectations are the outcome of the socialization process of each member of a given group—a process that begins in infancy and continues throughout life (Smoyak, 1968). A person's behavior is extensively influenced by the cultural orientation of his or her life group.

Culture dictates such behaviors as language spoken, foods preferred, and religious ceremonies practiced, and it specifies how each family member is treated, who is talked to and worked with, where the ill are cared for, how many children are acceptable within the family, and how children are reared. Yet, the individual is rarely consciously aware of the influence of culture.

Because no individual knows all the cultural definitions of his life group, variations can and do exist within groups. Such variations usually exist because of differences in age, religion, dialect spoken, gender role, socioeconomic background, geographic location of the group in the country of origin and the country of residence, history of the group, contact of the younger generation with older group relatives, or adoption by the group of values of the country of residence (Orque, 1981).

If a nurse from one group is caring for a patient from another group and the patient's expectations of health care are different from those of the nurse, an incongruence in socialization can be said to exist (Smoyak, 1968). The result is role conflict or ambivalence. Role ambivalence surfaces in the form of behavioral conflicts between patient reactions and the expectations of the health care provider

Armed with the knowledge of what to assess, the framework for assessment, suggestions for intervention, and guidelines for evaluation, nurses can develop an awareness of their own cultural orientation and that of their patients and will better be able to identify both similarities and differences. As a result, nurses may be more open-minded in providing care for persons from cultures other than their own, decreasing the possibility of illogical or premature generalizations and thereby preventing patient role conflict or role ambivalence (Deutsch, 1971).

CULTURE'S ROLE IN CHILDBEARING

Culture is especially significant in the childbearing process, because it defines the meaning of the experience and dictates how those involved are to react to the events (Clark and Affonso, 1979). In no known culture is pregnancy ignored or treated with indifference. Instead, it invariably elicits a variety of emotions and feelings. Cultural values and beliefs about childbearing touch every aspect of social life. It appears that all cultures have beliefs concerning appropriate behavior throughout pregnancy, labor and delivery, and the puerperium. Cultural patterning regulates such aspects as spacing of children, diet during pregnancy, support given the woman during childbearing, drugs allowed during labor, and immediate care of the newborn, as well as dictating attitudes about childbearing in general (Richardson and Guttmacher, 1967). To provide holistic, family-centered care, the nurse must, therefore, be aware of the woman's cultural orientation from preconceptual planning through the family's adjustment to the neonate.

SOCIETY'S EXPECTATIONS FOR BEHAVIOR

Individuals view pregnancy within the context of their cultural environment. All societies tend to regard pregnancy as a significant biological event and to ritualize it. They also recognize certain critical psychologic and social aspects of childbirth, including the parents' role during pregnancy, maternal emotional responses during pregnancy and labor, the father's role during pregnancy and labor, parental–infant bonding and attachment, and supporting behaviors expected from family and friends (Simmons, 1952).

Until recently, in the United States stress was placed on the physical event of pregnancy, whereas in primitive societies people tended to emphasize the psychosocial spheres. Pregnancy was strictly "women's work" in America. The expectant father had little to do with the pregnancy until the day of birth. His job was then to get his wife to the hospital, pace the hospital waiting room, and wait for the nurse's report on the sex and health of the infant and the health of the mother. It was rare for the father to be present at the birth (Shapiro, 1987). During modern times, however, this emphasis is shifting. More stress is being placed on prenatal preparation by parents through the use of childbirth preparation classes. Society expects fathers to play an increasingly large role both during pregnancy and birth, and in child-care. New meanings are being applied to the phrase "helping around the house." Yet, establishing psychologic and social rules in a society with a rapidly changing cultural pattern proves to be difficult, as the reader will see in the following sections.

Family Planning

There is a direct relationship between a country's industrial development and its economy. In turn, economic factors play a major role in how a culture views pregnancy and childbearing, and these views directly influence the group's acceptance of the concept of family planning. The United States provides an excellent example of a culture within which the economic factors of industrialization and inflation resulted in a major shift from a procreative imperative to a family planning concept.

The marital and procreative imperative was the accepted way of life in America after the Industrial Revolution and prior to the Second World War. Because sex was confined to marriage, everyone got married. The major functions of marriage were considered to be reproduction and childbearing. Those wanting to experience sexual pleasure were expected to fulfill certain duties and responsibilities. This suited the government, churches, and employers, who desired a rising birth rate for a pool of cheap labor. It also allowed the male to remain the breadwinner and kept male wages higher by preventing competition from female workers.

During this time, most of the jobs available to women were part-time temporary, and poorly paid. Married women who were working did so to supplement their breadwinner-husband's income or to purchase specific products deemed important for a decent standard of living (Harris, 1981). This pattern continued until the early 1960s.

A decisive break came in the early 1960s, with the beginning of the Great Inflation. At that time, many jobs specifically suited for women opened up. The jobs were either low-level information processing or low-level people processing. Most were situated within or dependent upon some branch of government or the bureaucracy of some large corporation. The call-up of women for duty in the service-job market resembled the call-up of women into manufacturing early in the Industrial Revolution, except that this call-up did not threaten the livelihood of the male worker. By this time, parents were finding it increasingly difficult to achieve or hold on to the middle-class standard of consumption without the help of the wife's income.

With the need for women to continue to work and the expense of raising children increasing, government and society realized that a rising birth rate could no longer be considered an asset. The need to plan for each additional child was stressed; the result was a reduction in the population growth. The fertility rate began a historic plunge, reaching zero population growth in 1972 and falling to an average of 1.8 children per woman by 1980. Generally speaking, in the United States, the lifetime, male-dominated, two-parent, multichild family has virtually ceased to exist (Harris, 1981).

Many societies still place great social and economic value on the woman's role as childbearer. Because women in traditional cultures have few means of increasing their self-esteem, the experience of pregnancy is considered to be the greatest opportunity for her to actualize her potential (Meleis and Sorrell, 1981). Child spacing practices therefore have strong cultural underpinnings that make it necessary to assess each person's attitudes concerning the value of children, the importance of the childbearing role, and the acceptance of the planning process.

Pregnancy

It is a natural biologic function for women to give birth, and most expectant mothers do not view themselves as being ill. Even so, many of the signs and symptoms a woman experiences during pregnancy would indicate illness under other circumstances, and these symptoms usually bring the woman in contact with health professionals. As a result, pregnancy is often labeled as an illness, and pregnant women are expected to adopt the role of patient. They are expected to act in an appropriate manner by seeking and accepting appropriate professional prenatal care (Bond and Bond, 1980).

Prenatal Management

The most prominent feeling about pregnancy is a sense of responsibility for the safe development of the fetus. This feeling is the basis for the many prescribed regulations and prohibitions of behaviors for both the mother and father. These regulations are based on the belief that the parents' values and practices will affect the fetus and will make the difference between a normal and a difficult birth outcome. In the United States, the value placed on a healthy outcome is probably the primary factor responsible for the woman's seeking of prenatal care, through either a physician, an outpatient clinic, or a hospital. Additionally, parents are expected to participate in the aforementioned childbirth education programs in order to assure as healthy an outcome as possible.

Intrapartal Management

Most cultures have conditions and techniques for giving birth that vary greatly from those practices found in Western societies (Johnston, 1980). Between 1906 and 1935, the event of childbirth in the Western world was moved from the home to the hospital. The routine use of sedatives, analgesics, and anesthesia accompanied this move. Subsequently, childbirth became labeled an "illness" and pregnant women became patients. In an attempt to correct the high maternal mortality rate, hospitals emphasized cleanliness, fewer persons present during labor and delivery, and techniques such as perineal shaving. Currently, the laboring mother is generally confined to bed for the major portion of her labor. Emphasis continues to be placed on constant maternal and fetal monitoring, no food or drink allowed the laboring mother, the use of an episiotomy and forceps for delivery, and a recumbent position for giving birth (Roberts, 1979).

It could be said that these practices continue for the safety of the baby and mother, but this is not necessarily true. In 1981, McVicar said that there were more women having babies in this decade that were in the low-risk category than ever before (Orr et al., 1987).

In most other cultures expectant mothers do not view themselves as ailing and, therefore, they support home deliveries, spontaneous birth without operational intervention, and (in many cultures) an upright position for delivery (Liu, 1979).

The use of medication during labor and delivery is not a new or modern practice. Many primitive cultures have used labor stimulants as well as drugs for pain relief during labor and delivery. The acceptability of the practice of using medication during labor is culturally controlled, and use of medication is a common practice in hospitals in Western societies.

In all known societies access to delivery is limited to a rigidly specified group of people. Most frequently, children and men are excluded (sometimes with the exception of the husband or a male childbirth specialist), as are women who have not themselves had children (Jordan, 1980). However, Western societies, including the United States, now stress the importance of the presence of the father during the labor and delivery process. It is the rare "American" husband or hospital that expects the father to be absent during labor and delivery.

Physical contact with the laboring woman remains of great significance in most cultures. Typically, the contact differs in terms of degree, type, and purpose. In the past, as well as in most primitive cultures, touch was generally used to relieve pain, support the position, or enhance uterine action. In the United States today, touch is most generally used as a means of communicating psychosocial support to the laboring woman and to provide relaxation, distraction, and pain relief (Hedstrom and Newton, 1986).

Postpartal Management

The majority of societies prescribe giving a great deal of indulgent care to the woman after delivery. In Western societies, the move is away from pampering and toward early postpartal ambulation, however. The new emphasis is on teaching soon after delivery, with the desired outcome being for effective, independent care of self and the newborn, and early dismissal from the hospital.

Management of the Newborn

Many cultures, both modern and primitive, emphasize physical closeness of the mothers and newborn soon after delivery. How a society views maternal–infant attachment, to a great degree, dictates the type of feeding promoted by the culture, immediate post-delivery care practices, and activities of immediate care of the newborn. In the United States, practices such as formula feeding, 4-hour scheduled feedings, and early weaning emphasized in the 1960s and 1970s reflected technological changes that changed the role of women. A recent return to "naturalism," though, has encouraged a move back to more traditional practices, including breastfeeding—usually "on demand" (Stanton, 1979)—and the continuance of nursing following the woman's return to work.

The mother is still the major care provider for the newborn in most societies, including the United States. Noteworthy exceptions are the black American family, where any relative may become the primary caregiver (May, 1979) and the Chinese in Taiwan, where the mother-in-law is the primary caregiver for some time following the birth.

Guidelines For Nurses

The pregnant woman's cultural background affects the way in which she reacts to health care regardless of the point at which she enters the health care system. The nursing process—assessment, planning, intervention, and evaluation—provides the nurse with a systematic method of determining the reasons underlying a patient's behavior and thereby allows the nurse to understand and respond appropriately.

Components of a Cultural System

Assessment of childbearing practices should focus on four components of a cultural system:

1. The *value system*, which prescribes conduct involving the notions of duty, desirability, and obligations.
2. The *kinship system*, which refers to categories of rights, duties, and obligations of role behavior in marriage and family life.
3. The *knowledge and belief system*, which defines the processes of conception, pregnancy, labor, and childbearing.
4. The *ceremonial and ritual system*, which provides the means for people to re-enact a part of their culture and allows for the incorporation of meaning into their daily lives (Aamodt, 1979).

These four systems function simultaneously.

Two tools for assessing the client's cultural orientation that incorporate these four components are the Kay-Galenic framework and the Newton framework.

The Kay-Galenic Framework

Margarita Kay (1982) combined her knowledge of organized behavior with a model developed by Galen in the second century after Christ to develop a framework for analyzing the childbearing experience. As an ethnographer (one who studies the races of mankind), Kay has, since 1965, been observing people and participating as much as possible in their daily lives. In so doing, she has established categories of behavior throughout the childbearing process that are common to all societies. She has discovered that cultures have distinctive differences in behaviors and beliefs within several categories that help distinguish them from one another.

Galen's model is based on the management of extrinsic (external to the body) factors that are common to all societies. These extrinsic factors include six categories for assessment:

1. Air and water.
2. Food and drink.
3. Sleep and wakefulness.
4. Movement, exercise, and rest.

5. Evacuation and retention.
6. Passions of the spirit or emotions.

The resultant Kay-Galenic framework provides a method of assessment that can help the caregiver determine the attitudes and beliefs underlying patient behaviors, thereby yielding an analysis of the woman's cultural orientation related to the childbearing process.

Prenatal Period

The Kay-Galenic framework suggests obtaining attitudinal and behavioral information to learn as much as possible about how a specific culture feels about pregnancy. The following questions can help with data collection for the prenatal period:

- Who is permitted to get pregnant?
- Should marriage precede pregnancy?
- What is the acceptable age range for pregnancy?
- By whom may a woman get pregnant?
- How many times should a woman be pregnant?
- How closely should her pregnancies be spaced?

A society's acceptance of pregnancy is based on the value it places on children and how it views the maternal role of childbearer. In societies where children are valued as assets and the role of childbearer is seen as a means for the woman to establish self-esteem, families are large. When the reverse is true, the nuclear family is comparatively small. The caregiver who strives to teach family planning to an Arab-American or Mexican-American family will probably become very frustrated, since those cultures place great value on children and on large families. The experience of pregnancy is considered to be the greatest opportunity for the Arab or Mexican woman to actualize her potential and to increase her self-esteem (Kay, 1979; Meleis and Sorrell, 1981). The opposite is true in China, where low value is placed on the woman's role as childbearer and emphasis is instead on the woman's ability to serve society as a worker. Pregnancies beyond the first-born are usually terminated by abortion (Iorio and Nelson, 1983; Wang, 1985).

In the United States, teenage pregnancies are on the increase: in 1983, 35 percent of sexually active females became pregnant before the age of 19 and, of these, 59 percent proceeded to delivery. Approximately 90 percent of adolescent mothers (both married and unmarried) kept their babies (Horn, 1983). Cultural beliefs about the prevention of pregnancy and contraceptives, the significance of being a mother at an early age, and the kinds of support systems available to them within their own social network, are influential in the adolescent becoming pregnant—and during their pregnancy (Mott, 1986). In Western nations, unwed mothers are able to raise their children with few repercussions, whereas the social and cultural climate of Taiwan, for example, makes life intolerable for the unwed mother (Wang, 1985); hence, most pregnancies are terminated.

A culture's acceptance of family planning is also dependent on its acceptance of planning processes in general. Most Arab-Americans are oriented to the present. Planning ahead has the potential of defying God's will and therefore bringing about unanticipated disappointments. When contraception is practiced, intrauterine devices (IUDs) or abortions are likely to be preferred (Meleis and Sorrell, 1981). In contrast, the overpopulation problem in China has led the government to encourage couples to bear only one child. If there is more than one pregnancy, 3–5 years are expected to pass between births (Iorio and Nelson, 1983).

Besides population concerns, socioeconomic background, marital status at first birth, and the degree to which the first child was wanted, greatly affect how quickly another pregnancy occurs. The age of the mother when she first gave birth is also important. In the United States, young women who gave birth to their first child at age 16 or younger are more likely to have a second child within 2 years than are those who were either aged 17–18 or 19–22 when they had their first child.

Using Galen's model, Kay incorporated pregnancy-related questions to form the Kay-Galenic framework, which can be used to identify cultural differences.

AIR AND WATER

- What is considered a desirable environment for the mother?
- Should air and water be hot or cold?
- What parts of the pregnant woman's body may be touched by water?
- What kind of water can be used?

Mexican-Americans believe that exposures to the forces of nature can cause childbearing complications. They believe, for example, that a pregnant woman can prevent her infant from being born with anomalies after she has been exposed to a lunar eclipse by wearing a *cinta*, a belt of keys, over her womb (Abril, 1977). The Vietnamese and the

Pueblo women of New Mexico believe that it is unhealthy for both mother and child to be in the prescence of the dying or to attend funerals. Indeed, the baby may cry inconsolably afterwards (Hollingsworth, Brown, and Brooten, 1980; Higgins, 1983).

Many Spanish-speaking people believe that the pregnant woman should avoid cool air that is in motion. Encouraging her to get fresh air if it is spring, fall, or winter may fall on deaf ears. Bathing is encouraged, but the water should never be cool (Kay, 1979).

FOOD AND DRINK

- What can the pregnant woman have?
- What must she have?
- What must she avoid?

Although pregnancy is considered a natural process by the Vietnamese, women observe certain taboos and special customs. The pregnant woman must eat nourishing foods and avoid "unclean" ones such as beef, dog, pork, and snake meat. Some of these foods are eaten in her native country. She should not smoke or drink. Prescribing a diet that stresses beef and pork would be very ineffective with Vietnamese women. However, pork is preferred in the postpartal period. Pueblo women also have certain taboos relating to food. For example, though herbs, medicines, and teas are thought to relieve the discomforts of pregnancy and enhance the pregnant woman's health, berries are not to be consumed because they are believed to cause birthmarks. Precautions regarding food must also be taken by the father, e.g. albinism is thought to be caused by the father eating the white leaf inside corn husks prior to conception (Higgins, 1983).

Many Spanish-speaking people classify foods, practices, and medicines according to the hot–cold theory. This theory stems from the ancient humoral typology that classifies body fluids as either hot or cold. A "hot" body state, for example, is counteracted by eating cold foods. Conversely, hot foods are avoided during pregnancy to prevent the fetus from being born with red skin or a rash; "cool" preparations are essential (Murillo-Rohde, 1980). Examples of hot and very hot foods to be avoided are white beans, chili, garlic, fish, pork, turkey, onion, potato, wheat bread, rice, chocolate, coffee, salt, sugar, honey, and sweet rolls. Examples of cold and very cold foods to be eaten are beef, lamb, rabbit, chicken, green beans, beets, peas, radishes, oatmeal, cucumber, limes, oranges, tomatoes, spinach, and mutton (Bringas and Chan, 1979). Milk is to be avoided, as it is believed to cause the fetus to grow too large, resulting in a difficult delivery. The nurse who is aware of this belief might consider an extra dietary supplement of calcium for Mexican-American mothers.

SLEEP AND WAKEFULNESS

- How much sleep should the pregnant woman get?
- In what position should she sleep?

Mexican-Americans believe that a pregnant woman tends to need more sleep but that if she gives in to the desire for extra sleep, she will have a difficult delivery. She is also expected to sleep on her back in order to protect the fetus (Kay, 1979). A knowledge of these attitudes will allow the nurse to understand why the Mexican-American mother with supine hypotension persists in lying on her back against the advice of the nurse and the physician.

MOVEMENT, EXERCISE, AND REST

- What movement is desirable?
- What is dangerous?
- What is prescribed?
- Is massage given?

The Vietnamese, like many other cultures (Hollingsworth, Brown, and Brooten, 1980; Turrell, 1985; Stern, Tilden, and Maxwell, 1985), believe that the pregnant woman should avoid all strenuous activity. She is also to act and talk at all times as if the fetus were observing her, thus carrying out a type of "prenatal education" by counseling the fetus in physical, moral, and intellectual activities (Hollingsworth, Brown, and Brooten, 1980).

To the Mexican-American, massage is an important part of prenatal care that helps fix the fetus in a position that is favorable for delivery (Kay, 1979).

EVACUATION AND RETENTION

- What attention is given to body excrement?
- What is believed to be healthy or pathologic in urination, defecation, sweating, salivating, or mucus secretion?

The pregnant Mexican-American woman "refreshes" herself repeatedly by taking milk of magnesia (1–3 tablespoons a day) or an antacid (2–4 doses a day) during the first two trimesters of pregnancy (Murillo-Rohde, 1980).

PASSIONS OF THE SPIRIT OR EMOTIONS

- What emotional expression is permitted?
- What parts of the body may be seen?
- Which parts may be touched by the mother, by her mate, and by the person giving health care?

The pregnant Vietnamese woman abstains from sexual intercourse during the later part of her pregnancy. A special bed is prepared in a relatively private part of the house designated by an astrologer as the place with the best protection against winds that might carry evil spirits (Hollingsworth, Brown, and Brooten, 1980).

The Jewish pregnant woman avoids planning for the baby in advance, fearing that if the Angel of Death even hears the infant's name prior to its official naming, the baby might be taken (die) (Bash, 1980). The nurse should not be concerned, therefore, when she discovers that the mother has not prepared the nursery, even in the third trimester.

Jewish, Mexican-American, and Arab-American pregnant women are expected to manifest modesty at all times. Many seek nurse-midwives because they do not want their bodies viewed by a strange man. Islamic law prescribes to women from India, Pakistan, and Bangladesh that there should be no physical contact between themself and any other man besides their husband. This can be overcome only if the health care worker is of a nationality or religion other than their own (Turrell, 1985). Special care should be taken to protect their privacy.

It is a belief among Hispanics, Amish, Hutterites, and both whites and blacks in the South that even the mother's superficial emotional states can affect the fetus. For example, feelings of hate for an individual may cause the infant to resemble that person, or if the mother sees someone having a seizure and feels pity for him, her child may suffer seizures. A similar resemblance may result if the pregnant woman worries about a loved one with a particular health problem (Johnston, 1980).

Intrapartal Period

In an effort to be supportive during the intrapartal period, it is important for the nurse to ask questions that will produce specific answers about how a certain cultural group feels regarding the labor process.

- What is believed to cause labor?
- When should labor occur?
- Where should labor take place?
- How long is labor perceived to last, and what length is desirable?
- Who can touch the laboring woman, how, and where?

For most traditional cultures, labor is expected to take place in the "home". Even in developed, industrialized countries, including the United States, women living in rural areas choose to labor at home. The trend, in general, is away from the hospital setting and toward birthing clinics or private homes.

In most traditional or primitive cultures, it is felt that the woman's body knows best—that given enough time, nature will take its course. Labor will progress to delivery without medical intervention. A wait-and-see attitude is taken (Jordan, 1980). Thus, attempts on the part of the physician to stimulate or manipulate labor may be met with great disapproval.

In many primitive cultures, touch is used to provide the laboring mother with physical support, massage (ranging from light tickling to a firmness intended to increase the force of uterine contractions), and compression of the abdomen to help express the fetus. It is usually the mother's helper who provides this touch, e.g. the husband, the mother's mother, or a midwife. In the Mayan culture it is the husband or a female attendant, in Cambodia it is usually the husband, and among the Hmong of Laos the husband physically supports his wife during both labor and delivery (Hedstrom and Newton, 1986; La Du, 1985). Many aspects of touch are now being taught in the United States.

Following the Kay-Galenic framework, cultural beliefs about the intrapartal period can be determined by asking questions in the six main categories.

AIR AND WATER

- Is air dangerous?
- Is a bath allowed?

The Mexican-American and the Vietnamese

woman is expected to continue to avoid cool air and cool water throughout labor.

FOOD AND DRINK

- What will retard the process of labor?
- What will encourage birth?
- What is considered dangerous?

The British custom is to have three meals a day during labor (Clark and Affonso, 1979). The Mexican-American laboring mother drinks chamomile tea to ensure effective labor and uncomplicated separation of the placenta (Kay, 1979). Pueblo women drink hot tea that is made from toasted juniper twigs and berries steeped in boiling water at the beginning of labor to relax the system (Higgins, 1983).

SLEEP AND WAKEFULNESS

- Should sleep between contractions be encouraged?
- Should medicine be taken to prevent wakefulness?

The Vietnamese woman in labor will not request pain medication and is expected to smile throughout the process. This is a reflection of Buddhist teaching, which prohibits the expression of strong emotions (Hollingsworth, Brown, and Brooten, 1980). In contrast, pain tolerance in Arab-American women seems low, and they moan, cry, and scream during labor and delivery. If pain medication other than epidural or spinal anesthesia (which they fear) is offered, it will readily be accepted (Meleis and Sorrell, 1981). This is also true of Nigerian women.

Mexican-American women believe that pain is to be endured with patience and that medication should not be taken to blot it out (Kay, 1979).

MOVEMENT, EXERCISE, AND REST

- What movement can be done during labor?

Laboring Southeast Asian and Mexican-American women prefer to walk around until the delivery is imminent (Gordon, Matousek, and Lang, 1980; Kay, 1979). The Mayan expectant mother (who lives in a society located on the peninsula of Yucatan, Mexico) prefers to labor and deliver lying crosswise in her matrimonial hammock (Jordan, 1980).

EVACUATION AND RETENTION

- May obstetric systems attend to evacuation in order to hasten birth?

Most traditional or primitive cultures do not approve of hastening labor in any way. Arab-American women might be fairly receptive to such labor manipulation, however, as they value treatments that are intrusive (Meleis and Sorrell, 1981).

PASSIONS OF THE SPIRIT OR EMOTIONS

- Is labor feared?

The Arab-American woman cries, moans, and screams during labor and delivery. She usually makes no attempt to prepare for childbirth and does not readily use breathing or relaxation techniques. Labor is an intense, frightening, and uncontrolled experience (Meleis and Sorrell, 1981). Nigerian women experience labor and delivery in much the same way. Trying to assist these women with modern breath control techniques can be very frustrating to the nurse whose cultural orientation dictates that the birthing experience should be endured with quiet control.

Birth

To learn more about how a specific cultural group feels about the birth process, the following questions should be addressed (Kay, 1982):

- Who can attend?
- Where should delivery take place?
- What is done to help with separation and expulsion of the placenta?
- What is done with the placenta?

Vietnamese husbands are not expected to participate in childbirth. A midwife attends to the birth in rural areas and a physician does so in urban hospitals (Hollingsworth, Brown, and Brooten, 1980).

The birth experience for Arab-American women is a female affair. A woman in labor wants her female relatives and friends present but not her husband or any other man (Meleis, 1981). The same is true for Mexican-American and Nigerian women.

Notable exceptions to the practice of male exclusion during labor and delivery are the Jewish and

Mayan cultures, where the woman's husband is expected to be present during the process. Whereas the Mayan husband is expected to see his mate suffer, the Jewish husband acts as his mate's advocate and protector, though he does not touch her during labor—a preset plan of verbal communication is arranged (Bash, 1980; Jordan, 1980).

For the Mayan expectant mother, delivery occurs in her matrimonial hammock in the home (Jordan, 1980). The Southeast Asian woman prefers to deliver squatting by the bed, whether at home or in the hospital (Gordon, Matousek, and Lang, 1980).

If medication is needed to contract the uterus in order to expel a retained placenta, many cultures advocate the use of fundal pressure or the inducement of vomiting instead.

Many cultures attach special meaning to the placenta and the caregivers should determine the desires of the mother and/or family regarding its disposal.

Postpartal Period

The following are key questions helpful in obtaining information about a specific culture's expectations regarding the postpartal period (Kay, 1982):

- When does the puerperium start and end?
- Is the postpartal woman secluded?
- If so, where?

The Hispanic mother observes a period of 40 days after the delivery during which she is not allowed to touch water, do heavy work, or have sexual intercourse (Murillo-Rohde, 1980). The Chinese mother is restricted to her home for a full month after the delivery to regain her strength. During this time she is cared for by family members (Iorio and Nelson, 1983).

In Arab-American families, children and relatives are expected to be part of all events and are encouraged to visit the new mother and baby as soon after the birth as possible (Meleis and Sorrell, 1981).

A maternity leave of absence from work is granted for 56 days after delivery in the Soviet Union. The leave may be extended if there were any complications during the delivery. The parents may decide whether the father or mother will take the majority of the postpartal leave (Gay, 1985).

In India, the wife returns to her parents' home and stays there for 40 days. The husband remains at his family home. The mother has no contact with other members of the family for she is considered to be unclean (Turrell, 1985).

Again, using Galen's extrinsic factors, Kay has suggested pertinent questions to ask during the postpartal period.

AIR AND WATER

- Is air desirable or dangerous?
- Where may air enter?
- How is the mother protected from air?
- When is a bath permitted?
- When may water be touched?
- Should water be hot or cold?
- What happens if the water taboo is ignored?

The Mexican-American mother's legs are placed together immediately after delivery to prevent air from entering the womb. She believes that the entry of air can cause the uterus to chill and that she must also protect her feet, head, and body from any cold air (Kay, 1979). The same is true for cold water, which should not be touched for 15 days after the delivery.

Southeast Asians believe that a bath taken prior to several weeks after delivery will lead to intestinal damage and will cause the mother to lose vital nutrients through her skin. Shampooing of the mother's hair is believed to cause the baby to "fall apart" and should not be done for several weeks after delivery (Hollingsworth, Brown, and Brooten, 1980).

Haitian-American women maintain a practice of baths, vapor baths, and dressing warmly during the postpartal period to become healthy and clean again after childbirth (Harris, 1987; Dempsey and Gesse, 1983).

FOOD AND DRINK

- What food and drink are required at this time?
- What foods and liquids are forbidden?

Hispanics avoid "cool" or "cold" foods to prevent the impediment of blood flow, which, it is believed, could prevent uterine involution (Murillo-Rohde, 1980).

Vietnamese mothers prefer rice, pork, and chicken during the postpartal period. They believe that salty foods and pork stews restore strength, that all foods should be physically hot to counteract heat loss that occurred during labor and delivery, and that physically cold foods are bad for teeth and increase heat loss. Because beef and seafoods are believed to cause itching of the episiotomy, they are forbidden until 6 months after delivery. Water is restricted, to prevent stretching of the stomach (Hollingsworth, Brown, and Brooten, 1980).

The Hmong of Laos believe that the postpartal woman should adhere to a strict diet of chicken cooked in water, rice, and black pepper. The diet is to be utilized for 30 days following the delivery (La Du, 1985).

SLEEP AND WAKEFULNESS

- What sleep is prescribed?

Most cultures encourage rest and sleep during at least the first few days following delivery.

MOVEMENT, EXERCISE, AND REST

- What movement is prescribed?
- What activity is forbidden?
- What rest is required and discouraged?

The Vietnamese discourage early ambulation, as it is believed to cause stretching of the stomach. Sexual relations are not resumed for 2–3 months after delivery (Hollingsworth, Brown, and Brooten, 1980).

Mexican-American mothers believe that they should remain in bed for at least 3 days after delivery and should not do heavy work for 40 days. Sexual intercourse is not allowed during these 40 days (Murillo-Rohde, 1980).

Many members of the black American culture continue the practice of bedrest for 10 days following delivery. The mother will follow the activity dictated by hospital practices then proceed to place herself on bedrest after discharge.

EVACUATION AND RETENTION

- What is done about lochia, its retention, and its disposal?
- What attention is given to the bowels and to the bladder?

In the Hispanic culture, "hot" foods are eaten to prevent the flow of lochia toward the head, which could result in nervousness or even insanity. They are also taken to fortify *la matriz débil* or "weak womb" (Murillo-Rohde, 1980).

The Vietnamese believe that sour foods, including salads, cause incontinence, so they are forbidden (Hollingsworth, Brown, and Brooten, 1980).

PASSIONS OF THE SPIRIT OR EMOTIONS

- Is it safe to express happiness over a new baby, or does this invite the "evil eye"?

Many cultures fear the evil eye, *mal ojo*. The Mexican-Americans, Arab-Americans, Nigerians, and Vietnamese believe that evil and sickness will befall the newborn who is praised but not touched at the same time by another, especially if that other is a stranger. Vietnamese parents often dress a newborn in old clothes to minimize its desirability and to prevent the spirit's jealousy (Hollingsworth, Brown, and Brooten, 1980).

Newborn Period

Using the Kay-Galenic framework, questions can be asked in each of the six categories to learn more about the specific culture.

AIR AND WATER

- When is the infant bathed?
- How, what parts of, and by whom is the infant bathed?
- What air is dangerous, what is desired, and where?
- How is the baby protected?

Many cultures ritualize the bathing and dressing of the newborn. As soon as the cord is cut, the Vietnamese mother bathes the baby in tepid water. Only after this first bath may the father see the baby (Hollingsworth, Brown, and Brooten, 1980).

As with the mother, the Mexican-American newborn is wrapped to protect its head, feet, and body from cool air.

FOOD AND DRINK

- When is the baby first fed?
- What is the baby fed?
- When is the baby given food other than milk?
- How is it prepared?

Most cultures continue the practice of breastfeeding, putting the baby to breast immediately following the delivery and allowing nursing as often as desired. Nursing is continued until the child is 1–2 years of age. An important point to remember with some Mexican-American mothers is that they will not put the newborn to breast until 3 days after delivery, as they believe that colostrum is "filthy" (Kay, 1979).

SLEEP AND WAKEFULNESS

- Where does the baby sleep?
- Where is the baby when awake?
- What is done to promote sleep?
- Should the baby sleep on its back or stomach?

The Vietnamese mother is expected to have the newborn with her at all times, although her mother-in-law will help her with the actual care (Hollingsworth, Brown, and Brooten, 1980).

MOVEMENT, EXERCISE, AND REST

- Is the baby swaddled?
- What exercise is permitted?

The Mexican-American newborn is tightly swaddled and a belly band, or *fajita*, is placed around the abdomen to prevent the umbilicus from bulging (Zepeda, 1982). In the Soviet Union, the infant is immediately tightly swaddled and the swaddling is secured with a heavy cord tied around the center of its body (Gay, 1985).

EVACUATION AND RETENTION

- What is considered normal?
- Are diapers used?
- How are they handled?

Some Haitian women believe in the practice of immediately giving the newborn a purgative made from red oil that comes from a plant called "maskreti" to clean the infant's insides (Harris, 1987).

PASSIONS OF THE SPIRIT OR EMOTIONS

- What expression is anticipated?
- How is it taught, reinforced, extinguished?
- How long is the infant allowed to cry?

In most traditional and primitive cultures, the baby's fussiness is responded to immediately, and the needs for food, warmth, cleanliness, and protection are anticipated through teachings from older relatives.

The Newton Framework

Niles Newton (1970) developed a framework for the assessment of cultural orientation based on her studies of behavioral patterns displayed during pregnancy, labor and delivery, and puerperium in many different societies (Richardson and Guttmacher, 1967). This framework includes the following areas of focus:

Prenatal

1. What is the meaning and the value of reproduction to the culture?
2. How is pregnancy viewed by the society?
3. How does the society place responsibility for fetal growth on the parent?

Intrapartal

1. What is the importance placed on birth?
2. Is birth viewed as an illness or a normal physiologic process?
3. Is birth a private or a social event?
4. Is birth viewed as an achievement or an event to be paid for?
5. What practices are prescribed regarding medication and nutrition?
6. What practices are prescribed regarding activity?

Postpartal

1. What type of support is acceptable and who is allowed to provide it?
2. What practices are prescribed regarding medication and nutrition?
3. What practices are prescribed regarding activity and household responsibilities?

Newborn

1. How do members of the culture view children and react to them?
2. What are the patterns regarding infant care?

Use of the Kay-Galenic and Newton frameworks in the assessment phase of the nursing process can further systematize the nurse's collection of subjective and objective data. The nurse can then apply meaning to patients' behaviors, leading to appropriate goal setting and intervention.

Nursing's Role

The following are suggested goals and interventions for nurses who wish to become more holistic in their care. This can be accomplished by becoming more aware of cultural differences and similarities between the nurse and his or her patients and by learning how to intervene appropriately.

1. Become aware of one's own cultural orientation and the relationship it has to one's own health beliefs and practices. If nurses are aware that they themselves come from a culture with a full set of beliefs on every subject, half the battle is won (Mead, 1956).

   Look closely at one's own behaviors when practicing self-care actions. Ask what beliefs and attitudes initiated the behaviors. Refer to Fig. 6–1 for examples of questions to ask in order to develop this awareness.
2. Learn about cultural groups different from one's own. Read available literature—books, journals, articles. Attend seminars and workshops about specific cultures or about some specific aspect of culture. Conduct a small-scale cultural profile of one's own community.
3. Identify the cultural orientation of clients. Apply the Kay-Galenic or Newton framework to each patient as a part of the data-collecting process. Use an interpreter if there is a language barrier.
   a. Use sign language. Point to each body part and act out action words.
   b. Use phrases that create pictures.
   c. Speak in simple terms—not louder.
   d. Monitor the patient's facial expressions (Pearson, 1986).
4. Compare one's own cultural beliefs and practices with those of individual patients. Look for similarities and differences.

   Use Orque's tool (see Fig. 6–2) to make comparisons of all aspects of culture. Be sure also to keep in mind the factors that account for variations within cultures.
5. Evaluate the effects that patients' beliefs and practices might have on the success of their health care. Williams and Jelliffee (cited in Johnston, 1980) suggest that cultural practices can be classified as having either beneficial, neutral, harmful, or uncertain effects on the success of the individual in reaching optimal health.

As objectively, and as open mindedly as possible, determine into which category the patient's health beliefs and practices fit. Those practices that have a beneficial effect should be supported. An example of a cultural practice that is beneficial and should therefore be supported is walking during labor. Those practices that have no obvious effect should be ignored. An example is the Mexican-American practice of binding the newborn's abdomen, which has no obvious effect on the newborn but is important to the mother. The practices that have detrimental effects should be modified, if possible. Several tribes in Africa, for example, place cow manure on the newborn's cord to keep it moist, which means that many newborns die of tetanus. In order to prevent infection but allow the mothers to practice their ritual, caregivers cut the cord long, invite the mothers to treat the cord with manure or dirt, then cut the cord (Higgins, 1983).

It is important to be aware that few practices fit neatly into one category or another. Many must be evaluated on a "more-or-less" basis. Nurses should avoid taking the attitude that any practice different from their own is automatically "wrong". A position of sensitivity and support should be maintained in order to provide humanistic care.

Culture Self-Awareness Questionnaire

Objectively answer the following questions:

1. What status and value do various members have within your family?
2. Within your family, how important is health compared to other needs and values?
3. How much a family matter is illness?
4. Do family health beliefs and practices clash with the teaching and practices of the health program?
5. What effect would hospitalization of various family members have on those who are left at home?

FIGURE 6–1. Questions nurses can ask themselves to increase awareness of cultural attitudes.
SOURCE: Adapted from Brownlee (1978).

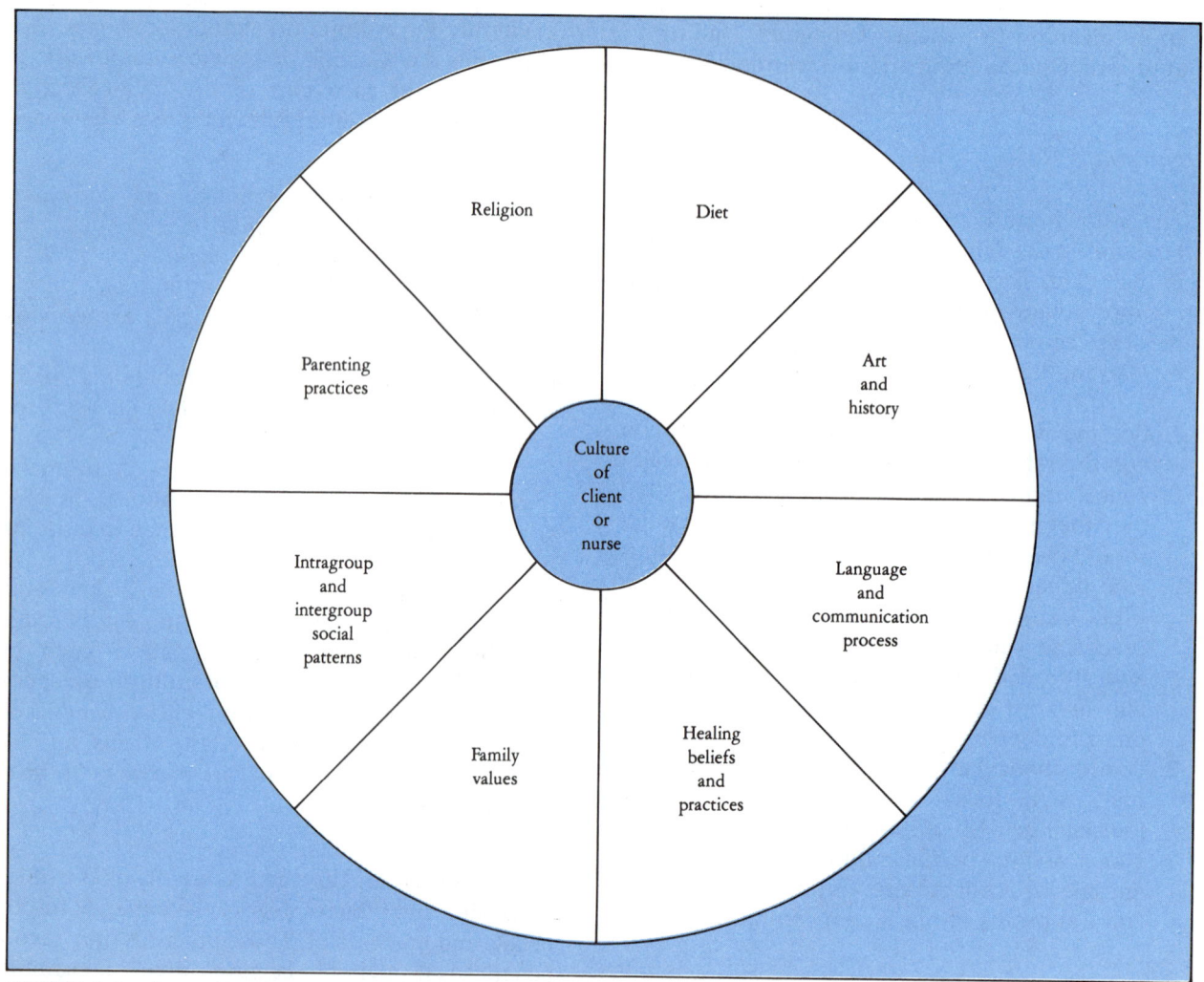

FIGURE 6–2. Cross-cultural assessment tool designed by Orque (1980) to be used in contrasting cultural variables of nurse and client.
SOURCE: Orque (1980).

SUMMARY

When nurses become aware of how their own cultural orientation affects their behaviors, they sensitize themselves to the need to assess the reasons for the behaviors and actions of their patients. They then become more aware of the differences and similarities between their own beliefs and practices and those of their patients. Understanding the cultural backgrounds of patients makes it easier for patients to communicate with the nurse, helps the nurse understand the reasons behind patients' behavior, and makes the nursing care more humanistic and personal. The result is greater satisfaction for both patient and nurse.

CASE PRESENTATION:

MEXICAN-AMERICAN MOTHER

Mrs. R.'s labor went almost unnoticed. She'd said nothing to the 7–3 shift nurses about being in labor, and she had never moaned or cried out. Only her grimacing and grunting alerted the 3–11 shift nurse of the presence of contractions.

Mrs. R., a Mexican-American (gravida 2, para 1), had been admitted to the antepartal unit approximately 24 hours earlier displaying all the signs and symptoms of pre-eclampsia. She was accompanied by her Mexican-American husband and their 2-year-old daughter. Mr. and Mrs. R. spoke very limited English, although Mr. R.'s ability was decisively better than his wife's. Mrs. R. was placed on strict bedrest and medications, with visitors limited to only her husband.

When it was determined that Mrs. R. was in labor, a vaginal examination was performed. As she was assessed to be 5–6 cm dilated, she was transferred to a labor room and her husband was notified. Despite attempts to involve Mr. R. in his wife's labor and delivery, he refused to participate and remained in her postpartal room with their daughter. He entered the labor room only when pressured to do so by the nurses and then only to translate the nurses' directions to his wife. Mrs. R. became agitated when her husband entered the room.

Mrs. R. delivered a 7-pound, 11-ounce baby boy. She was transferred again to her postpartal room. Mr. R. went home with their daughter, leaving the nurses to communicate with Mrs. R. as well as they could. Using sign language and simple words, the nurses were generally unsuccessful.

By the 3–11 shift the following day, it was apparent that there were problems. Mrs. R. had not drunk any of her water and had returned most of her meals untouched. When she was taken off bedrest after delivery, she remained in bed, much to the concern of the nurses. When the nurses set up Mrs. R.'s shower and encouraged her to take it, she smiled politely but refused to do so.

The nursery nurse who brought Mrs. R.'s baby to her exclaimed over all his black hair and his beautiful skin color. Mrs. R. became visibly upset, causing a hasty retreat by the nurse.

Worried, the nurses arranged a meeting with Mr. and Mrs. R. and a female interpreter. The ensuing discussion helped to unravel the reasons for Mrs. R.'s behavior.

Assessment

Using the Kay-Galenic framework, the nurse would have discovered the following Mexican-American beliefs and practices:

1. Labor is to be tolerated with patience and quiet acceptance.
2. The husband should not participate in labor and delivery.
3. Only "hot" foods and drinks are to be taken after delivery.
4. Ambulation is not encouraged until 3 days following delivery.
5. Water is not to be touched until 15–30 days following delivery.
6. The newborn will incur the "evil eye" if praised without the person touching it.

Goal

To have the patient's beliefs and practices be known to the health care providers, with resultant support and understanding.

Interventions

Contact an interpreter. Provide verbal and physical support and understanding of Mrs. R.'s practices and behaviors.

Evaluation

The effects of most of the Mexican-American practices identified are either harmless or unknown and will not have serious consequences if the nurse allows them to continue.

CASE PRESENTATION:

VIETNAMESE MOTHER

Mrs. N., a 22-year-old Vietnamese woman (gravida 1, para 0), had been in the United States for only a short time when she went into labor. She arrived in active labor at the birthing unit with her husband. The vaginal examination upon admission determined that she was 2–3 cm dilated. Neither Mr. nor Mrs. N. spoke much English.

Mrs. N.'s labor was difficult but she did not utter a sound. Her husband finally consented to remain in the unit but entered the labor room only when the nurses requested him to translate instructions to his wife. After 20 hours of labor, Mrs. N. was still only dilated to 5–6 cm, and it was decided that a cesarean section delivery would be necessary. Once Mrs. N. had returned to her postpartal room, Mr. N. left the nurses to communicate with his wife to the best of their ability.

Mrs. N. cooperated with the nurse's instructions to cough and deep breathe and turn from side to side, but she became agitated when the nurse set up a bedbath and began bathing her on the first postpartal day. She was even more upset on the second day.

By the third postpartal day, Mrs. N. was passing flatus and her i.v. and Foley catheter were discontinued. She could now be up in her room and in the hall. Mrs. N. got up to go to the bathroom, but when the nurse encouraged her to take a walk, she shook her head and refused. Because of lack of ambulation, on the evening of the third day, Mrs. N.'s abdomen distended with gas and she became very ill. A nasogastric tube was inserted and the I.V. was restarted. No one could understand what had happened.

Concerned, the nurses contacted an interpreter and held a conference with Mr. and Mrs. N. and the physician. The ensuing discussion was very enlightening.

Assessment

Using the Kay-Galenic framework, the nurse would have discovered the following Vietnamese beliefs and practices:

1. Labor is accepted quietly.
2. The husband should not participate in labor and delivery.
3. A bath taken earlier than several weeks after delivery results in intestinal blockage and loss of nutrients.
4. Early ambulation is discouraged as it causes stretching of the stomach.

Goal

To have the patient's beliefs and practices be known to the health care providers, with resultant support and understanding.

Interventions

Contact an interpreter. Provide verbal and physical support and understanding of Mrs. N.'s practices and behaviors.

Evaluation

When Mrs. N. was allowed to rest in bed and baths and showers were discontinued, she improved almost immediately. The knowledge gained in the conference also enabled the nurses to provide her with acceptable foods when she was allowed to eat.

REFERENCES

Aamodt, A. M. 1979. Culture. In *Culture, childbearing, health professionals*, ed. A. L. Clark. Philadelphia: F. A. Davis.

Abril, I.F. 1977. Mexican-American folk beliefs: How they affect health care. *MCN*. 2:168–173.

Affonso, D. D. 1979. Framework for cultural assessment. In *Childbearing: A nursing perspective*, eds. A. L. Clark and D. D. Affonso. Philadelphia: F. A. Davis.

Bash, D. M. 1980. Jewish religious practices related to childbearing. *J. Nurse-Midwifery*. 25:39–42.

Bond, J., and Bond, S. 1980. The sociology of maternity care. *Briefs*. 44(5):73–75.

Bringas, J. G., and Chan, T. Y. 1979. Spanish aid in clinical dietetics. *Nutrition in the life cycle*. 10–11.

Brownlee, A. 1978. The family and health care: Explorations in cross-cultural setting. *Social Work in Health Care*. 4(2):179–198.

Clark, A. L., and Affonso, D. D. 1979. *Childbearing: A nursing perspective*. 2nd ed. Philadelphia: F. A. Davis.

Dempsey, P. A., and Gesse, T. 1983. The childbearing Haitian refugee—Cultural applications to clinical nursing. *Public Health Report*. 98(3):261–267.

Deutsch, E. G. 1971. A stereotype—or an individual? *Nurs. Outlook*. 19:106–109.

Gay, J. 1985. Soviet health care: An American prospective. *JOGNN*. 14(2):156–159.

Gordon, V. C.; Matousek, I. M.; and Lang, T. A. 1980. Southeast Asian refugees. Life in America, part 2. *Am. J. Nurs*. 80:2031–2036.

Harris, K. 1981. Beliefs and practices among Haitian American women in relation to childbearing. *J. Nurse-Midwifery*. 32(3):149–155.

Harris, M. 1981. Why women left home. *Psych. Today*. 15(8):29–37.

Hedstrom, L. W., and Newton, N. 1986. Touch in labor: A comparison of cultures and eras. *Birth*. 13(3):181–186.

Higgins, P. G. 1983. Pueblo women of New Mexico: Their background, culture, and childbearing practices. *Topics Clin. Nurs*. 4(4):69–78.

Hollingsworth, A. O.; Brown, L. A.; and Brooten, D. A. 1980. The refugees and childbearing: What to expect, part 3. *RN*. 43:44–49.

Horn, B. 1983. Cultural beliefs and teenage pregnancy. *Nurse Practitioner* 8(8):35, 39, 74.

Iorio, J., and Nelson, M. A. 1983. China: Caring is the same. *Nurs. Outlook*. 31:100–104.

Johnston, M. 1980. Cultural variations in professional and parenting patterns. *J. Obstet. Gynecol. Neonatal Nurs*. 9:9–13.

Jordan, B. 1980. *Birth in four cultures*. Montreal: Eden Press Women's Publication.

Kay, M. A. 1979. The Mexican American. In *Culture, childbearing, health professionals*, ed. A. L. Clark. Philadelphia: F. A. Davis.

Kay, M. A. 1982. *Anthropology for human birth*. Philadelphia: F. A. Davis.

La Du, E. B. 1985. Childbirth care for Hmong families. *MCN*. 10(6):382–385.

Leininger, M. 1970. *Nursing and anthropology: Two worlds blend*. New York: John Wiley & Sons.

Liu, Y. C. 1979. Position during labor and delivery: History and perspective. *J. Nurse-Midwifery*. 24:23–26.

Liu, Y. C. 1983. China: Health care in transition. *Nurs. Outlook*. 31:94–99.

Mays, R. M. 1979. Primary health care and the black family. *Nurse Practitioner*. 4:10.

Mead, M. 1956, Understanding cultural patterns. *Nurs. Outlook*. 4:260.

Mead, M., and Newton, N. 1967. Cultural patterning of perinatal behavior. In *Childbearing: Its social and psychological aspects*, eds. S. A. Richardson and A. F. Guttmacher. Washington, D.C.: Williams & Wilkins.

Meleis, A. I. 1981. The Arab American in the health care system. *Am. J. Nurs*. 81:1180–1183.

Meleis, A. I., and Sorrell, L. 1981. Arab American women and their birth experience. *MCN*. 6:171–176.

Mott, Frank L. 1986. The pace of repeated childbearing among young American mothers. *Family Planning Perspectives*. 18(1):5–12.

Murillo-Rhode, I. 1980. Health care for the Hispanic patient. *Critical Care Update*. 7:29–36.

Newton, N. 1970. Childbirth and culture. *Psych. Today* 4(6):74.

Newton, N. 1979. Cross-cultural perspectives. In *Childbearing: A nursing perspective*, eds. A. L. Clark and D. D. Affonso. Philadelphia: F. A. Davis.

Orque, M. 1981. Cultural components. In *Maternity care: The nurse and the family*, ed. M. D., Jensen R.C.

Orr, J.; Neuberger, J.; Rowden, R.; Cumberlege, J.; and Flint, C. 1987. Retracing our cultural roots. *Nurs. Times*. 83(11):22.

Pearson, L. J. 1986. Ann Compian: Filling a need for culturally specific care. *Nurse Practitioner*. 11(7): 50, 55, 58, and 61.

Rackovsky, Rabbi I. 1980. Nurses, nursing, and culture. *Supervisor Nurse*. 11(7):20–21.

Richardson, S. A., and Guttmacher, A. F., eds. 1967. *Childbearing: Its social and psychological aspects*. Washington, D.C.: Williams & Wilkins.

Roberts, J. E. 1979. Maternal positions for childbirth: A historical review of nursing care practices. *J. Obstet. Gynecol. Neonatal Nurs*. 8(1):24–32.

Ruiz, M. C. J. 1981. Open-closed mindedness, intolerance of ambiguity, and nursing faculty's attitudes toward culturally different patients. *Nurs. Outlook*. 30:177–181.

Shapiro, J. L. 1987. The expectant father. *Psych. Today*. 21(1):36–42.

Simmons, L. W. 1952. Cultural patterns in childbirth. *Am. J. Nurs.* 52:989–991.

Smoyak, S. 1968. Cultural incongruence: The effect on nurses' perception. *Nurs. Forum.* 27:234–237.

Stanton, M. E. 1979. The myth of "natural" childbirth. *J. Nurse-Midwifery*, 24:25–29.

Stern, P. N.; Filden, V. P.; and Maxwell, E. K. 1985. *Culturally induced stress during childbearing: The Philipino-American experience.* Hemisphere Publishing Corporation.

Turrell, S. 1985. Asian expectation. *Nurs. Times.* 81(18):44–46.

Vernon, G. M. 1972. *Human interaction: An introduction to sociology.* 2nd ed. New York: Ronald Press.

Wang, J. F. 1985. Induced abortion: Reported and observed practice in Taiwan. *Health Care for Women International.* 6:383–404.

Zepeda, M. 1982. Selected maternal-infant care practices of Spanish-speaking women. *J. Obstet. Gynecol. Neonatal Nurs.* 11:371–374.

7

Ethics and Perinatal Nursing

BEHAVIORAL OBJECTIVES

Upon completion of this chapter, the reader should be able to:

- Differentiate between those issues that are ethical and those that are legal.

- Discuss the relationship between obligation and moral character.

- Define and discuss the principle of justice.

- Define and discuss the principle of autonomy.

- Define and discuss the principle of nonmaleficence.

- Define and discuss the principle of beneficence.

- Discuss the sanctity of life and quality of life principles.

- Apply the ethical principles to a case or dilemma and discuss their usefulness in moral decision making.

Surrogate mothers, artificial insemination, *in vitro* fertilization, genetic engineering, recombinant DNA, total *in vitro* gestation, fetal surgery, retrievable 1000 g infants—these are awesome times we live in; these are disturbing times we live in. Previous eras have not had the scientific know-how or the ability to tamper with the human reproductive and sexual processes in the ways that are presently or foreseeably possible. And the burden of our ability is that: "we can" does not mean "we ought to".

Whether or not we ought to act in a given way is the domain of *ethics*. *Normative ethics* is that branch of either philosophy or theology that examines norms of human conduct, in terms of what "ought" to be; a moral dilemma exists in any situation where two or more important and mutually exclusive norms (duties or values) conflict. The conduct in question might be a day-to-day decision that a nurse must make at the beside, or it might be a question of public or professional policy. Examples of the former include assisting at or counseling for abortions, and refusing to carry out orders to discontinue life support for an infant. Examples of the latter include the recent American Nurses' Association (ANA) policy on assisting in capital punishment and the California Nurses' Association policy on risk and duty in the resuscitation of patients with a communicable disease.

There is no question that our clinical capabilities have outstripped our moral reflection. Since the 1960s, however, there has been an escalating concern about the bioethical reflection that is past due in our health care decision making, and the nursing literature has reflected this general professional trend toward ethical analysis of cases and issues (Reich, 1978). The task of this chapter is to discuss the application of bioethical principles to the dilemmas that occur in perinatal nursing.

ETHICS: SOME BASIC CONCEPTS

Ethics is often used interchangeably with the term *morals*. While the distinction between the two is foggy, ethics is often considered the broader, more reflective term, while morals comprises more specific admonitions, traditions, or codes of behavior (Beauchamp and Walters, 1982), such as "Thou shalt not kill" and *"Primum non nocere"* (Jones, 1977).

One other aspect of the term *ethical* should be noted. Technically, this word is neutral, signifying neither right nor wrong, good nor bad. The term is commonly used to designate a morally appropriate act, and *unethical* connotes a morally wrong act. But *ethical*, rightly used, refers only to a class of actions or ideals and is a neutral term (Frankena, 1973). The same is true of the term *moral*. A "moral" action is not necessarily a right action. The designation "moral" refers only to the type of action being examined.

Ethics itself has two major divisions (metaethics and normative ethics) with a third division which, though related and important to ethics, is not a formal part of ethics. *Metaethics* is generally the province of professional ethicists, and deals with more ethereal questions such as "Why be good?" or "How do we know what is just?" *Normative ethics* deals with norms of obligation and value and is the principle ethical concern, in its applied form, of professionals. The focus of this chapter is that of applied normative ethics. Descriptive ethics describes what a given group believes morally or how they behave morally; descriptive ethics deals with *what is*, not what ought to be and thus is more properly the domain of psychology, sociology, anthropology, or history. That is not to say that descriptive ethics is unimportant or irrelevant, only that it is not regarded by ethicists as a formal part of ethics. Descriptive data can provide the data from which or over against which normative or metaethical studies proceed. Within nursing, the chief representatives of descriptive ethics are values clarification and moral development.

Ethics and Law

While *ethics* and *morals* may sometimes be used interchangeably, the same is not true for the terms *law* and *ethics*. The two disciplines do overlap, but they are not identical. An action may be held to be morally right but illegal, legal but morally wrong, and so on. Both law and ethics deal with what "ought" to be done, but they are not the same "ought". Law carries with it a coercive force (punishment) that is not found in ethics. The best that ethics has to offer by way of coercion is moral suasion, or consignment to purgatory, damnation, or Sheol.

Law and ethics differ in other ways. Law is generally minimalistic, while ethics goes further, dealing with ideals and supererogatory acts—that is, those acts that "go the second mile". Furthermore, law is legislated or promulgated for the maintenance, preservation, protection, and perpetuation of a given social group and the resolution of its conflicts. Ethics also has a social aspect; it governs relations among individuals and between groups and does have a social origin, at least in part. However, it is neither legislated nor created in the same way that law is (Frankena, 1973). Nor does it require of the individual only what the law requires; it exceeds the requirements of the law by being concerned with the moral character of the individual. The law requires only that the individual keep it, not that one be a virtuous person besides.

Obligation and Moral Character

Judgments about what is right or wrong behavior are called normative judgments of *obligation*. Such judgments tell us what we are obligated to do or not do. These actions are sometimes referrred to as good or bad, but the terms *good* and *bad* have a more precise ethical usage related to *norms of value*, not obligation. Norms of value are those qualities which are *good* or *evil* in persons (called *virtues* or *moral values*) or things or ends we ought to seek (called *nonmoral values*) (Fowler and Levin-Arift, 1987).

Norms of obligation tell us what is *right* or *wrong* to do, not what is good or evil in what we ought to be or value. Norms of obligation and norms of value, together, are essential to ethically right-making behavior. For, while "norms of obligation (whether teleological or deontological) tell us how to act, norms of value tell us what to be; the two are inseparable" (Crossley, 1979, p. 24). Thus, it is not sufficient to know what we ought to do. Nor is it sufficient only to be virtuous. Obligation and character must be linked. "Norms of obligation without corresponding character traits are useless; character traits without norms of obligation are directionless" (Crossley, 1979, p. 25).

BIOETHICS AND NURSING

Bioethics, or biomedical ethics as it is sometimes called, involves the application of general normative ethics to the more specific areas of health and the life sciences. Properly speaking, it is not a separate field in itself but a specialized inquiry into and application of general moral action guides to issues in health care. Bioethics is concerned with specific issues (such as abortion, fetal experimentation, and genetic engineering); foundational concepts (such as definitions of life, personhood, health, illnesss, and death); policy considerations (such as state or federal funding for abortions for poor women, the rights of the fetus, and the provision of contraceptives to minors); and moral limits to scientific inquiry and medical interventions in human lives. Thus, bioethics is a multifocused application of normative ethics to biomedical concerns.

Nursing ethics and medical ethics can be seen as subspecies of bioethics, or they can be seen as separate entities in themselves. However one chooses to define bioethics, it is not appropriate to view nursing ethics as a variant form of medical ethics; though there is some overlap in concerns addressed, medical ethics and nursing ethics are separate entities with distinctive traditions (see Fig. 7–1).

Nursing has always been concerned with ethics and education. In the 1896 articles of incorporation of what later became the ANA, the first substantive article stated:

> The object of the Association shall be: To establish and maintain a code of ethics, to the end that the standard of nursing education be elevated . . . (Associated Alumnae of Trained Nurses of the United States and Canada, 1896, p. 7)

Between its founding in 1900 and today, the *American Journal of Nursing* has published over 400 articles that specifically touch upon ethical concerns in nursing. Despite this historic and ongoing interest in ethics for nursing, however, bioethics *per se* has tended to focus upon the concerns of medicine alone.

The medically oriented bioethics literature is inadequate to meet the needs of nursing and nurses for an overtly simple reason: medicine is not nursing. It is morally relevant that the focus of the two professions is different. It has been said that medicine focuses on "cure" while nursing focuses on "care" (Massachusetts Nurses' Association, 1977). This distinction tends to imply that medicine gives no thought to care. While there are undoubtedly instances where this has seemed true, similar cases may also be found in nursing. It is perhaps better to say that medicine focuses on the diagnosis and treatment of disease—that is, on pathophysiology and psychopathology—whereas nursing focuses on the diagnosis and treatment of human responses to actual or potential health problems (American Nurses' Association, 1980). In other words, medicine is concerned with disease, while nursing is concerned with responses to disease and illness and with wellness, rather than with the disease itself.

There are other factors that make medical ethics less than optimal for nurses. One is the "obligation

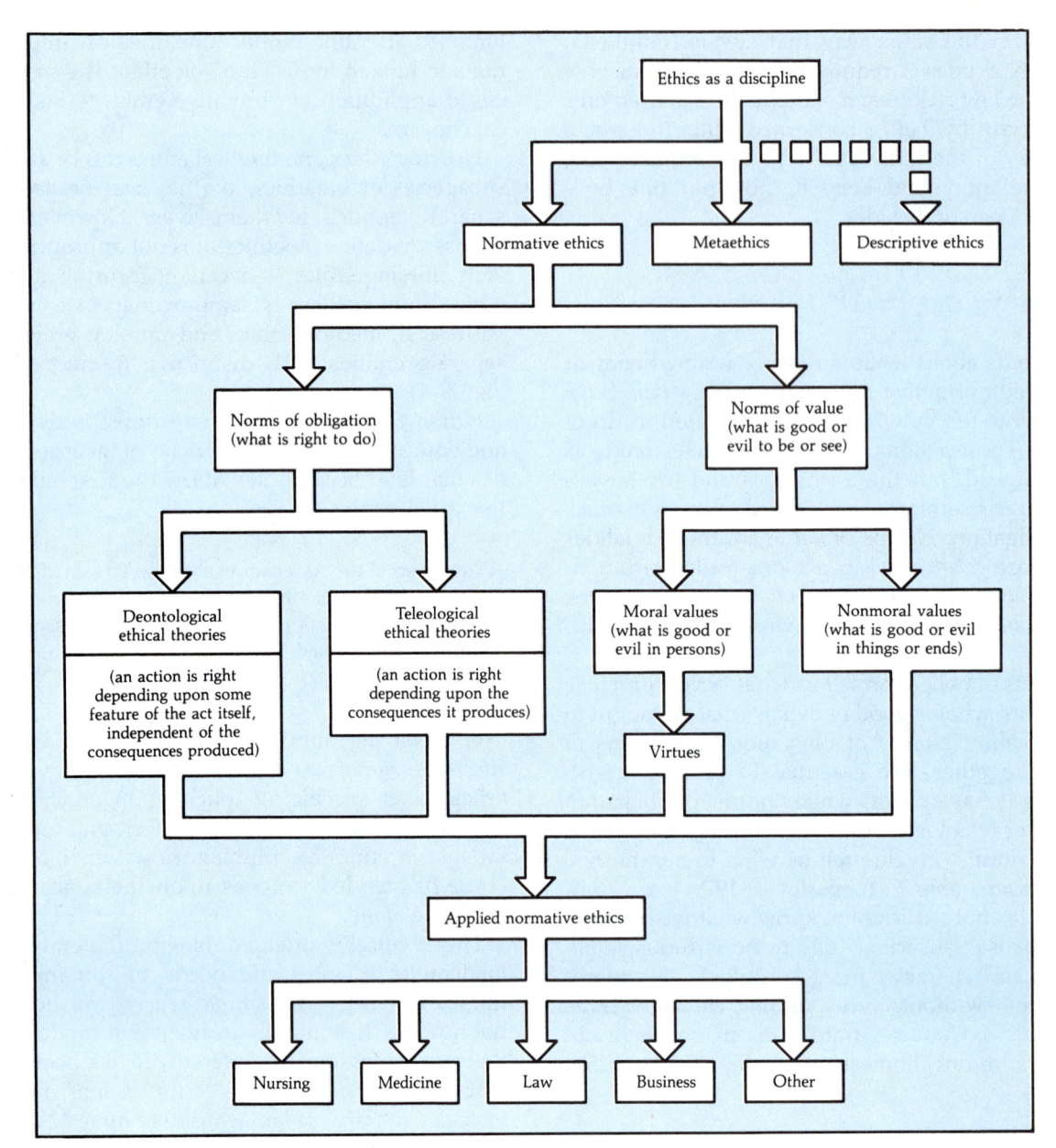

FIGURE 7-1. The role of ethics in nursing.

triad" of the nurse. As Jameton (1983) has pointed out:

> Nurses . . . work within a triangle of responsibilities—to the client, hospital and the physician. . . . In some settings, close teamwork exists; work is conducted with grace and respect for everyone involved. In other settings, ancient and momentous struggles for power, accumulated bitterness, frustration, and despair dominate negotiations over these functions (p. 17).

Physicians do not practice within such a triangle, and their decisions are often made unilaterally. Nursing is not at ease with vesting all or even most of the decision-making power in the professional. The codes for nurses, of both the ANA (1976) and the International Council of Nurses (1973), affirm that the nurse's first responsibility is to the client. Unfortunately, this philosophy often places the nurse in a difficult position with respect to the physician, the employer, or both. The nurse's decisions thus often reflect a compromise in ethical beliefs—a compromise brought about by social, political, economic, legal, and other "practical" concerns.

Ethical decision making in the practice setting

becomes a blend of personal and moral concerns. That is, whereas the nurse may decide to act in a way that is morally *acceptable*, he or she may not consider it to be morally *optimal*. It must be realized, however, that a nurse cannot make "purely ethical" decisions in the real context of practice. But it must also be realized that most clinical decisions have moral ramifications.

Pragmatic concerns are but one set of factors that influence ethical behavior. In order to function successfully within their profession, practitioners must accept and embrace the general moral norms and values of that profession. This is usually accomplished through the process of socialization. But the practitioner also brings to the profession a personal set of moral values, based on his or her personal philosophy and most deeply held beliefs. Upon occasion, these personal values may conflict with or seem strained by professional demands and values. In such situations, the professional may need to withdraw from the situation on moral grounds or alter the situation so that personal moral integrity will not be violated (Fig. 7-2).

Some values take precedence over those of science, health care, or the profession. When values conflict, the nurse generally opts for upholding his or her personal values; that is both right and fitting. In most situations, however, personal moral values, grounded in one's religion, philosophy, and culture, tend to impose additional constraints upon behavior rather than directly conflicting with professional values. For example, the nurse who maintains that abortion is morally wrong is morally obliged to refrain from participation in abortions. The value that the nurse expresses is a regard for the sanctity of human life. Nursing, as a profession, also affirms the value of human life. Any difference lies, in part, in how

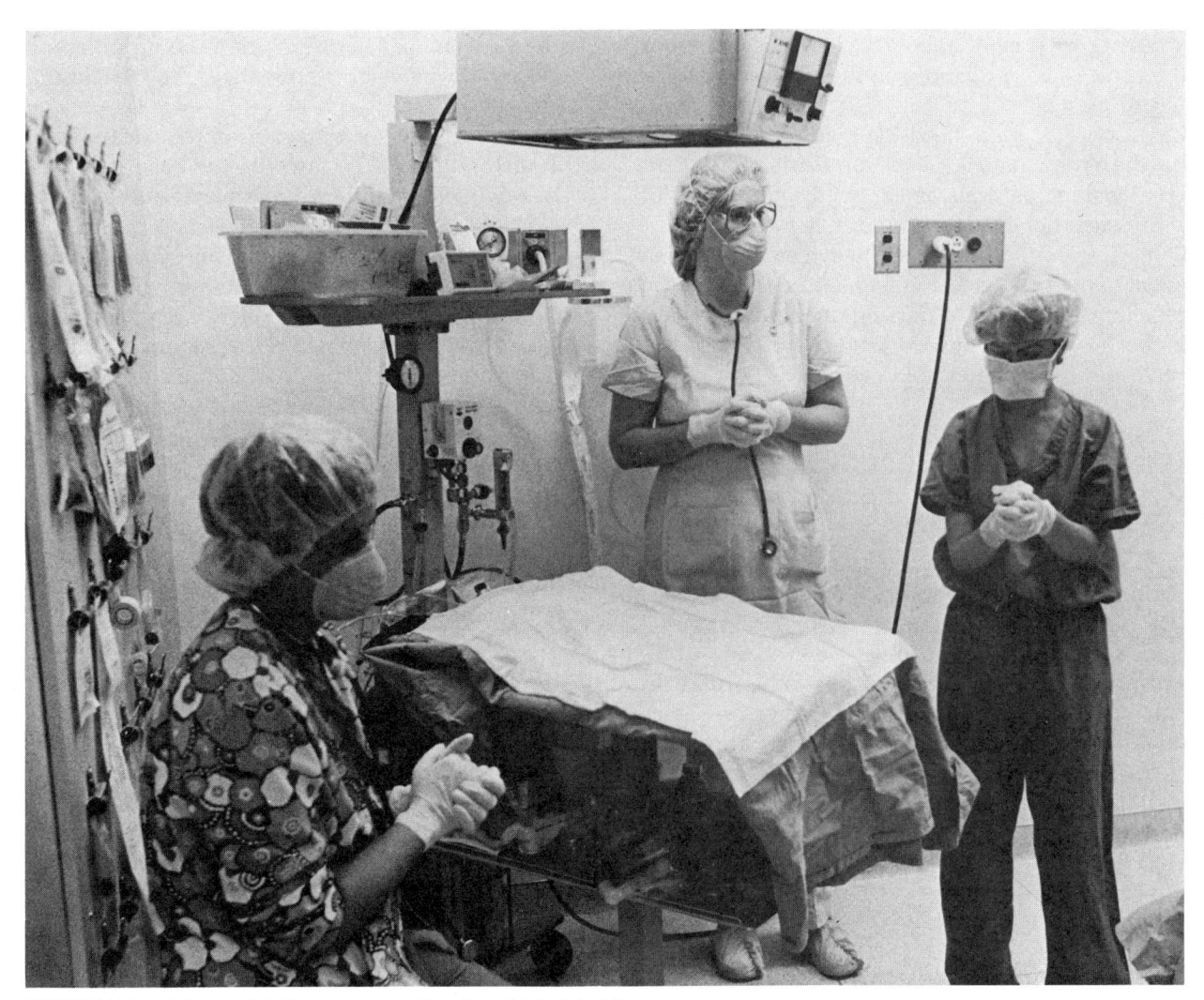

FIGURE 7-2. Labor and delivery team waiting for a high-risk delivery.

one defines human life; the Code for Nurses and the ethical tradition of the profession leaves this question open to individual interpretation. So the nurse who refuses to participate in an abortion, though perhaps at odds with hospital practice and voluntary associations for social reform, is not in conflict with professional moral values. Nevertheless, personal moral values have imposed an additional burden with regard to meeting the nurse's duties in practice.

Yet another factor that distinguishes medical from nursing ethics is the ways in which the two professions have grown. Nursing, though now a profession, has only recently moved from its roots in religious vocation. Even now, nursing retains perspectives that are religious or quasireligious in nature. Nursing's emphasis on the "dignity" and "sanctity" of human life is an example. Because of these origins, nursing retains an unusual regard for nurse–patient dialogue, empathy, and other aspects of a traditional understanding of caring.

Medicine, on the other hand, grew up in the academy. At least, that is, since its separation from the profession of theology in the secular universities of the 1200s (Shryock, 1959). This background has inevitably influenced the medical perspective on the moral nature of the professional–patient relationship, as well as on medicine's view of professional obligations and duties *per se*.

In view of the differences between the professions of medicine and nursing, and in view of the paucity of specifically nursing-oriented bioethical literature, much more work needs to be done in the area of nursing ethics.

TOOLS FOR DECISION MAKING: PRINCIPLES AND RULES IN BIOETHICS

Although there are a number of different ethical theories (deontological and teleological), moral decision making often relies on a few well-accepted principles and their derivative rules. In this section we introduce several major principles of bioethics and the moral rules that issue from them. Among the principles and rules we shall examine are justice, autonomy, nonmaleficence, and beneficence.

Justice

In common usage, the term *justice* refers to compliance with the law or to meting out the proper punishment for infractions. The concept of justice is actually much broader, and it is generally distinguished as having three major concerns: compensation, retribution, and distribution.

Nursing ethics is primarily concerned with distributive justice. *Distributive justice* deals with the proper distribution of harms and benefits in society, usually when conditions of scarcity exist. Discussions of distributive justice often have an economic concern, centering on the social distribution of wealth rather than on the distribution of services such as health care.

The principle of distributive justice would be used to examine issues at both the macroallocation (which includes public policy) and microallocation levels. Issues in macroallocation would include inequalities of distribution of prenatal care, federal funding of abortions through Medicaid, and decisions about allocation of monies to, say, prenatal and perinatal care in preference to such endeavors as heart transplants. The issue here is not whether abortion or other procedures are morally right but rather, given that abortions or funding or other services are available, how they shall be justly distributed.

Microallocation of scarce resources deals with the distribution of services at the case level, as when two fetal monitors are available and four are needed. Questions in microallocation would include: Which infant will be given the neonatal intensive care bed? Which mother will receive counseling or education? Which woman will be coached in the labor room? How vigorous will we be in using neonatal intensive care unit (NICU) resources for a particular low-birth-weight infant? (See Fig. 7–3.)

Selecting candidates for a treatment or other resource is properly divided into two stages. The first stage is preliminary selection, based upon medical or nursing criteria and on the resources needed. The second stage is the final selection from among the acceptable candidates (Childress, 1970).

The first stage of selection is properly the domain of the health professions. In some cases, acceptability is fairly clear-cut, but other situations of "medical acceptability" are more ambiguous. Childress proposes that "medical acceptability should be used only to determine the group from which the final selection will be made, and the attempt to establish fine degrees of prospective response to treatment should be avoided" (p. 343). He further holds that physicians should not choose between two medically acceptable patients when one appears to have a better medical outlook

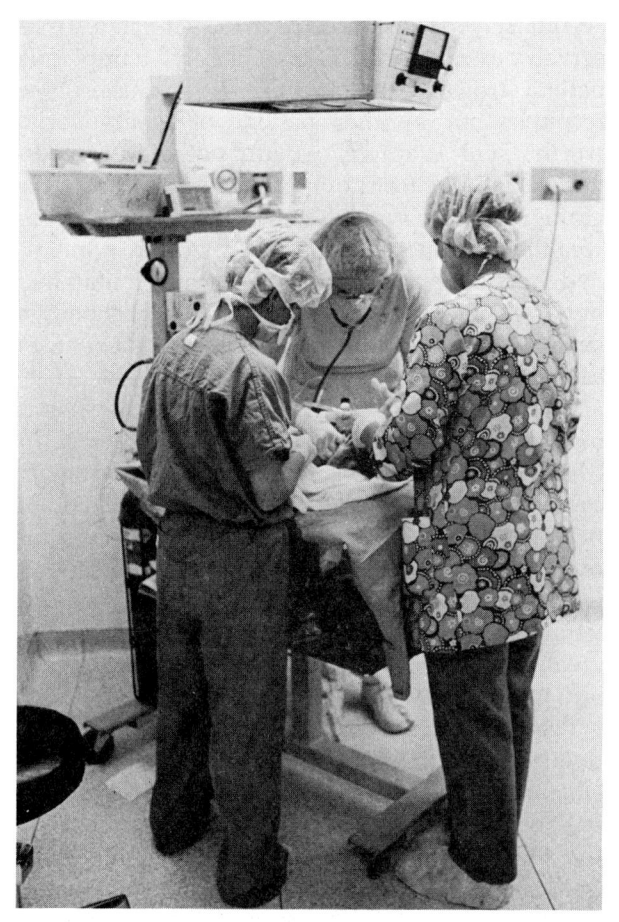

FIGURE 7-3. A team resuscitating critical newborn.

than the other. Nor would he accept anything more than a minimum consideration of psychologic or environmental factors. Those criteria "should be considered only when they are without doubt critically related to medical acceptability (e.g., the inability to cope with the requirements of dialysis which might lead to suicide)" (Childress, 1970, p. 344).

After the preliminary stage of selection, we come to the more difficult final selection. There are several alternative approaches to final selection. The first is to hold that "when not all can live, none should live, or at least no choices should be made between individuals, except when there are some who voluntarily relinquish their lives" (Childress, 1970, p. 344). Childress notes that, while perhaps a part of a heroic or saintly ideal of morality, this approach is ultimately "irresponsible . . . from several different standpoints, including society at large as well as the individuals involved" (p. 342).

The second alternative is to choose on the basis of the person's ability to pay for services. Veatch (1977, p. 237) deems this "one of the least defensible means of allocating lifesaving technology". There are several problems that make this position indefensible, including the inability of infants to pay for their care, the forces of society that have made women economically disadvantaged, and the fact that even "deserving" women are subject to financial difficulty through a variety of complex factors.

Another poor alternative is to attempt to make final selections on the basis of "strictly professional criteria". Such an approach would require the professional to be able to determine who would benefit most from nursing intervention. It also tends to leave the definition of *benefit* open and subject to individual interpretation. Furthermore, this perspective reduces moral decisions to questions of "scientific fact" and is also fundamentally based on a value judgment that gives primacy to "health" over other aspects of life and living.

Another approach is based on the vulnerability of the patient. That is, patients are selected on the basis of a perceived vulnerability related either to their status or to a special risk. The lifeboat ethic of ladies and children first reflects this perspective. Vulnerability, like benefit, is notoriously difficult to define. In addition, it is culturally or socially conditioned and often arbitrary. Because the motion of vulnerability involves labeling patients (whereas benefit does not), it is subject to abuse and can actually cause harm as well as benefit. That is, labels can be used either to deny or to permit special access to resources. For instance, the terms *unwed mother, abused spouse, child abuser, prostitute, lesbian mother, mentally retarded, rape victim,* and *gravida X para IX ab III,* can all be used to either harm or benefit the person so labeled; labels influence our decisions and actions as nurses.

From another perspective, the notion of vulnerability may be a reflection of what is called *compensatory justice.* In such cases, the individual's claim is based upon a social factor beyond the person's control that has contributed to the illness. Along the same lines, claims that are based on the weakness or helplessness of the individual, in the presence of a professional code or ethos that gives special regard to such persons (as in nursing) (Robb, 1900), may generally be considered to be sound moral claims. On the whole, however, this approach to microallocation is as problematic as the benefit approach. Regard for the weak can be incorporated into more useful approaches.

The next approach is based on criteria of social worth. In this approach, individuals are selected on the basis of an evaluation of their social worth, in either general or specific terms. It is usually a future-oriented criterion rather than one based on past contributions to society. This approach has major deficiencies. First, it would become necessary to weigh one person's social contributions against those of another. How are we to measure the value of aesthetic contributions to society (Charlotte Bronte) compared with political (Elizabeth C. Stanton) or professional (Florence Nightingale) contributions? If we perceive these evaluations to be simple ones, it is because of the hierarchy we have constructed in the values we hold.

A second difficulty with the social worth approach is its future orientation. This has two aspects: The future contributions of the individual, and the future needs or desires of the society. While a person's particular talents may lead us to believe that his or her contribution to society could be great, there is no guaranty that he or she would live to realize that potential, or, given a sufficiently long life, live up to that potential. Furthermore, today's potential contributions may be unnecessary or unwelcome tomorrow or may produce consequences other than those intended. Third, as Childress (1970) points out, a person's contributions are made within the context of his or her relational web, including his or her roles and functions in society. The social worth approach would

> in effect reduce the person to his social role, relations, and functions. Ultimately it dulls and perhaps even eliminates the sense of the person's transcendence, his dignity as a person which cannot be reduced to his past or future contribution to society (Childress, 1970, p. 316).

There are two other alternatives in microallocation. The first is the first-come, first-served (or "queue") approach, based upon "natural chance". The second is random selection, based upon artificial chance. According to Beauchamp and Childress (1979), none of the previously mentioned alternatives

> incorporate justice in the form of equality, equal access, and equal opportunity as well as [does] . . . the approach . . . which uses chance or queuing. . . . In a situation of life or death, equality may require queuing, lottery or randomization—whichever procedure is the most appropriate and feasible in the circumstances.

Almost everyone accepts the first-come, first-served principle; we do not generally "bump" one patient from treatment in order to use those resources for another patient of great "social worth". For example, we do not discharge an unwed mother from our prenatal education program in order to give her spot to a married, wealthier, or more famous woman. An unmodified queue approach does have its limitations, however; the very naturalness of natural chance is such that it is not always just and is sometimes capricious, wasteful, or imprudent.

Choosing by lottery in the second stage is a form of randomization, or artificial choice. In Childress's estimation, it is the method most capable of "preserv[ing] a significant degree of personal dignity by providing equality of opportunity" (1970, p. 348). He further maintains that while "not infallibly just . . . it is preferable to letting all die or saving only those who have the greatest social responsibilities or potential contribution" (p. 349).

Presupposing at least a limited queuing, randomized selection would not violate the relationship of trust established between the nurse and the patient; neither would it violate the provisions of the ANA Code for Nurses, nor the nursing ethos that maintains that patients are of equal moral worth. The patient knows that she will not be dumped by nursing so that care may be given to a more "attractive" patient. The patient's dignity and personhood are thus respected.

Selection by randomization does have its flaws, and it should not be employed without exception. But exceptions should be tightly controlled so as not to violate the ethical values that randomization preserves. When a lottery would create a "clear and present danger" to society because of the *loss* of an individual (*not* by reason of potential contribution), we may justifiably depart from selection by chance. Such situations are rare (Childress, 1970.

Suppose, however, that having been chosen for treatment, a patient refuses. Is it morally permissible for a patient to refuse needed counseling, education, or therapy? Here we must consider the princple of autonomy.

Autonomy

Ethics requires autonomous moral agents. *Autonomy* in ethics is the opposite of *heteronomy*, or the imposition of constraint (either internal or external), and is sometimes called *self-determination*. This is the sense in which Immanuel Kant used "autonomy": that an individual has the freedom and the power to bind himself to a universal law that is accepted on rational grounds; this is largely a concept of autonomy of will. To act from coercion, duress, habit, impulse, caprice, want, or strictly on orders, is to act nonself-legislatively, or heteronomously (Kant, 1976).

The principle of autonomy is related to the principle of *respect for persons*. Respect for persons means that others have the same right to make their own judgments as we have to make ours. That is, a person, because he or she is a person, has a right to rational self-determination (Downie and Telfer, 1969).

In nursing care, autonomy, respect for persons, and self-determination are at the heart of any consideration of the nurse–patient relationship. Patient autonomy is primarily protected through consent to treatment, referred to as *informed consent*. Respect for persons requires that patients be "fully informed" and "freely consenting". This means that the nurse utilizes his or her best clinical judgment in informing, counseling, and educating patients, taking into account each patient's status and communication skills. Patients are then free to determine which course of action would be best for them, in view of the way they define their own well-being. It is possible that the best medical or nursing decision might be wrong for a particular patient on moral grounds. Such patient decisions must be respected in so far as they do not compromise the nurse's moral integrity.

Postpartal Issues

Deferring discussion of prepartal and intrapartal issues for a moment, let us look at a few postpartal questions of autonomy. Take the example of a patient who refuses a blood transfusion, even though she will die without it. She refuses on religious grounds and is supported in this decision by her husband. This is one of a number of possible situations where the patient does not see "health" as the highest good. Other values—those of faith—are more fundamental than health. It is generally morally impermissible to attempt to subvert such a patient's moral value system and assert that the nurse's professional values (health, well-being) are more important than the patient's values (faith, obedience). Conversely, it is morally acceptable, though tragic, to affirm the patient's decision. (Note that the courts have also supported the legality of this decision.) If the professional overrides the patient's decision, whether by legal or other means (such as force), the patient (as unwilling participant) is absolved of religious guilt. Though this has traditionally been the case, more recent writings of members of one religious group have declared that the person who receives blood or blood products, *even by force*, remains responsible for violating a religious precept. In most instances, however, it is morally and legally permissible to force a transfusion upon an unwilling patient only when *not* doing so would seriously jeopardize another, as when the patient's children cannot be cared for if she dies.

Other postpartal issues in autonomy include compliance with treatments for complications, abstinence from intercourse in the immediate recuperative period, refusal of hematinics or other drugs, imbalance of activity and rest, poor nutrition, and refusal to return for a follow-up visit. Because these are areas of maternal volition and do not directly harm others, they usually fall within the sphere of permissible maternal autonomy, even if medically imprudent.

Prepartal Issues

The issue of autonomy presents a more difficult problem in the realm of maternity nursing than in other areas of practice. Ethics in nursing tends to maximize personal autonomy, even in instances where the results may be considered tragic. The line is drawn at the point where one person's exercise of personal autonomy would compromise the autonomy of another, or when one person's actions would harm another. That is to say, autonomy is not absolute. According to John Stuart Mill (1957):

> the sole for which mankind are warranted, individually or collectively, in interfering with liberty of action of any of their number is self-protection. His own good, either physical or moral, is not sufficient warrant (p. 9).

The complicating factor in prepartal maternal autonomy is, of course, the presence of the fetus. Although an organic part of the maternal body, the fetus is not solely that. And although another life or potential life, the fetus is not solely that either.

Many debates regarding maternal welfare and choice over against fetal welfare have erred in either one of two ways. Some argue for maternal rights to the exclusion of all concerns for the welfare of the developing fetus. Others argue exclusively for the rights of the fetus to the exclusion of all concerns for the pregnant woman. Such bipolar approaches are fraught with difficulties. Given this tension, what can be said about autonomy?

In cases where the prospective mother intends to carry the pregnancy to term, we would hope that her actions would reflect a concern for the welfare and well-being of the fetus. The mother ought not to knowingly and voluntarily engage in activities that carry a substantial risk of harm to the fetus. To some extent, risk is identified by research and is the responsibility of the health professional. Thus, patient education is of paramount importance. When research links smoking, drinking, drug taking, and other lifestyle behaviors to fetal and neonatal health, the nurse must communicate that information to the patient.

But patient education alone may not be sufficient. It is notoriously difficult for patients to stop smoking or drinking, for example, even in the face of a good reason to do so. The nurse's responsibility thus extends to assisting the patient to change her behavior, whether by referral (such as to a smoking cessation clinic) or by ongoing counseling or another nursing intervention. Caring, in the nurse–patient relationship, means assisting the patient to do those things that she cannot do alone.

In the moral realm, the mother who, out of ignorance, engages in activities that may potentially harm the fetus is not held to be morally culpable. However, with education comes moral responsibility. The mother who knowingly and perhaps deliberately or defiantly acts so as to harm the fetus is morally blameworthy. Most real-life situations, however, are not neat or clear-cut. Psychologic, economic, and other factors often play a part in determining what the pregnancy means to the woman; these factors are morally relevant and must be sorted out, too.

Other prepartal autonomy issues include prenatal diagnostic tests, bedrest, medication, and other treatments. Suppose a 41-year-old woman who was recently married has been determined to be pregnant for the first time, and physicians press her to sign a consent form for amniocentesis. She steadfastly refuses but is upset by the pressure to which she is being subjected. The nursing assessment determines that she has no intention of aborting if anything were to be discovered, does not feel a need for anticipatory knowledge of the status of the fetus, and does not want to know the fetus's sex. What is the responsibility of the nurse?

Of the 40 or more genetic diseases or conditions that may be discovered on amniocentesis, only a few are treatable. Although fetal surgery is possible, it is currently limited in its applications. Given the mother's intent, the presently limited scope of *in utero* treatment, and the fact that amniocentesis is not entirely without risk to the fetus, it is not morally required that the woman consent to the procedure. This does not yet answer the question of the nurse's role. With a primary responsibility to the patient, the nurse needs to be the patient's advocate both in guidance and counseling and with the physicians.

The Abortion Issue

We have been discussing cases of women who plan to carry the pregnancy to term. Now we turn to the issue of planned abortion. Abortion has been a topic of no mild controversy for centuries, producing an enormous body of literature. It is not within the scope of this chapter to discuss the ethics of abortion *per se*. There are, however, two major points that should be made here.

First, abortion is a legal reality in our pluralistic society. To say that it is legal is not to say that it is morally right. Nevertheless, it does mean that women cannot legally be denied an abortion on moral grounds if a hospital includes abortions among the services it provides. A nurse may decline to participate in abortions or proabortion counseling, but such withdrawal must be done *before* the fact. If there are procedures such as abortion that would violate the nurse's moral principles, the optimal time to make this known is at the time of employment, in writing. Abortion is a very important issue that the maternity or women's health nurse must grapple with and resolve if she is to provide consistent and effective treatment.

It must be recognized that moral discourse cannot do two things: (1) it cannot always prevent tragedy, and (2) it does not do away with disagreement, even among sincere and concerned persons. Nurses whose professional and even personal values are similar may still differ on the issue of abortion.

The second point to be made about abortion is that nursing is a *caring* profession. In cases where a patient makes a decision that the nurse disagrees with, the patient should not be abandoned or subjected to punitive measures. The nurse must be aware of the messages that she or he conveys to the patient, whether intentionally or unintentionally, and must seek to be a patient advocate in the true spirit of advocacy. Commonly, women who intend to abort or who plan to offer their child up for adoption are subtly punished by staff members. Despite a belief that abortion is morally wrong, some women find their life situation to be such that abortion is the least unjust course of action. Decisions for or against abortion are not easily made by the majority of patients. At times, patients have labored over decisions that health professionals have too easily dismissed as callous or self-interested. In short, nurses must remember compassion, empathy, openness, trust, and caring in their relationships with patients (see Chapter 43).

Other Issues

Several other issues fall under the rubric of the principle of autonomy. These include compulsory health programs, from public immunization through compulsory eugenics, research on human subjects, privacy, and confidentiality.

In compulsory health programs, the goals are to establish a minimum level of health for the general population, to contain potential or actual contagion, to eradicate specific diseases, and to improve or optimize public health. Examples in maternity nursing include PKU testing and instillation of erythromycin or silver nitrate drops in the eyes of neonates. In situations where noncompliance with compulsory programs endangers the health of others—as in treatment of sexually transmitted diseases—sufficient warrant can be found for requiring participation. Justification for such interference is based on principles of justice and autonomy, which afford maximum liberty compatible with like liberty for all (Rawls, 1971). Justification is not found on the basis of forcing patients to comply just because the treatment is considered beneficial. In the case of compulsory programs for infants, it is presumed that (1) the best interests of the neonate are being served, and (2) the infant would consent if he or she were able to do so.

Nursing research on human subjects is crucial to the advancement of clinical knowledge and techniques. Both therapeutic research and clinical trials are experimental interventions that will probably benefit the patient. Nevertheless, the patient must be informed of the experimental nature of the treatment, and consent must be obtained. In view of the probable benefit, consent is not usually a problem. Spousal consent is often obtained, on the presumption that the spouse has the best interests of the patient at heart or that the spouse would choose for the patient what the patient would choose were she able to do so.

Nursing research that is nontherapeutic, designed to advance scientific knowledge, to promote the common good, or to benefit people other than the patient himself, is a different kettle of fish. In this sort of research, it is generally held that we cannot risk another's well-being for the sake of a common good. When true consent cannot be obtained from a patient, or when consent is refused, research that is of no direct benefit to the patient should not be undertaken; even spousal consent is not acceptable here. Risk in nontherapeutic nursing research must be of the patient's own choosing. It has been reasonably argued that individuals have a duty to serve society by participating in nontherapeutic research. From a nursing perspective, however, it is more consonant with nursing values to argue that research on nonconsenting subjects is a direct violation of the nurse–patient relationship, which must be based upon trust. That trust, implied or stated, entails the belief that, while not absolute, patient autonomy should not be violated, nor should patients be used to nursing ends alone. This is a conservative approach and, as such, would include nontherapeutic nursing research involving the fetus.

Issues in confidentiality (the unauthorized release of patient information) and privacy (the unauthorized collection of patient information) also pertain to autonomy and respect for persons. To some extent, both confidentiality and privacy are myths (American Civil Liberties Union Foundation Project on Privacy and Data Collection, 1977). Most patients are unaware of the number of persons privy to the personal information on their chart and on reports. Our health care system has developed so that both confidentiality and privacy are ideals rather than a reality. For instance, in some hospitals charts are computerized and available to any staff person with a computer access code or key. Despite this situation, every effort must be made to maintain confidentiality and privacy in so far as is possible, especially in such cases as the lesbian mother who has conceived by means of artificial insemination, the surrogate mother who will be giving her baby up, or the couple who have conceived by means of artificial donor insemination. While the nurse must know the details of such cases in order to plan the care for the patient, he or she must spare no effort to maintain confidentiality and privacy.

Issues that arise in considerations of patient autonomy may also be examined from the perspective of the principle of nonmaleficence, often associated with the prime dictum of medicine, *primum non nocere*–"above all, do no harm" (Jones, 1977).

Nonmaleficence

Nonmaleficence is usually defined as the "avoidance of inflicting intentional harm or injury" and includes not putting the patient at *risk* of harm or injury. Nonmaleficence is a more stringent than *beneficence*, which is generally defined as an obligation to "do good" for another, whether by positive or negative acts. Some ethicists combine the two into one principle (beneficence), while others maintain that they are truly separate principles. For ease of discussion they will be treated as separate principles here.

Maleficence is the intentional infliction of harm or injury on another, whether actively or permissively, or the imposition of risk of harm. The principle of nonmaleficence prohibits intentional harm to patients but may allow some risk. Intentional harm is permissible only under rare and special circumstances, as in the forcible restraint of a violent patient. It is usually morally impermissible. Risk, however, may be imposed upon a patient if and only if greater patient care goals can justify the degree and probability of harm. Delivery by cesarean section is a good example. It is risky and harmful in itself, but the harm is unintended and the risk is outweighed by the hoped-for results.

The Nightingale Pledge (see Appendix A) exhorts nurses to refrain from harm; yet a number of interventions in perinatal nursing are inherently harmful or place the patient or fetus at risk of harm. For example, mandatory bedrest prior to delivery can and does negatively affect most of the maternal organ systems. The administration of analgesics during labor carries significant risk for both mother and delivering infant. Vaginal examinations may be a source of infection. Uterine massage induces pain. Separation of the infant and the mother may harm bonding. And restricting the father from the labor or delivery rooms may harm the marital or parental relationships.

The *principle of double effect* is sometimes useful in such situations. This rule is used in situations where an action will produce both harm and good. Its four conditions are (Dedek, 1976):

1. The action itself is good or at the minimum morally indifferent (neutral).
2. The good effect is not produced by means of the evil (harmful) effect.
3. Only the good effect, and not the evil (harmful) one, is directly intended.
4. The good effect proportionately outweighs the evil (harmful) effect, when the harmful effect is impossible to avoid.

An action in which good and evil effects are foreseen is permissible if and only if all four conditions have been met. This rule is generally most useful in situations of drug administration or proposed surgery.

Nursing is morally grounded in a respect for human life, which calls on us to honor, safeguard, maintain, and improve its bodily existence. This respect for life is touched upon, somewhat differently, in two principles: the sanctity of life principle and quality of life principle.

The Sanctity of Life Principle

According to the *sanctity of life principle* (SLP), life is sacred and of intrinsic value; we are obliged to preserve it. This principle also asserts that human lives are of equal value. It does *not* mean, however, that life should be preserved at any or all costs; such an approach is called *vitalism* and makes physical life an end in itself. Vitalism is actually a violation of the SLP, because it harms the dignity of the patient as a person. Vitalism is sometimes a faulty interpretation of the SLP, but too frequently it is a reflection of an inability to accept patient death except as a failure.

A proper understanding of the SLP is that life is sacred and cannot be terminated because of "defect". Furthermore, life has value that includes survival, freedom, and dignity, but it is not the highest good. Life is a relative value and our obligation to preserve it is also relative. It must not be absolutized, making it "life at any cost".

The Quality of Life Principle

The *quality of life principle* (QLP) is often placed in opposition to the SLP. It maintains that life under some conditions is not worth living and that the quality of life is as important as life *per se*. SLP supporters often accuse the QLP contingent of constructing a hierarchy of value of persons. They further charge that such an approach is subject to the caprice of the decision maker, is relative to the person who decides, disregards certain obligations and responsibilities, and is subject to great abuse in our pluralistic society. The sanctity of life camp is correct if the quality of life approach is based on social worth criteria. However, the QLP need not be understood in this way, nor must it be set against the SLP. *Both* are necessary to a sound understanding of life and to decision making with regard to life (see Fig. 7–4).

Combining the SLP and the QLP
The basic value that undergirds nursing care is the sanctity of life principle. However, modern medical science and technology have enabled us to prolong physical life, sustain individual cells, and harvest and maintain organs almost indefinitely. Such prolongation can profoundly violate our most fundamental personal and professional convictions about the nature, purpose, meaning, and dignity of human life. Merely because we *can* sustain an anomalous or marginally viable infant, *ought* we to do so? This is where we must combine, not counterpose, the SLP and QLP, understanding the SLP as the more fundamental principle for nursing. The QLP serves to modify the SLP, preventing a lapse into vitalism.

If we use the QLP to determine when instituting or continuing treatment would violate the SLP, we need criteria by which these determinations can be made. Ramsey (1978) argues that an "objective", "medical indications" policy is the best and safest approach, because quality of life determinations can ultimately open the door to active involuntary euthanasia. Based on the moral nature of the nurse–patient relationship, such euthanasia falls outside the bounds of what is morally permissible. (This point is supported by the ANA position paper on nursing involvement in capital punishment by lethal injection.) But a medical indications criterion is problematic, as we noted in our earlier discussion of microallocation. If quality of life criteria were not stated in such a way as to prevent active involuntary euthanasia, Ramsey would be correct (see Fig. 7–4).

McCormick (1978) rejects Ramsey's position and notes that "among objective conditions of the patient to be considered, one of the most crucial is the *kind of life* that will be preserved as a result of our interventions" (p. 32). McCormick has outlined five criteria for quality of life determinations. First, he maintains that life is a precondition for the realization of other values and achievements and is therefore to be preserved. Second, "the person is always an incalculable value, but . . . at some point continuance of physical life offers the person no benefit" (p. 34). Third, quality of life assessments are more broadly encompassed by the SLP. Fourth,

> Every *person* is of "equal value." But not every *life* is of equal value . . . we must avoid *unjust* discrimination in the provision of health care and life-supports. But not all discrimination (inequality of treatment) is unjust. *Unjust* discrimination is avoided if decision making centers on the benefit *to the patient* (p. 35).

Fifth, "life is a value to be preserved only insofar as it contains some potentiality for human relationships" (McCormick, 1974, p. 175). For McCormick, "the meaning, substance, and consummation of life is found in human relationships" (1974, p. 174). The extension of this point is that when the person can no longer enter into or maintain relationships because of her physical status, her life "becomes a negation of any truly human—i.e., relational—potential" (McCormick, 1974, p. 175).

Sanctity of life principle (SLP)
Life is sacred
Life has intrinsic value and dignity
Life is not the highest good, it is a relative good
Human lives are of equal value

⟵⟶

Quality of life principle (QLP)
Life under some conditions is not worth living
Quality of life is as important as sanctity of life

Vitalism ⟵ NOT

NOT ⟶ Social worth determinations

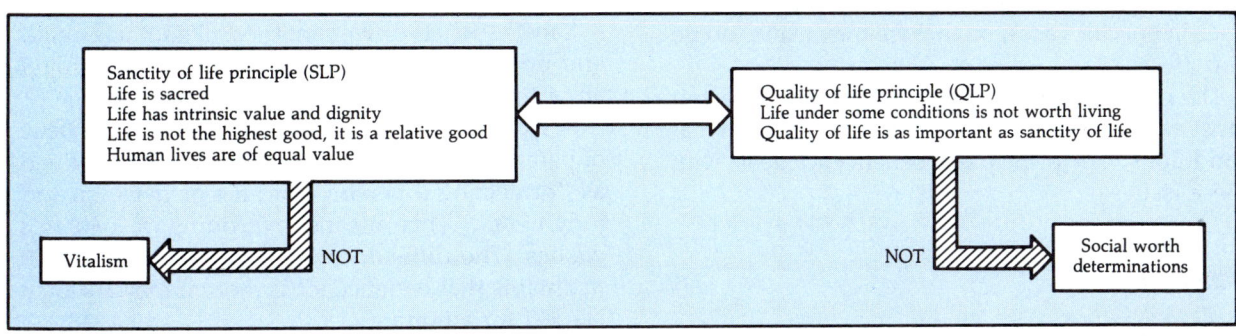

FIGURE 7–4. Sanctity versus quality of life.

The implications of this position for clinical care are:

1. All persons are of equal and inherent value and ought to be treated with due respect and dignity.
2. When we must err, we should err on the side of conserving life.
3. When continued treatment would assault the person's dignity, prove too burdensome for the patient, or merely prolong and increase pain, it is not morally *obligatory*.
4. Decisions should be made with the patient's participation and reflect the *patient's* true wishes and best interests.
5. In treatment decisions about infants and children, individuals who cannot consent, or those adjudged incompetent, the *patient's* best interests must be the basis for decision making.
6. If the patient wishes not to be treated, based upon her particular values and situation, nontreatment is morally permissible, even if life could otherwise be prolonged.

Again, McCormick (1978) writes (citing Veatch) that

> refusal of treatment may be considered reasonable "whenever they can offer reasons valid to themselves—that is, out of concern about physical or mental burdens or other objectives . . .

and that

> Treatment that conforms to such wishes and perspectives may be considered reasonable (morally appropriate), always allowing for legal appeal by physician [nurse] or hospital if a patient is judged to be frivolously jeopardizing life (p. 36).

These criteria do not directly answer the question of what to do about the salvageable infant with a poor prognosis for normalcy. Such cases must be examined individually, with the hope that these general rules will prove to be useful guidelines in specific cases, so that we may truly "do no harm".

The noninfliction of harm is a stringent duty; but must we also "do good"? And, if so, under what conditions? The principle of beneficence deals with these issues.

Beneficence

Ethics requires more of us than the law does. The principle of beneficence makes this apparent. It requires positive acts that will contribute to the well-being and welfare of others.

Beauchamp and Childress (1978) argue that the justification of beneficence as a duty is found in the social nature of human existence—that is, in social interactions, relationships, and interdependence. They divide beneficence into two main emphases: conferring good and balancing good.

As conferring good, beneficence is a duty, enjoined by the Nightingale Pledge (Gretter, 1896), in which the nurse promises to "devote myself to the welfare of those committed to my care" (see Appendix A). It is also found in the ANA Code for Nurses (American Nurses' Association, 1976). The principle of beneficence provides the moral justification for activities such as preventive health, health education for the public, nursing research, and public health measures such as water fluoridation.

When balancing benefits against costs and risks, beneficence involves using a principle of utility, as in cost-benefit analysis. Cost-benefit analysis need not refer only to money but may incorporate the measurements of risks versus present and future benefits. Such analyses should factor in "human values" and not be limited to economic values alone.

An example of an issue that has been subject to cost-benefit analysis is labeling of patients. Labels need not only harm; they may also benefit patients. When labels cost more than they benefit, they are morally unjustifiable. When they benefit without harm, they are morally justifiable.

Potter (1977) lists three criteria for labeling:

1. That the label treats persons as persons.
2. That it is not indelible—that is, it provides for its removal when the patient improves, grows, or changes.
3. That the label expands opportunities rather than constricts them—that is allows access to resources not open to others without that label.

Labels such as unwed mother, illegitimate child, and primipara are morally justifiable if and only if all of these three criteria are met.

A second major aspect of beneficence is the issue of paternalism. *Paternalism* may be broadly defined as "protecting a person from his or her own bad judgment". This means overriding a patient's wishes. The difficulty with paternalism is that it maintains that beneficence is more important than respect for autonomy.

Examples of paternalism include withholding information from a patient (such as that her infant has a birth defect or that fetal heart sounds have been lost); requiring bedside rails to be up for a postpartal patient who wants them down; performing a tubal ligation without consent or coercing a patient into consenting; incidental appendectomy during hysterectomy; and forced transfusions or other treatments.

Paternalism has strong and weak forms. Strong paternalism overrides truly voluntary and fully informed patient decisions. Weak paternalism occurs when the patient's capacity for judgments is so impaired that decisions may be considered nonvoluntary or when the patient is sufficiently uninformed or misinformed that decisions fail to reflect knowledge or understanding of the facts of the situation. Intense pain, psychotropic drugs, and hemorrhagic hypoxia fit this category. Please note that not all patient decisions under these conditions are nonvoluntary. Nursing assessment is vital under these circumstances.

Paternalism can be morally permissible in its weak form but is rarely morally justifiable in its strong form. That is, when either a patient's ability to give free consent, or her access to information is affected, nursing intervention to protect the patient is justifiable. However, when a patient is fully informed and freely consenting, the only justification for protective intervention is generally the prevention of harm to others.

The principle of beneficence is of particular importance to nursing. Nursing has a long and honorable history of doing good for others, even at great personal expense. Nursing has also had a history of placing beneficence before patient autonomy, although the pendulum has swung to the point where upholding patient autonomy is now interpreted as doing good. In this way, beneficence is built into the notion of patient advocacy.

SUMMARY

Nurses must be careful not to confuse issues of law, economics, or politics with those of ethics. They must also acknowledge that it is only a rare clinical decision that does not have moral ramifications. Our escalating technology and scientific knowledge, coupled with the increasing autonomy of nursing, have brought unprecedented and perhaps even unimaginable dilemmas to our practice.

If you read newspapers or listen to broadcast news, you will find many reproductive, maternal, or neonatal issues with tremendous moral implications: the sperm bank for Nobel Prize winners, the "Baby Jane Doe" case, surrogate mothers, Siamese twins (one of whom will die if they are separated), controversy over telling parents that their daughters seek contraception or abortions, the tremendously high teenage pregnancy rate, infants with defects who are left alive in utility closets or on doorsteps, and so on.

Ethical decision making is neither simple nor without cost. It can be made clearer and more certain, though, through the use of principles and rules. But principles and rules are insufficient unless coupled with habits of character—personal virtuousness—that enable nurses to do that which ought to be done. Obligation and virtue culminate in the moral aspects of the nurse–patient relationship, something that nursing has understood for centuries and that it affirms today in the ANA Code for Nurses.

REFERENCES

American Civil Liberties Union Foundation Project on Privacy and Data Collection. 1977. Medical records: The myth of personal privacy. *The Privacy Report.* 5(4):1–9.

American Nurses' Association, 1976. *Codes for nurses with interpretive statements.* Kansas City, Mo.: American Nurses' Association.

American Nurses' Association. 1980. *Nursing: A social policy statement.* Kansas City, Mo.: American Nurses' Association.

Associated Alumnae of Trained Nurses of the United States and Canada. 1896. *Minutes of the proceedings of the convention of training school alumnae delegates and representatives from the American Society of Superintendents of Training Schools for Nurses.* Harrisburg, Pa.: Harrisburg Publishing.

Beauchamp, T. L., and Childress, J. F. 1979. *The principles of biomedical ethics.* Oxford: Oxford University Press.

Beauchamp, T. L., and Walters, L. R. 1982. *Contemporary issues in bioethics.* Belmont, Calif.: Wadsworth.

Childress, J. F. 1970. Who shall live when not all can live? *Soundings.* 43(4):339–362.

Crossley, J. P., Jr. 1979. *The rise of value conflicts: Perspectives on ethical reflection.* Unpublished manuscript.

Dedek, J. F. 1976. Abortion. Ethical issues in nursing: A proceedings. St. Louis: Catholic Hospital Association.

Downie, R. S., and Telfer, E. 1964. *Respect for persons.* New York: Schocken.

Fowler, M. D. M., and Levine-Ariff, J. 1987. *Ethics at the bedside: A source book for the critical care nurse.* Philadelphia: J. B. Lippincott.

Frankena, W. F. 1973. *Ethics.* 2nd ed. Englewood Cliffs, N.J.: Prentice-Hall.

Gretter, L. 1896. *The Florence Nightingale pledge.* Unpublished manuscript.

International Council of Nurses. 1973. *1973 Code for Nurses.* Geneva: International Council of Nurses.

Jameton, A. 1983. *Nursing practice: The ethical issues.* Englewood Cliffs, N.J.: Prentice-Hall.

Jones, W. H. S. 1977. Selections from the Hippocratic corpus. In *Ethics in medicine,* eds. S. J. Reiser, A. J. Dyck, and W. Curran. Cambridge, Mass.: MIT Press.

Kant, I. 1976. *Foundations of the metaphysics of morals,* trans. L. White. Indianapolis: Bobbs-Merrill. (Originally published 1785.)

Massachusetts Nurses' Association. 1977. *The nature of professional nursing.* Boston: Massachusetts Nurses' Association.

McCormick, R. A. 1974. To save or let die: The dilemma of modern medicine. *JAMA.* 229:172–176.

McCormick, R. A. 1978. The quality of life—the sanctity of life. *Hastings Center Report.* 8(1):30–36.

Mill, J. S. 1957. *On liberty,* ed. E. Rapaport. Indianapolis: Hackett. (Originally published 1859.)

Potter, R. B. 1977. Labeling the mentally retarded: The just allocation of therapy. In *Ethics in medicine,* eds. S. J. Reiser, A. J. Dyck, and W. Curran. Cambridge, Mass.: MIT Press.

Ramsey, P. 1978. *Ethics at the edges of life.* New Haven, Conn.: Yale University.

Rawls, J. 1971. *A theory of justice.* Cambridge, Mass.: Belknap/Harvard University.

Reich, W. T., ed. 1978. *Encyclopedia of bioethics.* New York: Free Press.

Robb, I. A. H. 1900. *Nursing ethics: For hospital and private use.* Cleveland: E. C. Koeckert.

Shryock, R. H. 1959. *The history of nursing.* Philadelphia: W. B. Saunders.

Veatch, R. M. 1977. *Case studies in medical ethics.* Cambridge, Mass.: Harvard University.

8

Legal Issues in Perinatal Nursing

BEHAVIORAL OBJECTIVES

Upon completion of this chapter, the reader should be able to:

- Identify the sources of laws regulating nursing practice.

- Define the phrase "community standard of care".

- Relate professional society standards of care to contemporary practice.

- Identify mandates intrinsic to nursing practice acts.

- Discuss the legal parameters of practice for nurses in expanded roles in maternity and perinatal nursing.

- Discuss methods for ensuring patients' rights.

- Describe methods to ensure that patient records reflect standards of care.

- Define the nurse's responsibilities for documentation.

- Integrate the nursing process and legal requirements in practice.

- Develop a plan for providing informed consent for a nursing procedure.

- Describe the nurse's role in obtaining consent.

The profession of nursing continues to evolve to include more sophisticated patient care activities. In no other specialty has this been more evident over the past decade than in the field of perinatal nursing. It therefore becomes particularly important that perinatal nurses be conversant with the laws and standards regulating their practice. A thorough understanding of the interrelatedness of statutes, regulations, policies, standards of care, and case law should enable the nurse to analyze the legal aspects of proposed changes. Such an analysis will help ensure that change is accomplished in a planned way that reflects knowledge of what is necessary and what best serves the patient. Planned change should facilitate quality patient care, should be acceptable to the majority of the nurses in the specialty, and should maximize control by nurses of the evolution of their practice.

HISTORICAL BACKGROUND AND THE FRAMEWORK OF LAW

Because this text focuses on perinatal practice, this chapter will provide only an overview of general law as a framework from which to discuss pertinent perinatal legal issues. The reader is encouraged to explore other texts (see the suggested readings at the end of this chapter) that present and analyze general law more completely.

Figure 8–1 depicts the framework and interrelatedness of statutes, regulations, and common law and the sources of such law. *Statutes* are laws enacted by legislative bodies, either state or federal. Nurse practice acts are examples of statues. In most instances, statutes are broad and general and describe the legal boundaries for given situations. They may be likened to the policies of institutions and agencies.

By comparison, *regulations* are more specific and detailed. They are enacted by bureaucratic agencies for the purpose of explicating precise methods for implementing statutes. They tell nurses how to act and perform legally. They can be likened to the procedures of institutions and agencies. The disciplinary powers of nursing boards are examples of regulations.

Opportunities exist for nurses to influence the enactment and content of both statutes and regulations. Figure 8–2 depicts these opportunities. Public hearings are required prior to the adoption of both statutes and regulations at both the state and federal levels. It is strongly suggested that nurses become part of information networks through the offices of legislators, professional or specialty associations, or community groups. This involvement enables nurses to provide input and affect the law in its formative stages, which in turn facilitates the control of nursing practice by the nursing profession.

The last source of law is *common law*. Common law has its origin in three principal places: the courts, community practices, and attorney generals' opinions.

Common law established in the courts is often referred to as *case law*. Such law is the result of litigation and is accepted as precedent in reaching subsequent case decisions.

Community practices have come to be referred to as the *community standard of care*. They are the standards against which actual practice is measured. The concept of the "reasonable man" is often cited in this regard. According to this concept, the behavior of the individual should be

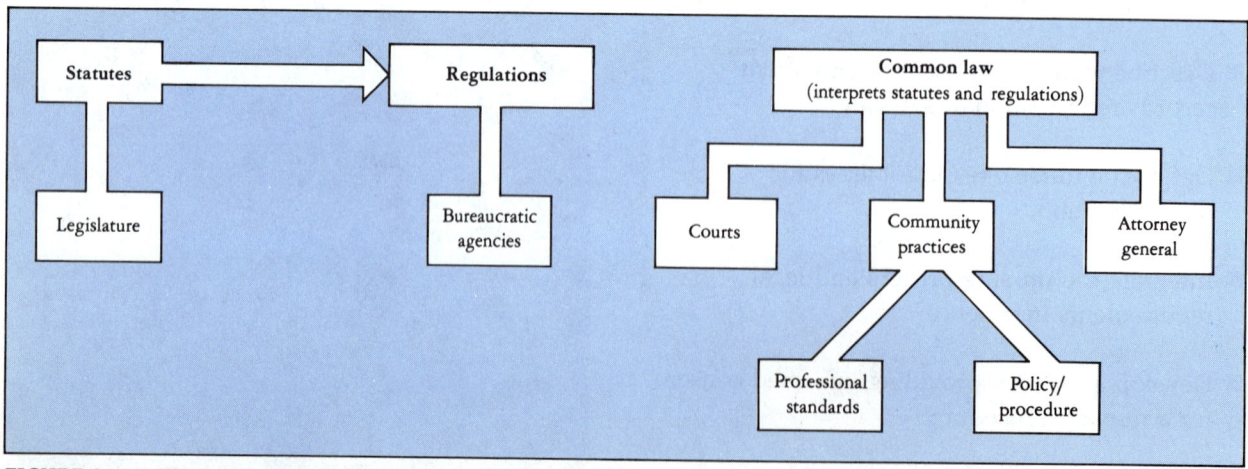

FIGURE 8–1. The origins and relatedness of laws.

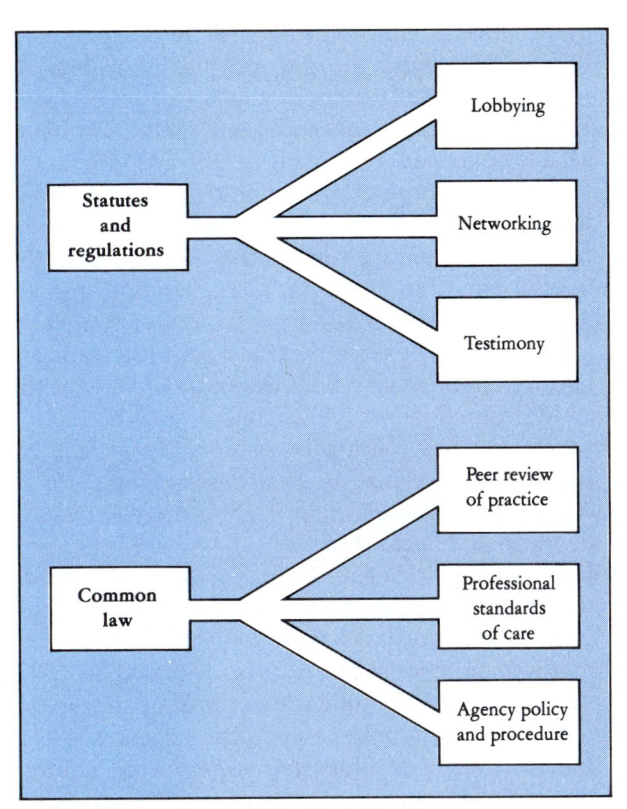

FIGURE 8-2. Opportunities for influencing the evolution of practice.

consistent with that of the reasonable, prudent person. Paraphrased, this means that the nurse's behaviors are analyzed against those of reasonable, prudent nurses.

Nurses were first held to a nursing, as opposed to a *medical*, standard of care in *Norton* v. *Argonaut Insurance Company*, in a decision rendered by a Louisiana Court of Appeals in 1962 (Ellis and Hartley, 1980). The extensive body of case law that has evolved since that decision makes it clear that the "reasonable nurse" standard will continue to be applied. It is helpful, therefore, for the nurse to ask how colleagues would approach a practice situation, to engage in discussions with colleagues, and to participate in formal and informal peer review of practices.

Although a nurse should never lose sight of the fact that he or she is always liable for his or her actions, it is comforting to know that the risk of actionable error is markedly diminished by adhering to the community standard of care. Contributing to and formalizing the community standard of care are the policies and procedures of the institution or agency in which the nurse practices and the standards of care developed and promulgated by professional and specialty societies.

Institutional or agency policies, in effect, determine what the nurse may do in that institution or agency. Procedures provide explicit detail as to how a task is to be performed. In actuality, policies and procedures are often the cornerstone of the community standard of care and, where they exist, will be central to case decisions. Nurses must be knowledgeable about the policies and procedures in their employment setting, adhere to them, and vigilantly ensure that they reflect the current state of practice.

Many of the policies and procedures commonly found in institutions, particularly hospitals, are mandated either in regulations or in standards promulgated by professional or specialty societies. The requirement for a policy that articulates the manner in which staffing patterns are determined is one example of a regulatory requirement for policy. The requirement for a policy that describes how the competency of nursing staff in cardiopulmonary resuscitation will be maintained is set forth in the Standards for Nursing Service of the Joint Commission for the Accreditation of Hospitals (JCAH). Greater specificity for perinatal nurses is to be found in both the Nurses Association of the American College of Obstetrics and Gynecology (NAACOG) Standards for Obstetric, Gynecologic, and Neonatal Nursing (Appendix B) and the American Nurses' Association (ANA) Standards of Maternal-Child Health Nursing Practice (Appendix C). Familiarity with both of these authoritative statements will enable nurses to examine their practice in light of standards agreed upon nationally.

The fact that such standards exist is of great legal significance because they tend to extend the "community" from the hospital or state to the nation. The standards can be used as a tool for evaluating one's own practice and may serve as a fulcrum for instituting improvements in agency or institutional standards of care.

Opinions issued by attorney generals are interpretations of law based on reviews of statutes and regulations. While such opinions are not law in the usual sense of the word, they are accorded the weight of law unless and until a court proceeding validates or negates them.

With this general overview of law as a framework, let us now focus on specific legal matters and issues of importance in perinatal nursing.

NURSE PRACTICE ACTS

The purpose of licensure for the professions is to protect the consumer. When nurses periodically reflect on the altruistic motive for licensure, it becomes clear that licensure is a force for establishing minimal standards of care in order to ensure safety for the patient or client. *Nurse practice acts* are mandates that enumerate those functions that every patient or client has the right to expect from every registered nurse. The changes that have occurred in nurse practice acts throughout the years are a reflection of the attention nurses have paid to this altruistic motive.

The first nurse practice act was adopted in North Carolina in 1903, and by 1923 all of the existing 48 states had licensure laws. These laws were said to be *permissive* in that they were voluntary: those who met certain standards could, by choice, be issued a license that would be registered with the state. There were no prohibitions against those without such licenses practicing the same as registered nurses, as long as they did so under the supervision of a physician.

The first *mandatory* licensure law was enacted in New York in 1947, and other states have followed suit over the years (Texas is the sole exception). A mandatory licensure law requires that all who wish to engage in the practice of registered nursing meet established standards and become licensed.

Beginning in the early 1970s, a nationwide movement had taken place to remove restrictions regarding diagnosis and treatment from nurse practice acts. This movement is believed to have had its origin in the concerns raised by nurses practicing in critical care units. It gained additional momentum with the evolution of other expanded roles in nursing, most specifically nurse practitioner roles.

Clarifying and expanding the scope of practice of *professional* registered nurses (RNs) quite naturally led to the analysis of the *educational* preparedness of RNs for the assumption of the functions articulated in practice acts. While practice acts continue to acknowledge dependent functions evolving from carrying out the physician's orders, it has become increasingly clear that strong foundations in the behavioral and physical sciences must be part of the basic education for the nurse to carry out such independent functions as nursing diagnosis and patient advocacy, particularly in the areas of disease prevention and health education. The American Nurses Association and major specialty associations (American Organization of Nursing Executives, Association of Operating Room Nurses, American Association of Critical Care Nurses, Nurses Association of the American College of Obstetrics and Gynecology) have agreed that a minimum of a bachelor's degree is required for entry into the practice of *professional* nursing. At least 10 states have already introduced legislation to bring this about and more than 25 are said to be formulating plans for the introduction of legislation. These efforts should clarify the overlapping functions of professional and technical nursing just as the efforts of the 1970s clarified the overlapping functions of medicine and professional nursing.

Nurses must examine closely both the statutory and regulatory sections of the licensure law in the state where they practice to determine whether the functions they perform are considered generic nursing acts or are medically delegated. *Fein v. Permanente Medical Group* (California 1981) established a clear legal precedent that nurses performing medically delegated functions will be held to the *medical* standard of care. Further, in states where licensure laws permit the performance of medical functions by nurses, detailed criteria, including, but not limited to, educational preparation, conditions under which the function is permitted, degree of physician supervision required (if any), and evaluation of competence are almost universally present.

This review of the changes that have occurred in nurse practice acts serves to reaffirm the commitment of nurses to the well-being of the patients and clients whom they serve. In all instances the changes that have occurred have enabled the patient and client to rest assured that his or her care will be given with due concern for basic minimal competency and in a safe manner.

EXPANDED ROLES IN PERINATAL NURSING

As an example of the growth of the profession made possible, in large part, by updating nurse practice acts, we now describe three expanded roles in perinatal nursing: clinical nurse specialist, nurse practitioner, and nurse-midwife.

Clinical Nurse Specialists

The role of the *clinical nurse specialist* was perhaps the first of the "expanded" roles in nursing. It evolved from the need of nurses to find a way to advance their practice without leaving direct patient care. In 1974 the American Nurses' Association Congress for Nursing Practice adopted a definition of clinical nurse specialist; it stated that master's level preparation is required in order to be called a specialist. Primary functions encompassed by the role of nurse specialist include patient care delivery, staff education, staff development, and research.

Some specialists in perinatal nursing have completed graduate curriculums that are broad and encompass the entire scope of perinatal care, including infant care. Others have focused more narrowly on a subspecialty area. The trend in practice, however, is for the specialist to operate rather broadly, since most agencies or institutions do not employ enough specialists to allow a focus on subspecialty issues.

Clinical nurse specialists have had their greatest impact on health care delivery in the contributions they have made to standardizing patient care. Standard care plans and standardized teaching plans are two examples. Such tools provide staff members with a basis for planning individualized patient care that is grounded in scientific principle and reflects careful research. Further, the additional knowledge acquired in graduate study in the areas of physiology and psychology make clinical nurse specialists invaluable resources to staff nurses when planning care in unusual, acute, or complicated cases.

In many institutions or agencies, the clinical nurse specialist may have joint clinical–administrative responsibilities. Some observers believe that having administrative authority facilitates implementation of clinical change. However, critics question whether the burden of administrative duty overshadows the attention to clinical activities; they prefer to see the specialist in an advisory or "staff" role free from line responsibility (Olsen, 1974). In any case, the improvements in standardized nursing care delivery that have occurred since the mid-1960s can almost exclusively be credited to the efforts of clinical nurse specialists.

Nurse Practitioners

Controversy continues to rage around the expanded role of *nurse practitioners*. It is a role that developed in response to perceived shortages of primary care physicians across the nation and out of the desire of nurses to have an opportunity to fully apply all they have learned. Continued controversy is fostered by the fact that no single nationwide standard for education exists: in some states a master's degree is required; in others, a bachelor's degree; and in others, special courses of variable length in addition to basic nursing education. The amount or degree of physician supervision also varies from state to state. Therefore, the responsibilities and legal authority are inconsistent.

Recent changes in nurse practice acts provide clear legal authority for the expanded role. Because specific methods vary from state to state, nurses are advised to review the wording of the legislation in their state.

Nurse practitioner functions include complete history and physical examination, episodic care for common or minor illnesses, long-term care for stabilized chronic illnesses, initial work-ups and partial management of prenatal and postnatal patients, well-baby care, family planning, and teaching and counseling (Bullough, 1975). In some states, the nurse practitioner role also includes attending the patient at delivery.

Most nurse practitioners differentiate the service they provide to patients from that of traditional medicine by focusing on their desire to work with the patient and family to achieve health maintenance and disease prevention. Because of their educational preparation in nursing, these practitioners teach and counsel rather than provide acute episodic care.

Nurse-Midwives

The American College of Obstetricians and Gynecologists (ACOG), the Nurses Association of the American College of Obstetricians and Gynecologists (NAACOG), and the American College of Nurse-Midwives adopted a statement in 1971 that articulated their common goal of improving and expanding the availability of health services to women. This statement allowed for the role of the nurse to be expanded so that nurse-midwives could practice.

Efforts to standardize the practice of *nurse-midwifery* have largely been made by the American College of Nurse-Midwives, which was formed in 1969. By accrediting educational programs of nurse-midwifery, the organization ensures standards of education. There has, however, been less standardization in establishing legal requirements and parameters nationwide. The American College of Nurse-Midwives states that the functions of the practitioner include responsibilities for the management and complete care of essentially healthy women and newborn during the childbearing process (Varney, 1980). There is a wide variety of state laws that govern how and even whether the practice is permitted. Nurses should become apprised of the laws in the states where they practice.

THE RIGHTS OF PATIENTS

Among the ways in which all nurses (and, most specifically, perinatal nurses) have applied the expanded authority of nursing to the goal of fostering patient advocacy has been ensuring patients' rights.

Trends in Patients' Rights

In 1959 the National League for Nursing (NLN) formulated a statement enumerating the rights of patients. Yet for many years after, health care providers, including nurses, continued to act as though they knew what was best for patients and made decisions for patients, often without offering alternatives. The human rights movement did much to alter this paternalistic behavior, and in 1973 the "Patient's Bill of Rights" was published (see Appendix D). Some states, including California and New York, have codified these rights in the regulations governing hospitals.

Although the nursing profession began the movement for human rights in the health care delivery system, the continuation of these efforts has almost exclusively been on the part of perinatal practitioners. Of particular importance in maternity nursing is "The Pregnant Patient's Bill of Rights and Responsibilities" published by the International Childbirth Education Association (ICEA). The preamble to this statement (see Appendix E) points out that additional rights must be accorded to the pregnant patient so that she may adequately attend to the considerations of *two* persons. In addition, Margaret Ribble (1965) has articulated what is tantamount to an infant's bill of rights in her book *The rights of infants*. This book provides guidance for nurses in their advocate role for those patients who cannot advocate for themselves. All practitioners are strongly urged to study this work.

Communication about Patients

The commitment of nurses to thorough, consistent care delivery can be strengthened through the application of certain key principles of communication. The major tool for communication about patients is the medical record.

Documentation

The role of nurses in patient record keeping is crucial, since nurses are able to provide, through the record, a 24-hour picture of the patient's progress. By accurate reporting of objective findings and subjective commentaries by the patient, each nurse can influence both the medical and nursing planning of the patient's care. Precise and concise documentation of significant details will (1) foster continuity of care as it guides other health practitioners, (2) enhance consistency in recognizing individual needs, and (3) promote cost-efficient, efficacious acts by care providers.

The nurse's responsibilities for documentation include recording what is seen, sensed, said, done, and achieved. A complete and detailed record is frequently the nurse's best defense in litigation. The chart often stimulates recall of specific instances and of the individual patient. However, it is hoped that avoiding lawsuits will not be the sole motivation for good record keeping. Rather, good charting should be viewed as an extension of good care. A chart that is complete will reflect the nursing process, nursing diagnoses, nursing acts in response to these diagnoses, and outcomes. Through quality assurance activities, charts can be used to determine compliance with the standard of care and can serve as the basis for education to improve or enhance standards of care.

It must be noted, however, that the medical record is a legal record. As such, it may become the "first line of defense" when disputes arise and it is accorded the weight of truth versus bias, memory, or perception of various members of the health team involved with the patient. Furthermore, the contents of the medical record, in accordance with the rights of patients, must be treated with confidentiality. Table 8–1 offers charting tips that will assist the nurse in ensuring that the record communicates necessary information, fosters continuity of care, and provides a clear statement of the patient's progress as well as a defensible legal record.

Part of ensuring that the record is legally defensible includes adequate attention to and documentation of consent.

Consent

The act of obtaining the patient's consent has become increasingly complicated by court rulings that consent that is not fully "informed" is not legally valid. Such rulings have defined *informed consent* in terms of the patient's right to know the

TABLE 8-1. Charting Tips

When You Chart, Do

1. Record your acts.
2. Record your observations.
3. Record the *outcomes* of your acts, where appropriate.
4. Record the patient's statements about her care or condition.
5. Be consistent; you *are* establishing a standard of care for yourself, your unit or service, and your hospital.
6. Avoid value judgments.
7. Avoid defensive statements.
8. Correct errors by drawing a single line through the erroneous entry and initialing the line.
9. Treat the record as *confidential*.
10. Adhere to your agency's or institution's requirements for record keeping.

---

nature of, the risks and benefits of, and the alternatives to a proposed treatment or procedure (Hershey and Bushkoff, 1969). Some state courts have indicated that informed consent is required only for *complex* procedures—that is, ones that are not commonly and easily understood. Without exception, where case law exists the courts have held that the dialogue that is required to obtain an informed consent remains the responsibility of the person who will actually perform the treatment or procedure. Thus, while the physician may delegate the responsibility for conducting all or part of the discussion with the patient, present case law indicates that the physician still retains the legal responsibility for ascertaining that the patient has full understanding. Furthermore, while the physician may lawfully delegate the performance of certain procedures and treatments to others, such as nurses, case law appears to still hold the physician responsible for ensuring that the patient is adequately informed. Thus, it seems reasonable to assume that the modern team approach to patient care can create problems when two or more practitioners are working with the same patient. The issue of the nurse's obligation to obtain informed consent cannot be ignored, although there is no present case law on this issue. It seems prudent for each practitioner to obtain consent for the particular procedure or part thereof that he or she will perform.

It should be kept in mind that if informed consent is to have meaning, the notion of *informed denial* must exist. That is, the constitutional right of self-determination encompasses the right to refuse. Court decisions have, to date, upheld the rights of patients and surrogates representing the patient's interests to refuse treatment and even to require its withdrawal. Attention is given in these decisions to the burden versus the benefit of the treatment. There is emerging controversy in perinatal nursing centers surrounding the fact that many believe conflicts exist between the rights of the mother compared to those of the fetus. Technological advances which enhance the ability to diagnose and treat the fetus are at the root of these controversies. Some favor seeking court orders to force treatment upon the unwilling pregnant woman. However, there is *no reported case* of a court imposing civil or criminal penalties for failing to seek a court's review of a competent adult's refusal of treatment.

In consent disputes, liability may arise from one of two causes: (1) the patient asserts a complete lack of consent (battery), or (2) the patient alleges a failure on the part of the caregiver to adequately disclose information related to the treatment or procedures (negligent nondisclosure; lack of informed consent). Care should be exercised to avoid coercion in obtaining consent. Full and open discussions with the mother during the prenatal phase regarding anticipated problems should clarify areas in which the clinician's attitudes and values are in conflict with the mother's. Transfer of care to a clinician who is not in conflict could forestall the use of coercion which arises due to the perceived critical or emergency nature of a problem. It is urged that where law is absent, the nurse use common sense. In the face of consistent court rulings, it can be said that to inform the patient can do no harm.

It must be noted that under the doctrine of *respondent superior*, the hospital *is* liable for the acts of its employees when these wrongful acts occur within the scope of employment. This fact does not provide the individual wrongdoer with immunity from personal liability, however. Further, the hospital has the right to recover from an employee any amount it is compelled to pay as a result of the employee's misconduct or error (Lasky, 1983).

It must always be remembered that a consent form is in no way informed consent. A consent form is merely documentation of the patient's agreement to undergo a procedure or treatment. The nurse who signs as a witness on such a form certifies that the person signed the form. *Informed* consent arises out of discussion of information about the nature of the procedure or treatment. Some hospitals have, in fact, ceased using consent forms altogether in favor of a note in the medical record that details what the patient was told (Holder and Lewis 1981).

Clearly, common sense and ethics should dictate that the nurse report to the physician immediately any information indicating that a patient lacks understanding of proposed treatments or procedures. It may also be necessary to report this finding to a hospital representative to protect the hospital from liability. The aim should be to increase the patients' understanding so that they can be active participants in decisions about their care.

CURRENT LEGAL CONTROVERSIES IN PERINATAL NURSING

The remainder of this chapter is devoted to highlighting some important controversies in the field of perinatal nursing care delivery for which law is still evolving.

These controversies stem from two sources: the rights of the unborn fetus and the rights of the (defective) newborn. Case law is sparse and statutes and regulations are generally imprecise. Certainly these matters will continue to occupy the minds and thoughts of ethicists for the foreseeable future. This chapter reflects current case law decisions. However, some decisions are still subject to appeal and the law is still formative.

A Fetal "Right to Life" Amendment

On January 22, 1973 the Supreme Court of the United States declared invalid all state laws that protected fetal life from the time of conception. The Court held that a woman's right to privacy is violated if she is not allowed to abort her unborn child. The Court could find no constitutional provision explicitly protecting the fetal right to life and, therefore, said no regulations on abortion are permissible in the first trimester of pregnancy, since the fetus is not a "person" within the meaning of the Constitution. The Court did, however, say that regulations governing abortions in the second trimester are permissible in order to protect the life of the pregnant woman. Further, regulations regarding abortion in the third trimester are permissible to protect the pregnant woman or the potential human life within the woman.

This decision prompted a movement for a constitutional amendment to recognize the fetal right to life. As evidence that most Americans oppose abortion, proponents cite the majority votes in both the House and Senate in 1976 to allot no federal funds to finance abortions unless the pregnant woman's health would be endangered (Smith, 1977).

Controversial revisions to both state and federal regulations in 1987 have further limited the use of funds for abortions to minors by requiring that consent for the abortion be obtained from the minor's parent(s). Heated debate and court appeals continue with the expectation that the constitutionality of these proposals will be challenged.

The nurse in perinatal practice should be familiar with the regulations regarding abortion in his or her state. In all states, the nurse has the right to refuse to participate in the performance of abortions. Many institutions and agencies provide a document on which the nurse can indicate his or her preference at the time of employment (conscience clause). If such a document is not available, the nurse who objects to participation in abortions should state this in writing and ask that the statement be placed in his or her personnel record.

The Rights of Defective Newborns

Dilemmas that arise regarding the rights of defective newborns seem to stem mainly from our imperfect and imprecise definition of *viability* (Swinyard, 1978). Regulations in many states provide that the "viable" fetus must receive the same consideration for medical treatment even if it is a result of a spontaneous or induced abortion. Obviously, an ethical dilemma occurs when the pregnancy is terminated by induced abortion because the fetus is known or believed to be defective. The nurse should focus on the words "consideration for medical treatment" and not assume that such regulations mandate "heroics". The agency or institution should, however, provide clear policy direction to its nursing staff for actions they are to take when a viable fetus is born and the physician is not present to provide medical consideration.

In some respects, even more troublesome are the questions that arise surrounding the care and treatment of defective newborns. The laws that do exist often seem to be in conflict with one another, especially with regard to the rights of parents to withhold or give consent to treatment compared to their obligations to care for their child, and the fine line that physicians must walk in determining a reasonable course of treatment while avoiding charges of infanticide when minimal treatment seems best. Ethical considerations weigh heavily in making such decisions and the law gives no clear mandate (see Chapter 7). Quality of life and the best use of limited resources are examples of related issues involved.

It is also not clear in the law what constitutes treatment. Is feeding treatment? Some federal authorities think that it is a basic right, whether treatment or not, and have attempted to forbid the withholding of food and water in hospital nurseries. Although these efforts have not been successful to date, the issues involved are by no means resolved. However, a 1982 Louisiana statute may have accomplished what federal authorities have failed to do (Hortz, 1983). This statute specifically accords to the parents and physician the right to discontinue medical and surgical intervention, including denial of nutritional support, when the infant has no reasonable chance of recovery. Further, the Louisiana Supreme Court has upheld this statute as constitutional. In another recent case in New York, the court upheld the rights of the parents to refuse consent for surgery on an infant born with spina bifida and hydrocephalus. There is a strong possibility that other states will enact statutes similar to the one in Louisiana, and the Federal Department of Health and Human Services has indicated its intent to reintroduce regulations on the subject of infant nutrition.

Perinatal nurses should involve themselves in the continuing debates about legal issues, since nurses are left to carry out the physicians' orders. If the law is to evolve in a way that will best serve the majority, lawmakers should have the input of those who carry it out. Laws that are ethically acceptable are best formulated through the broadest possible representation of the views of all involved in its formation.

AIDS

The so-called "black plague of the 80s" raises another level of potential conflict between the rights of the mother and those of the unborn fetus. Ultra-conservatives have taken the position that the woman with AIDS who knowingly becomes pregnant is, in fact, guilty of child abuse. Of perhaps more compelling concern to the majority of Americans and clinicians are the number of infants born to women in high-risk categories (sexually promiscuous and IV drug abusers) who are placed for adoption. What are the "rights to know" of the potential adoptive parents? Will they or anyone want to take these infants if the high-risk category is revealed? What if the mother refuses to have the HIV test herself and/or refuses to permit it for the infant?

Many believe that state laws, where they exist, do *not* preclude hospitals establishing HIV testing for *all* infants as a screening requirement and advocate this as an ethical and clinically valid obligation. This approach would be consistent with the Center for Disease Control's recent advocacy of "universal blood and bodily fluid" procedures for *all* patients in the hospital under the thesis that it is the patient about whom we have no data that places us at the greatest risk.

Some state laws do, however, expressly prohibit the release of the results of the HIV test (California) without the consent of the individual tested. Such laws were enacted at a time when it could be said that HIV positivity was not, in and of itself, *diagnostic* for AIDS. While this is technically still true, the percentages of those who are HIV positive, and who eventually go on to meet the criteria for AIDS, is rising and, it is predicted, will reach 100 percent by 1990.

SURROGACY

Legislation in abundance is under consideration due principally to the improvised nature of the agreements which have received widespread public attention. Several states propose the outright prohibition of surrogate agreements; others propose laws which would force the surrogate mother to release the infant to the father if the contract included independent legal representation for the surrogate mother; medical and psychological screening of the surrogate mother, the father-to-be and his spouse; and the right of the surrogate mother to choose her own doctor and to terminate the pregnancy if she so desired. New York state is considering the latter approach with the proviso that a judge review the contract prior to insemination. In this fashion, the rights of both the surrogate mother and the father-to-be would be guaranteed, while at the same time assuring a home for the baby.

Predictably, laws will be slow in coming since

inconsistencies with present contract, custody and adoption laws are almost assured. Unanswered questions still plague both society and the legislators who represent society: What about payment beyond the costs of care? If a court declares a surrogate mother unfit, what is its obligation to the children she may already have borne? What if neither the surrogate mother nor the father-to-be want the baby? Clearly, laws must evolve, but they must be carefully drafted to protect all parties concerned.

SUMMARY

Part of the difficulty that occurs when attempting to discuss the legalities of nursing practice is that nursing still exists as a poorly defined specialty, in spite of major gains in the past decade. Much of what was once the practice of medicine has become part of the practice of nursing. For example, today it is common practice for a perinatal nurse to perform vaginal examinations, insert intravenous needles in tiny infants, and interpret fetal heart rate monitor strips. All of these procedures were once considered the sole purview of the physician. These duties have shifted from the physician to the nurse because the hospital is increasingly being used as the main base of episodic health care, because it is the nurse who is present when the crisis occurs, and because the minute saved by having an educated practitioner present who can legally take definitive action may well become the minute that makes the difference between life and death.

In the days of the "captain of the ship" concept, it was assumed that the physician was responsible and liable for all acts relating to patient care. Now, however, we know and recognize the fact that each individual is legally liable for his or her own acts; responsibility thus often becomes an ethical concern. This change has been brought about by the growing complexity of practice with a corresponding increase in skills and numbers of health team members and a higher level of public awareness and sophistication.

It has been said that the picture of the devoted nurse providing humanitarian services for the patient, oblivious to the rest of the world, has faded, if in fact it ever did exist. The humanitarian or *ethical* aspects of nursing practice are now associated with the *legal* aspects of practice. The nurse today must function in a manner strongly modified by this new area of personal liability.

SUGGESTED READINGS

Bullough, B. 1975. *The law and the expanding nursing role.* New York: Appleton-Century-Crofts.
Cazalas, M. W. 1978. *Nursing and the law.* 3rd ed. Germantown, Md.: Aspen Systems Corporation.
Creighton, H. 1981. *Law every nurse should know.* 4th ed. Philadelphia: W. B. Saunders.
Streif, C. J. 1975. *Nursing and the law.* 2nd ed. Roseville, Md.: Aspen Systems Corporation.

REFERENCES

American Nurses' Association Executive Committee and the Standards Committee of the Division on Maternal–Child Health Nursing Practice. 1973. *Standards of maternal–child health practice.* Kansas City: American Nurses' Association.
Asnes, M. Surrogacy—What's Legal?; July, 1987; Condé Nast Publications.
Bash, D. B., and Gold, W. A. 1981. *The nurse and the childbearing family.* New York: John Wiley & Sons.
Bergerson, G. R. 1982. Charting with a jury in mind. *Nurs. Life.* 2:30–33.
Bernstein, A. H. 1982. Damage awards for wrongful birth and wrongful life. *Hospitals.* 56:65–67.
Besch, L. 1979. Informed consent: A patient's right. *Nurs. Outlook.* 27:33.
Bouvia v. Superior Court, (Cal 1986) 179 Cal. App. 3d 1127.
Bowes, W. A., and Selgestad, B. 1981. Fetal versus maternal rights: Medical and legal perspectives. *Obstet. Gynecol.* 58:209–214.
Bullough, B. 1975. *The law and the expanding nursing role.* New York: Appleton-Century-Crofts.
Cason, C. L.; Highfield, M. E.; and Hartfield, M. T. 1982. Clinical nurse specialist role development (research). *Nurs. Health Care.* 3:25.
Cazalas, M. W. 1978. *Nursing and the law.* 3rd ed. Germantown, Md.: Aspen Systems Corporation.
Creighton, H. 1981. *Law every nurse should know.* 4th ed. Philadelphia: W. B. Saunders.
Creighton, H. 1982a. Nurse practitioner in law for the nursing manager. *Nurs. Management.* 13:14–15.
Creighton, H. 1982b. The right of informed refusal. *Nurs. Management.* 13:48–49.
Cushing, M. 1982a. The legal side: Gaps in documentation. *Am. J. Nurs.* 82:1899–1900.
Cushing, M. 1982b. When medical standards apply to nursing practice. *Am. J. Nurs.* 82:1274–1276.
Cushing, M. 1983. The legal side: "Do not feed." *Am. J. Nurs.* 83:602–604.
Ellis, J. R., and Hartley, C. L. 1980. *Nursing in today's world: Challenges, issues, and trends.* Philadelphia: J. B. Lippincott.
Gruendemann, B., and Hesterly, S. 1973. *The surgical patient.* St. Louis: C. V. Mosby.
Haire, D. 1975. *The pregnant patient's bill of rights and*

responsibilities. International Childbirth Education Association, Inc., Committee on Health Law and Regulation, Minneapolis, Minn.

Harper, R. G.; Little, G. A.; and Sia, C. G. 1982. The scope of nursing practice in level III neonatal intensive care units. *Pediatrics*. 70:875–878.

Hershey, N., and Bushkoff, S. H. 1969. *Informed consent study*. Pittsburgh: Aspen Systems Corporation.

Holder, A. R., and Lewis, J. W. 1981. Informed consent and the nurse. *Nurs. Law & Ethics. 2(2)*.

Hollowell, E. C. 1983. Patient charting: The legal cornerstone of nursing. *J. Pract. Nurs*. 33:35–37.

Horan, D. J. 1982. Legally speaking: Infanticide: When doctor's orders read "murder." *RN*. 45(Jan.):75–86.

Hortz, J. F. 1983. One state's solution to the Baby Doe controversy. Imprint, Action Kit for *Hospital Law*, p. 23.

Kapp, M. B. 1982. Abortion and informed consent requirements. *J. Obstet. Gynecol*. 144:1–4.

Kolder, V. E., Gallagher, J., Parsons, M. T.: Court-ordered obstetrical interventions. *N. Engl. J. Med*. 1987; 316:1192–1196.

Landswirth, J.: Fetal Abuse and Neglect: An Emerging Controversy. Pediatrics, 1987; 79:508–514.

Lasky, P. 1983. *Hospital law manual*. Pittsburgh: Aspen Systems Corporation.

Mathieu, D.: Respecting Liberty and Preventing Harm: Limits of State Intervention in Prenatal Choice; *Harvard J. of Law and Public Policy* 1985; 8:19–52.

Nelson, L. J.: Clinical Ethics Report; May 1987; Vol 1 #5.

Nichols, M. E., and Wessels, V. G. 1977. *Nursing standards and nursing process*. Wakefield, Mass.: Contemporary Publishers.

Nurses Association of the American College of Obstetricians and Gynecologists. 1981. *Standards for obstetric, gynecologic, and neonatal nursing*. 2nd ed. Washington, D.C.

Olsen, L. 1974. The expanded role of the nurse in maternity care. *Nurs. Clin. North Am*. 9:459–466.

Patterson, P. 1982. Fetal therapy—Issues we face. *AORN*. 35:663–668.

Regan, W. A. 1982. Legally speaking: Assisting at abortions: Can you really say no? *RN*. 45:71.

Report of the Sixty-fifth Ross Conference on Pediatric Research. 1973. *Ethical dilemmas in current obstetric and newborn care*. Columbus: Ross Labs.

Ribble, M. 1965. *The rights of infants*. 2nd ed. New York: Columbia University Press.

Roberts, F. B. 1977. *Perinatal nursing*. New York: McGraw-Hill.

Robertson, J. A. 1982. The right to procreate. *J. Legal Medicine*. 3:333–336.

Roberston, J. A., and Fost, N. 1976. Passive euthanasia of defective newborn infants: Legal considerations. *J. Pediatrics*. 88:883.

Ruddick, W., and Wilcox, W. 1982. Operating on the fetus. *Hastings Center Report*. 12:10–14.

Sarner, H. 1968. *The nurse and the law*. Philadelphia: W. B. Saunders.

Smith, C. P. 1977. *The fetal right to life argument*. Silver Spring, Md.: Citizenship Enterprises.

State of California. 1980. *Business and Professions Code*, Chapter 6, Article 2, Section 2725.

Steinfels, M. O. 1978. New childbirth technology: A clash of values. *Hastings Center Report*. 8:9

Streif, C. J., ed. 1975. *Nursing and the law*. 2nd ed. Rockville, Md.: Aspen Systems Corporation.

Swinyard, C. A. 1978. *Decision making and the defective newborn*. Springfield, Ill.: Charles C. Thomas.

Tilbury, M. S. 1982. Legal aspects of the expanded role: Informed consent. *J. Contin. Ed. Nurs*. 13:5–9.

Trandel-Korenchuck, D. M., and Trandel-Korenchuck, K. M. 1978. How state laws recognize advanced nursing practice. *Nurs. Outlook*. 26:713.

Varney, H. 1980. *Nurse midwifery*. Boston: Blackwell Scientific Publications.

Whitehead v. Superior Court, (N Jersey 1987) 163 NJ: App. 1d 277.

Wiley, J. 1976. The nurse's legal responsibility in obstetric monitoring. *J. Obstet. Gynecol. Neonatal Nurs*. 5:775–785.

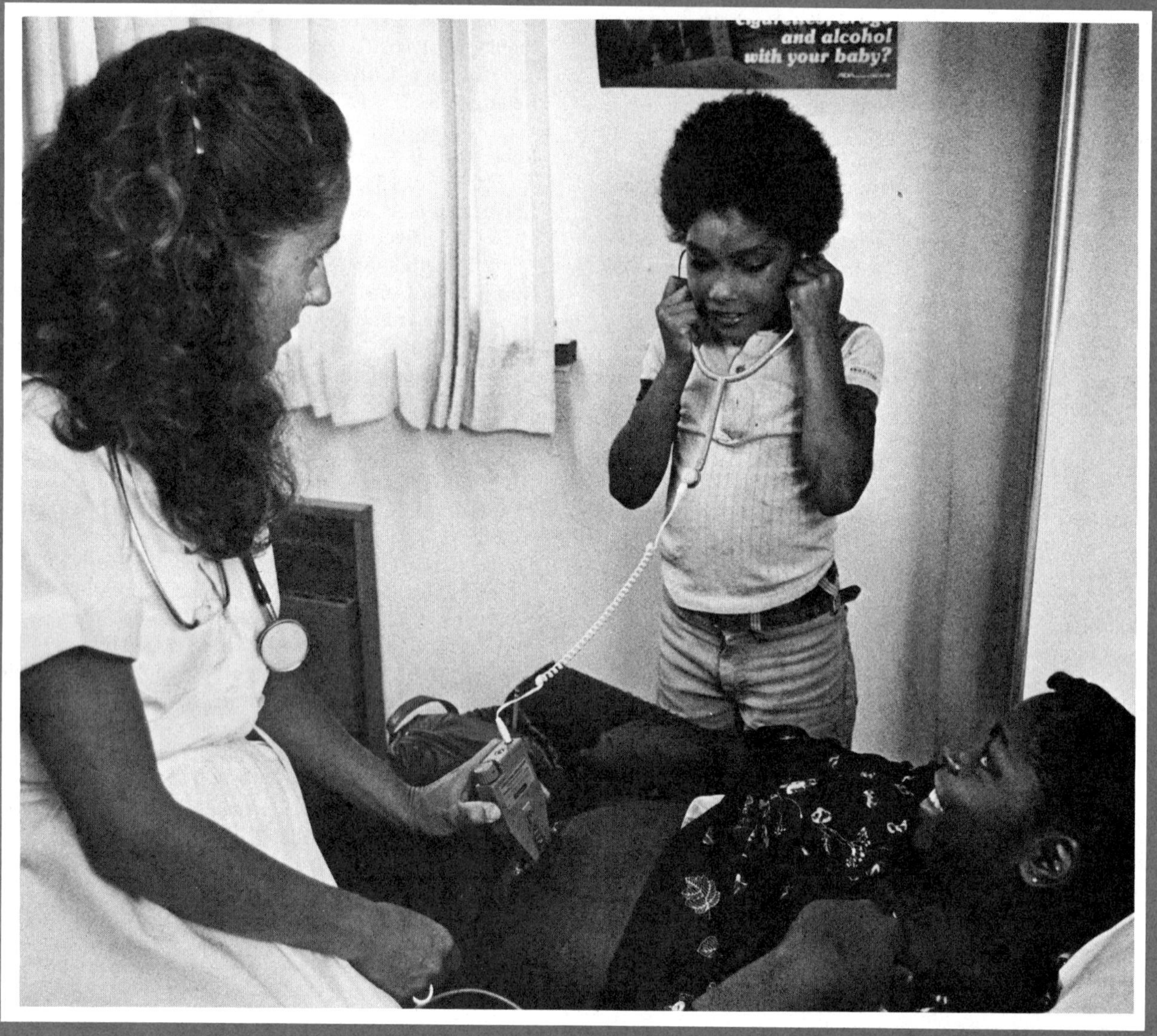
and alcohol
with your baby?

ated period, with the onset of labor at the end of that time. Due to its length and the vast developmental changes that occur during it, the prenatal period is often divided into three subperiods. The first, the period of the zygote or ovum, consists of approximately the first two weeks following conception. The second, the period of the embryo, extends from about the end of the second week through the end of the eighth week following conception. It is during this period that all the basic structures of the organism—internal and external—are formed. The third subperiod, that of the fetus, extends from the end of the second month of pregnancy through the termination of the pregnancy, usually at the end of the ninth month. During this time the organism's physical structure is refined, and it grows tremendously in size. Also, the organism gradually develops the capacity to sustain life outside the uterus.

UNIT TWO

CHANGE: THE PRENATAL PERIOD

9

Physiologic Changes in the Fetus

BEHAVIORAL OBJECTIVES

Upon completion of this chapter, the reader should be able to:

- Trace the normal gametogenetic processes of the male and female.

- Discuss the necessary events and phases of fertilization.

- Categorize the layers of the decidua and describe the fate of each during pregnancy.

- Describe placental development.

- Identify the three germ layers and the derivatives of each.

- Trace the developmental patterns of major embryonic and fetal systems during the 40 weeks of gestation.

- Identify the placental mechanisms of nutrient transfer and the factors affecting placental blood flow.

Each of us is unique. Each encounter with another human being reflects the uniqueness of the hereditary and developmental processes through which a single cell develops into a full-term infant. This chapter presents an overview of the process of conception and the establishment of the truly parasitic relationship between the mother and fetus. The placenta, the organ of exchange between mother and fetus, is followed through its developmental stages to its mature state. The products of conception and their development through embryonic and fetal stages are highlighted. Organ system maturation and functioning in the intrauterine environment are discussed. The student is encouraged to read this chapter once to gain a general understanding of the dynamic growth and differentiation that occurs in embryonic life, then return to the text a second time to identify the specific developmental events and when in pregnancy they occur.

OVARIAN AND ENDOMETRIAL CYCLES

In the mature female the interrelated *ovarian* and *endometrial cycles* occur simultaneously, one to produce an ovum for reproduction and the other to create a suitable environment where implantation and development can occur.

The reproductive cycle is mediated by the reciprocal actions of the neurohumoral and endocrine systems, specifically the hypothalamus, anterior pituitary, and ovaries. Ultimate control of the normal reproductive cycle lies with the hypothalamus.

Gonadotropin-releasing hormone (luteinizing hormone and follicle-stimulating hormone) is released from the hypothalamus. This releasing hormone acts upon the anterior pituitary to initiate the production and release of *follicle-stimulating hormone* (FSH) and *luteinizing hormone* (LH).

The ovaries contain specialized FSH and LH receptor cells. Once triggered, these cells cause increased follicle cell growth and hormone production. Apparently released simultaneously, FSH and LH work both independently and interdependently. The actions of FSH precede those of LH. FSH promotes the development of follicles within the ovary but cannot induce estrogen secretion by these follicles. LH, acting in conjunction with FSH, is responsible for stimulating not only estrogen secretion (responsible for the proliferative phase of the endometrial cycle), but also *ovulation* (release of the ovum from the follicle) and the structural changes associated with a ruptured follicle.

Approximately 18 hours after peak production of LH, ovulation occurs. Estrogen production is reduced and progesterone secretion is maintained.

The ruptured follicle changes structurally during the postovulation phase. *Luteinization* (vascularization, cell enlargement, and lipid accumulation) occurs, and the mass of follicular cells becomes the *corpus luteum*. These altered cells secrete large amounts of progesterone (responsible for the secretory phase of the endometrial cycle), which diminishes abruptly 7–8 days after ovulation. Involution of the corpus luteum occurs at this time, causing a decrease in progesterone and estrogen production.

The decrease in blood levels of these ovarian hormones triggers a response in the anterior pituitary. FSH production is initiated, followed by LH production. This leads to new follicular development and the beginning of a new reproductive cycle.

Both ovarian and endometrial cycles are composed of several overlapping phases. Table 9–1 and Figure 9–1 show these phases.

Follicular Development and Ovulation

Let's take a closer look at the ovarian cycle. The release of FSH stimulates growth and maturation of the follicle. Usually one follicle becomes mature enough to be released from the ovary during each cycle. However, several ova throughout the ovary undergo maturational changes each month.

The *oocyte* (immature ovum) within the *primary follicle* begins to increase in size under the influence of FSH. The cells surrounding it multiply and change to become cuboidal. These cells are known as the *follicular cells*. The development of the layers of follicular cells becomes eccentric (asymmetrical), and a fluid-filled space (the *antrum*) appears. This forces the oocyte and most of the follicular cells to one side (Fig. 9–2). A mucoid layer (*zona pellucida*)

TABLE 9–1. **Cyclic Changes in the Ovary and Endometrium**

Phase	Day	Influence
Ovarian cycle		
Follicular phase	1–14	FSH, LH
Luteal phase	15–28	
Endometrial cycle		
Menstrual phase	1–5	
Proliferative phase	6–14	Estrogen
Secretory phase	15–16	Progesterone
Ischemic phase	27–28	

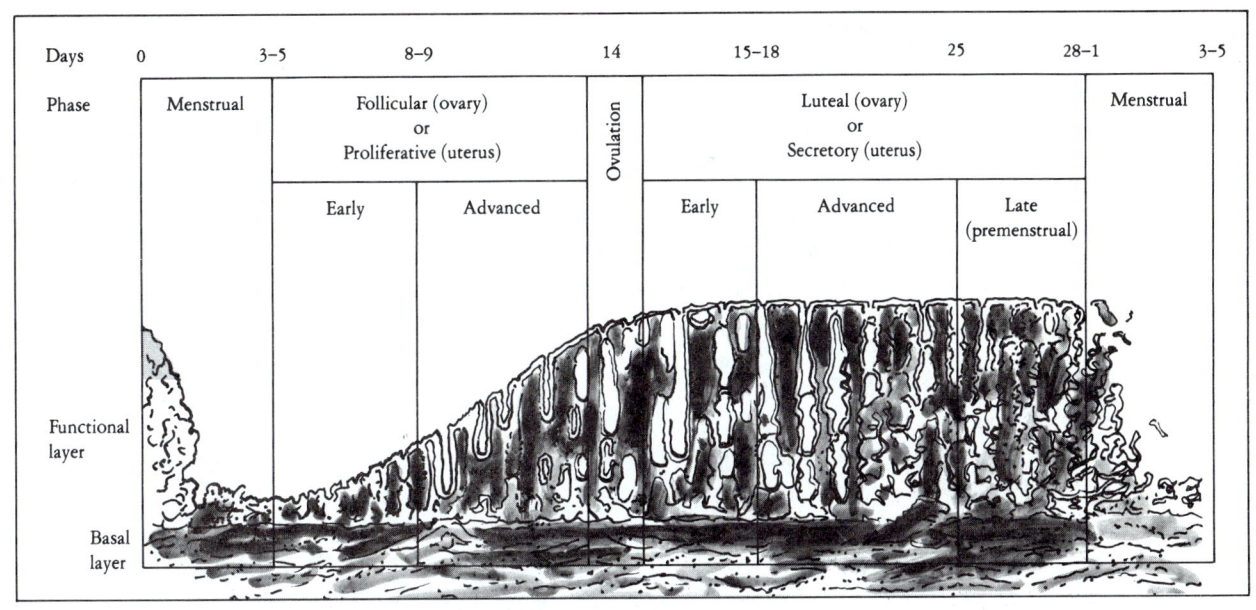

FIGURE 9–1. Cyclic changes in thickness and forms of glands and arteries of the endometrium during the ovarian cycle.
SOURCE: Pritchard, MacDonald, and Gant (1985).

forms around the ovum and remains intact until the ovum arrives in the uterus and following ovulation.

Under the synergistic effects of FSH and LH the follicle becomes a mature *graafian follicle*. At this stage, the follicular cells around the oocyte are identified as the *cumulus oophorus*. They project into the enlarge fluid-filled antrum (see Fig. 9–2). The *stromal cells* (the cell layers enclosing the antrum, cumulus oophorus, and oocyte), enlarge, and the surrounding capillary network is pulled closer.

During these changes, the stromal cells become two separate layers. The *theca interna* is a highly vascular group of hypertrophied cells that synthesize estradiol-17; the *theca externa* is avascular connective tissue.

At full maturity, the graafian follicle is large, measuring 5–10 mm. The oocyte has continued to grow steadily, with most of the increase occurring in the cytoplasm. Nutrient storage, in the form of yolk granules, constitutes most of this cytoplasmic increase.

Prior to ovulation, the *primary oocyte* initiates reduction division of the chromosomes, which decreases the number of chromosomes from 46 (the number found in somatic cells) to 23. This constitutes the first meiotic division; it will be completed at the time of ovulation.

During the maturation process, the graafian follicle moves toward the surface of the ovary. The ovarian and follicular walls are thin, and the follicle forms a blisterlike protrusion on the ovarian surface.

The ovum is extruded as the follicular and ovarian walls become thinner and eventually rupture. The production of proteolytic enzymes and prostaglandins facilitates this process. The cumulus oophorus and follicular fluid from within the antrum are carried along at the time of rupture.

The ovum is released at the fimbriated end of the fallopian tube. The egg is captured and pulled toward the tube, to be propelled down the tube toward the uterus by ciliary action.

At the time of ovulation, a small amount of *spotting* (midcyle bleeding) may occur. Vaginal secretions and discharge may increase. Basal body temperature usually increases slightly (0.25–0.5°C) and remains elevated through the endometrium's secretory phase. Occasionally, ovulation may be accompanied by pain *(mittelschmerz)* due to irritation of peritoneal tissue by follicular contents and blood.

Corpus Luteum

After ovulation the corpus luteum forms at the site of the ruptured follicle. Morphologic changes occur as a result of the continued presence of

162 CHANGE: THE PRENATAL PERIOD

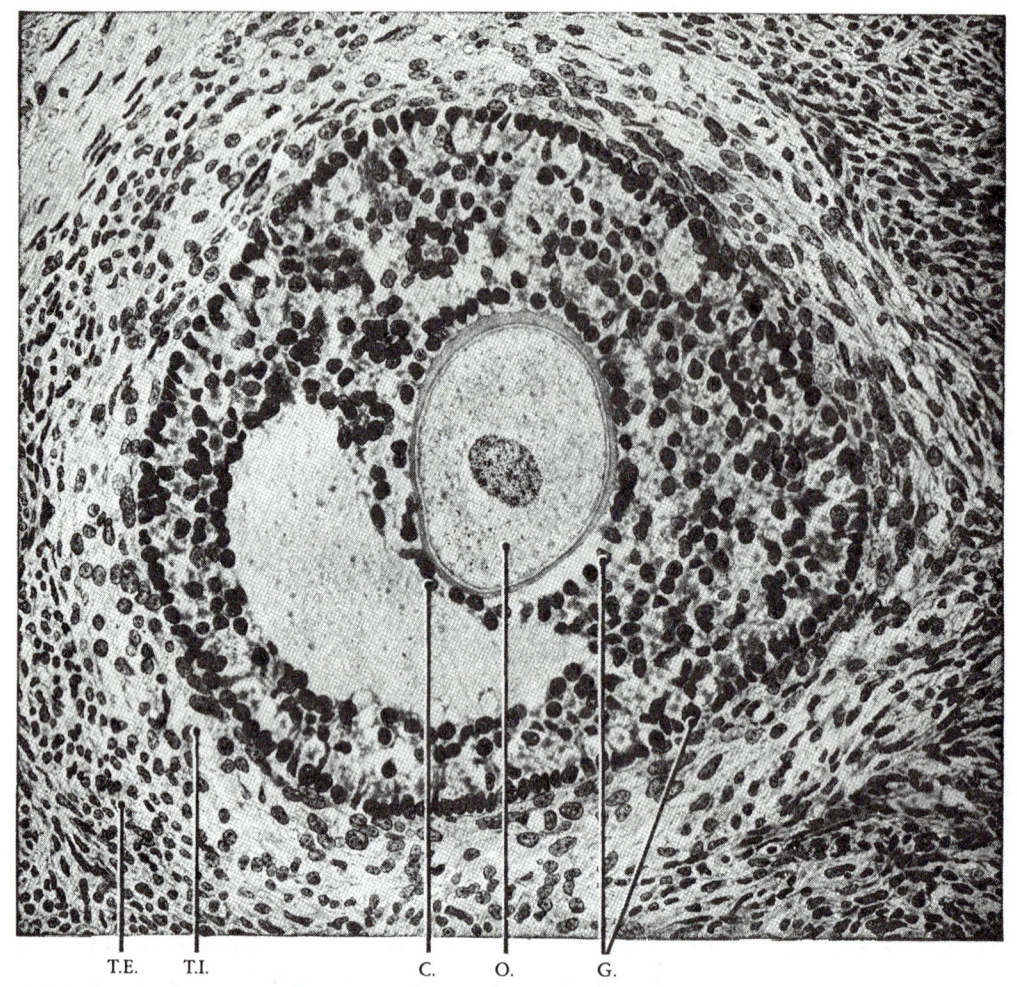

FIGURE 9–2. Graafian follicle approaching maturity. TE, theca externa; TI, theca interna; C, cumulus oophorus; O, ovum; G, granulosa cell layer.
SOURCE: Pritchard, MacDonald, and Gant (1985).

luteinizing hormone and its influence on the *granulosa (follicular) cells*. Once the follicle has collapsed and the antrum has been obliterated, the cells take on a golden color and secrete steroids.

The primary steroid released is progesterone. However, small amounts of estrogen are also produced. Vascularization increases, and at maturity the corpus luteum measures 1–3 cm in diameter.

If fertilization does not occur, regression begins around the 25th day of the cycle. Degeneration continues until scar tissue forms. Eventually, this is reabsorbed. During the scar phase the corpus is known as the *corpus albicans*.

If fertilization does occur, the corpus luteum undergoes hyperplasia in response to human chorionic gonadotropin (HCG). Progesterone secretion increases to maintain the pregnancy. Following implantation, the developing placenta assumes the maintenance role and the corpus luteum regresses.

Endometrial Cycle and Changes in Cervical Mucosa

Estrogens

At the completion of menstruation, estrogen levels are low. The endometrium is 1–2 mm deep, and the endometrial glands are narrow and straight. Cervical mucus is thick, opaque, and scant.

As the estrogen levels increase, the endometrium moves into the *proliferative phase*. Endometrial glands hypertrophy, becoming longer and more tortuous. The deep layers of the endometrium are compact and dense, while the upper layers are made up of large, loosely packed cells. These changes continue until just before ovulation, when the endometrium is six to eight times its minimum depth.

The cervical mucus becomes thin, almost watery, and clear under the influence of estrogen. This facilitates movement of spermatozoa. The pH becomes more alkaline (from pH 7.0 to 7.5), which is also more favorable to sperm survival. *Ferning* (a fernlike pattern in a specimen of dried cervical mucus) becomes very pronounced at ovulation.

Progesterone

Estrogen has primed the endometrium in the proliferative phase. Following ovulation estrogen has little further influence. However, progesterone causes epithelial folding as the *secretory phase* begins. Uterine glands become quite tortuous, secreting small amounts of uterine fluid. Stromal cells become edematous, and celluary hypertrophy occurs. Glycogen deposition increases within the tissues. These preparations provide an environment in which a fertilized ovum can develop. If fertilization and implantation occur, the endometrium continues this growth, increasing in thickness.

If fertilization does not occur, progesterone and estrogen levels fall rapidly as the corpus luteum degenerates. About 2–3 days before menstrual onset (corresponding to this regression of the corpus luteum) leukocytes infiltrate the stromal cells. There is a loss of tissue fluid and secretions stop, resulting in a decrease in endometrial thickness. Collapse of the arteries and glands produces small areas of epithelial necrosis.

The *ischemic phase*, characterized by arterial vasoconstriction and ischemia, occurs 4–24 hours prior to menstruation. The superficial layers of the endometrium become pale due to lack of blood flow. Vessel relaxation follows, leading to rupture of the smaller blood vessels and hemorrhage into the tissue.

This hematoma formation causes the endometrial layers to distend and rupture. Fissures develop, and the tissue detaches from the basal layer. The *menstrual phase* begins. The remaining basal layer provides the foundation for generation of the functional endometrium. Review Figure 9–1 to identify endometrial changes by phase and day.

Menstruation

Menarche is the age of onset of menstruation. Early cycles are usually anovulatory and can be very irregular. Most women begin to menstruate in their early teens (at 12–13 years of age) and settle into a regular pattern after 2–3 years.

The normal menstrual cycle is considered to be 28 days. However, cycles vary greatly. Numerous factors affect the cycle—for example, illness, fatigue, stress, temperature, and altitude. Therefore, cycle length depends on both the individual's normal cycle pattern and extraneous environmental conditions.

A woman with a cycle of normal length will experience approximately 400 menstrual cycles during her lifetime. Blood loss ranges from 40 to 60 ml/cycle, with an average iron loss of 0.4–1.1 mg/day (150–400 mg/year).

The menstrual fluid is not, however, composed of blood and blood products alone. Cervical and vaginal secretions are also discharged, along with mucus, bacteria, and cellular debris. Usually the drainage is dark red, and it may have a distinctive odor.

GAMETOGENESIS

In all human cells except the mature gamete (sex cell) there are 46 chromosomes. These chromosomes are found in pairs, with 22 pairs of *autosomes* and one pair of *sex chromosomes*. In the female, the sex chromosomes consist of two X chromosomes, while male cells contain one X and one Y chromosome. The 46 chromosomes determine the *genotype* (genetic make-up), *phenotype* (external appearance), and sex of each individual.

In order for fertilization to take place, *gametogenesis* (the production and development of mature gametes) must occur. This is the process by which the primordial germ cells change into mature reproductive cells. For both male and female cells this entails a reduction in the number of chromosomes from 46 to 23 (*diploid* to *haploid* number). This occurs through *meiotic division*. Meiotic division consists of two successive divisions in which genetic material can be exchanged between chromosomes and one chromosome of each pair is randomly placed in each sex cell (see Fig. 9–3).

Spermatogenesis

Gamete production in the male begins at puberty (about age 14) when the testes begin to release androgen. Gamete production involves two processes, spermatogenesis and spermiogenesis, both of which occur in the testes. *Spermatogenesis* is the

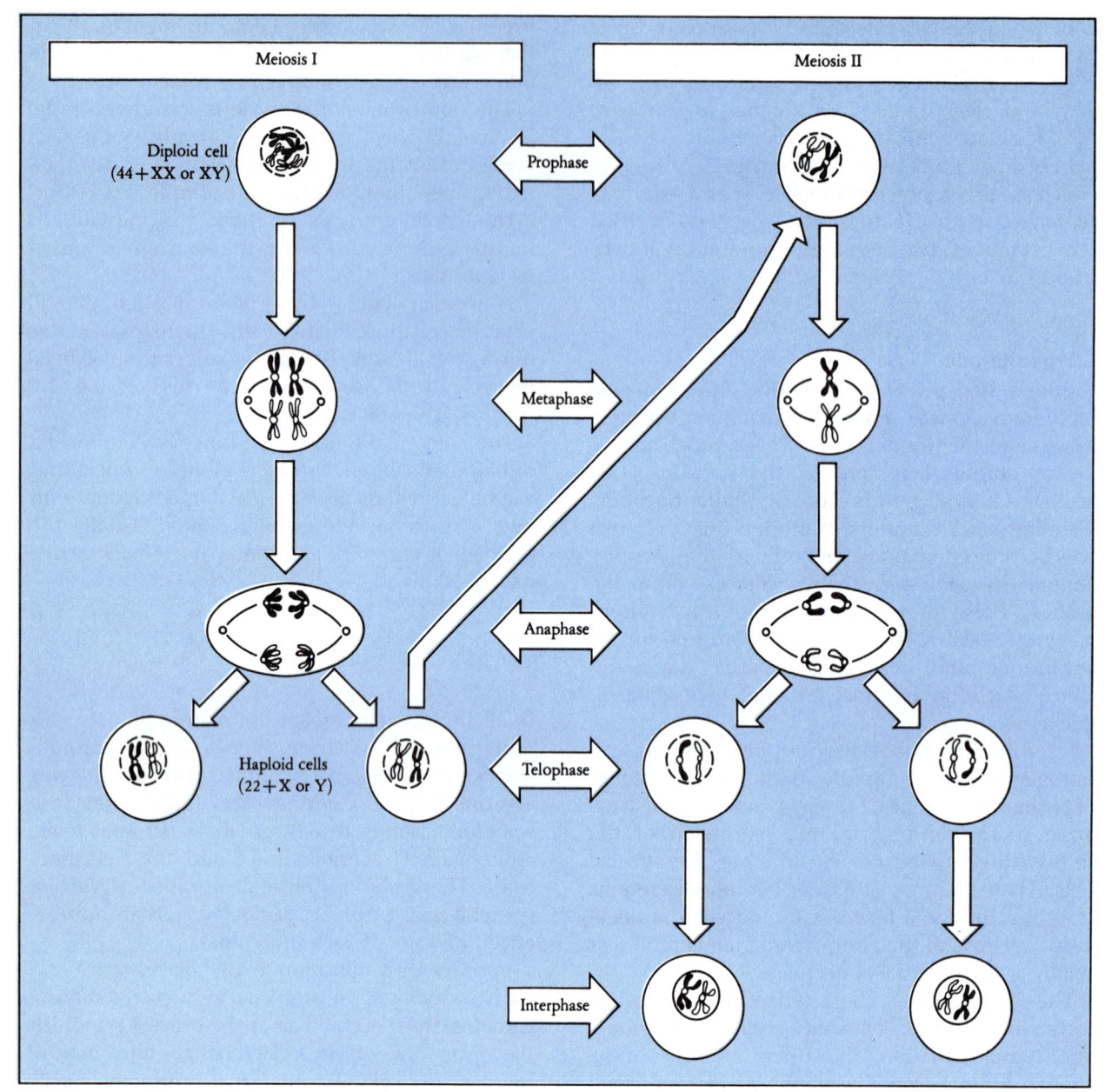

FIGURE 9-3. Meiotic cell division. Two pairs of chromosomes are identified. Each chromosome is made up of two halves, or *chromatids.*

reduction in the number of chromosomes, while *spermiogenesis* is the maturation of the spermatid (end product of spermatogenesis) into the highly specialized sperm cell with acrosome, head, neck, body, and tail (see Fig. 9–4). Once these two processes begin, they continue until old age.

Spermatogenesis occurs in the seminiferous tubules of the testes, where the diploid *spermatogonia* (primitive reproductive cells) undergo mitotic division. The spermatogonium begins to increase in size, and mitotic division stops. The reproductive cell is now referred to as a *primary spermatocyte.* The first meiotic division yields two haploid cells (secondary spermatocytes), each containing 22 autosomes and either an X or a Y chromosome. These two cells undergo the second meiotic division, yielding four spermatids. Each sperm takes approximately 64–74 days to reach functional maturity (Clermont, 1963; see Fig. 9–5).

Oogenesis

Oogenesis (female gamete production) begins in fetal life with the proliferation of *oogonia* (primitive reproductive cells). By a fetal age of 20 weeks there

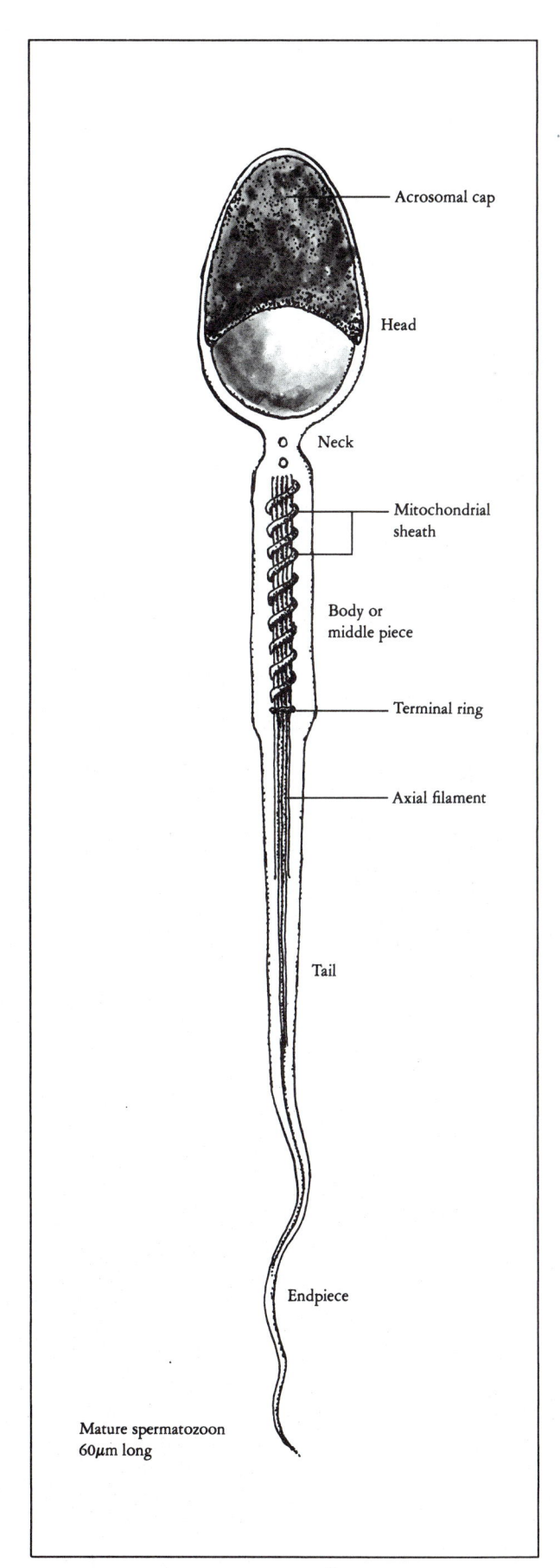

FIGURE 9–4. The mature sperm cell.

are between 5 and 7 million oogonia in the ovaries. All the ova that an individual will produce are present as oogonia by the fifth month of gestation (Byskov, 1982). These cells enlarge and become known as primary oocytes. A layer of follicular cells (the primordial follicle) develops around the oocyte, and the first meiotic (reduction) division begins. However, this division is halted just prior to the first meiotic metaphase (see Fig. 9–3), and the ovaries become dormant until puberty.

Degeneration *(atresia)* of some of these primitive follicles occurs during the rest of gestation, so that at the time of birth only 2 million oocytes remain. Atresia continues, so that by the time of puberty 400,000–500,000 oocytes are available for maturation and possible conception (Baker, 1982).

At puberty, follicle-stimulating hormone and luteinizing hormone begin to be released, causing further follicular maturation. A graafian follicle develops (see Fig. 9–6). At this time, the zona pellucida is formed and the primary oocyte is surrounded by several layers of cells. With each menstrual cycle, approximately 1000 oocytes go through maturational changes or atresia. Usually only one is released. This means that, on average, a woman has the capability of ovulating and potentially achieving pregnancy 400 times before, at *menopause*, the ova are gone and the ovary changes structurally and functionally.

Just prior to ovulation the first meiotic division is completed. The two cells produced are of unequal size, because of unequal division of the cytoplasm. The smaller cell *(polar body)* is deposited outside the cell membrane of the secondary oocyte and eventually degenerates there. The second meiotic division is initiated but stops to await penetration by the sperm. This division is also unequal, producing an ovum and a second polar body (see Fig. 9–5).

FERTILIZATION

Once the spermatids are transformed into the "true" sperm structure, they are set free in the *seminiferous tubules* and transported in the seminal fluid to the *epididymis* and *ductus deferens*. Here they are stored until discharge at ejaculation. Approximately 300–500 million sperm are released with each orgasm. They are transported to the vicinity of the cervix by peristaltic movements of the penis and vagina. Once released into the vaginal tract, the sperm can propel themselves. Flagellar movements of the tail assist the sperm in moving at a rate of 2–3 mm/min, depending on the alkalinity of the surrounding environment. The

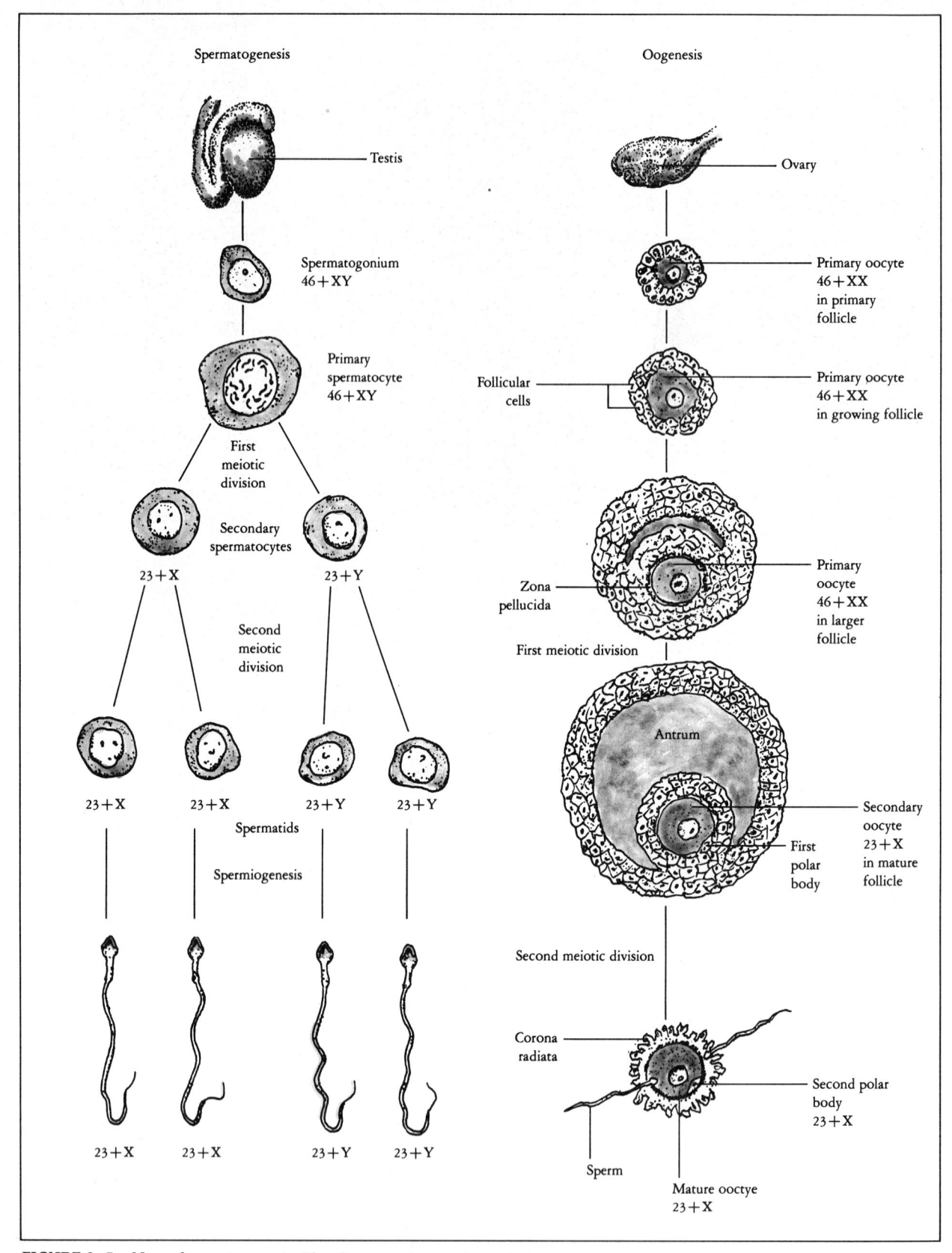

FIGURE 9-5. Normal gametogenesis. The chromosome complement of the germ cells is shown at each stage. Note that (1) following the two meiotic divisions, the diploid number of chromosomes, 46, has been reduced to the haploid number of 23; (2) *four sperm* form from one primary spermatocyte, whereas only *one* mature oocyte (ovum) results from maturation of a primary oocyte; (3) the cytoplasm is conserved during oogenesis to form one large cell, the mature oocyte (ovum).

SOURCE: Moore (1977).

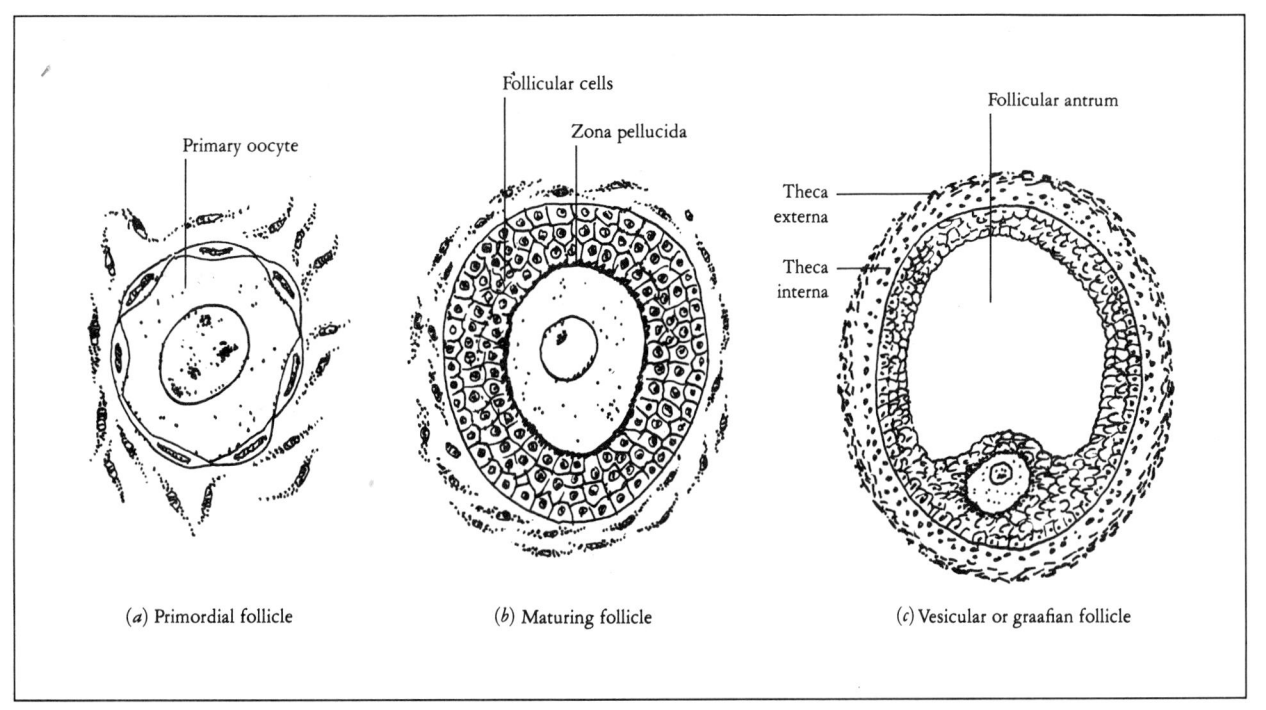

FIGURE 9-6. Changes occurring in the primordial follicle during the first half of the ovarian cycle. Under the influence of FSH, the primordial follicle (a) matures into the graafian follicle (c). The oocyte remains a primary oocyte until shortly before ovulation. During the last few days of the growing period, the estrogens produced by the follicular and theca cells stimulate the formation of LH in the pituitary.
SOURCE: Langman (1981).

pH of the semen is between 7.2 and 7.8. This is important for both mobility and protection against the acidity of the vagina, which has a pH of 5.7 (Harper, 1982).

Following ejaculation, the first sperm reach the cervical mucus in approximately 90 seconds. Midway in the menstrual cycle the mucus has thinned, being 99 percent water instead of the usual 89 percent. This improves the sperm's chances of penetrating the mucous plug. Five minutes after ejaculation, sperm can be found in the fallopian tubes. Only 200–500 sperm survive to reach the ovum (Harper, 1982).

Sperm are viable in the female genital tract for between 24 and 72 hours, after which degeneration occurs. The maximum likelihood of fertilization is probably within the first 24 hours, however. The ovum has a shorter life span. Degeneration begins soon after ovulation, and viability is only about 24 hours. Therefore, fertilization must occur within this time (Silverstein, 1980).

Before fertilization can take place, *capacitation* must occur. Capacitation consists of structural alterations that occur in the sperm after it enters the female genital tract. The time required for capacitation is approximately 5–7 hours (Langman, 1981).

Fertilization begins when a capacitated sperm penetrates the zona pellucida. It is completed when the chromosomes of the ovum and sperm unite, usually in the fallopian tube. The high levels of estrogen in the blood at the time of ovulation increase the contractility of the tube, facilitating ovum passage (Spence, 1982).

While only one sperm is required for fertilization, the others may contribute to the *acrosome reaction*, which allows the sperm to penetrate the *corona radiata* (the cells surrounding the released ovum) and the zona pellucida. Enzymes released from under the acrosomal cap dissolve the jelly cement between the cells of these two structures. In this way, the sperm separates the cells and creates a passageway to the ovum's cell membrane. The sperm attaches itself to the membrane and releases more enzymes, which create an opening in the membrane and allow the head and neck of the sperm to enter.

Once the sperm penetrates the ovum, the zona pellucida reacts by losing its permeability. This process is called the *zona reaction*. It prevents any more sperm from entering the ovum. At this point the second meiotic division resumes in the ovum. Then the chromosomes of both sperm and ovum are free to mingle and to align properly, completing fertilization. Figure 9-7 shows the phases of the fertilization process.

Once fertilization occurs and the chromosomes from the parents join, cell division can begin and further development is initiated. The results of fertilization are (a) restoration of the diploid number of chromosomes, (b) species variation, (c) genetic sex discrimination, (d) initiation of rapid mitotic division (cleavage).

The fertilized ovum is now called a *zygote*. Division of the zygote occurs in the first 30 hours and continues over the next 3 days (Moore, 1977). Now termed a *blastomere*, the conceptus travels toward the uterus. The zona pellucida remains intact to prevent the cells from adhering to the walls of the fallopian tube.

After dividing three to four times, the blastomere is a solid ball of cells *(morula)* and is ready to enter the uterus. The morula floats inside the uterus for 2-3 days, receiving nourishment from the thick mucus lining the uterine walls. The zona pellucida dissolves during this period and allows fluid to seep in between the cells of the morula. This separates the cells, creating a hollow ball called the *blastocyst*. At this time, two distinct layers of cells can be identified: an inner cell mass and an outer cell layer. The inner cell mass, or *embryoblast*, will yield the embryo, the amnion, and the yolk sac membranes. The outer cell layer, or *trophoblast*, will contribute the fetal component of the placenta. The loss of the zona pellucida allows implantation to begin (see Fig. 9-8).

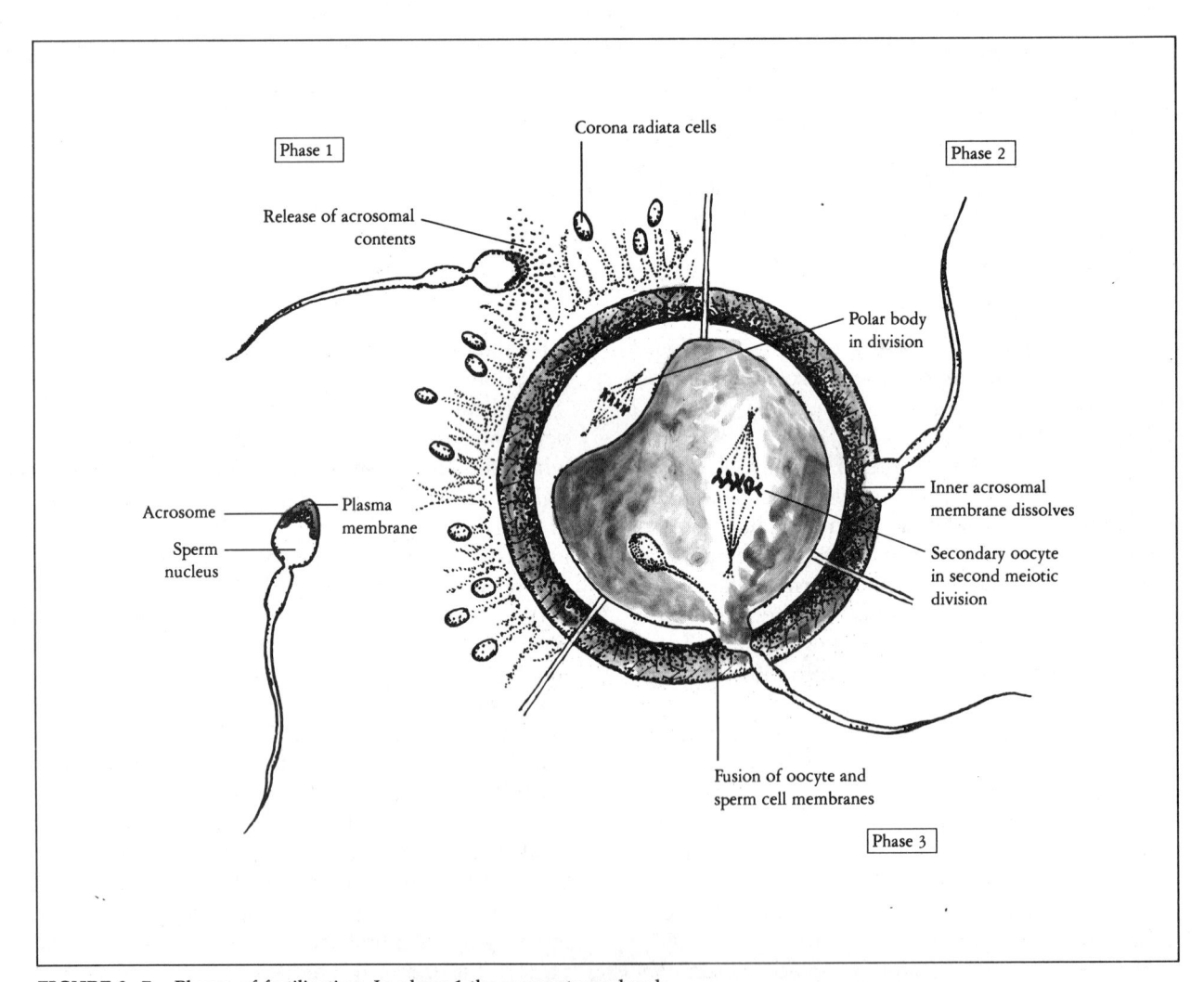

FIGURE 9-7. Phases of fertilization. In phase 1 the spermatozoa break through the corona radiata barrier. In phase 2 one or more spermatozoa penetrate the zona pellucida. In phase 3 one spermatozoon penetrates through the oocyte membrane, thereby losing its own plasma membrane.
SOURCE: Langman (1981).

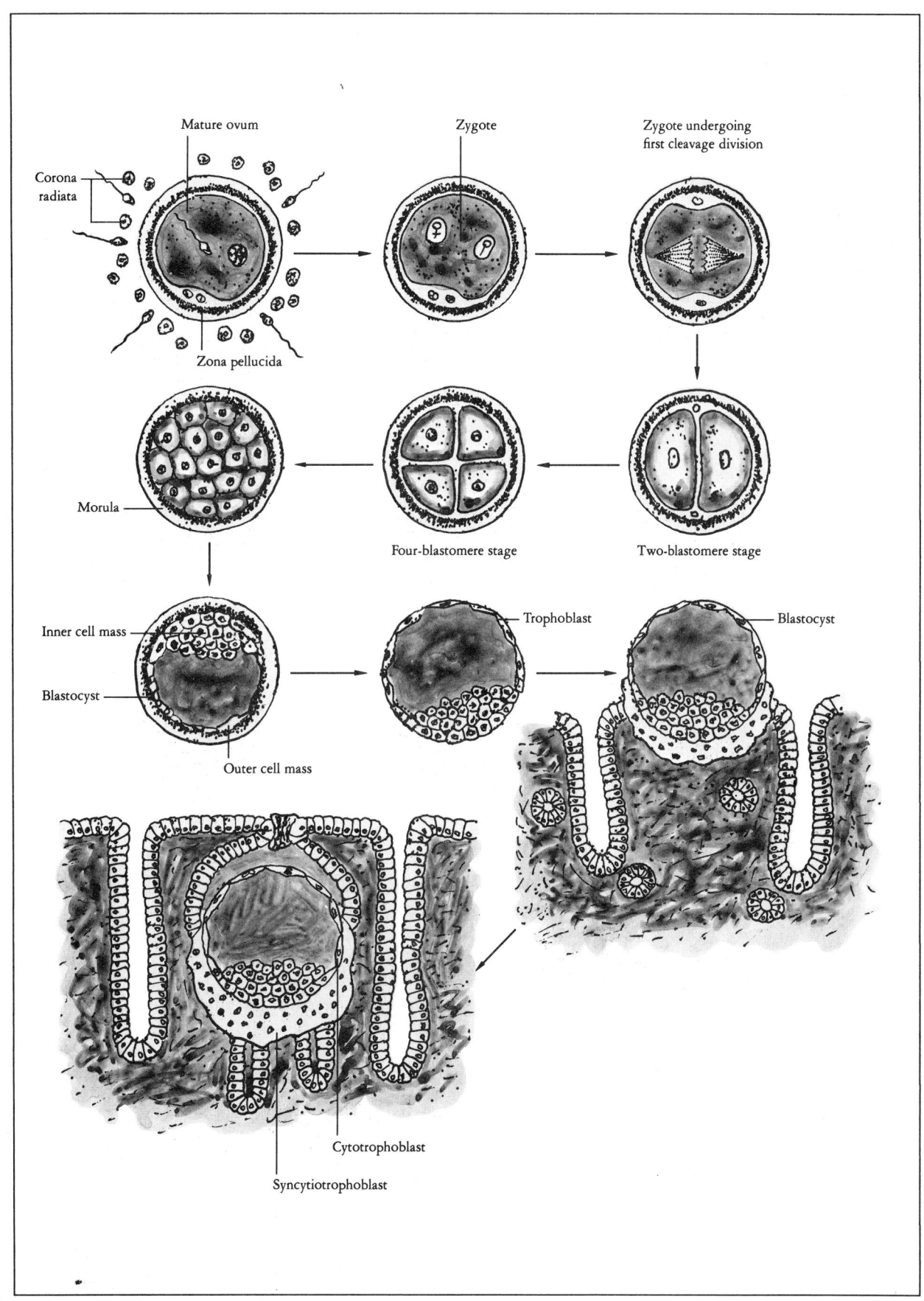

FIGURE 9–8. Stages of fertilization, cleavage, and implantation.
SOURCE: Snell (1983).

IMPLANTATION

Nutrient requirements increase as the conceptus grows and differentiates. Implantation allows these requirements to be met. The trophoblast usually attaches to the upper third of the posterior or anterior wall of the uterus. This implantation process normally occurs in the three steps: (1) attachment, (2) penetration, and (3) invasion and embedding. On the 5th day after fertilization the blastocyst adheres to the uterine wall. After this initial adherence, attachment spreads rapidly. Trophoblastic cells erode the associated uterine epithelium. This erosion process continues until the *embryoblast* is completely embedded on day 11.

THE DECIDUA

The vascularity and thickness of the endometrium increase greatly in preparation for implantation. Once implantation occurs, the endometrium is termed the *decidua*. The attachment and implantation cause the adjacent decidual cells to become engorged with glycogen and lipids. This response is called the *decidual reaction*. It quickly spreads from the site of implantation throughout the decidua. The swollen decidual cells release their contents during the erosion process to provide nourishment to the developing embryo.

The portion of the decidua that covers the embryoblast is called the *decidua capsularis*. This superficial layer thins as the embryo and amniotic cavity grow. As the embryo projects into the uterine cavity, the capsularis comes into contact with the other walls of the uterus, where fusion of the two layers occurs (fourth to fifth month of gestation). Once this happens, the uterine cavity is essentially eliminated.

The section of decidua that lies below the embryoblast is the *decidua basalis*. This becomes the maternal component of the placenta, contributing the vascular supply that serves the intervillous spaces between the chorion and the decidua basalis.

The decidua that lines the rest of the uterine cavity is the *decidua parietalis*. At birth, this layer is torn away as the placenta and chorion are expelled. The bulk of the decidua basalis is also shed with the placenta (see Figs. 9–9 and 9–10).

PLACENTAL DEVELOPMENT

When the embryoblast is partially embedded in the decidua (8th day), two distinct layers of cells can be identified in the trophoblast. The inner layer *(cytotrophoblast)* is a group of mononucleated cells, while the outer is multinucleated, due to the fusion of individual cells in this layer and the disappearance of distinct cell membranes. This multinucleated region is termed the *syncytotrophoblast*, or *syncytium*. It is responsible for the erosive nature of the trophoblast (see Fig. 9–11).

On the 9th day spaces, or *vacuoles*, appear in the syncytium. These fuse together to form *lacunae*, isolated spaces that will eventually develop into an intercommunicating labyrinth. The intervillous spaces will be derived from this system.

During the 11th and 12th days, the invading syncytium encounters the congested and dilated capillaries of the decidua. The syncytium enzymes break down walls of these vessels, and blood is released into the lacunae. Initially, venous blood is tapped and stasis occurs. Directional flow is established when the syncytium encounters the larger arteries (spiral arteries) and veins.

Once blood enters the lacunae, the embryo moves into a period of rapid cellular differentiation and growth because of the increased concentration of nutrients available. However, the growth increases the distance these nutrients must travel by diffusion to the embryo, establishing the need for a circulatory system in the fetus and placenta.

Between the 9th and 25th days of gestation the *chorionic villi* develop. The *chorion* (trophoblastic tissue) is the first placental membrane to form. It is the outermost embryonic membrane, enclosing the embryo, amnion, and yolk sac. Chorionic growth occurs radially around the embryo in fingerlike projections. These projections take on a fine villous appearance. Blood vessels eventually form within the villi, allowing physiologic interchange to occur between the fetus and the mother.

Initially the villi cover the whole chorionic surface. However, as the uterine cavity is obliterated, the intraluminal villi become compressed against the decidua parietalis. Ischemia sets in and is followed by degeneration of these villi. Those villi located beneath the embryo, in contact with the decidua basalis, continue to lengthen, developing an extensive surface for exchange. This is the *chorion frondosum*.

The villi develop into a treelike structure with numerous branchings, becoming a tangled, bushy mass. Certain branches make contact with the maternal decidua to become *anchoring villi*. Others float freely in the intervillous space, surrounded by maternal blood and conducting most of the exchange between fetus and mother (see Fig. 9–12).

The placenta continues to grow throughout

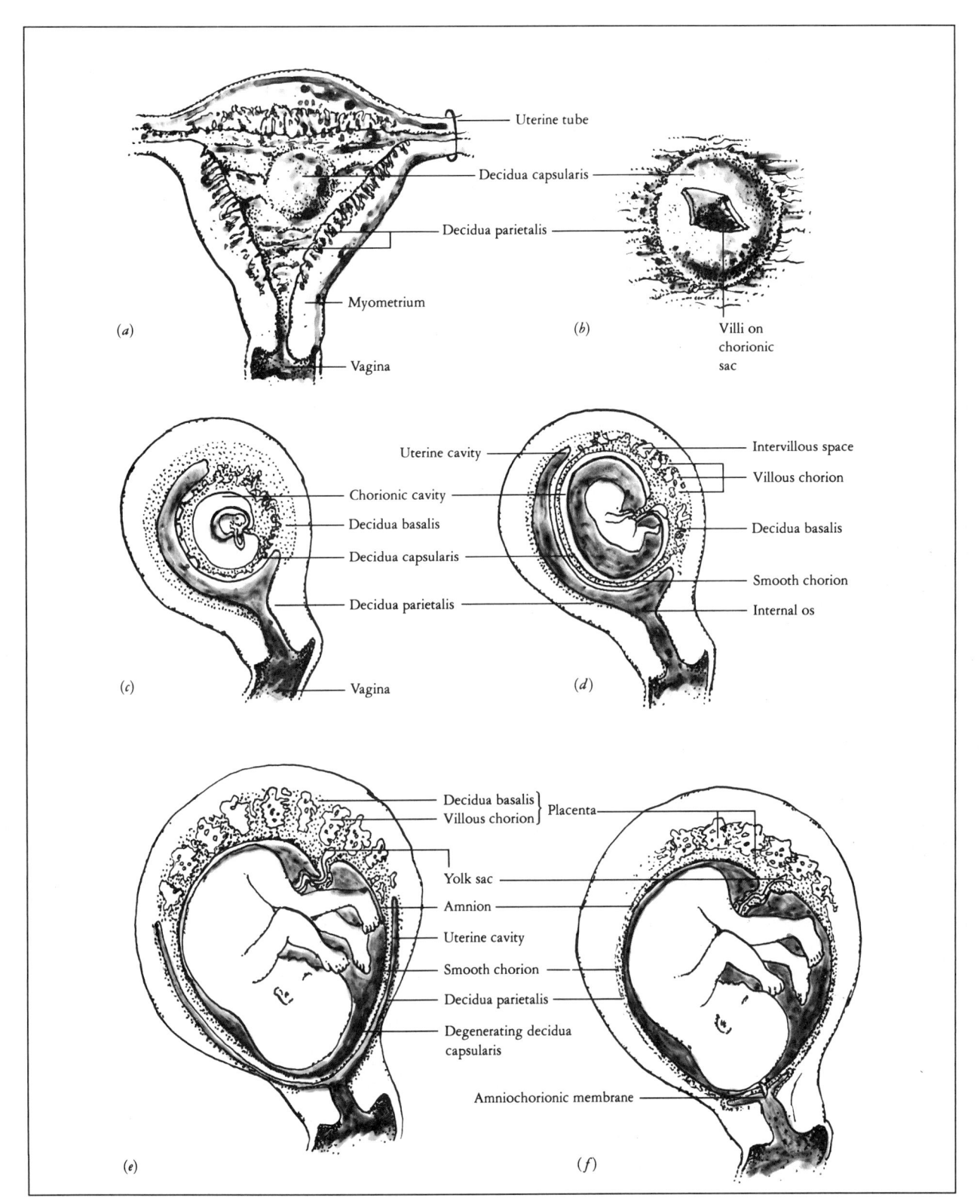

FIGURE 9-9. The maturing decidua. *(a)* Frontal section of the uterus showing the elevation of the decidua capsularis caused by the expanding chorionic sac of a 4-week-old embryo, implanted in the endometrium on the posterior wall. *(b)* The implantation site. The chorionic villi have been exposed by cutting an opening in the decidua capsularis. *(c–f)* Sagittal sections of the gravid uterus from the 4th to 22nd weeks, showing the changing relations of the fetal membranes to the decidua. In *(f)* the amnion and chorion are fused with each other, and the decidua parietalis is obliterating the uterine cavity. Note that the villi persist only where the chorion is associated with the decidua basalis; here they form the villous chorion (fetal portion of the placenta).
SOURCE: Moore (1977).

172 CHANGE: THE PRENATAL PERIOD

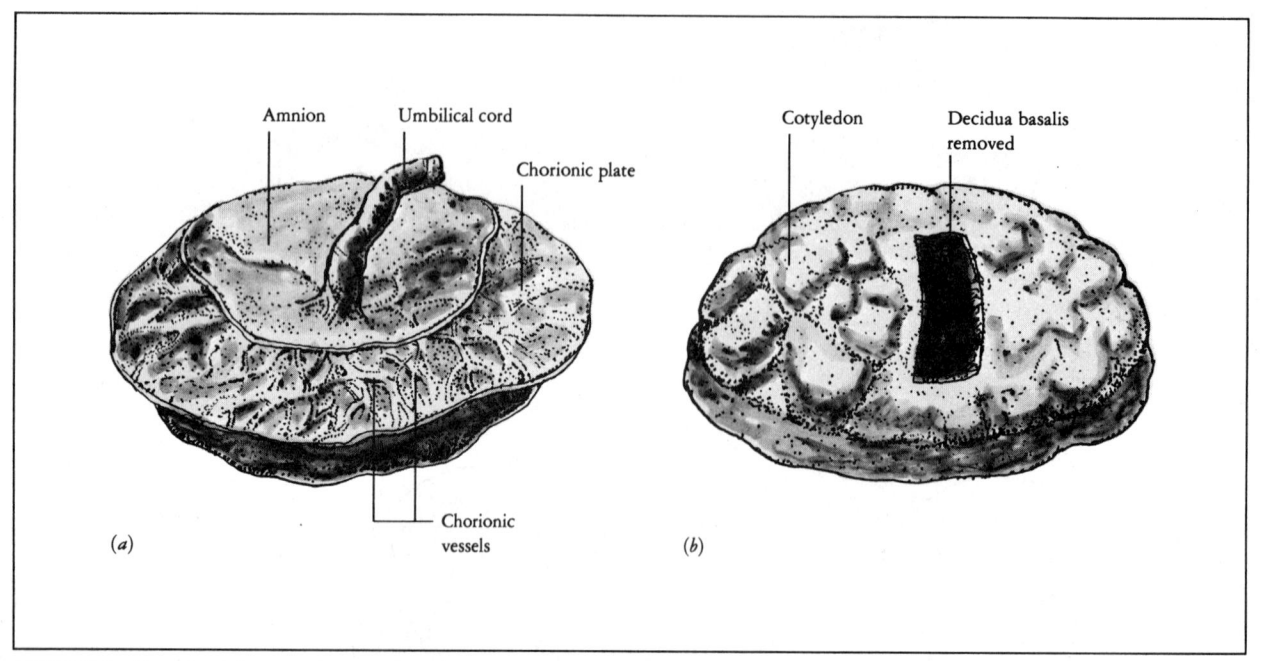

FIGURE 9–10. The full-term placenta shown from (a) the fetal side and (b) the maternal side.
SOURCE: Langman (1981).

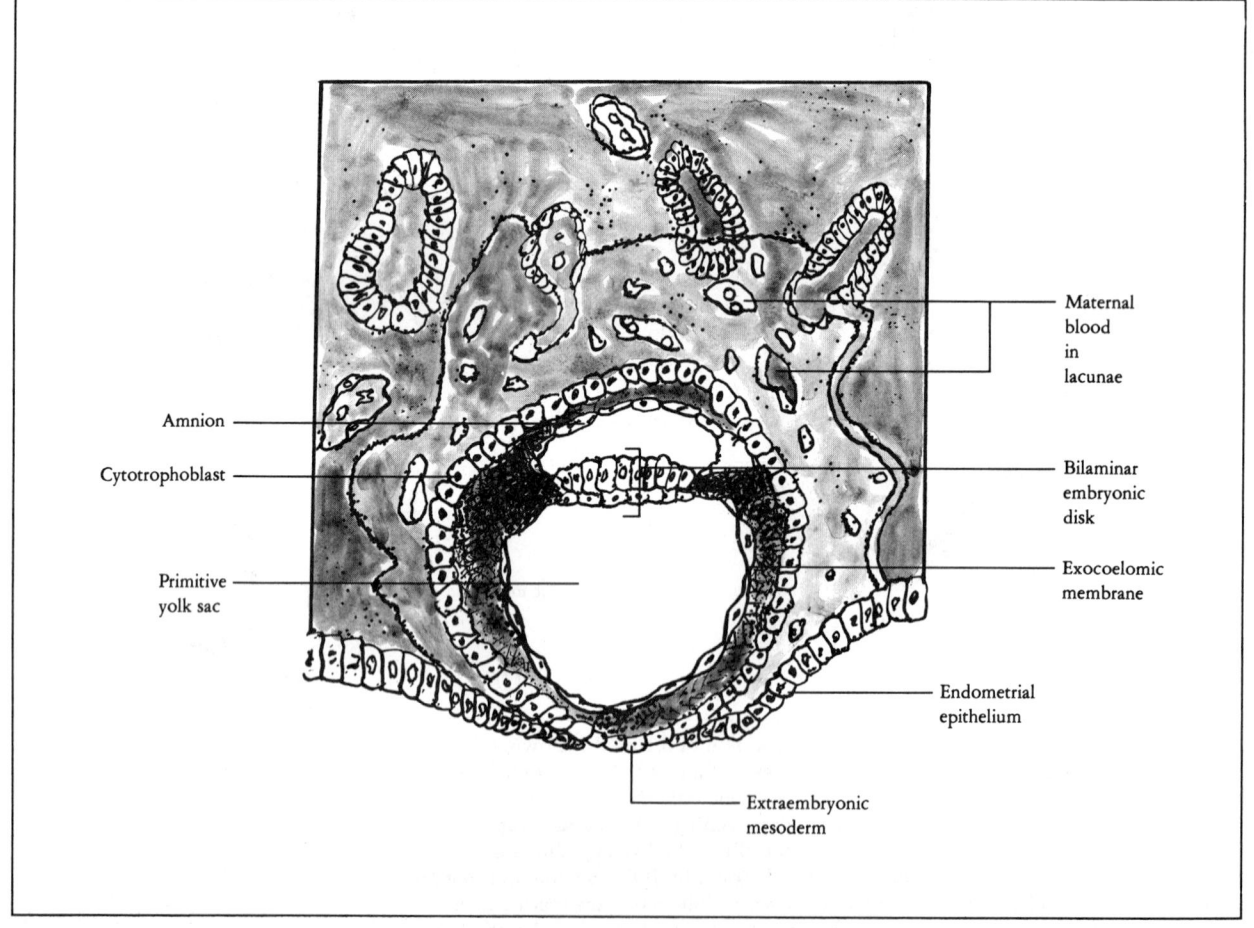

FIGURE 9–11. A section through an implanted blastocyst of approximately 9 days.
SOURCE: Moore (1977).

Physiologic Changes in the Fetus 173

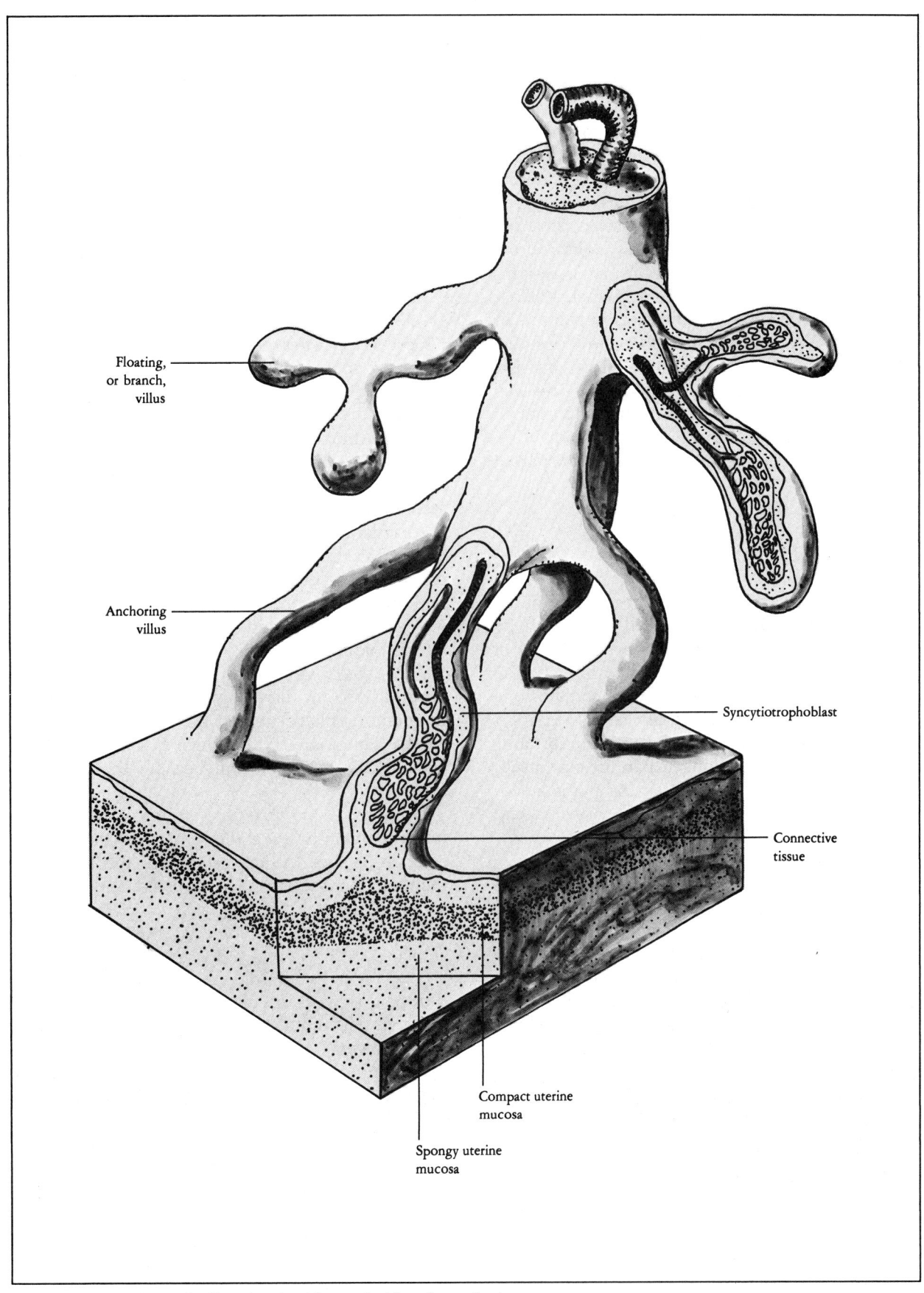

FIGURE 9–12. Placental villus after the 4th month. Note the anchoring villi and branch villi.
SOURCE: Tuchman-Duplessis, David, and Haegel (1980).

pregnancy, but no new villi are added after the 12th week.

After the 5th month of gestation the cytotrophoblastic layer disappears and a single layer of syncytium covers the villi. The placenta continues to grow in diameter and thickness until the 20th week. At this time, it will cover half of the uterine surface. Further growth is in thickness only. At 40 weeks' gestation, the placenta is discoid, 20 cm in diameter, and 3 cm in thickness. It weighs approximately 500 g (one-sixth of the fetal weight) (Tuchman-Duplessis, David, and Haegel, 1980).

The maternal surface of the mature placenta is rough and red. During the 4th month decidual septa form between anchoring villi, giving the placenta 15–20 lobules called *cotyledons*. The fetal surface, on the other hand, is shiny and gray in appearance because of the adherent amnion. Umbilical vessels can be seen through this transparent surface.

THE UMBILICAL CORD

The umbilical cord develops from the fusion of the yolk sac, the body stalk, the allantois, and its vessels. It usually attaches at or near the center of the placenta. At full term it is approximately 1–2 cm in diameter and 50–55 cm long. It contains one vein and two arteries that are enclosed in connective tissue called *Wharton's jelly*. It is tortuous because the vessels are longer than the cord itself. The umbilical cord functions as the pathway for physiologic exchanges between the placenta and the fetus.

EMBRYONIC DEVELOPMENT

Pregnancy is an average of 10 lunar months (40 weeks, 280 days) in length. The *embryonic period* is considered to be the 3rd through the 8th weeks. During this time the embryo gains its morphologic characteristics, distinguishing it as a human fetus, and establishes all the organs *(organogenesis)*. It is a period of prime importance, in that the embryo is most vulnerable to teratogenic events and major morphologic anomalies during this time.

The 2nd week of development is considered "preembryonic" and is a time of cellular differentiation and membrane establishment. The inner cell mass can be seen to differentiate into two types and layers of cells, the *endoderm* and the *ectoderm*. The embryo is a flat disk at this stage, known as the bilaminar germ disk. The endoderm can be thought of as the precursor of the inside of the embryo and the ectoderm as what will become the outside.

The amniotic cavity appears during this week as a space within the ectoderm. The ectodermal cells that lie next to the cytotrophoblast are termed *amnioblasts*. The ectodermal cells line the amniotic cavity, which initially lies above the embryo (away from the uterine lumen) (Langman, 1981). When the embryo folds to become a cylinder, the amnion encloses it in the amniotic sac (see Fig. 9–13).

Amniotic fluid provides a buoyant medium that (1) allows the embryo to develop symmetrically, (2) prevents adherence by the membranes to the growing embryo, (3) cushions against injury by equalizing internal and external pressures, (4) controls the temperature of the embryo, and (5) assists in musculoskeletal development by allowing free movement by the fetus. The amniotic fluid also provides data that aid in assessing fetal well-being.

Another cavity, the *yolk sac*, also becomes apparent during this stage of development. It is formed by a layer of endodermal cells that delaminates and moves outward into the chorionic cavity. The yolk sac is incorporated into the embryo during the lateral folding stage.

The *connecting stalk* can also be distinguished around the 13th day. The connecting stalk is the only embryonic tissue that traverses the chorionic cavity (Langman, 1981). Once blood vessels are established, this area will become the umbilical cord.

During this 2nd week the embryo grows slowly in comparison to the earlier growth of the trophoblast, reflecting the importance of the establishment of an efficient exchange system and the need for nutrients.

The 3rd week is a time of rapid growth. It coincides with the first sign of pregnancy, the first missed menstrual period. The major changes seen during this week occur as the bilaminar embryo becomes trilaminar, having three germ cell layers.

The *primitive streak* (a midline thickening in the ectoderm) develops and gives rise to cells that migrate between the ectoderm and endoderm. These cells will become the *mesoderm*.

The ectoderm will later give rise to the nervous system, skin, hair, nails, epithelium of the oral and nasal passages, and the salivary glands and mucous membranes of the nose and mouth. Most of the internal organs (kidneys, ovaries, testes, heart), the blood and blood vessels, and the lining of pericardial and peritoneal cavities are derived from the mesoderm. The endoderm contributes

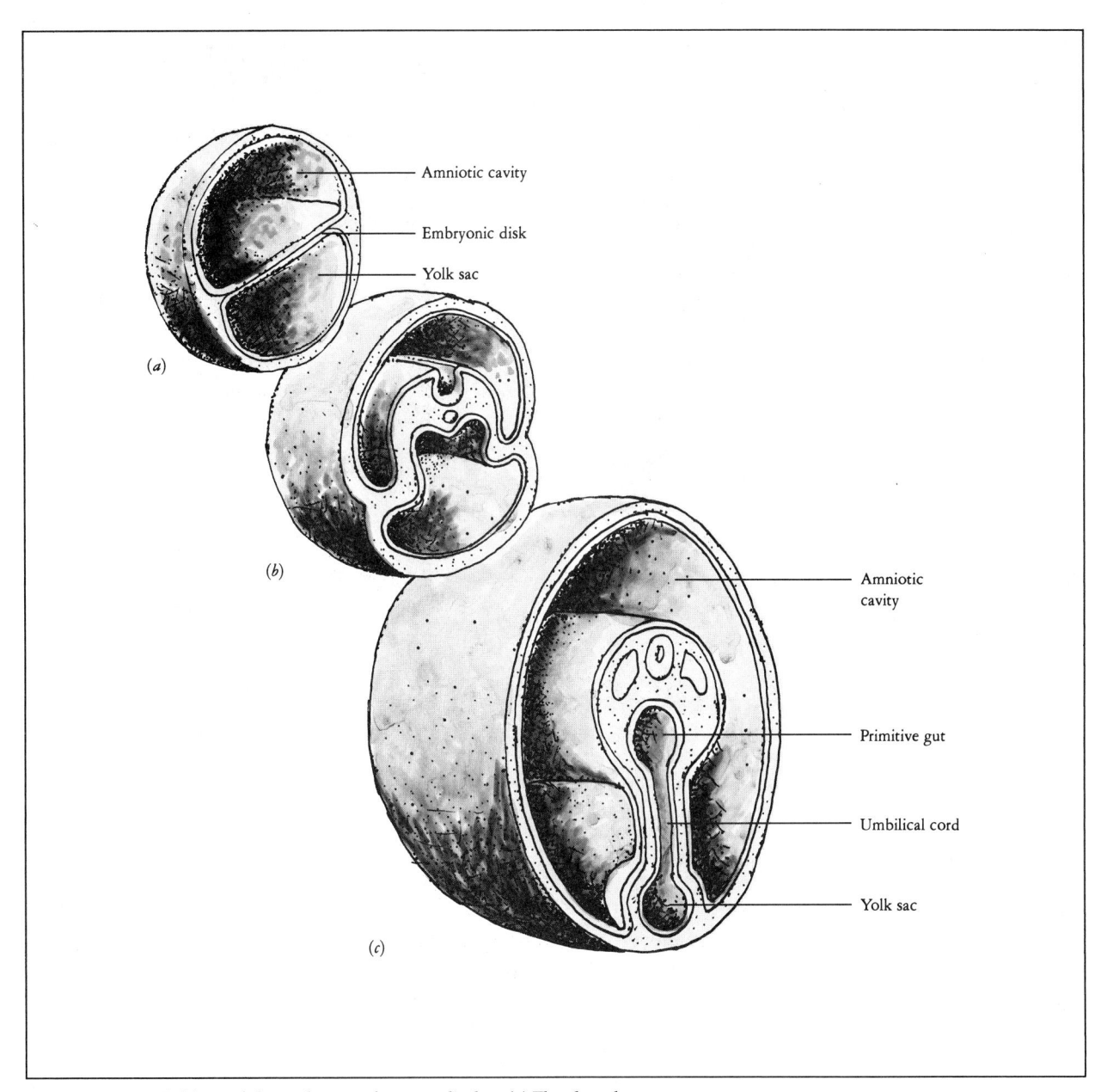

FIGURE 9–13. Folding of the embryo to form a cylinder. (a) The dorsal region thickens, especially on the midline; (b) the edges of the disk swing ventrally, carrying the amnion with them; (c) the embryo is surrounded by the amniotic cavity.
SOURCE: Tuchman-Duplessis, David, and Haegel (1980).

the epithelium for the digestive, respiratory, and urinary systems.

Embryonic development progresses in a cranial to caudal pattern. The embryonic disk becomes pear-shaped, with a broad cephalic end and a narrow caudal end. The *neural plate* forms along the midline of the ectoderm, developing into the cylindrical tube that becomes the definitive brain and spinal cord. Pairs of *somites* (body segments) develop parallel to the neural tube. Embryologists distinguish this stage of development by the number of somite pairs (see Figs. 9–14 and 9–15).

Blood vessels can be seen in the yolk sac and allantois. Those in the allantois later become the umbilical vessels. Blood vessels soon appear in the embryo and connect with the two cardiac tubes. These tubes will fuse together, and by the end of the following week the heart tube will be beating

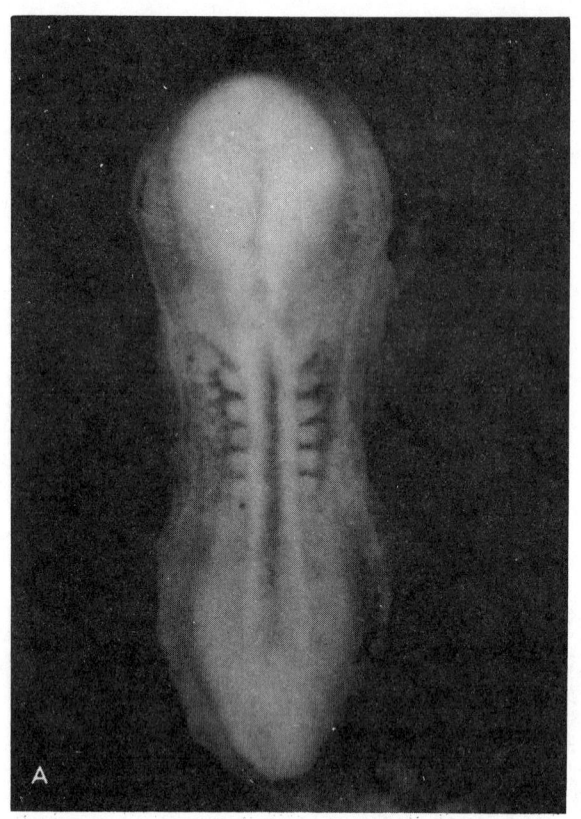

FIGURE 9-14. Embryos at about 22-23 days. In (a) the embryo is essentially straight, whereas the embryo in (b) is slightly curved.
SOURCE: Courtesy Professor Hideo Nishimura, Kyoto University, Japan.

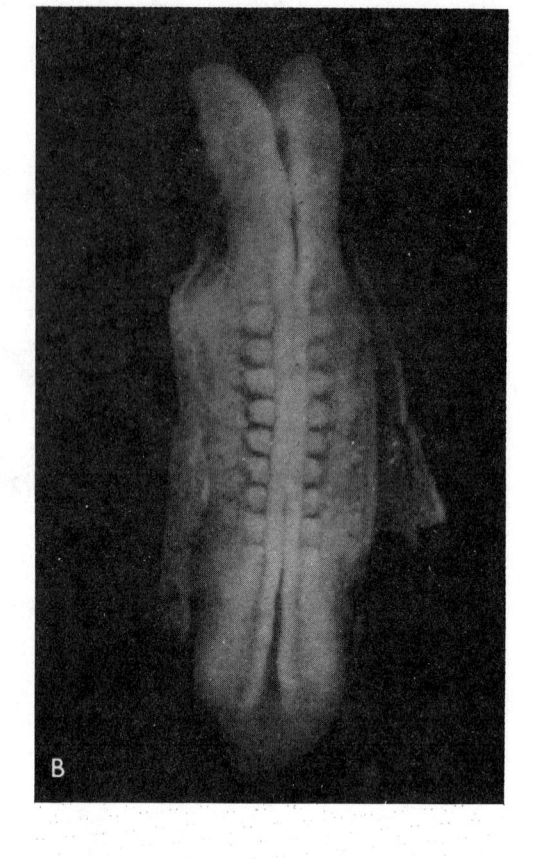

with a regular rhythm. Primitive blood cells are also being created so that nutrient exchange can occur.

During the 4th week the neural tube closes on both ends and the brain begins to enlarge rapidly. Initially the embryo is almost straight; the typical head to tail curvature occurs after brain enlargement. Arm and leg buds are only swellings at this point. The optic pits and lens placodes are clearly visible, although facial structures are not yet definitive. The *branchial arches*, which later give rise to the upper and lower jaw, are distinct.

Rapid head growth is the hallmark of the 5th week of gestation. The embryo now has the characteristic C-shaped body (see Fig. 9-16). The atrium has divided to partially partition the very prominent heart. The forelimbs begin to show, and the hand plates can be distinguished. The brain has five distinct areas, and cranial nerves are recognizable.

Limb differentiation continues during the 6th week. Finger rays can now be seen. The brain continues to be very large in proportion to the rest of the body. The trunk is beginning to straighten as it continues to develop. The face is more distinct. The jaws are visible, the nares and upper lip are formed, and the palate is coming together. The morphology of the heart is quite close to its final form as the valves begin to form. The liver is beginning to take over fetal blood cell production, and circulation is established.

During the last 2 weeks of the embryonic period, further facial development occurs. The eyes shift from their lateral positions to a more forward placement, moving closer together and becoming more distinct as retinal color is well established. Although the eyes are still open, eyelids are developing, the eyelids will fuse by the end of the 8th week. The mouth is formed as the tongue and palate are completed. The external ear is quite distinct, but upward migration has not occurred. The face is definitely human in appearance.

The limbs have undergone considerable change. Limb regions are distinct, and the wrist and elbow are flexed, letting the arms fall across the chest. Fingers are longer now, and the toes are clearly differentiated. The feet are approaching the midline, where they will be able to meet. Centers of ossification can be seen in certain bone areas.

The head is more erect and the neck is better developed. Neuromuscular development allows

Physiologic Changes in the Fetus

or at least begun, and the embryo now moves to the *fetal stage*. During the next 7 months the fetus will continue to grow and the existing structures will be refined. Organizational development of organ systems will improve the functioning of these systems. All this is in preparation for labor, delivery, and transition to the extrauterine environment.

Weeks 9–12

As the 9th week begins, the head is approximately half the length of the body. However, over the next 3 weeks the body will grow rapidly, doubling in length by the 12th week. Head growth begins to slow down. The neck lengthens and the chin is lifted off the chest. The face is very broad, with the eyes widely separated, and the ears remain low set. The nose is prominent and the chin is small. The eyelids are fused, not to open again until the

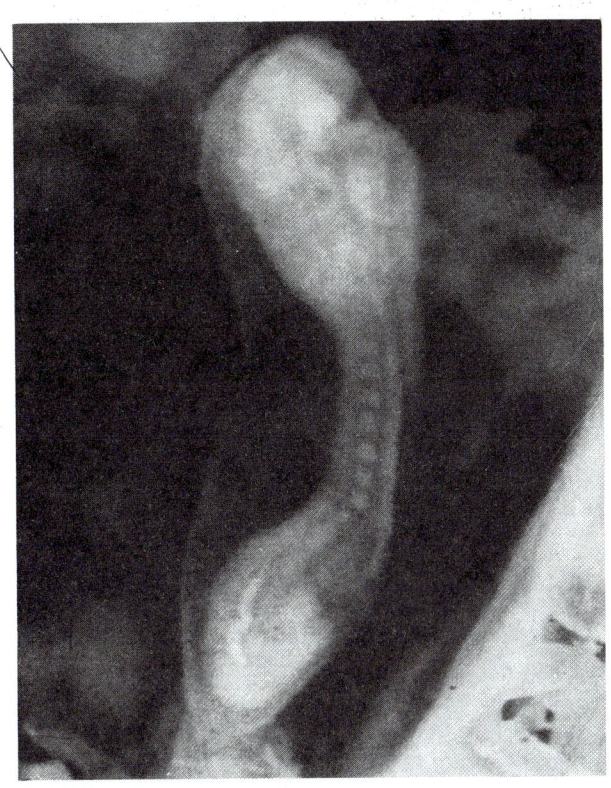

FIGURE 9–15. A 3.1-mm human embryo at about 24–25 days. The embryo lies within its amniotic sac and is attached to the chorion by the connecting stalk. Note the well-developed villi.
SOURCE: Courtesy Professor E. Blechschmidt, Director of the Institute of Anatomy, University of Gottingen, Federal Republic of Germany.

spontaneous fetal movements that can be discerned with ultrasound equipment.

During these weeks urogenital and gastrointestinal development has been significant. Initially, both systems ended in a single blind pouch, but now septa have divided the two structures. Structures of the kidneys and internal genitals are being laid down and refined. External genitals appear, but the sex of the embryo cannot be determined.

The gastrointestinal system has experienced rapid growth, forcing the small intestine to herniate into the umbilical cord. Continued elongation will occur over the next 2 weeks. The 10th week will bring intestinal migration with reentry into the abdominal cavity. The rectal passage is complete and the anal membrane is perforate.

FETAL DEVELOPMENT

By the end of the embryonic period all the major systems and external features are well established

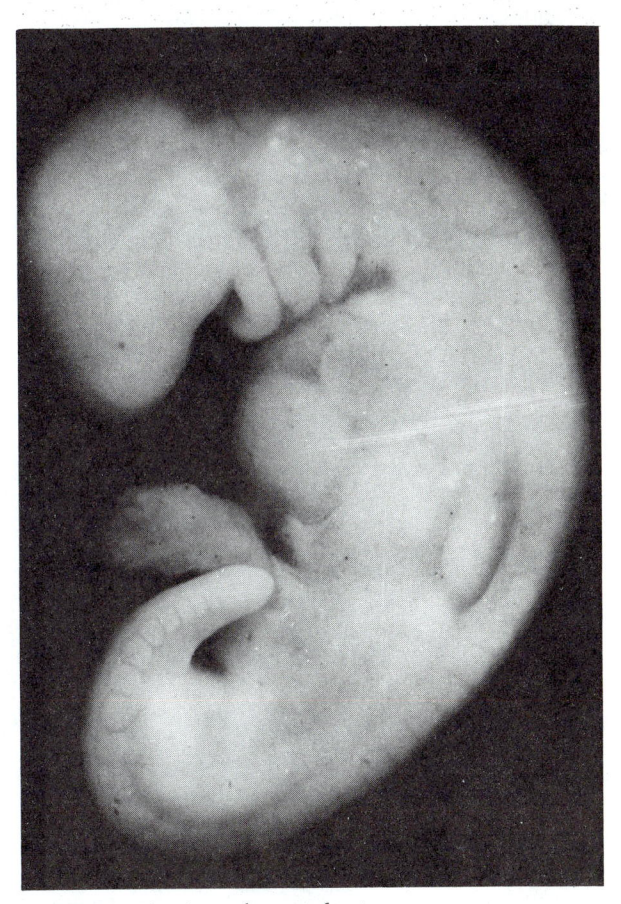

FIGURE 9–16. An embryo at about 28 days. The embryo has a characteristic C-shaped curvature, four branchial arches, and a visible arm bud. The head prominence is easily seen.
SOURCE: Courtesy Professor Hideo Nishimura, Kyoto University, Japan.

25th week. Fingernails are apparent. The intestines reenter the abdominal cavity, and the kidneys begin to secret urine. The fetus begins to swallow amniotic fluid as the buccopharyngeal and anal membranes rupture (the intestinal system is now open from the mouth to the anus). Bile is being secreted. The arms are disproportionately long, having reached their proportionate final length. The legs must develop and grow further to appear in proportion. Fingers are well defined, having developed enough to curl and make a fist. Faint lip movements can be seen, indicating the development of the sucking reflex. The external genitals differentiate fully by the 12th week. Crown-rump length is 50–80 mm, and fetal weight is 8–14 g (see Figs. 9–17 and 9–18).

Weeks 13–16

Rapid growth continues. The fetal skin is very thin and blood vessels can be identified easily. The eyes have moved to the front of the face, and the ears have migrated (due to neck and head growth) upward onto the side of the head. *Lanugo* (downy hair) can be seen on the body, especially on the head. More muscle and bone development has occurred, and the fetal skeleton is clearly visible with x-ray photography. The fetus is more erect. The lower limbs are now longer than the upper.

Fetal movements are more frequent (although the mother usually cannot feel them yet). Thumbsucking can be detected with ultrasound. Meconium is being produced in the intestine now that amniotic fluid is being swallowed. Brown fat deposition begins. Crown-rump length is 80–140 mm, and fetal weight is 14–200 g (see Fig. 9–19).

Weeks 17–20

Fetal movements are such that the mother is able to feel "quickening," and the heart rate is audible with a stethoscope. These signs can assist in affirming the delivery date and confirming the reality of the pregnancy for the mother.

The rapid growth begins to slow somewhat. Lanugo is clearly visible over the body, being heaviest over the shoulders. Head hair, eyelashes, and eyebrows are beginning to grow. Nails are now clearly visible on both fingers and toes (Fig. 9–20). The sebaceous glands have become active, and the fetus is covered with a greasy cheeselike substance known as *vernix caseosa*, which protects the fetus from the macerating effects of the amniotic fluid. Without vernix, epidermal tissue would become chapped and hardened. Lanugo may assist in holding the vernix caseosa to the skin.

Lung development has continued, and bronchial branching is essentially complete. Terminal

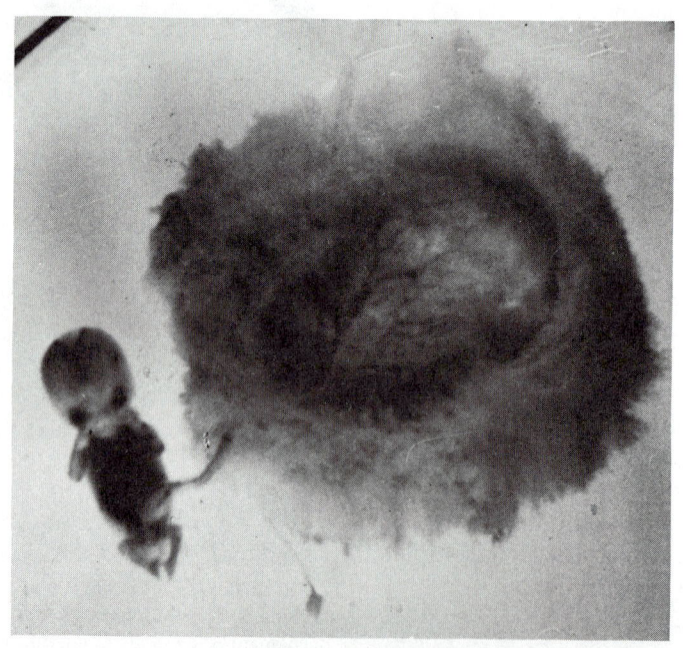

FIGURE 9–17. At week 9 the head is almost half the fetal length, the eyelids have fused, the fingernails appear, and the external genitals are differentiating.
SOURCE: Courtesy Landrum B. Shettles.

Physiologic Changes in the Fetus   179

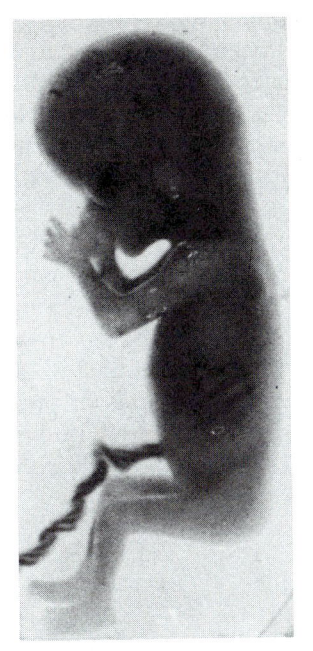

FIGURE 9–18. The fetus at week 12.
SOURCE: Courtesy Landrum B. Shettles.

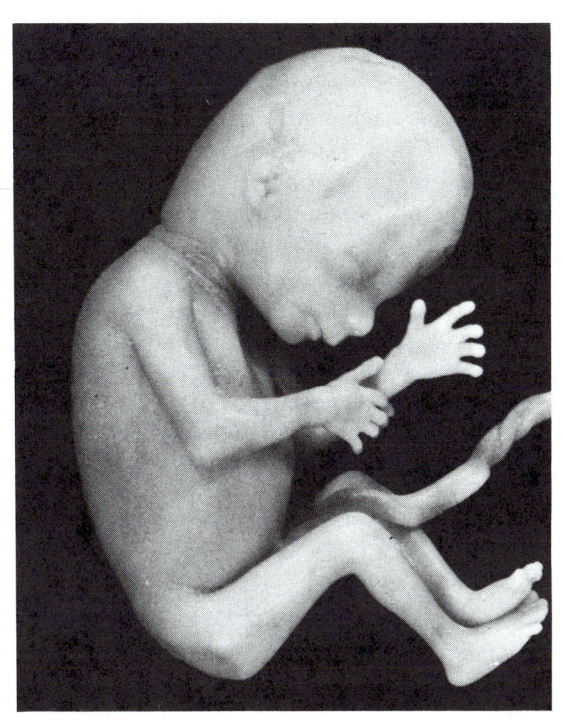

FIGURE 9–19. The fetus at 15 weeks. Brown fat is beginning to form.
SOURCE: Courtesy Landrum B. Shettles.

air sacs (future alveoli) are developing, and the pulmonary capillary bed is forming. Gas exchange in the lungs is not yet possible.

Weeks 21–24

Substantial weight gain occurs during weeks 21 through 24. The body begins to look correctly proportioned and plump. The skin is still wrinkled due to the lack of subcutaneous fat and red because the blood is visible in the capillaries. Skin ridges on the palms and soles form the individual's unique fingerprints and footprints.

Head hair is quite long, and eyebrows and lashes are quite distinct. The eye is structurally complete and the eyelid will be opening soon. The crown-rump length is 200–228 mm, and fetal weight is 300–780 g.

Weeks 25–28

The face and body have attained the general appearance they will have at the time of birth. The "old man" look is due to the red, wrinkled skin. Subcutaneous fat deposition will begin to fill out some of these wrinkles.

Extrauterine viability becomes possible at this stage, although mortality rates among infants born

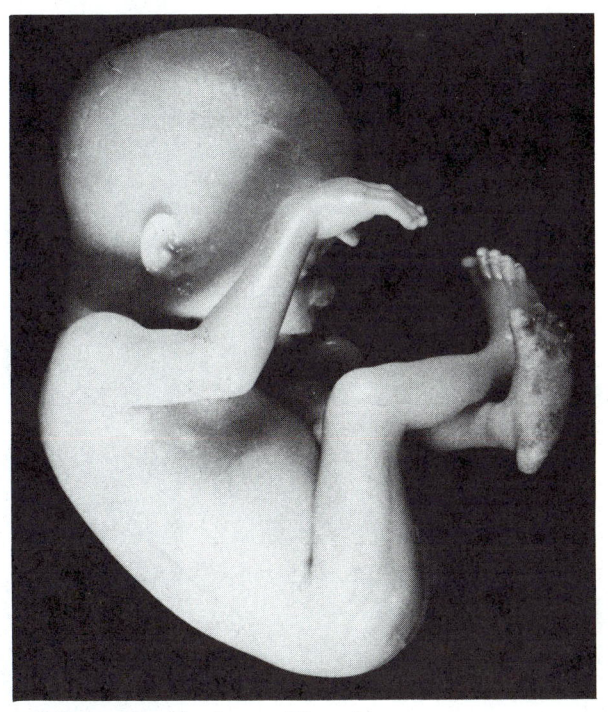

FIGURE 9–20. The fetus at 20 weeks. Eyelids, eyebrows, and fingernails are well developed at this age.
SOURCE: Courtesy Landrum B. Shettles.

this prematurely are very high. Respiratory failure is the leading cause of death. Lungs and pulmonary vasculature are not fully mature, but they can support gas exchange. Brain development has been rapid, and the nervous system can initiate rhythmic breathing movements (although it may have difficulty sustaining respirations for long periods) and can partially control body temperature (Moore, 1977).

The eyelids have unfused and now open and close under neural control. If the fetus is male, the testes have begun their descent into the scrotum. At 28 weeks crown-rump length is approximately 260–300 mm, and weight ranges from 1000 to 1200 g (see Fig. 9–21).

Weeks 29–32

Weight gain continues as fat and muscle tissue are laid down. Bones are fully developed but not completely ossified, making them soft and flexible. Mineral deposition increases during this period. The skin is less wrinkled and the fetus has a more "filled-out" appearance. The fetus has become pink as the thickness of the skin has increased. Fingernails extend beyond the tips of the fingers by 32 weeks. As a result, fine scratches on the skin are not uncommon. Crown-rump length averages 350 mm, and weight averages 2500 g.

Weeks 33–36

The fetus continues to fill out. Toward the end of this period growth begins to slow. Lanugo begins to disappear. Survival rates of prematurely born infants continue to increase with increasing gestational age. Crown-rump length averages 400 mm, and weight averages 3200 g.

Weeks 37–40

At 38 weeks, the fetus is considered full term. The skin is smooth and pink. Toenails have extended beyond the tips of the toes. Most of the lanugo has been shed; the shoulders and upper arms exhibit

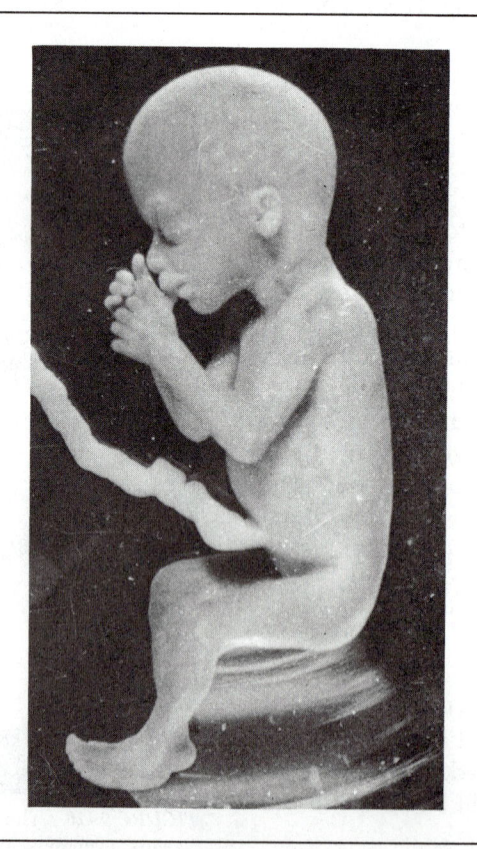

FIGURE 9–21. The fetus at 26–29 weeks.
SOURCE: Courtesy Landrum B. Shettles.

the last of this fine, downy hair. The testes have descended into the scrotum in the male, but in the female the ovaries remain high in the abdominal cavity until after birth.

The fetus fills the uterine cavity by this time and has assumed a "position of comfort". The extremities are well flexed. Because of the uterine cavity's pear shape, the fetus is usually in the head-down position. The chest is prominent, but its circumference is still about 2 cm less than that of the head. The nipples are well developed.

Myelination is in progress. Sleep–wake cycles have been established that will continue after delivery. The size of the fetus depends on genetic, nutritional, and environmental circumstances. Environmental considerations include age of the mother, number of preceding pregnancies, and whether this is a single or multiple pregnancy. Crown-rump length varies between 45 and 50 cm and weight ranges from 3000 to 3800 g. The female usually weighs less than the male.

ORGAN SYSTEM DEVELOPMENT AND FUNCTION

Having summarized embryonic and fetal development, we will now take a closer look at the development of individual organ systems.

Placental Function

To a large extent the pattern of development that occurs in the embryo is determined by the availability of nutrients. Prior to arrival in the uterus, the zygote relies on the large stores found in the cytoplasm of the large ovum. The endometrial secretions known as uterine milk provide nutrients to the morula through diffusion. These secretions, used while the morula floats freely inside the uterine cavity, are rich in glycogen. After implantation the developing embryo lies in a pool of nutrient-rich fluid made up of the broken down cells of the decidual.

The development of the chorionic villi and the blood vessels connected to the embryonic and fetal bloodstream bring the nourishment from the maternal bloodstream to the developing fetus. As the placenta ages, the membrane thins and the number of capillaries increases. These morphologic changes result in an efficient mechanism for transporting substances to meet the demands of the growing fetus. The placenta provides for the fetus through the transfer of gases, transport of nutrients, excretion of wastes, transfer of heat, and production of hormones. Therefore, the placenta assumes some or all of the functions of the respiratory system, gastrointestinal system, liver, kidney, endocrine system, and even the skin.

At term the placenta occupies approximately one-third of the uterine surface. Blood flow through the intervillous spaces is 700 ml/min, representing about 10 percent of the maternal cardiac output. Somewhere between 70 and 90 percent of that passes through the intervillous space to the fetus. The remainder meets the needs of the myometrium. Under normal conditions this vascular bed is maximally dilated, leaving little capacity for further dilation. Both hormonal and neuronal mechanisms can cause vasoconstriction and contribute to reduced blood flow. Bedrest is the one intervention presently available that can positively affect uterine blood flow. By decreasing the demands of other organ systems for circulation, bedrest enhances the flow to the uteroplacental unit.

Intervillous blood is supplied by the spiral arteries. Blood spurts out of these arteries under pressure and travels upward toward the chorionic plate. It then drifts downward toward the decidua to be drained by the venous system. The process is a relatively passive one.

Nutrient Transfer

There are several mechanisms of nutrient transfer: diffusion, facilitated diffusion, bulk flow, active transport, pinocytosis, and movement through breaks in the cell membrane.

Diffusion requires no energy and is based on movement along a high–low concentration gradient. Those substances transferred to and from the embryo by diffusion include oxygen, carbon dioxide, sodium, chloride, and fatty acids. Of all the transfer mechanisms, diffusion is the most important. When limitations occur in placental transfer, the first substances to be affected are the ones exchanged by diffusion. The two major deleterious fetal conditions associated with the placenta are asphyxia and intrauterine growth retardation. Both of these conditions are the result of alterations in diffusion.

Facilitated diffusion is also based on a concentration gradient; however, the rate at which a substance is transferred is in excess of what would cross the cell membranes by ordinary diffusion alone. The substances transferred are picked up by a carrier (a cellular substance such as sodium) at one side of the cell membrane and released at the opposite side. Glucose, the major fuel source for the fetus, is transported this way.

Active transport requires that a substance be transferred *against* a concentration gradient (moving from a low concentration to a high concentration). This requires the use of energy by the cells involved. Amino acids, water-soluble vitamins, and minerals are mobilized in this fashion.

Bulk flow is the mechanism by which water is moved. Large volumes of water, driven by an osmotic or hydrostatic gradient, move through micropores in the cell membranes.

Pinocytosis is required for the transport of large molecules such as globulins. A cellular vacuole engulfs the substance, moves it across the cell, and exudes it on the other side.

Breaks in the cell membrane of the fine villous structures of the placenta allow very large substances to enter the maternal circulation. Red blood cells are released this way.

Factors Affecting Uterine Nutritive Function
The factors that decrease blood flow to the uterus do so either by affecting pressure (the arterial pressure minus the venous pressure) or increasing vessel resistance. Uterine contractions are an excellent example of a factor that decreases blood flow. Contractions interrupt flow by pinching off the veins, thus reducing or eliminating outflow. The fetus must rely on either stored nutrients or those available in the blood remaining in the intervillous spaces. Usually, the full-term fetus is able to withstand this "normal" stress.

Prolonged contractions or a reduced blood flow to the uterus may interrupt the exchange of nutrients and waste products for an abnormally long time. This places the fetus at risk. Chronic hypertension or pregnancy-induced hypertension may decrease uterine blood flow through arterial vasospasm and increased vessel resistance. Compression of the vena cava can occur when the gravid uterus falls against that vessel. This will interfere with venous blood return to the mother's heart and with cardiac output. When cardiac output is reduced, less blood is available to the uterus and placenta. Vigorous maternal exercise can also decrease uteroplacental blood flow by shunting blood to those muscles under stress. Certain pharmocologic agents (that is, vasopressors) can also lead to vasoconstriction, thus interfering with nutrient exchange.

A chronic disturbance in uteroplacental blood flow may result in inadequate fetal growth and development, producing the syndrome known as *intrauterine growth retardation* (see Chapter 32).

Endocrine Function
Endocrine secretion is another function of the placenta. Hormones synthesized and secreted include the steroid hormones estrogen and progesterone, and the protein hormones *human chorionic gonadotropin* (HCG), *human chorionic somatomammotropin* (HCS), also called *human placental lactogen* (HPL), and *thyrotropin*. All of these hormones play important roles in the maintenance of the pregnancy and the support of embryonic development.

Fetal Nervous System

The nervous system, and indeed all fetal systems, develops in a series of precisely timed steps. It is in this way that specific connections between the nervous system and the target cells or organs are achieved.

Development begins during the 3rd week of gestation, when the mesodermal germ layer is derived from the ectoderm. Following this, *neurulation* begins. Neurulation is the transformation of the ectoderm overlying the *notochord* (a midline cord of tissue between the endoderm and ectoderm) into the neural tube. Neural tube formation occurs in three successive stage: the neural plate, the neural groove, and the neural tube.

The *neural plate* is a sheet of cells derived from the ectodermal germ layer. The notochord seems to induce differentiation of the neural plate around the 17th day of gestation. (The notochord will eventually form the vertebral column and cranium, the basis of the axial skeleton.)

The *neural groove* develops as the midline of the neural plate thickens and invaginates. This invagination causes the center line to drop down and the edges to turn upward, forming a groove.

Neural tube formation occurs as the invagination process continues, bringing the edges together. Eventually the edges meet and fuse. Once the tube is formed, the ectoderm is separate from the nervous system.

All three stages of neural tube development are present at the same time in different regions of the embryo. Closure of the tube begins on the 21st day in the middle region of the embryo. The fusion progresses rostrally (toward the head) and caudally (toward the tail) in a zipperlike fashion. Both ends of the tube remain open for a short period of time, with anterior closure occurring before posterior (see Fig. 9–22).

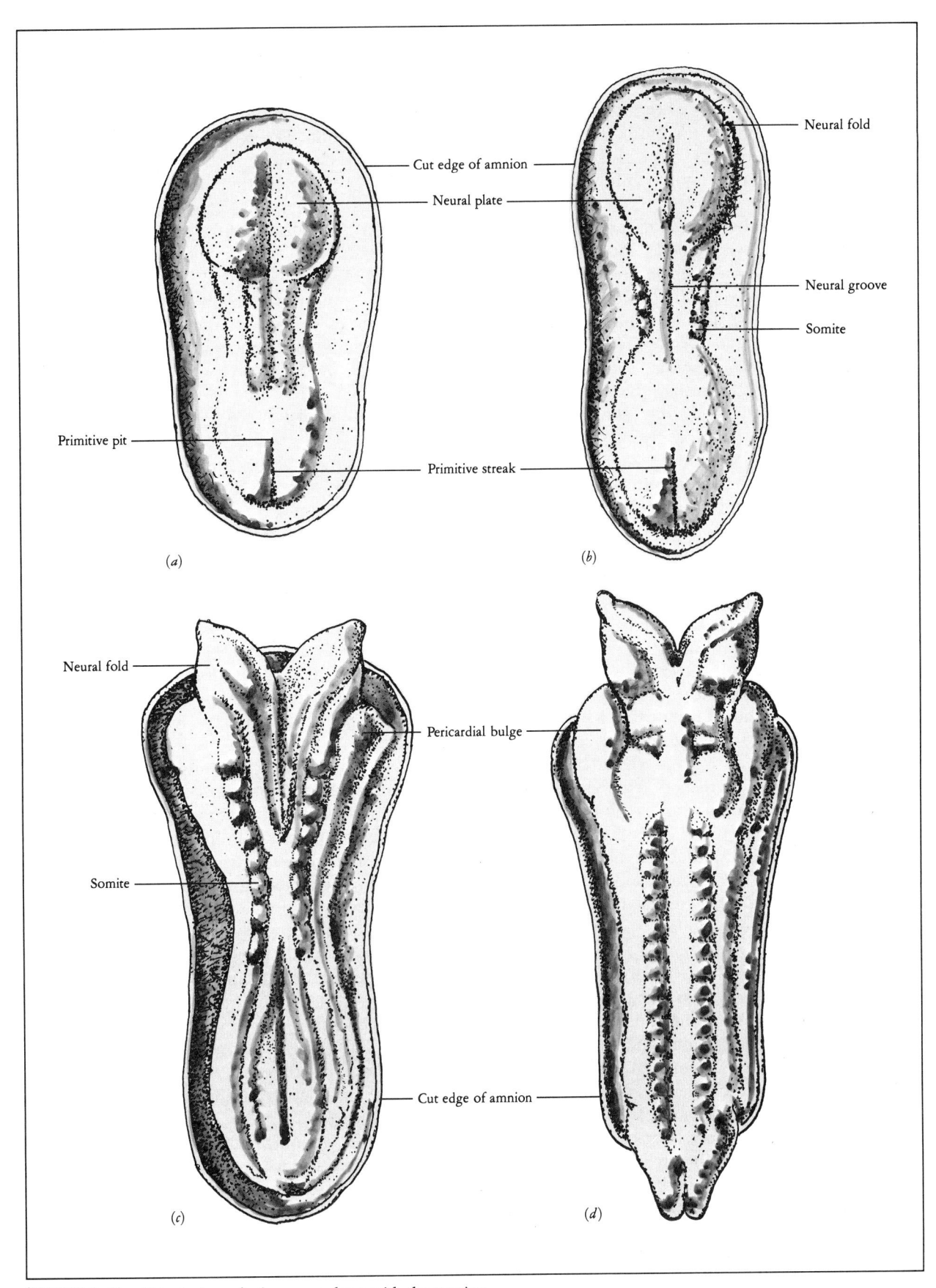

FIGURE 9-22. Dorsal view of a human embryo with the amnion removed. (a) The neural plate is clearly visible; (b) the somites, neural groove, and neural folds can be identified; (c) closure of the neural groove has begun; (d) the nervous system remains in contact with the amniotic cavity through the open ends of the neural tube.
SOURCE: Langman (1981).

Closure of the two ends of the tube is followed by rapid enlargement of the brain. This development contributes to the cervical and cephalic flexure that brings the embryo into the C-shape characteristic of this stage (see Fig. 9–16).

Histogenesis of the neural tissue begins once closure is complete; it involves multiplication of cells and differentiation of this tissue. This process continues for a relatively long time, especially in the higher cortical structures. The first peak in activity is found early in development: between 10 and 18 weeks there is a massive increase in the number of neurons. Beginning at about 30 weeks' gestation and continuing through the first postnatal year, another growth spurt occurs. At the end of this year, the final number of neurons (impulse conductors) will have been attained and glial cells (support and protection cells) will have been formed.

After histogenesis is complete, *myelination* begins. *Oligodendrocytes,* or *Schwann cells,* cover the axon, speeding neural impulses and decreasing the energy requirements for transmission. This is a lengthy process, beginning in the 4th month of gestation and reaching peak activity levels at birth. Myelination continues into adulthood. The first pathways to be myelinated are the sensory neurons of the peripheral nervous system.

Stage of myelination and maximum functional ability are positively correlated. This may explain the length of time required for psychomotor development in children.

The embryo exhibits sufficient neuromuscular development by $7\frac{1}{2}$ weeks to respond to stimuli through movement. The contralateral reflex response (bending the head away from the side stimulated) that appears at this early stage of development is initially associated with facial (perioral) stimulation. By 9 weeks the fetus is able to demonstrate full body response to the same stimulus, as well as spontaneous movements. These spontaneous movements are an indication of maturation of the medulla.

Medullary respiratory centers are responsive at $5\frac{1}{2}$ months, and the fetus can be respiratorily viable at the end of the 6th month. Sucking and grasping reflexes can be seen at 5 and 6 months respectively. These responses can be seen even in the anencephalic fetus, indicating that there is no cortical involvement in these reflexes.

Cerebral maturation begins in the 7th month of gestation. However, the process is a slow one, taking many years to complete. Dendritic and enzymatic development lead to the synchronous, coordinated responses indicative of maturation.

Obviously the fetus does not develop in a sensory vacuum. Filtered light and muted sounds are part of the environment. Kinesthetic input and touch, in relation to the uterine wall and other body parts, begin as soon as spontaneous movement becomes possible. It is not known whether this input is necessary for nervous system development. Development may be independent of stimulus input; however, other functional capabilities seem to be responses to endogenous and exogenous induction and processes.

Fetal Circulatory System

The heart is the first organ to function in the fetus, beginning to pump before development is complete. During the 3rd week of development two cardiogenic cords develop and fuse to form a single tube, the pericardial cavity. This tube begins to elongate. Both ends of the tube are held stationary, so that as the tube begins to lengthen the middle section begins to loop to the right. This bending on itself forms a U-shape and then an S-shape (Fig. 9–23). Peristaltic waves begin. At the end of the 4th week, these waves become coordinated contractions circulating blood through the embryo.

Separation of heart chambers begins during the 4th week and continues until the 7th week. This process divides the heart into the four characteristic chambers. Initially, the thickening subendocardial tissue (cushions) partitions the atrioventricular canals. These cushions grow toward the lumen of the heart from the dorsal (back) and ventral (front) walls. Eventually the cushions fuse.

The first of two septa begins to grow from the top of the common atrium toward the endocardial cushions. At the lower edge of this thin membrane (the *septum primum*) is an opening (the *foramen primum*) that allows continual mixing of blood in the atrium. This opening becomes progressively smaller as the septum primum and endocardial cushions develop.

Before this opening is obliterated, perforations appear in the upper portion of the septa. These perforations fuse together into a single opening, the *foramen secundum*. This allows for continued movement of blood across the atrium. Concurrently, the free edge of the septum primum fuses with the endocardial cushion.

At the end of the 5th week, another septum (the *septum secundum*) forms to the right of the septum primum. This is an incomplete partition that grows downward until it overlaps the foramen secun-

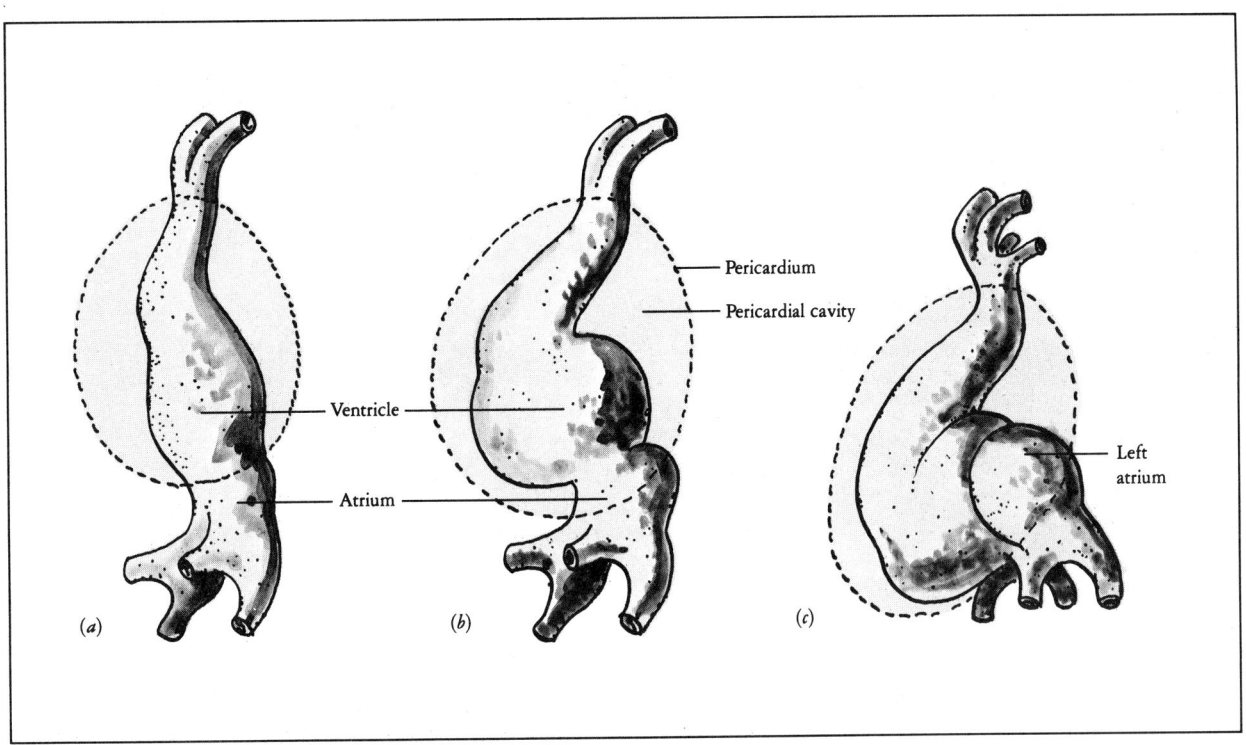

FIGURE 9-23. Formation of the cardiac loop. *(a)* At 8 somites; *(b)* at 11 somites; *(c)* at 16 somites. The broken line indicates the pericardium. Note how the atrium gradually assumes an intrapericardial position.
SOURCE: Langman (1981).

dum. This creates the flap valve needed for the newly formed *foramen ovale.* This flap valve allows right to left shunting of blood when the pressure in the right atrium is higher than the pressure in the left (see Fig. 9-24).

The first indication of ventricular septation occurs during the 4th week. A muscular ridge can be seen projecting upward from the apex of the common ventricle. Extensions of the endocardial cushions form the membranous portion of this septum. Ventricular separation is completed at the end of the 7th week, at which time the pulmonary trunk is aligned with the right ventricle and the aorta with the left.

The division of the single outflow tract *(truncus arteriosus)* into pulmonary artery and aorta occurs during the 5th week. Two ridges of tissue develop on opposite walls, growing inward until eventually they meet and fuse. This septum spirals upward, probably due to the flow of blood through the truncus while septation is occurring.

During the 6th week the mitral and tricuspid valves develop from tissue extensions of the endocardial cushions. After truncal septation is complete, the semilunar valves are formed.

In adult circulation blood passes from the right atrium to the right ventricle to the pulmonary artery to the lungs. Blood returning from the lungs goes to the left atrium, the left ventricle, and the aorta and then to the rest of the body. Embryonic circulation works in a parallel fashion. Blood from various parts of the body returns to the separate ventricles and is distributed to different organ systems.

The fetal lungs are fluid filled. The low arterial oxygen pressure causes pulmonary vasoconstriction, which leads to a high pulmonary vascular resistance. This results in a low-volume pulmonary circulation.

The systemic vascular resistance is low because nearly half of the descending aortic flow enters the placenta (450-600 ml/min). Here oxygen exchange occurs, and the blood then returns to the fetus via the umbilical vein. Diverted in the liver at the portal sinus, this oxygenated blood enters the inferior vena cava. This shunt allows the umbilical blood to bypass the hepatic microcirculation. After the blood enters the right atrium, one-third of this flow streams preferentially across the foramen ovale and into the left atrium.

Once in the left atrium this blood is combined with the pulmonary venous return, thereby reduc-

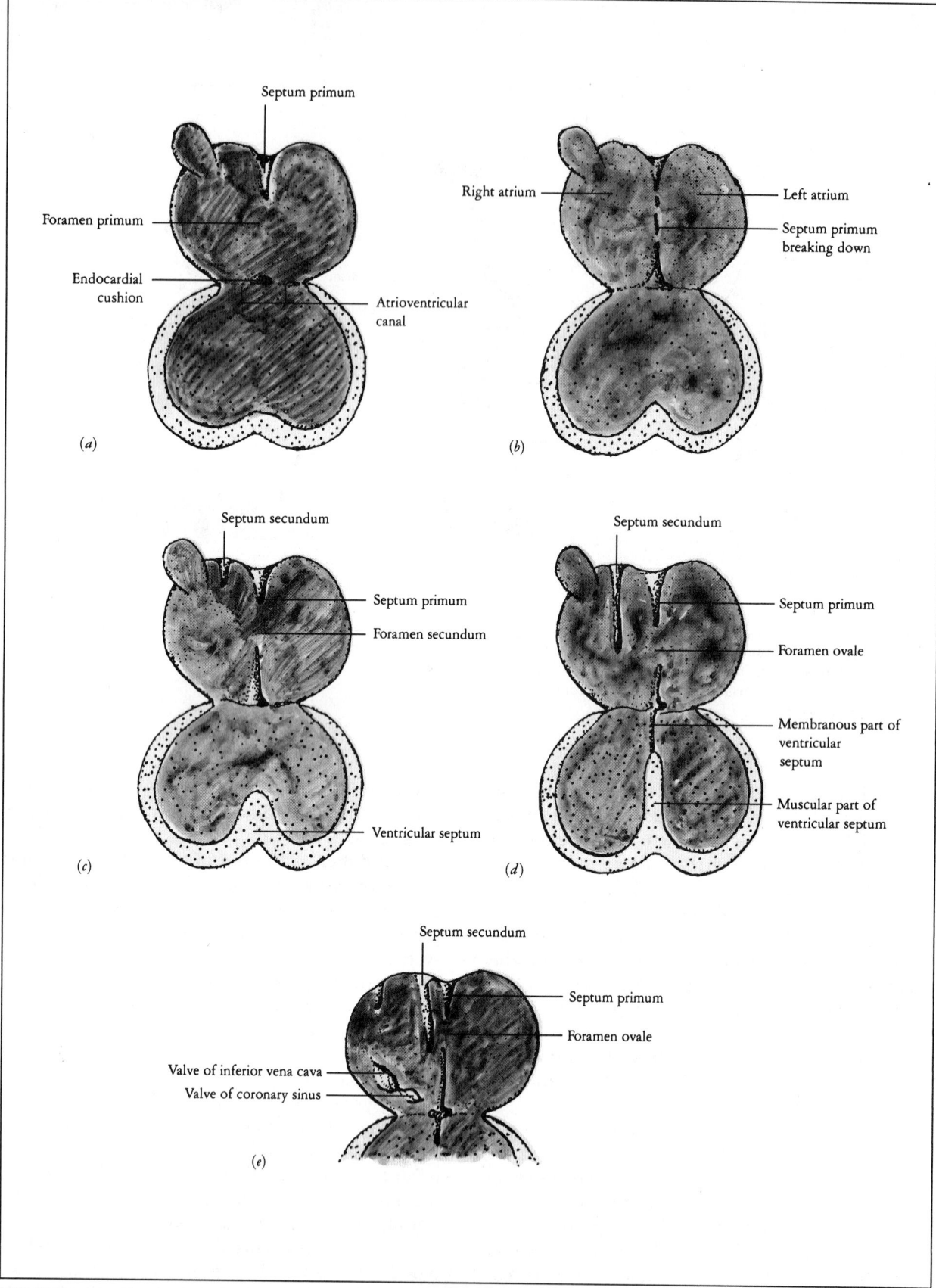

FIGURE 9-24. The division of the primitive atrium into right and left atria by the appearance of the septa. The fate of the venous valves is also shown, as is the appearance of the ventricular septum.
SOURCE: Snell (1983).

ing the pO_2 of the blood to about 26–28 torr (Rudolph, 1974). This blood is then pumped out of the left ventricle to the coronary circulation and upper body.

Deoxygenated blood returns via the superior vena cava to the right atrium. Here it mixes with the blood returning from the placenta (via the inferior vena cava) and enters the right ventricle. Very little crosses the foramen ovale. This mixture has a pO_2 of 16–18 torr (Rudolph, 1974) and is ejected into the pulmonary trunk. Most of this blood is shunted across the ductus arteriosus, however, and enters the descending aorta to service the abdominal organs and the lower body (see Fig. 9–25).

The fetus normally functions on lower arterial oxygen pressures than an adult does. However, there is little tolerance for hypoxic events. When hypoxic stress is encountered, the fetal heart rate falls, blood pressure rises, and there is a fall in cardiac output. In contrast, the adult usually compensates for hypoxia with increased cardiac output.

Fetal adaptation to hypoxia or asphyxia is accomplished through redistribution of blood flow. Placental blood flow is maintained, while flow to the gastrointestinal tract, skin, kidneys, and lungs is decreased. The heart, brain, and adrenal glands receive an increased proportion of cardiac output to compensate for the decreased oxygen levels in the blood. Through this redistribution the fetus acts to preserve those organs necessary for survival.

Fetal Renal System

Normal kidney development begins during the 3rd week of gestation with a movement of mesodermal cells away from the somites from the cervical region of the embryo all the way to the tail. These cells form the nephrogenic cord, from which three successive sets of kidneys will arise: the pronephrons, mesonephrons, and metanephrons. Movement through the successive stages is necessary for normal kidney development.

The *pronephrons* develop in the cervical region, appearing in the 4th week. Seven to ten solid or tubular cell groups grow from the nephrogenic cord. These are nonfunctional, primitive structures. The development is cranial to caudal in nature. Regression of the first clusters occurs before the total number of pronephron structures is established.

The pronephrons induce the development of the *mesonephrons*. As the pronephrons regress, the mesonephrons appear. These are larger, more complex structures located between the first and third thoracic segments. Eventually, 40 pairs of thin-walled tubules develop. Each tubule contains a primitive glomerular structure, a proximal tubule segment, and a distal tubule segment. The distal tubule connects to the mesonephric duct, which empties into the cloaca.

A total of 7–15 of these structures are functional at any one time. They remain functional until the end of the 4th month when the metanephric kidney (true kidney) begins to function. The mesonephrons contribute significantly to amniotic fluid production.

In the female, the mesonephrons have largely regressed by the end of the 3rd month. In the male, however, certain portions of the mesonephric structures remain to form the ducts of the epididymis, ductus deferens, and ejaculatory duct.

The *metanephrons* appear between the 31st and 34th days. The renal corpuscle and tubules originate from the cells of the nephrogenic cord (see Fig. 9–26). The excretory portion (collecting ducts, calix, pelvis, and ureter) take form from a specialized structure known as the ureteric bud, which develops off the mesonephric duct.

The ureteric bud branches off the mesonephric duct near its junction with the cloaca. The bud grows posterolaterally, entering the nephrogenic cord at the first to second sacral segments. Once the bud contacts the nephrogenic tissue (approximately the 8th week), it begins to branch dichotomously. The branches form the renal pelvis, the major and minor calyces, and the collecting ducts. The last generations of branching are associated with nephron induction.

The metanephric tubules are formed from clumps of cells around the tips of the bud branches. The clumped cells form a vesicle that becomes a tube, one end of which connects with the tip of the bud branch while the other end develops around the glomerulus, creating Bowman's capsule. Nephron induction stops at 32–35 weeks' gestation. Further growth of the kidney proceeds from the development of these nephrons, not from the development of new structures.

Hypotonic urine formation continues throughout fetal life. The urine is a major contributor to amniotic fluid formation and acts as a volume regulator. However, the kidneys are not vital for maintaining a homeostatic environment or for fetal survival.

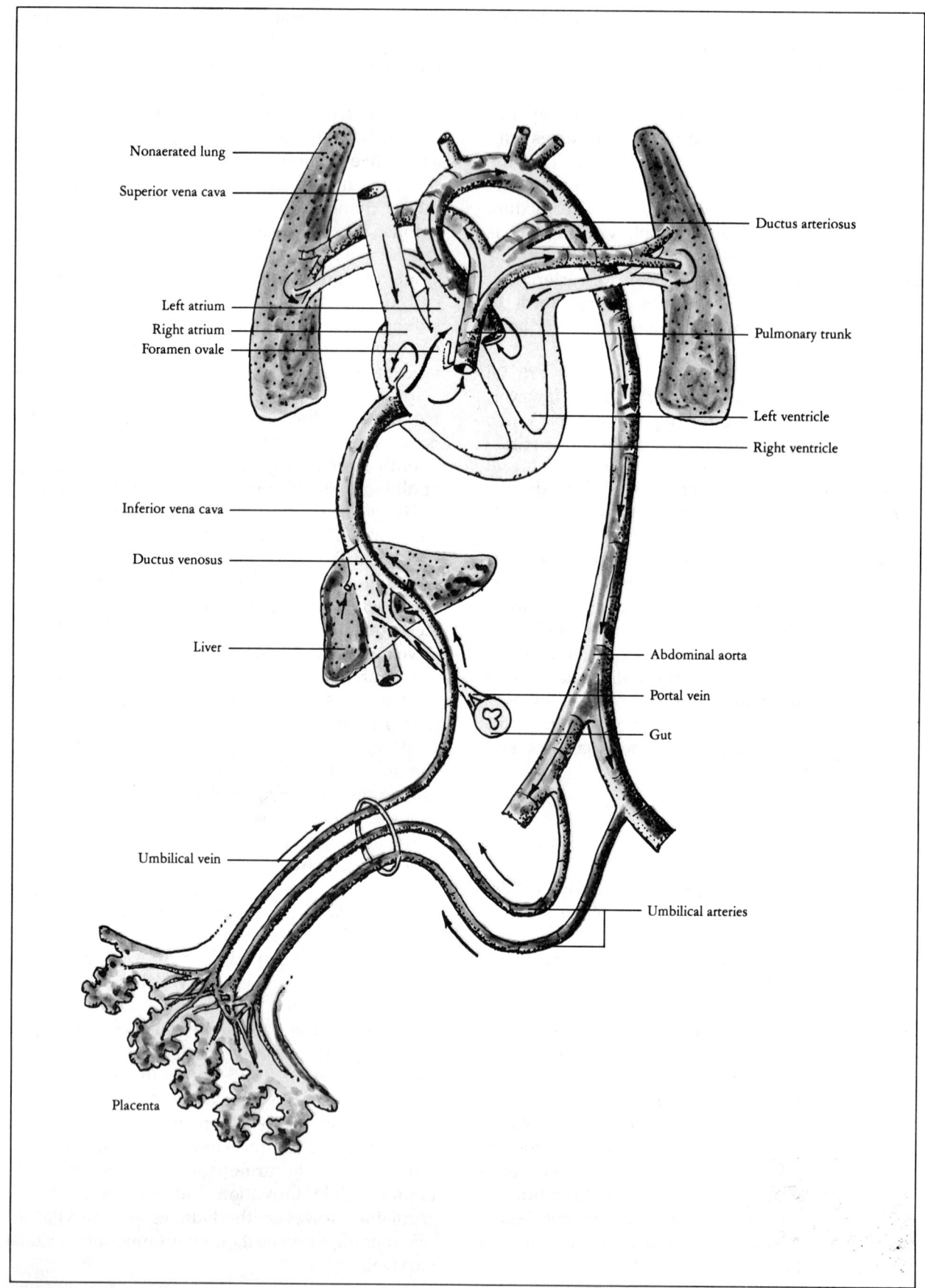

FIGURE 9-25. Fetal circulation.
SOURCE: Snell (1983).

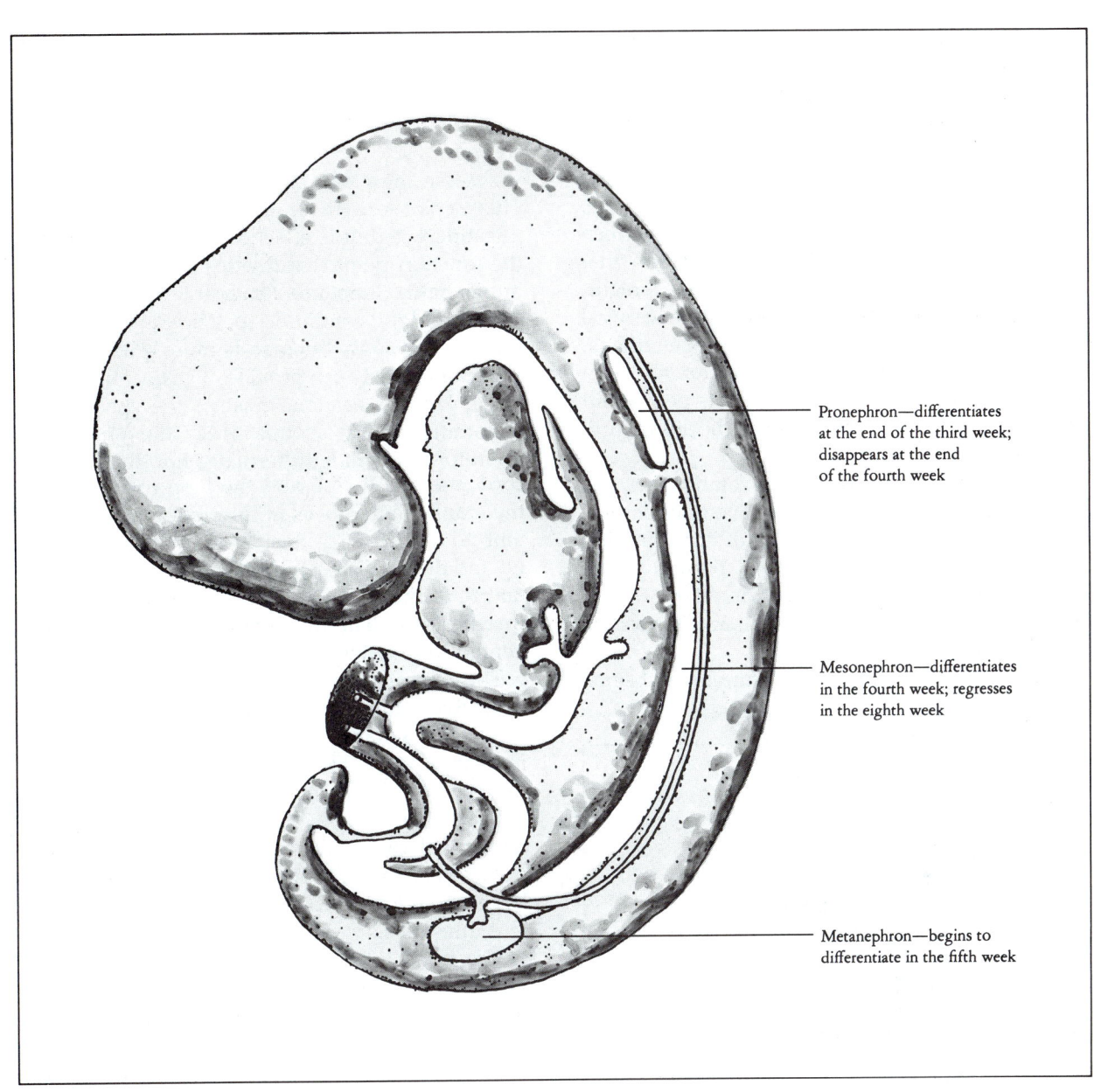

FIGURE 9-26. The development of the nephrogenic cord. The three primitive kidneys are shown together, although in reality they succeed each other.
SOURCE: Tuchman-Duplessis and Haegel (1974).

Fetal Gastrointestinal System

The endoderm, appearing during the 8th day, rapidly forms the yolk sac, which will be the basis for the digestive tract. When the lateral edges of the trilaminar embryonic disk fold to form a cylindrical body, part of the yolk sac is incorporated into the body. This forms the primitive gut, later to develop into the foregut, midgut, hindgut, liver, and pancreas.

At first the digestive system is a closed system, with a *buccopharyngeal membrane* covering the *stomodeum* (primitive mouth orifice) and a *cloacal membrane* covering the cloaca (anal pit). The cloaca eventually divides into the urogenital sinus and the rectum. Endodermal and ectodermal sheaths form the membranes. They are reabsorbed in the 4th and 9th weeks, respectively.

The pharynx, lower respiratory tract, esophagus, stomach, and duodenum (to the point where the common bile duct enters) develop from the *foregut*. At 26 days of gestation, the *laryngotracheal diverticulum* begins to develop. The septum that is created separates the trachea from the esophagus (see Fig. 9-27). The esophagus is a very short tube initially, but it rapidly increases in length to keep up with neck and thorax development. Between the 8th and 10th weeks the lumen is essentially obliterated with endothelial lining proliferation.

The esophagus, stomach, and intestine have a similar developmental process. Position, size, shape, and function mark the differences between these structures. The stomach is a dilation that forms toward the caudal end of the foregut. Initially, the stomach is located in the cervical region. It descends as the embryo lengthens. During this descent the stomach rotates in a clockwise direction until it assumes its permanent position. The enlarged liver forces the stomach to lie in an oblique direction.

The dorsal border (prior to rotation) of the stomach grows faster than the ventral border, thereby creating the curvature and increasing the stomach's capacity. At the cranial portion of the stomach, the fundus can be identified. These changes result in the definitive characteristics we know as the mature stomach.

The *midgut* (duodenum, jejunum, ileum) begins as a simple tube that has a wide communication with the yolk sac. The remnant of this connection is the *vitelline duct*. The initial growth of this tube parallels the curvature of the primitive spinal column. However, growth of the midgut soon progresses at a rate faster than that of the body. This rapid growth leads to a bending of the intestine where it is attached to the vitelline duct, the junction point that divides the intestinal loop into a cranial limb and a caudal limb.

The midgut continues to lengthen, forming a U-shaped loop that demands more room than the abdominal cavity can provide. The liver and developing kidneys assume most of the space in the abdominal cavity at this time (the 6th week). Therefore, the midgut herniates into the umbilical cord (see Fig. 9-28), and the loop rotates so that the cranial limb moves to the right and the caudal limb to the left (side to side orientation instead of up and down). The jejunum and ileum (the cranial limb) are the only portions of the small intestine that herniate. The duodenum and colon are prevented from entering the cord by retention bands.

The ongoing growth of the intestine leads to extensive coiling with the umbilical cord. Most of this growth happens in the cranial limb (small intestine), while the caudal limb (the large intestine) changes relatively little.

During the 10th week, the midgut reenters the abdominal cavity. Once initiated, this migration occurs very rapidly. The abdominal cavity is now large enough to accommodate the liver, kidneys, and intestines.

The small intestine is first to return. The jejunum fills the left side of the cavity and presses the descending colon along the left wall. The ileum fills the right side. The large intestine returns last. During reentry further clockwise rotation occurs. This 270-degree rotational process changes the original intestinal orientation to the definitive intestinal placement.

The last segment of the primitive gut to develop is the *hindgut*. The hindgut gives rise to the posterior half or third of the transverse colon, the descending colon, the sigmoid colon, the rectum, and the upper portion of the anal canal, and part of the urogenital system. The lower end forms the cloaca, a sinus composed of the allantois, urogenital sinus, and anorectal canal. The cloacal membrane initially maintains a closed system. Reabsorption of this membrane occurs during the 8th week, opening the digestive system to the amniotic cavity.

A wedge of mesenchymal tissue grow down-

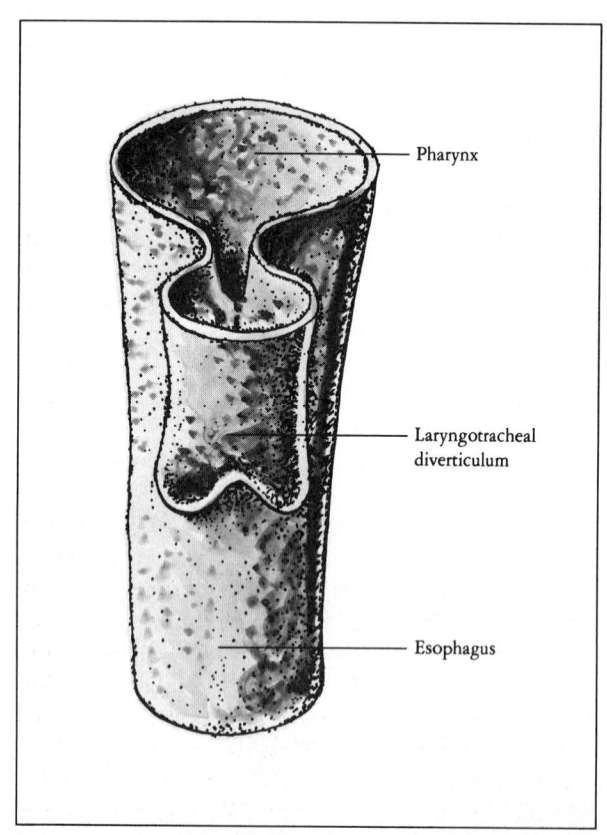

FIGURE 9-27. Septation of the foregut.
SOURCE: Snell (1983).

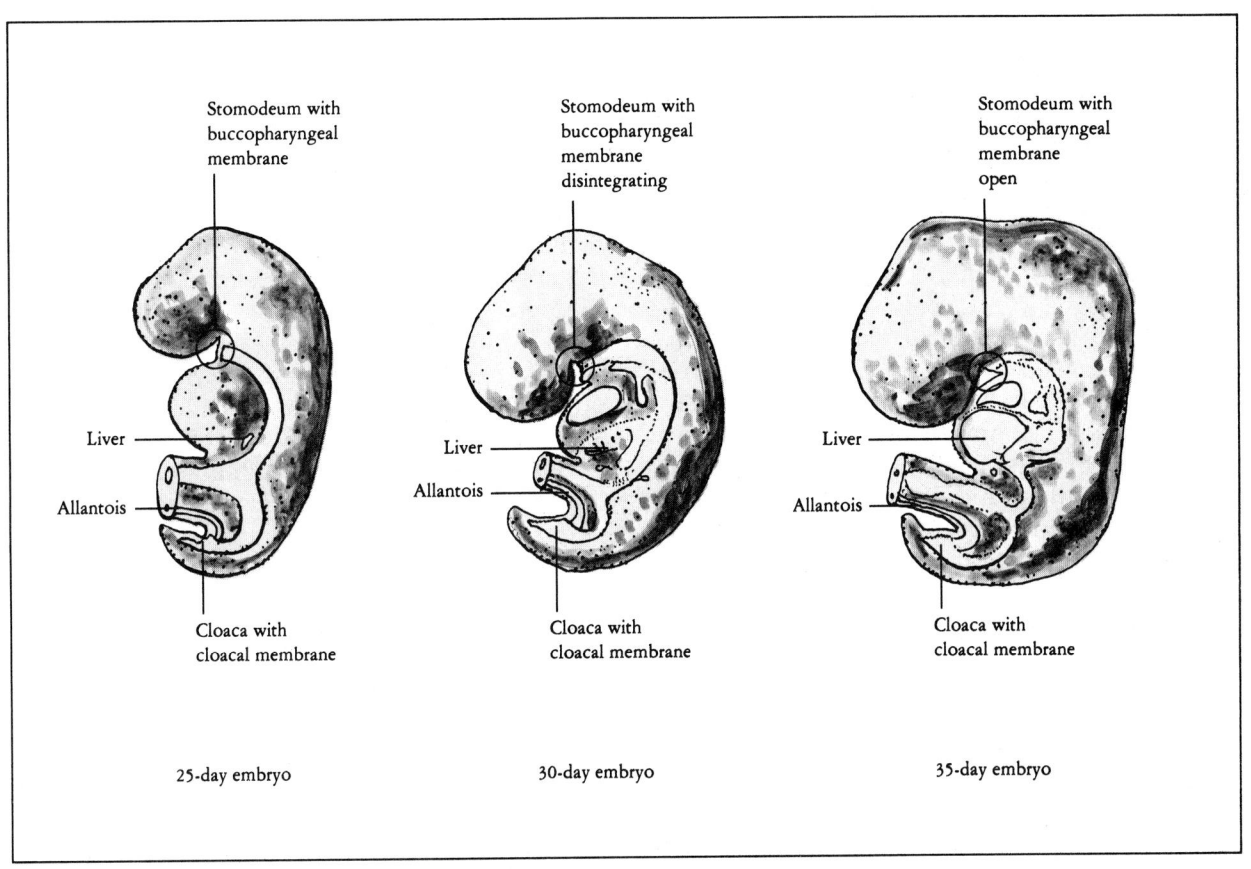

FIGURE 9-28. Embryonic development of the gastrointestinal tract: early stages.
SOURCE: Tuchman-Duplessis and Haegel (1974).

ward to eventually fuse with the cloacal membrane. This junction is the future site of the perineum. This urorectal septum divides the cloacal cavity into the primitive bladder and the anorectal canal.

The anorectal canal develops into the upper portion of the anal canal and rectum. The lower half of the anal canal is formed by an ectodermal depression that moves upward, to fuse eventually with the anal membrane (previously the cloacal membrane).

Gastrointestinal development and function characteristically progress from the proximal to distal portions. Motility also develops in this fashion. Intestinal peristalsis can be detected during the 13th week. Ganglionic cells are distributed throughout the intestine by 12 weeks (Siegel and Lebenthal, 1981), and swallowing can be seen as early as 11 weeks' gestation (even though sucking is not seen until 24 weeks) (Herbst, 1981). The exact mechanism stimulating the swallowing reflex is not known.

In the normal pregnancy, the volume of amniotic fluid increases proportionally with fetal age, length, weight, and placental weight. Pritchard (1985) documented full-term infants swallowing 450 ml of amniotic fluid (out of 850 ml) per day. Swallowing may contribute to the control of amniotic fluid production during fetal life. The injection of contrast material (dye) into the amniotic fluid demonstrates that gastric and intestinal motility increase with advancing gestational age (Koldovsky, 1978; Siegel and Lebenthal, 1981).

In the full-term infant gastrointestinal enzymes are present and functioning at appropriate levels. Raw materials are absorbed and then transformed into useful compounds by the liver or cells of the body. Once converted in the liver, these compounds are released into the bloodstream for transport to areas that need them. In a dual role, the liver also modifies toxic agents or end-product compounds in preparation for excretion in the bile.

In the fetus, these "normal" liver functions are unnecessary because the placenta allows maternal systems to maintain the homeostatic environment for the fetus. In an adaptive mode, the liver becomes a hemopoietic organ and is relatively uninvolved in bile formation (until the 5th month), glycogenolysis, or biotransformation of metabolic end products. Late in pregnancy, however, storage of essential nutrients does occur in preparation for the stress of transition. Hepatic glycogen begins to accumulate rapidly near term; 90 percent of it will be released within the first 2–3 hours following delivery (Thaler, 1981).

During pregnancy, the processing and biotransformation of fetal metabolic end products is in essence completed by the maternal system. The fetal and neonatal liver contains little smooth endoplasmic reticulum (where these processes occur), and the activities of the microsomal enzymes are greatly reduced or nondetectable (Thaler, 1981). Activation occurs once placental separation and gastrointestinal intake have been established.

Meconium can be seen in the small intestine during the 16th week, and it moves progressively toward the colon. This sticky, green-black stool is made up of mucus, bile, cellular debris, lanugo, gastrointestinal secretions, and vernix caseosa. All of these are ingested during swallowing of amniotic fluid. Normally, meconium is not passed until after delivery. Meconium-stained amniotic fluid may be an indication of fetal distress.

SUMMARY

Gametogenesis provides the unique germ cells necessary for species propagation and variation. The end result of fertilization (capacitation, acrosome reaction, penetration, and zona reaction) is the joining of paternal and maternal genetic material and the restoration of a chromosome number of 46 in the zygote.

Once fertilization takes place in the fallopian tube the zygote travels to the uterus to implant in the vascularized decidua. Placental development is rapid as the demand for nutrients increases. Once established, the parasitic relationship between mother and embryo allows for the differentiation and maturation of the conceptus.

Embryonic development is a time of differentiation and organogenesis. Every organ system is established, and the embryo take on the morphologic characteristics of a human being. The fetal period begins in the 9th week and is a time of maturation and refinement. The fetus prepares for labor and transition during the last months.

There are several methods of nutrient transfer across the placenta. Diffusion, facilitated diffusion, bulk flow, and breaks in the cell membrane do not require energy for transfer. However, active transport and pinocytosis require cellular energy for the movement of nutrients against a concentration gradient or across a cell.

Those factors affecting uterine blood flow (thereby creating potential danger for the fetus) either affect the blood pressure at the intervillous spaces or increase vessel resistance. This can alter nutrient transfer, especially the availability of oxygen, and place the fetus at risk for hypoxia (when there is insufficient oxygen) or intrauterine growth retardation (when substances for growth are not available).

Specific organ systems begin their development during the embryonic period and mature during the fetal period. However, it is evident that functional capacity (adult functioning) is usually not achieved prior to delivery. The transition to extrauterine life is the beginning of further refinement and activation of these organ systems. Maturation will occur at various stages in the development of the individual.

REFERENCES

Baker, T. G. 1982. Oogenesis and ovulation. In *Reproduction in mammals: Germ cells and fertilization*, eds. C. R. Austin and R. V. Short. Cambridge: Cambridge University Press.

Byskov, A. G. 1982. Primordial germ cells and regulation of meiosis. In *Reproduction in mammals: Germ cells and fertilization*, eds. C. R. Austin and R. V. Short. Cambridge: Cambridge University Press.

Clermont, Y. 1963. The cycles of the seminiferous epithelium of man. *Am. J. Anat.* 112:35.

Harper, M. J. 1982. Sperm and egg transport. In *Reproduction in mammals: Germ cells and fertilization*, eds. C. R. Austin and R. V. Short. Cambridge: Cambridge University Press.

Herbst, J. J. 1981. Development of sucking and swallowing. In *Textbook of gastroenterology and nutrition in infancy*, vol. I, ed. E. Lebenthal. New York: Raven Press.

Koldovsky, O. 1978. Digestion and absorption. In *Perinatal physiology*, ed. U. Stave. New York: Plenum Publishing.

Langman, J. 1981. *Medical embryology*. 4th ed. Baltimore: Williams & Wilkins.

Moore, K. 1977. *The developing human*. Philadelphia: W. B. Saunders.

Pritchard, J. A.; MacDonald, P. D.; and Gant, M. F. 1985. *Williams obstetrics*. 17th ed. New York: Appleton-Century-Crofts.

Rudolph, A. M. 1974. *Congenital diseases of the heart*. Chicago: Year Book Medical Publishers.

Siegel, M., and Lebenthal, E. 1981. Development of gastrointestinal motility and gastric emptying during the fetal and newborn periods. In *Textbook of gastroenterology and nutrition in infancy*, vol. I, ed. E. Lebenthal. New York: Raven Press.

Silverstein, A. 1980. *Human anatomy and physiology.* New York: John Wiley & Sons.

Snell, R. S. 1983. *Clinical embryology for medical students.* 3rd ed. Boston: Little, Brown.

Spence, A. P. 1982. *Basic human anatomy.* Menlo Park, Calif.: Benjamin Cummings.

Thaler, M. M. 1981. Liver function and maturation in the perinatal period. In *Textbook of gastroenterology and nutrition in infancy*, vol. I, ed. E. Lebenthal. New York: Raven Press.

Tuchman-Duplessis, H., and Haegel, P. 1974. *Illustrated human embryology*, vol. II: *Organogenesis.* New York: Springer-Verlag.

Tuchman-Duplessis, H.; David, G.; and Haegel, P. 1980. *Illustrated human embryology*, vol. I: *Embryogenesis.* New York: Springer-Verlag.

10
Physiologic Changes in the Maternal System

BEHAVIORAL OBJECTIVES

Upon completion of this chapter, the reader should be able to:

- Identify the signs and symptoms of pregnancy and state whether they are presumptive, probable, or positive indicators.

- Associate functional changes that may occur in pregnancy with related physiologic changes.

- State nursing interventions used when counseling a woman regarding minor discomforts experienced during pregnancy.

- Evaluate laboratory results and recognize normal values observed during pregnancy.

Change is inevitable throughout our lives, but never is it quite so pronounced as in pregnancy. The physiologic changes of pregnancy occur over 9 calendar months, or 40 weeks. In comparison to our life span, this is a brief period, yet it is a vitally important one.

Most women are aware of the possibility of pregnancy by the time they contact their physician. Diagnosis of pregnancy is usually, though not always, easy. Diagnosis is based upon (1) subjective or presumptive signs that bring the woman to her physician, (2) objective or probable signs, and (3) positive signs that are evident in advanced pregnancy.

Once pregnancy has begun, dramatic physiologic changes occur. This chapter discusses the phenomenal changes that occur during pregnancy and focuses on the physical effects on the pregnant woman.

SIGNS AND SYMPTOMS OF PREGNANCY

Signs of pregnancy are objective evidence perceptible to an examiner, while symptoms are subjective sensations of the patient.

Presumptive Signs and Symptoms of Pregnancy

Presumptive signs of pregnancy are often identified by the woman early in the gestation period. These signs include (1) cessation of menses, or *amenorrhea*, (2) breast changes and tenderness, (3) discoloration of the vaginal mucosa, and (4) an increase in skin pigmentation and the appearance of abdominal striae. The symptoms that may accompany these presumptive signs include (1) nausea, with or without vomiting, (2) increased frequency of urination, (3) perception of fetal movement, or "quickening," and (4) excessive fatigue.

Signs

CESSATION OF MENSES (AMENORRHEA) Cessation of menses is one of the earliest signs of pregnancy. Among nonpregnant women, the interval and duration of the menstrual cycle varies, with the average interval being 28 days. Cycles range from 15 to 45 days, and a woman's individual cycles can vary in length from one cycle to the next (Chaizze et al., 1968). The duration of each menses ranges from 2 to 7 days in most women. In healthy women with regular menstrual cycles, one missed menstrual period is suggestive of pregnancy. When the second cycle is missed, the probability is much stronger. Brief, scant bleeding may occur during pregnancy. This bleeding is normal and does not rule out the possibility of pregnancy.

Pregnancy may occur at various times throughout the life-cycle. It is not unusual for ovulation to occur prior to menarche, during the breastfeeding period before menstruation has resumed following a previous pregnancy, or prior to menopause. In counseling women about the possibility of pregnancy, it is important to discuss these issues.

Amenorrhea may result from conditions other than pregnancy, including anovulation, emotional disorders, environmental changes, and acute or chronic metabolic or systemic disorders.

BREAST CHANGES Early in pregnancy, many women experience tenderness and tingling in the breasts, especially in the nipple area. This results from breast engorgement caused by growth of the secretory ductal system. Many women also report changes in the pigmentation of the areola and the nipple, and enlargement of the sebaceous Montgomery's glands.

DISCOLORATION OF THE VAGINAL MUCOSA During pregnancy the vaginal mucosa, cervix, and vulva take on a dark bluish or purplish-red coloration caused by vasocongestion of the pelvic vessels. This is known as Chadwick's sign (some sources consider this a probable sign). This finding is not a conclusive indicator of pregnancy, because these changes are found in other conditions that include pelvic congestion.

INCREASED SKIN PIGMENTATION AND THE APPEARANCE OF ABDOMINAL STRIAE Hormonal changes in pregnancy are associated with common cutaneous manifestations. Darkening of the pigmentation of the nipple and areola may occur, especially in dark-haired women. Subcutaneous glands of the areola, the *Montgomery's glands*, become more prominent. A line between the symphysis and umbilicus, called the *linea alba*, may darken and then is called the *linea nigra*. Reddish and irregular stretch marks, or *striae*, may appear on the abdomen, buttocks, or breasts. Striae develop as a result of the breakdown of the underlying connective tissue. Some women develop a darkening of the skin over the forehead and cheeks. This is known as *melasma gravidarum*, or *chloasma gravidarum*, the "mask of pregnancy." This is also hormonally induced and will fade after pregnancy.

Symptoms

NAUSEA, WITH OR WITHOUT VOMITING Nausea, a common condition during pregnancy, is caused by changes in the gastrointestinal system. Symptoms may range from mild distaste for food to continuous nausea and vomiting. Because these symptoms often occur early in the day, the condition has been referred to as "morning sickness," but it can occur at any time of day. Symptoms usually begin approximately 6 weeks after the onset of the last menstrual period and continue for 6–12 weeks. Cessation is usually spontaneous, but in some instances nausea may continue throughout pregnancy.

INCREASED FREQUENCY OF URINATION Early in gestation the growing uterus exerts pressure on the urinary bladder, increasing the frequency of urination. As the enlarging uterus enters the abdominal cavity, this pressure subsides until late in pregnancy, when the fetal presenting part descends into the maternal pelvis and, again, frequency of urination increases.

PERCEPTION OF FETAL MOVEMENT The first perception of fetal movement, or *quickening*, is a feeling of fluttering movements. Quickening usually occurs between the 16th and 20th week after the onset of the last menstrual period, and the sensation of movement gradually increases in intensity. *Multigravidas* (women who have been pregnant before) generally become aware of fetal movements earlier than *primigravidas* (women pregnant for the first time).

EXCESSIVE FATIGUE Extreme fatigue commonly occurs in early pregnancy and persists throughout the first trimester. Fatigue occurs again toward the end of pregnancy as the woman gets larger and her weight increases.

Probable Signs of Pregnancy

Although certain objective changes, called probable signs of pregnancy, are more definite indicators than the presumptive signs and symptoms, they do not constitute differential diagnosis, or confirmation. These signs include (1) enlargement of the abdomen, (2) changes in shape, size, and consistency of the uterus, (3) changes in the cervix, (4) Braxton Hicks sign, (5) ballottement, (6) outlining of the fetus, and (7) results of endocrine tests.

ENLARGEMENT OF THE ABDOMEN Increasing size of the abdomen, especially when accompanied by amenorrhea during the childbearing years, is strongly suggestive of pregnancy. By the 12th week of gestation, the uterus can be felt in the abdomen just above the symphysis pubis. By the 20th week, the uterus is at the level of the umbilicus. Abdominal enlargement is more noticeable in multiparous women (women who have had viable fetuses before) than nulliparous women (those who have never borne a viable child) because of a decrease in abdominal muscle tone caused by previous gestations.

CHANGES IN SHAPE, SIZE, AND CONSISTENCY OF THE UTERUS Uterine changes occur within the first 3 months of pregnancy and can be noted during physical examination. At about 6–8 weeks after the onset of the last menstrual cycle, *Hegar's sign* becomes evident. Upon bimanual examination of the isthmus of the uterus, the area between the cervix and the body of the uterus is felt to be very soft, often to the extent that the cervix and the body of the uterus seem to be separated.

The uterus becomes irregular in shape during early pregnancy. By the 5th week of gestation, *Braun von Fernwald's sign* is apparent. This consists of irregular softening and enlargement of the uterus at the site of implantation. *Piskacek's sign*, an asymmetrical, softened enlargement of the uterine cornu due to placental development, may be present. Generalized enlargement of the uterus occurs by the 8th week, progressively increasing during pregnancy. At term, fundal height reaches approximately 38–40 cm.

CHANGES IN THE CERVIX By 6–8 weeks of gestation, the cervix softens considerably. This softening is referred to as *Goodell's sign*.

BRAXTON HICKS SIGN Painless, irregular uterine tightenings occur throughout pregnancy. These are normal physiologic contractions that are not associated with cervical changes. These contractions, called *Braxton Hicks sign*, are not a positive sign of pregnancy, because they can occur as a result of other physiologic processes as well.

BALLOTTEMENT During midpregnancy, the fetal volume is less than that of the amniotic fluid. When pressure is exerted on the uterus, the fetus will sink and then rebound to its original position. The examiner's finger can feel a tap as the fetus descends.

OUTLINING THE FETUS As the fetus grows, the outline of the fetal body can be palpated through the maternal abdomen (see Chapter 15). Myomas often feel like the fetal head or small part, thus confusing the diagnosis. Therefore, palpation of the fetal body cannot be considered a positive sign of pregnancy.

RESULTS OF ENDOCRINE TESTS Chemical tests for the presence of human chorionic gonadotropin in maternal plasma or urine are performed to diagnose pregnancy. None of these tests can provide a positive diagnosis because of the high incidence of false positives and false negatives.

Endocrine tests are based on the detection of human chorionic gonadotropin (HCG) in the maternal plasma and urine. A variety of immunoassay or bioassay techniques measure HCG in the body fluids. Many hormonal tests show a high percentage of false positives and false negatives. If circulating levels of luteinizing hormone (LH) are high, the LH cross-reacts with the antibody to HCG and may induce a false positive reaction in an assay sensitive to HCG. Tests that have lower sensitivity to HCG levels in order to decrease the LH influence may result in a high percentage of false negative results.

The radioimmunoassay (RIA) that employs antibodies against the beta subunit of HCG is specific for HCG and does not cross-react with LH. This test is so sensitive that it can diagnose pregnancy at least 1 week prior to expected menses after ovulation. The RIA for HCG is not as accurate as that for the beta subunit of HCG, but if done correctly, its accuracy reaches 100 percent.

HCG has antigenic properties that allow it to be identified by immunologic tests using the technique known as hemagglutination. This method can detect HCG in the urine 42 days after the beginning of the last menstrual period. This technique consists of exposing Gravidex (latex foam particles coated with HCG) to urine to which antiserum has been added. If the urine contains no HCG, agglutination occurs and the test is negative. If HCG is present, agglutination does not occur and the test is positive. A single drop of urine will give results in 2 min with approximately 92 percent accuracy. In the pregnosticon test, sensitive red blood cells are added to 8 ml of urine. The test is positive if no agglutination occurs. The test takes 2 hours to complete and is quite sensitive, resulting in a low false negative rate. (See Table 10–1 for tests currently used to diagnose pregnancy.)

Biologic tests for pregnancy have been used less often since the introduction of the immunologic tests. These tests take a long time to yield a result and are more expensive to conduct (see Table 10–2).

TABLE 10–1. *Tests Currently Used for Diagnosis of Pregnancy*

Test	Testing Time	Range of Gestation (Days)
Agglutination tests		
Slide	2 min	24–50
Tube	2 hours	24–48
Radioreceptor		
Qualitative	1 hour	12–22
Quantitative	3 hours	8–10
Radioimmunoassays		
HCG	24–36 hours	8–10
Beta–HCG (semiquantitative)	2 hours	7–14
Beta–HCG (quantitative)	24 hours	6–8
Enzyme Immunoassay		

SOURCE: Eskin (1981).

TABLE 10–2. *Biologic Tests for Diagnosis of Pregnancy*

Immunologic Test	Material Injected	Animal	Positive Result	Length of Time
Ascheim-Zondek	0.5 ml urine	Mouse	Hemorrhagic corpora lutea are observed in the ovaries	5 days
Friedman	10 ml urine	Female rabbit	Hemorrhagic spots are observed on the surface of the ovary	2 days
Hogben	1–2 ml urine	Toad	Ovulation occurs	6–12 hours
Mainim	urine	Male toad	Spermatozoa appear in toad's urine	2–5 hours

SOURCES: Hickman (1978); Pritchard, MacDonald, and Gant (1985).

The *home pregnancy tests* which are currently available are both accurate and sensitive. Many are based on the immunologic agglutination of sheep erythrocytes into a ring and they can detect pregnancy a few days after the missed period. The most recent tests using the monoclonal antibody technology detect the presence of HCG in the urine on the first day of the missed period.

Positive Signs of Pregnancy

The positive signs of pregnancy are *diagnostic* of pregnancy. That is, they are completely objective and are not present in any other physiologic state. They are usually present after the 3rd or 4th month of pregnancy. The three positive signs of pregnancy are (1) presence of the fetal heartbeat distinct from that of the mother, (2) perception of fetal movement by the examiner, and (3) recognition of the fetus by x-ray examination or of the embryo or fetus by sonogram.

PRESENCE OF THE FETAL HEARTBEAT The fetal heart can be heard by auscultation by 17–19 weeks of gestation in most pregnancies. With the ultrasound Doppler device, the heartbeat can be detected as early as 8–10 weeks of gestation (Taylor, 1971). With a fetoscope, the heart rate cannot be heard clearly until 18–20 weeks. The heart rate should be between 120 and 160 beats/min and must be counted simultaneously with the maternal pulse to make a definite distinction between them. Often the bounding maternal aorta is easily audible in the supine position, and its sound must be distinguished from that of the fetal heartbeat. Also, mechanical movement of the fetal heart can be detected by real-time sonography or fetal echocardiography by the end of the 2nd month of pregnancy.

Upon auscultation of the abdomen, other sounds may be detected. The *funic*, or umbilical cord, *souffle* is a sharp, whistling sound heard in synchrony with the fetal heart rate and caused by blood pulsating through the umbilical arteries. The uterine souffle is a soft, blowing sound heard in synchrony with the maternal heart rate. It is caused by the blood passing through the dilated uterine vessels. The maternal pulse may be very distinct. Caution must be taken in monitoring to differentiate between the maternal and fetal pulses. Heart tracings of the maternal pulse are common, especially when a preterm infant is monitored. If the maternal pulse is rapid, it may simulate the fetal pulse.

PERCEPTION OF FETAL MOVEMENT BY EXAMINER By the 20th week of gestation, the examiner can detect fetal movement by placing a hand on the maternal abdomen. Movement may vary from a faint flutter to more pronounced activity later in pregnancy. Fetal movements may also be visible as pregnancy progresses.

RECOGNITION OF THE FETUS ON X-RAY OR SONOGRAM The use of x-rays in diagnosing pregnancy is not common practice because of the possibility of gonadal damage and genetic abnormalities. Other factors also limit its diagnostic value. The fetal skeleton cannot be distinguished until the 16th week of pregnancy, and even then its detection depends on variables such as the thickness of the abdominal wall and the radiologic techniques used. X-ray examination is useful in confirming the death of a fetus or in differentiating the pregnant uterus from abdominal tumors.

Sonographic examination can demonstrate an intrauterine pregnancy. Ultrasound waves are passed through the maternal abdomen. Tissue density is visualized on a gray scale and is seen as a two-dimensional picture. By the 6th week of pregnancy, the gestational ring is easily identified, and fetal parts can be seen as early as 10 weeks (refer to Chapter 13).

Estimation of Gestational Age

Gestational age, or duration of pregnancy, can be estimated in several ways. The *menstrual age* is estimated from the first day of the last menstrual period (LMP). This is approximately 2 weeks before ovulation and fertilization occurs. The total length of gestation is about 280 days, or 40 weeks. This is also estimated as $9\frac{1}{4}$ calendar months, or 10 lunar months.

Although gestational age is most commonly estimated from the date of the last menstrual period, embryologists also count the length of pregnancy from the time of ovulation. The *ovulation age*, or *conception age*, is estimated from approximately 2 weeks following the first day of the last menstrual period. Estimated this way, the total length of gestation is 266 days, 38 weeks, $8\frac{3}{4}$ calendar months, or $9\frac{1}{2}$ lunar months.

Gestation is also divided into *trimesters*, three units of 3 calendar months each. Embryologic events are often associated with the trimester in which they occur.

It is most accurate to discuss gestation in terms of weeks rather than months, because of the difference between calendar and lunar months and because gestational events happen within short periods of time.

Various measurements and external characteristics are valuable in determining gestational age. These include measurement of the fundal height (McDonald's measurement), ultrasonic evaluation (crown-rump measurement and biparietal diameter of the fetal head), and assessment of physiologic changes during pregnancy.

EFFECTS OF PLACENTAL HORMONES

The syncytiotrophoblast (the outer, multinuclear layer of the trophoblast) synthesizes hormones that regulate metabolic changes during pregnancy. The protein hormones, *human chorionic gonadotropin* (HCG) and *human placental lactogen* (HPL), also called *human chorionic somatomammotropin* (HCS), as well as the steroid hormones, progesterone and estrogen, are produced by the placenta and have pronounced effects on maternal physiology.

Human Chorionic Gonadotropin

The glycoprotein HCG is similar to the luteinizing hormone (LH) and is secreted by the syncytiotrophoblast a few days after implantation, or during the 3rd week of pregnancy. HCG rises to peak levels in the plasma and urine by the 8th week of gestation and then declines to lower levels. The most apparent function of HCG is to maintain the corpus luteum during early pregnancy. HCG plays a role in the initiation of testosterone synthesis in the testes of the male fetus and in the ability of the trophoblast to develop specific immunologic properties to fight infection.

Human Placental Lactogen

Human placental lactogen (HPL), or human chorionic somatomammotropin, is produced by the trophoblast and may be detected as early as the 3rd week after ovulation. Its concentration rises steadily during the first and second trimesters. The concentration in maternal blood is approximately proportional to the size of the placenta.

Placental lactogen functions indirectly and directly in a number of metabolic activities, including (1) lypolysis and elevation of circulating free fatty acids, providing a source of energy for the mother and fetus and sparing both glucose and protein for fetal use; (2) the antiinsulin effect of HPL, leading to elevated maternal glucose and resulting in increased insulin secretion by the islets of Langerhans and mobilization of the source of amino acids to the fetus; and (3) the synergistic action with hydrocortisone and insulin, playing a role in the development of the alveoli of the mother's breast (lactogenic effect).

Estrogen

The numerous effects of estrogen during pregnancy include the following:

1. Enlargement of the uterus, breasts, and genitals.
2. Changes in fat deposition
3. Altered nutrient metabolism.
4. Changes in sodium and water retention.
5. Hematologic changes.
6. Vascular changes.
7. Stimulation of production of the melanin-stimulating hormone, which is responsible for hyperpigmentation during pregnancy.

Estriole is the primary estrogen produced by the placenta during pregnancy. The levels of estriole in the serum and urine increase during pregnancy and are used as indicators of fetal well-being.

Progesterone

Progesterone is produced by the corpus luteum during the first 2 months of pregnancy and by the trophoblastic cells of the placenta 8–10 days after conception. Levels of progesterone rise steadily throughout pregnancy.

Progesterone has the following functions in pregnancy:

1. Promotes development of the decidual cells in the endometrium to provide appropriate nutritive matter for the developing blastocyst.
2. Assists implantation.
3. Decreases contractility of the uterus.
4. Promotes development of the secretory ducts of the lobular–alveolar system.
5. Increases fat deposition.
6. Reduces gastric motility.
7. Increases sodium retention.
8. Affects respiration by increasing sensitivity of the respiratory center to CO_2.

CHANGES IN THE REPRODUCTIVE SYSTEM

Uterus

The progressive increase in the size of the uterus is the most easily observed distinctive sign of pregnancy. This phenomenal growth is partially due to the development of new muscle fibers early in pregnancy, but it is primarily due to the enlargement of preexisting muscle fibers. Cellular hypertrophy and the rapid growth of tissue are thought to be associated with the increased synthesis of *polyamines* (a number of nitrogen-containing organic compounds) (Russell and Durie, 1978). Polyamine levels measured in maternal urine during pregnancy increase with hypertrophy of the uterus. Uterine muscle cell size reaches seven to eleven times the length and two to seven times the width of muscle fibers of the nonpregnant uterus. This is a result of estrogen stimulation and distention caused by the growing fetus.

During pregnancy, the uterus is tranformed from a small, solid structure to a relatively thin-walled, muscular container capable of housing the fetus, placenta, and amniotic fluid. Over a relatively short period of time, the gravid uterus achieves a size 20 times greater than that of the nonpregnant uterus. The uterus increases from approximately 6.5 to 32 cm in length, from 4 to 24 cm in width, and from 2.5 to 22 cm in depth. The weight increases from 50 to 1000 g at full term. The total volume of the contents of the uterus at term averages about 5 l, but may be as much as 10 l or more, while the capacity of the nonpregnant uterus is 10 ml or less. Other uterine changes that occur during the early weeks are regarded as subjective signs of pregnancy and were discussed earlier in this chapter.

Throughout pregnancy the uterine wall changes in thickness and consistency. During the first few months, the uterine wall becomes considerably thicker, while losing the firmness and resistance characteristic of the nonpregnant state. As pregnancy advances, the uterine wall gradually thins to approximately 1.5 cm or less. The walls soften and are easily indented, as demonstrated by ease of palpation of the fetus through the maternal abdomen.

As the uterus grows, it undergoes changes in its shape. In the first few weeks, the pear shape is maintained, but as pregnancy advances, the fundus enlarges and becomes spherical. The uterus increases more rapidly in length than in width and assumes an ovoid shape. As the uterus enlarges, it is no longer solely a pelvic organ. It begins to displace the intestines laterally and superiorly and ultimately reaches almost to the liver. Discomfort is often felt as the broad and round ligaments are stretched by the tension exerted by the growing uterus.

The musculature of the uterus consists of three layers: (1) an internal layer extending over the fundus and into the various ligaments; (2) a dense layer of muscle fibers containing intermeshed blood vessels; and (3) an external layer consisting of sphincter-like fibers around the insertions of the tubes and the external os. The middle layer comprises the main portion of the uterine wall. Each cell layer interlaces with the one adjacent, forming a figure 8, resulting in constriction of the blood vessels during uterine contraction.

Early in pregnancy, irregular, painless uterine contractions occur. As pregnancy progresses, these contractions are palpable and easily detected. They are stimulated by increasing amounts of estrogen and increasing distention of the uterus. During each contraction, the uterus becomes firm to the touch and then returns to its relaxed state. These contractions were first identified by Braxton Hicks, after whom they are named. Such contractions occur sporadically and without regularity. Often in late gestation (38–40 weeks) they take on a more regular pattern and may become uncomfortable. Braxton Hicks contractions are not associated with cervical changes and often account for "false labor."

Cervix

The cervix consists primarily of connective tissue, with a small amount of smooth muscle (see Fig. 10–1). During pregnancy, the cervix undergoes pronounced softening and takes on a cyanotic appearance. These changes are a result of increased vascularity and edema of the cervix, as well as hypertrophy and hyperplasia of the cervical glands. The cervical glands occupy approximately half of the entire cervical mass at term as compared to the small fraction of the mass they occupy in the nonpregnant state. Progressive thinning occurs in the septa of the endocervical canal. The endocervical glands secrete a thick mucus that accumulates and obstructs the cervical canal, forming the *mucous plug*. The formation of the mucous plug helps to prevent ascending bacteria from entering the uterus. Loss of the mucous plug indicates that cervical dilation has begun. Hyperactivity of glandular tissue during

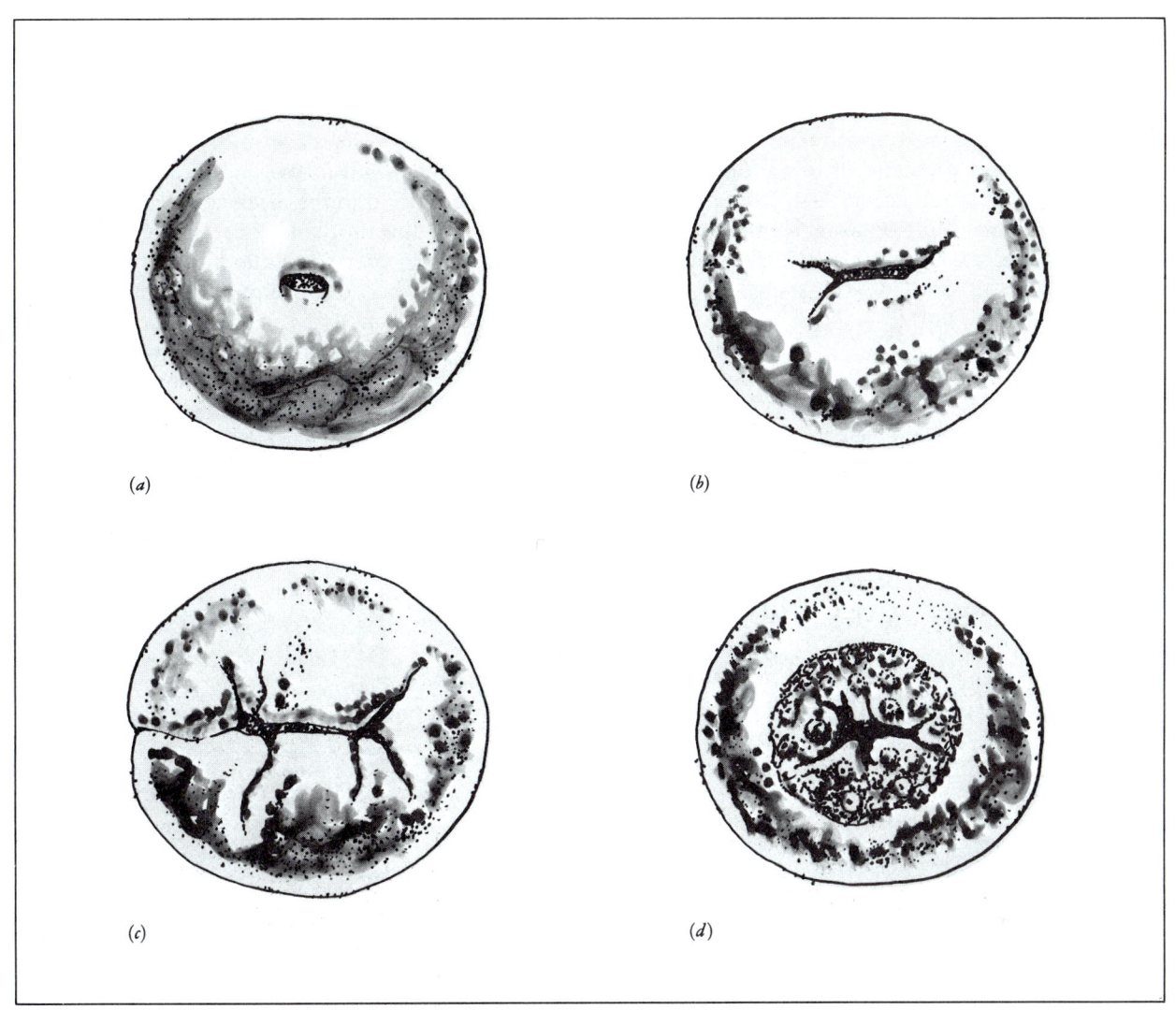

FIGURE 10–1. Common appearance of the cervix. (*a*) The nulliparous cervical os is small and either round or oval. (*b*) After childbirth the os has a slitlike appearance. (*c*) Difficult deliveries may tear the cervix, producing permanent lacerations. (*d*) Ectopion, often present in multigravidas, is a pinkish-red, bumpy tissue composed of columnar epithelium.

pregnancy is associated with normal physiologic mucorrhea, although an abnormal increase in mucous discharge may be indicative of cervical changes associated with the onset of labor.

Vagina

Changes similar to those that occur in the cervix during pregnancy also occur in the vagina. The increase in vascularity produces a characteristic bluish-purple color of the vaginal mucosa (Chadwick's sign). Estrogen-induced changes result in thickening of the mucus, loosening of the connective tissue, and hypertrophy of the smooth muscle cells. These changes cause an increase in the length of the vaginal wall and the perineal body to permit passage of the infant. Rugae, or folds of the vaginal mucosa, are prominent in nulliparous women but become less prominent with subsequent deliveries.

The vaginal flora consists of numerous leukocytes, no red blood cells, and a mixed bacterial colonization, with lactobacilli predominating. Vaginal secretions may contain bacteria, parasites, or neoplastic cells from the lower or upper genital tract. Leukorrhea is common during pregnancy. The discharge is normally thick and white, with an acid pH varying from 3.5 to 6, which serves to inhibit pathogenic colonization in the vagina. The pH is conducive to the growth of yeast organisms, and monilial vaginitis is a common vaginal infection during pregnancy.

The increased vascularity within the vagina and pelvic viscera results in an increased sensitivity and may heighten sexual interest and arousal during the second trimester. It is not unusual for spontaneous orgasm to occur. Also, some women may experience multiple orgasms for the first time due to the increased congestion, which results in a resolution period that is less complete.

Breasts

During pregnancy, breast changes are noted soon after the first missed menstrual period (see Fig. 10–2). After the second missed period, many women experience breast fullness, tenderness, and tingling. High estrogen and progesterone levels induce hypertrophy of the mammary alveoli. The breasts increase in size and become nodular. By the end of the 2nd month, characteristic changes occur in the nipple. The pigmentation darkens and the nipple becomes larger and more erectile. Montgomery's glands (hypertrophic sebaceous glands) become prominent within the primary areola. Venous congestion occurs in the breasts, especially in nulliparous women. A thick, yellowish fluid may appear after the 10th week of gestation and may be expressed with gentle massage. This secretion, called *colostrum*, thickens as pregnancy nears term. The breasts also increase in

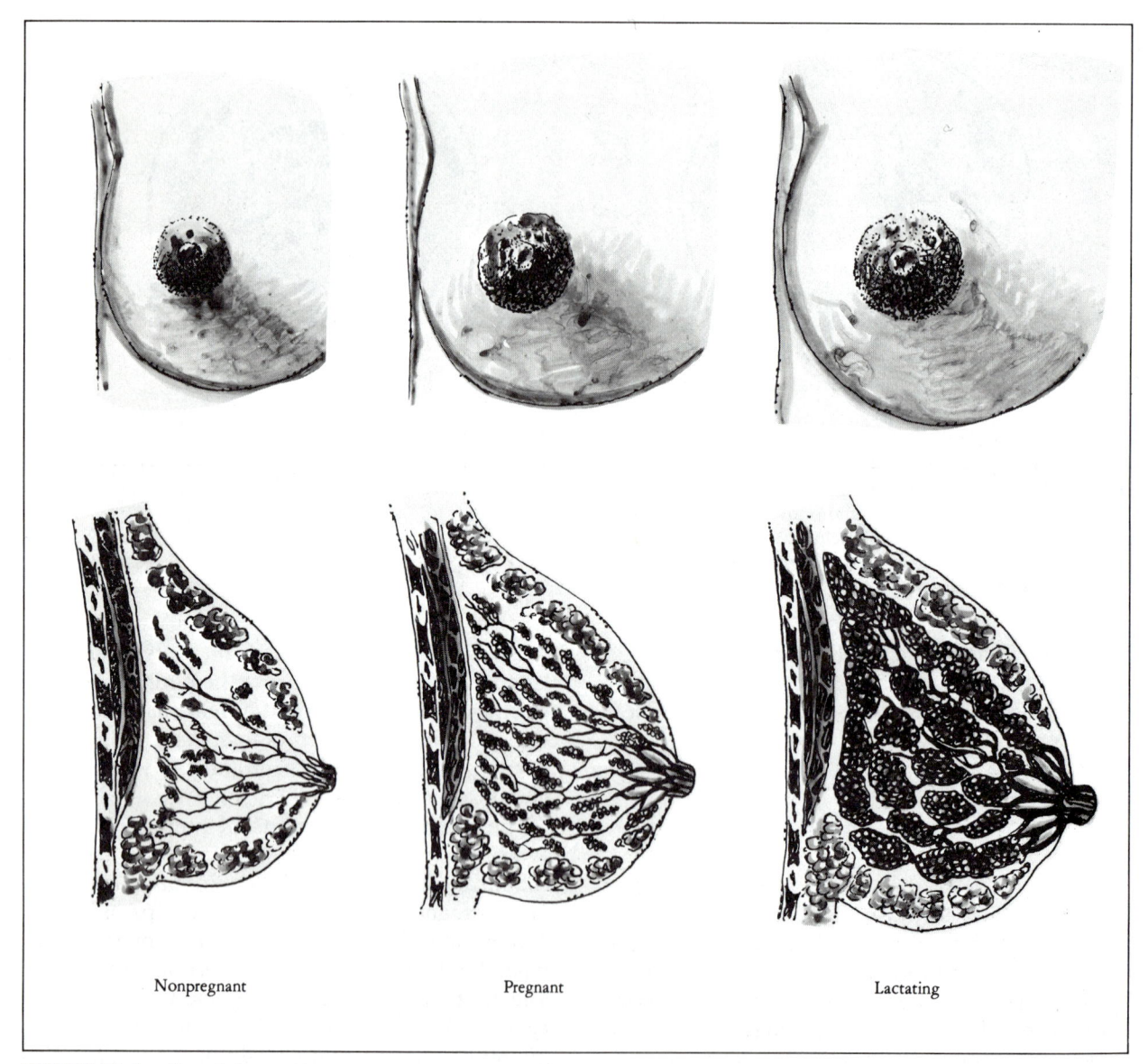

FIGURE 10–2. Breast changes in pregnancy.

size, and striae similar to those found on the distended abdomen may appear.

Perineum

The external structures of the perineum enlarge as a result of increased vasocongestion, increased vasculature, hypertrophy of the perineal body, and the fat deposition that occurs during pregnancy. The labia majora draw close together, covering the introitus in nulliparous women; after delivery, the labia majora separate again. Increased pelvic congestion, relaxation of the smooth muscle of the veins, the increasing pressure of the growing fetus, constipation, and obesity may cause varicosities of the perineum and rectum.

CHANGES IN THE CARDIOVASCULAR SYSTEM

During pregnancy, as the size of the uterus increases, the heart is slightly displaced upward and to the left, while at the same time it rotates slightly on its long axis. Slight cardiac enlargement and systolic murmurs may be normal during pregnancy.

Heart

As pregnancy progresses, the enlarging uterus displaces the heart upward and to the left, rotated slightly on its long axis. The apex of the heart is moved laterally from its position in the prepregnant state and the cardiac silhouette will appear enlarged. The extent of these changes will be dependent on the size of the uterus, strength of the abdominal muscles, and position of the abdomen and thorax. The cardiac volume increases by about 75 ml, or approximately 10 percent, as the pregnancy proceeds to term.

During pregnancy, cardiac sounds may be altered:

1. *Heart sounds.* An exaggerated splitting of the first heart sound is heard with increased loudness of both components. There are no definite changes in the second heart sound. There is a loud, easily heard third heart sound.
2. *Heart murmurs.* Systolic murmurs appear in 90 percent of pregnant women, disappearing after delivery. A soft, transient diastolic murmur is heard in 19 percent of pregnant women.

No changes are characteristically found on an electrocardiogram other than a slight deviation of the electrical axis to the left as a result of the change in the cardiac position during pregnancy.

Changes in Blood Pressure and Volume

Resting maternal pulse is approximately 10–15 beats/minute faster throughout pregnancy, returning to the normal prepregnancy rate after delivery. Blood pressure changes often occur during pregnancy, with a second trimester drop and then a rise closer to term. Any sustained increase of 30 mm Hg systolic or 15 mm Hg diastolic, after 20 weeks of gestation, may be indicative of pathology, which may result in the development of preeclampsia. Maternal position may significantly affect blood pressure. Supine hypotension may occur from pressure exerted on the vena cava by the gravid uterus. The left lateral recumbent position is optimal for maternal–fetal exchange and cardiac output during pregnancy. Blood pressure in the brachial artery is highest when sitting, lowest in the left lateral position, and intermediate in the supine position. Venous blood pressure does not change in the arms, but a steady and rather marked increase occurs in the legs. Blood flow in the legs is retarded during pregnancy, except in the left lateral recumbent position. This increase in venous pressure in the lower extremities accounts for *dependent edema*, which commonly occurs late in pregnancy. Development of hemorrhoids and of varicose veins in the legs and vulva is common during gestation.

Maternal cardiac output increases significantly during the first trimester and remains elevated during the second and third trimesters. The blood volume increases by 40–50 percent, reaching its peak at 30–32 weeks of gestation (Callander et al., 1974). This increase may be even greater in multiple pregnancies. The increased plasma volume supplies the hypertrophied vascular system that maintains the pregnancy and serves as a safeguard against excessive blood loss during delivery.

CHANGES IN THE RESPIRATORY SYSTEM

During pregnancy there is an accelerated production of red blood cells (RBC). The amount of increase depends on the amount of iron available. Because a large amount of iron is needed to maintain the pregnancy, iron supplementation is necessary. The pregnant woman requires 18–21 mg of iron each day. It is difficult to obtain this iron level through diet alone. Therefore, an oral supplement of 30–60 mg of iron is usually necessary to maintain hemoglobin levels in normal pregnancy. Although the number of RBC increases, the erythrocyte count will decrease because of physiologic hemodilution. The hematocrit (42% ± 5%) and hemoglobin (12–16 g/dl) values decline, resulting in the "pseudoanemia" of pregnancy. This decline is commonly seen during the second trimester, when the rapid expansion in blood volume occurs.

Leukocyte production increases during pregnancy. The white blood cell (WBC) count rises despite the increase in plasma volume. The average count is 10,000–11,000 WBC/mm^3, increasing dramatically in labor and the early postpartum period to as high as 25,000 WBC/mm^3.

Total plasma protein decreases during pregnancy to 3–3.5 g/dl (the normal level is 4–4.5 g/dl). This decrease is largely a result of the fall in albumin concentration. The decrease in plasma proteins produces an increase in the sedimentation rate (0–20 mm/hour).

The plasma fibrin level is increased as much as 40 percent at term, and the fibrinogen level increases approximately 50 percent (Pritchard, MacDonald, and Gant, 1985). The clotting time during pregnancy remains equal to nonpregnant clotting time (5–15 min) (Pritchard, MacDonald, and Gant, 1985; Byrne et al., 1981).

The body's physiologic adaptation to pregnancy is a response not only to support the growing pregnancy, but to reduce risks associated with the pregnancy. (See Table 10–3 for hematologic changes during pregnancy.)

During pregnancy both mechanical and biochemical changes may affect maternal respiratory function and gas exchange. Progressive enlargement of the uterus elevates the level of the diaphragm by approximately 4 cm. The thoracic cage increases in diameter and circumference to accomodate the lungs, although not enough to prevent a reduction in the residual volume created by the elevation of the diaphragm. Alterations in respiratory function are apparent between 20 and 24 weeks of gestation.

Respiratory rate, maximum breathing capacity, and vital capacity seem to be unchanged. However, oxygen consumption is greater, because the increase in circulating hemoglobin results in increased total oxygen carrying capacity. The tidal volume, minute ventilatory volume, and minute oxygen uptake increase as pregnancy advances.

The increase in the minute ventilatory volume is presumably caused by the stimulatory effect of progesterone. This hyperventilation produces a mild respiratory alkalosis. Metabolic compensation by renal excretion of bicarbonate partially offsets the expected pH change. The result is a slightly alkalotic pH in the arterial blood.

TABLE 10–3. *Hematologic Changes During Pregnancy*

Test	Nonpregnant Value	Pregnant Value
Hematocrit (average)	41.7	37
Hemoglobin	12–16 g/dl	>10 g/dl
Red blood cells (RBC) volume	1355 ml	1790 ml
White blood cells (WBC)	5000–10,000/μl	5000–12,000/μl 25,000/μl during labor
Plasma protein	4.0–4.5 g/dl	3.0–3.5 g/dl
Fibrinogen	200–400 mg/dl	300–600 mg/dl
Platelets	150,000–400,000/μl	150,000–400,000/μl

SOURCES: Pritchard, MacDonald, and Gant (1985); Byrne et al. (1981).

TABLE 10-4. Effects of Pregnancy on the Respiratory System

No Change	Increase	Decrease
Respiratory rate	Tidal volume	Functional residual capacity
Maximum breathing capacity	Minute ventilatory volume	Residual volume
Vital capacity	Minute O_2 uptake Arterial pO_2 Gradient between alveolar and arterial pO_2	Arterial pO_2

After the 24th week, thoracic breathing replaces abdominal breathing. Toward the end of pregnancy, many women experience slight dyspnea due to the pressure on the diaphragm (see Table 10-4).

CHANGES IN THE RENAL SYSTEM

During pregnancy, marked changes in structure and function occur in the kidney, ureters, and bladder. Changes in renal structure result from the activity of estrogen and progesterone, pressure from the gravid uterus, and an increase in blood volume. There is general dilation of the renal collecting system, which produces the physiologic hydronephrosis of pregnancy. The ureters elongate and become tortuous, with the right ureter tending to dilate more than the left late in pregnancy, perhaps because of obstruction by the enlarged uterus. The renal pelvis enlarges, probably due to the increase in renal vascular volume and blood flow occurring during pregnancy. Urinary stasis and vesicoureteral reflux occur as a result of the pressure of the gravid uterus on the pelvic brim. The increased urinary tract volume is probably the major cause of increased incidence of acute pyelonephritis with asymptomatic bacteriuria.

Increased urinary frequency occurs early in pregnancy until the uterus grows above the pelvis into the abdomen. It occurs again in late pregnancy as the gravid uterus descends into the pelvis once more. Pelvic congestion in pregnancy results in hyperemia of the urethra and the bladder. The bladder is pulled up out of the true pelvis by the growing uterus, and the urethra elongates. The bladder is susceptible to trauma and hemorrhage because of its increased vascularity. Bladder tone is decreased with an increased capacity of 1300-1500 ml. Overdistention and retention of urine is common in the postdelivery period.

Renal function changes during pregnancy as a result of hormonal activity, blood volume increases, and maternal posture and physical activity. The following changes in renal function are seen:

1. The glomerular filtration rate (GFR) increases as much as 50 percent by the second trimester, and this increase persists until term.
2. Renal plasma flow (RPF) increases in early pregnancy and then decreases in the third trimester, returning to nonpregnant values.
3. The increase in the GFR and the RPF induce changes in laboratory values and renal function tests. The results of the following tests might indicate a pathologic process in pregnancy, while indicating normal renal function in the nonpregnant state.
    a. *Creatinine clearance.* This is the most useful test of urinary function during pregnancy provided urine is collected accurately over the specified period of time. During the day, pregnant women tend to accumulate water in the form of dependent edema. At night, while in the recumbent position, the fluid is mobilized and excreted via the kidney.
    b. *Glucose.* Glucosuria is common during pregnancy due to the increase in glomerular filtration together with impaired tubular reabsorption capacity for filtering glucose. It is advisable to screen all pregnant women for glucose intolerance, because pregnancy is a diabetogenic state.
    c. *Protein.* Proteinuria may occur in women who have *orthostatic proteinuria* (proteinuria

only when erect). Protein should not exceed 300 mg/l in a 24-hour urine collection.

CHANGES IN THE DIGESTIVE SYSTEM

Several common discomforts in pregnancy are associated with physiologic changes in the gastrointestinal system.

Stomach, Esophagus, and Intestine

Nausea and vomiting, which occur primarily during the first trimester, may be in response to the secretion of HCG. Metabolic changes that affect carbohydrate metabolism, the presence of hepatitis, dehydration, or particular tastes or odors may also induce nausea or vomiting. Persistent vomiting beyond the first trimester or excessive vomiting at any time is termed *hyperemesis gravidarum*. It may be associated with emotional disorders as well as physical changes.

The influence of progesterone induces relaxation of the smooth muscle of the intestine, causing decreased motility. The rate of gastric emptying is decreased, esophageal regurgitation produces heartburn (pyrosis), and bloating and constipation result. Later in pregnancy the growing uterus displaces the stomach and intestines, resulting in positional changes in the viscrea. Herniation of the upper portion of the stomach may occur as a result of its upward displacement, causing a widening of the hiatus of the diaphragm. Hemorrhoids may also appear because of the pressure of the gravid uterus on the lower intestine.

Mouth and Teeth

The gums may become hyperemic, soft, and swollen during pregnancy. Mild trauma, even from brushing the teeth, may induce bleeding. High estrogen levels increase vascularity and induce connective tissue proliferation. There is no increase in saliva production, although ptylism may result from a decrease in unconscious swallowing associated with nausea. Pregnancy *epulides* (small, benign vascular lesions) may develop, but these regress spontaneously after pregnancy.

No significant changes occur in the teeth during pregnancy. Demineralization does not occur, and dental caries result only from poor hygiene.

Liver

During pregnancy minor changes occur in liver function. High levels of estrogen and progesterone produce symptoms of suppression of bile flow (cholestasis) and itching (pruritus gravidarum), with or without jaundice. These symptoms disappear after delivery.

CHANGES IN THE MUSCULOSKELETAL SYSTEM

The increase in weight and the shift in center of gravity during pregnancy cause marked changes in posture, balance, and walking. Progressive lordosis is characteristic of normal pregnancy. As the uterus extends anteriorly, the body compensates by increasing the lumbosacral curve, which shifts the center of gravity to the lower extremities. A compensatory curvature of the cervicodorsal region is required to maintain balance. A waddling gait is typical in pregnancy. A great amount of stress is put upon the ligaments and muscles of the middle and lower back and spine, causing backache and discomfort, especially during the third trimester. Aching, numbness, and tingling are occasionally felt in the upper extremities, presumably caused by anterior slumping of the neck and flexion of the shoulder girdle, which exerts traction on the ulnar and median nerves.

High levels of circulating hormones (steroid sex hormones and relaxin) and the increased elasticity of connective and collagen tissue cause relaxation and hypermobility of the pelvic joints during pregnancy. Separation of the symphysis pubis can occur, causing instability of the sacroiliac joint. Women experience increased difficulty in walking and may experience pain, which is exaggerated by obesity and multiple pregnancy.

Research has maintained that a calcium-poor diet will result in decalcification of the bone, while no change occurs in the teeth. Requirements for calcium and phosphorus are approximately 1.2 g/day. This is about 0.4 g/day above the needs in the nonpregnant state. A well-balanced diet is adequate to provide these essential elements.

CHANGES IN SKIN AND ASSOCIATED STRUCTURES

Significant changes occur in the skin during pregnancy.

Pigmentation

Hyperpigmentation is a commonly recognized sign of pregnancy. Estrogen and progesterone are primarily responsible for this change. The degree of change often depends on skin type. Fair-complexioned women will experience less pronounced changes than women with darker complexions. Generalized pigmentation changes may develop, but more commonly, localized areas of hyperpigmentation are seen on the nipples and areolae, umbilicus, linea alba (which becomes the linea nigra), axillas, and vulva and perineum. The mask of pregnancy, originally referred to as chloasma but now termed melasma, is a splotchy and irregular melanin hyperpigmentation that characteristically develops on the forehead, cheeks, temples, and upper lip. Preexisting pigmented moles (nevi) and freckles often darken during pregnancy. Some nevi may increase in size, and new nevi may appear. After pregnancy nevi usually regress.

Hair

An increase in hair growth during pregnancy is rare. When it has been observed, it has been associated with signs of virilization. Postpartum hair loss is very common. The cause is not known, but it is believed to be due to hormonal changes.

Connective Tissue

Striae gravidarum (stretch marks) commonly develop during pregnancy. They appear chiefly on the lower abdomen and the breasts. Initially, they are pinkish purple, later becoming white. They never disappear completely and leave depressed, irregular bands in the skin. Striae formation is related to skin stretching and the fragility of cutaneous elastic tissues associated with adrenocorticoid hyperactivity.

Blood Vessels of the Skin

During pregnancy, there is an increase in vascular permeability and proliferation brought about by progesterone. Local venous congestion occurs in the mucosa of the vestibule and vagina (an early sign of pregnancy). Edema, not associated with toxemia, is evident in nondependent areas. Arteriolar proliferation results in the formation of spider angiomas. Erythema (redness) occurs on the palms. Bright red elevations of the skin (*spider nevi*) may develop on the chest, neck, face, arms, and legs. Capillary hemangiomas may occur on the head and neck but are considered unusual below these areas. Small hemangiomas have been observed on the tongue, upper lip, and eyelid. The hemangiomas become smaller after delivery but do not recede completely.

Pregnancy may aggravate or improve skin problems. Often pregnancy imposes an unpredictable course on dermatologic disorders.

METABOLIC CHANGES

The demands of pregnancy result in a hypermetabolic state that ensures adequate growth and development of the fetus. The expectant mother must meet her own nutritional needs as well as those of the conceptus.

Weight Gain

Weight gain is probably one of the most often discussed topics in pregnancy. It is difficult to say how much weight should be gained. It may depend on the woman's weight and nutritional reserves at the time of conception. An average weight gain during pregnancy is about 25–30 lb (see Chapter 12).

Protein Metabolism

Protein demands increase during pregnancy. At term the fetus and placenta account for approximately 50 percent of the total increase in protein induced by pregnancy. The remainder is found in the uterus, breasts, and maternal blood in the form of hemoglobin and plasma proteins. Although plasma protein increases, the concentration of several plasma proteins decreases because of pregnancy-induced hemodilution.

Carbohydrate Metabolism

Carbohydrate needs are considerably increased. The fuel requirements of the growing fetus are met primarily by glucose, especially during the second half of pregnancy. Pregnancy is a diabetogenic state in which placental hormones function as insulin antagonists, rendering an increase in the availability of circulating glucose to be utilized by the mother and the fetus. Because of the increased glomerular filtration rate, small amounts of glucose may be excreted in the urine. A preexisting diabetic state can be significantly complicated by pregnancy, resulting in hyperglycemia and ketoacidosis.

Lactose is excreted in the urine late in pregnancy in association with breast development in preparation for lactation. Lactose can be distinguished from glucose in the urine—Dextrostix will identify glucose, but not lactose.

Fat Metabolism

Plasma lipids—including total lipids, cholesterol, phospholipids, neutral fat, lipoproteins, and amino acids—increase during the second half of pregnancy. Only a moderate amount of this lipid increase is laid down as fat stores. In pregnancy, starvation will cause ketosis because of the fast utilization of glucose and the resultant burning of fat for energy. The high blood levels and increased deposition of fat result partly from increased intake and partly from increased conversion of glucose to fat. Later in pregnancy, fat stores decrease with the increased nutritional needs of the fetus.

Mineral Metabolism

Requirements for iron increase considerably during pregnancy. About 1000 mg of elemental iron is needed for adequate maternal blood cell mass, hemoglobin synthesis, and increased tissue demands. Dietary intake is not adequate to meet the need for iron and, therefore, oral supplementation is necessary. The mother requires about 18 mg of iron each day. Iron transfer across the placenta goes only toward the fetus. Iron stores in the fetal liver will provide support during the first months of neonatal life until iron intake is adequate.

Daily requirements of 1.2 g of calcium and 1.2 g of phosphorus are met through a well-balanced diet in pregnancy. Circulating calcium and magnesium are slightly decreased because the lowered plasma protein concentration results in decreased binding capacity. Serum phosphorus levels remain within the nonpregnant range.

Water Metabolism

Pregnancy requires an increase in water to supply the fetus, placenta, amniotic fluid, and expanded maternal blood volume. At least 6.5 l of extra water is retained during a normal pregnancy. Fluid retention is due in part to increases in the adrenocorticosteroids, increased tubular reabsorption, retention of sodium, and circulatory stasis in the lower extremities.

Pitting edema, especially in the lower extremities, is a discomfort common in pregnancy. Unless associated with hypertension and proteinuria, edema has no adverse effect upon pregnancy. The use of diuretics is contraindicated and may result in dehydration, hyponatremia, or thromboembolism in the woman and electrolyte imbalance in the fetus.

CHANGES IN THE ENDOCRINE SYSTEM

Pituitary Gland

Estrogen causes slight enlargements of the anterior lobe of the pituitary gland during pregnancy. In isolated cases, this enlargement may be sufficient to compromise the optic chiasma and reduce the visual fields. Visual impairment subsides after delivery as the size of the gland return to normal.

The hormonal influence of the pituitary is necessary for pregnancy to occur, but the maternal pituitary is not essential for the maintenance of pregnancy. The anterior pituitary continues to produce the tropic hormones during pregnancy, but the amounts differ only slightly if at all from those produced in the nonpregnant state. Follicle-stimulating hormone (FSH), secreted by the anterior pituitary, stimulates growth of ova. FSH levels then fall to become clinically undetectable by the 10th day after ovulation and remain at these levels throughout pregnancy. Luteinizing hormone stimulates ovulation, and then LH levels fall in response to high levels of estrogen and progesterone. Suppression of the anterior pituitary seems to be caused by an increase in HCG, the concentration of which rises sharply about 10 days after ovulation and remains elevated until midpregnancy, when levels begin to fall. Levels of thyrotropin and adrenotropin, hormones that alter maternal metabolism, may increase slightly, while gonadotropin concentration is decreased. Melanotropic hormone production is increased and is responsible for the added pigmentation in pregnancy. Production of pituitary somatomammotropin (growth hormone) is suppressed. Production of prolactin, responsible for initiation of lactation, is increased and is maintained throughout lactation.

Oxytocin and vasopressin are secreted by the posterior pituitary. Oxytocin is responsible for initiation of uterine contractions and the stimulation of milk ejection from the breasts. Vasopressin causes vasoconstriction that results in increased blood pressure. It also has an antidiuretic effect and therefore plays a role in fluid balance. Vasopressin secretion is regulated by changes in plasma osmolarity and blood volume.

Prolactin is found in concentrations five times greater in pregnancy than in the nonpregnant state. The action of prolactin in mediating lactalbumin synthesis is inhibited during pregnancy by progesterone. Following delivery, with the removal of the influence of progesterone, lactation may proceed.

Thyroid Gland

Pregnancy induces a moderate enlargement of the thyroid, caused by hyperplasia of the glandular tissue and increased vascularity. The result is an increase in the rate of iodine metabolism. In pregnancy, the basal metabolic rate (BMR) increases as much as 25 percent at term. Most of this increase is the result of greater oxygen consumption, needed to support the metabolic activity of the mother and the fetus.

In pregnancy, elevated circulating thyroid hormone values are not indicative of a hyperthyroid state. The thyroxine-binding proteins of plasma, principally an alpha globulin, are increased, resulting in a greater iron binding capacity. This can be measured as increased protein-bound iodine (PBI) and butanol-extractable iodine (BET) in the plasma. The increase in circulating estrogen seems to be the major cause for changes in circulating levels of thyroid hormones and binding capacity. An elevated plasma thyroxine level and a lowered triiodothyronine (T_3) uptake are indicative of a high estrogen state. The level of unbound thyroxine, the true index of general metabolism, is relatively unchanged. In a normal pregnancy the thyroid continues to function normally.

Parathyroid Gland

Increased levels of the parathyroid hormone are observed. Parathyroid hormone increases plasma calcium (Ca^{2+}) as well as the formation of 1,25-dehydroxycholecalciferol, the physiologically active metabolite of vitamin D. As the need for calcium and vitamin D increases, the plasma level of parathyroid hormone is elevated. Tetany, due to calcium deficiency or phosphorus excess, is indicative of hypoparathyroidism. Hypocalcemia may play a role in the onset of preterm labor.

Adrenal Glands

In pregnancy there is slight hypertrophy of the adrenal cortex, but little change occurs in adrenal function. There is an increase in the concentration of circulating cortisol, but much of it is bound, resulting in only a slight elevation in free cortisol. Aldosterone secretion increases during pregnancy to protect against the natriuric effect (increases in the rate of secretion of sodium in the urine) of progesterone. The adrenal medulla shows no significant change in structure or function during pregnancy.

Pancreas

Early in pregnancy the hyperplastic islets of Langerhans increase insulin production. Placental hormones with insulin antagonists cause decreased tissue sensitivity to insulin, but glucose levels rise only slightly.

Glucose metabolism changes during pregnancy because of a lowered renal threshold, an augmented glomerular filtration rate (GFR), and reduced tubular reabsorption of glucose. Glycogen storage is decreased because of the need for circulating glucose for fuel. Women with a marginal pancreatic reserve may develop glucose intolerance or true diabetes during pregnancy.

CHANGES IN THE IMMUNOLOGIC SYSTEM

The developing fetoplacental unit within the maternal uterus is technically considered an allograft, a graft between two individuals of the same species but of different genotype. The tolerance of the allograft of pregnancy has generated theoretical speculation about the basic immune suppression mechanism involved. Proposed theories of the factors responsible for the acceptance of the pregnancy are listed here, along with the evidence against those theories.

1. *The fetoplacental unit lacks antigenic capabilities.* This theory must be discounted, because investigation has proven both that the embryonic

tissue is antigenic and that the fetus is capable of mounting an immunologic response to antigenic stimuli as early as the first trimester.
2. *The uterus is a privileged immunologic site, resistant to the normal rejection process.* This has not been substantiated. The fetus is able to develop without rejection outside the maternal uterus, as is seen in ectopic pregnancies.
3. *The maternal organism cannot generate immunologic rejection during pregnancy.* No differences in immunologic competence between pregnant and nonpregnant women have been found. During pregnancy, most antibodies evoke a host response.
4. *Barriers between fetal and maternal surfaces decrease antigenicity of the trophoblast.* The placental barrier is permeable in both directions.
5. *Nonrejection is mediated by an immunoglobulin acting as a serum-blocking factor.* This in not conclusive.

Viral and bacterial infections in pregnancy are associated with a higher incidence of morbidity and mortality than occurs in the nonpregnant state. A contributing factor may be the physiologic changes pregnancy induces in structure and function of various systems. For example, respiratory and urinary tract infections are more common during pregnancy. Changes in the body's defense mechanisms normally occur in response to pregnancy.

Resistance to infection encompasses a variety of components. Initially, the invading organism encounters some barrier during its entry; next, it comes in contact with nonspecific defenses; and finally it activates the host's immune system.

Both nonspecific defenses and the immune response may be classified as cellular or humoral. The activated T-cell lymphocyte is the principal effector in cell-mediated immunity, while humoral immunity results from the production of *antibodies* by the plasma cells. Antibodies belong to one of five classes of immunoglobulins. However, only three of these classes have any apparent role in antimicrobial immunity:

1. *IgG:* Most abundant of the antibodies; active in the serum and interstitial fluid; crosses the placenta.
2. *IgM:* A large molecule; will not pass into extravascular fluid or cross the placenta; remains in the serum.
3. *IgA:* Dominant antibody in secretions of the body's external and internal surfaces; found in breast milk or colostrum.

The *complement system* is a group of nine separate proteins that act sequentially to produce a biologic effect that helps with the removal of the pathogen. The various components of the immunologic system operate synergistically to produce this antimicrobial effect.

During pregnancy, maternal IgG is decreased due to placental transport. IgM and IgA levels do not change significantly, but complement activity increases.

Cellular immune response is decreased in pregnancy, resulting in high maternal susceptibility to viral infections. The total white blood cell count increases, but T-cell activity declines, reflecting depressed cellular immunity.

Physical barriers are important during pregnancy. The vaginal epithelium, cervix, and mucous plug obstruct ascending microorganisms from entering the uterine cavity. The fetal membranes represent an additional barrier, although bacterial infection can occur through intact membranes. Amniotic fluid also serves an antimicrobial function. When these barriers are gone, the uterus provides an ideal environment for bacterial proliferation.

MINOR DISCOMFORTS OF PREGNANCY

Along with the observable physiologic changes that occur during pregnancy come the minor discomforts often associated with these changes. As nurses, we provide not only physical care, but also emotional care. This chapter has provided an introduction to the "normal" changes in pregnancy, as a basis for distinguishing them from the abnormal. Physical change leads to an array of emotional reactions in all women during pregnancy. Every nurse working with maternity patients must be aware, sensitive, responsive, and supportive during this period of physical and emotional change. Table 10–5 summarizes the discomforts of pregnancy, their diagnosis, physiology, associated complications, and relief measures.

SUMMARY

Pregnancy imposes dramatic physiologic changes upon a woman's body. A thorough understanding of the normal events that promote change in pregnancy is essential as a basis for providing

Text continued on page 217

TABLE 10-5. Minor Discomforts of Pregnancy

Discomfort	Differential Diagnosis	Physiology	Associated Complications	Relief Measures
Nausea and vomiting—"morning sickness" occurs in 50%–60% of all pregnancies; often subsides after first trimester; may occur at any time during the day.	Gastrointestinal problems; gastritis; cholecystitis; pancreatitis; hiatal hernia; Meniere's disease	Gastrointestinal system: may be due to hormonal influence (possible HCG); may be associated with psychologic factors, especially if it continues beyond the first trimester	Dehydration; electrolyte imbalance; malnutrition; weight loss; ketosis; intrauterine growth retardation	Small, frequent feedings; avoid offensive odors of foods; avoid empty stomach; maintain good posture; eat dry carbohydrate foods; good oral hygiene; consult physician for intractable vomiting
Heartburn or acid indigestion	Hiatal hernia; toxemia; esophageal reflux; peptic ulcer	Gastrointestinal system: progesterone induces slowing of peristalsis, digestion, motility, and relaxation of the cardiac sphincter and delay in emptying time of the stomach; regurgitation into the esophagus; upward pressure by the enlarging uterus decreases capacity	Nausea and vomiting; decreased appetite; constipation (may be caused by antacids); changes in electrolyte absorption	Milk; chewing gum; antacids (do not use baking soda or Alka-Seltzer because of high salt content)
Ptylism (excessive salivation)	Drug stimulation; oral pathology; 7th cranial nerve damage; rabies	Gastrointestinal system: may be due to elevated estrogen levels; stimulation of the salivary glands by the ingestion of starch	Decreased nutritional intake; loss of fluids and electrolytes	Belladonna extract; chewing gum; mints; good mouth care; decreased starchy foods
Gingivitis and epulides (hyperemia, hypertrophy, bleeding, tenderness)	Gum disease	Gastrointestinal system: estrogen influences increased vascularity and proliferation of connective tissue	Dietary insufficiency; trauma to gums; infection	Gentle brushing; good mouth care

(continued)

TABLE 10–5. *Minor Discomforts of Pregnancy (continued)*

Discomfort	Differential Diagnosis	Physiology	Associated Complications	Relief Measures
Food cravings	Pica	Gastrointestinal system: cause probably culturally influenced	Dietary insufficiency	Discussion of folklore and beliefs; nutrition counseling; satisfaction of cravings while maintaining a balanced diet; report pica (cravings for strange foods, often not edible: laundry starch, clay, dirt) to physician
Constipation	GI obstruction; ileus; spastic colon; cancer of the colon; depression; myxedema	Gastrointestinal system: progesterone influence decreases motility; increased reabsorption of water and drying of stools; iron intake increases constipation; intestines are compressed by the growing uterus	Hemorrhoids; headaches; fatigue	Fluid intake (6 glasses of water per day); roughage in diet (bran, whole grains, vegetables, fruits); stool softeners or laxatives with consent of physician; moderate exercise
Hemorrhoids	Anal polyps; fissures	Gastrointestinal system: relaxation of the smooth muscle wall of the vessels; pressure of the gravid uterus and the presenting part; bearing down for bowel movements or during labor	Pain; constipation; bleeding; iron deficiency	Lying down on side to reduce pressure; avoiding constipation by increasing fluid intake; sitz bath; witch hazel compresses
Flatulence	Viral gastrointestinal enteritis; food intolerance; colitis	Gastrointestinal system: decreased tone and emptying time of the bowel; compression of the bowel by the gravid uterus	Constipation; abdominal pain	Avoiding gas-forming foods; bulk in diet; chewing slowly; small, frequent meals; exercise

TABLE 10-5. Minor Discomforts of Pregnancy (continued)

Discomfort	Differential Diagnosis	Physiology	Associated Complications	Relief Measures
Increased urinary frequency	Urinary tract infection; diabetes mellitus or insipidus; excessive use of coffee or tea	Renal system: vascular engorgement of the renal pelvis and altered bladder function due to hormonal influence; weight of the uterus decreases bladder capacity; presenting part applies pressure on the bladder	Insomnia; stress incontinence; hematuria	Limiting fluid before bedtime; consult physician for hematuria or burning sensation
Varicosities—may be in the legs, vulva, or perianal area	Thrombophlebitis; phlebitis; trauma	Cardiovascular system: relaxation of the walls of the blood vessels; pressure of the gravid uterus; pooling in the lower extremities; hereditary predisposition	Leg pain; edema; ulcers; orthostatic hypotension; faintness on standing if extensive	Avoiding long periods of standing or sitting; elevation of legs; rest periods; nonrestrictive clothing; exercise; weight control
Pedal edema	Toxemia; cellulitis; varicosities; renal problems; trauma	Cardiovascular system: decrease in venous return (posture aggravated); sodium retention; fluid retention	Discomfort	Avoiding standing for long periods; elevating feet; rest periods; support stockings
Dizziness	Hypotension; hypoglycemia; central nervous system damage; alcohol use	Cardiovascular system: postural hypotension due to hormonal influence; venous stasis in lower extremities later in pregnancy	Fainting; trauma; fetal distress if hypotension persists	Avoiding the following: standing for long periods, crowded rooms, warm areas, sudden changes in position, and hypoglycemia; moderate exercise; deep breathing; cool environment

(continued)

TABLE 10–5. Minor Discomforts of Pregnancy (continued)

Discomfort	Differential Diagnosis	Physiology	Associated Complications	Relief Measures
Supine hypotension	Severe hypotension; central nervous system damage; alcohol use	Cardiovascular system: compression of the vena cava by the weight of the gravid uterus when supine	Uteroplacental insufficiency; fetal distress; maternal and fetal hypoxia	Side-lying position (preferably left side); semi-Fowler's position with knees bent
Backache; joint pain; hypermotility of joints	Urinary tract infection; sciatica; referred gastrointestinal pain; disk problems; acute muscle strain; labor	Musculoskeletal system: exaggerated lumbar and cervicothoracic curve due to the shift in center of gravity as the uterus enlarges; relaxation of symphyseal and sacroiliac joints due to hormonal influence	Back strain; pain; difficulty walking or sitting; loss of balance	Good posture; back exercises; rest; heat to back; back rubs; using good body mechanics; firm mattress
Leg cramps	Thrombophlebitis; leg strain; cellulitis	Musculoskeletal system: pressure of the enlarged uterus compresses the nerves extending to the lower extremities; decrease in level of diffusable serum calcium or an increase in serum phosphorus	Tingling; numbness; loss of balance due to sensation changes	Dorsiflexing foot; avoiding pointing toes when stretching legs or lying in a prone position; avoiding excessive dietary intake of phosphorus in milk, cheese, or meat; increasing calcium intake (vitamin D may aid in the absorption of calcium)
Round ligament pain	Ectopic pregnancy; appendicitis; endometriosis; ovarian cyst; pelvic inflammatory disease (PID)	Musculoskeletal system: uterine enlargement causes stretching of ligaments	Dyspareunia; restricted mobility; insomnia	Exercise; adequate rest; pillow support for the abdomen; avoiding jerky movements; using good body mechanics

TABLE 10–5. Minor Discomforts of Pregnancy (continued)

Discomfort	Differential Diagnosis	Physiology	Associated Complications	Relief Measures
Dyspnea	Chronic lung disease; pulmonary emboli; pneumonia	Respiratory system: pressure from growing uterus limits expansion of lung; hormonal influence alters respiratory capabilities; hyperventilation occurs during pregnancy	Fatigue; restlessness; excessive hyperventilation; dizziness; fainting; insomnia	Semi-Fowler's position; elevation of head and shoulders on pillows when lying down; breathing techniques (deep chest breathing with arms elevated over head); good posture; avoiding overeating
Nasal stuffiness	Sinusitis; chronic infection	Respiratory system: increased vascularity induced by hormones	Chronic irritation; nose bleeding; insomnia	Reassurance that it will regress after pregnancy; sleeping with extra pillows
Headaches	Toxemia; hypertension; central nervous system damage; migraine headaches; eye disturbances	Neurologic system: tension; eyestrain; vascular engorgement; vasodilation; sinus congestion	Depression; insomnia	Rest periods; relaxation techniques; adequate nutrition
Mood swings	Psychologic disturbances; depression; metabolic imbalances	Neurologic system: physiologic changes in pregnancy; physiologic and metabolic changes; change in lifestyle; new priorities and responsibilities; ambivalent feelings toward pregnancy	Depression; resentment toward pregnancy	Open communication; reassurance; emotional support for both partners; adequate rest; adequate nutrition, supportive services
Periodic numbness or tingling in the arms or fingers	Nerve damage; trauma	Neurologic system: postural changes causing drooping of shoulders produces brachial plexus traction syndrome	Loss of movement; dropping objects	Good posture; back exercises; supportive bra; reassurance that discomfort will resolve after pregnancy

(continued)

TABLE 10-5. Minor Discomforts of Pregnancy (continued)

Discomfort	Differential Diagnosis	Physiology	Associated Complications	Relief Measures
Breast fullness and tingling	Ovarian cyst or tumor; intracranial tumor; chronic cystic mastitis	Integumentary system: hypertrophy of the mammary gland; increased vascularity and pigmentation; increase in size of nipple and areola caused by hormone stimulation	Breast discomfort	Wear well-fitting bra with good support—may need to be worn 24 hours; avoid breast stimulation
Spider nevi	Metabolic changes	Integumentary system: increased estrogen causes dilation of small networks of arterioles; they appear as red, spiderlike points on the skin over the neck, thorax, face, and arms		Reassurance that they will fade after pregnancy; may not disappear totally
Palmar erythema (may accompany spider nevi)	Metabolic changes	Integumentary system: reddish mottling of skin over palms and inner fingertips caused by hyperestrogenism		Reassurance that this will return to normal after delivery
Melasma or chloasma (face); linea nigra (abdomen)		Integumentary system: hyperpigmentation of skin over face, causing "mask of pregnancy", and darkening of linea alba on the abdomen		Reassurance that this will decrease after pregnancy
Leukorrhea	Vaginal infection: *Trichomonas vaginalis*; *Candida albicans*; *Neisseria gonorrhea*; monilial vaginitis	Reproductive system: hormone stimulation increases production of cervical mucus by the hypertrophic and hyperactive mucous glands	Pruritis; odor; discomfort	Good hygiene; perineal pads; vinegar and water douche; cornstarch; reassurance

TABLE 10-5. Minor Discomforts of Pregnancy (continued)

Discomfort	Differential Diagnosis	Physiology	Associated Complications	Relief Measures
Braxton Hicks contractions	Labor; fibroids; fetal movement; gas pain	Reproductive system: uterine muscle contraction due to hormonal influence commonly occurring throughout pregnancy at irregular intervals	Regular contractions may cause premature cervical changes; discomfort; insomnia	Rest, lying on left side; reassurance
Insomnia	Use of central nervous system stimulants; excessive fear or worry	Anxiety; fetal activity; musculoskeletal discomfort; dyspnea; increased urinary frequency	Fatigue; poor nutrition; psychologic stress; depression	Relaxation techniques; massage; warm milk; herbal tea; pillows for support; warm bath before retiring
Fatigue	Anemia; infectious disease; heart disease; emotional distress	May be due to increased hormone production	Depression; lack of exercise; insomnia; loss of appetite	Rest periods; adequate nutritional status; emotional support and reassurance

good prenatal care. With knowledge of these normal physiologic changes, a nurse can provide information, support, and counseling, and can assist in early detection of abnormal conditions that may occur during pregnancy. This chapter has provided a foundation from which to expand an understanding of the physiologic events that affect the course and outcome of pregnancy.

REFERENCES

Byrne, C. J.; Saxton, D. F.; Pelikan, P. K.; and Nugent, P. M. 1981. *Laboratory tests—implications for nurses and allied health professionals*. Menlo Park, Calif.: Addison-Wesley.

Callander, R.; Garrey, M. M; Govan, A. D. T.; and Hodge, C. 1974. *Obstetrics illustrated*. 2nd ed. Edinburgh: Churchill Livingston.

Chaizze, L.; Brayer, F. T.; Macisco, J. J.; Parker, M. P.; and Duffy, B. J. 1968. The length and variability of the human menstrual cycle. *JAMA*. 203:377.

Eskin, B. A. 1981. Diagnosis of pregnancy. In *Principles and practice of obstetrics and perinatology*, eds. L. Iffy and H. A. Kaminetzky. New York: John Wiley & Sons.

Hickman, M. A. 1978. *An introduction to midwifery*. Oxford: Blackwell Scientific.

Pritchard, J. A.; MacDonald, P. C.; and Gant, N. F. 1985. *Williams obstetrics*. 17th ed. Norwalk, Conn.: Appleton-Century-Crofts.

Russell, D. H., and Durie, B. G. M. 1978. Polyamines as biochemical markers of normal and malignant growth. In *Progress in cancer research and therapy*, vol. 8. New York: Raven.

Taylor, E. S. 1971. *Beck's obstetrical practice*. Baltimore: Williams & Wilkins.

11

Psychologic and Emotional Changes of Pregnancy: Mother and Family

BEHAVIORAL OBJECTIVES

Upon completion of this chapter, the reader should be able to:

- Define the concept of developmental crisis.

- Describe the concept of pregnancy as a developmental crisis.

- Describe the psychologic changes of pregnancy.

- Describe the development of maternal identity during the three psychologic trimesters.

- Discuss the expectant father's experience during pregnancy.

- Discuss the nurse's role regarding the psychologic needs of the family during pregnancy.

From the moment the woman first realizes she is pregnant, the pregnancy exerts a profound impact on the woman herself and, to some extent, on every person with whom she has a significant relationship. The pregnancy and the child it promises stimulate and necessitate dramatic changes in the woman and her family system which are life-long and irreversible. The entire family has to undergo psychologic and interactional changes as well as changes in the physical space within the household. The pregnancy represents a developmental crisis for the mother and father of the unborn baby because they must develop a new identity for themselves as parents of this baby. Any other children in the family also enter a new phase in their lives, that of older siblings. The woman's announcement that she is pregnant might also mean that extended family members will have to begin to see themselves in new roles as well—grandparents, aunts, uncles, etc. Although only the expectant mother experiences the physical pregnancy, to some extent the entire family is pregnant. All relationships and roles within the family system must be realigned to make a place for the expected child. In order to care for the pregnant family effectively, the nurse must understand the nature of the psychological experience of the pregnancy as well as the physical course of pregnancy.

This chapter examines some of the changes experienced by the family during pregnancy. It focuses on the mother's experience, because her response to the pregnancy is seen as central to the entire process. Then it examines the experiences of the father and the family. The last section of the chapter deals with the nurse's role regarding the psychological adaptation of the family during pregnancy.

THE CONCEPT OF A DEVELOPMENTAL CRISIS

A developmental crisis occurs when a person's progression through life brings her to a period of significant maturational change. Such periods of change create disorganization in the person's self-concept, identity, and patterns of behaving. A developmental crisis entails changes in the person's life roles—either significant changes in an existing role, or a new role (or "status") is added. It is a period in which the new role is integrated into the person's concept of self, and new ways of behaving according to the expectations of the role ("role behaviors") are learned. The way she used to behave are no longer as effective or appropriate, but she is not quite sure how to behave nor is she completely comfortable performing the new behaviors. As a result, during a developmental crisis, the person's life is in a period of disequilibrium; in fact, it could be said that a great deal of the element of "crisis" is due to the disequilibrium the person experiences. She finds herself no longer what she was but not yet what she is to become. She feels lost, anxious, confused, unsettled, and frequently nostalgic for the way life used to be.

The intensity of the experience of a developmental crisis and the length of developmental crises may vary. Within a particular individual's life, some developmental crises may be experienced more intensely than others; for example, adolescence is typically a very intense experience. Moreover, the intensity of the experience of a particular developmental crisis may vary from one time to another for the individual going through it. The length of developmental crises varies, from a period of several months, as in the case of pregnancy, to several years, as in the case of adolescence.

Developmental crises can be initiated by a variety of factors, but all have to do with the individual's phases of growth and development. Some developmental crises are initiated by factors which are almost entirely sociocultural, such as marriage. More commonly, developmental crises can be initiated by physical factors such as adolescence or pregnancy. The physiological changes, however, initiate psychologic and sociocultural changes as well. The physiologic changes in the individual's body cause her to begin to see herself in a new light, changing to some degree how she has behaved in the past. Other people observe these changes and begin to see her differently and to expect her to behave differently than she had before the changes became apparent. The individual has to alter the way she interacts with the world and the world has to alter the way it interacts with her. Therefore, the individual's developmental crisis is not hers alone, but also involves other people with whom she has significant relationships. She has to learn the requirements of this new role in life, and other people have to make a place for the individual's new role in their concept and expectations of her.

Developmental crises and the role changes they require occur whether the individual has chosen willingly to make the change, as in the case of a planned pregnancy or marriage, or whether the change simply "happened" to the individual, as in the case of an unplanned pregnancy or adolescence. Nevertheless, once the individual has begun to make the transition from one way of being to another, she never can go back to the way she was before. Just as puberty makes permanent changes in the individual's body and mind, pregnancy, even if it ends in miscarriage or stillbirth, makes permanent changes in the woman's body, and more important, in the way she sees herself. The very fact of having begun the period of change in and of itself represents a permanent change in the person's self-system.

A developmental crisis represents a period of time in which the person undergoing change is between what she was and what she is to become. It is a time in which the new role and role requirements are being learned. She has the chance to explore, learn, and practice the skills required of her in the new role and to integrate the role into her concept of herself. This period of time is considered a "moratorium" which provides a transition period in which the individual can explore the new role and its implications more fully, and can perform some of the role behaviors in situations which allow her the opportunity to practice and make mistakes without risking censure by the social group (Erikson, 1956). Like an actor on the stage, the person has to learn a role in order to perform it appropriately.

Learning role behaviors also occurs in other ways. The individual may have had some opportunity to learn about the new role by playing the opposite, or "alter" role, or through play (Mead, 1934). For example, a little girl learns something about being a mother by being mothered herself and has opportunities to practice the adult roles while playing with her dolls (see Fig. 11–1). People also learn something about life roles by observing others in the roles. Preadolescent children, for example, learn what being a "teenager" means by observing adolescents going about the business of being teenagers.

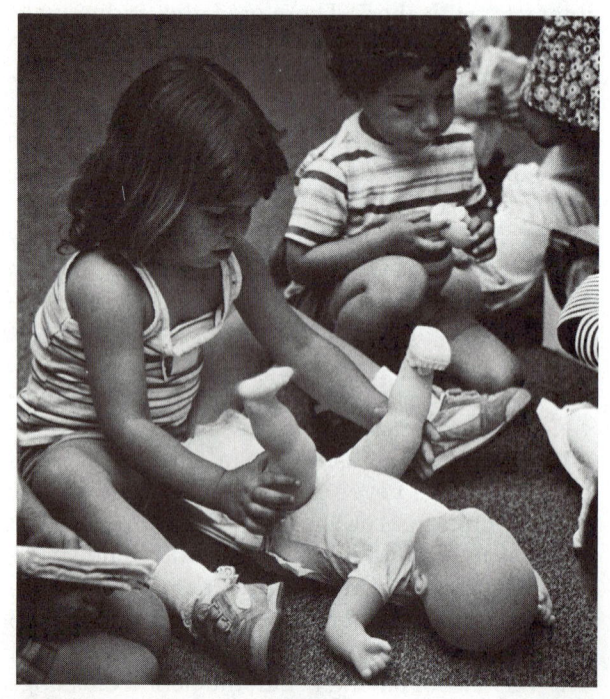

FIGURE 11–1. Through doll play, little girls learn about motherhood.

An important part of assuming a new role is being accepted into the new role by other people. The individual usually has achieved something that indicates that she is ready to move into a new role, such as the development of secondary sexual characteristics or receiving an engagement ring. Sometimes the role change is facilitated by cultural practices, or "rites of passage," by which the social group acknowledges that the individual has moved into a new stage in life and ritualistically moves her into it. A good example is the engagement period preceding marriage. The entire engagement period, especially the final days before marriage, are marked by numerous celebrations and social gatherings that appear to assist the group and the individual to change their perception of her. The celebrations and parties which take place give the social group the opportunity to "approve" the coming marriage by giving gifts and sharing special foods.

Some of these cultural practices also seem to be aimed at giving the person the chance to relinquish old roles which would be contradictory to the new role. One example is the "bachelor party" in which the groom-to-be and his friends "mourn" his transition from being a bachelor to being a married man. Another significant cultural acknowledgement of the newly married individual's role change is the fact that there is a special title for each spouse—"bride" and "groom"—which indicates the social group's awareness that they are not yet established in their new roles. By performing such rites of passage, the social group confers the new role upon the individual and expects her to begin to act accordingly. The social group probably will continue to allow some "mistakes" as the individual sets about performing the new role behaviors, as long as she does not violate important social rules. As time goes by, however, the social group will expect increasingly closer adherence to the role behaviors. Should the individual not adhere to the social expectations of her in the new role, social sanctions may be brought to bear on her.

PREGNANCY AS A DEVELOPMENTAL CRISIS

Pregnancy is one example of a developmental crisis because it requires a substantial alteration in life roles and identity reformulation for each of the parents (Rubin, 1975). The first pregnancy represents the couple's transition from being childless and possible "newlyweds" to being parents. They each have to change the way they see themselves and each other as well as their combined image as a couple. With the coming of an infant, they no longer will be as free to come and go as they please. They will have new and heavier responsibilities—socially, financially, and psychologically. Their time-frame will change because a child represents a real and living investment of themselves in the future. Their way of thinking about themselves, their relationship, and the world must change because of the new life they are bringing into it.

Pregnancy also indicates or implies that the parents are to become truly adults. Adulthood is attained when the individual has satisfactorily resolved the issues of adolescence and has acquired a sufficient sense of identity, a knowing of who she is, and is able to assume a place as a responsible member of society by becoming committed to a career, marriage, and parenthood. Pregnancy causes each parent to become aware that they are adults, they can "no longer find their way back . . . to childhood" (Jessner, Weigart, and Foy, 1970). Parenthood also brings a firmer commitment to another person, the child, than any other type of relationship can bring. Marquart (1976) has noted the "permanency of parenthood: One can divorce a spouse, but not one's own child." In other words, pregnancy marks an irrevocable life change, a commitment on the part of each of the parents to the coming infant, and places them quite definitely in the responsible world of adulthood.

Pregnancy represents a period which could be considered a moratorium, because the couple are no longer childless, in the true sense of the word, but they are not yet parents. Pregnancy provides the couple a period of time in which they can explore, rethink, and learn in order to become capable parents of the infant when it is born. Pregnancy terminates in a culturally sanctioned "rite of passage", the birth itself, with its attendant ritualistic practices and ceremonious acknowledgements of the change in role of the parents.

It should be understood that the biologic fact of pregnancy does not necessarily mean the parent or parents automatically will take on the psychologic, social, and cultural role of parenthood. Parenthood in the psychologic, social, and cultural sense is a *willingness* to rear a child; an individual can reproduce without actually becoming a parent. For example, the biologic father may never be aware that he has sired a child, or he may not choose to assume the parental role for that child. Likewise, the biologic mother may decide to terminate the pregnancy or give the child up for adoption.

It is also quite possible for an individual to become a parent in the psychologic, social, and cultural sense without ever having been pregnant. The identity reformulation necessary for parenthood appears to be more difficult for the adoptive parent, however, because of the absence of the biologic changes which occur during actual pregnancy. Adoptive parents' adaptation to parenthood appears to be complicated further by the absence of the time provided by pregnancy in which to go through some of the changes necessary to become a parent. Although adoptive parents may have wanted a child for some time, the time between learning that they are going to get a child and receiving the child may be only a matter of a few days.

Pregnancy is a "period of constant psychophysiologic change and upheaval" for each of the parents (Jessner, Weigart, and Foy, 1970). Colman and Colman (1972) observed that couples experience a certain amount of stress as a result of the changes that are taking place and will be taking place in their lives whether they are expecting the first, second, or third baby.

Additional stress is experienced by the mother who is not married or does not have a stable relationship with a partner. This mother will have to deal with all the adaptations and changes of pregnancy in a situation that may not be acceptable to her friends or family. In addition, she may have to make decisions about whether to keep the pregnancy and keep the infant; if she plans to keep the child, she must decide how she will maintain the child on her own.

The second pregnancy also represents a developmental crisis for the family. The parents have adjusted to the idea of themselves as mother and father of one child. With a second pregnancy, they have to come to terms with the idea that their exclusive relationship with the first child must be altered, and they must become parents of another infant as well. They have to deal with their fear that they might not be able to love another child as much as they love the first one, and their vague suspicion that in some way they are betraying the older child by deciding to have another one, a feeling which Rubin (personal communication) has compared to bigamy. Moreover, the parents have to help the older child deal with an impending significant change in his or her own life, that of becoming an older sibling, sharing his parents with someone else, and having to relinquish a favored and unique place as the only child. The parents may recall how they felt in a similar situation when they were children, how they may have resented the arrival of a sibling, and they may want to do all they can to lessen the impact on the older child.

Just as psychologic parenthood must be attained as the infant and parents develop and mature, being the parent of one infant does not automatically make them parents of the next infant. The process and evolution of parenthood has to be reworked with each child (Rubin, 1967c; Grubb, 1980).

Pregnancy also affects people who are not members of the nuclear family. Anyone who might be expected to take part in the care or rearing of the anticipated child will have to make some changes in their roles.

During pregnancy, the mother is biologically in the process of becoming a mother. Every physiologic system of her body is affected. The biologic changes stimulate and assist her in the psychologic work of becoming a mother. Because the infant is growing within her body, the mother is much more involved and committed to the process of becoming a parent. The infant is hers before it is any one else's—a part of her body and absolutely dependent upon her. Unlike other people who are affected by the anticipation of the infant, the situation is always with the mother, and her experience is much more encompassing and dramatic. Pregnancy brings about changes which indicate development and maturation of the woman as she grows psychologically, as well as physiologically, toward becoming a mother.

PSYCHOLOGIC CHANGES OF PREGNANCY FOR THE WOMAN

Rubin (1967a, 1967b, 1967c, 1970, 1975, 1984) has explored extensively the woman's subjective experience during pregnancy and childbearing. She divides pregnancy into three "psychological trimesters" based on clearly observable changes in the woman's experience and response. These psychologic trimesters are "in harmony with the biological changes" of pregnancy and are seen as developmental stages in the psychologic work of pregnancy (1970, p. 502), while the purposes of the biologic processes of pregnancy are developing a healthy baby and establishing lactation, and the purposes of the psychologic processes of pregnancy are to become a mother of this particular child and to attain an identity of herself as the mother of this child (Rubin, 1984).

The First Trimester

The woman's psychologic work of pregnancy does not begin with conception. There is a period of 2–4 weeks during which conception, nidation, and some of the early physiologic changes have begun before the woman misses a menstrual period. The missed period initiates the early exploration which characterizes the work of the first psychologic trimester of pregnancy. Thus the psychologic processes of pregnancy encompass about 1 month less than do the biologic processes. The woman is not actually "psychologically pregnant" until she is certain that she has conceived.

A great deal of the woman's psychologic work during the first trimester is devoted to the attempt to determine, for sure, whether she is pregnant, because "there is nothing there: nothing demonstrable can be seen, heard, or felt, even indirectly, by anyone" (Rubin, 1970, p. 503). Because she has no definite proof that she is pregnant and her amenorrhea is not being caused by some sort of illness, the woman begins to search her own body for indications that she is pregnant. Rubin sees the woman's turn toward her own body for verification of the pregnancy as the beginning of the introversion which is so characteristic of the pregnant woman. The woman's body gives her vague data in the form of changes in her breasts, changes in the way she feels, nausea, and occasionally, weight gain. The scale can offer the woman important information: in the early months, weight gain can indicate the presence of a baby, and later, her capacity to make a big, healthy baby (Rubin, 1970).

Since the woman has so little to substantiate or verify the fact that she is pregnant, the opinions of other people become important to her. The obstetrician's diagnosis is probably tentative, though helpful in her data search. However, she needs to have others who are closer to her, such as her husband and her mother, acknowledge her pregnancy. Such an acknowledgement helps to make the pregnancy more real to the woman herself.

The focus of the woman's work during the first psychologic trimester is not the baby. The baby, as such, does not exist for her. Her reality consists of the *question* of whether or not she is pregnant. Her focus is on herself, and her efforts to answer the question of pregnancy and to adjust to the fact that she is *probably* pregnant.

As time goes by, the woman becomes increasingly convinced that she is probably pregnant and there is the sense of surprise and pride in her feminine accomplishment. Nevertheless, she also is dismayed because "now" is just not the right time in her life for a pregnancy, regardless of how much the pregnancy may have been desired and actively sought (Rubin, 1970). She finds herself thinking, "It's nice to have a baby, but not now." Pregnancy is something that has happened to her, and at this point, she is not entirely convinced that she likes the idea.

The woman begins to do what Rubin (1970) calls a "cost analysis", in which she weighs the benefits of pregnancy and her current situation against the costs of having an infant at this particular time in her life. She finds herself in a nebulous, uncertain situation, with abstract and intangible benefits. What she has to give up is very real—the pregnancy means that she will have to make some important changes in her life. She will possibly have to alter career goals. Babies and pregnancies are expensive, so the family financial situation will be affected. Furthermore, she probably will be unable to work for a while, if she has been employed. And, should she decide to return to work after the baby is born, she will have to find someone to care for the infant and will have to pay for such care.

The time of the pregnancy looms before her, lengthy and insurmountable. The 7–8 months stretching before her seem like a prison sentence, empty and boring (Rubin, 1970).

The Second Trimester

The woman enters the second psychologic trimester when she perceives fetal movement (Rubin, 1970). The fetus's gentle movement within her body is a definite message that says to the mother, "Yes, I am here." Fetal movement provides an important turning point in the woman's psychologic work: it tells her there is life within, there is a presence. The question of whether she is pregnant is answered by something within her own body—the fetus itself.

Along with fetal movement come other pieces of information which confirm the woman's pregnancy. The uterus has grown sufficiently to move out of the pelvis into the abdominal cavity and to begin to make its presence noticeable to the external world. Her clothing start to feel tight across the tummy and she needs a larger bra for her growing breasts. Other people begin to talk about "when the baby comes"; even people who she has not told she is pregnant begin to treat her in a special way. Other people's response provides the woman with continued important reinforcement and verification that there is an infant. Technological devices provide additional data that there is truly an infant within. She may hear the fetal heart sounds or see the fetus's vague shape with ultrasound, but it is the fetus's own movement within her body which provides on-going, day-to-day proof that it is there and alive.

The term "quickening", which has been used to indicate the first perception of fetal movement, can also be used appropriately to describe the woman's response to the experience. The pace of her psychologic work quickens. She becomes "actively pregnant" and she begins to feel that there is so much to do and not enough time in which to do it (Rubin, 1970).

A great deal of the woman's activity during the second psychologic trimester, particularly during the last half, reflects the creative process going on within her body. The mother is interested in how well she is able to produce a baby and begins to do things which will help make a big healthy baby. She eats foods which will nourish the baby and help it grow strong. She welcomes the opportunity to go to the obstetrician and be weighed, for each weight gain is seen as an indication that the baby is growing. During this psychologic trimester, the woman welcomes weight gain; she attributes all the weight she gains to her baby, so weight gain means that her baby is doing well. The physician's admonitions against gaining too much weight may go unheeded due to her pleasure in feeding her baby and seeing proof that her baby is growing.

The woman behaves as though her involvement in the biologically creative process of making a child is so encompassing that it spills over and is expressed in other creative tasks. She typically becomes involved in traditionally feminine creative activities such as cooking special foods and making or choosing special clothing.

The second trimester is a pleasant time for the mother. She looks good, her skin glows, her hair is lustrous. She feels good and feels good about herself. She is happy and content. She develops a narcissistic love and pleasure in herself that "erases the boundaries between the I and the thou" (Deutsch, p. 162). The woman loves the infant as a part of herself. Furthermore, since it is the presence of the child within which has caused her to feel so good about herself, her good feelings include the infant. As her feelings of pleasure and love toward the infant grow, the mother experiences an increased need for more information about it.

With the second trimester, the woman's attention shifts from herself and the question "Am I pregnant?", to the pregnancy and the affirmation, "I truly am pregnant." As the pregnancy becomes prominent in her mind, her focus shifts to the baby and its condition (Rubin, 1970). She becomes increasingly introspective, her attention is withdrawn from what is outside to what is inside and what it means.

The woman's increasing withdrawal of attention from the outside world is accompanied by a constriction of her social space (Rubin, 1970). She becomes more selective in her social relationships, restricting those which are not relevant to her changing situation. At the same time, her social sphere broadens to include people who are relevant to her situation. She seeks out other pregnant women or women who have recently given birth, and she begins to seek increased or renewed contact with her own mother (Rubin, 1967a, 1970).

When the woman first begins to experience fetal movements, she describes them and her perceptions by saying, "It's like . . .", finishing the sentence by comparing the fetus to a butterfly, a fish, or the like. The fetus is an "it", rather amorphous and vague. As the second trimester progresses, the mother needs to know even more about this strange individual who is inside and a part of herself, unknown yet known. The primagravida wonders what an infant is like. To have an infant of her own is an unknown. The multigravida knows what children are like and has one or more of her own, but she does not know what *this* child is like. The mother begins to search her environment as well as her own body for information that will help her develop a concept of the infant she carries. She examines her perceptions of the baby's movements and her body's physiologic responses to the pregnancy and uses the information to form ideas about her baby's characteristics. She carefully examines baby pictures of her mate, herself, and her other children, developing ideas of what related babies looked like. She becomes very aware of children in the environment and studies them—how they look, how they act, and how their mothers respond to them (Rubin, 1967a, 1970, 1984).

She wonders what it will be like to be the mother of this infant. In order to begin to form a picture of the infant and of herself as its mother, the woman, like any one beginning a relationship with someone new, needs to know the sex of the other person because not knowing the baby's sex gives the situation an uncomfortable ambiguity. She cannot interact with an "it", she needs to know whether the other person in this important relationship is a male or a female (Rubin, 1970). Again, the woman examines her own body for information that will help her answer her question. She may use one or more of the many "folk" methods for determining the baby's sex and fantasizes about being the mother of a girl or a boy (Rubin, 1970). Often, although the woman may want to have a boy as a gift for her partner or family, she secretly prefers a girl, like herself (Rubin, 1972).

As the second psychologic trimester progresses and the baby grows, fetal movements, which had been so indefinite, become increasingly apparent. The mother begins to be able to distinguish the various fetal parts. Her efforts to learn about her child continue. Her introversion and feelings of special love and concern for the child intensify. The infant becomes increasingly real and present to her. A sense of alienation develops in response to other people's persistent references to "when the baby comes"; for the mother, the baby is already "there", not an entity that will appear at some point in the future. To the woman, her infant child is ". . . here and now, an awareness restricted to herself alone which produces a sense of pleasure in exclusive and intimate possession . . ." (Rubin, 1970). These feelings toward her child bring about the mother's increasing protectiveness toward it and her accompanying sense of vulnerability.

The Third Trimester

The third psychologic trimester is ushered in by the woman's dramatically intensified sense of vulnerability, which typically occurs during the 7th month of biologic pregnancy. This vulnerability arises from her feeling that anything so precious and valuable as her baby can be injured, lost, stolen, or insulted by careless, malevolent, or envious forces or individuals (Deutsch, 1944; Rubin, 1970, 1984). She feels that she has to protect her infant from all these potential dangers. Her baby and her body which surrounds it become vulnerable to danger. However, the fetus's growth is making it project into space, and her body becomes less capable of enclosing and protecting it (Rubin, 1984).

The woman responds to her increased sense of vulnerability by becoming more and more cautious. She carefully studies the environment for danger and avoids situations and people that pose potential dangers. She avoids revolving doors, buses, frisky children, fast drivers, and open spaces in her efforts to protect her infant and herself. She tends to retreat to her home, where she worries about burglars and intruders. She ventures out only when necessary, and when she does go out she tries to control the circumstances as much as possible in order to avoid danger. She may insist on having fire and burglar alarms installed in her home and may compulsively check all doors and windows each night to assure herself that they are locked and secure. A large dog that she has never allowed to stay indoors might suddenly be invited indoors, particularly at night.

Her efforts to avoid danger lead the woman to limit her contacts with other people and she becomes lonely and isolated (Rubin, 1970). She is likely to feel that her situation is very unique; no one in the world feels as she does and no one really understands. As a result, she feels even more isolated.

The woman's 7th-month vulnerability can be a difficult time for the baby's father as well. The woman sees her partner as the one person who can be with her in her efforts to protect the infant and herself. She will try to persuade him to stay home with her as much as possible. She wants him to drive her places and go with her on errands she formerly did alone. The father does not share her sense of vulnerability, and it is impossible for the woman to explain it to him. The man deals with her fears by explaining that she has nothing to worry about, that her fears are groundless, and in fact, rather silly and illogical. He may not respond well to her need to have him nearby. In her vulnerable state, the woman may fear that she will lose her mate or that he will desert her, either emotionally or physically.

During the absences of her mate, the woman likes to be in the company of other "safe" people. She may persuade her mother, a sister, or a close friend to stay with her when her mate is gone. Or she may go to the person's home and stay for hours. When she goes for prenatal visits, the woman may linger long after her examination because she feels safer close to the physician and nurse. She might openly express her wish that the "doctor will just keep me" when she goes for her prenatal visits. The hospital and clinic seem like secure havens in the midst of such a dangerous world.

The 7th month is probably the most difficult month of pregnancy (Rubin, 1970). The woman senses that she is alone in a very difficult situation and that no one really cares, appreciates, or understands her predicament is at its peak; her experience during the 7th month can become almost intolerable. The 7th month vulnerability predisposes some women to premature labor as an attempt to find a way out of the situation. The woman's desire for a big, healthy baby possibly helps counteract her urge to get out of such an unpleasant predicament. Rubin believes that "the woman goes into labor from the seventh month on" (personal communication, 1974, 1975), as she experiences numerous periods of "false labor" which may be physiologic expressions of her desire to "get it over with".

By the 8th biological month of pregnancy the woman has more or less come to terms with her situation, even though it continues to be difficult. She still feels vulnerable, in fact the physical changes which contributed to her vulnerability are increasing. The baby is continuing to grow, her body is more and more difficult to maneuver in space—through doors, up and down stairs, in and out of chairs. However, the woman seems to have decided that she has to find a way to live with her situation, and she manages to do so. As a result, the woman's emotional experience during the remainder of the third psychologic trimester of the pregnancy, although difficult, is less painful (Rubin, 1970).

The woman's relationship with the baby within takes on a new character in the third psychologic trimester. The baby is no longer passive and inert. She and the baby are now interdependent and interrelated. The woman's perception of the fetus is like "an inner organ . . . a part of self", but, the fetal movements, which are more vigorous and frequent, call her attention to the fact that the baby is not a part of self (Rubin, 1984). The mother has the rather bewildering situation of being simultaneously one with and separate from the fetus. The vigor of the fetal movements contribute to another important alteration in the mother's response: the fetal movements become less welcome. Fetal movements no longer are perceived as the fluttering of a butterfly or some other delicate and delightful creature, because their intensity and frequency cause them to begin to be perceived as prods, pokes, jabs, and occasionally even bites and scratches. The fetus's movements, which had been sweet reminders and messages, become painful and intrusive, angry expressions of the baby's crowded conditions. The mother continues to love the infant she carries and she continues to feel as one with it; however, its presence within is becoming problematic and unpleasant.

The due date, or expected date of confinement

(EDC), becomes very important and is the focus of a great deal of the woman's psychologic work during this trimester. To the woman, the calculated EDC will be the *exact* day when her baby will be born. As the woman gets closer to the actual date of the EDC on the calendar, the greater the EDC seems to loom and to influence her behavior. The EDC becomes an "overriding, preeminent engagement", in that all the woman's life activities and all her thinking are in terms of this date. The approaching EDC tends to speed up and organize the woman's efforts as she becomes intensely involved in her plans and preparations for her "engagement" (Rubin, personal communication 1974).

The third trimester woman anticipates and fears the EDC. On one hand, the pregnancy is becoming so uncomfortable that she begins to wish, or even to be convinced, that the baby really is due earlier than the physician had calculated. It is not uncommon for the woman to believe that her baby is due 2–4 weeks sooner than the EDC (Rubin, 1984). On the other hand, she feels that time seems to be going so fast. In fact, as the EDC approaches, time seems to be going *too* fast. There is so much to do and so little time in which to do it. Nevertheless, had she a choice, she would not choose to move the EDC backward in time and give herself more time to accomplish what she wants to accomplish, she wants the pregnancy to have ended by the designated date (Rubin, 1984).

The ambivalence about the EDC also reflects the third trimester woman's intensely ambivalent feelings about labor and delivery. Although labor and delivery promise relief from the trials and tribulations of pregnancy, they may pose a threat to her own welfare and the welfare of the baby. Popular literature, folk stories, and word-of-mouth are filled with examples of the dangers of labor and delivery. She knows that women can die during childbirth, so she may view her forthcoming labor and delivery as a very real threat to her own life. In addition, she becomes more aware of the possibility that the child she carries may be defective in some way, making her fearful of the first time she will see her baby.

During this trimester the woman is troubled by nightmares which reflect her fears for herself, her baby, and her fears of labor and delivery. She dreams that the baby she carries within is some sort of hairy monster or has some horrible deformity. She dreams that she herself is exploding, being ripped apart or otherwise annihilated (Deutsch, 1944; Rubin, personal communication, 1974). Awake or asleep, she dreads labor and delivery because then she will either live or die, and she will find out just what kind of child her body is producing. The spurts of energy which other people see so charming in the pregnant woman are really a response to her feelings of vulnerability, her fears, and her nightmares. She keeps busy doing things so she will not have as much time to worry and brood, thinking if she gets tired enough, perhaps she will be able to sleep and not have the awful dreams (Rubin, 1970). What the woman does during her spurts of energy further reflects her primitive fear of death, that she "won't be coming back". She cleans her house until it shines, she cooks and freezes meals for her family because she is not sure she will survive labor and delivery.

The third psychologic trimester is not a pleasant time for the mother. She is uncomfortable, awkward, angry, frightened, and lonely. Where her psychologic work regarding the pregnancy during the first psychologic trimester had been "Am I pregnant?", and during the second had been "Yes, I am pregnant!", in the third psychologic trimester, she responds, "I'm pregnant all right. There's no doubt about it. I'm getting tired of it and I never want to be pregnant again!"

Weight gain takes on a new meaning during the third psychologic trimester. Pounds that had been a welcome confirmation of feminine functional ability in the second trimester now become a source of despair. Since the woman tends to attribute all the weight gained to the baby, she may perceive the baby as being too large for her to continue to contain within herself. It threatens to become so large that there is no more space left and it seems that her body might explode from overdistension. The baby inside becomes so large that she has trouble breathing. Its pressure causes her ankles to swell, and she worries about the loss of functional abilities, such as the ability to walk upstairs without becoming winded. She feels "as big as a barn". No longer does she feel pretty, and her conversations reflect her increasingly poor self-concept.

The woman's changed perception of the baby within and the discomforts she experiences during the last few weeks of pregnancy serve an important function. Were the wonderful feelings of the second psychologic trimester to continue, the woman would never want to make the psychologic changes necessary to terminate the pregnancy. She would stay pregnant, the treasured infant safe within her body forever.

TABLE 11–1. The Psychologic Trimesters of Pregnancy

Parameters	First	Second	Third
Focus	Self	Baby	Labor and delivery; safety of self and baby
Response to being pregnant	"Am I pregnant?" "Is there a pregnancy?"	"I am pregnant!" Pregnancy is wonderful!"	"No doubt about it, I'm pregnant and I'm tired of it; I don't want to be pregnant again."
Affective response	Waiting, unsure, scared, moody	Pride, joy, pleasure, looks good, feels good	Despairing, fearful, vulnerable, trapped; becomes angry and hostile
Baby	Not there	Baby and self are one	Baby and self are one; begins to separate from pregnancy; wants baby in outside world
Weight	Not much weight gain; disappointed because weight gain would help verify pregnancy	Weight gain means baby is growing/thriving; she's a good mother	Too much; baby is too big; "I'm fat, too big"
Time	Time is empty	Time is present	Time is unbearable; time is running out
Space	Begins to become introverted, examines own body to determine whether she is pregnant	Introversion, inward focus; restricts social sphere; attention on mothers and children	Introversion further restricts space because of vulnerability

It is as though nature is seeing to it in advance that the imminent separation from the child should not be so painful (psychologically) for the mother . . . [The mother's discomforts] transform the fetus into an alien being . . . the relationship with the child is split . . . [the polarity between herself and the infant is established and strengthened, and] . . . the enemy (the child within) must get out in order to reappear as a precious friend in the outside world" (Deutsch, 1944, pp. 221, 222).

Table 11–1 summarizes some of the important characteristics of the woman as she goes through the psychologic trimesters of pregnancy.

DEVELOPMENT OF MATERNAL IDENTITY

The period of pregnancy allows the woman to become a mother biologically. Becoming a mother psychologically does not occur automatically at the end of pregnancy. The achievement of a firm concept or identity of herself as a mother, in the sense that she is comfortable in the role, occurs considerably later than the birth of the child (Rubin, 1967c). Pregnancy does, however, give the woman some time in which to begin to resolve the developmental crisis before her and to begin the process of taking the role as mother of this infant into her self-system.

As a rule, the woman deeply and sincerely wants to be a mother to her child and expends a great deal of effort toward that goal during the pregnancy and after the birth of her child. The woman's efforts aimed at becoming a mother, referred to as *maternal identity development*, are initiated by and develop in direct relation to the biologic progression of the pregnancy and childbearing. Becoming a mother is not instinctive; it is the result of efforts involving psychologic, social, cognitive, and affective elements (Rubin, 1984). Maternal identity development is specific to each child. In other words, having achieved an identity of self as the mother of one infant does not mean that this identity will transfer itself to a subsequent infant. The process of taking on the identity of mother has to be reworked with each infant, although it tends to be more streamlined when the woman has given birth to several children.

THE PROCESS OF MATERNAL ROLE TAKING

There are five operations involved in the process of maternal role taking that provide a framework for understanding how the woman resolves the developmental crisis accompanying pregnancy: (1) mimicry, (2) role play, (3) fantasy, (4) introjection–projection–rejection/acceptance, and (5) grief work (Rubin, 1967a, 1984). Together they represent a progressive movement into an integration of self in the new role.

Mimicry

Mimicry is an active operation in which the woman searches the environment and her memory for other people who are or have been in the role she is working to attain, and then examines their behaviors and imitates them (Rubin, 1967a). Women who are working to achieve a role through mimicry carefully examine and mimic every remembered or observed characteristic and behavior in their earnest effort to learn what it is like to be what they themselves are trying to become. They act like a person who has achieved the role. Mimicry can be observed, for example, in the behavior of the woman who is still in her first trimester of pregnancy but begins to wear maternity clothes. She is dressing like someone who is, without question, pregnant. She herself is not quite sure, but the clothing provides assurance and an opportunity to feel as though she really is pregnant.

Role Play

Role play is acting out what a person in the sought role actually does in particular situations. Role play is the earliest form of role behavior (Rubin, 1967a). The woman actually tries the role in a situation with another person, and observes that person's response in order to evaluate her ability to perform the role behavior. For example, a pregnant woman might offer a young child a piece of candy or a cookie in order to try the role of "self-as-mother-in-giving". A woman who is expecting her second child might seek out situations in which she could care for another child and see how she functions as "self-as-mother-of-two". The mother commonly involves her mate in role play, with the two of them interacting in some sort of parental situation with a recipient of the role functions. They might offer to babysit for a friend's infant, or they may get a kitten or a dog to see how well they are able to care for and nurture something small and dependent.

Fantasy

Fantasy involves cognitively "trying on for size" varieties of possible role situations (Rubin, 1967a). Fantasy takes place in thought rather than in behavior and represents a deepening involvement in the role because the woman is considering how it will be for herself. Fantasy occurs by way of fears, wishes, dreams, and daydreams. Many fantasies have to do with the characteristics of the infant the woman carries, and as a result, fantasies increase markedly after the woman begins to become aware of fetal movement.

Fantasies stimulate the woman to act. She may express her fantasies directly, or in the case of fearsome fantasies, the woman's behavior may express her attempts to assure herself of reality, that her fantasies are not true and will not be. Planning, data gathering, and attempts to learn about her internal process, the baby, labor and delivery may result from fantasy. In addition, fantasy has a great deal to do with the vulnerability which becomes so dramatically apparent during the 7th month of pregnancy.

Introjection-Projection-Rejection/Acceptance (IPR/A)

This process resembles mimicry in that the mother-to-be searches the environment for people who are in the sought role and examines their behavior. However, IPR/A involves more than merely copying a behavior. Because the woman has been building up a repertoire of role expectations for herself, she has something against which to assess the role performance she observes in others. The behavior of others is taken in (introjection), to be examined for "fit" against her own role expectations. She quickly imagines herself performing in that way (projection), and makes a judgment about the behavior based on how well it fits with her own developing sense of what is right for her in the role. If the fit is good and the behavior seems appropriate for her, it is accepted; if the fit is not good and the behavior seems inappropriate, it is rejected. IPR/A implies that the woman has been involved in exploration of the role long enough to have formed some emerging concept of self in the role, and has had accumulated some experiences, partly as a result of her role play, against which to make a judgment. On some occasions IPR/A affirms and verifies other courses of action the woman may already have chosen; on others, it provides her the opportunity to learn new ones. IPR/A tends to bind role traits more firmly into the woman's system. IPR/A allows the woman's emerging concept of herself in the role to be evaluated by examining the behavior of a model. Accepting the behavior of the model serves to either affirm her own opinion of how a particular behavior should be performed, or it helps her learn more about the role. Rejection of the behavior of another allows the woman to consolidate her beliefs about the role.

An identity of self-as-mother is the goal and the result of the woman's mimicry, role play, fantasy, and introjection–projection–rejection/acceptance. The mother's progress toward comfort within the role is indicated by her use of the word, "I", and use of the present tense in referring to role behaviors. For example, saying "I am . . .", "I like . . ." reflects some comfort with the role. However, the role of mother implies the existence of a child. The child during pregnancy is real and present, but it is present in a different way than a child who is in the external world. What the woman does to and with the infant in reality is very limited. As a result, the woman cannot be expected to have a firm identity of herself in the role of mother of this particular child until some time after the child is born (Grubb, 1980).

Grief Work

Grief work is an operation that has to do with giving up those elements of the former self which would be in conflict with the new role. It involves recalling and reviewing those conflicting elements and loosening attachments to them. A certain amount of sadness or nostalgia is usually involved in the process because the person knows she can never go back and be that way again. Loosening attachments to elements of the former self results in a gradual elimination of certain behavior patterns, and eventually may lead the person to give up certain old roles entirely. Most grief work probably is never finalized, it is only brought to some sort of resolution, as is the grief work in the loss of a loved one. Grief work allows the woman to disengage from elements of the former self and put them away in order to make room for and move into her new identity as mother of this infant (Rubin, 1967a).

MATERNAL TASKS

From the foregoing, it is evident that although the pregnant woman becomes introverted and restricts her participation in certain social interactions, she is very active cognitively as she devotes her attention to understanding and learning new role behaviors in order to become a mother (Rubin, 1975). In addition to her movement toward taking on the identity of mother, she also works to reorder the immediate external world for herself and her child and explores some elements of her own emerging relationship with her infant. The totality of the woman's psychologic work of pregnancy has been grouped into four "maternal tasks": (1) seeking safe passage for self and baby through pregnancy, labor, and delivery; (2) securing acceptance of the baby and herself as pregnant by significant persons in her family; (3) learning to give of herself; and (4) binding-in to the unknown baby.

The woman works on all these maternal tasks throughout the pregnancy. One task may predominate at a particular time and another task at another. However, each task is significant and is essential to her becoming a mother to the infant within, and making her world ready for its birth. If there is a substantial lag in one of the tasks, there will be lags in the other tasks as well, and the successful completion of the pregnancy may be compromised (Rubin, 1975).

Seeking Safe Passage for Self and Baby

Seeking safe passage receives most of the mother's attention throughout the pregnancy. Unless she can be reasonably sure of the continued safety and survival of herself and her baby, she cannot attend to the other maternal tasks. Ensuring safe passage includes seeking obstetrical care and adherence to prescribed or recommended practices that will contribute to a healthy outcome of the pregnancy, like taking prescribed prenatal vitamins, eating a balanced diet, and getting enough rest. The woman's efforts to ensure safe passage also might include adherence to other practices which might be considered superstitious or "folk" practices, no matter how well educated she might be. She might avoid such things as raising her arms over her head in order to keep from getting the umbilical cord wrapped around the baby's neck, or she might confess that she is afraid to "tempt fate" by being too hopeful about the outcome of the pregnancy. Some women engage in practices that appear to be a direct reflection of the ancient fear of attracting the attention of the "evil eye". The woman does not want to take a chance that she might inadvertently do something to harm her child. She is vulnerable to superstitious behavior because what is going on within is unknown and mysterious, but extremely important.

The woman's work on the maternal task of seeking and ensuring safe passage for herself and her baby changes over the three psychologic trimesters of pregnancy. In the first trimester, she is concerned about herself. Is she really pregnant or is she ill? In the second trimester, her growing attachment to the child within makes her become protective toward it. It is her attachment to the child which brings her for prenatal care. The woman seeks safe passage in the third trimester because she is concerned about herself and the baby. She and the infant are one, and whatever threatens the safety of one threatens the safety of the other. Moreover, she fears the coming labor and delivery because of what she may learn about her child and for what might happen to herself. Thus, seeking safe passage in the first trimester is for pregnancy care, in the second trimester it is for baby care, and in the third it is for "delivery care".

Securing Acceptance

Lack of acceptance of the infant by significant others may seriously threaten the outcome of the pregnancy. The woman who does not feel that the coming child is welcomed and accepted by people who are important to her is particularly at risk for complications of pregnancy. Rubin observes that securing acceptance is a condition "necessary to produce and sustain the energy for all the other tasks". The maternal task of securing acceptance involves a reworking of psychologic, social and physical space within the family constellation to make a place for the coming child (Rubin, 1975).

The reworking of relationships within the family involves a loosening of all bonds within the family so they can be realigned to make a place for the coming infant. The addition of a new family member will affect all intrafamilial bonds; each person's relationship with every other person will be affected. The loosening and realignment of bonds is a difficult and somewhat painful process because it requires, to varying extents, relinquishing some elements of the former relationship in order to make place for another person. The woman expecting her first child, for example, has to rework her relationship with her mate so that he will be willing to give up his exclusive relationship with her and make a place in their lives for their child. She needs to feel that her mate wants the child and is willing to make the sacrifices required of him. A woman who is pregnant with her second baby has to loosen and realign the exclusive relationship with her first child. She has to begin to alter her concept of that child as "the baby", and begin to move him into the position of older brother or sister. This realignment of the mother's relationship with the first child continues to be a problem postpartum (Grubb, 1980).

The woman's work on the maternal task of securing and ensuring acceptance by significant others has an observable progression throughout the three psychologic trimesters of pregnancy. In the first trimester, the woman's efforts are primarily to secure acceptance of herself as pregnant. This acceptance serves several purposes. It helps her in her "cost analysis" of pregnancy, in which she examines the gains offered by the pregnancy against the costs entailed in making such a dramatic alteration in her lifestyle. The acceptance of her pregnancy by significant others helps to affirm the fact that she is pregnant. In addition, it has been suggested that the lack of such acceptance is associated with complications of pregnancy, such as preterm labor and low birth weight (Richardson, 1981, 1987; Ramsey, Abell, and Baker, 1986).

In the second psychologic trimester, the mother's focus shifts to the infant within. She fantasizes how it will be in certain situations, how it might fit into her family as a son or daughter to her mate, as a grandchild to her parents, or as a sibling to her other children. She hopes the family will be pleased.

The father's pleasure and successful participation in role-play with the mother serves as a boost in the mother's work on the task of securing acceptance by this significant person. His participation indicates that he is willing and able to take on the role as father to the coming infant. The mother also may place herself and the older child in a role-play situation in order to observe the older child's response to a younger child. If the older child seems to be interested in the young child and is willing to interact with it in the role-play situation, the mother receives some assurance that the child will be willing to accept the coming sibling. The woman who appears to be most content and pleased with herself during the second psychologic trimester is the one whose pregnancy and coming infant are happily accepted by her family, including her mate, her other children, and her extended family (Rubin, 1975).

The third psychologic trimester can pose some problems for the woman in her efforts to secure acceptance of the infant by significant others. These problems occur if the family wants a child with particular characteristics, e.g. if the family strongly desires a particular sex. The mother wishes to gratify their desire, but more important, she fears that they might reject an infant who does not fulfill family requirements. If they so strongly desire a girl, could they, and would they, accept a boy? Will they accept *this* infant? To the pregnant woman, the more willing the family seems to accept the infant she carries unconditionally, the less they are seen as potentially rejecting the child, and because she and the child are as one, rejecting her. The less willing the family to accept the child, the greater she perceives their rejection of it and of her (Rubin, 1975).

The family's acceptance of the coming child is also indicated by their willingness to make the physical space accommodations necessary to make a place for the infant within the household. The coming of the infant requires that some space be rearranged. Possibly someone will have to give up his or her old bed so the baby will have a place to sleep. The mother, as the coming baby's advocate, does all she can to make these transitions easier for everyone involved. She may, for example, spend more time decorating and arranging the older child's new room and moving him or her into it from the nursery than she spends arranging the nursery for the baby. Her mate's willingness to become involved in the redecorating tasks will also be perceived as evidence of his acceptance or rejection of his child.

The willingness of significant others to accept the coming infant affects the developing mother–child relationship (Richardson, 1981, 1987). Evidence that others accept herself as pregnant and accept the baby she carries provides the mother with energy and enhances her motivation to establish her own relationship with her baby. The woman herself and society expects her to accept the child she carries unconditionally whether or not she is actually pleased with it. Such unconditional acceptance is considered an inherent part of maternal behavior. Her family's willingness to accept the infant will have a considerable influence on the mother's ability to accept and mother it.

Learning to Give of Self

Giving is an inherent and pervasive part of being a mother, during both childbearing or childrearing. The giving of mothering requires that the woman give of her own physical self as well as of her psychologic and emotional self. The experience of being required to give of herself begins with pregnancy, when the woman has to permit the child to use her body and change her body and her image of herself. She has to give up some of her hopes and plans, and change parts of her lifestyle in order to accommodate the coming infant. Moreover, she eventually has to come to terms with the hazards of labor and delivery in order to "give birth". Maternal giving does not end when the child is born; although its nature may change it continues throughout the remainder of her life (Rubin, 1975).

Giving is not something the mother knows how to do instinctively, it has to be learned. She has to explore the meaning and essence of giving in order to learn how to give. The pregnancy extracts its toll from the woman's body, so in one sense her physical giving during pregnancy takes place without her voluntarily choosing to permit it. The woman does have the choice, depending on her own personal beliefs, of whether to permit the physical giving of pregnancy to continue. It is the voluntary giving essential for the child to thrive that the woman has to learn and be able to do on a day-to-day basis, especially after the baby is born.

Since giving of self is one of the most pervasive of maternal behaviors and one of the most socially idealized characteristics of maternal behavior, it is actively explored as a part of the woman's efforts to take on the identity of self as mother. The mother's exploration of giving is easiest to see in role play: the woman places herself in situations where she can explore her effectiveness as one who gives things, typically food and care, to another. If the proposed recipient of the gift is willing to take the gift and makes good use of the gift by eating or enjoying it, the woman's opinion of herself in that behavior is enhanced and her efforts to take on the role are given a boost.

She explores giving to the infant by eating foods that are healthful, thereby giving the infant things that will make it grow big and strong. She also eats "fun" foods such as cakes and cookies in order to symbolically give the infant foods that it will like. The woman explores maternal or nurturant giving by preparing or making things, such as food or clothing. For example, she might prepare some special food then feed (give) it to her mate in order to experience the act of making and giving something to someone who is important to her. The woman in the second psychologic trimester also explores the meaning of giving by being given to or receiving (Rubin, 1975). The symbolic value of the gift is more important to her than the actual value of the material object. The object's value is in the fact that it represents the giver's interest, time, and acceptance of the woman herself and her situation.

The exhaustion and feelings of depletion of the third trimester arise, in part, from the woman's feelings that she is physically "given out", due to the toll extracted on her body by the pregnancy. Her physical depletion causes her to feel she needs to be given to. The gifts she is given, or extracts from other people, particularly her mate, provide her with additional inputs of psychologic energy to carry on with the pregnancy. Such gifts represent the other person's concern and continuing interest in her. During the vulnerable 7th-month, the gifts of companionship the woman receives from other people are more valuable than the objects she may receive. Other people's willingness to give her their time and their company provide her with some relief and help her deal with her fears.

During the third trimester, the woman explores the threats awaiting her during labor and delivery. She knows that labor and delivery hold the threat of loss of intactness and pain. She might have to give the ultimate gift during labor and delivery, her own life, in order to give birth. The mother's examination of the maternal task of giving during the last few days and weeks of pregnancy, therefore, involves a careful weighing of the possible costs to herself of giving birth. "One does not give or give-in generously to a loss of intactness, a loss of life" (Rubin, 1975).

Binding-In to the Unknown Baby

Maternal binding-in is the dynamic process of attachment and interconnection with the infant that begins in the prenatal period. Binding-in is never completed, even in the neonatal period, nor is it static. Binding-in does not just happen. Maternal binding-in is an attachment that constantly grows and changes as the individuals in the relationship grow and change, and so the relationship is perpetually in a state of becoming. Binding-in includes but goes beyond love for the other in the relationship because the interconnection with the other endures even when love is severely taxed and when anger or hostility are directed toward the other.

Maternal binding-in is an increasing personalization and individuation of the child which is stimulated and sustained by the presence of the child. In order to bind-in, the mother has to locate the child with its present characteristics and take it into her self-system. Concurrently, she has to locate herself in relation to the infant as its mother. Therefore, maternal binding-in has two halves: binding-in to the infant and binding-in to self as mother of the infant.

Binding-in, like the other maternal tasks, has a progression over the three trimesters of pregnancy. In the first trimester, the woman cannot bind-in to the infant because the infant, as such, does not exist. Instead, the woman first has to bind-in to the idea that she is pregnant (Rubin, 1975).

The process of binding-in to the infant is given an enormous boost during the second psychologic trimester. The woman feels wonderful during the second trimester and attributes the way she feels to the infant within. Her positive feelings contribute greatly to her developing attachment to the child she carries, because the narcissistic love she experiences includes the child as a part of herself. She develops a secret, romantic love toward the child and a sense of "we-ness", an exclusive, special relationship between herself and the infant that no one else can share or appreciate. These special feelings toward her infant cause the mother to seek more information about it in order to know all its qualities and characteristics (Deutsch, 1944).

The woman's growing attachment to the infant within leads to the vulnerability seen in the 7th month. She feels that she has something extremely valuable inside, her love toward the child has become a possessive love, and what one possesses can be taken away. She begins to fear that something terrible could happen to the infant and she becomes very protective. As described earlier, this vulnerability and the growing pregnancy combine to move the woman toward becoming uncomfortable and unhappy about being pregnant.

With the progression of the third trimester, the woman's binding-in to the child appears to come to a standstill of sorts. Her love for the infant endures, but her attention turns more toward the pregnancy, which is becoming increasingly hateful, unpleasant, and tiresome. She feels increasingly unattractive, cumbersome, uncomfortable, and big. She loves the child but hates the pregnancy and her hatred for the pregnancy helps her begin to "bind-out" from the pregnancy and become willing to take the risks to be "delivered" from the pregnancy and rejoin her infant in the outside world. The maternal task of binding-in increases in intensity again in the neomaternal period, beginning slowly and speeding up when the woman begins to see the baby respond to her and her care.

The maternal tasks are not put aside at the end of pregnancy. Although their expression changes following the birth of the infant, they continue to be an important element of the woman's relationship to the child and the world for the remainder of her life as the child's mother. Safe passage becomes a concern about the child's growth, development, and well-being. The mother continues the task of seeking and ensuring acceptance of the child by significant others by such things as teaching her child to be polite, sharing the child's picture with relatives, and encouraging interactions between the child and the rest of the family. Giving continues in the many expressions of nurturance, concern, and care that typify motherly behavior. Binding-in continues to be worked upon as the child grows and goes through the various phases of development. Table 11–2 summarizes the characteristics of the maternal tasks during the three psychologic trimesters of pregnancy.

THE FATHER'S EXPERIENCE

The experience of pregnancy is not limited to the woman alone. It affects her entire family and social support system. Because the mother is the individual whose physical status and psychologic system

TABLE 11–2. *Maternal Tasks During Pregnancy by Psychologic Trimesters*

Task	First	Second	Third
Safe passage	Concern about self. Alerted, something is "not there," "Am I sick or am I pregnant?"	Concern about baby. Care of and for baby. "Is my baby all right?"	Concern about self and baby. Seeking delivery care. "Will I and my baby safely go through labor and delivery?"
Securing acceptance	Works on acceptance of herself as pregnant	Works on acceptance of her baby. Task not as important because of own pleasure in pregnancy	Works on acceptance of this baby, as it is
Giving	Cost analysis: "What do I have to give up?" "Can I give up all that I have to?"	Works on meaning of giving. What does gift symbolize? Care/love. Learns to give by being given to	Feels "given out." Feels she cannot give any more. Extracts gifts from others
Binding-in	Binds in to idea of self as pregnant. Baby is not real	Attachment to baby. Secret, romantic love between self and baby. Feels good—attributes it to baby. Seeks messages from baby	Carries a valuable treasure. Becomes fearful—what one treasures/possesses can be taken away. Hates being pregnant but wants her baby

SOURCE: Rubin (1975).

are most affected by the pregnancy, the medical establishment has tended to focus its attention on the mother and more or less ignore the rest of her family. Family members, however, are important because their response to the pregnancy and the coming child will affect the success of the pregnancy, the success of the mother–infant interaction, and the infant's future as well.

The father's life, in particular, is profoundly affected by the pregnancy. "Pregnancy constitutes an important developmental challenge for the prospective father, which . . . brings about internal upheaval and change." At the same time as the man faces having to change his own identity so he can become a father, he has to adapt to a relationship with his mate which is also changing. Moreover, he has to try to adapt to the woman's changeable emotional state and respond to her through all phases of the pregnancy (Cath, Gurwitt, and Ross, 1982; Clinton, 1986).

Although the father's experiences and needs during pregnancy have not been explored as extensively as have the mother's, to some extent his experience appears to mirror and parallel the mother's experience. His experience and responses tend to lag behind the mother's, however, probably because he does not undergo the same biologic participation as the mother.

Marquart (1976) and Herzog (1982) have studied the experiences and needs of expectant fathers and report some findings which suggest that the father goes through a progression of responses which could be compared to Rubin's concept of the maternal psychologic trimesters of pregnancy. For example, the fathers reported that when they learned that their wives were pregnant, they went through a period of fairly intense ambivalence about the situation. The men in Herzog's study became more narcissistic and increasingly preoccupied with their own insides, a behavior that seems comparable to the mother's turn inward during the pregnancy. They strongly felt the need and desire to nurture and care for their mate and the infant she carried. There was a blurring of the men's perceptions of the distinctions between themselves and the infant, and between themselves and their mates.

Fathers frequently respond to their partner's pregnancy by experiencing physical or emotional symptoms. This phenomenon is called "couvade syndrome" and is more likely in fathers who are more involved affectively with the pregnancy and when there are other stressors, such as economic difficulties or the father's illness prior to the pregnancy. Physical symptoms vary widely and include nausea, anorexia and other gastrointestinal symptoms, musculoskeletal and skin symptoms, colds, and weight gain or loss. Emotional symptoms experienced by expectant fathers include depression, anxiety, irritability, nervousness, and concern about their own health (Colman and Colman, 1973; Leibenberg, 1969; Herzog, 1982; Clinton, 1986).

Perception of fetal movements may have an important effect on the father as well as the mother. Being able to feel the baby move within his partner's body, even though the father is not able to feel the movements until considerably later than is the mother, changes the fetus from an idea to a reality. Although this experience makes the father feel pleased and happy, his ambivalence about the pregnancy appears to remain. In fact, awareness of the reality of the infant can stimulate intensified feelings of envy toward the woman for her creative abilities. Furthermore, the father may become aware that he fears that his unique relationship with his mate is being threatened by a possible rival. Being able to feel the baby moving within his mate's body has another effect in that it helps the father begin to separate the baby from his concept of his wife and his concept of himself—in other words, the blurring of the distinctions between self, mate, and child which occurred earlier in the pregnancy begins to change after quickening (Gurwitt, 1982; Diamond, 1986).

Like the work of the pregnant woman, the expectant father's psychologic work to come to terms with his changed and changing identity involves a reworking of past and present significant relationships. The father reexamines and reevaluates his relationships with his mate, his siblings, and his own parents. This phenomenon has been observed to occur at about the 15th to 25th weeks of the pregnancy and involves the father's attempts to "sort things out" with his family of origin, especially his own father. The man's efforts to take on the role of father include turning toward his own father and exploring his relationship with him, and reviving and reestablishing contact with the idealized father of his childhood (Diamond, 1986).

The father may experience fears during the last 2–3 months of the pregnancy, which have to do with the welfare of his mate and the unborn infant. This concern about his mate and child may make him susceptible to superstitious beliefs and practices. He may feel that powerful forces are at work and come to regard his mate's body and what is going on within it as almost magical. He may fear that the pregnancy will somehow change or harm his mate. Fathers also report feeling much more protective toward their wives and unborn babies at about the same time as they notice the mother responding more protectively toward the unborn infant (Gurwitt, 1982; Marquart, 1976; Diamond, 1986).

Part of the father's experience during pregnancy is a response to the changes in the woman, rather than in response to the pregnancy itself. Some of the father's experience, therefore, can be seen as reactions to the woman's psychologic trimesters. For example, the father may feel inadequate and helpless when faced with his mate's moodiness during the first and third psychologic trimesters. The woman's increasing introversion and her narcissistic pleasure in herself during the second trimester serve to make the father feel left out and lonely (Strichler, Bowden, and Reimer, 1978). Her fear, anxiety, and hostility during the third trimester may be very threatening and frustrating to him and his sense of competence.

The expectant father has some additional responses to the pregnancy that can be problematic. The area of sexuality, for example, can be a problem due to the rather sudden changes in both of the parents' desire for intercourse once they learn that they are expecting a baby. Learning that his mate has conceived tends to make the man feel particularly potent and pleased with himself. This feeling of potency tends to make him desire coitus even more. In addition, his insecurity in this new situation may make him need the closeness of intercourse for reassurance. On the other hand, some fathers avoid intercourse when their mate is pregnant because they are afraid of harming the baby or the woman, or because of a primitive fear of "contaminating" the woman and the pregnancy. Some fathers see the fetus as a third-party "observer" during coitus. Because she is so introverted, the woman may be unable to respond to her mate as fully as she might. Some women notice increased sexual desires during pregnancy, especially the second trimester, but most have diminished desire for intercourse, although they have increased needs to be held and nurtured by their mates (Swanson, 1980; Reamy and White, 1985).

The fathers in Herzog's (1982) study reported feeling increased needs for coitus; they also felt deprived that their own sexual needs were not being met. The difference between the sexual needs of the woman and the man due to the pregnancy, as well as their changing sexual needs during the pregnancy, can become a serious problem for the couple and their relationship unless they are able to communicate openly and honestly with each other.

Financial concerns are a feature of the expectant father's response to the pregnancy. He becomes aware of the increased financial needs of his family and may feel that the burden of providing for the family will be his alone. Financial worries tend to remain with the father during the pregnancy and during the postdelivery period as well.

The man's efforts to take-in the new identity of self as father also appear to be similar to the mother's. The men in Marquart's (1976) study reported that they became more interested in interacting with other men who were already fathers or were themselves expectant fathers and that the topic of pregnancy become important in their conversation. This response by the father is similar to the pregnant woman's interest in the new role that causes her to seek out other women who have had children or are pregnant in order to observe them and talk to them about the subject of pregnancy and childbearing. As indicated earlier, Rubin (1967a) has observed that expectant fathers are frequently involved in the pregnant woman's efforts to take-in the role of mother through the operations of fantasy and role play. The father's participation probably serves not only to assist his mate in her efforts but also helps the man in his own work taking in the role of father. Sherwen (1986) examined the dreams and fantasies of expectant fathers and noted the similarity to those of expectant mothers. Fathers' fantasies and dreams reflect anxiety about their ability to provide and care for their family and their fear for the welfare of their partner, their baby, and themselves. They also fantasize about happy family gatherings that include the expected baby.

There may also be some counterpart to the maternal tasks in the father's psychologic work during the pregnancy. The man's increased protectiveness toward his mate and unborn child have already been noted. This protectiveness might be an indication of the "paternal task" of assuring safe passage. There are also indications that the father works on safe passage, e.g. the father feels responsible for being sure that the woman will be transported safely and efficiently to the hospital when she begins labor. He assists her in and out of cars and low chairs and generally becomes more considerate and concerned about her welfare while she is pregnant with his child. He cooperates to some degree in her need for increased protection during her intense vulnerability by seeing to it that additional locks are installed on the doors, by checking the windows to be sure they are closed, and by going outside to check for burglars when she hears a noise.

The father appears to seek acceptance of the unborn infant by helping to inform extended family members of the pregnancy and helping to choose a name for the baby. A lot of his involvement in acceptance appears to have to do with being one of the most important individuals in the mother's life who will be called upon to accept the child. The father has to indicate his acceptance by becoming involved in the preparation of the physical place for the child within the household and by stating and demonstrating his willingness to accept the infant.

The father's willingness to accept his partner's pregnancy may be crucial in her decision to maintain the pregnancy and can affect its outcome. His response to her changing body, his tolerance of her moods and her introversion, as well as his participation in preparing for the baby provide important reassurance and support and can lead to an increased closeness between the couple (Hobfall, Nadler, and Leiberman, 1986).

The expectant father's exploration of giving primarily has to do with coming to terms with what he will have to give up. In this regard, Rubin commented that the expected father's psychologic work tends to remain in the first trimester because so much of what he has to do concerns "cost analysis", which takes place in the woman's first trimester. The expectant father has to give up his exclusive relationship with his mate. He may feel that the growing fetus literally and figuratively comes between them, and he has to come to terms with the fact that this is the way his life will be in the future. The baby will be there and will definitely interfere with the couple's former way of relating to each other. He will have to give up some of the peace and quiet in the household, some of his privacy, and some of his social and financial freedom. He will have to act in new and more responsible ways, and will have greater responsibilities.

The father will also have to do a great deal of giving to his mate. The pregnant woman is very needful and her mate is usually the person to whom she looks first to meet some of her needs. Throughout the pregnancy and into labor, delivery, and the postpartal period, he will have to give her time, attention, comfort, companionship, concern, and relief. It is not surprising that fathers frequently feel deprived, and that they continue to feel deprived well into the postpartal period (Grubb, 1980).

The father's binding-in to the unborn infant is different from the mother's. The unborn baby is always with the mother, frequently reminding her of its presence and reality; such is not the case with the father. The mother has many experiences with the unborn infant and more input from it with which to begin to form an attachment; the father's opportunities are more limited. As a result, the father's binding-in to the infant is much less active than the mother's. The man who is actively striving to take in the new role of father is usually pleased to receive information which will help him "know" the infant, and he will participate in the woman's role play and fantasy although he does not tend to initiate much of this behavior himself. Because he does not have the numerous opportunities to know the coming baby that the mother has, the father's concept of the baby remains somewhat nebulous, the infant not entirely real. Once the father can see the infant, his binding-in to the child begins in earnest.

Expectant fathers have more *choice* in terms of the degree of involvement and their response to their partner's pregnancy (Herzog, 1982). They do not have the biologic changes and stimuli which seem to create a more predictable response by the woman. Various "styles" of response by fathers have been identified, which include (1) the "observer" father, who remains more distant, a bystander; (2) the "expressive" father, who responds intensely and sees himself as a full partner in the pregnancy; and (3) the "instrumental" father, who responds by attempting to "manage" the pregnancy, focusing on tasks (May, 1982a, 1982b).

Diamond (1986) proposes a seven-stage sequence of prospective fatherhood:

- *Stage 1: Getting ready* is that period when the couple has decided to try to conceive.
- *Stage 2: Conception* is the period when conception has occurred and has just been diagnosed. The father's response is typically a mix of joy, pride, upheaval, and conflict.
- *Stage 3: The first trimester* marks the beginning of the expectant father's developmental crisis. It is characterized by his work on relationships with the partner as well as his family of origin; the

emergence of physical and emotional "couvade" symptoms; and an increased identification with self as a child being nurtured by mother and father.
- *Stage 4: Midpregnancy* occurs approximately between weeks 15 and 25 and is characterized by the emergence of the fetus in the family constellation. Fetal movements and sonography confirm the baby's life and reality for the father and stimulate ambivalence, envy of the woman's creativity, and an upsurge of creativity in his job or other projects.
- *Stage 5: The turn toward one's father and fathering* occurs at approximately the same time as Stage 4. Stage 5 seems to provide time for the man to work through old difficulties with his own father and reestablish connections with him. A successful conclusion of the work at this stage appears necessary for the father to intensify his involvement with his partner and the pregnancy during the remainder of the pregnancy.
- *Stage 6: Toward the end of the second trimester* is less well defined, but is characterized by the father's thinking about the infant as a specific sex and separate from himself and his partner. There are fantasies in which the fetus is aggressive or intrusive and the father experiences hurtful, sadistic feelings toward the baby or the partner which might be frightening to him because of the implication of abuse.
- *Stage 7: The last trimester* is characterized by more orientation toward the reality of the coming birth, increased empathy with his partner, role-play, and a sense that something awesome and magical is happening. The father becomes more intensely involved in getting things ready for the birth, and more observant of children and childrearing.

THE SIBLING'S EXPERIENCE

The older sibling does not truly come to terms with the reality of the coming child during the pregnancy. Instead, the baby becomes a reality when it is born and begins to make an impact on the older child's life. Nevertheless, the pregnant woman is aware that the older child will be making a significant change in his or her own life and begins to try to move the child into that position in order to lessen the stress the child will surely feel when the new baby arrives.

Because she is the adult in the situation and thus able to foresee some of the impact of the new baby on older children, the mother tries to initiate the changes in the older children's roles. In order to begin to help the other children move into their new roles, however, the mother first must change her own concept of each of the children. Each child will be affected by the birth of the baby, each will move one space higher in the age rank of the family, but it is the child who is next older than the unborn baby who will be affected most. The mother's concept of this next older child will be altered most dramatically by having a new baby. The mother will encounter difficulties in changing her concept of this child from "baby" to "older child", because this child still is the baby and will be so until the new baby is born and takes over the "baby" position (Grubb, 1980).

Expectant parents engage in various strategies designed to assist their older children to come to terms with the fact that there will be a new baby in the family. They talk about the baby, they allow the child to listen to the fetal heart sounds, (see Fig. 11–2) and encourage the child to feel the fetus move; they might move the older child into their new room with its new bed, which they are informed is because they are growing up; they call the child's attention to babies and encourage the child to interact with babies; and, in general, they attempt to help the child accept the idea that the new baby will be an asset to the family. The older child's response will be affected by the efforts and attitudes of the parents, and on the child's own developmental level.

The toddler is not able to understand that there will be a new baby. The toddler appreciates and enjoys the interactions with the parents which have to do with the baby because their attention is so intense. The child may learn various responses which please the parents, such as patting the mother's abdomen and saying "Baby", but the toddler is not able to make the connection between the word "baby" and the future arrival of a sibling.

The preschool age child is better able to make the connection that there will be a new baby in the family some day. The child can participate in family spatial rearrangements in preparation for the baby and can understand that the baby is "in a special place in mommy's tummy". The preschooler tends to like babies and probably will think a new baby in the family is a good idea. However, to the preschool age child, "someday", if it is not now, does not exist. The child's orientation to the present makes "someday" unreal, so the baby and its expected arrival will also be unreal.

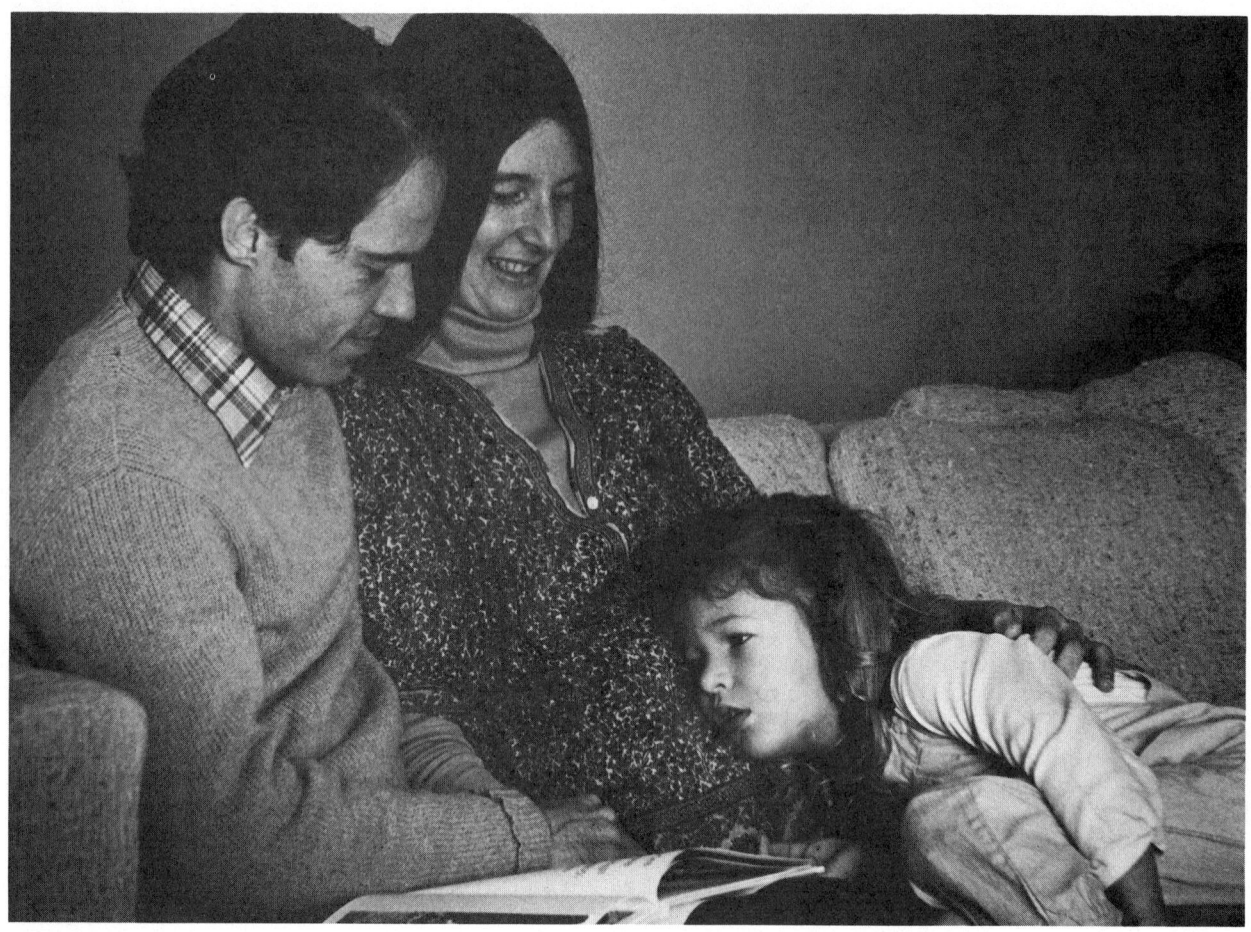

FIGURE 11–2. Expectant parents can actively plan strategies to prepare the older child

The school age child will be able to understand better that there will be a new baby in the family and when this event will occur. The school age child likes babies and enjoys being around them. He or she will look forward to becoming a big brother or sister, being a babysitter, and helping mother care for the new baby (see Fig. 11–3).

The child who is a teenager may have problems dealing with the idea that mother is pregnant again. The teenager understands when the baby will arrive, where it is, and more important, how it got there in the first place. Because the teenager is so involved in coming to terms with his or her own sexuality, the idea that the parents are sexual beings may be difficult to comprehend or accept. A mother who is pregnant is a sharp reminder that the parents are sexually active. As a result, the teenager may react with anger or embarrassment to the pregnancy: a baby may be all right, but a pregnant mother may not be all right.

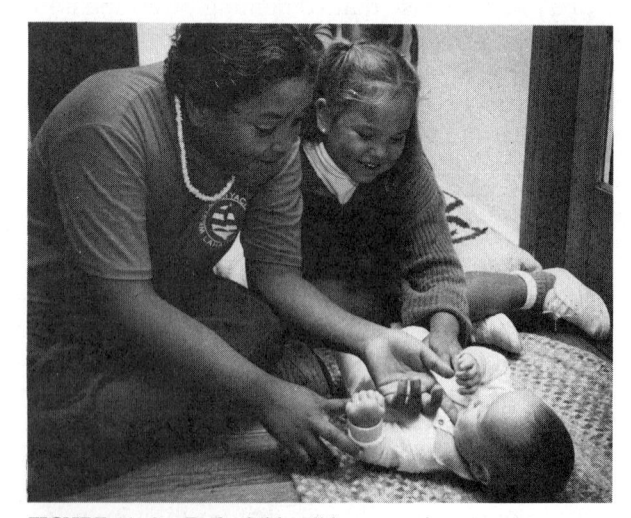

FIGURE 11–3. Each child will be affected by the birth of the baby.

THE GRANDPARENTS' EXPERIENCE

Grandparenthood is something that happens to people due to a choice made by their children. Becoming aware that he or she is going to become a grandparent can create a developmental crisis for the person. Becoming a grandparent can mean that the person will be one of the "older generation" and have to come to terms with the fact that he or she is now old enough to have children of childbearing age. Grandparenthood means that there will be changes in the relationship with their own children. The child will be more independent of his or her parents. Their concept of their child will have to change to include the fact that the child is becoming a parent. And they will be reminded of their child's sexuality.

The grandparent's response to their child's pregnancy will depend on several factors. Their own age at the time grandparenthood begins is important. Grandparents who no longer are capable of reproducing may have to deal with this reminder of their loss of that important capacity and their own advancing age. Grandparents who are still capable of bearing children are less likely to feel threatened. In addition, they might have children of their own at home who are keeping them busy being parents. The grandparents' response will also depend on (1) how well they have mastered their own developmental tasks, (2) their comfort with their own sexuality, and (3) their past relationships with their own grandparents, parents, and children.

Although they impact on each other, adapting to grandparenthood and adapting to aging are different. In fact, some of the loss and lowered self-esteem experienced with aging can be compensated for by grandparenthood (Severino, Teusink, and Bernstein, 1986). Several tasks have been identified as a part of the developmental phase of grandparenthood:

1. Self-esteem regulation, i.e. deriving a sense of self as a bridge between generations, and as a source of security and knowledge.
2. Reworking of previously unresolved conflicts, particularly those concerning separation–individuation from their own parents, their response to their own pregnancies and the birth of their children, and separation from their own children.

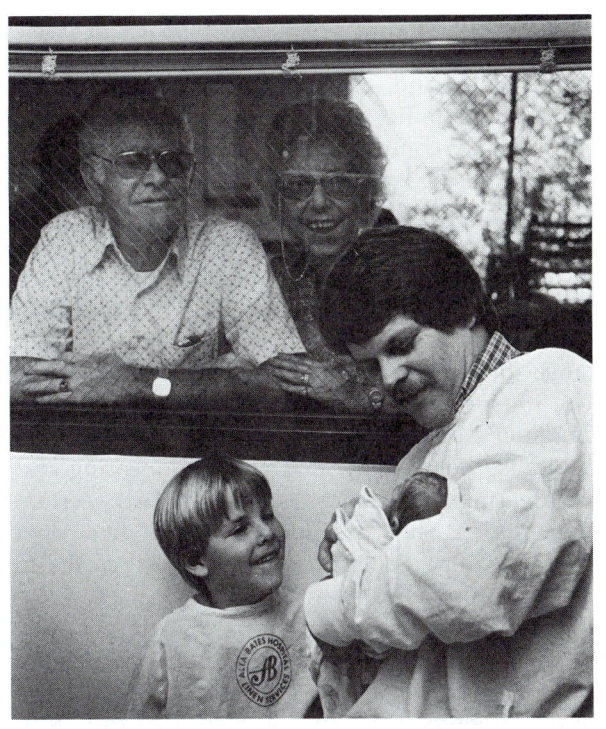

FIGURE 11–4. The experience of becoming a grandparent varies with age.

3. Identifying with their own child as a parent and their own parents as grandparents (see Fig. 11–4).
4. Resolving the symbolism of grandparenthood, such as the view of grandparenthood as a part of aging and eventual death of self.
5. Reworking grandparent–grandchild bonds with the birth of each new grandchild (Severino, Teusink, and Bernstein, 1986).

The arrival of each new grandchild will stimulate a degree of developmental crisis for the grandparents, particularly those who are geographically and/or psychosocially close to the parents and involved with their grandchildren (Sprey and Matthews, 1982).

It appears likely that the *maternal* grandmother and the *paternal* grandfather will have the most pronounced response to the pregnancy. In the expectant parents' efforts to take on their new life roles, they turn to their same-sex parent so they can rework, examine, and understand what it means to be a father or mother. The expectant parents will probably seek a somewhat intensified relationship with the same-sex parent in order to reexperience being parented as they learn how to parent.

Although the experience of being prospective grandparents can be gratifying, it can also create ambivalence and discomfort. For example, the middle-aged father can become jealous of his son and sexually competitive with him in an effort to defend himself against the experience of being old. Each of the expectant mother's parents may react intensely to the pregnancy because of their concern about the welfare of their daughter and her baby. The mother of the pregnant woman may have an experience which is more dramatic because she identifies with her daughter's situation. The prospective grandmother identifies with her daughter's ongoing experience, but the situation can cause her to relive her own childbearing and childrearing experiences and to rework certain elements of her relationship with her own mother—in particular, how her mother reacted to her being pregnant.

The pregnant woman's turn toward her own mother affects the prospective grandmother's relationship with her daughter in several ways. The pregnant woman has an increased need to experience nurturing and mothering by her own mother. The pregnancy allows the mother and her daughter a new opportunity to work on certain elements of their past relationship and possibly establish a more satisfactory relationship for the future. As she turns toward her mother in her present situation, the pregnant woman has the opportunity to learn more about the role of mother by observing her own mother's role performance. As a result, the prospective grandmother becomes a powerful model for the pregnant woman in her efforts to take in the new role.

THE NURSE'S ROLE

In dealing with the psychologic needs of the family which is expecting a baby, the nurse is the best instrument for data collection, analysis, and intervention. Because of the nurse's background in the physical, psychologic, and social sciences, the nurse, more than any other member of the health care team, is able to see the individual and the family holistically, as an interacting, interdependent system. The nurse's understanding of what might be expected to occur and the nurse's willingness to listen, to take time, to question gently, and to care, provide data which can be used to meet the needs of the family. These characteristics, in and of themselves, can also provide relief and support to the pregnant woman and her family.

The nurse is usually the health care worker who is in the best position to be informed about the family's adaptation to the pregnancy and coming infant. The ability to know the family and understand its roles, relationships, and communication patterns well enough to assess the effectiveness of familial adaptation requires that the nurse have a continuing and stable relationship with the pregnant woman and some of the other family members. Nurses in prenatal clinics, obstetricians' offices, prenatal and prepared childbirth classes, or community health settings are in the best position to assess the family.

Various guidelines or tools have been developed which can be used to assist the nurse in the assessment of the psychologic adjustment of the pregnant family. The nurse should be cautious in using tools to assess the family's response to the pregnancy. The tools cannot reflect the total picture of the family's response because the nuances of emotional and psychologic responses simply cannot be reduced to detection by a "tool". Although tools can be helpful when collecting data, the best data collection device is the alert, skilled, and caring nurse (see Chapter 15).

Based on the careful assessment of the available information about the family's response to the pregnancy, the nurse arrives at a nursing diagnosis concerning their situation. The nursing approach to the psychologic needs of the family during pregnancy has as its goal a family which is able to adapt to the changes in life roles and situations so that they do not experience undue stress, and are ready and able to meet the tasks and adjustments required of them in the postdelivery period.

Various strategies can be used to assist the family as it strives to adapt to the pregnancy and the changes in family roles and relationships. Most hospital and health care facilities provide prenatal classes designed to help the parents learn about the characteristics of babies, how to care for them, and what they can expect in the postpartal period. Other classes are available which help prospective parents prepare physically and psychologically for the actual experience of labor and delivery.

Both prenatal and prepared childbirth classes offer another benefit in that they bring several pregnant couples together and provide an informal "group therapy" setting in which parents can discuss some of their experiences with pregnancy and their changing lives. The nurse teaching the classes should be alert to the need for, and able to deal with, the parents' concerns (see Chapter 14).

Some health care facilities also offer classes for the couple who are contemplating pregnancy.

These classes were originally designed to meet the needs of the woman who had been involved in a career for several years before considering a pregnancy, but are helpful for other women and their partners as well.

Health care facilities may offer classes which assist the other members of the family in their adjustment to the pregnancy and coming child. Sibling classes can give children information on fetal development, characteristics of the newborn, changes in the child's own role, what to expect while the mother is in hospital, and give the child a chance to practice some simple baby care techniques with a doll. In addition, sibling classes can give the parents some guidelines for preparing the older child for the arrival of the baby (see Fig.11–5).

Maternity centers which permit the family to be present during the labor and delivery frequently provide some sort of preparatory classes for each person who will be with the mother during the intrapartal and postpartal periods. If the parents want to have the older child present during the intrapartal experience, the nurse must be sure that the child has a fairly clear concept of what will occur and that someone, not the mother or father, will be present during the intrapartum whose only responsibility is to assist the child in dealing with the experience.

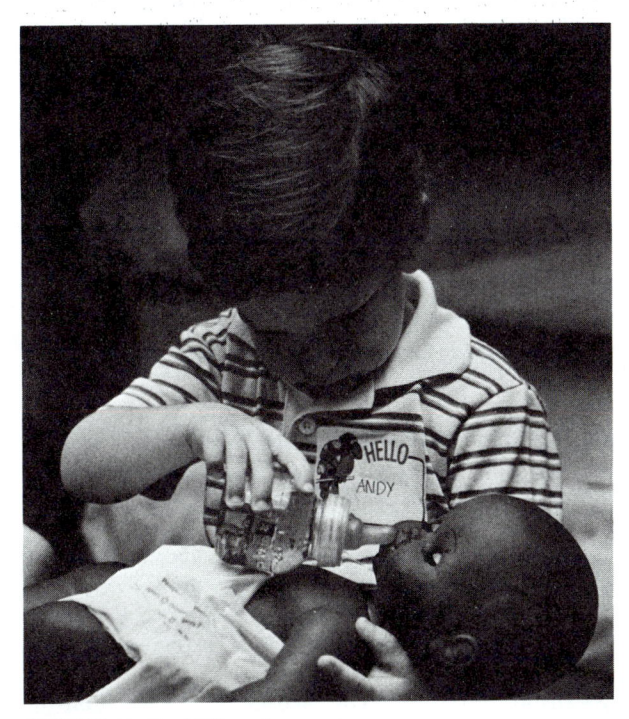

FIGURE 11–5. Sibling classes give the child an opportunity to practice baby care techniques.

Grandparent classes are becoming increasingly popular with consumers and health care agencies. Grandparent classes may offer information on changing birthing and parenting practices; how to support a woman during labor, delivery, and breastfeeding; tips on being a "welcome grandparent"; and information about the physiology of labor and delivery. Grandparent classes can provide tours of the maternity unit and give grandparents the opportunity to view a film about childbirth (Horn and Manion, 1985). In addition, grandparent classes can provide a forum in which grandparents can work on their own changing roles and self-concept.

The nurse uses other techniques to help the family deal with their response to the pregnancy. The nurse can serve in an advisory capacity or as a person who can sit down with the family and help them work through some of the difficult periods. The nurse might also refer the family to other health care workers as the need arises. For example, the nurse might refer the family to appropriate government agencies for financial assistance or to a psychologist or social worker for more intensive emotional and psychologic support. In order to make appropriate referrals, the nurse needs to know what is available in the community and how to help families take advantage of the community's resources.

The nurse dealing with the pregnant woman must always keep in mind the fact that the entire family system is pregnant. Each family member's response may have an effect on the outcome of the pregnancy. The nurse should strive to maintain an awareness and ongoing assessment of family responses and interactions. It is important that the pregnant woman's emotional state be assessed continuously. It also might be worthwhile to conduct an assessment of the father's response directly, rather than by way of the woman's report. Grandparents should ideally be included in the process of family assessment and intervention. In addition, guidance and support should be offered to parents in their efforts to assist their older children to get ready for the new baby.

SUMMARY

The ultimate goal of the psychologic work of pregnancy for the entire family is one of binding-in. Each family member has to bind-in to the coming child to some extent.

The family structure is altered during the pregnancy, but the process of adapting has only begun.

Though the adaptation process continues after the baby's birth, total adaptation is never achieved totally. Roles and relationships within the family will continue to change throughout the lifetime of the family.

The birth of a baby is a very important event in the lifetime of the family, and it necessitates significant changes in every person and every relationship within the family structure. The pregnancy and the birth of the baby precipitate crises in family identity. By the nature of their training and expertise, nurses are in an ideal position to assist the family as it works through these crises.

REFERENCES

Cath, S. H., Gurwitt, A. R., & Ross, J. M. (1982). *Father and child: Developmental and clinical perspectives.* Boston: Little, Brown.

Clinton, J. F. (1986). Expectant fathers at risk for couvade. *Nursing Research, 35*(5), 290–295.

Colman, A. D., & Colman, L. (1973). *Pregnancy: The psychological experience.* New York: Herder and Herder.

Deutsch, H. (1944). *The psychology of women, vol. 2: Motherhood.* New York: Grune and Stratton.

Diamond, M. J. (1986). Becoming a father: A psychoanalytic perspective on the forgotten parent. *The Psychoanalytic Review, 73*(4), 41–64.

Erikson, E. H. (1956). Ego identity and the psychosocial moratorium. In *New perspective for research,* eds. H. Witmer and R. Kotinsky. Washington, D.C.: U.S. Department of Health, Education, and Welfare.

Grubb, C. (1980). Perceptions of time by multiparous women in relation to themselves and others during the first postpartal month. *MCN, 9*(4), Monograph 10.

Gurwitt, A. R. (1982). Aspects of prospective fatherhood. In *Father and child: Developmental and clinical perspectives,* eds. S. H. Cath, A. R. Gurwitt, and J. M. Ross. Boston: Little, Brown.

Herzog, J. M. (1982). Patterns of expectant fatherhood: A study of the fathers of a group of premature infants. In *Father and child: Developmental and clinical perspectives,* eds. S. H. Cath, A. R. Gurwitt, and J. M. Ross. Boston: Little, Brown.

Hobfall, S. E., Nadler, A., & Leiberman, J. (1986). Satisfaction with social support during crisis: Intimacy and self-esteem or critical determinants. *Journal of Personality and Social Psychology, 51*(2), 296–304.

Horn, M. & Manion, J. (1985). Creative grandparenting: Bonding the generations. *Journal of Obstetrical Gynecological and Neonatal Nursing, 14*(3), 233–236.

Jessner, L., Weigert, E., & Foy, J. L. (1970). The development of parental attitudes during pregnancy. In *Parenthood: Its psychology and psychopathology,* eds., E. J. Anthony and T. Benedek. Boston: Little, Brown.

Liebenberg, B. (1969). Expectant fathers. *Child and Family, 8*(2), 265–278.

Marquart, R. (1976). Expectant fathers: What are their needs? *Am. J. Mat. Child Nurs., 1*(1), 32–36.

May, K. A. (1982a). The father as observer. *MCN, 7,* 315–322.

May, K. A. (1982b). Three phases of father involvement in pregnancy. *Nursing Research, 31,* 337–342.

Mead, G. H. (1934). *Mind, self, and society,* ed. C. W. Morris. Chicago: University of Chicago Press.

Ramsey, C. N., Abell, T. D., & Baker, L. C. (1986). The relationship between family functioning, life events, family structure, and the outcome of pregnancy. *The Journal of Family Practice, 22*(61), 521–527.

Reamy, K., & White, S. E. (1985). Sexuality in pregnancy and the puerperium: A review. *Obstetrical and Gynecological Survey, 40*(1), 1–13.

Richardson, P. (1981). Women's perception of their important dyadic relationships during pregnancy. *MCN, 10*(3), 159–174.

Richardson, P. (1987). Women's important relationships during pregnancy and the preterm labor event. *Western Journal of Nursing Research, 9*(2), 203–222.

Rubin, R. (1967a). Attainment of the maternal role, part 1: Processes. *Nursing Research, 16*(3), 237–245.

Rubin, R. (1967b). Attainment of the maternal role, part 2: Models and referrents. *Nursing Research, 16*(4), 342–346.

Rubin, R. (1967c). The neomaternal period. In *Current concepts in clinical nursing,* ed. B. Bergenson. New York: C. V. Mosby.

Rubin, R. (1970). Cognitive style in pregnancy. *Am. J. Nurs., 70*(3), 502–508.

Rubin, R. (1972). Fantasy and object constancy in maternal relationships. *MCN, 1*(2), 101–111.

Rubin, R. (1975). Maternal tasks in pregnancy. *MCN, 4*(3), 143–153.

Rubin, R. (1984). *Maternal identity and the maternity experience.* New York: Springer-Verlag.

Severino, S. K., Teusink, J. P., & Bernstein, A. E. (1986). Overview: The psychology of grandparenthood. *Journal of Geriatric Psychiatry, 19*(1), 39–55.

Sherwen, L. N. (1986). Third trimester fantasies of first-time expectant fathers. *Maternal-Child Nursing Journal, 15*(3), 153–170.

Sprey, J., & Matthews, S. H. (1982). Contemporary grandparenthood: A systemic transition. *Annals of the American Academy of Political and Social Science 4660, 466*(Nov), 91–103.

Stichler, J. F., Bowden, M. S., & Reimer, E. D. (1978). Pregnancy: A shared emotional experience. *Am. J. Mat. Child Nurs., 3*(3), 153–157.

Swanson, J. (1980). The marital sexual relationship during pregnancy. *J. Obstet. Gynecol., Neonatal Nurs., 9*(5), 267–270.

12

Maternal Nutrition

BEHAVIORAL OBJECTIVES

Upon completion of this chapter, the reader should be able to:

- Describe to a client the reason for specific nutrient increases in pregnancy and lactation

- Discuss the Recommended Daily Allowances for pregnant and lactating women.

- Briefly discuss the role various nutrients play during pregnancy.

- Explain the importance of the client interview.

- Describe the tools used during nutrition assessment.

- Identify biochemical tests used to assess nutritional status.

- Explain the importance of the daily food guide.

- Describe optimum patterns of weight gain during pregnancy for different prepregnancy weights.

- State several nutritional risk factors and why they are considered to be risk factors.

- Discuss some ethnic and cultural influences on eating behavior.

Food, as the source of all nutrients, is essential for life and growth. Without an adequate supply of food, the fetus or newborn cannot grow and develop normally (Worthington-Roberts, Vermeersch, and Williams, 1985). Therefore, good nutrition during pregnancy and lactation is of profound importance. Furthermore, the mother can change her behavior to improve her nutrition, affecting both the infant and herself. The nurse as a change agent in maternity settings can assist mothers in planning the change toward optimal nutrition and lactation. By careful use of the nursing diagnosis and intervention, nurses promote optimal health. Behavioral and lifestyle changes in nutrition made at this time can be longlasting, and the nurse can facilitate these changes. This chapter will discuss the importance of nutrition during pregnancy and the postpartum period and review specific nutrient requirements. Also included is an examination of the nutrition assessment process and its component parts which include the patient interview, biochemical tests, anthropometry, and assessment of risk. Finally, this chapter will address factors that can influence the diet of pregnant and postpartum women and how the nutritional care plan can take these factors into account.

HISTORICAL PERSPECTIVES

Nutritional recommendations for mothers have been communicated by families, communities, and cultures throughout recorded history. Each group has had specific recommendations or restrictions for the pregnant woman, very few of which were based on scientific investigation or well-controlled studies. Tradition, fear, and myth contributed significantly to these messages about nutrition and pregnancy until the 1900s.

Since that time, with increased knowledge of biochemistry and human reproduction, there have been significant gains in the understanding of the nutritional aspects of pregnancy. Studies carried out in the two World Wars concluded that starvation or near starvation, especially during the third trimester, affected the size of the newborn (Keys et al., 1950).

However, it was not until the 1960s that it was recognized that nutrition was an important factor in pregnancy outcome. In an effort to more clearly understand the problem, the National Research Council's Committee on Maternal Nutrition undertook a 3-year study to describe the effects of nutritional factors in pregnancy (Food and Nutrition Board, 1970). Their report organized and presented information related to weight gain, adolescent nutrition during pregnancy, and the effect of nutrition on toxemia of pregnancy.

In 1969, a White House Conference on Food, Nutrition, and Health developed a policy statement calling for a national commitment to maternal nutrition. The Panel wrote:

> There must be a national affirmation that every woman has the right to high quality and high standard health care. This includes a food intake that will prepare her for and carry her through a healthy pregnancy and childbirth and permit her infant to flourish. It affirms that the basic right to adequate nutrition is an inseparable part of the basic right to health care and that women require and are entitled to sufficient amounts of nutritious food (White House Conference on Food, Nutrition, and Health, 1969).

Following this commitment, several government programs were developed to support good nutrition during pregnancy for low-income women. It was recognized that low birth weight and prematurity, especially among the low-income population, was contributing to the high U.S. infant mortality rate. Nutrition became a focus of activity in health professional task forces, and guidelines for nutritional assessment and intervention were published by the American Dietetic Association in collaboration with the American College of Obstetrics and Gynecology (1978).

During the 1980s many states began to develop prenatal care programs that integrate nutrition and nutrition services into the health care plan. These programs usually have a nutritionist as a member of the health care team and the nurse works closely with all care providers to develop the health care plan (Fig. 12–1). The nurse provides nutritional information to the client and assists with behavioral changes that will improve the patient's choices of foods and her diet.

THE IMPORTANCE OF NUTRITION IN PREGNANCY

The growth and development of an entire individual is the nutritional task of pregnancy. The rapid rate of growth and the differentiation of cells and tissues require a substantial increase in nutrients, which are derived from the pregnant woman's food intake. In order to sustain this growth, the maternal systems must increase their effectiveness and efficiency.

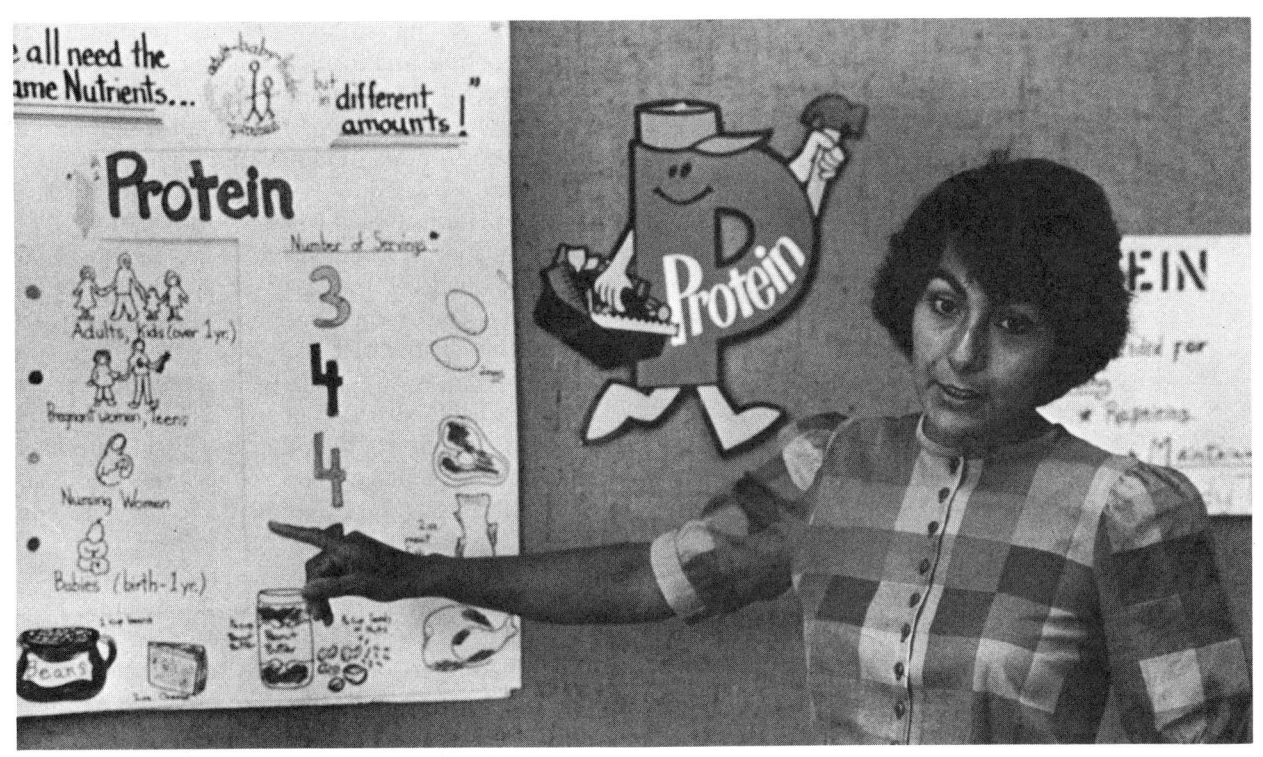

FIGURE 12–1. Nutritionist discussing importance of protein with a group of pregnant women.

For many years researchers have attempted to demonstrate through scientific studies the relationship of nutrition during pregnancy and the health of the newborn. These studies generally fall into a few categories. The first are the epidemiologic studies which review populations for correlations between nutritional factors and birth outcomes. One such study, carried out in the 1960s, examined over 44,000 birth records and found that birth weights increased as the weight gain during pregnancy increased, indicating a definite relationship between the nutritional status of the mother and the health status of the newborn (Naeye, 1979).

A second group of studies that relates nutrition to birth outcome are the diet deficiency studies. Both excesses and deficiencies of nutrients can cause specific congenital malformations. Seller (1987) proposes that major changes in nutrients during embryonic development can cause disturbances resulting in congenital malformations. If these changes occur during the last stage of growth, the effects are not as apparent. As an example of a congenital defect that may be affected by nutrient intake, Seller (1987) refers to studies examining the relationship between neural tube defects and diet.

Actually, studies are now pointing to the importance of nutrition prior to conception and its effect on the outcome of the pregnancy. Caan et al. (1987), in a study of mothers who had short intervals between pregnancies, found that birth outcomes were improved when the women received the nutritious foods offered through the WIC program (Fig. 12–2). These foods were given during the postpartum period following the previous birth and were continued until 5–7 months postpartum. The birth weights and birth lengths of the babies were significantly higher when the mothers were provided with the supplemental foods (California Department of Health Services, 1987).

Nutrition during lactation is also very important. During pregnancy the body generally stores 2–3 kg of fat for lactation. Usually used in the first 5 months of lactation, these stores create a buffer for the mother as the caloric demands of breastfeeding are great. However, a poor diet may result in a decrease in breast milk volume as well as affect the quality of fats and the levels of some vitamins and minerals (California Department of Health Services, 1987).

Although studies may conflict about the degree to which nutrition affects pregnancy outcome and lactation, all authorities recognize the value of good nutrition. Healthy babies and mothers are derived from well nourished populations. On that fact there is no dispute.

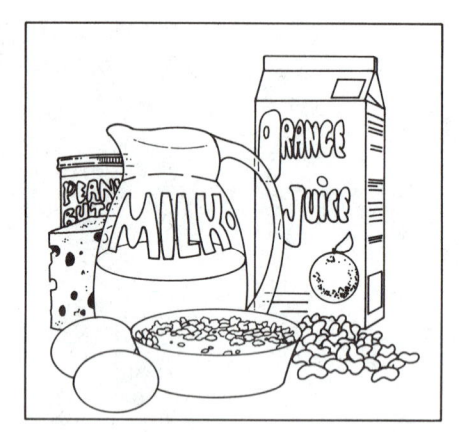

FIGURE 12-2. Food groups for protein requirement.

NUTRITIONAL NEEDS

How much of which foods does the pregnant woman need? She needs to have nutrients in her body available to the fetus and herself for optimal growth, maintenance, and storage.

The Food and Nutrition Board of the National Research Council has published a list of the basic nutrient requirements for pregnancy and lactation as well as for nonpregnant women, men, and children. These basic requirements are called the Recommended Daily Allowances (RDAs) and are calculated to meet the needs of practically all healthy people and include a margin of safety. The RDAs for the adult woman are calculated for an average woman who is 5 ft 4 in tall weighing 120 lb. These recommendations are reviewed periodically and updated as research in the field of nutrition indicates. Although the RDAs cover many nutrients, recommended levels have not been established for all essential nutrients and the Food and Nutrition Board has listed what are called the "Estimated Safe and Adequate Daily Dietary Intakes of Selected Vitamins and Minerals" (Food and Nutrition Board, 1980). Examples of nutrients which are included in this list are such essential nutrients as copper, fluoride, and sodium. Because the requirements for all nutrients are not known a varied diet is essential.

Table 12-1 lists the RDAs for the pregnant woman in different age groups while Table 12-2 shows the same RDAs for nonpregnant women for comparison. The RDAs may vary according to age groups and the RDAs for pregnant adolescents (ages 11-18) are higher than for adults—specifically protein, vitamin D, calcium, and phosphorus. Niacin requirements are higher for girls aged between 11 and 14 than for those aged 15-18.

Unfortunately, many women and teenagers do not meet the RDAs in their regular diets. Ideally,

TABLE 12-1. *Recommended Dietary Allowances for Pregnant and Lactating Women*

| | Age | | | | |
	11-14	15-18	19-22	23-50	Differences for Lactation
Energy, kcal	2500	2400	2400	2300	+200
Protein, g	76	76	74	74	−10
Vitamin A, RE	1000	1000	1000	1000	+200
IU	5000	5000	5000	5000	+1000
Vitamin D, µg	15	15	12.5	10	same
Vitamin E, Q-TE	10	10	10	10	+1
Ascorbic acid, mg	70	80	80	80	+20
Niacin, mg	17	16	16	15	+3
Riboflavin, mg	1.6	1.6	1.6	1.5	+0.2
Thiamin, mg	1.5	1.5	1.5	1.4	+0.1
Vitamin B_6, mg	2.4	2.6	2.6	2.6	−0.1
Folacin, µg	800	800	800	800	−300
Vitamin B_{12}, µg	4	4	4	4	same
Calcium, mg	1600	1600	1200	1200	same
Phosphorus, mg	1600	1600	1200	1200	same
Iodine, µg	175	175	175	175	+25
Iron, mg	18+	18+	18+	18+	+6
Magnesium, mg	450	450	450	450	same
Zinc	20	20	20	20	+5

SOURCE: Food and Nutrition Board (1980).

TABLE 12-2. Recommended Daily Dietary Allowances for Women (nonpregnant)

	Age			
	11-14	15-18	19-22	23-50
Energy, kcal	2200	2100	2100	2000
Protein, g	46	46	44	44
Vitamin A, RE	800	800	800	800
IU	4000	4000	4000	4000
Vitamin D, μg	10	10	7.5	5
Vitamin E, α-TE	8	8	8	18
Ascorbic acid, mg	50	60	60	60
Niacin, mg	15	14	14	13
Riboflavin, mg	1.3	1.3	1.3	1.2
Thiamin, mg	1.1	1.1	1.1	1.0
Vitamin B_6, mg	1.8	2.0	2.0	2.0
Folacin, μg	400	400	400	400
Vitamin B_{12}, μg	3	3	3	3
Calcium, mg	1200	1200	800	800
Phosphorus, mg	1200	1200	800	800
Iodine, μg	150	150	150	150
Iron, mg	18	18	18	18
Magnesium, mg	300	300	300	300
Zinc	15	15	15	15

SOURCE: Food and Nutrition Board (1980).

the diet should conform to the RDAs before pregnancy, so that additional needs are not impossible to achieve. During pregnancy and lactation there are increased requirements for protein, iron, and folacin as well as other vitamins and minerals. There is also a significant increase in energy needs. Energy is measured in kilocalories (kcal) but is commonly known simply as calories.

Energy

Although calorie needs during pregnancy and lactation will be discussed in the section under weight gain, it is worth noting that this is an important and critical requirement during pregnancy and lactation. The number of calories needed varies with the individual and the RDA, for kilocalories do not have a margin of safety since it is assumed that increasing kilocalories is not generally a problem.

Protein

Protein is needed for fetal growth and maternal storage from the 2nd month of pregnancy. The protein requirement is an additional 30 g daily, although the amount needed may vary depending on the type of proteins selected. The RDA is based on a diet of at least one-third animal proteins. If protein from vegetable sources is predominant in the diet, the protein is less complete, that is, missing some essential amino acids, and the requirements are greater.

In the American diet, protein intake is generally sufficient and approaches or exceeds the RDA. For example, the protein requirement during pregnancy of 74 g/day can be met if the woman consumes an average piece of chicken (leg and thigh), a hamburger (4 oz) and three 8-oz glasses of milk over the course of the day (Fig. 12-3).

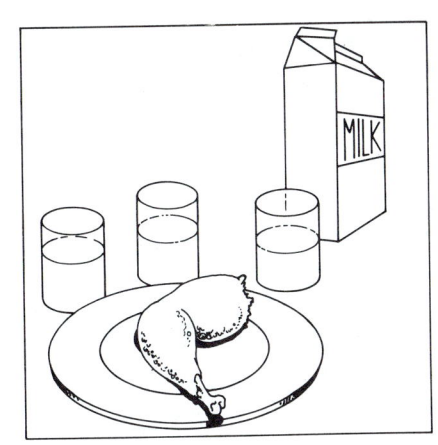

FIGURE 12-3. WIC program foods.

Iron

Increased iron needs result from the increase in maternal blood supply and from the increase in the need for the placenta and fetus. A nonpregnant woman's normal diet supplies moderate amounts of iron, which may not meet the RDA of 18 mg/day. Added to that is the increased need during pregnancy which often cannot be met through diet alone. During lactation an additional 5–6 mg/day over the prenatal requirement is recommended because of the amount of iron that is needed in maternal milk. Consequently, the iron levels of most women are often low, and 33–50 percent of pregnant women have low hematocrits if iron supplements are not used. Therefore, it is recommended that 30–60 mg of supplemental iron be prescribed during pregnancy, postpartum and during lactation.

Only approximately 10 percent of the iron in food is actually absorbed and the rate of absorption is dependent on several factors (Food and Nutrition Board, 1980). For example, studies have shown that when either ascorbic acid (vitamin C) or an animal or fish protein is present in the meal, iron absorption is increased. Therefore, many nutritionists recommend that a patient drink orange juice with their meals. It is known that iron from animal sources is absorbed more completely than iron from vegetables sources. The intake of a large quantity of one mineral, such as zinc, at the same time as iron decreases iron absorption. Excessive quantities of dietary fiber also promote decreased iron absorption by binding minerals in the stool. These competing factors are important to recognize when counseling women who have inadequate stores of iron in their bodies. Table 12–3 lists some food sources of iron.

TABLE 12–3. Examples of Food Sources of Iron

Liver[a]
Beef[a]
Fortified breakfast cereals[a]
Enriched grains
Dark meat poultry
Eggs
Spinach
Canned or dried beans, peas and lentils

[a]These foods are very high sources of iron.

Calcium, Phosphorus, and Magnesium

The requirements for these three minerals increase by 50 percent in pregnancy and lactation (see Table 12–1). Calcium is important not only for bone and teeth development of the fetus and the infant but also blood clotting, normal muscle action, and other metabolic activities (Williams, 1985). Working to the advantage of the pregnant woman is the fact that vitamin D, parathyroid hormone, estrogen, and progesterone improve maternal absorption of calcium and result in an increase in the maternal bone mass. However, the pregnant and lactating woman still must make a conscious effort to increase her intake of high calcium foods since the RDA of 1200 mg is often difficult to meet. Dairy products such as milk, cheese, and yogurt are excellent sources of this essential mineral. Table 12–4 includes some foods that are considered to be good dietary sources of calcium.

Phosphorus is available in many common foods and is closely associated with calcium in the body. Like calcium it is involved with bone growth, but, unlike calcium, phosphorus deficiency seldom occurs. However, a high intake of phosphorus can upset the calcium–phosphorus balance and cause a subsequent loss of calcium. Phosphorus is present in milk and milk products as well as lean meats. Excess phosphorus is now entering the American diet through processed foods and soft drinks (Williams, 1985).

Magnesium is also a component of bone and is involved in a variety of metabolic functions

TABLE 12–4. Dietary Sources of Calcium (provides 250–300 mg of calcium)

Milk, 8 oz
Cheese (hard and semi-soft), $1\frac{1}{2}$ oz
Cottage cheese, 2 cups
Ice cream, $1\frac{1}{2}$ cups
Yogurt, 8 oz
Pudding, 8 oz
Tofu (if made with a calcium salt), 7 oz
Sardines, 6 medium
Salmon, canned, $\frac{1}{2}$ cup
Mackerel, canned, $\frac{1}{2}$ cup
Broccoli, collard greens, mustard greens, kale, $1\frac{1}{2}$–2 cups cooked

SOURCE: Adapted from California Department of Health Services (1987).

including carbohydrate and protein metabolism (Williams, 1985). Foods rich in magnesium are vegetable proteins, whole grains, nuts, and bananas.

Zinc and Iodine

The RDA for zinc increases to 20 mg during pregnancy and to 25 mg during lactation. Given that the regular American diet is low in zinc the pregnant or lactating woman must pay particular attention to the inclusion of zinc in her diet. The importance of zinc can be attributed to the fact that it is an essential component in many cell enzyme systems (Williams, 1985). The best food sources of zinc are meats, eggs, and seafood, especially oysters. Other good sources of zinc include legumes and nuts.

Iodine is important for thyroid hormone synthesis and the requirement is elevated during pregnancy and lactation. The American diet generally has more than sufficient iodine to meet these needs, especially since iodized salt is widely used.

Fat-Soluble Vitamins

Certain vitamins are soluble in fats and are stored in the body. These vitamins include vitamins A, D, and E. The need for vitamin A during pregnancy increases to 1000 I.U. (International Units) and is even higher during lactation (1200 I.U.). Vitamin A is essential for a variety of body functions and during fetal development it is critical for epithelial tissue formation, bone and teeth growth, and cell development (Williams, 1985).

Vitamin A can be formed by the body from the precursor beta-carotene, which is found in plants, or is available from animal sources as vitamin A. Deep yellow and dark green vegetables and fruits are excellent plant sources of beta-carotene, while liver and eggs are good sources for the pre-formed vitamin A. Also, butter and fortified margarines contain some vitamin A. Women should have little difficulty in making certain that their diets during pregnancy and lactation have sufficient amounts of vitamin A. Excessively large intakes of vitamin A, called megadoses, that are over 50,000 I.U. can be harmful during pregnancy. There have been cases reported of congenital malformations during pregnancy when mothers have taken megadose supplements of this vitamin. Because vitamin A is fat-soluble and therefore is stored in the body, it theoretically may lead to such effects on the developing fetus.

Vitamin D, another fat-soluble vitamin, is intricately involved in calcium and phosphorus metabolism. During pregnancy and lactation the requirement increases due to the demand from fetal skeletal development, but the need can be met by consuming milk, which is fortified with vitamin D. There are only a few good food sources of vitamin D (yeast and fish oil) but exposure to ultraviolet rays (sunlight) will result in the synthesis of the vitamin in the skin.

As an antioxidant vitamin E slows down the breakdown of cells by oxygen. A further 2 International Units is added in pregnancy to the 8 International Units recommended for nonpregnant women, even though deficiencies are very rare. Vegetable oils as well as meat, fish, eggs, and leafy green vegetables are good sources of vitamin E.

Water-soluble Vitamins

Unlike the fat-soluble vitamins, which are stored for long periods, water-soluble vitamins must be regularly supplied. If excessive amounts are taken, they are mostly excreted in the urine. During pregnancy, there are increased requirements for many of the water-soluble vitamins, the largest increase being folacin.

During pregnancy the need for folacin, also called folic acid, doubles to 800 µg/day since folacin is critical for DNA synthesis. When one realizes the enormous quantity of DNA that must be produced not only to develop the embryo into a full-sized newborn but also to increase the maternal support structures, it becomes apparent as to why the demand for folacin is so great during pregnancy. It may be difficult to meet the RDA when eating a regular American diet and, therefore, folacin supplements are recommended during pregnancy. Although the requirements during lactation are less, there is still a 25 percent increase over the nonpregnant RDA and supplementation is usually continued. Folacin deficiency during pregnancy can cause megaloblastic anemia and may be associated with other conditions including congenital malformations (Sellers, 1987).

This B-complex vitamin is very important during pregnancy and lactation and women should be encouraged to eat foods high in folacin, including green leafy vegetables, asparagus, liver, and orange juice. Table 12–5 contains a more complete list of foods rich in folacin.

TABLE 12-5. Dietary Sources of Folacin (provides 75 µg of folacin)

Broccoli, $\frac{3}{4}$ cup cooked
Asparagus, $\frac{1}{2}$ cup cooked
Lettuce greens such as endive and romaine, 1 cup
Peas, $\frac{3}{4}$ cup (unless canned)
Liver, 2 oz
Dried beans cooked, 1 cup
Peanuts, $\frac{1}{2}$ cup
Orange juice, $\frac{3}{4}$ cup
Oranges, 2 medium
Cantaloupe, $\frac{1}{2}$ medium
Tomato juice, $1\frac{1}{2}$ cups

SOURCE: Adapted from California Department of Health Services (1987).

Other B vitamins, including B_6, niacin, riboflavin, and thiamin, are important in key metabolic activities that relate to energy production and tissue synthesis (Williams, 1985). Therefore, the Recommended Daily Allowances are increased during pregnancy and lactation and these B vitamins are usually included in the regular prenatal supplement. Good sources of thiamin include beef, pork, enriched or whole grains, and legumes. An excellent dietary source for riboflavin is milk, while niacin can be found in meats and enriched grains.

Vitamin B_6 (pyridoxine) is involved in a variety of metabolic functions including protein, fat and carbohydrate metabolism. Deficiencies during pregnancy have occurred and can be corrected with supplements (Williams, 1985). Some women may start their pregnancy with low levels of B_6 if they had been using oral contraceptives. Oral contraceptives have been found to increase the need for B_6 in some women and supplements are sometimes recommended.

Supplementation

The physiologic demands of pregnancy and lactation, arising from both the growing fetus and infant and the maternal metabolic needs, result in an increased need for a wide variety of nutrients. Many of these needs can be met by increasing certain foods in the diet that are rich in these nutrients. These changes in eating behavior by the patient require careful planning and supplements are routinely prescribed to ensure adequate intake. A supplement should contain at least 30–60 mg of iron, 400–800 µg of folacin and the RDAs of vitamins C, D, E, B_6, and other B vitamins. Zinc is added because of the high requirement during pregnancy and is supplemented at the RDA level of 20 mg. Calcium is usually added to prenatal supplements but should not be higher than 250 mg, since in larger doses it may inhibit absorption of iron and zinc (California Department of Health Services, 1987). Calcium supplements made from bone meal, dolomite, or oyster shells are not recommended as they may be contaminated with harmful substances such as lead or mercury (Roberts, 1983).

NUTRITIONAL ASSESSMENT

All pregnant and lactating women require an assessment of their nutritional status regardless of income and education. The nurse's task in nutrition assessment is to define the patient's nutrient needs during pregnancy and lactation, assess the patient to identify any deficits, and develop a nutritional plan with the patient to improve her diet. This assessment should preferably be done at the patient's first prenatal visit by either the nurse or, if one is available, the nutritionist or dietitian.

The Health Care Team

The nurse is a member of the perinatal health care team that may include the medical provider (physician or midwife), social worker, nutritionist, and health educator. Often the nurse is the first health professional to see the pregnant patient and may be the first to learn of any nutritional problems. Sometimes a nutritionist is available for nutritional assessment and case management but often one is not available, or available only for high-risk patients, such as diabetic women. Therefore, it is essential that the nurse understands the nutritional requirements of pregnancy and lactation and is familiar with the process of nutritional assessment.

Nutritional Risk Factors

There are certain conditions or factors that may identify a woman as being nutritionally at risk. Some of these factors are:

1. Adolescence
2. Short interconceptual interval

3. Low income
4. Overweight
5. Underweight
6. Inadequate weight gain
7. Excessive weight gain
8. Anemia
9. Smoking, alcohol use, or drug addiction
10. Pica
11. Breastfeeding during pregnancy
12. Poor diet
13. Medical conditions such as diabetes, kidney dysfunction

These risk factors alert the nurse to special needs that the patient may have which can adversely affect the pregnancy. This information can be added to that from the physical examination, nutrition history, anthropometric measurements, and biochemical tests to determine the overall nutritional status of the patient. Recommendations can then be made to the patient for changes in her behavior and diet.

The Client Interview and Nutritional History

The client interview remains the most valuable beginning for patient care of any type. It is through the interview that the nurse can learn about the patient's diet and any other factors that may influence her nutritional status such as cultural background, education, and family structure. It is therefore critical that the interview be conducted in a careful and supportive manner so that as much information as possible can be elicited (Fig. 12–4).

During the interview the nurse will collect information about the patient's diet, also called the nutrition history. This information is used as the basis for making a dietary assessment, that is, evaluating the diet for adequacy as well as to determine if the client is ingesting excessive amounts of high-calorie foods or non-nutritive substances. The nurse may also be able to identify from the history any food aversions, intolerances, or allergies. Based on the assessment the nurse and patient will jointly develop a behavior change plan to bring the diet up to recommended standards.

The interviewing process is the key to not only collecting the information that the nurse needs but also to establishing the trust that is necessary for the patient to be willing to make behavioral changes. Introducing oneself and stating interest

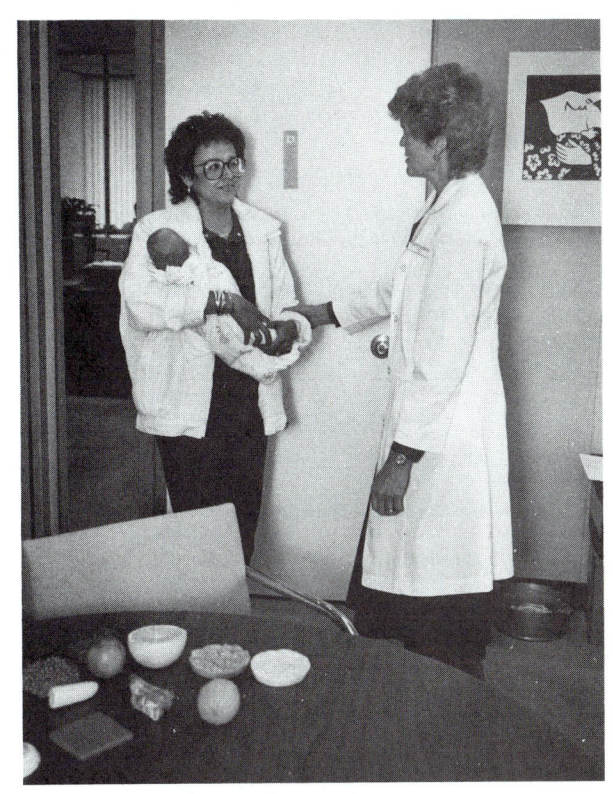

FIGURE 12–4. Nurse greeting client with newborn for nutritional history.

and concern begins a relationship and stimulates motivation.

There are many aspects to the nutrition interview, other than simply gathering verbal information, that can affect the success of the interview. One component that can affect the outcome is nonverbal communication used by both the client and nurse (Snetselaar, 1983). The nurse needs to be aware of this type of communication and be ready to utilize it in the interview as it can assist her in a successful outcome. The following are some examples that Cormier and Cormier (1979) give of nonverbal communication:

Client Behavior	Possible Meaning
Leans forward	Readiness to provide information
Low voice	Reluctance to provide information

Another critical component of the interview is listening, especially listening by the nurse. By carefully listening to the patient the nurse can show her interest and be assured of hearing correctly. Developing good listening skills will aid

State of California—Health and Welfare Agency
Department of Health Services

NUTRITION QUESTIONNAIRE
FOR PRENATAL WOMEN

Name: _____ I.D. No.: _____ Date: _____

Please answer the following questions by checking the appropriate box or by filling in the blank. "Y" means "yes" and "N" means "no." Answer only the questions which apply to you. All information is confidential.

FOR OFFICE USE ONLY

1. a. How many times have you been pregnant? _____
   b. If you have children, list their names, birthdates, and birth weights below.

   Name, Birthdate, and Birthweight   Name, Birthdate, and Birthweight
   _____   _____
   _____   _____
   _____   _____

2. Do you now have or have you ever had any of the following?

Y N		Y N		Y N	
☐ ☐	Abnormal pap smear	☐ ☐	Kidney disease	☐ ☐	Premature infant
☐ ☐	Allergy/asthma	☐ ☐	Liver disease/hepatitis	☐ ☐	Infant weighing less than 5½ lb.
☐ ☐	Anemia	☐ ☐	Tuberculosis		
☐ ☐	Cancer	☐ ☐	Miscarriage	☐ ☐	Infant weighing 9 lbs. or more
☐ ☐	Diabetes	☐ ☐	Preeclampsia/eclampsia		
☐ ☐	Heart disease	☐ ☐	Multiple pregnancy	☐ ☐	Infant with medical problems
☐ ☐	Herpes	☐ ☐	C-section delivery		
☐ ☐	High blood pressure	☐ ☐	Hemorrhage during/after delivery	☐ ☐	Infant death
☐ ☐	Intestinal problems			☐ ☐	Other_____

3. Do you now have, or have you had any of the following?

Y N		Y N		Y N	
☐ ☐	Nausea	☐ ☐	Diarrhea	☐ ☐	Stress
☐ ☐	Vomiting	☐ ☐	Heartburn	☐ ☐	Cold, Flu
☐ ☐	Constipation/hemorrhoids	☐ ☐	Leg Cramps	☐ ☐	Other illness _____

4. a. Before this pregnancy, what was your usual weight?
      _____ Pounds   _____ Don't know
   b. If you have been pregnant before, how much weight did you gain during your last pregnancy?
      _____ Pounds   _____ Don't know
   c. How much weight do you expect to gain during this pregnancy?
      _____ Pounds   _____ Don't know
   d. Have you ever been:
      _____ Underweight   _____ Overweight

5. a. How often do you exercise (besides housework, child care)? _____
   b. What types of exercise(s) do you do? _____

6. Do you crave anything?   ☐ Yes   ☐ No
   If yes, what: _____

7. During your pregnancy, have you wanted to eat any of the following?

Y N		Y N		Y N	
☐ ☐	Ice/freezer frost	☐ ☐	Laundry starch	☐ ☐	Plaster
☐ ☐	Cornstarch	☐ ☐	Dirt or clay	☐ ☐	Other: _____

8. Are there any foods that you avoid eating?   ☐ Yes   ☐ No
   If yes, which food(s)? _____
   Why? _____

FIGURE 12–5. Nutrition questionaire.

NUTRITION QUESTIONNAIRE FOR PRENATAL WOMEN (Continued)

FOR OFFICE USE ONLY

9. Are you now on any of these special diets?
   - Y N Diabetic
   - Y N Low fat
   - Y N Low salt
   - Y N Weight loss
   - Y N Other: _____
   If yes, who suggested the diet? _____

10. a. Are you a vegetarian? ☐ Yes ☐ No
    b. If yes, do you consume milk products (milk, cheese, yogurt) and/or eggs? ☐ Yes ☐ No

11. a. During this pregnancy, are you taking the following?
    - Y N Prenatal vitamins/minerals
    - Y N Iron
    - Y N Other vitamins/minerals
    - Y N Aspirin
    - Y N Antihistamines/cold remedies
    - Y N Laxatives
    - Y N Other nonprescription drugs
    - Y N Birth control pills
    - Y N Other prescription drugs
    - Y N Marijuana
    - Y N Other drugs
    b. Is your doctor/clinic aware you are taking medications or drugs? ☐ Yes ☐ No

12. How many cups of the following liquids do you drink per day?
    ____ Water   ____ Sodas with sugar   ____ Coffee
    ____ Juice   ____ Diet soda, diet punch   ____ Tea
    ____ Milk   ____ Punch, Kool-Aid®   ____ Other: _____

13. a. How often do you drink beer, wine, hard liquor, or mixed drinks? _____
    b. When you drink, how much do you drink? _____
    c. Which type of alcoholic beverage do you drink most often? _____
    d. During this pregnancy, how many times have you had more than four drinks on any single occasion? _____

14. How many cigarettes do you smoke each day?
    ☐ Do not smoke
    ☐ Less than ½ pack/day (10 or less cigarettes)
    ☐ More than 1 pack/day (more than 20 cigarettes)
    ☐ ½—1 pack/day (11–20 cigarettes)

15. What was the highest grade or year of regular school you have completed?
    ☐ Elementary School   ☐ High School   ☐ Four-Year College
    ☐ Junior High School   ☐ Two-Year College   ☐ Graduate School

16. Do you live: ☐ Alone   ☐ With own family   ☐ With other people

17. Do you have access to a working stove, refrigerator, and oven? ☐ Yes ☐ No

18. Who does the following for your household:
    a. Plan meals   ☐ Self   ☐ Other
    b. Buys food   ☐ Self   ☐ Other
    c. Prepares food ☐ Self   ☐ Other

19. Which best describes the type and amount of food in your household?
    ☐ Enough of the kinds wanted
    ☐ Enough, but not always the kind wanted
    ☐ Sometimes not enought
    ☐ Often not enough

20. Are you receiving any of the following?
    ☐ Food Stamps   ☐ Medi-Cal   ☐ Other: _____
    ☐ WIC   ☐ AFDC/Welfare

21. a. How do you plan to feed your baby?
    ☐ Breastfeed   ☐ Both breast and formula
    ☐ Formula feed   ☐ Other: _____
    b. Have you ever breastfed or tried to breastfeed before? ☐ Yes ☐ No
    c. If yes, how long did you breastfeed? _____
    d. Why did you stop breastfeeding? _____

Reviewed By: _____

in building the trust relationship that is critical to the successful nurse–patient interaction. Recognizing the nurse's interest, clients will increase their own interest and will pay attention to the nurse.

Assessment Tools

Information about the patient's diet, behaviors and other factors that can affect her nutrition are collected utilizing several different forms. During the interview the nurse may administer a *nutrition questionnaire* or have the patient complete it while she is waiting to see the physician. An example of a nutrition questionnaire is shown in Fig. 12–5 and consists of questions about the patient's behavior and past history that may affect her current nutritional status. Next, the patient would complete a *dietary intake form*, which again may be filled out by the patient or by the nurse. If the patient completes it herself the nurse needs to make certain that clear instructions are given and then she must check the form for accuracy.

The dietary intake can take several forms. One type, called the *24-hour recall* method, requires that the patient either write down or tell the interviewer everything that she has eaten during the last 24-hour period. This method has the advantages that it is relatively easy to remember what one ate during the previous day and it is a fairly fast and accurate method. Table 12–6 lists recommended instructions for the patient who is completing the recall herself.

Another type of intake is the *food diary record*, where the woman records after she has eaten what was consumed. It may cover 2 days, 1 week, or some time period in between. This method has the advantage that it may more closely approximate the patient's usual diet since it covers more than 1 day. It also does not rely on memory but it does require that the patient consistently complete the form after each meal or snack. A major drawback to this method is that the patient may alter what she eats as a result of needing to record it. A third technique is called the *food frequency list*. It consists of a list of foods that contain nutrients needed during pregnancy and lactation and the patient tells the nurse which foods she eats and how frequently.

It is recommended that all patients complete a nutrition questionnaire and a dietary intake. Combining the food frequency list with a 24-hour recall format, as suggested by Williams (1985), is the most practical method for the diet history.

TABLE 12–6. *Patient Instructions for Completing a 24-hour Recall*

1. Please write down everything, all foods and liquids, that you consumed during the last 24 hours . . . from the time you awakened yesterday morning until you went to sleep yesterday evening.
2. Use measuring cups or spoons to describe the amount. For example:
   1 cup cornflakes
   $\frac{1}{2}$ cup milk (whole)
   1 tsp. sugar
3. Tell what is in a mixed food. For example:
   1 cup stew ($\frac{1}{4}$ cup meat, $\frac{1}{4}$ cup potato, $\frac{1}{4}$ cup gravy)
4. Remember to write down what is used in preparing the food. For example:
   Coated in batter
5. Remember to write down all the extras such as butter, jelly, and sugar.
6. Remember to write down snacks and drinks between meals.

SOURCE: Adapted from California Department of Health Services (1987).

The interviewer will soon learn that there are some aids that can assist the patient in recalling what foods she has eaten. Williams (1985) suggests that patients recall their activities during the day and then use this information to assist them in recalling what they have eaten. The questions that the interviewer asks can also assist the patient in recall. For example, if the patient states that she had a slice of toast the nurse would elicit more information by asking what type of bread, was it a normal size, did it have anything on it, if so, was it a teaspoon size pat of butter, etc. Many nutritionists use food models to assist patients in determining portion size. These food models are accurate replicas of common foods in actual sizes. If a patient, for example, has eaten spinach, the nurse may show her a food model of spinach in a half-cup portion and the patient can determine if her portion was the same.

Daily Food Guide

Once the information from the nutrition interview has been gathered, analysis begins. The diet is compared with the RDAs described earlier but, for convenience, the diet is assessed according to a recommended *daily food guide*. The guide has several categories of foods and if foods are eaten from each category according to the recommendations, then the patient will meet the Recommended Dietary Allowances for the majority of nutrients. The daily food guide may vary according to its source as there is not total agreement on what is both practical for the client and what will meet her nutrient needs. Table 12–7 is one example of a daily food guide for pregnant and lactating women. It is important to remember that varying the diet is essential for meeting the majority of nutrient requirements.

Many patients find it useful to see a *sample meal plan* which gives them an example of a balanced diet. Table 12–8 shows a sample diet for a pregnant woman that follows the daily food guide. Also useful for the patient to take home with her is a booklet explaining nutrient requirements during pregnancy and lactation, the daily food guide, and other information about nutrition. These booklets are available from a variety of sources including state and county health departments and the March of Dimes.

Most of the responsibility for improving the diet rests with the patient herself. However, there are several ways in which the nurse can influence the patient and increase her compliance with the recommended changes. Listed below are some suggestions (California Department of Health Services, 1987):

1. Involve the client in active participation.
2. Individualize advice so that it is specific to personal preferences and lifestyle.
3. Reinforce suggestions in regularly scheduled follow-up visits.
4. Be empathetic, warm, show interest, and demonstrate genuine concern.

Biochemical Tests

Nutritional assessments from dietary histories may reveal shortcomings in the diet but there are several biochemical tests that can indicate existing nutritional deficiencies. Biochemical tests can also uncover other abnormalities that may affect the pregnancy outcome.

Certain tests are used to test for nutritional anemias which may be caused by a deficiency in iron, folacin, or B_{12} (San Francisco Department Health, 1987). Nutritional anemias have been linked to complications of pregnancy (Garn et al., 1981). The most common type of anemia in pregnancy is iron deficiency. Since anemia occurs with some frequency during pregnancy, blood

TABLE 12–7. *Daily Food Guide for Pregnant and Lactating Women*

Food Group	Number of Servings
Milk and milk products	4 (serving size of 1 cup, milk, $1\frac{1}{2}$ oz cheese)
Protein foods	4, recommended 1–2 servings of vegetable protein (serving size of 2 oz meat, fish, poultry or 2 eggs; 1 cup cooked beans, 2 oz peanut butter, $\frac{1}{2}$ cup nuts or seeds)
Grain products	6 servings (serving size of 1 slice bread, $\frac{1}{2}$–$\frac{3}{4}$ cup of cereal, $\frac{1}{2}$ cup of rice, $\frac{1}{2}$ cup of pasta, 1 tortilla)
Vitamin C, fruit, and vegetables	1 serving ($\frac{3}{4}$ cup orange juice, $\frac{1}{2}$ grapefruit, $\frac{1}{2}$ cup broccoli, $\frac{1}{2}$ green or red pepper)
Dark green vegetables	1 serving ($\frac{3}{4}$ cup cooked spinach, broccoli, brussel sprouts, leafy greens, dark green lettuce)
Other fruits and vegetables	2–3 servings

SOURCE: Adapted from March of Dimes (1986).

TABLE 12–8. *A Day's Sample Menu for Pregnant Women*

Breakfast:	orange juice, bran flakes with peaches, milk
Morning snack:	peanut butter on whole wheat toast, milk, fruit
Lunch:	vegetable juice, egg salad sandwich with lettuce, tomato slices, 2 oatmeal cookies
Afternoon snack:	cup of yoghurt, carrot sticks
Dinner:	chicken, carrot, raisin, and apple salad, baked potato, broccoli, apple juice
Evening snack:	crackers with cheese, milk, dried apricots

SOURCE: Adapted from March of Dimes (1986).

tests to measure hematocrit and hemoglobin levels are performed on all pregnant and postpartum women. The Mean Corpuscular Volume (MCV) test, which is the average volume of red blood cells in a sample, is another method for evaluating the presence of anemia and can assist in determining if the anemia is due to an iron deficiency or is caused by a drop in folacin levels. However, if both deficiencies are present, the MCV may not be helpful. B_{12} deficiency is much rarer and is most likely to be seen in patients who are strict vegetarians, since animal foods are the chief source of B_{12} (California Department of Health Services, 1987). It is recommended that hemoglobin, hematocrit, and MCV tests be performed at the first prenatal visit, at the beginning of the third trimester and again at the postpartum visit. Table 12–9 gives guidelines for evaluating the results of these tests (San Francisco Department of Health, 1987).

Urine is routinely checked for protein and glucose using a simple and quick test. High levels of protein may indicate preeclampsia, a condition of elevated blood pressure that occasionally occurs during pregnancy. (Preeclampsia is explained further in Chapter 30). During pregnancy there is an increased incidence of diabetes called gestational diabetes which needs to be carefully controlled to avoid serious consequences for the fetus. Approximately 3–5% of all pregnant women develop gestational diabetes. (See Chapter 30 for more information on diabetes during pregnancy.) If either protein or glucose levels in the urine is abnormal, further tests are usually performed to determine the cause of the abnormal test results.

Often gestational diabetes begins later in pregnancy. Since it is critical to screen for this condition, a *glucose tolerance test* is generally administered at 24–26 weeks gestation for all pregnant women to test for gestational diabetes (San Francisco Dept. of Health, 1987). This procedure tests for elevated blood glucose levels after the patient has followed a prescribed diet that includes a specific amount of carbohydrates.

A physical exam should be a part of a complete nutritional evaluation. Table 12–10 lists some clinical signs of inadequate nutrition although these conditions can be caused by other factors.

Anthropometric Assessment

Anthropometry refers to the measurement of physical characteristics such as weight and height. Since prepregnancy weight and weight gain during pregnancy are useful predictors of outcome, weight measurements are essential in prenatal care. The nurse needs to determine the patient's percent of desirable weight for height in order to determine if the patient was underweight or overweight prior to becoming pregnant. Table 12–11 lists desirable weight for height. Weight and height should be measured at the initial prenatal visit. Weight should be measured at each subsequent visit.

Weight Gain and Weight Control

How much weight the pregnant woman should gain has been the subject of great debate. As early as 1889, a German physician recommended high-protein, low-carbohydrate, fluid-restricted diets to reduce the birth weight of infants born to mothers with contracted pelves (Hytten and Leitch, 1971). Even in the early 1970s, many physicians were still assuming that a limited weight gain reduced complications. However, in the 1960s several studies found that an increase in maternal weight resulted in an increase in the birth weight of the offspring. A landmark report, *Maternal Nutrition and the Course of Pregnancy* (Food and Nutrition Board, 1970), concluded that an average weight gain during pregnancy of 24 lb is desirable.

Current research is focusing on what the recommended weight gain should be for different categories of pregnant women. The recommendations are based on prepregnancy weight and are as

---

TABLE 12–9. *Definitions of Nutritional Anemias*

Test	Mild/Moderate Deficiency	Severe Deficiency
Hemoglobin (Hbg)	<11.0 g	<10.0 g
Hematocrit (Hct)	≤33.0%	≤30.0%
MCV	<77.5 or >97.5	<75.0 or >100.0

SOURCE: San Francisco Department of Health, 1987

TABLE 12–10. Significant Clinical Signs in Nutritional Evaluation

Body Area	Clinical Signs that may Indicate Poor Nutritional Status	Possible Nutritional Implications
Hair	Dull, dry, sparse, or shedding	Multiple nutrient inadequacies may be present (e.g. protein and vitamin deficiencies)
Face	Swollen or edematous	Protein deficiency (albumin) or sodium excess with resultant water retention
	Pale	Iron and protein inadequacies
Eyes	Pale conjunctivae	Iron deficiency
	Redness of membranes; redness and fissuring of eyelid corners	Vitamin B complex inadequacies, especially of riboflavin
	Dryness of membranes; dullness of cornea	Vitamin A deficiencies
Lips	Swollen, red cracks at the sides (cheilosis)	Vitamin B complex inadequacies, especially of riboflavin
Tongue	Bright red or swollen	Vitamin B complex inadequacies or GI disorders
	Pale	Iron deficiency
	Papillary hypertrophy	Multiple nutrient inadequacies
Teeth	Carious or missing	Excessive intake of carbohydrate (sucrose) or alcohol, poor hygiene, or multiple nutrient inadequacies (e.g. calcium)
Gums	Bleeding	Vitamin C deficiency with resultant true or conditioned scurvy
Glands	Thyroid enlargement (goiter)	Iodine inadequacy or toxicity
Abdomen	Edematous	See Face
Skin	Dry, flaking, or scaly	Vitamin A or B complex deficiencies
	Petechiae (small purple spots or hemorrhages under the skin)	Vitamin C deficiency
	Poor turgor or tone; pressure scores	Multiple nutrient inadequacies, especially of protein and vitamin C
	Xanthomas (fat deposits under the skin, around joints, and under the eyes)	Increased serum levels of LDLs or VLDLs with resultant hyperlipoproteinemia
Nails	Brittle, ridged, or spoon-shaped	Iron deficiency
Extremities	Muscle wasting	Macronutrient inadequacies (carbohydrate, fat, and protein) with resultant marasmus
		Protein deficiency with resultant kwashiorkor
	Edematous	See Face
Nervous system	Mental irritability and confusion; burning and tingling of hands and feet (paresthesis); loss of position and vibratory sense; weakness and tenderness of muscles (may result in inability to walk); decrease and loss of ankle and knee reflexes	Chronic nutrient inadequacies, especially B complex (e.g. thiamin) deficiencies; excessive intake of alcohol or drugs

SOURCE: California Department of Health Services (1987).

TABLE 12–11. *Desirable Weight for Height (Weight without clothes and height without shoes for women 25 and older)*[a]

Height (in)	Desirable Weight (lb)	<90% Desirable Weight (lb)	>135% Desirable Weight (lb)
58	106	94	144
59	109	97	148
60	112	100	152
61	115	102	156
62	119	106	162
63	122	109	166
64	126	112	171
65	130	116	177
66	134	119	182
67	138	123	188
68	142	126	193
69	147	131	200
70	151	134	205

[a]For women between 18 and 24 years, subtract 1 lb for each year less than 25.
SOURCE: Adapted from California Department of Health Services (1987).

follows (adapted from San Francisco Department of Health, 1987):

1. 30+ lb for underweight women (<90 percent of standard weight).
2. 24–30 lb for normal and moderately overweight women.
3. 15–20 lb for obese women (>135 percent of standard weight).

Underweight women, that is those weighing less than 90 percent of the standard weight, tend to have babies of lower birth weight than women who are heavier (Abrams and Laros, 1986). The nurse will need to evaluate the underweight woman's diet carefully and make recommendations to assure sufficient calorie as well as nutrient intake. Ideally, the underweight woman who is planning to become pregnant should try to increase her weight prior to becoming pregnant.

Studies have shown that weight gain during normal pregnancy follows the pattern shown in Fig. 12–6. During the first trimester the weight gain is generally 2–4 lb. Thereafter, the gain is approximately 1 lb/week. Figure 12–6 has three distinct curves, each one for the different categories of prepregnancy weight described above. The nurse plots the weight gain at every prenatal visit on the chart according to the week of gestation with the prepregnancy weight being the starting point or zero. The prenatal weight gain grid is a useful tool for recognizing weight gain problems but small variations around the average curve are considered normal. By showing the patient her weight gain on a chart the nurse can further the patient's understanding of what a normal weight gain is.

Women who lose more than 5 lb in the first trimester, or are at less than prepregnancy weight at 14 weeks gestation, are considered to be at increased risk and should be carefully evaluated and counseled. The same is true for women who gain less than 2 lb during any month in the second or third trimester. Inadequate maternal weight gain has been linked to low birth weight and perinatal morbidity and mortality (Committee to Study the Prevention of Low Birthweight, 1985).

Excessive weight gain during pregnancy, assuming there is no underlying medical condition, usually does not compromise the outcome. However, it may result in obesity in the postpartum woman which can lead to the development of obesity-related diseases such as diabetes. Therefore, a woman who gains in excess of 9 lb/month or more than 2.2 lb/week should be counseled and her diet reviewed. It needs to be stressed that *dieting* during pregnancy *should be avoided* and that the goal is a more gradual weight gain. Nutritionists are concerned that when calorie intake is restricted to the point where fat stores are burned, then Ketosis can result. This condition has been associated with impaired fetal development (Food and Nutrition Board, 1980).

Patients often have a better understanding of the

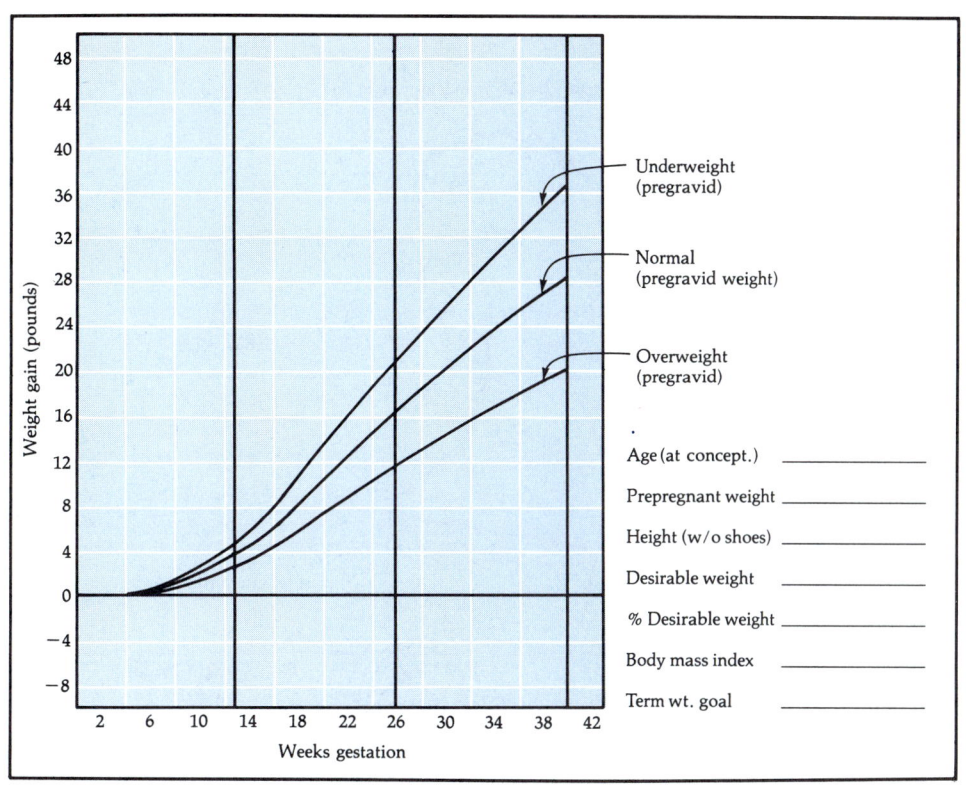

FIGURE 12-6. Prenatal weight gain grid.

importance of gaining weight during pregnancy when they understand where the extra weight goes. As Fig. 12-7 shows, the fetus, placenta, and amniotic fluid contribute less than half of the optimal weight gain. An important component of the weight gain are the maternal stores which provide essential energy during lactation. Not only are extra calories needed to provide for the weight gain shown in Fig. 12-6, but the increase in calories is also needed to meet the energy requirements of pregnancy. Therefore, the RDA for pregnancy includes an additional 300 kcal which may vary according to the individual's requirements.

Weight Control During Lactation and Postpartum

There is a significant increase in the RDA for calories when a woman is lactating. This increase results from both the energy requirements for the production of milk and the calorie content of the milk itself. There is also a large increase in fluid needs, up to 4 liters of liquid daily, and there is a corresponding increase in thirst.

The nutritional requirements vary with the amount of milk produced. After establishment, the milk supply is about 600-700 ml daily. This amount varies depending on the baby's needs and if the baby is being supplemented with other foods. It is estimated that 900 kcal are needed to produce 1 liter of human milk (Gibbs and Seitchik, 1980). About one-third of those calories come from maternal stores (stored during pregnancy) and the remainder must be supplied by the diet. Consequently, mothers report and studies show that even with the RDA increase of 500 kcal, lactating mothers use some existing body fat and weight in milk production (Blackburn and Calloway, 1976).

The postpartum woman who is not breastfeeding needs to lose excess weight *gradually*. An appropriate rate of weight loss is between 1 and 2 lb/week. The new mother has many demands, including taking care of the newborn and recovering from the stress of delivery, that may cause fatigue, which should not be compounded by a restrictive diet. The postpartum woman should continue to follow the daily food guide and continue her prenatal supplements for at least 2-3 months postpartum, even if she is not lactating.

Where does the 24 pounds of weight go?

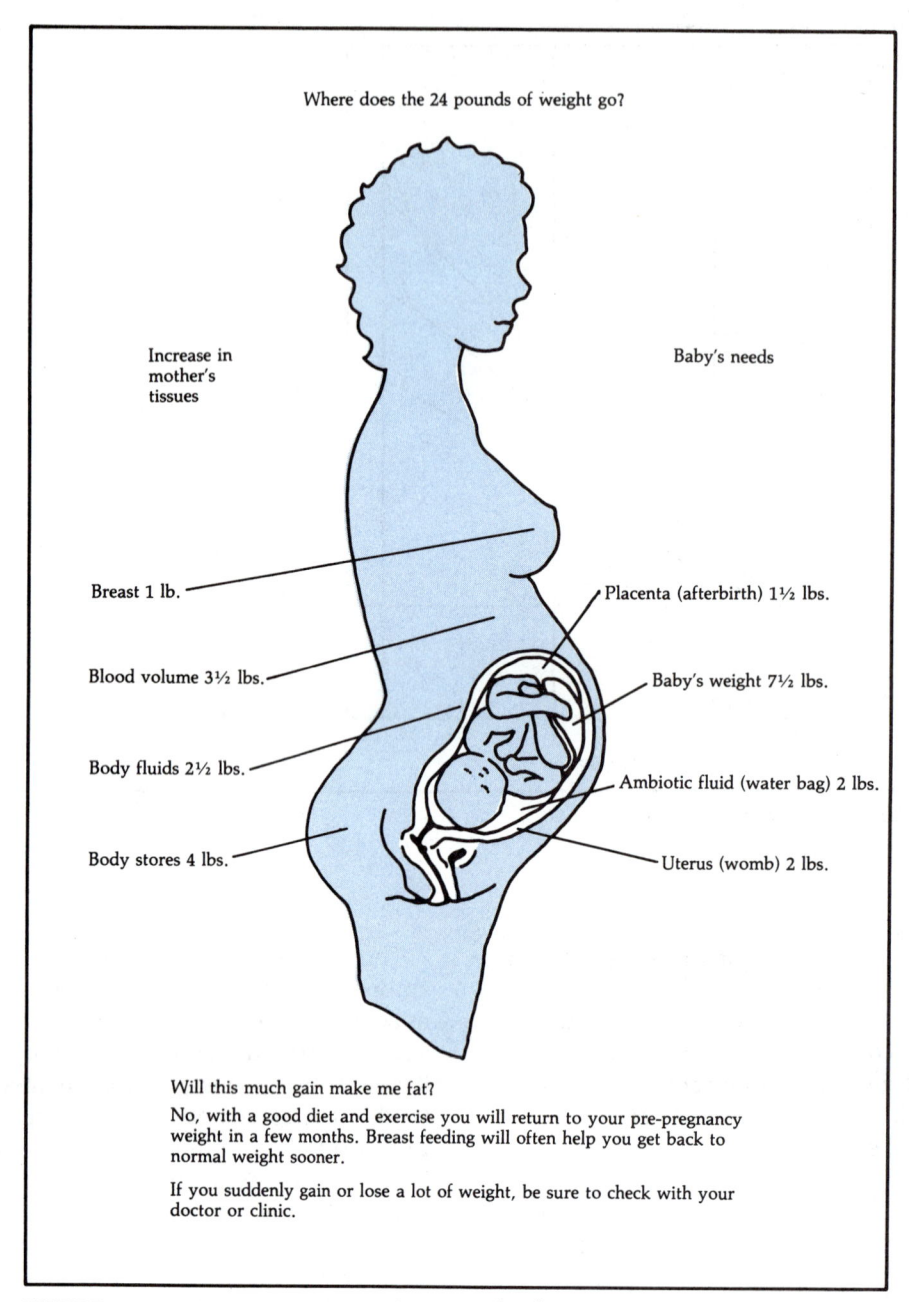

Increase in mother's tissues
- Breast 1 lb.
- Blood volume 3½ lbs.
- Body fluids 2½ lbs.
- Body stores 4 lbs.

Baby's needs
- Placenta (afterbirth) 1½ lbs.
- Baby's weight 7½ lbs.
- Ambiotic fluid (water bag) 2 lbs.
- Uterus (womb) 2 lbs.

Will this much gain make me fat?
No, with a good diet and exercise you will return to your pre-pregnancy weight in a few months. Breast feeding will often help you get back to normal weight sooner.
If you suddenly gain or lose a lot of weight, be sure to check with your doctor or clinic.

FIGURE 12-7. Maternal weight gain shown graphically.

NUTRITIONAL RISK FACTORS OF PREGNANCY

Some of the nutritional risk factors listed warrant further discussion, so that the nurse can be aware of why they are considered to be risk factors which may compromise pregnancy outcome.

Teenage Pregnancies

One risk factor that has received a lot of attention and is of growing concern is adolescent pregnancy. Although Chapter 38 has been devoted to a discussion of this topic the nurse needs to be aware of the nutritional requirements of the teenage mother. McArney (1985) reports that teenage mothers have over twice the incidence of babies of low birth weight than other age groups. The major concern during pregnancy is that the young adolescent is still growing at the same time that her fetus is developing, and this "conflict" may contribute to the high percentage of babies of low birth weight (Frisancho, Matos, and Flegel, 1983). Furthermore, Frisancho, Matos, and Flegel found that teenagers need to gain more weight than do older women to produce a child of average birth weight.

Table 12-1 lists several RDAs that are higher for adolescents than for older women. These include an increased need for calories, protein, vitamin D, calcium, and phosphorus. Since the teenage diet may not be optimal and often includes "fast foods," snacks, and skipping of meals, the nurse needs to work closely with the teenage patient to improve her diet.

Spacing of Pregnancies

Both short interconceptual intervals (<12 months between delivery and conception) and breastfeeding during the current pregnancy are nutritional stresses that may lead to less than optimal nutritional status (California Department of Health Services, 1987). With short spacing between births there may be a depletion of the mother's stores of many nutrients. Breastfeeding may cause serious competition between the nutrient demands of pregnancy and lactation.

Low Income

Low income is considered a risk factor because, in addition to not being able to afford to buy food, women may not have adequate cooking facilities or may be homeless and lack family support. There are several government programs that can provide assistance including the Federal Food Stamps Program and Women, Infant and Children. WIC, which provides high nutrition foods as well as nutrition counseling for low-income women, has been shown to reduce the incidence of low birth weight and premature infants (Stockbauer, 1987).

Weight Control

Women who are obese at the outset of pregnancy may be more prone to developing complications such as gestational diabetes. They may also be at the margin of nutritional status as a result of frequent dieting and other poor dietary practices. Compounding these factors is the woman's fear of gaining excessive weight during pregnancy. Women in this group need to be counseled about the importance of proper weight gain during the course of their pregnancy.

Smoking, Alcohol, and Drugs

Chapter 40 addresses substances consumed by pregnant women that may adversely affect the growing fetus. It is well established that smoking during pregnancy leads to low birth weight and other complications. Ingesting alcohol during pregnancy can also result in serious complications including fetal alcohol syndrome. Therefore, the nutrition questionnaire or other components of the medical interview should include questions concerning smoking, drinking alcoholic products, and using drugs.

Pica

Another important risk factor is the practice of eating non-nutritive substances such as clay, laundry starch, ice, or dirt. This practice is called *pica* and there is an increased incidence of pica among certain groups, especially low-income women of the southern United States. Pica should be discouraged as it can result in an inadequate intake of essential nutrients. There may also be toxic substances, such as lead, in the non-food item that can seriously affect the fetus (Committee on Nutrition of the Mother and Preschool Child, 1982). The nutritional questionnaire administered to pregnant and lactating women should include a question about pica.

INFLUENCES ON EATING BEHAVIOR: PROMOTING OPTIMAL NUTRITION

Ethnic Influences

People tend to eat as they did in their childhood. In pregnancy, ethnic influences may be exaggerated in the hope that what has worked for generations will work to produce a healthy baby in this case. However, the mother's ethnic background may not be indicative of her food practices as many people sample food from various cultures regularly.

In the United States there is great ethnic and cultural diversity. Table 12–12 lists some major ethnic groups in the United States.

TABLE 12–12. Major Cultural Groups in the United States

Chinese Americans (by region of origin because of differences in customs)
Mainland China
    Northern region (Mandarin)
    Inland region (Szechwan)
    Central coastal region (Shanghai)
    Southern region (Cantonese)
Taiwan
Hong Kong
Ethnic Chinese from Vietnam

Japanese Americans

Native Americans
    By cultural groups, e.g. Navajo, Pueblo, Eskimos, and others
    By tribe:
        Approximately 250–300 major tribes remain, varying in size
        Tribes in a cultural group share certain practices relating to eating, health, and other activities but retain many distinctive characteristics

Spanish-speaking Americans (Hispanic Americans)
Mexican Americans
    Settled immigrants
    Migrant workers
Spanish Americans
    Descendants of early Spanish settlers
Puerto Ricans
    Permanent residents
    Temporary residents who come to continental U.S. for work
Cubans
People from any other Spanish-speaking countries in Central and South America and the Caribbean

Southeast Asians
Vietnamese
    Cambodians
    Laotians

Filipinos

SOURCE: Adapted from Suitor and Crowley (1984).

One example of an ethnic food practice is the classification of foods into hot and cold groups (Nutrition Education Committee, 1986). The Chinese classify pregnancy as Yin (cold) and, therefore, hot (Yang) foods should be eaten to counterbalance. Cold foods such as milk are avoided during pregnancy. Interestingly, the Hispanic classification system labels pregnancy as a hot state (California Department of Health Services, 1987). Table 12–13 illustrates how Puerto Ricans classify foods and illnesses according to the hot–cold classification system.

Most cultures believe that certain foods can positively or negatively affect the fetus and that unusual food preferences, such as pickles and ice cream, are to be expected from a pregnant woman. Some women believe that an unsatisfied craving or an overindulgence in a food can cause a birthmark. As an example, red birthmarks are thought to be caused by overeating or an unsatisfied desire for strawberries (Gulick, Franklin, and Elinson, 1986).

Many individuals of Native American, Asian, and black cultures, as well as some Caucasians, cannot digest lactose, the main sugar found in milk. This condition, called *lactose intolerance*, can cause intestinal gas, cramps, or diarrhea if milk or a milk product is consumed. Some women have compensated for the lactose intolerance by including other foods in their diet that provide calcium such as canned fish, tofu, and other milk products that can be more easily tolerated such as cheese or buttermilk. There is also commercially available a product that, when added to milk, can break down the lactose so that it can be digested. However, most women have not compensated for those foods lacking in their diets and many pregnant and lactating women with lactose intolerance may not meet the RDA for calcium.

Cultural Influences

A common cultural dietary alternative is the vegetarian lifestyle. Whether the impetus for vegetarianism is religious (Seventh Day Adventist or Zen Buddhist) or societal (concern about expense or land use), the pregnant vegetarian must devote extra attention to her diet in order to fulfill her nutritional needs.

Lacto-ovovegetarians do not eat animal tissue but do include milk and eggs in their diets. Strict *vegans* will not eat any animal flesh or products and their diet consists of only plant foods. During pregnancy and lactation the vegetarian needs to

TABLE 12-13. The Hot-Cold Classification Among Puerto Ricans

	Frio (cold)	Fresco (cool)	Caliente (hot)
Illnesses or bodily conditions	Arthritis Menstrual period Pain in the joints	Colds	Constipation Diarrhea Pregnancy Rashes Ulcers
Medicine and herbs		Bicarbonate of soda Linden flowers Milk of magnesia Nightshade Orange flower water Sage Tobacco	Anise Aspirin Castor oil Cinnamon Cod liver oil Iron tablets Penicillin Vitamins
Foods	Avocado Banana Coconut Lima beans Sugar cane White beans	Barley water Whole milk Chicken Fruits Honey Raisins Salt cod Watercress Onions Peas	Alcoholic beverages Chili peppers Chocolate Coffee Corn meal Evaporated milk Garlic Kidney beans

SOURCE: Nutrition Education Committee, 1986

pay close attention to her diet as certain nutrients may not be present in the quantities found in animal sources. Protein requirements, which increase during pregnancy, are more difficult to meet and the pregnant vegetarian needs to be aware of complementary proteins. Since plant foods do not contain all essential amino acids, the vegetarian must combine proteins, mixing those that are missing one amino acid with others that have the missing amino acid. This process results in what are called *complementary proteins* and the process is described in detail by Lappe (1982) in *Diet for a Small Planet*, an excellent resource for vegetarians and the nurse who is working with vegetarian patients. Examples of complementary proteins evident in the diets of ethnic groups are:

1. Mexican Americans—corn tortillas with kidney beans.
2. Middle Eastern—whole wheat or bulgar wheat with soybeans and sesame seeds.
3. Southern United States—rice and red beans.

A pregnant vegan needs to consume her 74 g/day of protein from grains, cereals, and other plant sources. Consequently, she will receive few extra calories from low-nutrient foods such as candy and other sweets. Table 12–14 gives an example of one meal from which approximately 26 g of protein are consumed, one-third of the daily requirement.

Other possible deficiencies faced by the strict vegetarian include vitamin D, riboflavin, vitamin B_{12}, and calcium. These nutrients are contained in milk and the vegetarian must include other sources of these nutrients in her diet such as soy milk. Still, B_{12} needs to be added to the diet as well as iron and zinc. Calories may also not be adequate in the diet of a vegan and the nurse needs to monitor her patient's weight gain carefully. Most vegetarians know a great deal about their diet, often more than the nurse, but the nurse can help them learn about the particular nutrient needs of pregnancy. In summary, the pregnant vegetarian should follow the daily food guide for pregnant women using a guide for complementary protein

TABLE 12-14. Lunch Supplying One-third of the Daily Dietary Needs of a Pregnant Vegan

Food	Amount	Protein (g)	Calories
Potato salad	1 cup	7	250
Sliced tomato	1	1	25
Sweet pepper	1 cup	pepper—1	75
Stuffed with beans and oats		beans—14	210
		oats—2.5	65
Tangerine	1	1	40
		26.5	665

sources, include milk or soy milk in her diet, and take a supplement that includes at least B_{12}, iron, and zinc.

Common Discomforts During Pregnancy

There are conditions that occur during pregnancy that may be uncomfortable for the pregnant patient. Some of these discomforts, outlined below, may be reduced or alleviated through nutrition management.

Nausea and Vomiting

Nausea and/or vomiting, which is especially common during the first trimester of pregnancy, can be very distressing. Although sometimes called morning sickness, it can occur throughout the day and can even lead to weight loss. Table 12-15 suggests some methods that may reduce or eliminate nausea.

Heartburn

Heartburn is a common complaint during pregnancy and becomes more of a nuisance as the fetus grows and presses against the stomach. Many women find that they can reduce or avoid the incidence of heartburn by following certain suggestions. These suggestions include avoiding coffee and cigarettes, since they increase stomach acidity, and avoiding foods that are related to the patient's heartburn. Women should not lie down or bend over sharply right after eating and, for those who are very prone to heartburn, they should sleep with their head slightly elevated.

Constipation

Many women experience constipation during pregnancy as a result of the intestinal tract decreasing in motility. Other factors that may contribute to constipation include irregular eating habits, stress and an increase in calcium and iron in the diet (Coalition for the Medical Rights of Women, 1987). To avoid constipation women should try the following:

1. Drink at least 6–8 glasses of liquid each day.
2. Do daily exercise.
3. Add fiber to the diet, including prune juice, whole grains, and fruits.
4. Stimulate a bowel movement by drinking hot or cold liquid when stomach is empty.

Leg Cramps

Some women are prone to leg cramps which can be caused by a deficiency of calcium or magnesium

TABLE 12-15. Recommendations for the Management of Nausea and Vomiting During Pregnancy

1. Before rising in the morning, eat soda crackers
2. Arise slowly from bed avoiding sudden movements
3. Eat small frequent meals so that the stomach is not empty for long
4. Avoid greasy or fatty foods
5. Avoid strong odors especially while cooking
6. Drink liquids between meals rather than with food

SOURCE: Coalition for the Medical Rights of Women (1987).

(California Department of Health Services, 1987). The nurse, working with the patient, should make certain that sufficient sources of calcium and magnesium are included in the diet and that the diet is not excessively high in phosphorus from soda pop and excessive protein. Sometimes leg cramps appear not to be related to nutritional status or can be avoided if the patient does not point her toes when stretching.

BEYOND PREGNANCY AND LACTATION

The U.S. Department of Agriculture (1985) published recommendations for improving the American diet called *Dietary Guidelines for Americans.* These guidelines promote changes in American eating habits that may reduce the incidence of certain diseases such as obesity and heart disease. Women who have been recently pregnant may be interested in making these changes in their diets as they are now aware of the importance of nutrition and its effect on health and well-being. They are also in a position to influence the eating behavior of their families and may bring about positive changes that are long lasting.

The *Dietary guidelines* make recommendations about reducing the consumption of certain potentially harmful substances such as alcohol and the excessive intake of fat, sugar, calories, and sodium. It also encourages individuals to make certain that there are adequate amounts of fiber and complex carbohydrates (starch) in their diets. The following is a summary of the recommendations from the *Dietary guidelines:*

1. Eat a variety of foods.
2. Maintain desirable weight, i.e. limit calorie intake and exercise regularly.
3. Avoid excessive fat, saturated fat, and cholesterol, i.e. limit fried foods and reduce whole milk dairy products by replacing butter with margarine, whole milk with skim or low fat, etc.
4. Eat more starch and fiber, i.e. increase whole grain breads and cereals and replace less nutritious foods with these.
5. Avoid too much sugar, i.e. reduce the amount of sweets and sweetened foods, including candy, cakes, and soft drinks.
6. Avoid too much sodium, i.e. reduce the amount of table salt used and reduce or avoid high sodium foods such as preserved meats, some cheeses, and potato chips.
7. Avoid too much alcohol, i.e. pregnant women should not ingest alcoholic beverages, including beer and wine.

SUMMARY

Good nutrition during pregnancy is an important component of prenatal care. The nurse can assist the patient in making changes in her diet and eating behavior that will provide an optimal nutritional environment for the developing fetus and the newborn. This chapter has discussed the importance of nutrition, the nutritional requirements of pregnancy and lactation, and factors that may influence eating behavior such as ethnic and cultural lifestyles. Also explained was the process of nutrition assessment, whereby the nurse interviews and evaluates the client's diet and eating patterns. The interview is a critical component of the health care plan, as it is here that the nurse establishes the relationship between herself and her client that will allow her to facilitate change.

It is anticipated that the good eating habits that are begun during pregnancy and lactation will be carried on throughout the patient's life. Also, our educated patient will teach these to her family and she will in turn influence their nutrition and behavior and, eventually, the nutritional behavior of their children.

REFERENCES

Abrams, B. F., and Laros, R. K. 1983. Prepregnancy weight, weight gain, and birth weight. *Am. J. Obstet. Gynecol.* 154(3):503–509.

American College of Obstetrics and Gynecology, Committee on Nutrition. 1978. *Nutrition in maternal health care.* Chicago: American College of Obstetrics and Gynecology.

Blackburn, M. W., and Calloway, D. H. 1976. Energy expenditure and consumption of mature, pregnant and lactating women. *J. Am .Dietet. Assoc.* 69:29–36.

Caan, B.; Horgan, D. M.; Margen, S.; King, J. C.; and Jewell, N. P. 1987. Benefits associated with WIC supplemental feeding during the interpregnancy interval. *Am. J. Clin. Nutr.* 45(1):29–41.

California Department of Health Services, Maternal and Child Health Branch. 1987. *Nutrition during pregnancy and the postpartum period: A manual for health care professionals.* (Review Draft.)

Coalition for the Medical Rights of Women. 1987. *Natural remedies for pregnancy discomforts.* California Department of Health Services, Education Program Assoc., Inc.

Committee on Nutrition of the Mother and Preschool Child, *Food and Nutrition,* Board Commission on Life Sciences, National Research Council. 1982. *Alternative dietary practices and nutritional abuses in pregnancy—summary report.* Washington, D.C.: National Academy Press.

Committee to Study the Prevention of Low Birthweight, Division of Health Promotion and Disease Prevention, Institute of Medicine, National Academy of Sciences, 1985. *Preventing low birthweight.* Washington, D.C.: National Academy of Sciences.

Cormier, W. H., and Cormier, L. S. 1979. *Interviewing strategies for helpers: A guide to assessment, treatment and evaluation.* Monterey, Calif.: Brooks/Cole.

Food and Nutrition Board, Commission on Maternal Nutrition. 1970. *Maternal nutrition and the course of human pregnancy.* Washington, D.C.: National Academy of Sciences.

Food and Nutrition Board, Committee on Dietary Allowances, National Research Council, 1980. *Recommended dietary allowances.* 9th rev. Washington, D.C.: National Academy of Sciences.

Frisancho, A. R.; Matos, J.; and Flegel, P. 1983. Maternal nutritional status and adolescent pregnancy outcome. *Am. J. Clin. Nutr.* 38(Nov.): 739–746.

Garn, S. M.; Ridella, S. A.; Petzold, A. S.; and Falkner, F. 1981. Maternal hematologic levels and pregnancy outcomes. *Seminars Perinatalogy.* 5(2):155–162.

Gibbs, C. E. and Seitchik, J. 1980. Nutrition in pregnancy. In *Modern nutrition in health and disease,* 6th ed., eds. R. S. Goodhart and M. E. Shils. Philadelphia: Lea and Febigar.

Gulick, E. E.; Franklin, C. M.; and Elinson, M. 1986. Food beliefs and food behaviors among minority pregnant women. *J. Perinatology.* 6:197–202.

Hytten, F. E., and Leitch, I. 1971. *The physiology of human pregnancy.* 2nd ed. Oxford: Blackwell Scientific.

Keys, A.; Brozek, J.; Henschel, A.; Michelson, O.; and Taylor, H. L. 1950. Growth and development. In *The biology of human starvation,* vol. 2. Minneapolis: Minneapolis Press.

Lappe, F. M. 1982. *Diet for a small planet.* 10th anniversary edition. New York: Ballantine Books.

McAnarney, E. R. 1985. Adolescent pregnancy and childbearing: New data, new challenges. *Pediatrics.* 75(5):973–975.

March of Dimes Birth Defects Foundation. 1986. *Recipes for healthy babies.*

Naeye, R. L. 1979. Weight gain and the outcome of pregnancy. *Am. J. Obstet. Gynecol.* 135(1):3.

Nutrition Education Committee for Maternal and Child Nutrition Publications. 1986. *Cross-cultural counseling: A guide for nutrition and health counselors.* United States Department of Agriculture. Department of Health and Human Services.

Roberts, H. J. 1983. Potential toxicity due to dolomite and bonemeal. *Soc. Med. J.* 76(5):556–559.

San Francisco Department of Health. 1987. *Perinatal nutrition protocols.* San Francisco perinatal forum nutrition committee.

Seller, M. J. 1987. Nutritionally induced congenital defects. *Proc. Nutr. Soc.* 46:227–235.

Snetselaar, L. G. 1983. *Nutrition counseling skills.* Rockville, M.: Aspen Publications.

Stockbauer, J. W. 1987. WIC prenatal participation and its relation to pregnancy outcomes in Missouri: A second look. *Am. J. of Public Health.* 77:813.

United States Department of Agriculture. Department of Health and Human Services. 1985. *Dietary Guidelines for Americans.* 2nd ed. Home and Garden Bulletin No. 232.

White House Conference on Food, Nutrition, and Health. 1969. Final Report of Panel II-1: Pregnant and Nursing Women and Young Infants. December 1969.

Williams, S. R. 1985. *Nutrition and diet therapy.* 5th ed. St. Louis: Times Mirror/C.V. Mosby.

Worthington-Roberts, B. S.; Vermeersch, J.; and Williams, S. R. 1985. *Nutrition in pregnancy and lactation.* 3rd ed. St. Louis: Times Mirror/C.V. Mosby.

13

Prenatal Diagnosis and Fetal Well-being

BEHAVIORAL OBJECTIVES

Upon completion of this chapter, the reader should be able to:

- Identify currently used techniques for prenatal assessment of fetal well-being.

- Determine appropriate prenatal screening techniques for selected clients who have been categorized as high risk.

- Differentiate parental genetic or health history indications for various prenatal screening techniques.

- Develop an understanding of the risks, benefits, and side-effects of various prenatal screening procedures.

- Define nursing duties with regard to the high-risk childbearing couple undergoing prenatal screening for fetal well-being assessment.

Diagnostic tests of well-being can give health care providers and pregnant couples much needed information about pregnancy status. No one test is sufficient to diagnose the viability of a pregnancy or its chances of ending with a normal labor and delivery course. However, selective use of the tests can predict both placental insufficiency and the ability of the fetus to survive in the extrauterine environment. Since maternal morbidity and mortality from childbearing is relatively low at present, today's focus is on ways to decrease fetal death and illness. Although the fetus appears to mature best in the intrauterine environment, the proper timing of delivery depends on placental adequacy as well as the ability of the fetus to tolerate the outside world.

The prenatal screening techniques discussed in this chapter include sonography, CAT scan, x-rays, amniocentesis, genetic screening and counseling, fetal monitoring, assays of placental enzymes and hormones, and fetoscopy. Additionally, the recent screening techniques of percutaneous umbilical blood sampling (PUBS), placental grading, and chorionic villus sampling (CVS) will be considered in the range of prenatal techniques available to pregnant couples.

SONOGRAPHY

Definitions and Indications

Sonography (ultrasound) is frequently used for high-risk clients if a placental abnormality (previa or hydatididiform mole), fetal growth retardation, polyhydramnios, or another high-risk factor is suspected (see Table 13–1; Thompson, 1978). Sonography can also be used to determine fetal death, fetal anomaly (e.g. hydrocephalus), gestational age, or the existence of a multiple pregnancy. Diagnosis of multiple pregnancy alerts the health care team to the increased high-risk status of the mother. Frequently, sonography is used concurrently with the procedure of amniocentesis to decrease the risk of placental and fetal injury from the amniocentesis procedure. Additionally, with knowledge of a fetal abnormality from a sonogram, a couple and the health care team can modify delivery of an infant if needed and plan for the child's future care.

Procedure and Interpretation

By the use of high-frequency sound waves (above 20,000 cycles/sec) sonography can diagnose a pregnancy as early as 5 weeks. At that time the gestational sac can be visualized, because it is fluid filled, echo free, and surrounded by a solid uterine wall. High-frequency sound waves can be produced in a variety of ways, but one commonly used method employs piezoelectric crystals. When an electric current passes over these crystals, they vibrate at ultrasonic frequencies. Vibrations on the crystal surface produce an electric charge, which is amplified and recorded as light impulses, making fetal and uterine structures visible on an oscilloscope. The crystal acts as a receiver to detect returning echoes, which are then converted to electric energy. Like a light, sonography can be directed to a beam and focused. A transducer (in which the crystals are located) is moved across the pregnant abdomen in many different directions and planes. The transducer is moved from pubis to fundus and then transversely to get an accurate picture of the uterine contents (Fig. 13–1). Often, conductive jelly is placed on the client's abdomen to improve conduction of the sound waves used in sonography (Thompson, 1978). When performed according to protocol and for specific medical conditions, sonography appears to be a safe procedure (Levine and Schenker, 1985).

Diagnostic sonography can be carried out by any of three different sonographic methods:

1. The A-mode method allows the distance between interfaces within a body to be measured and thus is a one-dimensional system.
2. The B-mode (B-Scan) method provides an outline of structures in cross-sectional (two-

TABLE 13–1. High-Risk Factors for Fetal Well-being

Factors That Place a Fetus at Risk

Maternal characteristics
  Age: under 17 or over 35
  Parity: nulliparity or more than 5 pregnancies
  Socioeconomic status: poverty
  Chronic illness: anemia, diabetes, heart disease, hypertension, renal disease
  Acute illness: urinary tract infection, viral infection, toxoplasmosis
  Undernourishment

Obstetric complications
  Third trimester bleeding
  Toxemia
  Premature labor
  Prolonged pregnancy

Genetic factors
  Family history of genetic abnormalities
  Ethnic risk: e.g. Tay-Sachs disease, sickle cell disease or trait, fetal–maternal blood-type incompatibility

SOURCE: Cranley (1978).

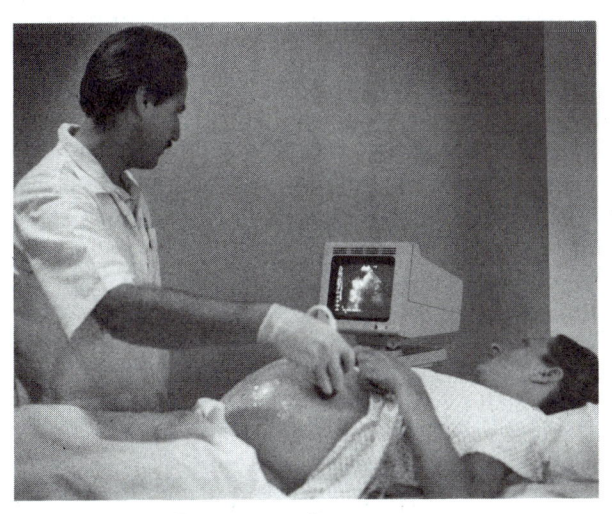

FIGURE 13–1. Expectant mother receiving a sonogram.

dimensional) form and converts echoes to dots for display. This method can show variations in tissue density and consistency.
3. The real-time method is the most recently developed form of sonography and the most advanced.

Many health care practitioners use only real-time (dynamic) sonography, because an entire field can be scanned sequentially to show movement of a structure (the baby's heart beating, a fetal leg moving, etc.). With real-time sonography, gestational age can be estimated rather accurately (within 2–3 weeks) by measurement of fetal crown-rump length, biparietal diameter (BPD), thoracic circumference, or a combination of these measurements. Term pregnancy can be diagnosed quite accurately if a fetal biparietal diameter of at least 9.5 cm is calculated. The BPD is the largest transverse diameter of the fetal head.

The sooner the sonogram is carried out (after 5 weeks following the last normal menstrual period), the more accurate the sonograph scan. Also, by the second trimester, sonography can be used to estimate fetal weight, and with sequential sonograms throughout the rest of the pregnancy, a diagnosis of intrauterine growth retardation can be made. Placental abnormalities can also be detected by sonography. In fact, sonography has almost completely eliminated the use of x-rays to locate a placenta (Thompson, 1978). Sonography aids in the assessment of placental thickness and size. Placentas are thicker in erythroblastosis fetalis, some viral diseases, and diabetes. On the other hand, placentas are smaller in small-for-gestational-age (SGA) babies, in poorly controlled diabetics, and postmaturity, a condition in which placental calcifications may be seen (Ragan, 1978).

Fetal abnormalities, particularly of the large structures (head and trunk), can also be visualized with sonography. Once abnormalities have been detected, amniocentesis or fetal blood sampling can be used to further identify possible chromosomal anomalies (Vintzileos et al., 1987). Ectopic pregnancies can also be ruled out if a sonogram shows an intrauterine pregnancy. If there is intra-abdominal pathology (for example, liomyoma or an ovarian cyst) that makes abdominal examination difficult, sonography can help confirm an intrauterine pregnancy. During the first trimester, when so many fetuses are aborted, serial sonograms at 1-week intervals can show fetal growth or degeneration (Thompson, 1978). In high-risk situations such as maternal diabetes or Rh sensitization, scans may be carried out to show fetal growth and well-being. With the improvement of sonography in the future, it may be possible to predict fetal weight and the possibility of placental insufficiency based on the amount of amniotic fluid. Sonography may be able to detect fetal activity accurately and relate that to gestational age (Epstein and Frigoletto, 1983).

Real-time sonography makes it possible to estimate fetal breathing movements (FBMs). Real-time sonography produces a dynamic picture and allows a count to be made of apneic and respiratory periods of the fetus. FBMs of 5 min or more in a 30-min period indicate fetal well-being (Marshall, 1979). However, the absence of FBMs is not a reliable sign of fetal difficulty, since FBMs are sensitive to other influences that are impossible to measure. Although this check for fetal well-being needs further investigation, some studies of prenatal monitoring have shown that SGA babies and babies delivered by cesarean birth because of fetal distress have few FBMs.

Nursing Roles

If a physician or nurse-midwife routinely uses sonography for prenatal care, counseling about the procedure should be given at the first prenatal visit. A thorough explanation of the procedure should include a discussion of the risks and benefits. Client questions should be answered and partner participation should be encouraged.

Often clients are encouraged to drink a large amount of fluid (approximately 500 ml) prior to coming for the examination, since a full bladder repositions the uterus and cervix for better visibility. The client is supine during the procedure and may face the sonography screen if she desires. Throughout the procedure, the nurse should explain and interpret what is being shown on the sonographic screen. If the test indicates fetal well-being, and if it is allowed through agency policy, the client may be provided with a Polaroid picture of one of the sonogram pictures. This can serve as the first picture in the baby book.

CAT SCAN

Definitions and Indications

In today's care of the maternity client, there is a dispute as to whether computerized axial tomography (CAT) or sonography is of greater value in prenatal screening. Both CAT scanning and sonography offer cross-sectional tomographic images of body anatomy, and both can assist in the interpretation of abdominal contents and structures. Therefore, both the CAT scan and sonography can be used effectively for obstetric and gynecologic procedures.

CAT scanning is a radiographic technique in which an x-ray source irradiates a body part with an encircling arc (Jaffe and Simonds, 1978). Detectors absorb and count the amount of radiation that penetrates the body part. A CAT scan is superior to sonography in showing organ outlines without interference from air or bone (Jaffe and Simonds, 1978). It is more efficient for organ visualization of obese clients (subcutaneous fat delineates organs), whereas sonography gives a better picture of thin clients. Sonography can detail a small area; a CAT scan can show a large area but without as much specificity as sonography (Gorham, 1978).

Procedure and Interpretation

A CAT scan can produce a three-dimensional image by use of a machine known as a scanner. No special preparations are needed for a CAT scan, although some physicians have their clients take nothing by mouth (NPO) for approximately 6 hours prior to the procedure. This is done to prevent the potential problem of aspiration, since some clients become nauseated from the contrast medium (frequently iodine in base) used in the examination. For an abdominal examination, the client is placed into an opening of the scanner and reminded to be very quiet during the scanning. The scanner takes pictures in a cross-sectional plane by using small beams of x-rays that pass from one side of the abdomen to the other side. A computer calculates the amount of radiation absorbed by different body tissues and can produce a printout of photographs that show different tissue densities. The scan takes about 1 hour to complete, and the client can usually return to normal activities almost immediately after the procedure. Although a CAT scan can be helpful in identifying abdominal masses, other diagnostic aids are often of equal value in identification and involve fewer risks of radiation exposure.

Ionizing radiation is used in a CAT scan, and therefore the procedure cannot be considered completely safe for a childbearing woman (Gorham, 1978). However, if in the physician's and client's minds, the benefit of using a contrast medium in a CAT scan to depict a pelvic abnormality outweighs the risks, then a CAT scan may be utilized to aid in the diagnosis of an illness. The CAT scan can be used without contrast medium to diagnose hydrocephalus in the fetus if sonography shows some evidence of this condition.

Nursing Roles

The CAT scan procedure can be quite frightening for a client. The machine is complex and powerful looking. The client is asked to be almost enclosed by it. Nursing support and education about the procedure, its risks, and its benefits are needed. Since the client is often alone in the scanning room during the scan, she may become quite anxious. It may make the client more at ease to know that assistance is readily available through intercom contact with the CAT scan operator.

X-RAYS (RADIOGRAPHY)

Definitions and Indications

The increasing use of sonography has allowed many clients to avoid exposure to ionizing radiation for prenatal diagnosis. Sonography can accurately show fetal head circumference and can also be used to assess pelvic dimensions to predict ease of labor and delivery. Because controversy still exists about the cumulative effect of radiation exposure on the fetus and the pregnant client, many physicians elect to avoid radiologic pelvic examinations unless the potential benefits of x-rays clearly exceed the perceived side-effects. Other physicians avoid radiologic exposure altogether once they have received information about childbearing status. Although its use in early pregnancy has been limited, amnioscopy of fetography can allow viewing of gross fetal structures. With the instillation of a contrast medium into amniotic fluid, a fetal outline can be visualized on x-ray film.

X-rays are most useful when fetal skeletal problems are suspected. If sonography indicates possible anencephaly, a flat x-ray is recommended to offer additional diagnostic information that will allow a decision for pregnancy termination (Epstein and Frigoletto, 1983). Although its use is decreasing, x-ray pelvimetry can also be useful for the diagnosis of a breech presentation and the need for a cesarean delivery. Before sonography became so popular, x-rays were used to assess fetal age by looking at the long-bone epiphyses. If the distal femoral ossification centers are visualized, the fetus is generally believed to be of at least 36 weeks of gestation. Visualization of the proximal tibial centers indicates an approximately 40-week fetus.

Procedure and Interpretation

Radiographic exams of the pregnant woman are conducted with abdominal shielding that still allows visualization of the desired anatomic part. Radiographic examinations allow detailed visualization of a part of the body while blurring other peripheral areas. Many nurses and physicians are expert at interpreting x-rays to diagnose disease and physical abnormalities.

The effect of radiation is generally believed to be cumulative and, therefore, unnecessary exposure to radiologic procedures must be avoided during pregnancy. Radiation doses for pregnant women must be minimized, because the fetus may be up to 10 times more sensitive than the adult to the production of radiation-induced leukemias (Hufton, 1979). There is also a risk of genetic damage, since both mother and baby are exposed to gonadal irradiation. The earlier the embryo is in its development, the more harmful radiation can be. There may be a critical developmental time when organogenesis is negatively affected by radiation exposure. Because radiation may be lethal for a very early fetus, many x-ray labs follow a 10-day rule for abdominal x-rays of women. This rule recommends that x-rays be carried out during the first 10 days of menses, when pregnancy is least likely to exist.

Mortality after the perinatal period and up to 6 years of age was not increased among the Japanese fetuses of the Second World War that were exposed to sublethal doses of radiation. Considerable uncertainty still exists as to the specific amount of radiation required to cause tissue damage. The risk of embryonic or fetal tissue receiving a lethal or sublethal dose of an x-ray (approximately 5 rads), which would cause congenitally determined handicaps, would probably be less than 1 case per 1000 births (Hufton, 1979). A single rad represents the radiologic amount that a woman would receive on a single radiographic abdominal examination. With improved radiographic techniques, the risk of inducing fetal malformations or cancer by radiographic examination may be less than it was a decade ago.

Nursing Roles

As in any other radiographic procedure, the nurse must assess client concerns and needs related to the x-ray procedure. Many clients may have heard of the need to avoid x-rays while pregnant and may need to express concerns about the use of x-rays in the diagnostic workup. Risks and benefits can be discussed with the client, and the physician should be notified of the client's anxieties. Appropriate interdisciplinary communication can reduce client concerns about the use of x-rays.

AMNIOCENTESIS

Definitions and Indications

One of the most valuable means of assessing fetal well-being or problems is by the analysis of amniotic fluid obtained by the technique of amniocentesis—the gathering of amniotic fluid cells via uterine puncture (Research McGill, 1980). Over 70 of 2300 genetic diseases known to affect humans can be diagnosed by amniocentesis. With continuing progress in radioimmunoassay and genetic study techniques, such biochemical testing will most likely become more sophisticated.

Knowledge of basic enzyme defects is invaluable in genetic counseling (Summer, 1982). Over the past 80 years, 521 autosomal recessive diseases have been identified, and in 160 of these, enzyme disorders have been discovered (Summer, 1982).

In many of these cases, amniotic fluid analysis can determine whether specific enzymes are lacking and can thus point to the existence of a fetal biochemical abnormality (see Table 13-2).

Biochemical abnormalities include the storage diseases (e.g. lipid, amino acid, and mucopolysaccharide abnormalities), neural tube defects (NTDs), trisomy 21 (or Down's syndrome), hemophilia, and Duchenne's muscular dystrophy. Amniocentesis can also detect sickle cell anemia. Fetal DNA samples can be retrieved from amniotic fluid and then tested for abnormal genes that cause a particular defect. Cytogenetic and biochemical studies are successful for diagnostic purposes in 99 percent of amniocenteses performed for chromosomal disorders and single gene effects (Summer, 1982). Amniocentesis adds a 1 percent risk to the probability of spontaneous abortion and an additional 1 percent risk to the developmental of neonatal problems. In 2–5 percent of the cases, insufficient fluid is obtained. In another 5–10 percent the cells from the amniotic fluid do not grow well enough to allow diagnosis of fetal genetic problems (Gray, 1982).

A total of 1 in 50 children is born with a physical defect resulting from a genetic abnormality that

TABLE 13–2. Genetic Disorders That Can Be Detectable by Amniocentesis

Disease	Measurable Enzyme (or other) Defect	Prenatal Diagnosis[a]
Abetalipoproteinemia	Apo-β-lipoprotein	Probable
Acatalasia	Catalase	Possible
Adenosine deaminase deficiency	Adenosine deaminase	Yes
Adrenogenital syndrome	Various steroid hydroxylases	Yes
Adrenoleukodystrophy[b]	C_{26} fatty acid accumulation	Possible
Argininosuccinicaciduria	Argininosuccinase	Yes
Aspartylglucosaminuria	β-Aspartylglucosamidase	Possible
Cerebellar ataxia, juvenile	Hexosaminidase A and B	Possible (some)
Chediak-Higashi syndrome	Unknown (intracellular inclusion body)	Possible
Cholesterol ester storage disease	Acid lipase	Possible
Chronic granulomatous disease[b]	NBT reduction	Yes
Citrullinemia	Argininosuccinic acid synthetase	Yes
Cystic fibrosis	MUGB hydrolysis	Yes
Cystinosis	Cystine accumulation	Yes
Ehlers-Danlos syndrome, type IV	Lack of type III collagen	Possible
Ehlers-Danlos syndrome, type V[b]	Lysyl oxidase	Possible
Ellis-van Creveld syndrome	Femur growth	Yes
Epidermolysis bullosa	Skin biopsy microscopy	Yes
Fabry's disease[b]	Ceramidetrihexoside glactosidase	Yes
Familial hypercholesterolemia	LDL cholesterol receptors	Yes
Fanconi's syndrome	Chromosome breakage	Yes
Farber disease	Ceramidase	Yes
Finnish nephrosis	α-Fetoprotein level	Yes
Fucosidosis	α-Fucosidase	Yes
Galactokinase deficiency	Galactokinase	Yes
Galactosemia	Galactose-1-phosphate uridyl transferase	Yes
Gangliosidosis, generalized (G_{M1}, Type I)	β-Galactosidase	Yes
Gangliosidosis, juvenile (G_{M1}, Type II)	β-galactosidase	Yes
Gangliosidosis, juvenile (G_{M2})	Partial deficiency of hexosaminidase A	Possible
Gaucher's disease	Glucocerebrosidase	Yes
Glucose-6-phosphate dehydrogenase deficiency[b]	Glucose-6-phosphate dehydrogenase	Possible
Glutaric aciduria, Type II	Glutaryl-CoA carboxylase	Yes

SOURCE: Golbus (1982).
[a]Yes = prenatal diagnosis accomplished; probable = enzyme activity present in normal amniotic fluid cells; possible = enzyme activity present in normal skin fibroblasts.
[b]X-linked.
[c]Autosomal dominant.

TABLE 13-2. Continued

Disease	Measurable Enzyme (or other) Defect	Prenatal Diagnosis[a]
Glycogen storage disease, Type II (Pompe's disease)	α-1, 4 Glucosidase	Yes
Glycogen storage disease, Type III	Amylo-1,6-glucosidase	Probable
Glycogen storage disease, Type IV	Branching enzyme	Probable
Glycogen storage disease, Type VIII	Phosphorylase kinase	Possible
Hemoglobinopathies	Synthesis of abnormal hemoglobin	Yes
Hemolytic anemia VIII	Triosephosphate isomerase	Probable
Hemophilia A[b]	Factor VIII deficiency	Yes
Hereditary coproporphyria	Coproporphyrinogen oxidase	Possible
Histidinemia	Histidase	Probable
Homocystinuria	Cystathionine synthetase	Probable
Hunter syndrome[b]	α-L-Iduronic acid-2 sulfatase	Yes
Hurler's syndrome	α-L-Iduronidase	Yes
Hyperammonemia, Type II	Ornithine carbamyl transferase	Probable
Hyperargininemia	Arginase	Probable
Hypercholesterolemia[c]	HMG-CoA reductase	Yes
Hyperlysinemia	Lysine-ketoglutarase reductase	Possible
Hyperthyroidism	Reverse triiodothyronine level	Possible
Hypervalinemia	Valine α-ketoglutarate transaminase	Possible
Hypophosphatasia	Alkaline phosphatase	Yes (some types)
Hypothyroidism	Reverse triiodothyronine level	Yes
I-cell disease	Nonspecific lysosomal enzymes	Yes
Ichthyosis, epidermolytic hyperkeratosis[c]	Skin biopsy microscopy	Yes
Ichthyosis, lamellar	Skin biopsy microscopy	Yes
Isovaleric acidemia	Isovaleryl-CoA dehydrogenase	Yes
Ketotic hyperglycinemia	Propionyl-CoA carboxylase	Yes
Krabbe's disease	Galactocerebroside β-galactosidase	Yes
Lactosyl ceramidosis	Lactosyl ceramidase	Possible
Lesch-Nyhan syndrome[b]	Hypoxanthine guanine phosphoribosyltransferase	Yes
Lysosomal acid phosphatase deficiency	Lysosomal acid phosphatase	Yes
Mannosidosis	α-Mannosidase	Probable
Maple syrup urine disease	Branched-chain ketoacid decarboxylase	Yes
Maroteaux-Lamy syndrome	Arylsulfatase B	Yes
Meckel syndrome	α-Fetoprotein level	Yes
Menkes syndrome	Copper incorporation	Yes (some)
Metachromatic leukodystrophy	Arylsulfatase A	Yes
Methylmalonic aciduria	Methylmalonyl-CoA mutase	Yes
Methyltetrahydrofolate methyltransferase deficiency	Methyltetrahydrosulfate methyltransferase	Possible
Methyltetrahydrofolate reductase deficiency	Methyltetrahydrofolate reductase	Possible
Morquio's syndrome	Chondroitin sulfate N-acetylhexosamine sulfate sulfatase	Possible
Mucolipidosis I (sialidosis)	α-Neuraminidase	Yes
Mucolipidosis III (pseudopolydystrophy)	Multiple lysosomal enzymes	Possible
Mucolipidosis IV	Electron microscopy	Yes
Mucopolysaccharidosis VII	β-Glucuronidase	Possible
Myotonic dystrophy[c]	Linkage analysis in some families	Yes
Neural tube defects	α-Fetoprotein level	Yes
Niemann-Pick disease	Sphingomyelinase	Yes
Nucleoside phosphorylase deficiency (with immunodeficiency)	Nucleoside phosphorylase	Probable
Ornithine α-ketoacid transaminase deficiency	Ornithine α-ketoacid transaminase	Probable

[a]Yes = prenatal diagnosis accomplished; probable = enzyme activity present in normal amniotic fluid cells; possible = enzyme activity present in normal skin fibroblasts.
[b]X-linked.
[c]Autosomal dominant.

(continued)

TABLE 13–2. Continued

Disease	Measurable Enzyme (or other) Defect	Prenatal Diagnosis[a]
Ornithinemia (gyrate atrophy of retina)	Ornithine aminotransferase	Probable
Orotic aciduria	Orotidylic pyrophosphorylase and decarboxylase	Possible
Osteogenesis imperfecta (severe AR form)	Femur growth	Yes
Osteopetrosis	Bone density	Probable
Phosphohexoisomerase deficiency	Phosphohexoisomerase	Yes
Placental sulfatase deficiency[b]	Placental sulfatase	Yes
Porphyria, acute intermittent type[c]	Uroporphyrinogen I synthetase	Yes
Porphyria, congenital erythropoietic type	Uroporphyrinogen III cosynthetase	Yes
Porphyria, variegate type	Protoporphyrinogen oxidase	Probable
Pyruvate decarboxylase deficiency	Pyruvate decarboxylase	Yes
Pyruvate dehydrogenase deficiency	Pyruvate dehydrogenase	Possible
Refsum disease	Phytanic acid α-hydroxylase	Probable
Sandhoff's disease	Hexosaminidase A and B	Yes
Sanfilippo syndrome, type A	Heparin sulfatase	Yes
Sanfilippo syndrome, type B	N-Acetyl-α-D-glucosaminidase	Yes
Scheie's syndrome	α-L-Iduronidase	Possible
Severe combined immunodeficiency disease[b]	T-cell incompetence	Possible
Sickle cell disease	Linkage with DNA polymorphism	Yes
Sulfite oxidase deficiency	Sulfite oxidase	Probable
Tangier disease	Apo-A-I-lipoprotein	Probable
Tay-Sachs disease	Hexosaminidase A	Yes
α-Thalassemia	Decreased synthesis of α-chain hemoglobin	Yes
β-Thalassemia	Decreased synthesis of β-chain hemoglobin	Yes
Vitamin B$_{12}$ metabolic defect	Vitamin B$_{12}$ coenzyme	Possible
Von Willebrand's disease[c]	Factor VIII deficiency	Yes
Wiskott-Aldrich syndrome[b]	Microthrombocytes	Possible
Wolman's disease	Acid lipase	Yes
Xeroderma pigmentosum	UV endonuclease	Yes

[a] Yes = prenatal diagnosis accomplished; probable = enzyme activity present in normal amniotic fluid cells; possible = enzyme activity present in normal skin fibroblasts.
[b] X-linked.
[c] Autosomal dominant.

could have been diagnosed by amniocentesis (Johnson, 1982). With the high success rate of amniocentesis in diagnosing fairly common genetic aberrations, there is no doubt that amniocentesis will continue as a viable prenatal diagnostic tool. The use of amniocentesis is increasing by 10–15 percent each year, but is falling short of reaching all eligible women (Gray, 1982). One study showed an annual increase of 43 percent in women over the age of 35 using amniocentesis during 1972–1983 (Naber, Huether, and Goodwin, 1987). Particularly for poor and rural women, amniocentesis is often economically or geographically inaccessible. In addition, these women may not perceive amniocentesis as an acceptable part of prenatal screening.

Various factors must be considered in scheduling an amniocentesis. The length of gestation is one important factor because it affects the amount of amniotic fluid present. If the fetus is at significant risk for having a specific disorder, amniocentesis can provide information to parents and physicians about whether the fetus is affected. If the risk of the disorder is greater than the risk of amniocentesis (currently calculated at 0.5 percent), amniocentesis will probably be chosen as part of the prenatal care. Once amniocentesis results are known, the parents have information that will enable them to make the decision to continue or terminate the pregnancy. Also, if amniocentesis is carried out early in the pregnancy, a decision may be made to treat the affected fetus *in utero* or after birth.

Amniocentesis is considered to be part of routine prenatal diagnosis in several cases. In many institutions, amniocentesis is carried out on pregnant women who will be at least 35 years of age by delivery time. At age 35, the chance of significant cytogenetic abnormality (primarily trisomy 21, or Down's syndrome) is 1 in 80; this figure greatly exceeds the risk of abortion or fetal demise due to amniocentesis. After age 40, the risk of significant cytogenetic abnormalities increases to 1 in 60, and at age 45 the risk is 1 in 20. Although no strong evidence exists for advanced paternal age causing fetal cytogenetic abnormality, in as many as 25 percent of cases of trisomy 21, the father may have contributed an extra chromosome. Amniocentesis is also recommended for a client who has had a previous pregnancy involving a fetus with chromosomal abnormality, neural tube defect, or in cases where the parents have a known genetic defect. In trisomy 21 the recurrence rate is 1–2 percent (Johnson, 1982).

Amniocentesis is also recommended in cases in which one of the parents is a known translocation carrier. One in 500 phenotypically normal persons carries a balanced chromosomal translocation, i.e. several chromosomes have interchanged parts without a deficiency or overproduction of genetic material (Milunsky, 1979). Such a translocation in a parent creates a genetically imbalanced infant. Some single-gene disorders (often X-linked and, thus, sex-determined) can be diagnosed by amniocentesis and fetal sex determination. Hemophilia and Duchenne's muscular dystrophy are both single-gene, sex-linked recessive disorders. In instances of recessive trait transmission, the chances of a trait appearing in a particular child are 25 percent. In the case of infant boys, the recurrence rate of a sex-linked disorder is also 25 percent. This percentage is arrived at as follows: there is a 1 in 2 chance that the child will be a boy, and there is a 1 in 2 chance that a boy will be affected with the disease. Biochemical disorders in previous children are also indications for an amniocentesis. More than 100 of these disorders can be identified by amniotic fluid analysis of lipid (Tay Sachs),

TABLE 13–3. *Recurrence Risks of Selected Anomalies*

	Example	*Mechanism*	*Risk*
Single defect			
Disruption	Porencephalic cyst	?Vascular rupture	Sporadic
	Gastroschisis	?Vascular rupture	Sporadic
Deformation	Calcaneovalgus	Multifactorial or uterine constraint	2–3%
	Equinovarus	Multifactorial or uterine constraint	2–3%
	Craniostenosis	Multifactorial or uterine constraint	Sporadic
Dysplasia	Hemangioma	?	Sporadic
	Presacral teratoma		Sporadic
Malformation	Cardiac defect	Multifactorial	2–5%
	Cleft palate	Multifactorial	2–5%
	Neural tube defect	Multifactorial	2–5%
	Hydrocephalus	Multifactorial	2–5%
	Omphalocele	?	Sporadic
Multiple defects			
Disruptions	ADAM sequence	Amniotic rupture	Sporadic
	Thalidomide syndrome	Teratogen	Sporadic
Deformations	Potter sequence	Renal agenesis, etc.	Usually sporadic
Dysplasia	Chondrodysplasia	Recessive gene	25%
		Dominant gene	50%
		X-linked gene	25%
	Marfan syndrome	Dominant gene	50%
	Neurofibromatosis	Dominant gene	50%
Malformations	Down's syndrome	Chromosomal nondisjunction	1%
	Down's syndrome	Chromosomal translocation	5–15%
	Cleft palate and lip pits (Van der Woude syndrome)	Dominant gene	50%
	Pierre Robin sequence (isolated)	?	Sporadic
	Beckwith-Wiedemann syndrome	Recessive gene	25%
	De Lange's syndrome	?	Sporadic
	VATER association	?	Sporadic

SOURCE: Wilson (1982).

TABLE 13–4. *Epidemiologic Observations About Neural Tube Defects*

Category	Specific Observations
Geographic variation	Highest frequency in the British Isles (especially in Ireland, Scotland, Northern Ireland, and Wales); parts of Pakistan, northern India, Egypt, and the Arab Countries. In the United States, frequency is highest in the east and south and lowest in the west. The frequency is lowest in Finland, Japan, and Israel
Racial/ethnic differences	High frequency among Irish and Sikhs. Low frequency among blacks, most Orientals, and Ashkenazi Jews
Seasonal cycles	Higher in spring conceptions; lowest in fall conceptions in the United States and Europe, with the reverse seen in Australia
Time variation	Epidemic-like waves in cycles; overall decline in past decade
Sex	An excess of female patients is found in both anencephaly and spina bifida, with more of a difference in anencephaly
Birth order	First-born children at highest risk, second-born children at lowest risk, with risk rising beyond third born
Maternal age	Young teenagers and women older than 35 years of age are at highest risk
Pregnancy history	Excess of women with miscarriage in pregnancy immediately preceding pregnancy with neural tube defect has been noted
Socioeconomic status	Frequency of neural tube defects is higher in lower socioeconomic classes
Maternal diabetes mellitus	Women with diabetes mellitus have a higher frequency of children with neural tube defects
Family history	Presence of certain congenital anomalies and other neural tube defects in first-, second-, and third-degree relatives increases risk of neural tube defects; previous child with neural tube defect increases risk for subsequent pregnancies
Maternal drug exposure in pregnancy	Valproic acid and aminopterin have been known to cause neural tube defects in offspring, as can maternal alcohol abuse

SOURCE: Cohen (1987).

carbohydrate, amino acid, and mucopolysaccharide metabolism (see Table 13–3; Johnson, 1982).

Amniocentesis can also be carried out to measure the level of alpha-fetoprotein (AFP), which is elevated in neural tube defects (NTDs) such as spina bifida and anencephaly. If there is a family history of NTDs (parents, siblings, and children of these persons), AFP level determination by amniotic fluid analysis is recommended (Hogan and Cheng, 1978). First synthesized by the yolk sac and fetal liver at about 6 weeks' gestation, AFP reaches peak levels at about 13 weeks' gestation. The amount of AFP noted in the maternal serum reaches its highest serum level at 30 weeks' gestation and then declines by the end of pregnancy (Haddow, 1982). Determination of the AFP level can give parents additional specific information about an affected infant and can help couples plan for pregnancy termination if the choice of raising a defective infant is not an option for them.

In a family that may be at risk for NTD, a maternal serum AFP and a sonogram are recommended. In cases of an elevated AFP and a normal sonogram, amniocentesis may need to be performed to further identify a NTD (Lindflors et al., 1987; see Tables 13–4 and 13–5). NTD can be expected to reoccur in 2 percent of affected families (Johnson, 1982). With an elevated AFP (sometimes eight times normal), the chances of the fetus having an NTD increase to 21 percent. At 15 weeks' gestation, normal AFP is approximately 18.5 mg/ml of amniotic fluid. AFP levels are elevated when there has been fetal leakage or hemorrhage into the amniotic fluid or if there is a multiple pregnancy. Amniocentesis can also increase fetal AFP, so a maternal blood sample for AFP should be taken prior to the test to prevent an erroneous interpretation of amniotic fluid AFP (Haddow, 1982).

A new test for acetylcholinesterase (AchE) has been developed to diagnose NTDs with greater accuracy than the measurement of AFP amniotic fluid or serum levels can provide. AchE is more fetus-specific than AFP and originates from the fetal CNS or exposed nerve terminals of the developing fetal nervous system. High AchE levels

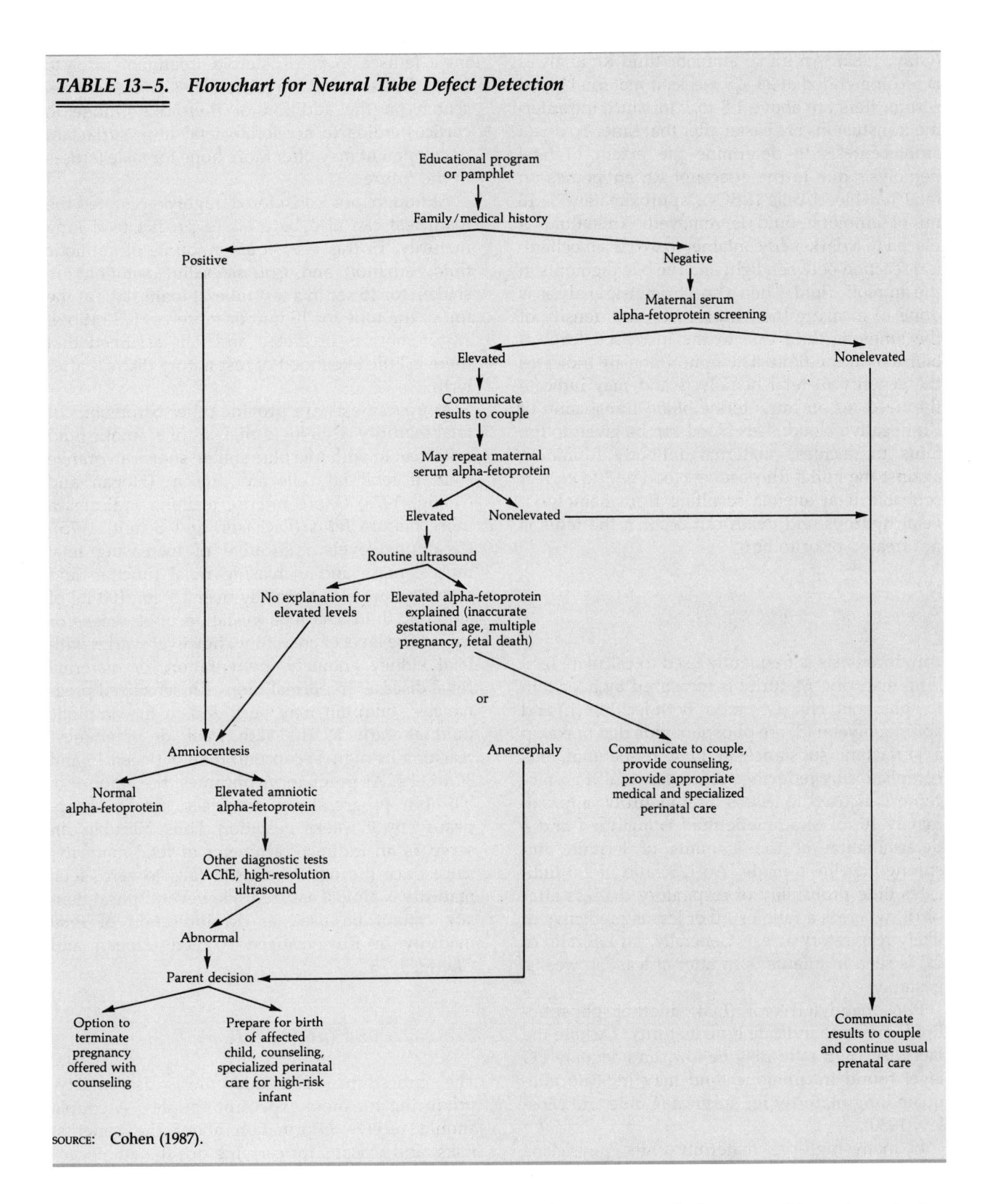

TABLE 13–5. Flowchart for Neural Tube Defect Detection

```
                    Educational program
                      or pamphlet
                           ↓
                    Family/medical history
                    ↙               ↘
              Positive              Negative
                                       ↓
                              Maternal serum
                              alpha-fetoprotein screening
                              ↙               ↘
                          Elevated          Nonelevated
                             ↓
                        Communicate
                        results to couple
                             ↓
                        May repeat maternal
                        serum alpha-fetoprotein
                           ↙        ↘
                      Elevated    Nonelevated ──────────────┐
                         ↓                                   │
                    Routine ultrasound                       │
                      ↙         ↘                            │
         No explanation     Elevated alpha-fetoprotein       │
         for elevated       explained (inaccurate            │
         levels             gestational age, multiple        │
                            pregnancy, fetal death)          │
                                      or                     │
                                                             │
  ↓                                                          │
  Amniocentesis                  Anencephaly   Communicate to couple,
   ↙        ↘                                  provide counseling,
Normal    Elevated amniotic                    provide appropriate
alpha-    alpha-fetoprotein                    medical and specialized
fetoprotein    ↓                               perinatal care
          Other diagnostic tests
          AChE, high-resolution
          ultrasound
               ↓
           Abnormal
               ↓
          Parent decision  ←───────────────
           ↙         ↘
    Option to     Prepare for birth              Communicate
    terminate     of affected                    results to couple
    pregnancy     child, counseling,             and continue usual
    offered with  specialized perinatal          prenatal care
    counseling    care for high-risk
                  infant
```

SOURCE: Cohen (1987).

indicate an NTD; lower levels than expected may be caused by recent fetal death (Haddow, 1982).

Amniocentesis should be offered to highly anxious pregnant women who may have been exposed to radiation or drugs in the prenatal period and are concerned about possible embryonic developmental defects. At about 22 weeks' gestation the procedure can be used to test for Rh-positive (Rh+) antibodies and bilirubin levels in a known Rh-negative mother who has a high antibody titer

(Gray, 1982). An initial amniotic fluid Rh analysis is recommended at 24–25 weeks if maternal blood serum titers are above 1:8 to 1:16, since intrauterine transfusions are easier after that time. To do an amniocentesis to determine the extent of fetal hemolysis due to the effects of Rh antibodies on fetal red blood cells (RBCs), approximately 5–10 ml of amniotic fluid is removed. This fluid is placed in a darkened container to avoid a biochemical reaction between light and the bile pigments in the amniotic fluid. Then a spectrometric analysis is done to measure the increased optical density of the amniotic fluid due to the increased level of bilirubin in the fluid. The optical density indicates the severity of fetal hemolysis and may indicate the need for an intrauterine blood transfusion of Rh-negative blood. This blood can be given to the fetus to decrease maternal antibody formation against the initial Rh-positive blood and to correct probable fetal anemia resulting from hemolysis. Fetal hydrops and death can occur if the fetus is not treated prior to birth.

Assessment of Fetal Maturity

Amniocentesis is frequently used to calculate fetal lung maturity. Maturity is measured by a lecithin to sphingomyelin (L/S) ratio. Both lecithin (L) and sphingomyelin (S) are phospholipids that make up a surfactant substance in lung tissue that aids compliance by reducing surface tension. If amniocentesis is used to assess lung maturity, approximately 10 ml of amniotic fluid is analyzed and a determination of the amounts of lecithin and sphingomyelin is made. An L/S ratio of 2:0 indicates little probability of respiratory distress after birth, whereas a ratio of 1:0 or less is predictive of likely respiratory arrest. Generally, an L/S ratio of 2:0 is seen in infants born after at least 36 weeks' gestation.

Phosphatidylglycerol (PG), another phospholipid, may also indicate lung maturity. Despite the fact that a L/S ratio may be low, an adequate PG level found in amniotic fluid may indicate adequate lung maturity for survival (Golde and Mosley, 1980).

In many high-risk maternity units, physicians are using corticosteroids to medicate mothers in premature labor (28–34 weeks' gestation) who have low L/S ratios. Celestone or Decadron is commonly used to encourage more fetal surfactant development and to decrease the probability of respiratory distress syndrome once the fetus is delivered. Female fetuses respond better than male fetuses to corticosteroid treatment prior to birth (Epstein and Frigoletto, 1983). Current research on the addition of thyroid hormone to corticosteroids to accelerate fetal lung surfactant development may offer more hope for male fetuses in the future.

Although not considered highly accurate, the foam test can also be used to predict fetal lung maturity. In this test, equal amounts of amniotic fluid, ethanol, and isotonic saline solution are shaken for 15 sec in a test tube. If foam stays at the top of the tube for 10 min or more, an L/S ratio of 2:0 or more is predicted and it is assumed that there is little likelihood of respiratory distress after birth.

Amniocentesis can provide other barometers of fetal maturity. Cytologic analysis of amniotic fluid cells treated with nile blue sulfate shows an orange stain if fetal fat cells are present (Hogan and Cheng, 1978). More intense staining indicates a more mature fetus (Dickason and Schult, 1975). Creatinine levels, indicative of increasing fetal muscle mass and increasing renal function and maturity, are also normally over 1.7 mg/100 ml of amniotic fluid at a fetal gestation of 35 weeks or more. The level of creatinine, however, varies with fetal kidney anomaly, dehydration, or maternal renal disease. In normal, non–Rh-sensitized pregnancies, bilirubin may be found in the amniotic fluid as early as the 12th week of pregnancy, reaching its highest concentration between 16 and 30 weeks. As pregnancy continues, the amount of bilirubin progressively decreases, finally disappearing by 38 weeks' gestation. Thus, bilirubin can serve as an indirect barometer of fetal maturity, since once the optical density falls to zero, fetal maturity is almost assured. However, optical density cannot be used as an indication of fetal maturity in Rh-sensitized women (Hogan and Cheng, 1978).

Procedure and Interpretation

The procedure of amniocentesis is anxiety-producing for most expectant couples. A couple should receive information about the benefits, risks, and reasons for carrying out the amniocentesis before the procedure is done. To allay some of the couple's anxieties, the nurse should answer questions and concerns throughout the preparation, the procedure itself, and the aftermath of the amniocentesis. Since results of the procedure are not known for up to 1 month, a supportive health care team is essential in helping the couple adapt to the waiting and to the possible outcome of a positive amniocentesis (a chromosomal abnormality). With a fetal abnormality found in the amniotic fluid analysis, the couple must make a decision to maintain or abort the pregnancy. Most physicians agree that amniocentesis must be completed by 20 weeks' gestation to allow a safe termination of the pregnancy if that is the decision of the couple. An abnormal karotype is found in approximately 1–2 percent of amnioscenteses (Johnson, 1982). Many couples who have an abnormal fetal karotype elect to abort the fetus. Many of these couples are referred by their primary physician to a genetic counseling service to aid in pregnancy termination and family planning.

Most physicians do a sonogram prior to amniocentesis to aid in confirmation of fetal gestational age, location of the placenta, and identification of multiple gestation. A sonogram prior to amniocentesis increases the chances of an effective tap, decreases pregnancy, laboratory and delivery complications, decreases risk of injury to the fetus, and decreases the chance of a bloody amniocentesis sample (Johnson, 1982). Blood in the sample can cause a false increase in fetal AFP, decrease amniocentesis cell growth, and affect the interpretation of the amniocentesis. Many physicians also recommend using abdominal palpation prior to amniocentesis to determine fetal parts, because the greatest amount of amniotic fluid will be found close to the small parts of the fetus.

Amniocentesis is a sterile surgical procedure (Fig. 13–2). The site of needle insertion is "prepped" with a Betadine (povidone-iodine) solution. An informed consent must be signed by the client after she has been told of the benefits and risks of the procedure. Hogan and Cheng (1978) recommend that if the client is less than 20 weeks' pregnant, she should not void prior to amniocentesis. The full bladder will help to hold the uterus steady and out of the pelvis. After 20 weeks' gestation, the client should be encouraged to empty her bladder prior to the abdominal tap.

A local anesthetic may or may not be given in the abdominal wall prior to insertion of the needle used to collect the amniotic fluid. The client can be warned that she may feel a cramping discomfort for 1–2 sec, since the uterus may respond to the needle insertion. A stylette is then inserted into the needle and is used to collect the amniotic fluid. Fluid is placed in a test tube, labeled with the client's name, and sent to the lab. If the fluid is to be analyzed for bilirubin levels, the tube of fluid should be collected in a darkened room under indirect light (flashlight), immediately wrapped in aluminum foil and then sent to the lab.

Amniocentesis side-effects are rare; they include transient nausea and vomiting (Johnson, 1982). Good cell growth is usually obtained with approximately 18–20 ml of amniotic fluid from a pregnancy of at least 16 weeks. There are about 12,000 cells/ml of amniotic fluid by 16 weeks of pregnancy. However, only a few of these cells can be cultivated to produce sufficient growth to allow an amniocentesis test result.

At 16 weeks of gestation, approximately 200 ml of amniotic fluid is present in the amniotic sac. Johnson verifies that aspiration of brown fluid may represent a previous bleed, but this is not a negative indicator unless an elevated AFP is also noted. Meconium-stained fluid is also not interpreted as adverse to fetal viability.

Fathers should be allowed to be present at the amniocentesis procedure so they can offer support and later guidance to their spouses. Once the amniotic fluid is collected, the Betadine is washed from the abdomen to prevent a skin burn and an adhesive bandage is generally placed over the puncture site. Vital signs are monitored before and after the procedure. In some cases of an Rh-negative mother with a negative titer, a vial (300 mg) of Rhogam can be given prior to completion of the amniocentesis procedure. This prevents formation of maternal Rh-positive antibodies. Pregnant women can resume their daily routine after an amniocentesis, although they should be warned about some transient cramping. In many outpatient settings, a post-amniocentesis client is placed on a fetal heart monitor (FHM) to assess fetal and uterine contraction activity. The monitoring is generally discontinued 2 hours after amniocentesis if no negative effects have been noted. Clients should be advised to report any vaginal spotting, fluid loss, severe cramping, or fever. These symptoms may represent maternal complications of infectious amnionitis, hematoma, bowel or bladder injuries, premature labor, spontaneous abortion, or placental puncture (Ward, 1983). Although research is limited on the potential effects of fluid loss as a result of amniocentesis, fetal limb abnormalities and respiratory difficulties may be relevant to this fluid loss during the second trimester of pregnancy (Finegan, 1984).

Nursing Roles: Genetic Counseling

Physicians overestimate the risks of amniocentesis and so may not offer that service to many of their

(a)

(b)

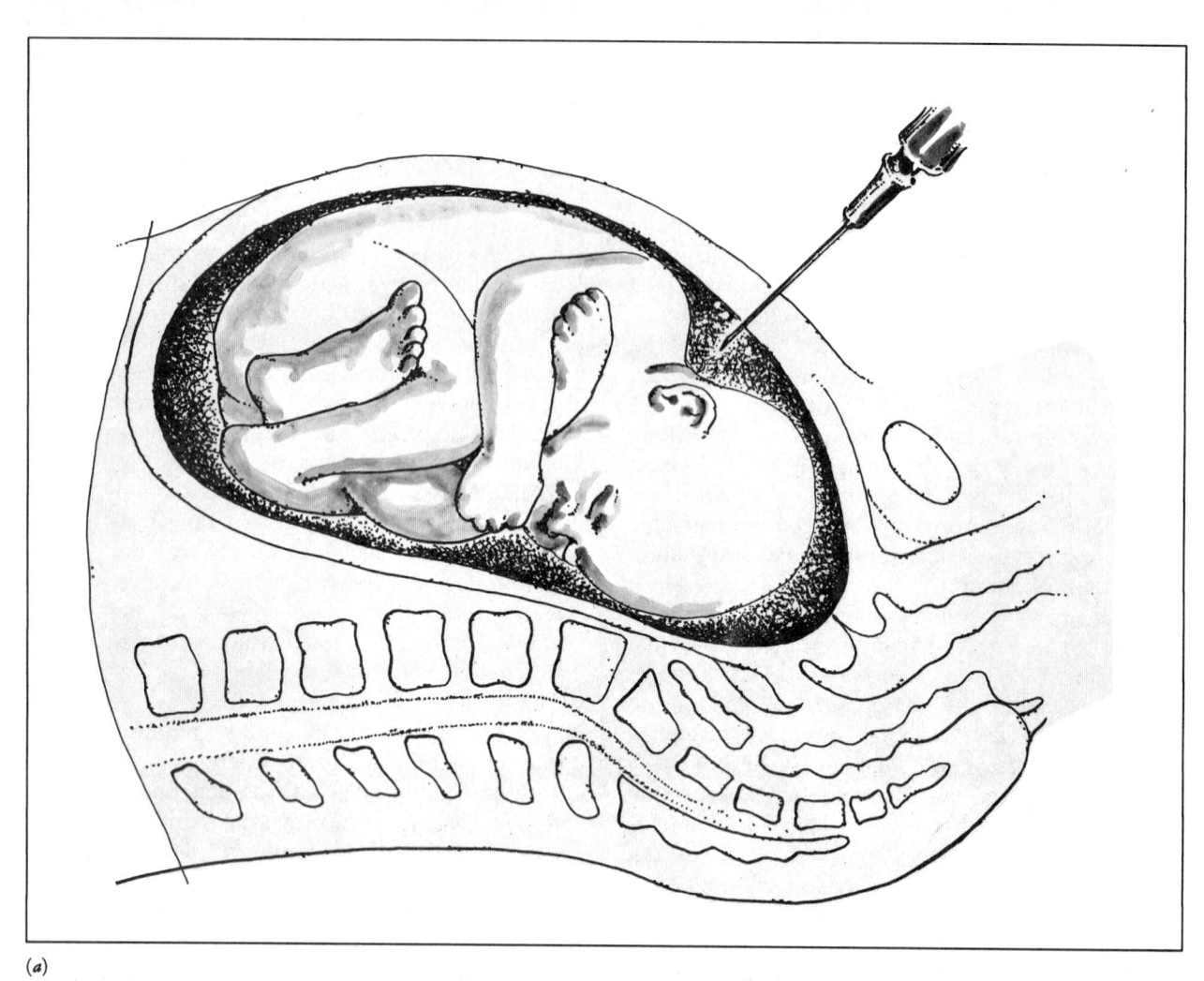

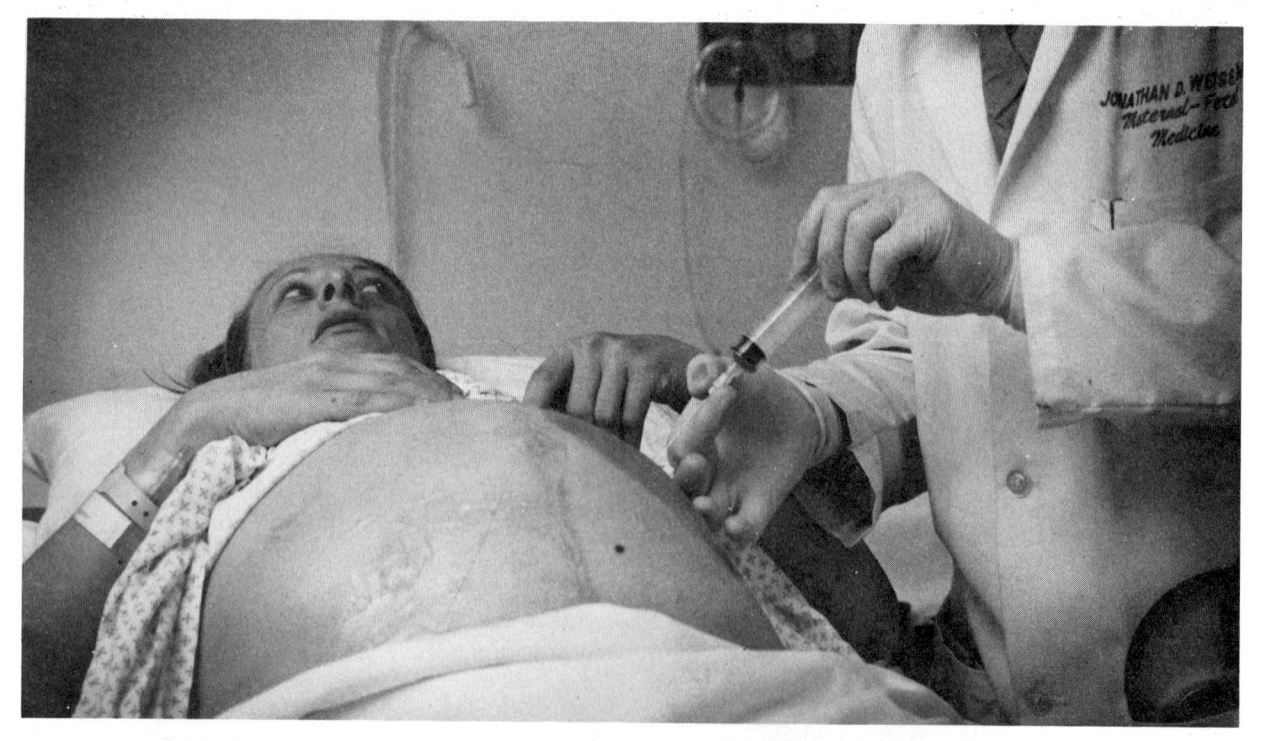

FIGURE 13–2. The technique of amniocentesis. (*a*) Note the location of the needle in relation to the infant. (*b*) Woman having amniocentesis done.

pregnant clients. However, the number of requests for genetic prenatal diagnosis has increased. Many of these requests have come from individual couples who have heard of the service but have not been offered amniocentesis by their physician. On the other hand, low-income groups do not seem to know about genetic diagnosis facilities and do not use these places as much as those individuals with higher incomes.

Once the results of the amniocentesis indicate an affected fetus (a positive amniocentesis), a physician should refer the couple to a genetic counseling service if this has not already been done. Even without an amniocentesis, physicians have the responsibility to refer childbearing clients to genetic services if a family history indicates a genetic abnormality, e.g. couples with a history of cleft palate, cleft lip, NTD, or congenital hip dislocation. These diseases are thought to be caused by multifactorial inheritance or by a combination of a minor gene defect and factors in the environment. The environment may well play a role in the demonstration of some of these defects, since their incidence can vary with the season of the year, family socioeconomic status, and birth order of the child. NTDs occur more frequently in Great Britain than in the United States, and more cases are seen in which conception occurred in the spring and early summer (Haddow, 1982). Other factors also seem correlated with NTDs (Cohen, 1987). The existence of a previous child who is deaf, blind, or retarded may point to previous antenatal infection, alcohol ingestion, or radiation exposure rather than genetic inheritance. Regardless of the etiology of the problem, however, genetic counseling can provide assistance to couples in sorting out how to prevent a repetition of an earlier defect (see Fig. 13-3; Kearney, 1978).

It is important that a couple in any genetic counseling situation understand the terminology used. For example, a couple must understand the meaning of diagnosis, prognosis, and occurrence of risk factors. Often showing pictures of what a child will look like with a particular condition assists parents in starting to understand the impact of a genetic disease. Exploration of family planning options, long-term complications, recurrence rates, and the infant's effect on the family system will allow the couple to more fully understand the problem. The genetic counseling sessions must be appropriate to the needs of the couple in exploring options aimed at a decision to abort or to maintain the pregnancy. After amniocentesis, a selective abortion is a second-trimester procedure. The methods used to abort in the second trimester may also contribute to the psychologic trauma of pregnancy termination. Also, little time may exist (1 week) between the time a couple learns of a fetal diagnosis and the time a decision must be made about what to do about the pregnancy. It is crucial

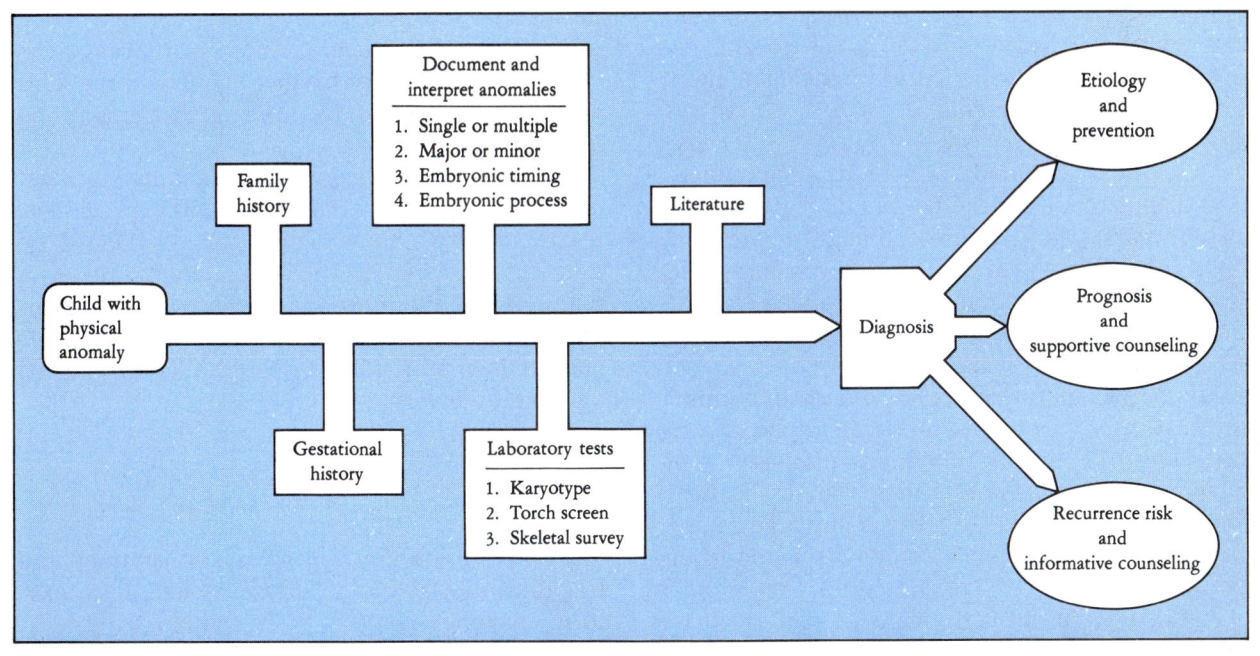

FIGURE 13-3. Steps in the evaluation of genetic abnormality in a pregnancy.
SOURCE: Wilson (1982).

that empathic support and straightforward information be given to couples throughout this highly emotional decision period (Adler and Kushnick, 1982). The use of the nursing process in working with affected couples in identifying nursing diagnoses, expected outcomes, goals, and interventions to meet those goals is needed to optimally meet a couple's needs at this time of crisis.

FETAL MONITORING

Definitions and Indications

The advent of external fetal heart monitoring (FHM) over the past decades has given health care practitioners additional screening information for prenatal diagnosis. The use of FHM in conjunction with other screening procedures (sonography, amniocentesis, and placental enzyme–hormone studies) can frequently provide insight into fetal maturity and well-being in pregnancies defined as high risk because of maternal age, disease, or previous maternity history. FHM is an accurate method of distinguishing the fetal heart tones (FHTs) from uterine activity or fetal movement.

Procedure and Interpretation

External FHM is dependent on the Doppler principle. A transducer sends out a continuous beam of high-frequency sound waves, which is directed through the maternal and fetal tissues and reflected back by moving parts of the fetal heart (Hon, 1968). Movements of fetal heart valves change the sound wave frequencies. These changes are transmitted to a transducer, amplified, and displayed on an exernal monitor graph. The client wears a belt on the abdomen where fetal heart tones (FHTs) are best heard. Frequently, oil, water, or water-soluble gel is applied to the transducer to increase the signal accuracy (see Fig. 13–4; Lojek and Yunek, 1978).

Photocardiography can also be used to monitor the FHTs. This procedure uses a microphone-type transducer that assesses the mechanical energy of fetal heart sounds. Photocardiography is sensitive to environmental and fetal activity and is best used when the client and fetus are quiet in a non-labor situation.

Frequently, health care personnel will want to monitor fetal heart tones and uterine activity concurrently. Uterine activity can be monitored with a specialized transducer called a tocodynamometer (see Fig. 13–5). A uterine contraction or activity causes the tocodynamometer to produce an electric signal. This signal is transmitted to the FHM and is recorded at the same time as the FHTs. The client wears a belt with the tocodynamometer on the fundal part of the uterus to monitor uterine irritability and contractions (Lojek and Yunek, 1978). It is important for the nurse to evaluate the record of FHTs relative to uterine activity. A baseline FHT is assessed over a 10-min period in the absence of uterine contractions. Usually, a baseline fetal heart rate (FHR) is between 120 and 160 beats/min. Fetal tachycardia (above 160 beats/min) may represent maternal infection, impending premature birth, maternal hyperthyroidism, or fetal cardiac arrhythmias. Fetal bradycardia (fewer than 120 beats/min) without deceleration is often associated with congenital heart lesions. A prolonged fetal bradycardia may be a sufficient indication to deliver a baby early. Persistent bradycardia is usually considered ominous, particularly when bradycardia follows the completion of a uterine contraction. On the other hand, some fetal heart rate (FHR) decline, a result of parasympathetic and vagal response, is expected with the start of a uterine contraction. Once the peak of the contraction is reached, the heart rate begins to return to the baseline. FHR decelerations frequently occur as a result of changed paO_2, $paCO_2$, and pH levels of fetal blood, and they often reflect reduced oxygen delivery to the fetus. Uteroplacental insufficiency, seen with maternal high blood pressure, oxytocin use, anemia, or diabetes, can also markedly disrupt oxygen delivery to the fetus and thus demands quick nursing assessment and intervention.

Two antepartal diagnostic tests utilizing FHM are the contraction stress test (CST) (previously termed the oxytocin challenge test, OCT) and the nonstress test (NST) or fetal acceleration determination (FAD). Both tests can give invaluable information about fetal well-being and fetal ability to sustain low morbidity and mortality in a usual labor and delivery.

Nonstress Test

The NST is noninvasive, less time consuming, and less uncomfortable than the previously used oxytocin challenge test (OCT). In the NST, the heart rate of the fetus is measured relative to the stress of fetal movement. Fetal heart acceleration is ex-

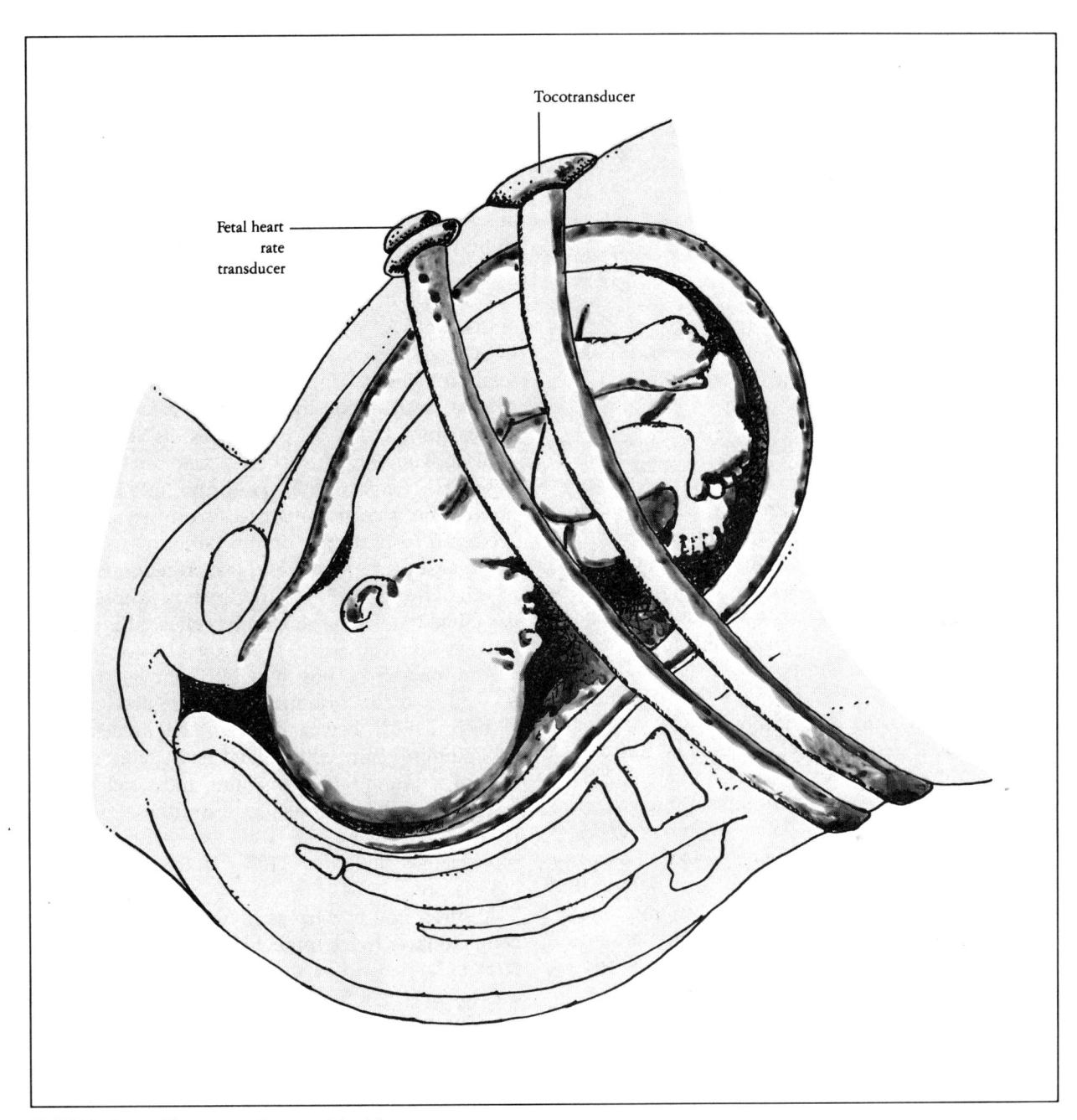

FIGURE 13–4. Placement of external fetal heart monitoring equipment. Before placement of the belts, the fetal position is palpated and the fetal heart found. Conductive gel is applied to the fetal heart rate transducer and tocotransducer and then put on the mother's abdomen for optimal sound.
SOURCE: Lieber (1980).

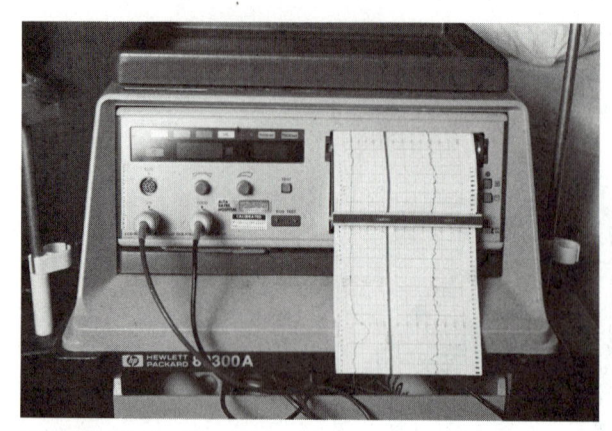

FIGURE 13-5. External fetal heart monitor with tocodynamometer recording FHTs.

pected with fetal activity. An acceleration in FHR is a transient increase of 15 beats/min (bmp) from a baseline FHR. If the fetal nervous system is intact, acceleration should occur (see Fig. 13-6). If accelerations do not occur, the client should be queried about possible medications that she is taking that might make the fetus sleepy (see Fig. 13-7). An informed consent should be signed by the client prior to the procedure. If little fetal activity is noted on the FHM screen, fetal activity may be initiated by an auditory stimulus of approximately 2000 cycles/sec. This stimulus can be supplied by a transducer applied to the lower maternal abdomen; the positive and expected response is a 15-sec or longer acceleration of the fetal heart rate of at least 15 beats/min within 5 sec of the stimulus. Sometimes, rubbing the maternal abdomen initiates fetal activity. In some clinics, clients scheduled for an NST are encouraged to fast and then drink orange juice immediately before the test. Many fetuses become more active with the increased level of intrauterine glucose. A client can be of considerable assistance in conducting the NST, since she can be placed on the FHM and then instructed to punch a button connected to the machine when she feels fetal movement. The FHM graph will then show both the FHR and a peaked line indicating when the mother perceived fetal movement.

The NST is invaluable because it is noninvasive, can be interpreted immediately, can be used with most pregnant clients, and is relatively easy and inexpensive to do. Unlike the CST/OST which may take several hours, the NST takes 20-40 min. In addition, the NST can give information that shows the need for additional monitoring (e.g. CST/OST or sonogram). This test may be expensive. Many times NSTs are not covered by insurance, and the nurse should communicate that fact to the client.

The NST is usually carried out between 32 and 36 weeks of gestation and may be done on a weekly basis in some high-risk pregnancies (e.g. clients with diabetes, high blood pressure, or suspected fetal growth retardation). If the NST is done for postmaturity, it should be done weekly after 40 weeks' gestation (Fig. 13-8).

NSTs are evaluated as reactive, nonreactive, or sinusoidal. A reactive pattern is a negative test. FHR accelerations are irregularly spaced relative to fetal movement (Fig. 13-9). Three to five periods of fetal movement in a 40-min FHM period is satisfactory, but a better test results when every fetal movement causes an acceleration in fetal heart rate (Lieber, 1980). The amplitude and duration of the accelerations are also important. Two accelerations within a 10-min period that increase by at least 15 beats/min and last 20 sec constitute a reactive (negative) NST, and the fetus is presumed to be healthy. This test may be repeated in 1 week for reevaluation.

A nonreactive (positive) NST shows frequent fetal movement without fetal heart accelerations (Schifrin, 1979). Fewer than two FHR accelerations in a 10-min span, with a fetal heart rate acceleration of less than 15 beats/min, and accelerations lasting less than 15 sec, is indicative of an unhealthy fetus (Fig. 13-10; Lieber, 1980). Many physicians schedule an OCT to follow if a positive NST is present.

A sinusoidal pattern is a suspicious test result characterized by definite FHR accelerations with fetal movement, but the number and amplitude are lower than for a reactive NST (2-5 accelerations/min and acceleration of 5-10 beats/min; Lieber, 1980). There may be no consistent fetal response to contractions and there may be minimal or absent beat-to-beat variability of the FHR. This pattern is frequently evaluated as ominous and may be due to fetal distress or anemia or maternal medication. The client needs further evaluation and additional testing (see Figs. 13-8, 13-9, and 13-10) by the prenatal care team.

Contraction Stress Test/Oxytocin Challenge Test (CST/OCT)

The CST/OCT can be very helpful in assessing the circulatory-respiratory reserve of the fetoplacental unit. Frequently, the test is administered after the

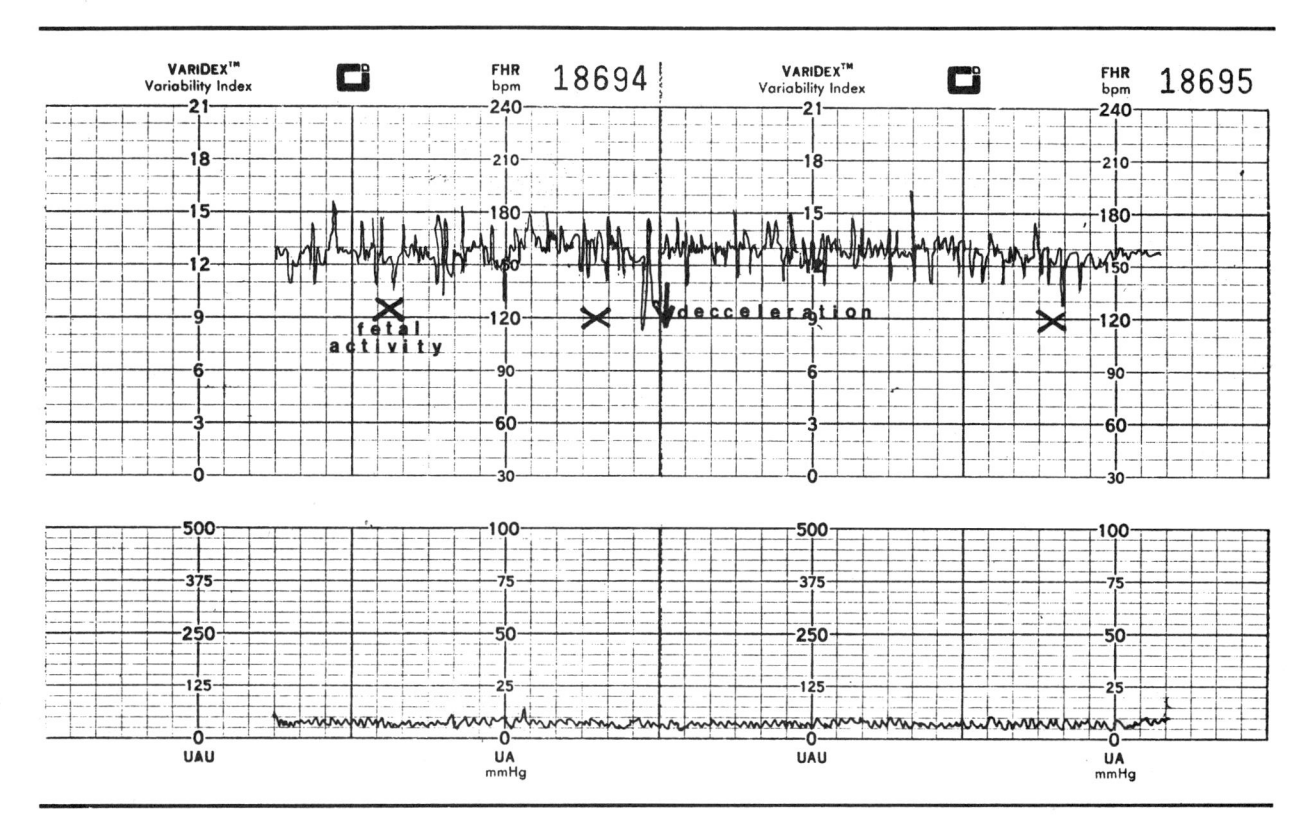

FIGURE 13-6. Reactive nonstress test consisting of a number of irregularly traced accelerations associated with fetal movements.
SOURCE: Lieber (1980).

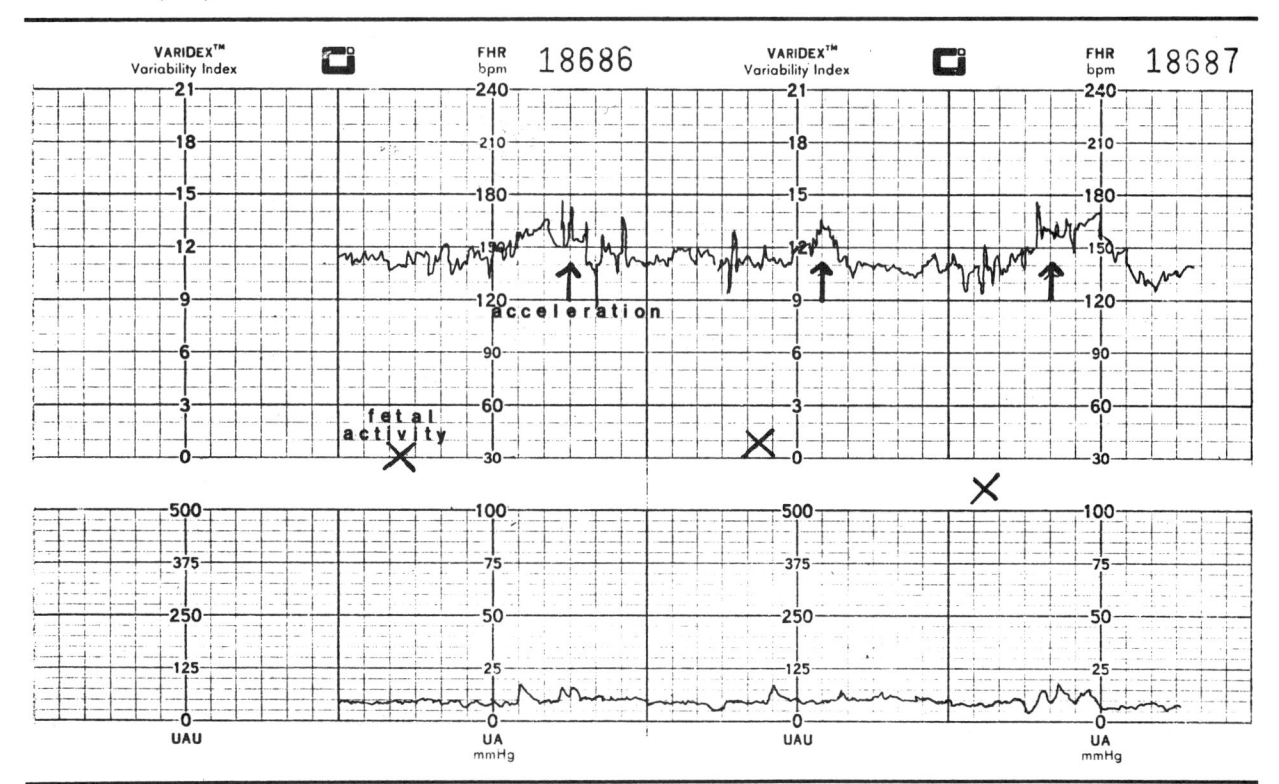

FIGURE 13-7. Nonreactive nonstress test showing fetal activity with no accelerations.
SOURCE: Lieber (1980).

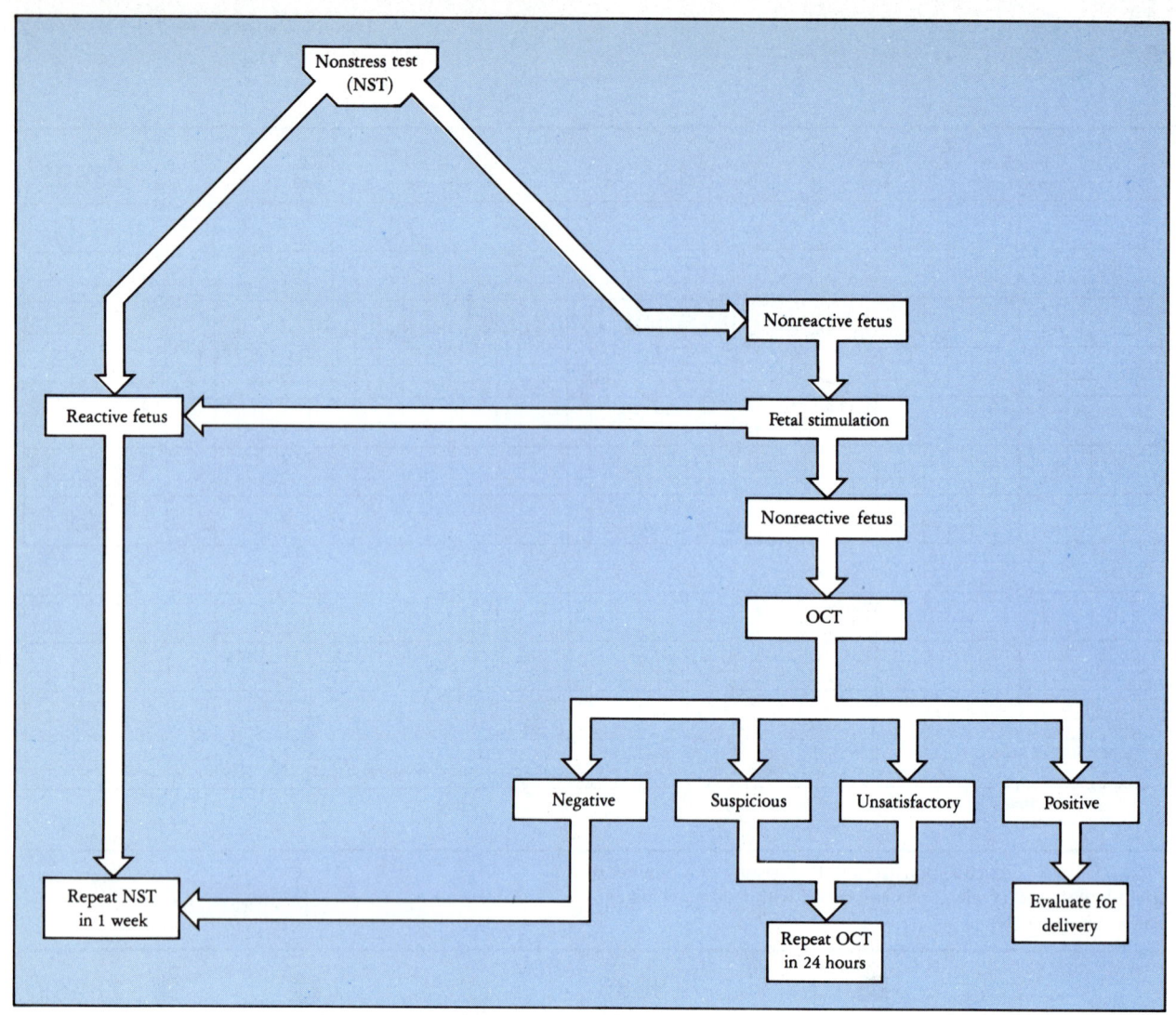

FIGURE 13-8. Actions based on nonstress test results.
SOURCE: Kopf (1978).

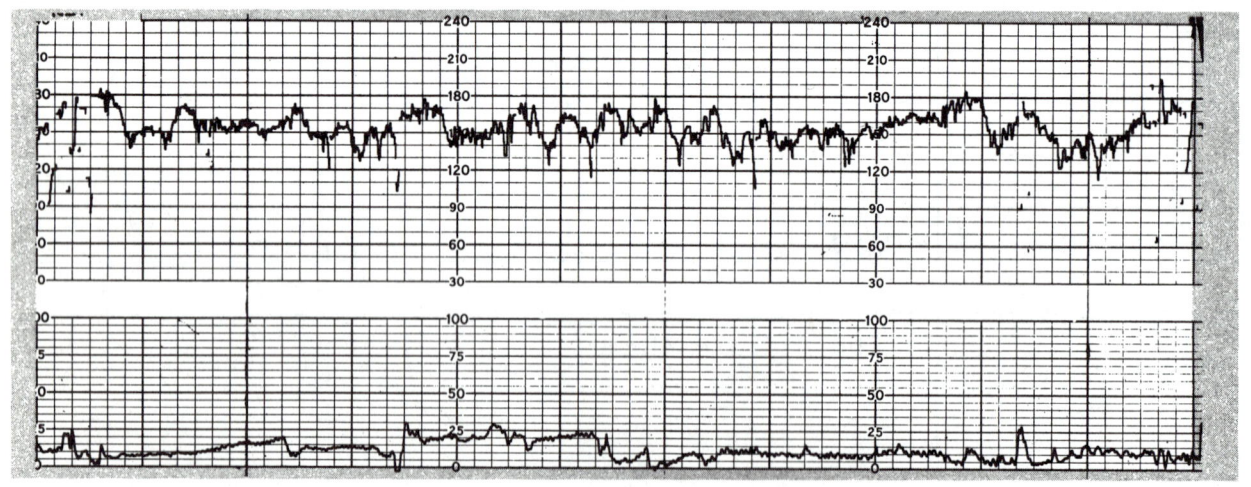

FIGURE 13-9. Reactive (negative) nonstress test (NST). A reactive NST shows two or more FHR accelerations that are of at least 15 beats/min, last 15 sec or more, are associated with fetal movement, and occur in a 10-min period; *or* five or more FHR accelerations of 15 beats/min lasting 15 sec, in a 20-min period. Note frequent FHR accelerations of more than 15 beats/min, lasting 15 sec.
SOURCE: Kopf (1978).

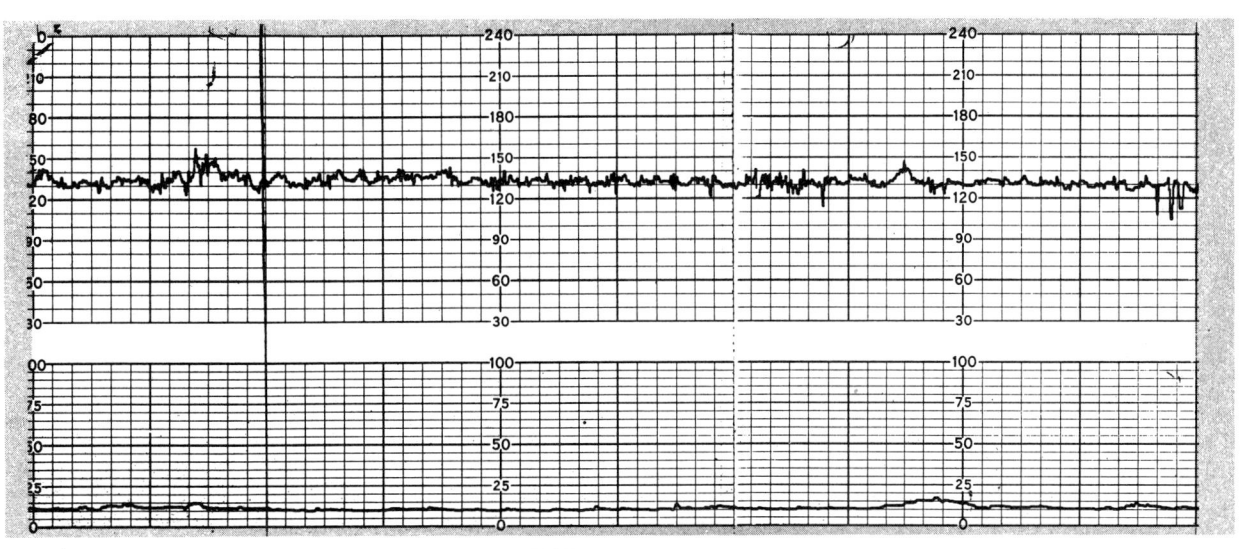

FIGURE 13–10. Nonreactive (positive) nonstress test (NST). A nonreactive NST shows less than two FHR accelerations of less than 15 beats/min, lasting less than 15 sec, and associated with fetal movement during a 10-min period; *or* less than five FHR accelerations of less than 15 beats/min, lasting less than 15 sec over 20 min. Two FHR accelerations are shown here. Because only one meets the criteria for a reactive fetus, the fetus is considered nonreactive.
SOURCE: Kopf (1978).

28th week of pregnancy if the physician suspects placental insufficiency. The test is also given to women who have had nonreactive NSTs or minimally reactive NSTs with poor FHR variability. If the fetus responds poorly to the CST/OCT, little placental reserve exists, and intrauterine hypoxia in labor is predicted. Fetal hypoxia is expected when the fetus has initial tachycardia and persistent FHR deceleration in labor. The exact value of the CST/OCT as a diagnostic tool is still debated, but a negative test generally rules out the need for intervention and a positive CST/OCT correlates well, but not absolutely, with uteroplacental insufficiency.

In one type of CST, the OCT, oxytocin (Pitocin) is given intravenously to induce uterine contractions. In another type of CST, the nipple stimulation contraction test, a pregnant client massages her breast nipple to stimulate uterine contractions. Three or more contractions in a 10-min period satisfy a good response to nipple stimulation (see Table 13–6). Generally, nipple stimulation has been shown to be safe and effective in initiating uterine contractions for a CST (Gantes, Kirchkoff, and Work, 1985; Marshall, 1986).

Since uterine contractions decrease uterine blood flow, fetal heart monitoring is done to assess fetal heart rate activity relative to uterine contractions in a CST. If the administration of oxytocin in 1 liter of intravenous fluid is to be used for an OCT, the client must sign an informed consent for the procedure. The client is placed in a semi-Fowler's position and on the left side during the OCT procedure to avoid compression of the vena cava by the enlarged uterus; in either maternal position, FHM can be done during the test. Fetal baseline heart rate and uterine activity are assessed for 30 min on the FHM before oxytocin is given. Since fetal sleep–wake cycles can last up to 20 min, an initial check of fetal activity over 30 min will ensure an accurate estimate of intrauterine fetal response without oxytocin. Frequently, a vaginal examination is carried out to check for cervical effacement and dilatation. The nurse should check for cord compression prior to oxytocin administration. This can be done by the Hillis procedure. In this technique, the nurse applies fundal pressure toward the client's feet; this causes the fetal chin to be compressed against the chest. The cord will be compressed, and the FHR will fall; with the release of fundal pressure, however, the FHR will return to normal (Diamond, 1978).

If the client does not have any uterine contractions or FHR deceleration with fetal activity in the 30-min observation time, an OCT is begun by administering oxytocin to stimulate uterine contractions. In most hospitals, oxytocin is given via the double-setup ("piggyback") procedure. Oxyto-

TABLE 13–6. Nipple Stimulation Contraction Stress Test: Nursing Guidelines

Purpose
To provide a safe and effective method for obtaining a contraction stress test with nipple stimulation while avoiding hyperstimulation and potential fetal distress.

Rationale
- Hyperstimulation may result in fetal distress with a prolonged deceleration of the fetal heart rate.
- Contractions should be of sufficient strength and duration to decrease uterine blood flow and stress the fetus.
- The left lateral position may decrease the possibility of hyperstimulation.
- Intermittent stimulation with rest periods may decrease the incidence of hyperstimulation and increase success of testing.

Policy
1. The test may be accomplished by having the woman brush her palm across one nipple through her clothes.
2. The procedure and fetal monitor should be explained to the woman and her partner and consent obtained.
3. Urine testing for protein and glucose may be done.
4. A contraction stress test requires in a 10-min period three contractions that are palpable to the operator with a duration of at least 40 sec. The tracing must be interpretable for both fetal heart rate and uterine activity.
5. The antepartum testing nurse may do the initial interpretation, but the physician of record must provide the final interpretation, preferably before the woman is discharged.

Procedure
1. Apply the external monitor with the woman in the left lateral position, and obtain 15–20 min baseline strip. Evaluate per nonstress test criteria and presence of spontaneous uterine activity.
2. Instruct woman to brush one nipple with her palm and continue stimulation for 2 min until a contraction is noted. During the contraction, discontinue stimulation until uterus is relaxed. Resume stimulation until the 2-min time period is ended; then rest for 5 min. Repeat process until test is completed or 40 min has elapsed before initiating oxytocin.
3. The contraction must be of at least 40 sec duration and palpable to the operator.
4. Blood pressure should be taken every 10 min during testing.
5. The woman's name, expected date of confinement, physician, date, reason for testing, position, blood pressure, strength of contractions, and final interpretation should be documented on the strip.

Fetal Distress
1. If uterine hyperactivity precipitates a deceleration of the fetal heart rate:
   - discontinue nipple stimulation;
   - maintain left lateral position;
   - give oxygen per mask at 6–7 l/hour;
   - notify physician.
2. In the presence of tachysystole and/or a tetanic contraction without a deceleration of the fetal heart rate:
   - discontinue nipple stimulation;
   - maintain left lateral position;
   - oxygen is unnecessary;
   - observe fetal heart rate carefully;
   - wait until uterine hyperactivity decreases to baseline frequency before discharging the patient;
   - fetal monitor strips should be safely maintained as part of the medical record.

SOURCE: Marshall (1986).

cin is placed in 1000 ml of 5 percent dextrose in water alongside another 1000 ml of unmedicated 5 percent dextrose in saline (normal saline solution for diabetic women). Should the client over-respond to the oxytocin, the infusion can be stopped by clamping that bottle's tubing, and the other bottle of unmedicated fluid can be infused. Often an intravenous infusion pump is used to monitor the small amount of oxytocin being infused for the OCT. Although hospital protocols vary, usually 1 ml (10 units) of oxytocin is placed in 1000 ml of intravenous fluid. This amount is sufficient to cause uterine contractions of some frequency. An expected response would be for a client to have three contractions in a 10-min period with each contraction lasting about 40–60 sec. In many hospitals nurses are required to monitor the client's response to oxytocin constantly because clients may respond in varying ways to the medication. If a client is not responding to the oxytocin by having uterine contractions, the nurse may increase the infusion rate according to the hospital's protocol—usually 3 drops/min every 15 min until the expected response is obtained. Throughout this time, the client is on the FHM, and maternal vital signs are monitored every 15 min to prevent complications.

It should be hospital policy that a professional

nurse remain in a client's room while oxytocin is being administered. This is because the medication is quite potent and may cause overstimulation of the uterus (see Fig. 13–11). Over-stimulation of the uterus (too frequent contractions without adequate time for uterine relaxation) can cause uteroplacental insufficiency. This necessitates immediate nursing assessment and intervention. With uterine contractions occuring closer than 2 min apart, or lasting longer than 90 sec, the oxytocin is generally discontinued to allow uterine relaxation.

In a CST/OCT, three kinds of deceleration patterns are possible. In a Type I deceleration (uniform decelerations, negative test), the fetus responds uniformly with a heart rate decline at the onset of the uterine contraction (see Fig. 13–12). Contractions last as long as 40 sec and are often as frequent as every 3 min. Type I deceleration is expected with fetal head compression. In Type II deceleration (late decelerations), a fairly constant decline in the FHR occurs after the peak of the contraction. Type II deceleration indicates a positive CST/OCT and usually suggests uteroplacental insufficiency. The FHR usually returns to its baseline, but the return may be delayed and may cause fetal hypoxia. In Type III deceleration, variable FHR declines are found, and the FHR may never get above 80 beats/min due to cord compression after an adequate contraction pattern has been noted. Type III decelerations (variable decelerations) are ominous and require additional health care team assessment and evaluations (e.g. repeat CST/OCTs and 24-hour estriols; see Fig. 13–13).

According to several authors, there are various problems associated with the use of the CST/OCT. The results are sometimes in error; 25 percent of positive OCTs were false in one study (MacDonald and Pritchard, 1976). Also, since there is a slight risk of starting labor with the use of oxytocin or uterine stimulation, the CST/OCT cannot be used with clients who have had previous cesarean births or premature labor, or who have placenta previa, multiple pregnancy or hydramnios.

Nursing Roles

In both the NST and CST/OCT, a calm and relaxed atmosphere is important for test accuracy. Many times, directions can be given about the test beforehand, which can decrease the mother's anxiety about her baby. Although the subject has not been researched extensively, maternal anxiety (stress response) may disrupt the usual FHR and lead to inaccurate results. One might imagine that maternal production of epinephrine in the stress response could cause lowered blood flow to the uterus and could thus be related to an altered FHR pattern. It might prove helpful in decreasing maternal anxiety if the same experienced nurse

FIGURE 13–11. Potential hyperstimulation of the uterus. Note that the tracing shows insufficient rest periods between contractions, flattening of the baseline, and beat-to-beat variability with acceleration of fetal heart rate.
SOURCE: Lojek and Yunek (1978).

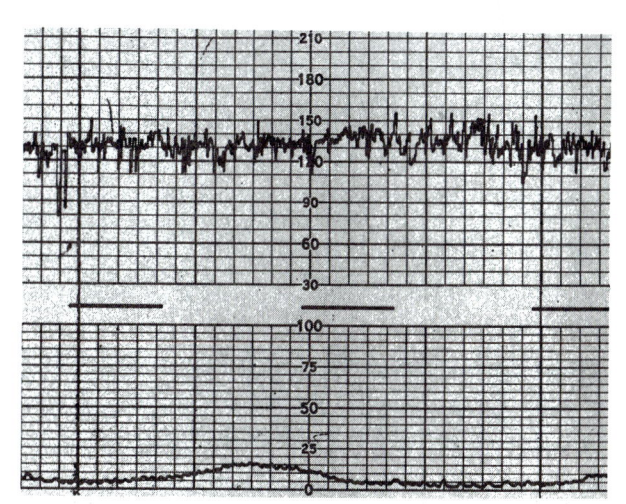

FIGURE 13–12. A negative oxytocin challenge test (OCT). During two uterine contractions, there are no late decelerations in FHR. FHR accelerates with fetal movement, which provides proof of fetal well-being.
SOURCE: Sethi (1978).

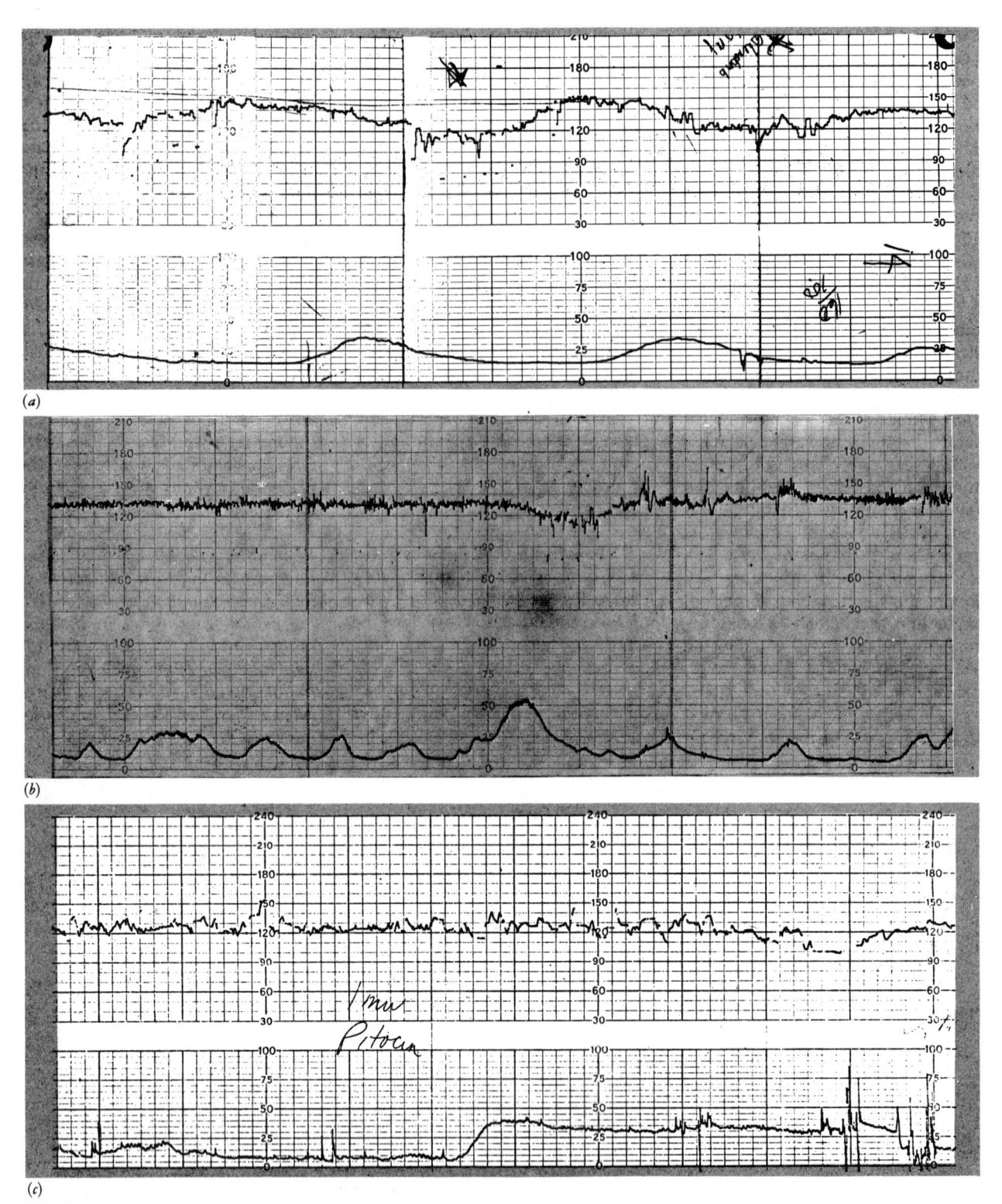

FIGURE 13-13. Nonnegative oxytocin challenge tests. (*a*) Positive OCT. Shown here are three consecutive late decelerations with contractions within 10 min. FHR occurs after peak of contraction, a late deceleration that is an ominous sign. (*b*) Suspicious OCT. There was audible late deceleration with one of the three contractions in 10 min. OCT was repeated within 24 hours. (*c*) Unsatisfactory OCT. This could not be interpreted accurately and, therefore, was repeated the next day. Note hyperstimulation of the uterus after the administration of 1 mU of oxytocin.

SOURCE: Sethi (1978).

could be present to do all CST/OCTs and NSTs. Particularly for a client having several tests, the opportunity to establish rapport with the screening nurse would be beneficial. Having a special room for conducting both the stress and nonstress tests might be helpful, since environmental noise or the psychologic effect of being in the labor unit might negatively affect test accuracy. Above all, humanistic approaches must be used and close contact with the client must be maintained. Meeting the emotional, communication, and informational needs of the client is crucial. In many cases, having a partner or significant other provide support during the CST/OCT and NST may be helpful, because the client has an assistant to help her remember her role in the test.

In the process of conducting the CST/OCT and NST, the nurse must monitor the client's response to the procedure closely. Maternal blood pressure and pulse and FHR should be checked at least every 15 min before the test, during the test, and after it is completed. The fetal outline and lie should also be assessed prior to the test, so that the FHM equipment can be applied accurately. In many cases, after an CST/OST the client remains connected to the FHM for at least 30 min to show any uterine activity relative to FHR. Most of the oxytocin in the body is quickly metabolized during this time. Possible problems with maternal hypotension can be prevented by encouraging the client to rest on her left side; this facilitates uteroplacental hemodynamics and minimizes the chances of a false test reading. Some clinics allow the NST client to sit in a recliner with her head elevated at 45 degrees. For some people this seems to be more relaxing than lying in bed. If the nurse notices any signs of uteroplacental insufficiency (e.g. hypotension, Type II decelerations, or rising baseline FHR), she or he should stop the oxytocin infusion, give nasal oxygen, encourage the client to lie on her left side, and improve hydration by increasing unmedicated intravenous fluid infusion at the levels prescribed by hospital protocol. Monitoring equipment should be checked throughout the test to ensure that it continues to function properly. The graphs from the FHM should become part of the prenatal record and should be sent to labor and delivery once a client is admitted. Information from previous CST/OCTs and NSTs may provide valuable information and alert labor and delivery nurses to the client's potential delivery problems.

Although FHM can give much significant information about the response of the fetus to uterine activity, some clients find the experience of "being tied to a machine" disturbing. Resistance to FHM might decline if the health care team were to prepare the client by explaining the FHM (how it works and what the risks and benefits are) early in prenatal care and showing her a working monitor without her being personally attached to it. Recent attempts to monitor clients "wirelessly" have been somewhat successful, and this sort of telemetry FHM may be part of future prenatal monitoring. In telemetry, a transducer could conceivably send a fetal heart rate signal to a central station while the client is up and about outside of the hospital. At the present time, however, there are problems with receiving accurate FHR signals from a distance. Only with technologic improvement will FHM by telemetry become a useful procedure.

FETAL BIOPHYSICAL PROFILE

The fetal biophysical profile is another test that provides a basis for clinical management and serves as a predictor of pregnancy outcome. This test has been shown to be as accurate an index of fetal condition as the nonstress test, and most major medical centers in the United States are now using it. The five major biophysical variables that are assessed by real-time ultrasound are:

1. fetal breathing movements (FBM);
2. fetal movements (FM);
3. fetal tone (FT);
4. qualitative amniotic fluid volume (AFV); and,
5. the NST.

Antepartum assessment of risk to the fetus based on observation of these biophysical activities yields immediate results, does not require perturbation of the intrauterine environment, is independent of accurate gestational dating, and produces results specifically related to the fetus being observed.

The concept of having the pregnant woman monitor fetal movement (FM) has gained increased acceptance as a determinant of fetal viability. A woman can feel in control of her pregnancy by participating in this inexpensive and noninvasive procedure to monitor her fetus' well-being (Gantes et al., 1986). A client who has not felt movement or who perceives a decrease in movement of a usually active fetus can be encouraged to notify her

TABLE 13–7. Fetal Biophysical Variables

Test	Normal	Abnormal
Nonstress test	Two or more fetal heart rate accelerations of at least 15 beats/min in amplitude and at least 30 sec duration associated with fetal movement(s) in 20-min period	One or less fetal heart rate acceleration of at least 15 beats/min and 30 sec duration associated with fetal movement in 40 min.
Fetal breathing movements	The presence of at least one episode of fetal breathing of at least 60 sec duration with a 30-min observation period	The absence of FBM or the absence of an episode of FBM of at least 60 sec duration during a 30-min observation period.
Gross fetal body movements	The presence of at least three discrete episodes of fetal movements within a 30-min period. Simultaneous limb and trunk movements were counted as a single movement	Two or less discrete fetal movements in a 30-min observation period
Fetal tone	Upper and lower extremities in position of full flexion. Trunk in position of flexion and head flexed on chest. At least one episode of extension of extremities with return to position of flexion and/or extension of spine with return to position of flexion	Extremities in position of extension or partial flexion. Spine in position of extension. Fetal movement not followed by return to flexion. Fetal hand open
Amniotic fluid volume	Fluid evident throughout the uterine cavity. Largest pocket of fluid greater than 1 cm in vertical diameter	Fluid absent in most areas of uterine cavity. Largest pocket of fluid measures 1 cm or less in vertical axis. Crowding of fetal small parts

SOURCE: Manning, Platt, and Sipos (1980).

physician for further assessment (real-time sonography can be used to detect fetal movements). In many cases, FMs are correlated highly with estriol levels and may be more predictive of fetal viability than estriol levels (Sadovsky, 1979). Although more research needs to be carried out to determine the significance of FMs and delivery outcome, such movements are known to vary according to maternal glucose level, time of day, and maternal smoking patterns (Richardson, 1983).

In the biophysical profile, each biophysical variable is given a score of 2 if it is normal or a score of 0 if it is abnormal. Table 13–7 lists criteria for determining normality. A planning score of 10 is correlated with a decreased incidence of low Apgar scores at 5 min (see Fig. 13–14), a decreased incidence of fetal distress in labor (see Fig. 13–15), and a decreased incidence of perinatal mortality (see Fig. 13–16). An average of 10 min is required to measure the four ultrasound variables (Manning, Platt, and Sipos, 1980).

PLACENTAL HORMONES AND ENZYMES

Definitions and Indications

Placental hormone levels can serve as valid indicators of placental adequacy and therefore can give information about fetal viability. Several placental hormones have been isolated. Both estriol and human placental lactogen (HPL) are important in diagnosing placental insufficiency and fetal well-being. Usually a variety of enzymes and hormones are assessed to give information about adequacy of the fetoplacental unit.

Early research indicated that pregnant women excrete large amounts of estriol, a breakdown product of estrogen. Later, the placenta was identified as the source of estriol. At term, 25 percent of circulating estrogen is estriol (Diamond, 1978). The well-being of the fetus can be monitored by checking maternal serum levels and urinary

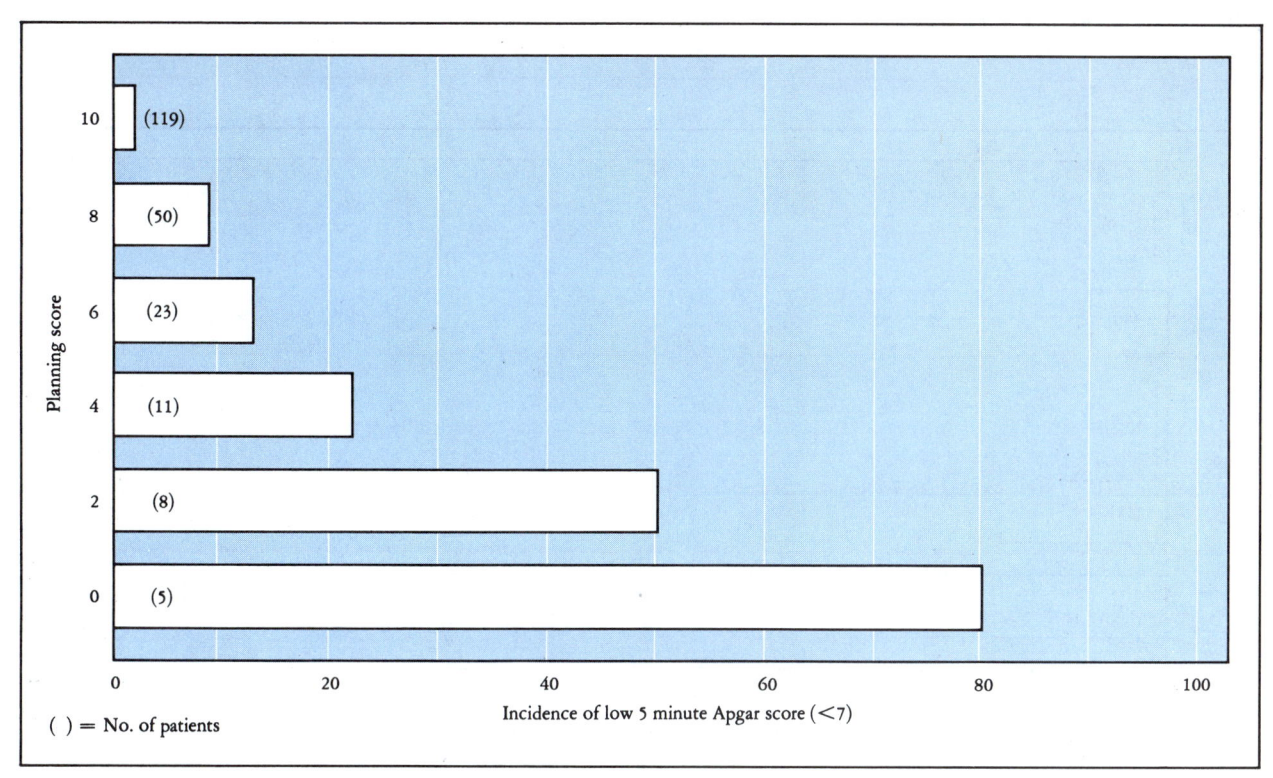

FIGURE 13–14. The relationship of a fetal biophysical variable score to the incidence of low 5-min Apgar scores. A 47-fold increase in the incidence of low Apgar scores is observed between a score of 10 (all normal) and 0 (all abnormal).
SOURCE: Manning, Platt, and Sipos (1980).

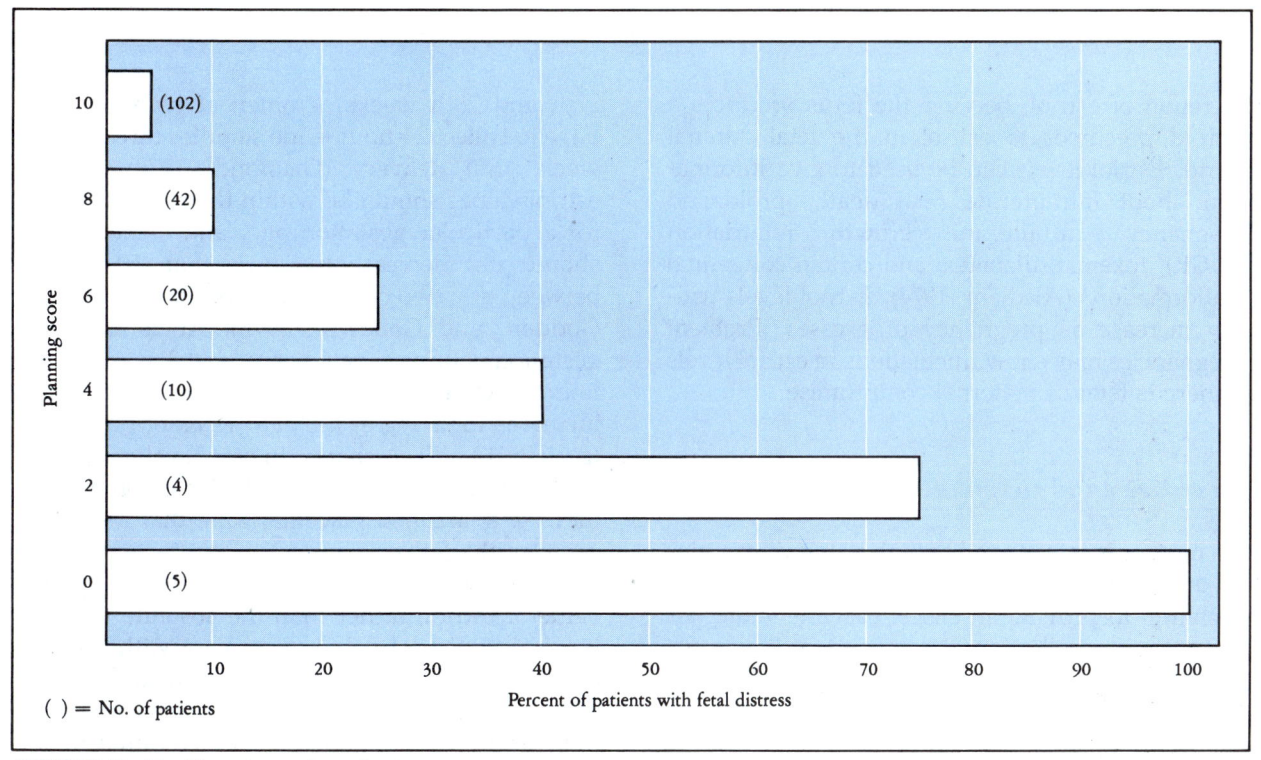

FIGURE 13–15. The relationship of a fetal biophysical variable score to the incidence of fetal distress in labor. A 37.5-fold increase in the incidence of fetal distress was observed between a score of 10 (all normal) and 0 (all abnormal).
SOURCE: Manning, Platt, and Sipos (1980).

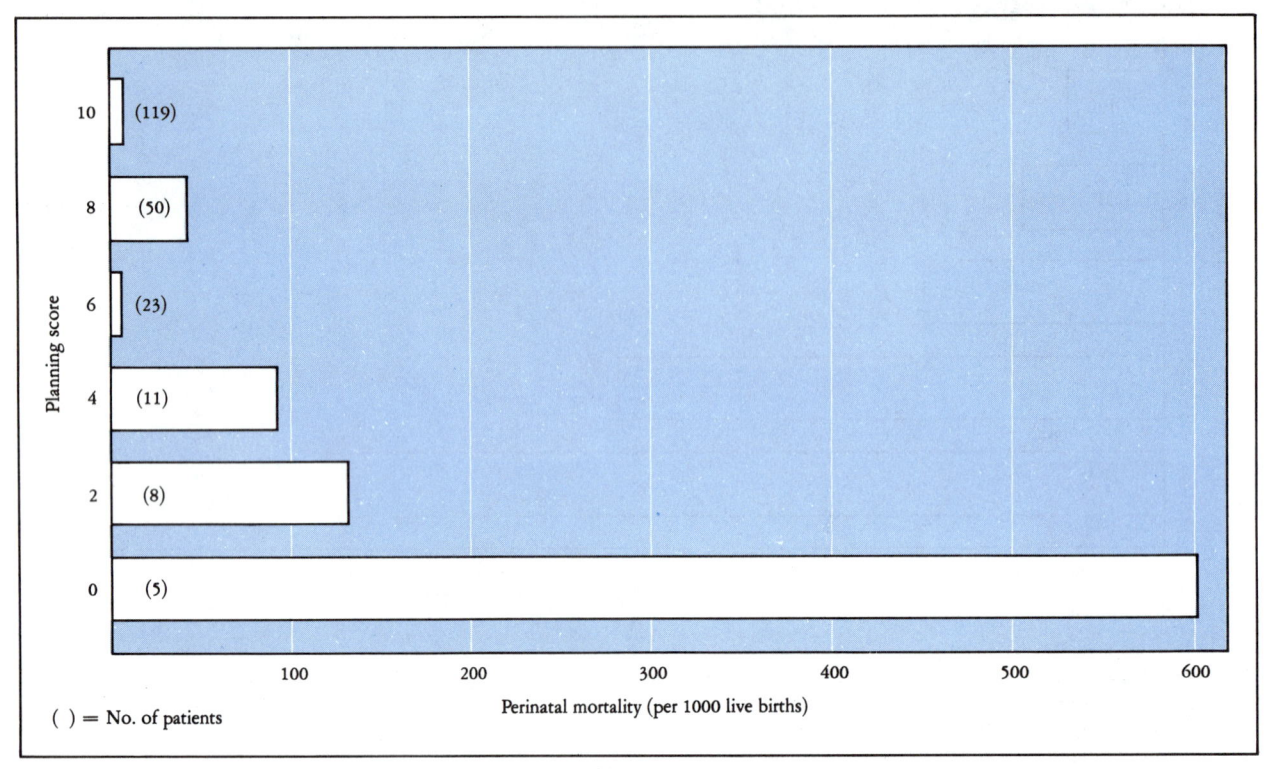

FIGURE 13–16. The relationship of a fetal biophysical variable score to perinatal death.
SOURCE: Manning, Platt, and Sipos (1980).

excretion of estriol, because the fetus produces a steroid precursor to estriol in the fetal adrenal gland. Estriol levels can be used to give information about intrauterine fetal death, prolonged pregnancy, intrauterine growth retardation (IUGR), toxemia, diabetes, and certain congenital malformations (Aladjem, 1974). Estriol levels usually increase as pregnancy progresses. Problem pregnancies may show fluctuations in estriol levels if there is fetal or maternal compromise.

Procedure and Interpretations

If a mother is categorized as high risk, two samples of urine are collected around the 26th week of gestation to provide an estriol baseline value. As 24-hour urine collections are needed, a client must be instructed to save all urine voided within that time period. Most hospital protocols instruct the client to discard the first urine voided in the 24-hour period but to save all other urine for the time period. Collected urine should be refrigerated or stabilized with a preservative in the bottle that the client receives from the clinic or hospital. Urine specimens are then collected weekly during the 27th and 28th weeks. Women at high risk may have to collect 24-hour urine samples three times a week until delivery (Diamond, 1978). Sample estriol values should be within the range expected for a particular gestation age, and estriol values should not decrease by more than 50 percent between any two consecutive specimens (Chance, Godden, and Goodwin, 1976). At 28 weeks of gestation, a urinary value of at least 8 mg estriol/24 hours is expected for fetal well-being. This value increases to 26 mg at the 38th week of pregnancy (see Fig. 13–17). A change in estriol values outside the range expected for a particular gestation may indicate a changed placental state that may compromise the fetus.

It is important to remember that the trend of the value of estriol, rather than the absolute value, is important. Estriol values may vary with the reliability of the collector, maternal drug therapy, bedrest, and the possibility of an incomplete 24-hour urine collection. Serial estriols, rather than a single value obtained by one 24-hour urine collection, are needed to interpret whether placental inadequacy exists. This insufficiency may be predictive of poor fetal response to labor and delivery. However, a low estriol level that increases consis-

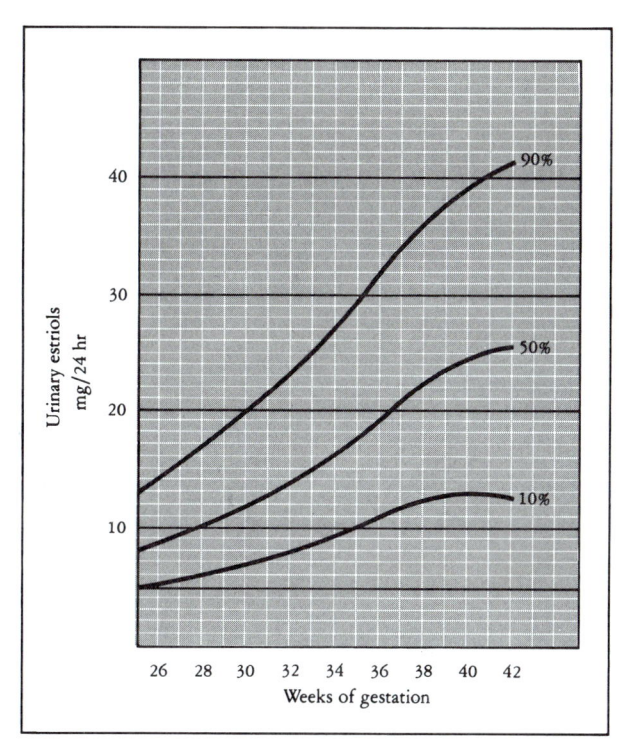

FIGURE 13–17. A 24-hour urinary estriol chart. It provides easy reference for interpreting values from the laboratory and a convenient way to record test results in the prenatal chart.
SOURCE: Burosh (1976).

tently over gestation may instead reflect a small baby in an intact placenta.

Plasma estriol values can also be obtained. These are positively correlated with urinary estriols and are easier to collect. Daily variations in plasma estriol are to be expected. Circadian rhythms also affect the amount of plasma estriol collected. Therefore, blood samples for estriol should be collected at about the same time every day (Patrick et al., 1980). Maternal renal efficiency, the reliability of the collector, the accuracy of the chemical method used to interpret the test, maternal laxatives, maternal medications (methenamine mandelate, corticosteroids, and antibiotics), and impaired fetal renal and adrenal function can all affect daily estriol levels. If kidney clearance problems invalidate urinary estriol assay values, serum estriol values may be more accurate.

Human placental lactogen (HPL), or human chorionic somatomammotropin, is secreted by the trophoblast of the placenta. HPL is closely related to pituitary growth hormone and may help prepare the breasts for lactation. HPL may help to make glucose accessible to the fetus, ensuring adequate nutrition to the rapidly growing fetus. HPL also increases lipolysis, making fatty acids available to the fetus for energy (Josimovich, 1974). A specimen for HPL analysis can be collected by a venipuncture. The test is relatively inexpensive, and it takes approximately 3 hours to obtain results. HPL levels rise as pregnancy progresses and then slowly fall after delivery (Heys, 1978).

Nursing Roles

The psychologic and familial impact of 24-hour urine collection can affect the efficiency of collection. It may be stressful for some families to collect human waste, and clients should be encouraged to ventilate these feelings. The need to remember that all urine for 24 hours must be saved in the bottle is also a stressor. Keeping the bottle under the toilet may increase the chances that a complete specimen will be received. In highly anxious clients, written instructions that thoroughly explain the test, its risks and benefits, and the interpretation of results may alleviate some of the anxiety. In many client situations requiring 24-hour urine collection, estriol screening is done to assess placental adequacy, and possible stress effects of the test must be considered. During the stress response, the anxious mother produces epinephrine and norepinephrine. This response can increase the maternal blood pressure and decrease placental perfusion. More congenital defects, fetal asphyxia, and neonatal deaths possibly due to placental inadequacy are noted among women who are perceived as highly anxious during pregnancy as compared to women who do not appear as worried about their pregnancies (Ascher, 1978).

FETOSCOPY

Definitions and Indications

The technique of fetoscopy is so new to the prenatal diagnosis arena that only selected specialized medical centers in the United States use it (Golbus, 1982). Because of the relative lack of availability of the procedure, and the specialized equipment and physician training required, fetoscopy at present is quite expensive.

Currently, fetoscopy is used to collect fetal tissue samples to obtain diagnosis of fetal disease. The fetal tissue samples are analyzed by electron microscope. Diseases such as hemoglobinopathies (hemophilia, thalassemia, sickle cell anemia) and hereditary skin diseases (genodermatoses, granulomatous diseases) can be detected by fetoscopy but generally cannot be isolated by sonography or the analysis of amniotic fluid. Generally, no biochemical abnormality exists in hemoglobinopathies and, therefore, current amniocentesis is inefficient in detecting fetal disease. Epstein and Frigoletto (1983) state that today's ability to carry out DNA sequence analyses on amniotic fluid cells has made fetoscopy unnecessary to diagnose fetal hemoglobinopathies.

Fetoscopy is a complex technique requiring specialized equipment and specialized competency of the physician doing the procedure. Many years were spent in perfecting an instrument that would require a fetoscopy incision no larger than that required for amniocentesis (Research McGill, 1980). Finally, a needlescope (a 1.7 × 150 mm straight view endoscope) was developed that has proven to be efficient in the technique of fetoscopy. The needlescope is effective because of its double cannula structure, which allows a fibroscope and a sampling needle to be used side by side (see Fig. 13–18).

Procedure and Interpretation

Fetoscopy is a sterile procedure. The client's abdomen is prepared with povidone-iodine solution, and local anesthetic infiltration is used prior

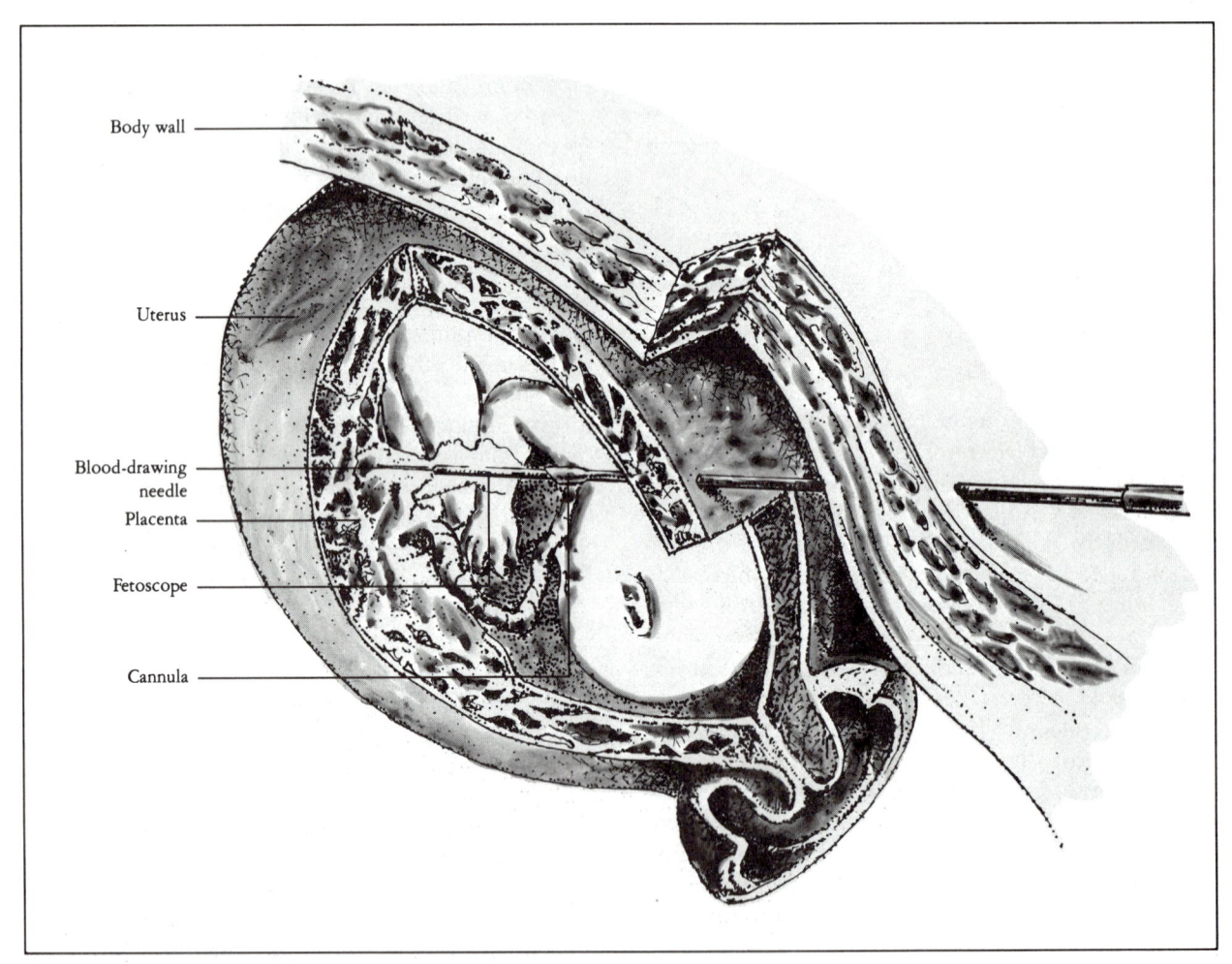

FIGURE 13–18. The technique of fetoscopy. Fetoscopy is being used in a few centers to obtain blood and tissue samples when suspected abnormality cannot be diagnosed from amniotic fluid analysis. A fiberoptic scope is passed through a cannula in the anterior wall of the uterus under ultrasonic guidance. Fetoscopy alone carries a 5 percent risk of fetal loss; risk from biopsy is not established.
SOURCE: Golbus (1982).

to the fetoscope equipment insertion. It is recommended that the client be supine and have received intravenous diazepam (Valium) to sedate both the baby and the mother (Elias and Esterly, 1981). With sonography guidance, the small needlescope is then introduced into the client's uterus through the anterior wall (Golbus, 1982). Real-time (dynamic) sonography prior to needlescope insertion can aid in the location of the placenta, visualization of fetal parts, confirmation of fetal age, and estimation of the depth of the amniotic cavity (Research McGill, 1980). The physician's knowledge of these factors ensures a more efficient fetoscopy.

Once the needlescope is inserted into the uterus, fetal blood samples are taken slightly above the junction of the umbilical cord and the placenta (Elias and Esterly, 1981). This puncture site is desirable because fetal blood is found more easily at the junction of cord and placenta. Tissue samples can also be collected from the fetal body (usually the buttocks, thorax, or back) with a pair of forceps that fits through the cannula of the needlescope. Bleeding from the punctured fetal vessel stops soon after the needle is removed; how soon bleeding stops may depend on amniotic fluid pressure, elasticity of the fetal vessel wall, or amniotic fluid coagulation factors (Research McGill, 1980).

Fetoscopy is best used at approximately 16–20 weeks of gestation and is most appropriate if fetal disease is suspected because one or both parents are disease carriers. Because the needlescope allows the physician to get close to the well-developed fetal parts at this time in gestation, blood and tissue samples can be collected to aid in the diagnosis of fetal disease. In the case of thalassemia, McGill Laboratories research shows that chromatography can be used to identify hemoglobin chains whose absence may reflect fetal thalassemia.

However, many physicians consider fetoscopy to be a research procedure and one that is not to be as routinely used as amniocentesis. For example, physicians note that fetoscopy requires complex obstetrics in a genetic diagnosis field that is just now evolving. There is a 5 percent chance of aborting after a fetoscopy; it is not currently known how many fetoscopies can be carried out before a woman increases her chance of aborting dramatically. This makes use of the procedure questionable (Golbus, 1982). In addition, there are risks of bleeding from the insertion of the needlescope, infection, fetal injuries, amniotic fluid leakage, and premature birth. The development of more refined sonography and other noninvasive techniques may decrease the use of fetoscopy with its inherent risks.

Nursing Roles

As with other prenatal diagnostic procedures, the use of fetoscopy demands an accounting of the benefits and the risks involved in the procedure. If it is known that one or both parents carry a life-threatening disease, the benefits of fetoscopy may outweigh the risks of doing the procedure. The nurse must assess the already existing knowledge base of the parents and their desire to learn more about the reasons for doing the fetoscopy. Once the fetoscopy is done and results of the test are known, the nurse should be supportive of the couple in decisions about whether to maintain the pregnancy. There may be the need for additional emotional support for the couple electing to continue the pregnancy and thus to raise an affected infant. If parents know they are carrying an afflicted infant, referral to an appropriate helping agency or peer support group may also be a nursing duty. Frequently, a peer support group can help couples define their parenting goals and can assist in their attainment of the desired parenting role.

Because of the invasiveness of the procedure, couples considering a fetoscopy will undoubtedly be anxious. The nurse must be emotionally supportive of the couple in their decision to participate or not in the procedure. Husbands and wives need to be encouraged to talk about their fears and to express concerns to the health care team. It is important that the nurse show empathy during the procedure to help the couple incorporate fetoscopy into the prenatal screening course and to make the couple aware of the nurses's unconditional support, which they may need once the fetoscopy sample results are known. In addition, the nurse can serve in an educational role by instructing couples about complications that may arise after the fetoscopy, complications that would also be associated with amniocentesis or any other invasive procedure into the uterus.

PLACENTAL GRADING

Definitions and Indications

Sonography has allowed sophisticated assessment of placental maturation. Although placental maturity alone cannot predict fetal lung maturity accurately, assessment of a mature placenta along with biparietal diameter measurements of a fetal head and a fetal abdominal circumference can be valuable in assessing fetal maturity (Harman et al., 1982; Seeds, 1984). Grading of placental tissue ranges from a score of 0 (immature) to a score of 3 (mature) and may prove significant with further research in diagnosing intrauterine growth retardation problems. Grading, along with the recently approved procedure of nuclear magnetic resonance (NMR), which can be used to assess pelvic blood flow and placental infarction, can also add to knowledge about fetoplacental adequacy in pregnancy.

Procedure and Interpretation

The process of sonography is used to allow placental grading by the physician. Relevant information under the topic of sonography in this chapter should be considered in the process and interpretation of placental grading.

Nursing Roles

Relevant nursing roles in placental grading include those listed under the topic of sonography. Further interpretation of the placental grading results may be needed by the client after the physician has explained grading findings. Nursing staff may participate well in this form of client education throughout the prenatal course.

CHORIONIC VILLUS SAMPLING

Definitions and Indications

Chorionic villus sampling (CVS) is done as early as 9 weeks of pregnancy to detect genetic disease. The test, currently available in only a few perinatal centers in the United States, can be used for women over age 35 or in couples who have experienced or have a history of genetic disease. Compared to amniocentesis, CVS can be carried out approximately 6 weeks earlier in the pregnancy. However, the risk of spontaneous abortion is greater for CVS (1–3 percent) as is the risk of infection when compared to the risks in amniocentesis.

Due to the present experimental nature of CVS, couples opting for this prenatal test receive extensive preprocedural teaching, information, and support about CVS. An informed consent is signed by the couple after they state understanding of the benefits, risks, and limitations of CVS. In many cases, long-term follow-up of the pregnancy and fetus is implied in consenting to the procedure so that research data can be collected to improve CVS outcomes for future CVS clients.

Procedure and Interpretation

Under the guidance of sonography, a sterile catheter is introduced into the cervix of the pregnant woman to collect a small sample of chorionic villi (fetal portion of the placenta). Although not as frequent, transabdominal CVS may be carried out with good efficacy if transcervical aspiration is contraindicated (Bambati, Oldrini, and Lanzani, 1987); (Figs. 13–19 and 13–20) surgical asepsis similar to that during an amniocentesis is maintained throughout the procedure due to the risk of infection. Routine cleaning of the cervix and vagina and a gonorrheal culture are carried out to decrease the risk of infection. Once the cells (villi) are collected, they are placed in culture media and then sent immediately to a genetic center for analysis. The karotype of the fetus as well as any diagnosis of fetal abnormalities similar to those identifiable by amniocentesis can then be deter-

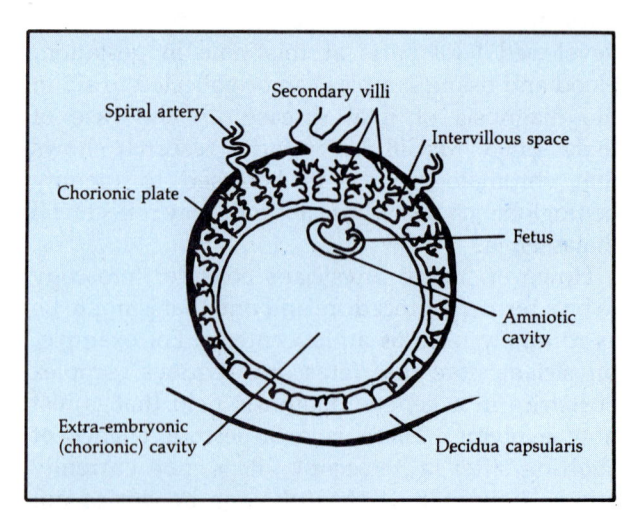

FIGURE 13–19. The human embryo at approximately 6 weeks gestation. At the embryonic pole, the villi are numerous and well-formed; at the abembryonic pole, the villi are fewer in number and less well-developed.

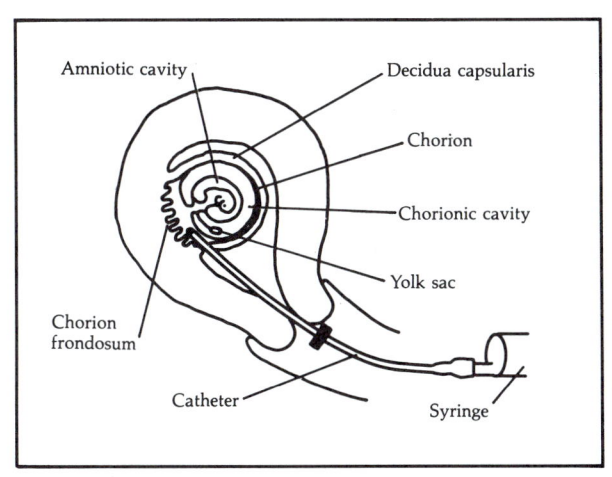

FIGURE 13–20. The uterus at 10 weeks gestation with biopsy catheter in position.
SOURCE: Hogge et al. (1986).

mined by a skilled genetic team. Although an AFP level can be obtained by amniocentesis, it is not possible to obtain this type of sample in a CVS. Although some collected villi grow rapidly to allow a karotype determination in several days, most cells do not gain a distinct appearance needed for genetic analysis until approximately 2 weeks after initial collection. Usually, 1 month is needed to grow amniotic fluid cells sufficiently to allow interpretation of a fetal karotype and possible fetal genetic abnormalities.

Possible negative effects of CVS include infection, spontaneous abortion, intrauterine fetal death, intrauterine growth retardation, or hematoma. Although there do not appear to be any effects of CVS on fetal movements (Boogert, Mantingh, and Visser, 1987), clients need to be warned to report any vaginal spotting, fluid loss, uterine cramping, or fever. These symptoms may indicate maternal complications necessitating medical attention.

Nursing Roles

The experimental nature of CVS may make some couples more anxious about the procedure. Anticipatory guidance by the health care team and active support of couples in their decision to use or not to use the CVS as a genetic testing procedure is needed.

Because CVS can determine a genetic abnormality early in the pregnancy (possibly before the pregnancy "shows"), couples may feel greater freedom in electing abortion at a fairly safe time of pregnancy should an abnormality be detected. On the other hand, if the fetus has a healthy genetic makeup, couples may feel renewed joy about the pregnancy. These couples indeed may be very receptive to prenatal education which could focus on optimal nutrition, avoidance of substance abuse, and serial prenatal care.

If couples elect to continue a pregnancy with the knowledge of a fetal defect, they can be appropriately guided through the pregnancy. These couples can be assisted to make decisions about labor and delivery care and early childhood care unique to their child's defect (i.e. need for a cesarean due to a neural tube defect and referral to a child development center).

Because CVS is still considered experimental, many insurance companies may not cover the cost of the procedure. There is some evidence that the cost of CVS may be up to 20 percent cheaper than that of an amniocentesis (Marchese et al., 1986). However, most couples will need support in the financial expense of a CVS, currently estimated to cost about $1200.

PERCUTANEOUS UMBILICAL BLOOD SAMPLING (PUBS)

Definitions and Indications

PUBS is a procedure which allows blood sampling of the fetus to diagnose problems which may later be incompatible to life. For example, in the Rh-negative mother carrying an Rh-positive fetus, antibodies produced by the mother may cross the placenta and destroy fetal red blood cells. The fetus may become anemic in this hemolysis and faces death if fetal hemoglobin reaches a dangerously low level. Other babies may live to birth but later die due to severe anemia which produces heart failure. PUBS can serially monitor the hemolysis inherent in this situation.

Unlike fetoscopy which carries a 4–5 percent risk of fetal loss, PUBS is safer (Garcia-Barrio, 1987). PUBS can also be carried out from the 17th week of pregnancy on and can be used to test for a variety of blood disorders (hemophilia, sickle-cell) or when other tests show the fetus to be oxygen starved (Hsieh et al., 1987). PUBS can be used to test for many defects observed in amniocentesis. Because actual blood is collected in PUBS, a faster chromosomal analysis (3 days) than amniocentesis can be obtained; sometimes, 2–4 weeks is required to get the results of chromosomal studies with amniocentesis. However, amniocentesis is easier to do for most obstetricians than PUBS and probably will remain a leading prenatal test for a long time to come (Garcia-Barrio, 1987).

Procedure and Interpretation

PUBS was first used in France in 1983 (Garcia-Barrio, 1987). The procedure requires that a fine needle be introduced through a pregnant woman's uterus into the fetal vein of the umbilical cord. Fetal blood is collected from this cord and analyzed for abnormality (e.g. Rh type, RBC, etc.). PUBS can be used to give fetal blood transfusions or other transfusions to aid fetal viability. Due to the complexity of the procedure, sonography is used to monitor the process of PUBS and is particularly important in an active fetus. The process usually takes about 8 min, although the infusion of blood to a diagnosed anemic infant may increase the length of the procedure to about 40 min (Garcia-Barrio, 1987).

In the PUBS procedure, sometimes local anesthesia is administered prior to the actual blood sampling. Many clients have reported the sensation of a "pin prick" when the needle was inserted into the abdomen. Clients are treated as out-patients and may resume their usual activities the day of the procedure. Some clients may receive medication to decrease uterine contractions and/or a course of antibiotics to prevent infection after a transfusion. The risks of the PUBS procedure include infection, excessive cord bleeding, premature labor, and placenta previa. Therefore, PUBS is used only where the benefits of the procedure outweigh its risks (Garcia-Barrio, 1987).

Nursing Roles

Like many of the recent prenatal tests now technologically available, clients will need anticipatory guidance and support by nursing staff if PUBS is to be part of prenatal monitoring. In some cases, several PUBS may be done to monitor fetal viability and, thus, active support by nurses is critical to allow couples psychologic and physical comfort with the procedure. Education about the risks of the procedure and the need for clients to report side-effects of PUBS needs to be provided by nursing staff. With a known fetal problem, nurses can assist couples in preparing for the labor and delivery of a perhaps vulnerable infant, and for infant care after birth.

Nurses can also share in the joy of couples who may have a fetal problem diagnosed and treated by PUBS and thus be quite healthy at delivery. For example, it is conceivable that PUBS may in the future be able to diagnose a low thyroxin level in a fetus, thus allowing intrauterine treatment and prevention of a mentally retarded child (Garcia-Barrio, 1987).

SUMMARY

The field of prenatal diagnosis is rapidly growing into a specialized division of maternity care. Over the past 30 years, numerous technologic advances have permitted nurses and other health care professionals to view the fetus and its environment without significantly increasing the risk of loss of the fetus. With further advances in prenatal screening, it can be predicted that superior noninvasive techniques will be developed to assess fetal well-being and to treat affected fetuses *in utero* prior to birth. It is anticipated that the cost of various prenatal screening techniques will decrease and that private insurance companies will cover these procedures as part of their comprehensive maternity services. With lower costs and insurance coverage of screening techniques, holistic maternity care can become a reality for many more childbearing families.

In the meantime, nurses need to consider their roles in the prenatal diagnosis arena. Despite increasingly more complex maternity technology, nurses will have to demonstrate more humanistic skills and strategies to meet consumer demands for more compassionate maternity care. Through knowledgeable use of the nursing process as part of prenatal screening, nurses can and will make a difference in providing "caring," individualized client approaches.

REFERENCES

Adler, B., and Kushnick, T. 1982. Genetic counseling in prenatally diagnosed trisomy 18 and 21: Psychological aspects. *Pediatrics.* 69(1):94–99.

Aladjem, B., ed. 1974. *Clinical perinatology.* St. Louis: C.V. Mosby.

Ascher, B. H. 1978. Maternal anxiety in pregnancy and fetal homeostasis. *J. Obstet. Gynecol. Neonatal Nurs.* 7(8):18–21.

Bambati, B.; Oldrini, A.; and Lanzani, A. 1987. Transabdominal chorionic villus sampling: A freehand ultrasound-guided technique. *Am. J. Obstet. Gynecol.* 157(1):134–137.

Boogert, A.; Mantingh, A.; and Visser, G. H. 1987. The immediate effects of chorionic villus sampling on fetal movements. *Am. J. Obstet. Gynecol.* 157(1):137–139.

Craney, M. S. 1978. Fetal and Maternal Monitoring Antepartal Fetal Assessment. Part I. *Am. J. Nurs.* 78:2098–2102.

Chance, G. W.; Godden, J. O.; and Goodwin, J. W., eds. 1976. *Perinatal medicine*. Baltimore: Williams & Wilkins.

Cohen, F. L. 1987. Neural tube defects: Epidemiology, detection, and prevention. *J. Obstet. Gynecol. Neonatal Nurs.* 16(2):112.

Burosh, P. 1976. Serial Estriol Determinations in High Risk Pregnancies: Implications for Primary Care Nursing. (pictorial) JOGNN.5.:34–40.

Diamond, F. 1978. High-risk pregnancy screening techniques. *J. Obstet. Gynecol. Neonatal Nurs.* 7(6):15–20.

Dickason, E. J., and Schult, M. O. 1975. *Maternal and infant care*. St. Louis: McGraw-Hill.

Elias, S., and Esterly, N. B. 1981. Prenatal diagnosis of hereditary skin disorders. *Clin. Obstet. Gynecol.* 24:1069–1087.

Epstein, M. F., and Frigoletto, F. D. 1983. Today's view in maternal and fetal medicine. *Patient Care.* 17(1):105–121.

Finegan, J. A. 1984. Amniotic fluid and midtrimester amniocentesis: A review. *Am. J. Obstet. Gynecol.* 91(8):745–750.

Gantes, M.; Kirchkoff, K. T.; and Work, B. A. 1985. Breast massage to obtain contraction stress test. *Nursing Research.* 34(6):338–341.

Gantes, M. et al. 1986. The use of daily fetal movement records in a clinical setting. *J. Obstet. Gynecol. Neonatal Nurs.* 15(5):390–393.

Garcia-Barrio, C. 1987. PUBS: A new prenatal test. *Am. Baby.* XLIX(7):49–51.

Golbus, M.S. 1982. The current scope of antenatal diagnosis. *Hospital Practices.* 17(4):179–186.

Golde, S. H., and Mosley, G. H. 1980. A blind comparison study of the lung phospholipid profile, fluorescence microviscosimetry, and the lecithin/spingomyelin ratio. *Am. J. Obstet. Gynecol.* 136(2):222–227.

Gorham, J. 1978. Relationship between ultrasound and computed tomography in whole-body scans. *Applied Radiology.* 7(1):127–137.

Gray, C. 1982. Prenatal diagnosis: The demand is increasing. *Can. Med. Assoc. J.* 126(1):64, 66, 70–71.

Haddow, J. E. 1982. Screening for spinal defects. *Hospital Practices.* 17(1):128–138.

Harman, C. R., et al. 1982. The correlation of ultrasound placental grading and fetal pulmonary motivation in five hundred sixty-three pregnancies. *Am. J. Obstet. Gynecol.* 143(8):941–943.

Heys, R. F. 1978. Placental insufficiency. *Briefs.* 42(1):11–13.

Hogan, K., and Cheng, D. T. 1978. The role of the nurse in amniocentesis. *J. Obstet. Gynecol. Neonatal Nurs.* 5(5):24–27.

Hogge, J. S., et al. 1986. Chorionic villus sampling. *J. Obstet. Gynecol. Neonatal Nurs.* 15(1):25.

Hon, E. H. 1968. *An atlas of fetal heart patterns*. New Haven, Conn.: Harty Press.

Hsieh, F. J. et al. 1987. Percutaneous ultrasound-guided fetal blood sampling in the management of nonimmune hydrops fetalis. *Am. J. Obstet. Gynecol.* 157(1):44–49.

Hufton, A. P. 1979. Radiation dose to the fetus in obstetric radiography. *Brit. J. Radiol.* 52:735–740.

Jaffe, C. C., and Simonds, B. D. 1978. Computed tomography and ultrasound of the abdomen. *Applied Radiology.* 7(1):81–91.

Johnson, M. 1982. Indications and techniques for genetic amniocentesis. *J. Reproduc. Med.* 27:557–559.

Josimovich, J. B. 1974. Human placental lactogen: Further evidence of placental mimicry of pituitary function. *Am. J. Obstet. Gynecol.* 120:550–552.

Kearney, B. 1978. Genetic counseling. *Australian Family Physician.* 7:803–811.

Kopf, R. 1978. Fetal and Maternal Monitoring: Nonstress test (pictorial). Part VI. AJN 78:2115–2117.

Levine, A., and Schenker, J. G. 1985. On the safety of diagnostic ultrasonography in obstetrics and gynecology. *Rev. Environ. Health.* 5(2):129–134.

Lieber, M. T. 1980. Nonstress antepartal monitoring. *MCN.* 5:335–339.

Lindfors, K. K., McGahan, J. P., Tennant, F. P., Hanson, F. W., and Walter, J. P. 1987. Midtrimester screening for open tube defects: Correlation of sonography with amniocentesis results. *AJR.* 149(1):141–145.

Lojek, R. M., and Yunek, M. J. 1978. Intrapartal fetal monitoring. *Am. J. Nurs.* 78:2102–2109.

MacDonald, P. C., and Pritchard, J. A. 1976. *William obstetrics*. 15th ed. New York: Appleton-Century-Crofts.

Manning, F. A.; Platt, L. D.; and Sipos, L. 1980. *Am. J. Obstet. Gynecol.* 136:787–795.

Marchese, C. A., Viora, E., Campogrande, M., and Carbonara, A. O. 1986. Cost-effectiveness ratio of chorionic villi biopsy for the prenatal diagnosis of chromosomal observations as compared to amniocentesis. *Ric. Clin. Lab.* 16(4):533–538.

Marshall, C. 1986. The nipple stimulation contraction stress test. *J. Obstet. Gynecol. Neonatal Nurs.* 15(6):459–462.

Marshall, K. 1979. Studies of infant breathing. *Briefs.* 42(1):3–6.

Milunsky, A. 1979. *Genetic disorders and the fetus*. New York: Plenum Press.

Naber, J. M.; Huether, C. A.; and Goodwin, B. A. 1987. Temporal changes in Ohio amniocentesis utilization during the first twelve years (1972–1983) and frequency of chromosomal abnormalities observed. *Prenat. Diagn.* 7(1):51–65.

Patrick, J., Challis, J., Campbell, K., Carmichael, L., Natale, R., and Richardson, B. 1980. Circadian rhythms in maternal plasma cortisol concentrations at 30 to 31, 34 to 35, and 38 to 39 weeks' gestational age. *Am. J. Obstet. Gynecol.* 136(3):325–334.

Ragan, W. D. 1978. Placental localization. *Perinatal Care.* 2(7):33–38.

Research McGill. 1980. Fetoscopy: A new technique for prenatal detection of genetic diseases. *Respiratory Care.* 25(2):255–258.

Richardson, B. S. 1983. Fetal activity: Measure of well-being. *Contemp. Obstet. Gynecol.* 22(3):211–228.

Sadovsky, E. 1979. What do movements of the fetus tell about its well being? *Contemp. Obstet. Gynecol.* 12(6):59–70.

Schifrin, B. S. 1979. Rationale for antepartum fetal heart monitoring. *J. Reproduc. Med.* 23:213–221.

Seeds, J. W. 1984. Impaired fetal growth: Ultrasonic evaluation and clinical management. *Obstet. Gynecol.* 64(4):577–584.

Sethi, S. 1978. Fetal and Maternal Monitoring Oxytocin Challenge Test. (Pictorial). Part V. AJN 78:2112–2115.

Summer, G. K. 1982. Development in genetic and metabolic screening. *Family & Community Health.* 4(4):13–30.

Thompson, H. E. 1978. Ultrasound introduction: The methods. *Perinatal Care.* 2(2):6–12.

Vintzileos, A. M., Campbell, W. A., Nochinson, D. J., and Weinbaum, P. J. 1987. Antenatal evaluation and management of ultrasonically detected fetal anomalies. *Obstet. Gynecol.* 69(4):640–660.

Wilson, G. N. 1982. Recurrence Risk of Malformations. *Journal of Reproductive Medicine.* 27(a):607–612.

14

Methods for Childbirth Preparation

BEHAVIORAL OBJECTIVES

Upon completion of this chapter, the reader should be able to:

- Discuss the history of prenatal education.

- Discuss various methods that promote relaxation during childbirth, noting advantages and disadvantages.

- Differentiate the Bradley and Lamaze methods of childbirth preparation.

- Discuss key elements for presentation of content in prenatal classes.

- Discuss the three phases of the expectant father's involvement in prenatal classes.

- Identify the role of the nurse in childbirth education.

A changing trend in childbirth education is the rise in the number of childbirth educators. The professional nurse should assume leadership in the role of health educator, basing the plan of care for the client on a thorough assessment in which the scientific approach dictates planning and action. When this education is complete, pregnancy and childbearing are more likely to be positive experiences for the mother and her family. The information obtained also tends to promote continued learning, with a resultant improvement in parenting skills.

Prenatal education is education that improves the health of the expectant mother, the developing baby, and their family. This education may be provided to the expectant mother on an individual basis or to groups of expectant mothers and their support persons with similar educational needs.

Prenatal classes may be taught before pregnancy, or early or late in pregnancy. Those classes that expectant couples attend late in pregnancy tend to focus on the upcoming birth and are usually referred to as childbirth classes. However, the content of childbirth classes frequently includes more than childbirth information only.

As knowledge about the effects of the birth on families has increased, so has the number of individuals enrolling in classes. Grandparents and children who will attend the birth of a sibling are examples of new groups for whom prenatal classes are taught. Groups have formed to promote prenatal education for parents. One of these is the National Association of Parents and Professionals for Safe Alternatives in Childbirth (NAPSAC).

HISTORY OF PRENATAL EDUCATION

In the nursing textbooks of the early 1900s, statements can be found regarding the role of the nurse in prenatal education of the expectant mother. The nurse was directed to "acquaint the patient with the phenomena of beginning labor," and at the same time was cautioned that it was not necessary for the mother "to be acquainted with the process of labor and its various complications" (DeLee, 1915, p. 96). While making home visits, nurses were directed to teach the pregnant woman about dress, diet, and mode of life during pregnancy. As times have changed, the focus of what the nurse should teach, as well as to whom, has also changed.

Prior to the Second World War

Before the Second World War, prenatal and childbirth education was sporadic, unorganized, and primarily done by female family members. Physicians offered limited information, based on the philosophy that the physician would manage all problems and that the woman should not worry.

One exception to this was work done by the Maternity Center in New York. As early as 1920, the center encouraged pregnant women to get early prenatal care and to enroll in classes that promoted health during pregnancy. This organization still provides leadership in prenatal education and childbirth programs. Teaching aids used in prenatal classes developed by the Maternity Center Association are still available, as is a referral service that helps couples locate services and facilities matching their desires. Many couples choose to deliver at the Maternity Center Association's homelike childbearing center, which is staffed by midwives (see Chapter 34). The Maternity Center has been a leader in improving the childbirth experience in the United States.

Following the Second World War

In 1946 the American Red Cross issued a unit of curriculum entitled *Mother and Baby Care and Family Health* as the second part of its home nursing program. This curriculum provided impetus for expanding prenatal education classes throughout the United States (Kernodle, 1949).

Childbirth education classes today are based on concepts imported from Europe in the 1940s and 1950s. These classes are eclectic in nature, utilizing concepts from many theories. The most influential methods of childbirth are those of Grantly Dick-Read, Fernand Lamaze, and Robert Bradley. We will discuss these approaches briefly here and explain them in greater detail later in the chapter.

The Influence of Dick-Read

In England during the 1930s and 1940s a physician, Grantly Dick-Read, spoke and wrote about the disadvantages of medical interventions such as anesthesia and the use of forceps. He conceptualized the idea that fear and anticipation of pain in a laboring woman resulted in increased tension, which led to increased pain and fear with future contractions.

The premise of Dick-Read's childbirth education method was the reduction of the fear–tension–pain cycle. He reasoned that reduction of fear could be accomplished through education about the childbirth process. Tension could be reduced by teaching the woman exercises to improve muscle tone and physical relaxation. The use of a controlled respiratory pattern helped the woman work effectively with her contractions. Dick-Read suggested that a prepared mother have someone with her through labor. Ideally, this person would have practiced with the expectant mother and would be able to help her cope with labor. He also identified the value in allowing the mother to see her baby immediately after birth, believing that this practice would promote the mother's feeling of success.

Dick-Read emphasized the avoidance of "unnatural aids" (that is, analgesia) in the childbirth process. He wrote *Childbirth Without Fear* (1944).

Dick-Read began touring the United States in the 1950s to spread his message. Although his ideas were received with skepticism, the Maternity Center Association became a prime supporter of this method. Classes based on his ideas became available, and many women benefitted from the exercises and education provided by the program.

The Influence of Lamaze

In 1950, Fernand Lamaze, a French physician, became interested in the Russian approach to childbirth. Lamaze and his associate, Pierre Vellay, promoted the Pavlovian theory of conditioned response as it applied to childbirth in the Western world.

Dr. Lamaze published *Painless Childbirth* in 1958. An American mother, Marjorie Karmel, who had experienced a Lamaze birth, published *Thank You, Dr. Lamaze* in 1959. These two books helped the American public understand the method. In the 1960s, through the efforts of Elizabeth Bing, author of *Six Practical Lessons for an Easier Childbirth* (1967), and Irwin Chabon, author of *Awake and Aware* (1966), regular classes for Lamaze preparation were established in New York City. These authors were influential in founding the American Society for Psychoprophylaxis in Obstetrics (ASPO) in 1960. ASPO is still active in the education and certification of childbirth educators to promote the psychoprophylactic approach to childbirth.

The International Childbirth Education Association (ICEA), which was also formed in 1960, promotes the Lamaze method and stresses the positive aspects of childbearing and parenting.

The basic premise of Lamaze is that the mind (psyche) can be trained for prevention (prophylaxis) of pain in labor. A coach, usually the expectant woman's husband or significant other, practices with the woman and attends the labor and birth. The woman learns neuromuscular control, relaxation, and specific breathing patterns that help her to cope with labor. The naturalness of pregnancy and childbirth are emphasized. The prepared woman is conscious and can participate effectively.

In early efforts to promote Lamaze's and Dick-Read's approaches, the naturalness of the birth process was stressed. The terms "natural childbirth" and "painless childbirth" were interpreted by skeptics as negating the use of obstetric advances such as newer anesthetics and medical intervention. Overzealous instructors promoted the idea of "going natural" to the couples who attended classes. At delivery, many of these couples were unable to meet the goal of an "all natural" delivery and found lack of support from the health care team. They experienced disappointment and guilt during the postpartum period. The Lamaze method was criticized for producing this feeling of failure in the mother. Information regarding medication and medical techniques is now discussed in Lamaze classes. Couples are encouraged to be knowledgeable and flexible and to participate actively in decisions regarding medical interventions necessary during labor and delivery.

Today, Lamaze's technique is a frequently utilized approach to childbirth. Over the years class content has changed, slower breathing techniques are taught, and classes emphasize the fact that the couple is part of the childbirth team. The classes incorporate information relevant to new techniques in obstetric care as well as parenting (see Appendix F for a list of resource groups).

The Influence of Bradley

The Bradley method is often called *husband-coached natural childbirth*. The American Academy of Husband-Coached Childbirth certifies teachers in this method. The method, developed by Robert Bradley, stresses relaxation, a quiet environment, and slow, deep breathing techniques throughout labor and delivery. The exercises to promote relaxation are taught to the couple over a number of months during pregnancy. Bradley's approach is based on what he observed in animal births: painless birth in quiet solitude with physical relaxation almost to the state of sleep. Bradley (1965) has written *Husband-Coached Childbirth*, which is used as a foundation for his classes.

The Influence of Kitzinger

The psychosexual method of childbirth education is a new method, introduced in the 1970s. Sheila Kitzinger, who wrote *The Experience of Childbirth* (1978), believes that pregnancy is a maturational crisis and that the childbirth experience can be psychotherapeutic, freeing the woman from sexual inhibitions that create marital tension. Developed in England, Kitzinger's method is based on Dick-Read's earlier work. Exercises are described in terms of physiologic processes and working in harmony with the body (Hassid, 1978). She teaches women to "swim" over the wave of a contraction by relaxing the mouth and jaw. The relaxation of the jaw is linked with the relaxation of the perineum on the theory that when the woman is smiling, with jaw relaxed, by association she allows the perineum to relax.

Kitzinger calls this method psychosexual because she sees sexuality as encompassing part of family relationships. The woman is taught to focus on the use of sensory memory. Exercises that promote conscious use of the pelvic floor muscles to facilitate descent of the infant are taught.

Cesarean Birth Classes

In the 1970s, as the number of cesarean births began to increase, classes to prepare parents for this kind of birth became more widely available. These classes are designed to reduce anxiety, decrease the need for medication, support the couple in choosing to be together for the birth, and prepare the couple for the course of recovery following birth. Many of these classes provide support and referral to cooperating physicians and hospitals should the couple seek to have a vaginal birth following the cesarean birth of a previous child.

Hypnosis and Yoga

Nurses should become aware of other methods that promote psychoprophylaxis during childbirth and for which there are prenatal classes. Two of these are hypnosis and yoga.

In the hypnosis method, the woman is prepared prenatally, through frequent hypnotic induction sessions, to relax and feel either diminished pain or no pain during labor and delivery upon hearing post-hypnotic suggestions or cues. The woman is put into a trancelike state by an obstetrician trained in hypnosis. There are two main disadvantages of the method: (1) the father is usually not present during the labor and delivery, and (2) the woman must be brought out of the trance in order to interact with the baby.

Yoga enthusiasts support its practice throughout the prenatal period as a way to relax during pregnancy and then to cope with labor and delivery. Yoga techniques of relaxation, concentration, and breathing are similar to techniques used in other childbirth methods.

CHILDBIRTH CLASSES

The benefits of childbirth preparation for mothers have been summarized as follows:

1. Lessened pain and anxiety.
2. Reduced medication needs.
3. Shorter labors.
4. Increased personal control.
5. Psychologic benefits of high personal assessment of their experiences.
6. Anticipation of a challenge and enjoyment of the joint effort with a coach.
7. Acknowledgment of one's resourcefulness with improved ability to cope.
8. Positive feelings about labor and the new baby (Genst, 1981).

In addition, couples attending a childbirth series frequently become resources for each other during the childrearing years, and they develop increased consumer skills in dealing with the health care delivery system (Fig. 14-1).

Theories that have been applied in psychoprophylaxis include (1) the gate theory of pain control (see Chapter 18), (2) Pavlov's theory of conditioned response, and (3) stress reduction through controlled relaxation. In addition, cognitive rehearsal of the labor and delivery experience can give couples a chance to be desensitized and to feel that they can master the real experience.

Couples have been found to benefit from information that prepares them for the sensations they will experience during labor and delivery. Patients who receive information regarding the sensations of intrapartal procedures may have less anxiety, and their expectations may be more consistent with their actual experiences than those who receive only procedural information (Hartfield, Cason, and Cason, 1982).

The Bradley Method

With the Bradley method of childbirth, classes begin in early pregnancy. In the first classes physical exercises that will aid in delivery or relieve discomfort are taught. There is a series of 12–15 classes throughout the pregnancy, depending on the

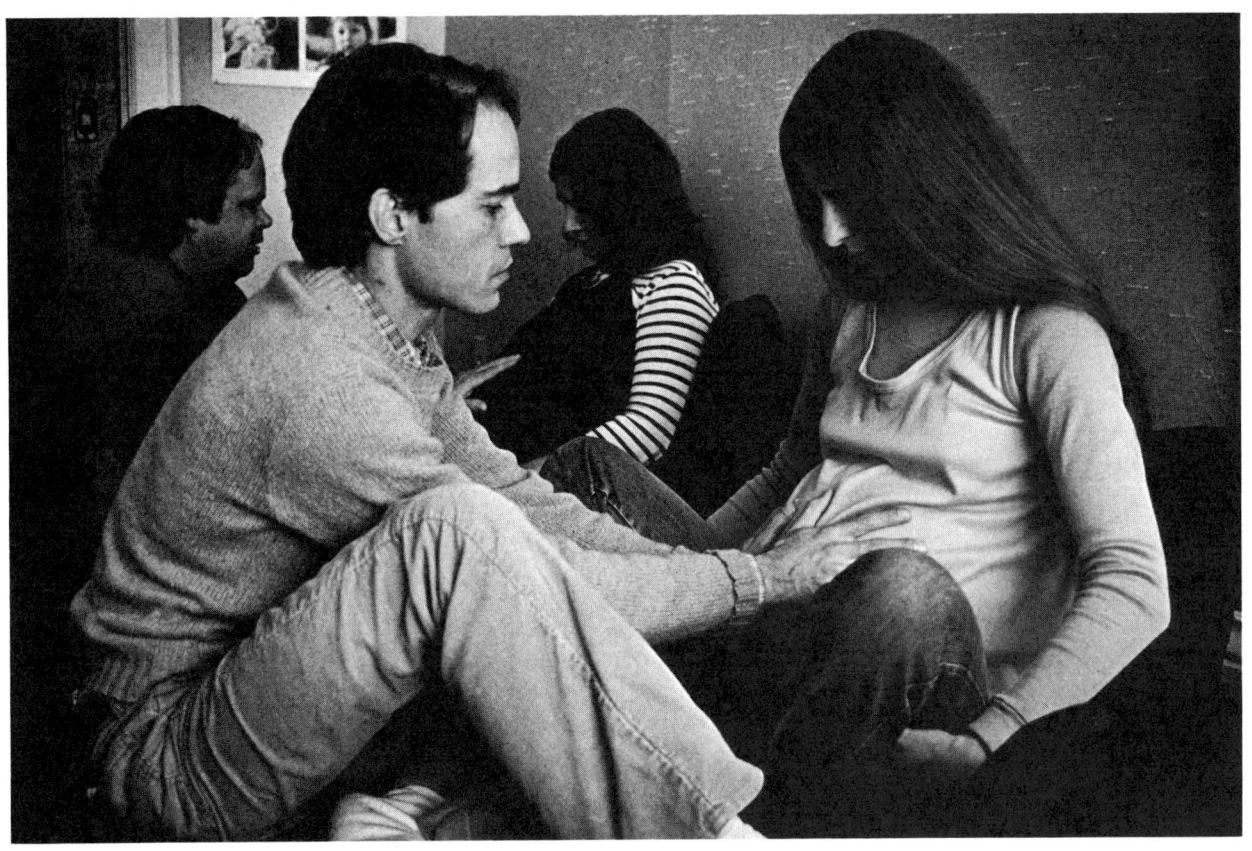

FIGURE 14-1. The partner provides a great deal of psychologic and emotional support.

needs of the couple. Most classes are concentrated in the last trimester, with couples attending weekly classes of 2–4 hours in length. Physical exercises include the pelvic rock, Kegals, and stretching of the legs and back (see Chapter 22).

The process of labor and delivery is thoroughly discussed. The couple are assisted in learning to respond to each other, so that the support person is totally familiar with the woman and can assist her to relax. The couple are encouraged to use relaxation techniques that they have used in the past. They are taught to practice the technique of massage daily, beginning with the extremities and working inward to the heart. This helps the woman relax completely. The coach talks quietly to the woman, describing scenes that promote relaxation. Soothing tones are encouraged. The woman assumes the most comfortable position, usually a sleeping position, and closes her eyes to relax completely. This seems easiest for couples whose past relationship has been calm, relaxing, and low-keyed. While couples are not taught to concentrate on breathing patterns as in the Lamaze method, a deep, rhythmical, abdominal breathing pattern has been found to be useful. Couples are encouraged to be "in touch" with their body's feelings and not to be frightened of the feelings experienced during labor and delivery.

In addition, as in other childbirth education classes, couples are taught consumer advocacy skills, including approaches they might utilize during the birth experience. The classes stress touring birth facilities and interviewing prospective physicians to find those with compatible philosophies, so that when couples strongly state their desires they will not meet with resistance from the health care team, resulting in lack of support and disappointment in their experience.

The partner must provide a great deal of psychologic and physical support for the Bradley method to succeed. Couples who have a close relationship have been found to have a better chance of success.

Some disadvantages of this method include the following: (1) preparation does not provide couples with enough coping strategies for use during labor and delivery, and (2) most women cannot relax throughout labor. Probably one of the strongest advantages of the Bradley method is that, since there are no set patterns that have to be followed during labor, the couple does not face the problem of failure to breathe correctly. The problem of failure to achieve has been criticized as a characteristic of other prepared childbirth approaches.

The Lamaze Method

Lamaze childbirth preparation classes begin in the last trimester of pregnancy, usually 6–8 weeks prior to the expected date of delivery. There are 4–6 classes in the series. The expectant mother and coach attend weekly classes, usually 2–4 hours in length.

The entire process of labor and delivery is discussed, so couples become familiar with the anatomic and physiologic process. Exercises such as those in the Bradley method are taught and practiced. Couples are encouraged to use techniques of relaxation to cope with the stress of labor and delivery (Fig. 14–2). *Neuromuscular-controlled relaxation*, which conserves energy, improves oxygen utilization, raises the pain threshold, and shortens labor, is taught and practiced daily. The couples practice so that the woman can replace restlessness and loss of control with useful relaxation, *effleurage* (light massage), and breathing patterns. Planned activities help to inhibit the perception of discomfort during labor contractions by the use of a conditioned response.

Relaxation is practiced so that the woman is able to relax and to conserve energy during labor. The coach can sense tension and with a verbal and touch command can promote relaxation. The woman concentrates on relaxing each part of her body until it feels limp or "heavy" to her. A command to contract an arm, a leg, or a combination of limbs gives the woman practice in concentration on relaxing while part of her body is tense. When the coach tells the woman to relax that portion that she has tensed up, she practices a response that will be useful when she tenses in labor. The woman learns to differentiate and isolate various muscle groups. Concentration on relaxing and developing mind control over muscle groups requires diligent daily practice by the couple. Such practice helps to condition the

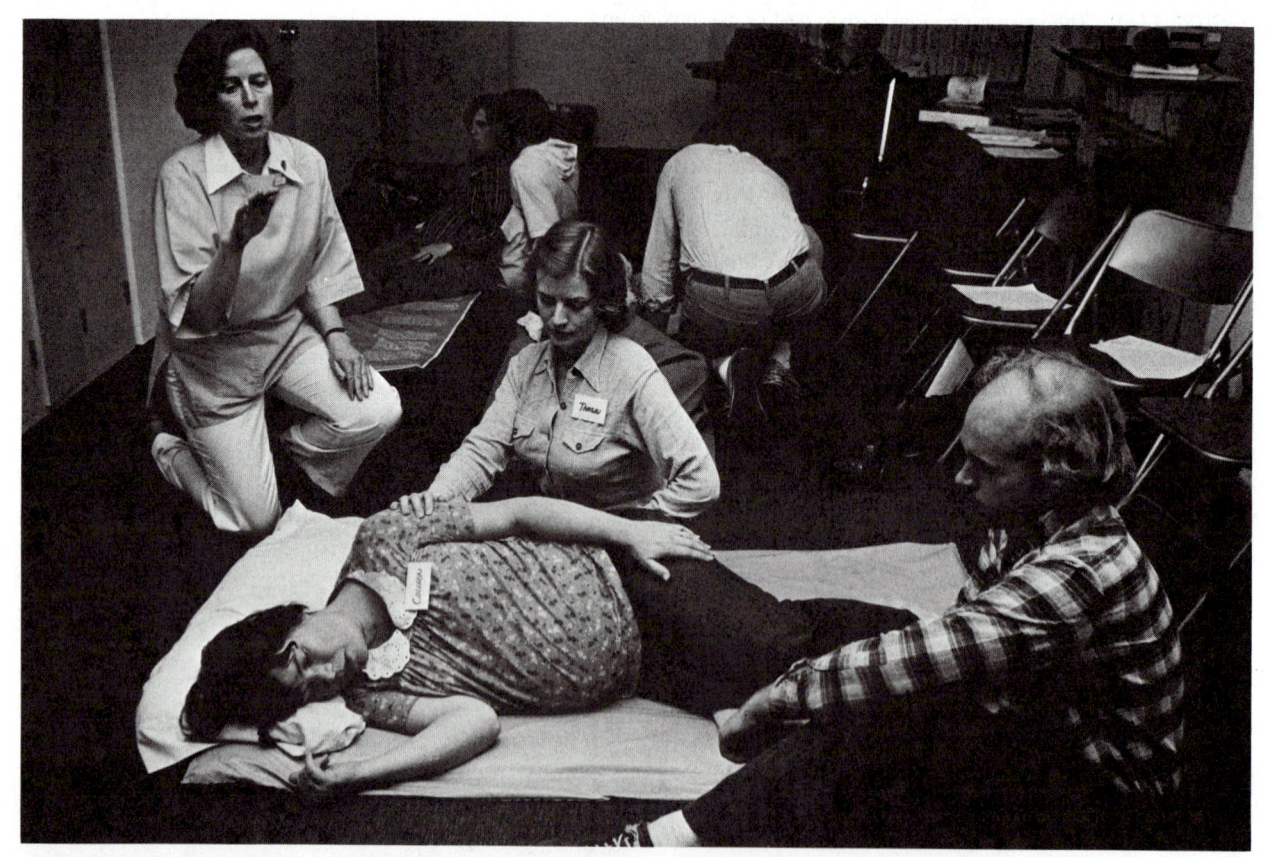

FIGURE 14–2. The coach and pregnant couple practice techniques of relaxation during pregnancy.

couple to use this technique automatically during labor.

Breathing patterns should be done while the woman is relaxed. Her eyes should be open and focusing on a particular point (any visual object that will help her to keep her visual sense active, distracting her from thinking about the contraction). At the beginning of each contraction, as well as at the end, the woman takes a cleansing breath. This is a deep breath, producing full chest expansion and lasting approximately 6–8 sec. The cleansing breath at the end of the contraction is part of the learned, conditioned response that acts as a signal that she has coped with the contraction. It also promotes a patterned response of relaxation between contractions. The coach is taught to time the contractions and quietly tell the woman each time 15 sec has gone by until the contraction ends.

In an effort to cope with the varying degrees of intensity of the contractions as labor progresses, the couple learns three main types of breathing:

1. *Slow, chest breathing.* In early labor, when the woman can no longer ignore a contraction or relax through the contraction, the breathing pattern is a deep, slow, chest pattern. Using the diaphragm and chest wall, the woman takes 6–8 slow, deep breaths over a period of 60 sec. The inhalation and exhalation should be even and of the same depth. This breathing is used for as long as the woman feels she is coping well and staying relaxed during the contractions. This deep slow breathing pattern is best utilized at 3–4 cm cervical dilation.
2. *Accelerated panting.* When the cervix is 4–7 cm dilated, the breathing is altered from a deep, slow, chest pattern to a shallower breathing pattern. In the middle of the contraction, accelerated panting is used; inhalation or exhalation should occur every 4 sec.
3. *Pant-blow breathing.* Pant-blow breathing is reserved for 7–10 cm dilation. This is a very shallow pattern that minimizes diaphragm and chest movement at a rate of one breath per second. While exhaling, the woman makes a sound of "he," which helps to keep the exhalation shallow. With every fifth exhalation instead of "he" the woman blows a short shallow puff just sufficient to make a candle flame flicker. Changing this pattern helps the woman concentrate on the breathing rather than on the strong contractions. One variation is changing the pattern from four short breaths out and a blow on the fifth exhalation to a 4-3-2-1-1-2-3-4 pattern of short breaths before the short blow. Another variation that requires intense work with the coach is a variation in which the coach calls a number between 1 and 6. The woman in labor does that number of short breaths with exhalations making the "he" sound. On the next exhalation while she is blowing, the coach calls another number between 1 and 6. She proceeds to do as many inhalation/exhalations as called, blowing while the coach calls another number. This continues until the contraction ends. The speed of breathing increases and depth decreases as the contractions get stronger and closer together.

There are two main types of breathing practice for the pushing stages of labor:

1. The most commonly used pattern is one in which the mother takes two cleansing breaths followed by 1–15 sec of breath holding, during which she pushes vigorously with the contraction. She continues to take short but deep breaths and to hold each breath for as long as she can until the contraction ends. The coach counts out loud the number of seconds she is holding the breath.
2. The other breathing pattern is one in which the woman takes two deep breaths at the start of the contraction and then on the third breath begins gentle pushing, letting the air of the last breath out in short puffs that would cause a candle flame to flicker. This method reduces the risk of rupture of small blood vessels in the mother's face and sclera. The coach counts the number of seconds the woman works with the breath and begins the count at 1 again when she takes a new deep breath to work with the rest of the contraction.

Research to support one breathing type over the other as being safer for mother and baby is inconclusive. Therefore, both types are taught and used, depending upon the condition of the mother and fetus, the effectiveness of the mother in pushing, and the preference of the obstetrician or midwife.

As new research identifies more effective techniques, breathing patterns will be altered so that labor and delivery are as easy and safe as possible. The nurse must be aware of new breathing patterns and regional differences in ways to work with the couple in labor. In early labor the nurse should find out what breathing patterns the couple have been taught. The couple should then demonstrate the techniques so that the nurse can help them work with the patterns as they have adopted them.

KEY ELEMENTS OF PRENATAL EDUCATION

Timing and Location

Prenatal education can occur in any setting in which the nurse encounters an expectant mother. This could be in a private office, an outpatient clinic, a school, or an occupational setting.

The mother should be in optimal health prior to conception. Education regarding nutrition, venereal disease, effects of drugs, infections, environmental influences, sexual intercourse, and genetic counseling should be made available to individuals of childbearing age (see Chapter 15).

The period from time of conception to confirmation of the pregnancy is a highly significant time in terms of ensuring optimal embryonic and fetal development. By the time a woman suspects that she is pregnant because of a missed menstrual period, she may already be 2 weeks pregnant. Many women are told that the first prenatal visit to a physician or clinic should be after missing two menstrual periods, at which time a woman may be 6 weeks pregnant.

The importance of early prenatal education cannot be overemphasized. Education should begin prior to conception, preferably as a part of adolescent health care, since fetal organ development is usually complete before the first prenatal visit (Brann and Cefalo, 1983).

Women of childbearing age should be educated about the importance of sound nutrition, rest, and the avoidance of harmful agents such as alcohol, tobacco, caffeine, other drugs, and x-rays, whose influence on the developing fetus should be emphasized.

Target

Although the mother is the primary target of prenatal education, it is necessary to identify her family and support system and to provide these individuals with relevant prenatal education. Grandparents and children in the family also benefit from prenatal education. When the expectant mother is unmarried, the choice as to whether she attends classes with couples should be hers.

Structure

Various encounters with health professionals can provide prenatal education for the pregnant woman. The health team responsible for the woman's care should use a planned approach to meet the identified needs of the patient and family.

Various checklists are used to ensure that at least a minimum number of topics have been discussed with the expectant couple (Bretschneider and Minetola, 1983). Such an approach prevents unnecessary repetition. The nurse must be cautious in the use of checklists, as this can prevent the development of an individualized plan for patients.

The nursing process begins with assessment at the initial prenatal visit. The nurse should gather significant data about the woman's physical, psychologic, emotional, and social status at every prenatal visit. The plan of care should be refined as assessment data changes.

A relationship that fosters trust is more likely to result if the same nurse sees the patient at each visit. Trust helps to ensure a thorough assessment. Information that an expectant mother is reluctant to share may be very significant, and she may share it only after trust has developed between patient and nurse.

If the nurse is working with expectant couples, once their educational needs are established a plan of care can be developed to meet those needs. The nurse should discuss with the couple what options are available to them. Options such as individual or group classes and type of classes should be reviewed. A couple makes many choices in early pregnancy—the type of infant feeding they will use, childbirth classes they will attend, the type of birth experience they want, and postpartum parenting classes they will attend. The nurse must stay up to date to inform expectant couples of the classes and birth experiences available in their area. By belonging to childbirth-related groups, reading local newspapers, and attending meetings with those involved in prenatal education, the nurse can increase his or her knowledge about what is available for patients. Nurses will find that attending the classes to determine content, teaching style of the instructors, basic goals, and theories provides valuable information for supporting their clients. Helping the couples develop wise consumer skills in choosing classes is part of the role of the nurse. Couples should be encouraged to compare similar classes for credentials and philosophy of the instructors, cost, length of the classes, enrollment numbers and location.

Economics

The economic condition of the nation and its people has an impact on the structure of prenatal education. While individualized prenatal education would be ideal, the cost is prohibitive. Therefore, much prenatal education is taught to groups of expectant couples. As unemployment and the cost of living rise, fewer people spend money on "nonessentials."

Financial costs of prenatal education are usually supported in one of three ways:

1. Fees are paid directly to the independent instructor teaching the class.
2. Fees are paid to the institution that employs the instructor.
3. Fees are included in the total cost of the services of the clinic or physician providing the patient's care.

Large group classes can be a financial asset to hospitals. The nurse who teaches such classes frequently receives pay at her regular pay scale while the institution reaps the profits. If tuition is charged, the cost to the expectant couple ranges from minimal fees to as much as 10 percent of the physician's bill.

Types of Classes

Because of economic factors, there has been a steady increase in the numbers and types of classes taught in hospitals. Classes are usually taught by nurses employed by the hospital. These classes teach the couple what to expect at the hospital where they will deliver. The obstetricians and pediatricians who practice at the hospital usually support the hospital classes.

In the hospital-based classes, the expectant couple become known to the nurses who will be caring for them during the childbirth experience. The patient's prenatal nursing record is updated and used by each nurse who cares for them.

Most expectant couples enrolled in private classes are referred to those classes by their physician. Independent instructors must maintain effective communication with prenatal care providers, usually physicians or midwives, and the personnel of the places where couples plan to give birth. The expectant couple and health care team should provide information to the independent instructor regarding changes in procedures. Any pertinent information regarding the couple and their wishes, fears, and concerns should be communicated to the rest of the health care team. Many instructors have developed forms, completed by the couples, that describe their self-identified desires and needs for the pregnancy, birth, and postpartum period. This information should be added to the patient's record for continuity of care. Information usually requested as a type of "wish list" may include:

- Desire to attend prenatal classes.
- Choice of method for feeding the baby.
- Care of the newborn: circumcision, supplementary water, demand feeding, and rooming in.
- Desires for childbirth: place, support persons, use of a birthing bed or birthing chair, and positions for delivery.
- Procedures that are considered acceptable or unacceptable: episiotomy, intravenous fluids, monitors, enemas, and perineal shave.
- Choices of medication and anesthesia.
- Procedures desired after birth: breastfeeding on the delivery table, a Leboyer bath, and bonding.
- Length of hospital stay for mother and baby.
- Desire for sibling visitation.
- Special dietary needs.
- Desires regarding a support person.
- Anesthesia if cesarean section should be necessary.

Although the expectant couple may complete such a list early in pregnancy, they should revise it as their needs and desires change. The nurse can check the list and help the couple determine how they can best achieve their goals. It is important for the couple to share this list with their physician to determine whether their requests are realistic. Should their choices not be available, the couple can make adjustments so they will not be disappointed.

Assessment of Learning Needs

Assessment of the expectant couple's motivation, learning needs, readiness to learn, language, and cognitive ability is essential (see Chapter 24).

The prenatal educator should be aware of the problem of selective learning and retention. This occurs in any educational experience—the learner hears or retains only that information that reinforces past experiences, perceptions, knowledge, and motivation. Many couples have heard accurate information and have practiced exercises correctly in class. However, they also receive additional information from reading and listening to others' experiences. Time dulls the memory, so that when they are ready to use the technique or information from the class, the couple may remember it incorrectly. Active practice of procedures and positive feedback from the instructor contribute to a more successful prenatal learning experience.

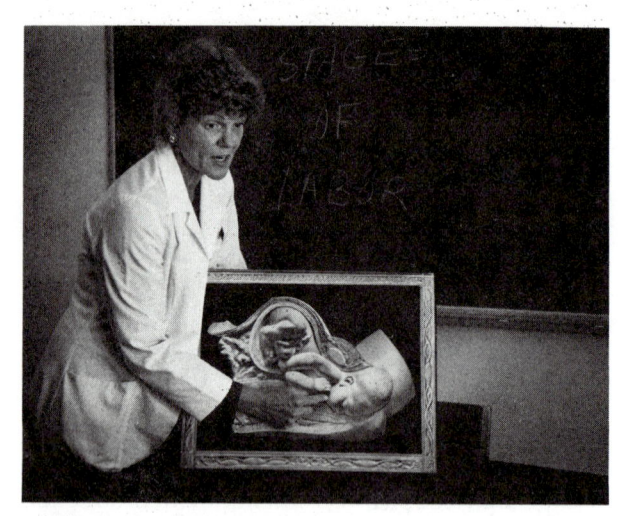

FIGURE 14–3. The use of charts is an effective teaching strategy in discussing the labor process.

Teaching Strategies

Various teaching strategies have been used to involve expectant couples in the learning process during prenatal classes. The teacher varies the technique based on whether the content is psychomotor, affective, or cognitive in nature. Sentence completion and drawing a picture of the expectant mother (self or significant other), and writing about the expected birth have been reported as techniques to promote expression of feelings, or affective learning (Harris, Dombro, and Ryan, 1980; Bretschneider and Minetola, 1983). Self-assessment of strengths and desires helps couples to better understand each other and their experiences. Games and role play are also useful strategies for affective learning. Demonstrations and return demonstrations are used for psychomotor learning and for the development of skills. Lectures, group discussions, and audiovisual aids (Fig. 14–3) such as slides and films are useful for content presentation and cognitive learning objectives. The nurse should carefully choose strategies that produce positive outcomes and that decrease the expectant couple's fear and anxiety.

Content

The nurse should consider the educational level, cultural background, socioeconomic status, and philosophic base of the expectant couple in planning course content.

The course should definitely include content areas related to choices the expectant couple must make. Such topics as breastfeeding versus bottle feeding, circumcision, and appropriate layette items can be included. The nurse is cautioned against the attitude that while the expectant parents are a captive audience they should be taught everything there is to know about pregnancy, childbirth, and parenting. Baby bathing may be better taught after the baby arrives. If it is taught during a prenatal class, the skill may be forgotten by the time it can be put to use.

The content of the class may vary. Feedback from the couples gives the nurse valuable data from which to modify the course to meet the learner's needs.

A list of specific content taught in prenatal classes was produced from a 1980 survey of childbirth educators conducted by the Nurses Association of the American College of Obstetricians and Gynecologists. The results identified eight categories of content that are appropriate to include but that are not always taught: (1) exercise, (2) diet, (3) drug use, (4) normal processes of growth and development, (5) potential problems such as birth defects, (6) family relationships, (7) postdelivery care of the neonate, and (8) coping strategies for dealing with the health care system. As a result of this survey, guidelines for childbirth education were developed that will help to standardize content (Susmor and Grossman, 1981).

Prenatal content will change as research provides concrete evidence of the benefits of patients having knowledge. Such evidence has been cited in two recent studies. Women in labor are less upset, bothered, or disturbed in their reactions to fetal monitoring when they are told about the monitoring in prenatal classes and when they see the monitors while touring the labor and delivery areas (Beck, 1980). Similarly, cesarean-birth parents whose preparation includes information about the entire procedure have fewer unmet needs than couples who do not receive the information (Fawcett, 1981).

Periodically, the prenatal educator should review each content area to determine its validity for inclusion in the classes. The updating of content occurs on a regular basis as new techniques and treatments are developed. This evaluation helps to ensure that the couples receive pertinent, useful education.

Fathers' Needs

Fathers are beginning to be recognized as having unique needs that can be met through specific objectives of prenatal classes. Careful and complete assessment of the father's past experiences, feelings, expectations, and learning ability will aid the nurse in meeting his needs. The assessment should include whether the fathers are experiencing any physical or psychological symptoms. Addressing these symptoms may allow the childbirth educator to reduce the anxiety of the fathers, thereby increasing their ability to support the mother (Strickland, 1987). Some fathers report pressure from other fathers who have attended births. The idea that only "macho" men can attend and that those who are less masculine cannot has influenced some fathers to attend classes. Other fathers have received pressure from expectant mothers to attend classes. The prenatal educator should assess the motivating factor for the father's attendance.

In view of research findings, assessment of the father's needs in prenatal classes should be carried out (see Chapter 37). Three phases of first-time fathers' involvement in pregnancy have been identified: announcement, moratorium, and focusing.

Announcement lasts from the first suspicion of pregnancy to a few weeks after confirmation. In this phase the father has not integrated pregnancy as a part of his life.

Moratorium is characterized by emotional distance and postponement of involvement in the pregnancy. Depending on the father's readiness for the pregnancy, moratorium usually lasts from the 12th to 15th week of pregnancy to late in the second trimester.

Focusing frequently begins when the father feels the baby's movement. It involves a sense of excitement and involvement, and the process of redefining the man's roles and defining his future status (May, 1982).

To intervene appropriately, the prenatal educator must determine which stage the father is in. Preparation of the father for the stages of response to the process of labor and delivery will enhance the father's self-esteem. These stages are (1) the excitement of early labor, (2) the doubt of mid-labor, (3) the immersion or self-absorption of transition, (4) the exertion of pushing, and (5) the power and pride of achievement at birth. If a father understands before labor the feelings he is likely to experience, his ability to support his wife during labor and delivery will be increased (El Sherif, McGrath, and Smyrski, 1979).

Encouraging and strengthening the father's belief in what he already knows about the woman he is going to support promotes his feelings of being prepared. Positive feedback to the father regarding his activity is essential to help him feel prepared and to reduce his feelings of uselessness.

Fathers should be allowed the opportunity to express their fears and doubts as well as to anticipate their joy. They need an opportunity to adjust to the role of fatherhood. They should be reassured that the nursing staff will offer support and assistance (see Chapter 37).

SUMMARY

Prenatal education is an integral part of the nursing care of the pregnant woman and the people who support her. Ideally, prenatal education begins prior to conception.

The two most common childbirth preparation strategies are the Lamaze and Bradley methods. The focus of prenatal education is to prepare the pregnant woman and the person who will support her during labor and delivery. Complete knowledge of the processes of labor and delivery as well as the ability to relax during contractions are the goals of these classes.

The nurse uses the nursing process to meet the prenatal educational needs of the pregnant woman and her family. The nurse who provides prenatal education needs to be flexible and to communicate effectively. As an advocate for change in the health delivery system, the nurse promotes positive experiences for the expectant couple regardless of their culture, age, educational level, or socioeconomic status. The nurse has a responsibility to keep abreast of the latest scientific advances in related fields. The role of the nurse in prenatal education is one of responsibility whch provides both challenges and rewards.

REFERENCES

Beck, C. T. 1980. Patient acceptance of fetal monitoring as a helpful tool. *J. Obstet. Gynecol. Neonatal Nurs.* 9:350–353.

Bing, E. 1967. *Six practical lessons for an easier childbirth.* New York: Grosset & Dunlap.

Bradley, R. 1965. *Husband-coached childbirth.* New York: Harper & Row.

Brann, Jr., A. W., and Cefalo, R. C., eds. 1983. *Guidelines for perinatal care.* American Academy of Pediatricians and American College of Obstetricians and Gynecologists.

Bretschneider, J. U., and Minetola, A. C. 1983. Another look at early-pregnancy classes. *MCN.* 8:268–273.

Chabon, I. 1966. *Awake and aware.* New York: Dell.

DeLee, J. B. 1915. *Obstetrics for nurses.* 4th ed. Philadelphia: W. B. Saunders.

Dick-Read, G. 1944. *Childbirth without fear.* New York: Harper & Row.

El Sherif, C.; McGrath, G.; and Smyrski, J. T. 1979. Coaching the coach. *J. Obstet. Gynecol. Neonatal Nurs.* 8:87–89.

Fawcett, J. 1981. Needs of cesarean birth parents. *J. Obstet. Gynecol. Neonatal Nurs.* 10:372–376.

Genst, M. 1981. Preparation for childbirth—evidence for efficacy. *J. Obstet. Gynecol. Neonatal Nurs.* 10(2):82–85.

Harris, R.; Dombro, M.; and Ryan, C. 1980. Therapeutic uses of human figure drawings by the pregnant couple. *J. Obstet. Gynecol. Neonatal Nurs.* 9:232–237.

Hartfield, M. T.; Cason, C. L.; and Cason, G. J. 1982. Effects of information about a threatening procedure on patients' expectations and emotional distress. *Nurs. Research.* 31:202–206.

Hassid, P. 1978. *Textbook for childbirth educators.* San Francisco: Harper & Row.

Karmel, M. 1959. *Thank you, Dr. Lamaze.* Philadelphia: Lippincott.

Kernodle, P. B. 1949. *The Red Cross nurse in action, 1882–1948.* New York: Harper & Row.

Kitzinger, S. 1978. *The experience of childbirth.* 4th ed. New York: Pelican/Penguin.

Lamaze, F. 1958. *Painless childbirth.* London: Burke.

May, K. A. 1982. Three phases of father involvement in pregnancy. *Nurs. Research.* 31:337–342.

Strickland, O. L. 1987. The occurrence of symptoms in expectant fathers. *Nurs. Research.* 36:184–189.

Susmor, J. L., and Grossman, E. 1981. Childbirth education. *J. Obstet. Gynecol. Neonatal Nurs.* 10(3):155–160.

15

The Role of the Nurse in the Prenatal Period

BEHAVIORAL OBJECTIVES

Upon completion of this chapter, the reader should be able to:

- Discuss the concept of health promotion and its relationship to the growth and development of a healthy fetus and newborn.

- Explain the purpose of assessing the general health and reproductive history of the pregnant woman.

- Explain the purpose of a complete physical assessment of the pregnant woman, including abdominal palpation and performance of Leopold's maneuvers.

- Discuss the reasons for assessing the psychologic status of the pregnant woman in relation to parenthood.

- Describe a plan for health promotion throughout the pregnancy.

Prior to the turn of the century, few women sought out doctors or nurses for advice or care during their pregnancies, because they believed pregnancy and childbirth to be normal physiologic processes. Although this belief is not incorrect, statistics show that health care does improve the general outcome for both the woman and her baby. In fact, the earlier in pregnancy health care is begun, the more likely it is that there will be a favorable outcome (Niswander and Gordon, 1972; U.S. Department of Health and Human Services, 1981).

Currently available data show major progress has been made over the past several decades in improving the outcome. The infant mortality rate in 1950 was 29.2 per 1000 live births and in 1983 it was 11.2 per 1000 (National Center for Health Statistics, 1985). The utilization of prenatal care by black and white women has also seen an improvement in the last decade. However, in 1972 only 50 percent of black women compared to 70 percent of white women began prenatal care in the first trimester. During the 1970s both groups increased their early utilization of prenatal care by approximately 10 percent. This trend of improvement appeared to stabilize by 1982 at levels far below those of other industrialized countries (Ingram, Makur, and Kleinman, 1986).

Nurses were among the first health care professionals to recognize that assessment of the health status of women early in their pregnancy is important. Early in the twentieth century visiting nurses in cities in the northeast worked diligently to ensure that pregnant women had better nutrition, better working conditions, better spacing of their children, and earlier access to the health care system. Nurses were the leaders in providing prenatal care to pregnant women.

PRECONCEPTUAL COUNSELING

Nurses continue to be leaders in the care of the childbearing family. They have recognized that, ideally, preparation for parenthood should begin months and years before conception occurs. Today, growing public awareness of the early establishment of good health habits and the maintenance of health may make this ideal a reality. Nurses can do much to promote this ideal. There are reports on a series of regional conferences initiated by the Executive Committee of the ANA Council on Maternal–Child Nursing. These conferences of perinatal specialists were designed to look at strategies to increase access to prenatal care as one way to lower infant mortality. The major concern of the participants was the need to improve access to prenatal care and their major recommendation was that *all* pregnant women be ensured access to timely, comprehensive, high-quality maternity care. In the future, healthy women bearing healthy babies may become the standard as women actively plan and prepare for parenthood.

Nurses are in an ideal position in the health care system to affect the health status of women in the childbearing population. Dividing childbearing women into two groups, those actively involved in the health care system and those who are not, will help make clear how the nurse can influence the health habits of women to achieve the goal of healthy babies.

Many of the women who are infrequent users of the health care system are adolescents. These young women are not actively seeking parenthood but are exploring the dimensions of their physical and psychologic being. This exploration may lead to unplanned conception (Erickson, 1963; Bell, 1970; Zelnick, 1979; Hyde, 1982). Approximately 1 million adolescents become pregnant every year, and the Center for Disease Control (1977) estimates that 70 percent of all teenage pregnancies are unintentional (see Chapter 38).

Women in this group may not have had a complete health assessment since they entered school at age 5 or 6, unless they have been actively involved in organized sports activities that require a physical examination. And while they may value good health, they are most likely to think of it as a given, not something they must work at to maintain.

Nurses can have an impact on this group through education (Palmer and Lewis, 1976; Jordan and Valle, 1978). School nurses can explain the need for developing habits that will promote health—eating nutritious meals, getting rest and exercise, taking responsibility for individual actions, and caring about others. They can explain the importance of achieving physical and emotional maturation before becoming parents. They can help these young women value the concept of all babies being planned. Community health nurses can take advantage of their position to speak to adolescents in a variety of youth groups. They can initiate health care promotions that will reach out to young women who may not be actively involved in specific groups. All nurses who care about the health of future generations should get involved with adolescents—they are the parents of tomorrow.

The second group of women are those already involved in the health care system in some way. They may have recently had a baby. They may have sought health care out of a concern that they were pregnant and found they were not. Or they may have been seeking contraception. Regardless of the reason, the nurse has immediate and excellent access to this particular group—a group aware of and concerned about the possibility of parenthood. These women are in a state of readiness regarding the importance of planning for the children they will have. The nurse becomes an enabler and guide. The nurse can teach the importance of health and its effect on the future health of the baby and can encourage maintenance of good health habits and the abandoning of harmful habits. The nurse can help each woman think about preparing for the conception of her baby the way many women now prepare for the process of childbirth.

The preconceptual woman must learn that having a baby should be at least a year-long process. First, the woman should understand the importance of assessing the state of her own health and readiness for parenthood. Questions she might ask herself are:

1. Am I in a good nutritional state?
2. Is my weight within normal range?
3. Do I exercise regularly?
4. Am I using drugs or medications, drinking, or smoking?
5. Am I happy being me?
6. Am I enjoying my life just as it is?
7. Why do I want a baby?

Once she has answered these and similar questions for herself, is satisfied that having a baby is an important goal for her now, and is in a physically and emotionally healthy state, she is ready to begin to plan for when she would like to conceive.

It would be wise to plan for a possible conceptual date at least 3 months in the future. These 3 months should then be used to correct bad health habits and establish good habits, including the recording of important information (such as menstruation dates, exposure to illness, times of intercourse, and ingestions of prescriptive and over-the-counter medications). This concentration on maintaining and improving health status will help ensure a healthy beginning for the baby.

It is at least 2–3 weeks after conception before the woman suspects she is pregnant. The pregnancy is not generally confirmed until the embryo is 4–6 weeks old. By then the major organ systems are formed; the heart is beating, and if there are going to be major morphologic abnormalities, they have already occurred. It is a little late for the pregnant woman to begin wondering what might be done to prevent the baby's earliest exposure to alcohol, x-rays, drugs, and other chemicals when she is already 2 months pregnant.

NURSING ASSESSMENT OF THE PREGNANT PATIENT

Health History

The major purpose of the initial visit of the maternity patient, other than to confirm the fact of pregnancy, is to establish a database for future health care. If the maternity patient has been utilizing the health care system for preconceptual care, much of the baseline data important in health care and counseling during pregnancy will already have been accumulated. This availability of health data for a particular woman in the nonpregnant state (blood pressure, weight, nutritional status, menstrual record, emotional status, absence of chronic illnesses, and so on) ensures that changes in her overall health status will be recognized early. Conversely, when a maternity patient arrives for her initial visit never having been seen before, blood pressure at 124/82, a weight of 121 lb, and the date of her last menstrual period uncertain, it is impossible to determine accurately her current health status as it relates to this pregnancy. Was her prepregnant blood pressure 124/82, or was it 94/60? Was her prepregnant weight 121, or was it 105? Is she 6 weeks pregnant or 10 weeks pregnant? The answers to these questions make a significant difference in the kind of health intervention the nurse would plan to ensure a healthy outcome for the pregnant woman and her baby.

A thorough and accurate health history is vital to the continued health care of a maternity patient. In many ambulatory health care settings it is the role of the nurse to be historian, data gatherer, counselor, and educator. In situations where it is not, the nurse may want to establish this role for himself or herself. The nurse in the ambulatory maternity health care setting is likely to be the most constant member of the health care team. It is important to the comfort of the maternity patient and her adherence to recommended health measures that the nurse establish a trust relationship with her. The nurse can encourage the beginning of this relationship on the first visit during the taking of the health history.

Content of the Health History

The health history for a maternity patient should contain the same information that is collected for

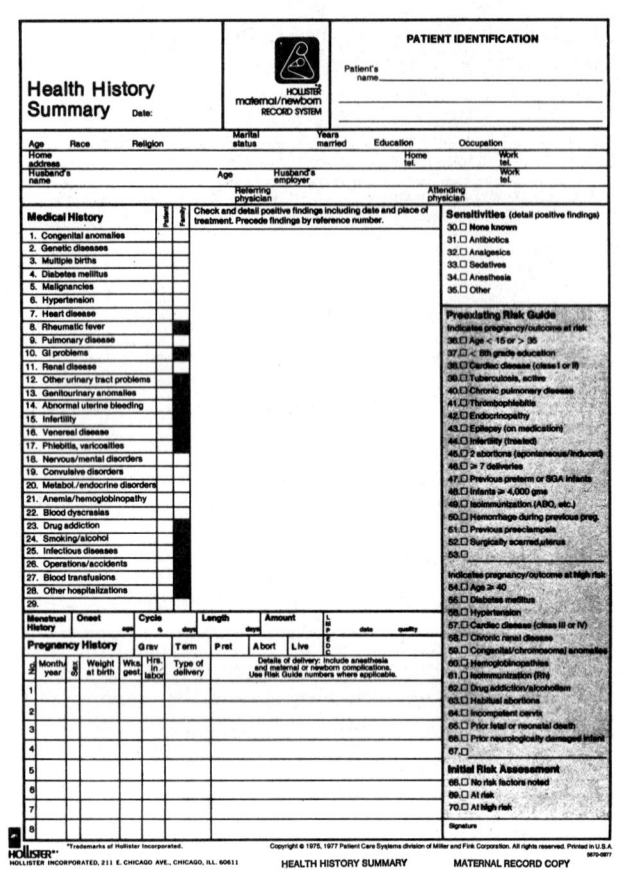

FIGURE 15–1. A sample health history form.

any patient (see Fig. 15–1). Some chronic illnesses, particularly diabetes, heart disease, and severe anemias, are known to have specific effects on pregnancy. The presence or absence of these conditions should be ascertained; if present, they should be carefully assessed. Other factors in the general health condition that should be noted include chronic lung problems such as asthma, chronic urinary tract infections, ulcers, varicosities and phlebitis, seizure disorders, allergies and drug sensitivities, thyroid disease, hepatitis and gall bladder disease, and major accidents or surgeries.

It is also important to collect data that will have a particular bearing on the woman's reproductive health throughout the pregnancy and childbirth and on the health of her unborn baby. These data include the woman's prepregnant health status—blood pressure, weight, use of alcohol, drugs, or tobacco, etc.—and her menstrual history—menarche, description of her normal periods, date of her last *normal* menstrual period (LNMP), and use of contraceptives prior to pregnancy.

Of equal importance is the woman's previous reproductive history. A pregnant woman is referred to as *gravida*. This term and the number accompanying it, such as *gravida* 2, refers to the total number of times a woman has been pregnant, regardless of the outcome of those pregnancies. The word *para* is frequently used to denote, at least partially, the outcome of the pregnancies. *Para* is defined as the number of pregnancies that have ended in the delivery of an infant weighing at least 500 g or more than 20 weeks' gestation whether dead or alive. A multiple birth is considered as *one parity*. Based on this definition it is difficult to determine the impact of a woman's previous parity with any degree of accuracy. For example, a woman pregnant for the fifth time who has delivered one baby at term, one at 36 weeks, one at 34 weeks, has had one miscarriage at 10 weeks, and has three living children would be described as a gravida 5, para 3, or G/P = 5/3.

A more accurate way of describing a woman's pregnancy record is the use of a five-digit numbering system referred to as G/TPAL. Because it denotes the outcome of each of the pregnancies, it is becoming the most widely adopted method nationwide. The letter G stands for *gravida*. The number of babies born at term (alive or dead) is given by T, the number of babies born preterm (alive or dead) is given by P, the number of pregnancies ending in abortion is given by A, and the number of children currently living is given by L. Using this shorthand method for the woman in our example, the nurse would record the pregnant woman at 5/1213. When she delivers this baby at term and alive, it will be 5/2214.

To further clarify the use of the two systems, here is another example: A woman is pregnant for the fourth time and her previous pregnancies ended with one term infant and two miscarriages at 12 and 16 weeks, and she currently has one living child. Using the gravida/para system, she would be recorded as a gravida 4, para 1; using the G/TPAL system she would be 4/1021. She delivers this pregnancy at 34 weeks—twin boys alive and doing well. Using the gravida/para system she would be gravida 4, para 2 (remember, para counts only the pregnancies delivered viable—not the number of babies). Using the G/TPAL system, she would be 4/1223.

Data should also be collected on the health of the father of the baby. Although this factor will not influence the health of the pregnant woman directly, it may affect the outcome for the baby.

The accumulation and weighing of health history data will allow the nurse and other health care providers the best opportunity to anticipate potential problems, provide appropriate health care throughout the length of the pregnancy, and support the maternity patient regardless of the course of her pregnancy.

Taking the Health History

The nurse may use a variety of methods and forms to obtain the initial health history on a maternity patient. As long as the nurse is familiar with the format, comfortable with her or his role, and concerned about the patient's well-being, the results should be the same. To make the patient comfortable, it would be wise to provide a quiet, private room for the history taking. This room should be one where the patient and nurse can sit face to face without barriers. The patient should be fully clothed, and the nurse should provide an atmosphere of interest and caring.

The nurse should begin with the patient's current situation: "Tell me about yourself. Why did you come? How are you feeling? How would you like me to help you?" Answers to these questions should be listened to intently. By the time these three questions have been answered completely, the nurse may have obtained most of the health history needed. Additional historical data can be added easily by direct questioning.

It is important to remember that getting an accurate and complete health history takes time (an average of 30–60 min) and concentration. A knowledge of human nature is important in getting an accurate accounting of critical information. An example of a nurse trying to establish the date of the last normal menstrual period demonstrates this:

NURSE: When was your last menstrual period?

PATIENT: I'm not really sure. Let's see. Today is December 15th. I usually get my period around the end of the month. Hmmm . . . I don't remember having my period in November.

NURSE: What were you doing at Thanksgiving? Did you have your period then?

PATIENT: Ummm . . . Oh, no, I'm sure I didn't. We went to Mike's folks for Thanksgiving—no, I didn't get my period then.

NURSE: What about October . . . Halloween? Do you remember getting your period then?

PATIENT: No . . . No, I'm sure I'd remember if I did. Mike and I went to a costume party dressed as rabbit. Hmmm—funny when you think about it now! Oh, that's right, I do remember having my period in September. My birthday is the end of September and Mike wanted to take me out to supper. We didn't go because I didn't feel very well. Yes, that's when I had my last period.

As long and convoluted as this conversation seems, it got results. When a patient is not planning on becoming pregnant, she may not be a very good historian. She may not understand or recognize the importance of all that has been happening to her and how it could affect her unborn baby. If she had been planning and preparing for the pregnancy, she could have been keeping a preconceptual and early pregnancy history. And if she had made a visit to her health care provider to confirm her state of health prior to conceiving, most of the baseline data would already be in her record.

General Health Assessment

Following the completion of the health history, the nurse should proceed to collect physical data that will establish the current health status of the pregnant woman. At the initial visit the nurse should take the patient's temperature, pulse, respirations, blood pressure, height, and weight (Figs. 15–2 and 15–3). If the patient was seen preconceptually, the current findings should be compared with those recorded previously. If not, the nurse should obtain the preconceptual weight and blood pressure by asking the patient.

General Appearance

During the time the nurse is taking the history and beginning the physical assessment, observations should be made about the patient's general appearance. The nurse should develop an overall impression of the health/illness status of the patient. The initial physical assessment of a pregnant woman should be the same as for any woman. During the first trimester of pregnancy very little physical change will be noted in any of the major systems with the exceptions of the reproductive system, the breasts, the bladder, and the possible nausea and vomiting associated with early preg-

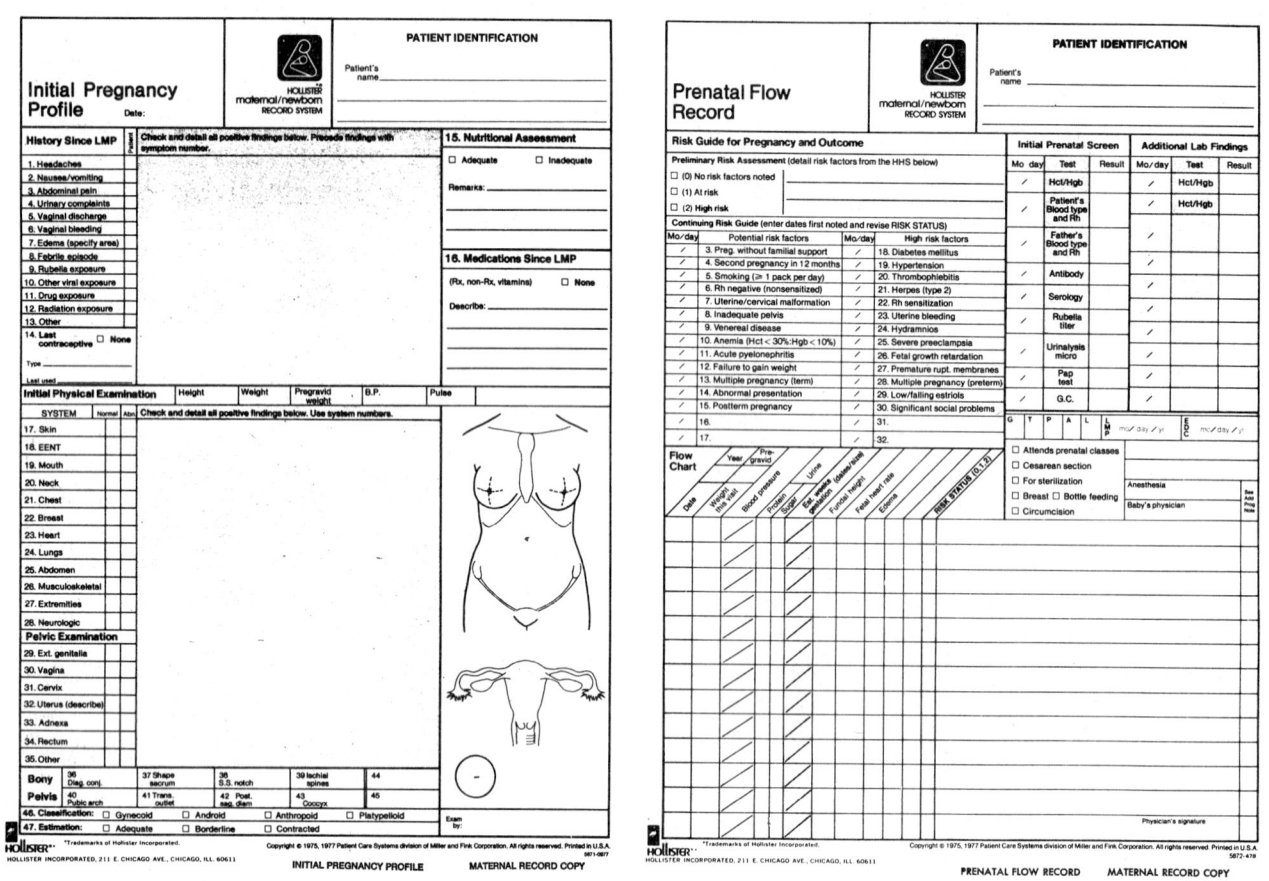

FIGURE 15-2. Health assessment forms used during prenatal visits. *Left:* Pregnancy profile; *right:* flow record.

nancy. By the second trimester changes may be noted that are normal for the pregnant woman and are a result of the impact of the rapidly enlarging uterus.

Blood Pressure

Regular blood pressure measurements are an important tool in assessing the continuing health of a pregnant woman. The blood pressure in a healthy pregnant woman during the first trimester should remain the same as it was in her nonpregnant state. During the second trimester, a slight drop may be noted in the healthy pregnant woman.

The blood pressure should be taken with the patient in a left lateral position, as blood pressure in a pregnant woman is lowest in this position. For maximum accuracy over time, the blood pressure should not be taken until the pregnant woman has had a period of rest after arriving at the clinic (to allow for relaxation and stress reduction), the blood pressure should always be taken on the left arm, with the pregnant woman in the same position each time, and the nurse should always record the manner in which the blood pressure is taken (to prevent inaccurate conclusions about blood pressure changes based on the manner in which the blood pressure was obtained).

The nurse should always record the *systolic pressure* as the number at which the first sound is heard when releasing pressure from the cuff. The *diastolic pressure* is recorded when a muffling sound is heard. The number may also be recorded at which no sound is heard, producing a reading such as 110/68/40 (Malasanos et al., 1981). It is inaccurate and can be dangerous to record only when sound is first heard and when sound is no longer heard, creating a reading such as 110/40.

A blood pressure rise of 30 mm Hg systolic or 15 mm Hg diastolic after 20 weeks of gestation may indicate the onset of preeclampsia. This concern about the degree of rise rather than an absolute number is why a baseline blood pressure prior to pregnancy is so important in providing appropriate health care to the pregnant woman. In addition

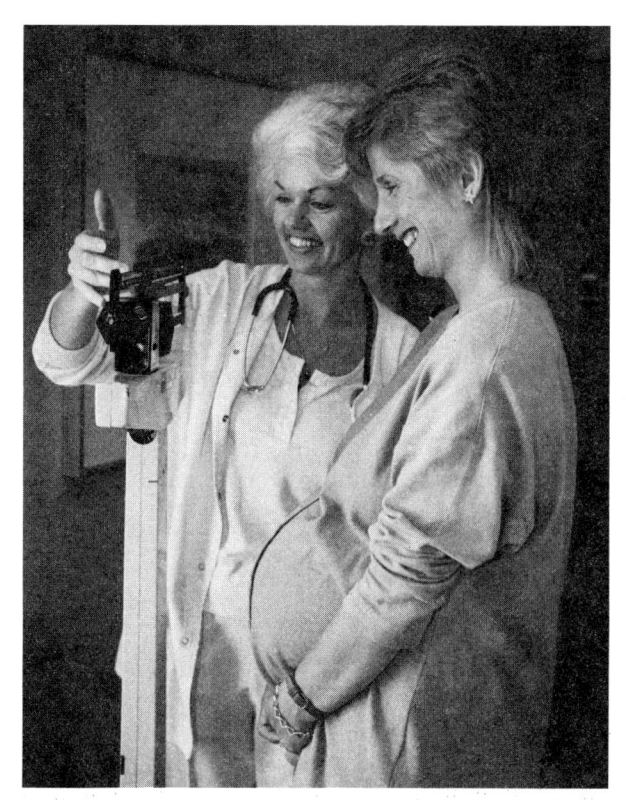

FIGURE 15-3. Part of the assessment process is obtaining current health data, such as weight gain.

to taking a regular blood pressure reading at each return visit, the nurse in the ambulatory prenatal care setting should consider doing a "roll-over" test between the 28th and 32nd weeks of pregnancy. This test for predicting preeclampsia is done by taking one blood pressure reading with the pregnant woman in a left lateral position, then having her roll onto her back, letting her rest for 5 min, and retaking her blood pressure while she is in the supine position. The test is considered positive, or indicative of the possible development of preeclampsia, if the diastolic blood pressure is 20 mm Hg greater in the supine position than in the left lateral position. If this test is positive, it is approximately 90 percent accurate in predicting the later development of some degree of preeclampsia (Gant et al., 1978). Women with a positive roll-over test need close monitoring and should probably be scheduled for more frequent prenatal visits than the average healthy pregnant woman.

Body Fluids

The collection of body fluid samples may also be done at this time. Blood is obtained by venipuncture for serology, hemoglobin, hematocrit, typing and Rh, and rubella titer. Sickle cell screening and titer and an antibody screen are done if their desirability is indicated.

In addition, although still relatively rare among pregnant woman, testing for the HTLV-III virus may be carried out. Pregnant women with AIDS have been reported and with extremely poor maternal and perinatal outcomes. Several hundred instances of perinatally transmitted AIDS have occurred. Pregnancy may seriously exacerbate the disease in women and there are reports in the literature of pregnant women dying within a few weeks of initial diagnosis, versus a mortality for nonpregnant patients of 30 percent during hospitalization for the first opportunistic infection. (Minkoff et al., 1986; Jensen et al., 1984; Pitchanik, Fischl, and Spira, 1983; Rawlinson et al., 1984). The nurse should be familiar with and utilize infection control guidelines similar to the precautions for general hepatitis B when performing the venipuncture and handling the equipment.

A urine sample is collected for a pregnancy test (if not already performed) and for glucose and albumin testing. A "clean catch" urine specimen will be needed if culture and sensitivity tests are to be done. The culture and sensitivity testing may not always be done, but increasingly health care providers are finding this procedure useful in diagnosing "silent" urinary tract infections that may cause problems during the pregnancy (Mocarski, 1980). Treatment that is begun early may well prevent miscarriage or premature labor later in pregnancy.

Lungs and Heart

Auscultating the heart and lungs and palpating the chest, back, and throat may uncover problems with the heart, lungs, and thyroid gland that were not revealed by history. However, pregnancy itself will change the respirations from abdominal to costal, increase the respiratory rate, and elevate the diaphragm, particularly from the second trimester on. Other normal changes may be noted in the cardiovascular system beginning in the second trimester. These changes include an increase in the pulse rate, a slight fall in the blood pressure, and a grade II systolic murmur in as many as 90 percent of all pregnant women (Pritchard, MacDonald, and Gant, 1985). And by the third trimester the nurse, when taking an apical pulse, may note the displacement of the point of maximal impact to the left and upward because of the enlarging uterus pushing upward. In addition, palpation of the throat and thyroid gland may reveal a normal enlargement of the thyroid gland by 50 percent due to hyperplasia. This hyperplasia is consistent with an increase in the basal metabolic rate normally seen in pregnant women.

Other Aspects of Physiology

The extremities should be assessed for varicosities and findings should be compared with the patient's personal and family history of varicosities and phlebitis. The pregnant woman should also be questioned about patterns of bowel and bladder elimination. The enlarging uterus will cause increased frequency of urination, particularly early in the first trimester and later in the third trimester, because of pressure on the bladder. Bowel patterns may change and constipation may be more of problem during the last trimester, as a result of the pressure of the enlarging uterus and of the high levels of progesterone. Dental caries should be cared for by a dentist, and the pregnant woman should understand that the old myth of losing a tooth for each pregnancy is just that—a myth.

Health Habits

Because of the damage that can be incurred by the fetus if the mother smokes, drinks, or abuses controlled substances, a prenatal nurse should ask questions to try to elicit specific information about these habits (see Chapter 40). These questions may be included as part of the nutritional history or 24-hour diet recall. If not, they should be asked at some point during the initial visit. The nurse may find out what the pregnant woman drinks by asking a direct but nonjudgmental question such as "I'd like you to tell me what you have had to drink in the last 24 hours . . . juice, water, milk, beer, coffee, soft drinks, tea, whiskey, cocktails?" This can be followed with a question about whether she drinks any of these liquids and how frequently. The pregnant woman is less likely to hide this important information when asked in this fashion than if she is asked about the intake of alcohol separately. This type of information may also be elicited while asking about bladder habits.

Similarly, data about medication and drug intake can be obtained by asking the woman about problems related to her food intake and bowel habits, such as: "Do you ever have incidents of being sick before or after you have eaten? Do you ever take medication for it? What kind? Do you take any other medications? Have you ever used a laxative? Have you taken any drugs that increased or decreased your appetite? Do you drink any special herbal teas?" With such questions the nurse may learn that the patient is a frequent user of sodium-based antacids or potent laxatives, or the nurse may discover that the patient has been trying to lose weight by taking amphetamines or other stimulants (prescription or illegal). The patient may reveal to the nurse that she has tried marijuana or cocaine as she describes how much better food tasted or how it increased her appetite. Or she may tell the nurse about specific teas she drinks to help her during her pregnancy.

The establishment of the nurse–patient trust relationship is essential to the compilation of accurate, honest, and meaningful data necessary for the nurse to help the patient and her unborn baby to a healthy outcome.

Assessment of the Breasts

A thorough and careful examination of the breasts is an important component of the overall initial physical assessment of the pregnant woman. It provides an opportunity for the nurse to ascertain whether the patient understands and performs self-breast examinations and to instruct her if she does not. In addition, changes in the breast may be one of the first and most evident presumptive signs of pregnancy. Some of these changes include increases in size, vascularity, and tenderness, reports of tingling and enlargement, and darkening of the areolas and nipples. Increased tenderness and tingling may be noted as early as several weeks after conception, while increases in size and vascularity may occur as early as 2 months after conception. The pregnant woman may also report leakage of colostrum as early as the end of the first trimester.

Breast examination provides an excellent opportunity for questioning the woman about whether she is planning to breastfeed her baby. Although she may not have made a decision about breastfeeding by the first visit, the nurse can encourage her to think about it and can serve as a resource person as she decides. There are a few important points the pregnant woman should be aware of in making the decision to breastfeed and in preparing for the breastfeeding experience.

First, it is important to her future success that she be committed to the idea of breastfeeding and really want to do it for herself as well as for her baby. It is also important that she have the support and encouragement of her husband or the significant other in her life. If there is a conflict between her desire to nurse and her husband's wishes for her, breastfeeding is likely to be unsuccessful.

Secondly, it is helpful for the woman to begin preparation for breastfeeding during the prenatal period. Wearing a properly fitting bra, for example, is important to comfort and overall preparation. The nurse should recommend that she buy at least two nursing bras in her current larger size. The size of bra she needs during the last two trimesters is the size she will continue to need until lactation ends.

Important to the physical preparation for breastfeeding is the mental and emotional preparation. A woman who is uncomfortable exposing and touching or handling her breasts will have a difficult time nursing her baby no matter how much she desires to be successful.

In assisting the pregnant woman to prepare for the breastfeeding experience, the nurse may also refer the woman to the nearest chapter of the La Leche League. This group of nursing mothers with certified leaders are experienced in breastfeeding and provide education and support to the woman both during pregnancy and postnatally (see Chapter 21).

Assessment of the Abdomen

Careful observation, palpation, and auscultation of the pregnant woman's abdomen is vital. The woman should first empty her bladder to reduce discomfort during palpation. She should be helped into a reclining position with her head elevated somewhat and her knees gently flexed. This position takes pressure off the abdomen and reduces tension from the lower back muscles. It also helps in preventing supine hypotension. Scars noted on the abdomen should be checked against historical information about surgeries or accidents. If there are discrepancies, the reason for the scars should be ascertained.

The nurse should assess the condition of abdominal muscle tone and should encourage the pregnant woman to maintain good overall muscle tone. Exercises that strengthen the abdomen and lower back will, in particular, relieve the stress caused by an enlarging uterus. In assessing muscle tone, attention should be paid to the presence or absence of hernias and to the condition of the skin. Presence of *striae* (stretch marks) and the *linea nigra* (dark line down the center of abdomen) should be noted (Fig. 15-4). Although nothing can be done to prevent or modify these marks, reassurance regarding their normalcy will help the pregnant woman cope.

Much of the assessment of the abdomen is done to compile information about the length of the gestation and the lie, presentation, and position of the fetus.

Length of Gestation

Assessment of fundal height will not, by itself, tell the examiner the length of gestation. However, the height of the fundus (top of the uterus) when correlated with other data (LNMP, quickening, date FHTs were first heard) will increase the accuracy in determining the week of gestation. Prior to measuring the height of the uterus the nurse should explain to the patient what is being done. While explaining, the nurse should gently place her or his hand on the pregnant woman's abdomen. As the patient is getting accustomed to the touch of the nurse's hands, the nurse can also be collecting data on the tone, irritability, consistency, and contractibility of the uterus. Fetal movement may also be felt by the examiner.

The nurse should then proceed to measure the distance of the uterus from the symphysis pubis to the fundus. There are several ways to measure this distance, and each varies in its accuracy and its correlation to gestational age of the fetus. The least accurate but easiest and most readily applied method is fingerbreadth measurement. In this method the nurse measures the distance of the fundus in relation to abdominal landmarks (see Fig. 15-5). This measurement is recorded in fingerbreadths from the symphysis pubis, the umbilicus, or the xiphoid process of the sternum. For example, the nurse locates the fundus and measures it at one fingerbreadth below the umbilicus (recorded as 1Fb ↓ U or U/1FB). This measurement would correlate with approximately 20 weeks' gestation. Inaccuracies using this method are a result of the differences in the width of examiners' fingers and individual variation in distances between the abdominal landmarks. Table 15-1 will help the nurse judge estimated gestational age using the fingerbreadth method.

The use of calipers provides the most accurate measurement of fundal height. One point of the caliper is placed on the superior border of the symphysis pubis and the other point is placed on the top of the fundus. The distance in centimeters at the apex of the calipers should equal the gestational weeks, after 22-24 weeks of gestation. Calipers are rarely used, however, because a tape

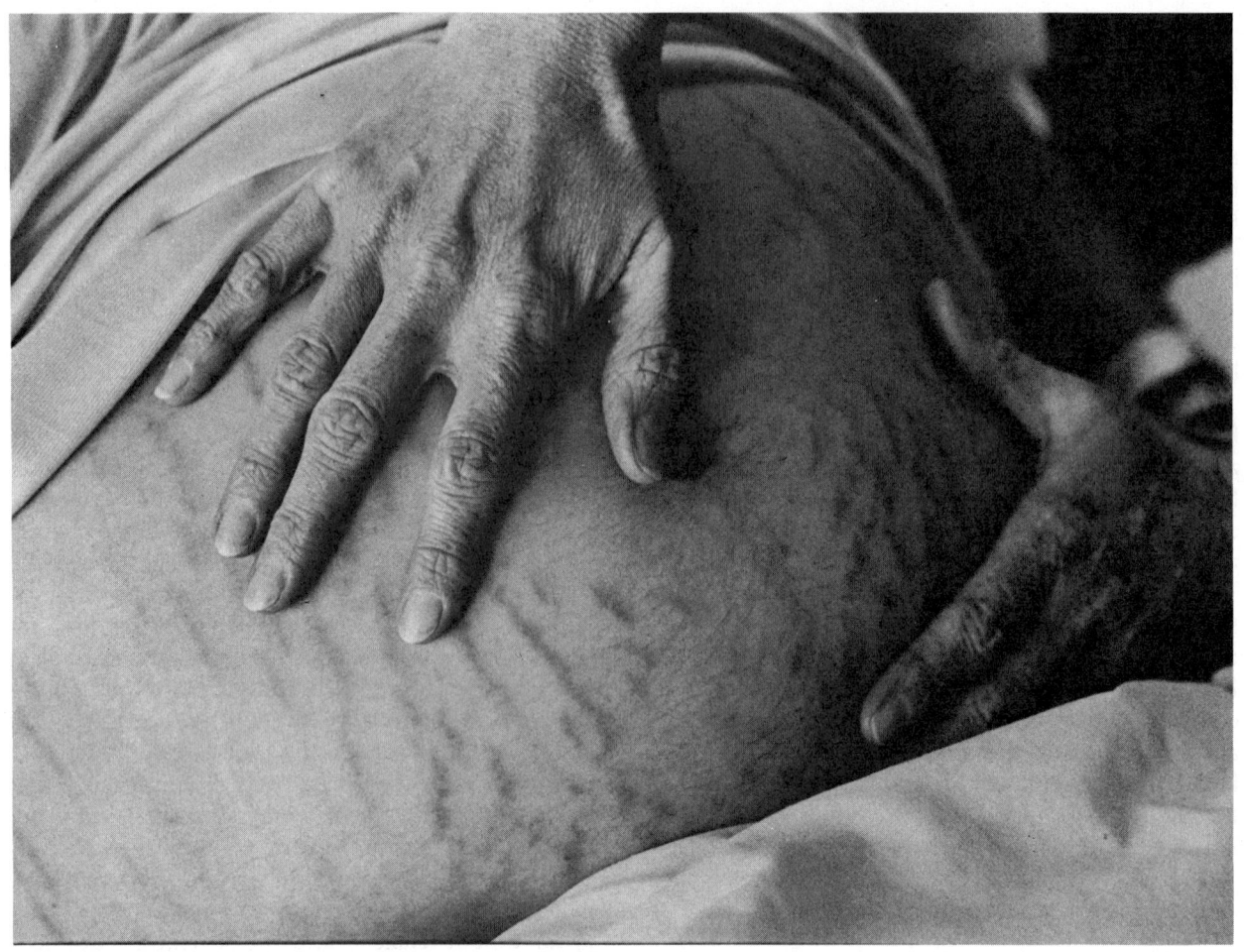

FIGURE 15-4. Abdominal striae should be noted.

measure will provide similar data and is more portable.

There are two methods of measuring fundal height using a tape measure. The more accurate is to place the end of the tape at the superior border of the symphysis pubis and to run the tape up the midline of the abdomen cover the curve of the uterus to the top edge of the fundus. As with the calipers, the number in centimeters at the top of the tape should equal the gestation in weeks after 22–24 weeks. The second method using the tape measure is to hold the end of the tape at the superior border of the symphysis pubis and, holding the other hand at right angles to the abdomen at the upper border of the fundus, to stretch the tape between the two hands. The number of the tape below the fingers of the top hand is then used to calculate the week of gestation mathematically. Before the fundus reaches the umbilicus, 4 cm is added to the measurement on the tape to get the week of gestation. After the fundus reaches or exceeds the level of the umbilicus, 6 cm is added to the measurement on the tape to get the week of gestation (Varney, 1987).

The accuracy of gestational week determination is increased (regardless of the method used) if the pregnant woman has good abdominal muscle tone, if the same examiner does the assessment each time, and if the same method of assessment is used each time. It is also vitally important that the nurse always record not only the gestational week determined but the method used to reach the determination. This will prevent error and confusion if different people are involved in this part of the assessment.

Nichols (1987), in a comprehensive report on dating pregnancy, supports the necessity of not relying on fundal height as a major factor in determining gestational age. In her classification system, uterine size/fundal height is ranked as level 3 data and can only be counted on to be accurate within a margin of 3 weeks. Nichols found no valid evidence to equate number of centimeters of uterine height with weeks of gesta-

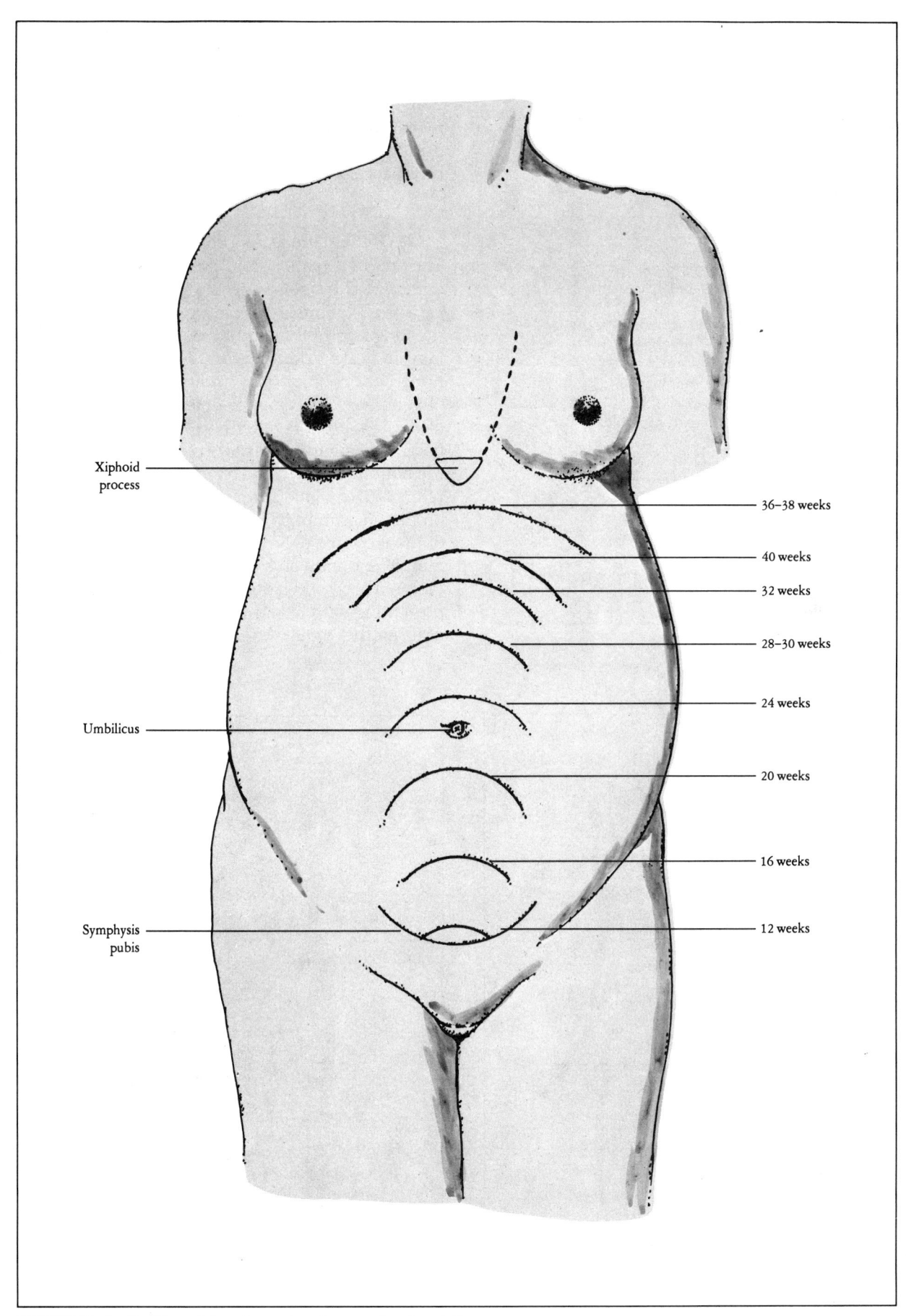

FIGURE 15-5. Position of the uterus at various weeks of gestation.

CHANGE: THE PRENATAL PERIOD

TABLE 15–1. Fundal Heights and Estimated Gestation

Fundal Height	Weeks
At level of symphysis pubis	12
Halfway between symphysis pubis and umbilicus (usually about 4 fingerbreadths above symphysis pubis)	16
1–2 fingerbreadths below umbilicus	20
1–2 fingerbreadths above umbilicus	24
One-third of distance between umbilicus and xiphoid process	28–30
Two-thirds of distance between umbilicus and xiphoid process	32
1–2 fingerbreadths below xiphoid process	36–38
2–3 fingerbreadths below xiphoid process if lightening occurs	40

tion. Level 1 data, specifically the last normal menstrual period (LNMP), gathered by the nurse during the history is the most accurate indication of expected date of delivery.

Lie, Presentation, and Position

The lie, presentation, and position of the fetus are determined by palpating the pregnant abdomen. *Lie* is the relationship of the long axis of the fetus to the long axis of the mother. A long ovoid contour may indicate a longitudinal lie, while a broader horizontal contour may indicate a transverse or oblique lie. *Presentation* is determined by that part of the fetus that is entering the pelvis first. If the head is coming first, it is a *cephalic presentation*; if the bottom is first, it is a *breech presentation. Position* refers to the relationship of a predetermined point on the presenting part to the front, sides, and back of the mother's pelvis. The occiput is the predetermined landmark on a well-flexed cephalic presentation. The abbreviation for the position of a fetus presenting with its occiput in the left inguinal area of its mother would be LOA (left occiput anterior).

FIGURE 15–6. Step 1 of Leopold's maneuvers.

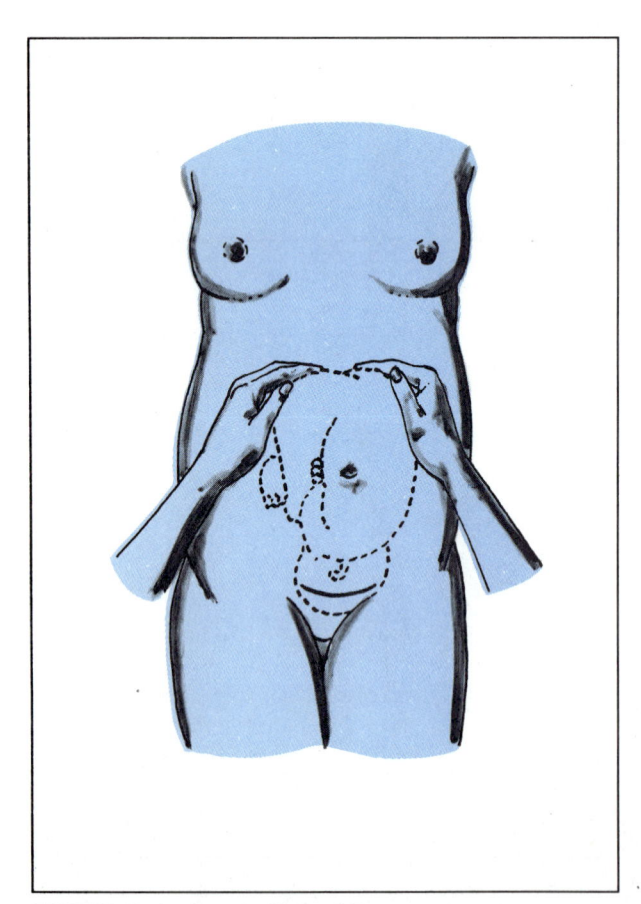

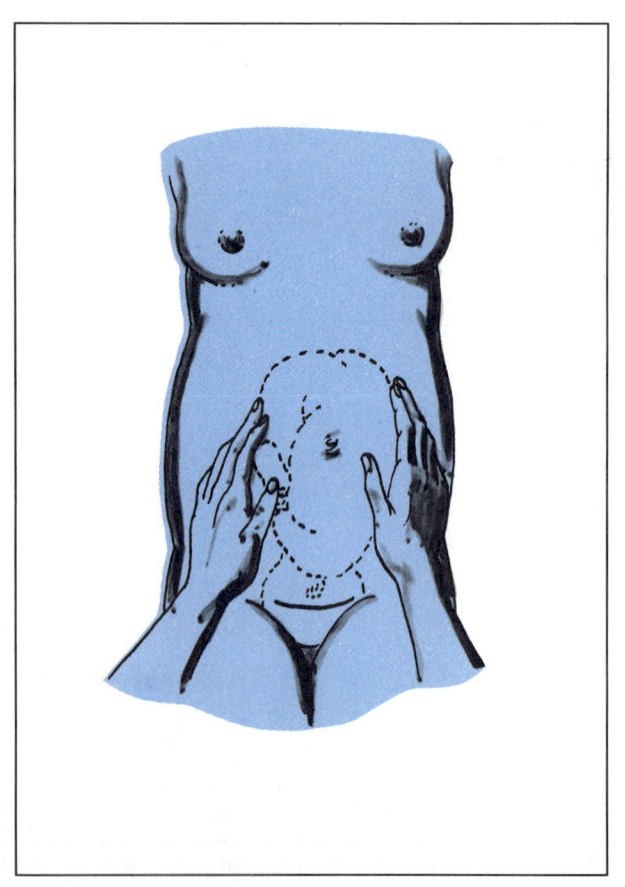

FIGURE 15–7. Step 2 of Leopold's maneuvers.

Fetal lie, presentation, and position are illustrated and discussed in greater detail in Chapter 16.

Although a given nurse may determine lie, presentation, and position in a variety of ways when palpating the abdomen of a pregnant woman, it is preferable for the less experienced nurse to follow a pattern or set of prescribed steps in determining position. This pattern is called *Leopold's maneuvers,* or the *abdominal touch picture.* When palpating the abdomen, the nurse should remember to use the flat palmar surfaces of the fingers. A pregnant abdomen should never be poked or kneaded like a mound of bread dough. Rather, the nurse should always use gentle, but firm, pressure.

In the first step of Leopold's maneuvers (Fig. 15–6), the nurse faces the patient and places both hands on the abdomen with fingertips nearly touching, cupping the hands around the part of the fetus in the fundus of the uterus. The firmness, roundness, and ballottement of the part of the fetus grasped in the nurse's hands aids in the determination of presentation. If the fetal part is rounded and somewhat soft and when moved the whole fetus moves, it is probably a breech in the fundus (cephalic presentation). If the fetal part is round and hard and moves independently of the rest of the fetus, it is probably the head (breech presentation). The information gathered in this step should be put together with information gathered in Step 3 to make a final determination of presentation.

In Step 2 (Fig. 15–7) the nurse, still facing the patient, places her or his hands on either side of the pregnant abdomen. Holding one hand steady, the nurse applies pressure against the fetus with the other hand. The hand applying the pressure can feel the resistance of the fetus. If the resistant part is long, smooth, and firm, it is the back of the fetus. If the resistant part is bumpy with nodules, indentations, and angles, the nurse is feeling the arms, legs, and knees (small parts) of the fetus. As the fetus gets older, the nurse may even feel movement on this side while palpating. If the back is felt more easily on the anterior portion of the abdomen and the small parts on the flank, the fetus is in an anterior position. If the back is felt more deeply into the flank and the small parts are

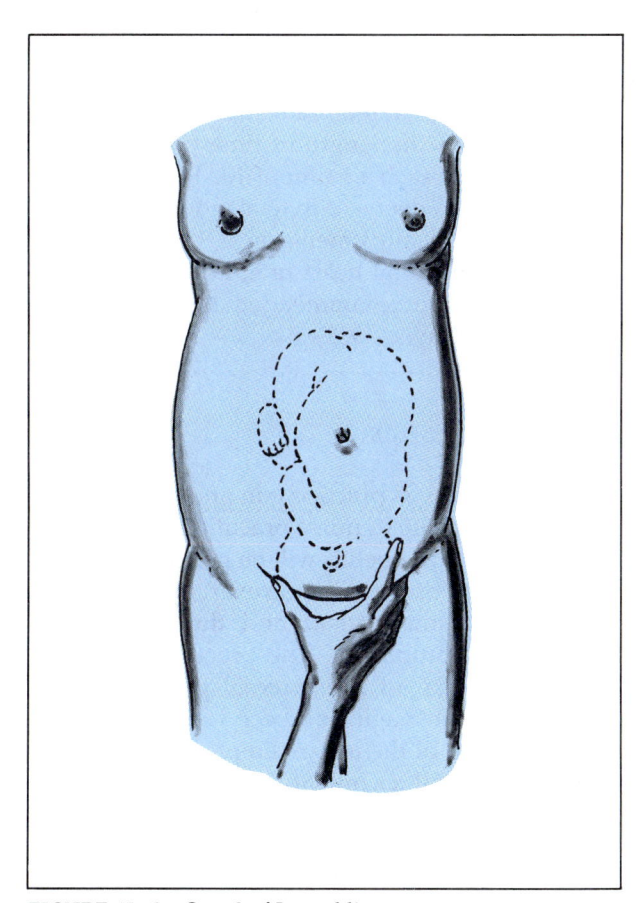

FIGURE 15–8. Step 3 of Leopold's maneuvers.

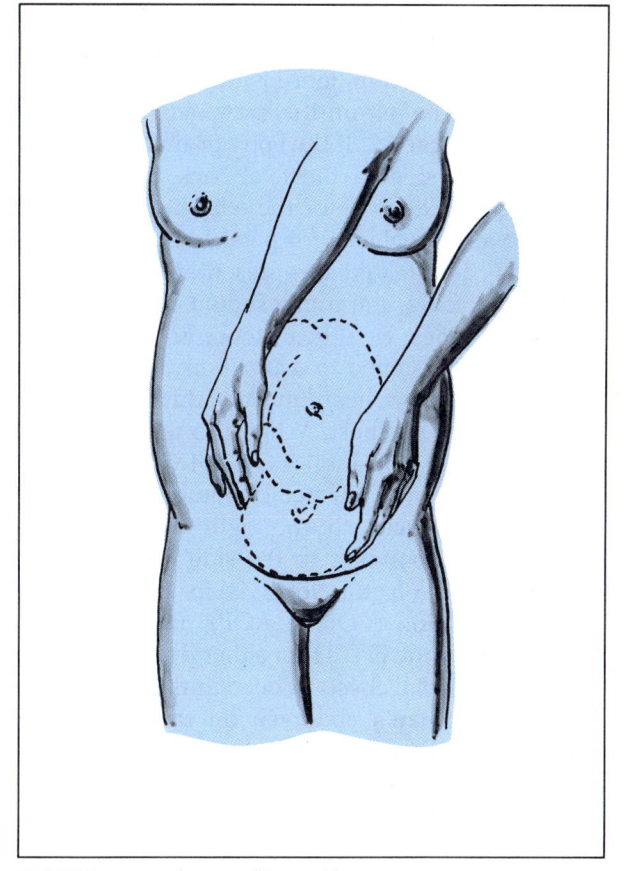

FIGURE 15–9. Step 4 of Leopold's maneuvers.

felt in the anterior part of the abdomen, the fetus is in a posterior position.

In Step 3 (Fig. 15–8) the nurse, again still facing the patient, takes the thumb and middle finger of the examining hand, holds them in a broad, arched, pincerlike position at right angles to the abdomen, and gently but firmly presses down just above the symphysis pubis, grasping the fetal part that lies beneath. If the fetal part is hard and rounded and can be moved independent of the mass in the fundus, it is the fetal head. If it is soft and rounded and when moved causes movement of the whole fetus, it is the breech. The examiner may wish to place the other hand gently on the fundus to compare the densities and the movement of the fetal mass.

The fourth step (Fig. 15–9) helps confirm the information gathered in Step 2 and assists the nurse in determining how far into the pelvis the presenting part has descended. In this step the nurse faces the patient's feet and places his or her hands on either side of the lower abdomen just above the symphysis. Sliding both hands along the fetus with fingers attempting to dip into the pelvis, the nurse ascertains the side of the cephalic prominence. One hand will slide down along the side and into the inguinal area under the symphysis pubis; the other hand will hit a bony prominence above the symphysis. In a well-flexed fetal head this bony prominence is the fetal brow. The brow should be felt on the same side as the fetal small parts in Step 2. If the bony prominence is felt on the same side as the fetal back in Step 2, it indicates an extension of the fetal head that may cause severe problems if it persists during labor.

Having determined the presentation and position of the fetus, the nurse should auscultate the fetal heart tones. Fetal heart tones are heard more readily when listened to over a bony prominence. Therefore, they are heard most readily through the fetal shoulder or chest. When the fetus is in the anterior cephalic position (LOA or ROA) the nurse should listen over the fetal shoulder below the mother's umbilicus to the right or left of the midline corresponding to the side on which the back was felt. If the fetus is in the posterior cephalic position (LOP or ROP), the nurse will probably hear the FHTs best either directly midline (through the fetal chest) or deep in the flank of the pregnant woman's abdomen on the side corresponding to the side on which the fetal back was felt. If the FHTs are heard best above the pregnant woman's umbilicus, a breech presentation is usually indicated.

Fetal heart tones normally range between 120 and 160 beats/min. They will accelerate with fetal movement. Fetal heart tones can first be heard using a fetoscope at 18–20 weeks' gestation. If an ultrasonic fetal heart monitor (Doppler) is used, the fetal heart can be heard as early as the 8th to 10th week. Because these dates are useful in determining the week of gestation, they should always be carefully and accurately recorded.

It is becoming increasingly evident that a valuable aid in assessing the health of the fetus, in addition to the fetal heart tones, is the frequency and pattern of fetal movement. A wide range of individual variations in daily fetal movement has been observed. Pregnant women have been found to be 76–90 percent accurate in their counting, and the "safety valve" is that the majority of women tended to undercount. The use of daily fetal movement assessment should be begun before 36 weeks of pregnancy to get an adequate baseline, but not so early that the pregnant woman loses her motivation. The gestational age at which fetal movement assessment should begin should be individualized depending on the risk factors in the pregnancy. The recommended counting pattern is for the mother-to-be to use a modified Cardiff method. This requires the woman to choose a time of day that is convenient for her and begin counting the number of fetal movements. When she has counted 10 fetal movements, she records this along with the length of time (i.e. 30, 60, 90 min) it took to reach a count of 10. The movement alarm signal is a decrease in fetal movement to less than three fetal movements in a 12-hour period with an audible fetal heart rate. Daily fetal movement counts are recommended for all postdate pregnancies (Davis, 1987).

Pelvic Examination

Unless the nurse is practicing in an expanded role as a nurse-midwife or nurse practitioner, the actual examination of the pelvis will be performed by the physician. The nurse will, however, be responsible for preparing the patient and the examination room for the procedure. The procedure includes visual inspection of the external genitals, visual inspection of the vagina and cervix using a speculum, palpation of the internal reproductive organs during bimanual examination, palpation of the bony pelvis, and collection of specimens for laboratory testing.

When setting up the exam room, the nurse

should ensure the privacy of the patient. The examining table should be positioned so that the foot of the table faces away from the door opening into the hallway. A gown and drape should be provided for the patient. Throughout the procedure only the part of the body that is being examined should be exposed. In addition, the nurse should arrange the necessary supplies on a stand for easy access and an orderly, smooth examination. These supplies usually include gloves, a speculum, water-soluble jelly, slides and culture media, an Ayer's spatula (see Fig. 15-10), and long cotton-tipped swabs for obtaining cells for the Pap smear and cultures for infection if indicated.

The nurse should be aware that a woman may or many not report an irritating vaginal discharge when an infection is present. Many vaginal infections, *Chlamydia* in particular, may be asymptomatic in 5-30 percent of women. Laboratory testing of a specimen of the secretions from the cervix is the principal diagnostic tool. Infants born to mothers with an active chlamydial infection may acquire an inclusion conjunctivitis that can cause chronic eye disease that leads to conjunctival scarring and superficial corneal vascularization (Loucks, 1987; Marvin and Slevin, 1987; Sweet, 1985). It is imperative that the nurse question the possibility of vaginal infections during history taking, and during the time of the pelvic exam

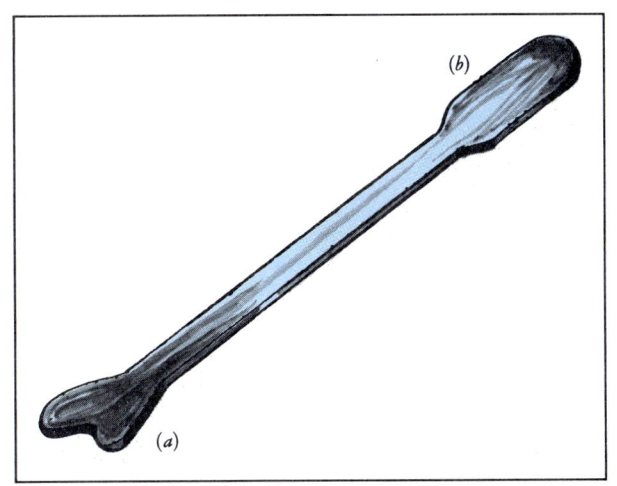

FIGURE 15-10. An Ayer's spatula. A specially designed wooden or plastic spatula with two ends, one (a) for obtaining cells from the squamocolumnar junction of the cervix and the other (b) for obtaining cells from the posterior fornix of the vagina for the Pap smear.

have available the variety of materials necessary to test for the specific vaginal infections the primary health care attendant may request.

The pelvic examination is usually the most anxiety-producing part of the initial visit for the patient. Prior to the examination the nurse should carefully explain the procedure and answer all questions. The patient should be asked to empty her bladder to reduce discomfort during the procedure. Once the patient is undressed and gowned, the nurse should assist her on to the table, with the aid of a footstool. The head of the examining table should be raised at approximately a 45-degree angle, which reduces stress on the back muscles, decreases pressure on the vena cava, and allows the patient eye contact with the examiner. When the patient has been assisted into the lithotomy position, the nurse should ensure the draping provides good cover.

Throughout these preparations for the pelvic examination, the nurse should be concentrating on helping the patient to relax. The nurse should ask the patient what makes her feel comfortable and should support her in relaxing. The nurse may explain each step during the examination so the patient understands what is happening and what is expected of her. As the examination is being conducted, the nurse should continue her assessment of the patient. She should accumulate information about how the patient copes with unfamiliar or stressful procedures and how she handles discomfort. This information can then be used throughout the pregnancy to make future procedures and unknown experiences easier for the patient to manage.

When the pelvic examination is completed, the patient should be given disposable wipes to clean the external genitals, assisted from the table, and allowed to dress in private. When the patient is once again in street clothes, she should be afforded some time with the examiner to get any last-minute questions answered, receive reassurance about her current state of health, and obtain instructions regarding health maintenance during the remainder of her pregnancy.

PSYCHOSOCIAL/ EMOTIONAL ASSESSMENT

Assessment of the patient's psychosocial/emotional status begins when the initial history is being taken. As data are collected about the patient's physical status, they should also be collected about the patient's psychosocial/emotional status.

Broad areas of concern in assessing a pregnant woman's psychosocial/emotional status are:

1. Was the pregnancy planned? If not, is the baby wanted now?
2. Is the patient married or involved in a stable, ongoing familial relationship? Does she have the support and approval of her significant others?
3. What is her economic status? Is she working? Will she continue to work? How does she see her pregnancy and work meshing?
4. How does she feel about her impending motherhood—excited, accepting, dismayed, anxious, angry?
5. How does the baby's father feel about the pregnancy and the mother of his child? Are they sharing a warm, supportive relationship? How does he feel about impending fatherhood—excited, accepting, dismayed, anxious, angry? Is he working?
6. What kind of support system does the pregnant couple have? Are they close to their parents, siblings, and other relatives? Have they established a place for themselves in the broader community? Do they have others who will support them throughout this pregnancy and come to their assistance if needed?

The above questions are of particular importance when the nurse realizes that the rate of battering and abuse of pregnant women is estimated to be on average 20–25 percent, and in one study the rate was as high as 54 percent. The evidence also suggests that the first experience of battering and abuse for the woman may actually have begun during the pregnancy. For those women who report being battered and abused prior to pregnancy, the intensity and/or frequency may increase during pregnancy. Some of the abuse appears to be directed at the pregnant abdomen and/or the genitals and twice as many miscarriages occur to the battered women than to nonbattered women. The overwhelming number of these reported abuses occur at the hands of the spouse or father of the baby (Helton, 1986; Campbell, 1986; Bradshaw, 1987).

Much of this information will be volunteered by the patient during taking of the initial history if the nurse is warm, caring, and listening attentively. Other data may be accumulated through direct questioning and observation of the patient during the initial and subsequent visits. Understanding the patient's psychosocial/emotional adjustment to this pregnancy will help the nurse in planning appropriate support for the pregnant woman throughout the pregnancy (see Chapter 11).

The pregnant woman may have certain questions regarding her sexuality during pregnancy. It is the role of the nurse to provide information to the couple before unnecessary concerns develop. The couple needs to understand that the effect of pregnancy on sexual desire varies. Sexuality during pregnancy may be influenced by many factors: the couple's relationship, their knowledge and attitudes about sexual activity during pregnancy, and physical or medical constraints (Weinberg, 1982). Figure 15–11 illustrates typical patterns of interest in sex during pregnancy, and Fig. 15–12 shows sexual desires, anxieties, and reassurance from the beginning of pregnancy through the postpartum period.

An important note to remember is that if data about the patient's psychosocial/emotional status are important to gather, they are important to chart. When information is transferred to the hospital staff prior to admission for delivery, or to the community health nurses at any time throughout the pregnancy, the accumulated data on the psychosocial/emotional status should be communicated as well as the physical status.

MAINTENANCE AND PROMOTION OF HEALTH FOR THE PREGNANT PATIENT

For the past several decades the schedule of visits for a pregnant patient after the initial visit has been based on the month of her pregnancy. This schedule was designed when health care personnel could do little in the way of assessment or intervention during the early part of pregnancy. Because there seemed to be little they could contribute to the health of the pregnant patient, they did not need to see her very frequently. Health care providers believed they could more easily influence the outcome as the pregnancy neared term and therefore saw the pregnant patient more frequently at this time. This schedule of visits is still followed by many providers of prenatal health care. During the first 6 months the pregnant patient is seen monthly, during the 7th and 8th months she is seen every 2 weeks, and during the 9th month every week.

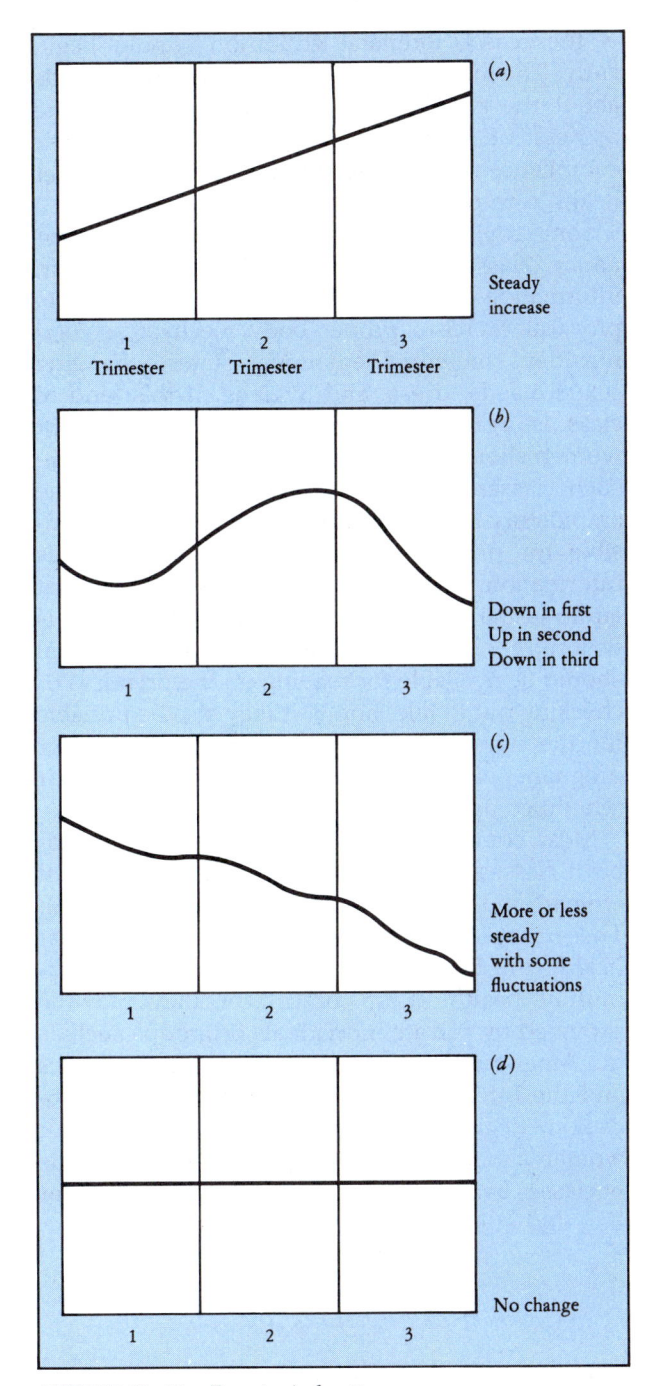

FIGURE 15-11. Four typical patterns of interest in sex during pregnancy. SOURCE: Bing and Coleman (1977).

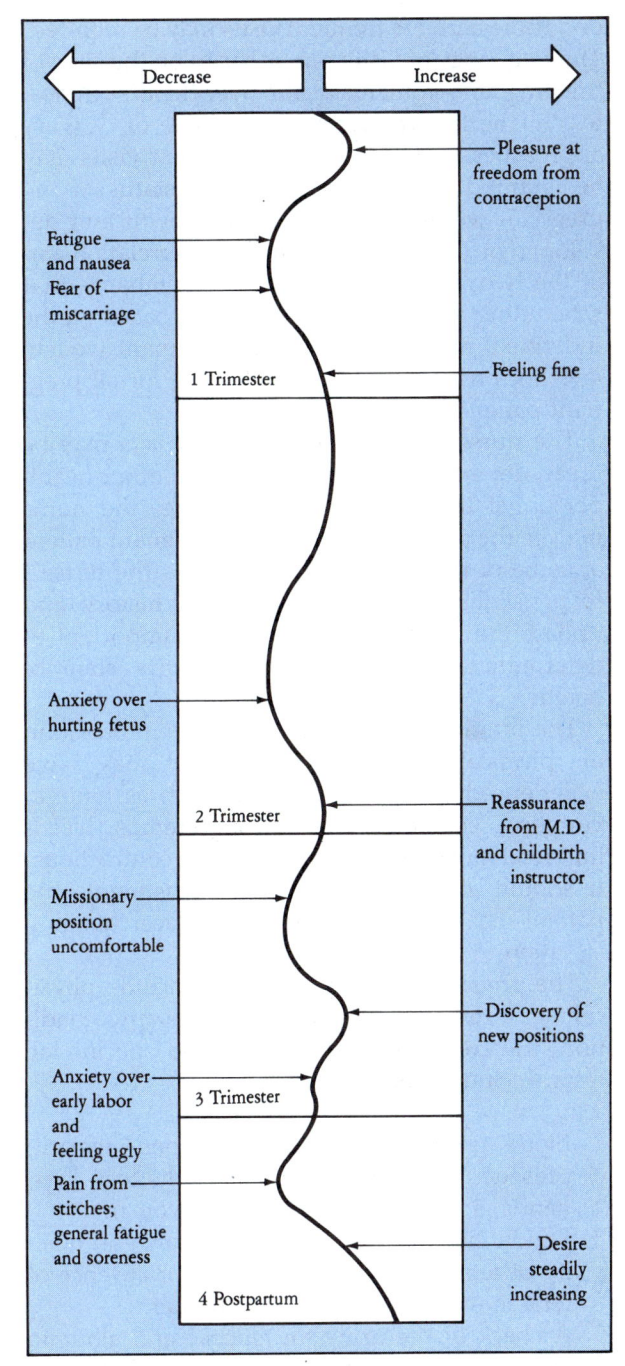

FIGURE 15-12. Desires, anxieties, and reassurance during pregnancy and postpartum. SOURCE: Bing and Coleman (1977).

As the boundaries of medical and health science have expanded and as more has been learned about fetal development and the effects of the pregnant woman's state of health on the outcome of the pregnancy, ideas about the "routine" schedule of prenatal visits have been changing. Health personnel are increasingly recommending frequent visits during the first trimester, to allow time for thorough evaluation of the health status of the pregnant woman and the embryo or fetus. These visits provide multiple opportunities for the establishment of a trust relationship and for health teaching early in the pregnancy.

As the pregnancy progresses through the second trimester, less frequent visits may be required. The frequency of visits can be based on the state of the pregnant woman's health over the first trimester. In the last trimester, as the date of delivery approaches, a return to more frequent visits may be required to monitor the health status of the pregnant woman, the continued growth and development of the fetus, and the interrelationship of the two. The major point to remember is that scheduling of return visits should be based on the individual needs of a particular pregnant woman and not on a preconceived schedule for all pregnant patients.

The nurse's role during prenatal visits may be great, depending on the demands on other health personnel in the ambulatory setting, the nurse may be the only person to see the pregnant patient at some of the visits. It thus becomes the nurse's responsibility to collect an interim history and update the basic vital physical data important to determining the patient's and fetus's state of health.

The interim history should include information on physical symptoms the patient may have experienced since her last visit, such as nausea, vomiting, edema, headaches, leg cramps, bleeding, fetal movement, lightening, and contractions. It should also cover emotional adjustments the patient has been making to her everchanging situation.

The physical assessment should include physical measurements of the pregnant woman's condition, the condition of the fetus, and specific lab tests. Included should be:

1. Blood pressure, pulse, respirations, weight, presence or absence of edema in the feet, legs, hands, and face of the pregnant woman.
2. Fundal height, position of fetus, rate and quality of fetal heart tones, presence or absence of fetal movement felt by the examiner.
3. A check of the urine for glucose and albumin (repeat hemoglobin or hematocrit when indicated and antibody titers as indicated for rubella and Rh).

These data should be carefully recorded, compared with previous data, and reported to the appropriate health care provider if significant.

Continuing Prenatal Education

The pregnant woman's immediate need to understand the changes that are occurring in her body, in her emotional state, and in her developing baby is the reason prenatal education should begin early. The more the pregnant woman understands about the changes she is experiencing and the process of pregnancy, the better will be her compliance with the regimen recommended by her health care providers.

Some communities have developed "early pregnancy" classes. These series of classes may contain information on positive health habits, appropriate physical exercise, proper body mechanics, good nutrition, mercurial emotional states, changing sexual needs, dress, and hygiene. If this kind of class is available in the community, pregnant women should be referred. In communities where such classes are not available, the nurse in the ambulatory maternity care setting must be responsible for providing pregnant women with this information. Some settings are designed so that audio-visual aids can be used while the patient is waiting for her appointment. Reading material should be available for reading on the premises or checking out to take home. It may also be possible for the nurse to set up small group classes for pregnant women to attend before or after their scheduled appointments.

Most communities now have prepared childbirth classes available to any interested pregnant woman and her support person (Sumner, 1976). These classes may be associated with a particular health care facility (doctor's office, hospital, community health nurse' office), or they may be provided by private individuals or groups such as the American Society for Prophylaxis in Obstetrics and the International Childbirth Education Association. Regardless of the provider, the pregnant woman should be encouraged to review the kinds of classes available, select the most appropriate for her, and attend.

Development of Relationships

Pregnancy is a time of change. It is certainly a time of physical change, and it is usually a time of emotional upheaval as well. Pregnancy has been referred to as a period of crisis. But a crisis is not necessarily a negative force. With appropriate support and guidance, it can be a time of great positive, personal growth (Caplan, 1957; Coleman and Coleman, 1977).

Much of the emotional support and guidance the pregnant woman needs will be provided by the nurse. The nurse is the first of the health care providers to establish a relationship with the pregnant woman, during the taking of the health history. At each subsequent visit the nurse inquires about how the patient feels, emotionally and physically. Much of what the woman learns about her state of health, the changes she is going through, and the recommended health regimen during her pregnancy comes from the nurse.

It is important for the nurse to have a deep appreciation of the changes the pregnant woman is going through. During the first trimester, the woman is resolving her feelings about being pregnant. She is being forced to come to grips with the fact of the pregnancy and her impending motherhood. She is looking at the father of her baby from a new perspective. He is no longer just her husband, lover, friend—he is now the father of her child. As she sorts through these feelings and impressions, she may have a need to talk about them with an objective, outside professional. The professional frequently chosen by the pregnant woman is the nurse.

Often the woman is ambivalent about the immediate fact of pregnancy, even when the pregnancy has been planned. The nurse needs to note the initial reaction to the confirmation of the pregnancy and continue to remain alert to the changes in the emotions of the woman as the pregnancy progresses.

By the second trimester most woman have come to accept the fact of pregnancy and have decided how they will cope with their coming motherhood. They are working through their change of status (daughter to mother, girl to woman) and are beginning to assume the responsibilities that go with their changing status. During this period, the nurse will find the pregnant woman more goal-directed. She is busy making plans for her new infant and the period after childbirth. She is asking the nurse for support as she practices her new role of mother. The nurse can assist the woman in this growth by encouraging her to make decisions and by acknowledging her efforts to take charge of her life and that of her unborn child.

Learning more about her unborn baby may help the pregnant woman feel more in control. It is useful to the woman to understand the physical growth and development of the fetus. The nurse can explain this to her while showing her where the baby's buttocks, head, and limbs are in the course of the abdominal touch picture. Discussing the baby's physical characteristics and feeling the baby's bottom and limbs can help the pregnant woman begin to identify her fetus as a real baby. Explaining to the pregnant woman some of the physical attributes (ability to hear, hiccup, suck its thumb, respond to touch) will heighten this perception of the fetus as a baby. The father of the baby and any siblings should also be educated about the baby and should be present at prenatal visits to hear the FHTs whenever possible.

It is also important for the nurse to help the woman become familiar with her unborn baby as an individual. Explaining that even before birth her baby is establishing an individual activity pattern helps the woman in her adjustment to the baby after birth. The woman who perceives her unborn baby as an individual capable of reacting to the surroundings will make a quicker and more realistic adjustment to her baby after the birth.

As the woman moves into the third trimester of her pregnancy, she cannot ignore the reality of impending childbirth. During this trimester the nurse should continue providing emotional support and reassurance. The woman needs to hear that she is competent and capable of being a "good" mother. She will talk about how she was mothered and will want to discuss how she will care for her child. She will be asking for confirmation and acceptance of herself in the role of mother. The nurse who has listened to the woman attentively throughout the pregnancy and has recognized her positive role changes should be able to provide that confirmation. If the woman has problems coping with the changes of pregnancy and the assumption of her new role, the nurse should recognize this and help the woman seek out appropriate resources for the resolution of these feelings.

The nurse should encourage the woman and her support person to attend prepared childbirth classes. Attending such classes supports the couple's preparation for parenthood—they are working together toward a common goal. Discussion of how they will support each other during childbirth may facilitate a discussion of how they will support each other as parents. Working together as a team to have this baby will help them understand how they can work together to rear the child.

Throughout the course of the pregnancy it is as important for the nurse to document the emotional status of the pregnant woman as it is to record the physical changes. The nurse should have an excellent understanding of the woman's perceptions of herself as a mother, her constellation of support persons, how she uses her support system, and how she asks for help, and the nurse should share this information with other health care providers involved in the pregnant woman's care.

Occasionally, the nurse will feel overwhelmed by a pregnant woman who needs a great deal of support and seeks to receive all of it from "her" nurse in the ambulatory care setting. If the nurse has been attentive to the needs of the woman, this dependency should be detected before the nurse feels overcome. The nurse should never feel diminished if it becomes apparent that an individual patient needs more support than one caregiver can provide. Although it is the nurse's responsibility to provide emotional support and guidance as needed, sometimes additional support is required. It then becomes the responsibility of the nurse to arrange for referral and to maintain good communication with the referral source.

ANTICIPATORY GUIDANCE

Evaluation is vital to anticipatory guidance. The nurse must evaluate the progress of the woman throughout the pregnancy. Where has she been? Where is she going? How is she coping with the physical and emotional changes? The nurse must have an excellent understanding of the physical and emotional needs of a pregnant woman and the ability to communicate clearly to meet those needs.

The nurse must be at least one step ahead of the pregnant woman, anticipating the next physical or emotional change the patient will experience. It is of minimal value to the woman to learn in childbirth classes during the last 8 weeks of pregnancy how to minimize the backaches and cope with the mood swings she has been experiencing since the first trimester.

Guidance and support need to be offered unconditionally throughout the pregnancy. The need for guidance and support may vary from woman to woman and will certainly vary from time to time for an individual woman. The nurse must be alert to these changing needs for support and evaluate the kind of support and guidance that will be most appropriate at a particular time for an individual woman.

The education required to help women understand prenatal changes should be spaced evenly throughout the length of the pregnancy. Attempting to teach everything the woman might need to know early in pregnancy will only frustrate the teacher and overwhelm the learner. For the most effective utilization of the prenatal education the nurse may provide, the pregnant woman must desire that information. The nurse will need to utilize adult learning theory to evaluate learner readiness, individual learning style, and appropriate methodology to present the information.

SUMMARY

Historically, nurses have been the leaders in recognizing the need for prenatal care and in providing for that need. The recognition of the importance of early, high-quality prenatal care has led nurses to a beginning involvement in preconceptual health care, teaching, and counseling.

Nurses are the most consistent members of the health care team in the ambulatory maternity care setting. Their initial and continuing assessment of the physical, psychosocial, and emotional status of the pregnant woman and her fetus is vital to a healthy outcome. Nursing interventions based on the findings of assessment are important in making the pregnancy a pleasant and rewarding experience for the pregnant woman and her family. The warm and caring nurse who has a broad knowledge of pregnancy and a deep understanding of human nature will be able to provide the guidance needed as the family goes through the prenatal period. The quality of prenatal care a woman receives can dramatically alter the outcome of her pregnancy.

REFERENCES

Bell, R. P. 1970. Parent–child conflicts in sexual values. In *Readings in child development and personality*, eds. P. H. Mussen, J. J. Conger, and J. Kagan. New York: Harper & Row.

Bing, E., and Coleman, L. 1977. *Making love during pregnancy*. New York: Bantam Books.

Bradshaw, M. 1987. Attitudinal abuse toward the pregnant woman. *Holistic Nurs. Prac.* 1:1–12.

Campbell, J. C. 1986. Battering during pregnancy. *Am. J. Nurs.* 86:910–913.

Caplan, G. 1957. Psychological aspects of maternity care. *Am. J. Public Health.* 47:25–31.

Center for Disease Control, U.S. Department of Health and Human Services. 1977. *Teenage childbearing and abortion patterns—United States*. Washington, D.C.: U.S. Government Printing Office.

Coleman, A., and Coleman, L. 1977. *Pregnancy: The psychological experience*. New York: Bantam Books.

Davis, L. 1987. Dating pregnancy: Gathering and using a reliable data base. *J. Nurse-Midwifery*. 32:195–204.

Erickson, E. H. 1963. *Childhood and society*. 2nd ed. New York: W. W. Norton.

Gant, N.; Worley, R.; Cunningham, F.; and Whalley, P. 1978. Clinical management of pregnancy-induced hypertension. *Clin. Obstet. Gynecol.* 21(2):397–409.

Helton, A. 1986. Battering during pregnancy. *Am. J. Nurs.* 86:910–913.

Hyde, J. S. 1982. *Understanding human sexuality*. 2nd ed. New York: McGraw-Hill.

Ingram, D. D.; Makur, D.; and Kleinman, J. C. 1986. National and state trends in use of prenatal care, 1970–1983. *Am. J. Public Health.* 76:415–423.

Jensen, L. P.; O'Sullivan, M. J.; Gomez-del-Rio, M.; Setzer, E. S.; Gaskins, C.; and Penso, C. 1984. Acquired immunodeficiency (AIDS) in pregnancy. *Am. J. Obstet. Gynecol.* 48:1145.

Jordon, C. V., and Valle, S. L. 1978. Teenage health consultants. *Synergist.* 7(2):43–47.

Loucks, A. 1987. *Chlamydia:* The unheralded epidemic. *Am. J. Nurs.* 87:920–922.

Malasanos, L.; Barkauskas, V.; Moss, M.; and Stoltenberg-Allen, K. 1981. *Health assessment.* 2nd ed. St. Louis: C. V. Mosby.

Marvin, C., and Slevin, A. 1987. Chlamydia—cause, prevention and cure. *MCN.* 12:318–321.

Minkoff, H.; deRegt, R. H.; Landesman, S.; and Schwarz, R. 1986. *Pneumocystitis carinii* pneumonia associated with acquired immunodeficiency syndrome (AIDS) in pregnancy: A report of three maternal deaths. *Obstetrics & Gynecology.* 67:284.

Mocarski, V. 1980. Asymptomatic bacteriuria—a "silent" problem of pregnant women. *MCN* 5(4):238.

National Center for Health Statistics. 1985. Advance report of final mortality statistics, 1983. *Monthly Vital Statistics Report.* 34:6–7.

Nichols, C. 1987. Dating pregnancy: Gathering and using a reliable data base. *J. Nurse-Midwifery.* 32:195–204.

Niswander, K. R., and Gordon, M. 1972. *The women and their pregnancies.* DHEW Publication No. NIH 73-379. Washington, D.C.: U.S. Government Printing Office.

Palmer, B. B., and Lewis, C. E. 1976. Development of health attitudes and behaviors. *J. School Health.* 46:401–402.

Pitchanik, A. R.; Fischl, M. A.; and Spira, T. J. 1983. Acquired immune deficiency syndrome in low-risk patients: Evidence for possible transmission by an asymptomatic carrier. *JAMA.* 250:1310.

Pritchard, J. A.; MacDonald, P. C.; and Gant, N. F. 1985. *Williams obstetrics.* 17th ed. New York: Appleton-Century-Crofts.

Rawlinson, K. F.; Zubrow, A. B.; Harris, M. A.; Jackson, U. C.; and Chao, S. 1984. Disseminated Kaposi's sarcoma in pregnancy: A manifestation of acquired immune deficiency syndrome. *Obstetrics & Gynecology.* 63:25.

Sumner, G. 1976. Giving expectant parents the help they need: The ABC's of prenatal education. *MCN.* 1:222.

Sweet, R. L. 1985. *Chlamydia,* group B streptococcus and herpes in pregnancy. *Birth.* 12:17–24.

U.S. Department of Health and Human Services. 1981. *Better health for our children: A national strategy.* Volume III—*A statistical profile.* DHHS Publication No. PHS 79-55071. Washington, D.C.: U.S. Government Printing Office.

Varney, H. 1987. *Nurse-midwifery.* Boston: Blackwell Scientific.

Weinberg, J. S. 1982. *Sexuality, human needs, and nursing practice.* Philadelphia: W. B. Saunders.

Zelnick, M. 1979. Sex education and knowledge of pregnancy risk among U.S. teenage women. *Family Planning Perspectives.* 11:355–357.

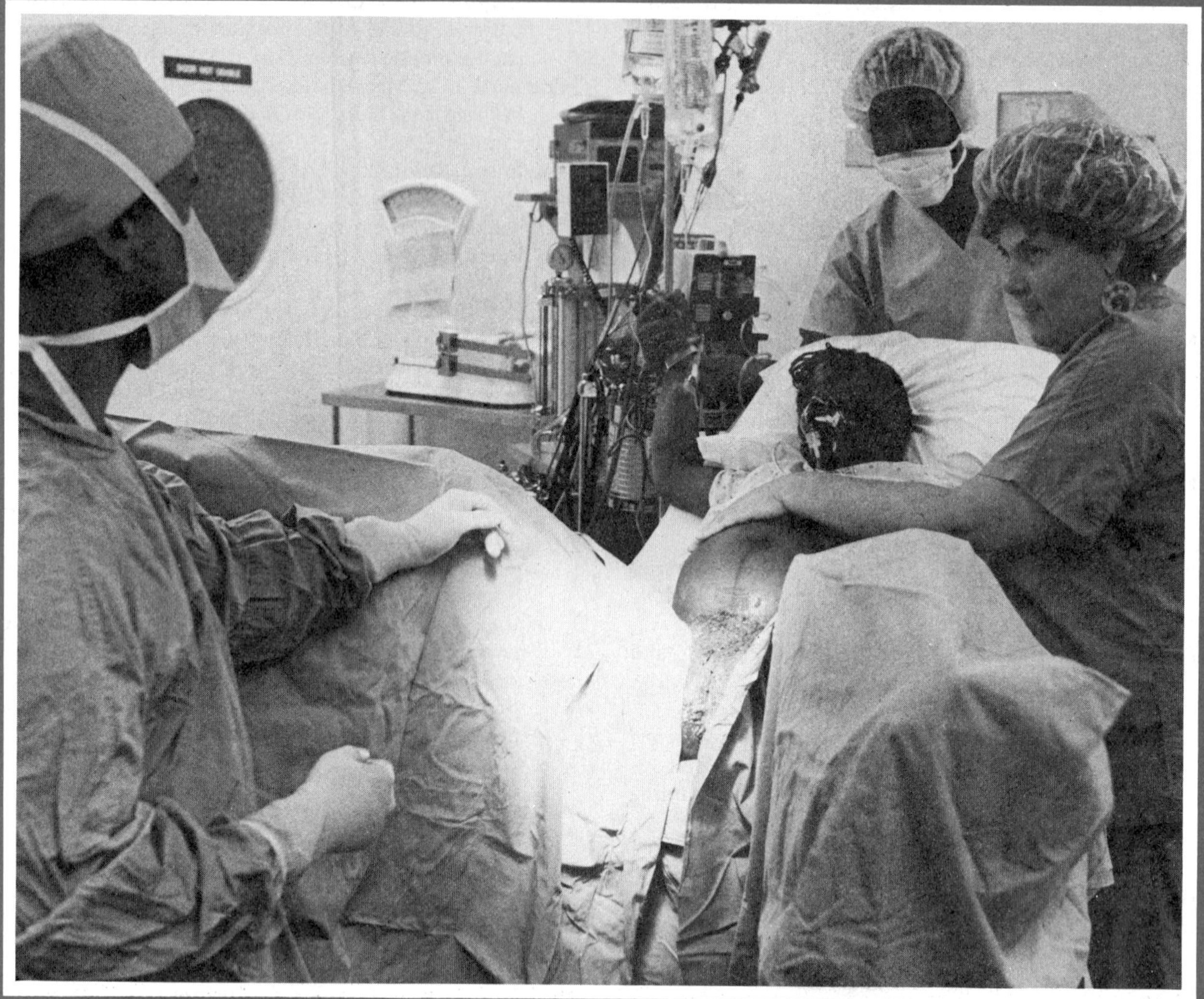

UNIT THREE

CHANGE: THE INTRAPARTAL PERIOD

16

The Labor Process: Change in the Mother and Fetus

BEHAVIORAL OBJECTIVES

Upon completion of this chapter, the reader should be able to:

- Discuss the physiologic activities that contribute to the onset of labor.

- Describe the biophysical changes that occur in the woman during each stage of labor.

- Identify the cardinal movements of the fetus during labor.

- Describe the relationship between the pelvic characteristics of the woman and the fetus during labor.

- Identify maternal and fetal attributes that influence the progress of labor.

- Differentiate between true and false labor.

Despite the fact that reproduction has occurred since the human species came into being, understanding of this intricate process continues to grow. In the past 25 years, knowledge of fetal development and maternal physiologic changes which take place at birth has expanded. Knowing more about the normal labor process makes it easier to identify deviations and to incorporate the handling of these deviations into clinical practice.

This chapter focuses on two areas: (1) the change process in the female body which culminates in the birth of a new life; and (2) the change in the body of knowledge surrounding labor and labor practices.

Labor can be viewed by women as an exhilarating and rewarding event in itself or as a mere means to an end which must be endured. Wider understanding of the process holds out the possibility that more women will experience labor and birth as a joyous experience.

Covered in this chapter are the currently held theories of labor and its physiology, a description of maternal and fetal adaptations, and the nature of normal labor.

THEORIES OF LABOR ONSET

During pregnancy, the human fetus is sustained and well protected within the uterus. The mother provides all the necessary nutrients and removes the waste products necessary to assure growth while managing to maintain the homeostasis necessary for her own functions. The successful transition from intrauterine to extrauterine life requires that the fetus be mature enough to adapt to the enormously different conditions of life in air rather than in fluid, with no placenta to provide nutrients and handle wastes. The mother must also be able to expel the fetus from the uterus without endangering herself or the fetus in the process. Both are vitally involved in the process of birth. How this is accomplished in the human species is not known precisely. The exact mechanism of the onset of labor remains unknown. It is now recognized that the factors that trigger the initiation of labor vary from one species to another.

Results found with rabbits, for example, indicate that withdrawal of progesterone secondary to the decline of the corpus luteum will trigger labor, but such results have not been duplicated in humans. However, in the last 10 years great progress has been made in the interpretation of definitive biochemical events, leading to a greater understanding of human reproduction. The following statements summarize the findings of current research on the onset of labor:

1. Initiation of labor varies from one species to another.
2. Studies focusing on hormonal influences have failed to identify the initiator of labor in humans.
3. Multiple factors seem to be involved in the process, each having an essential role in the maintenance of gestation and in initiating or supporting labor.
4. The process in humans may be one that extends over a period of time (days or even weeks) before labor is actually established.
5. The mother and fetus are involved in the triggering of the labor process.

The popular factors considered to be involved in the delicate balance of this process are presented in Table 16–1, along with the research findings, proposed theory, and proposed function of each factor in the labor process.

Researchers continue to postulate on the interaction and interrelationship of maternal and fetal hormones in the process of labor, and the identification of the triggering factor.

BIOPHYSICAL CHANGES IN THE MOTHER DURING LABOR

Just as the triggering mechanism from the onset of labor may well take place over a period of time, so, too, many of the maternal activities of the labor process begin early to prepare for the climax of the childbearing experience. Let us review the changes that occur in the woman during labor.

Labor is the process or series of mechanisms by which the products of conception—fetus, placenta, and membranes—are expelled from the uterus through the birth canal. It involves the expulsive musculature of the uterus but more significantly calls for the complete participation of the woman and her fetus. Ideally, normal labor involves the expulsion of the fetus in the vertex presentation and occurs sometime between the 38th and 42nd weeks of gestation.

Uterus

Primarily a muscular organ, the uterus consists of a corpus and a cervix which are different in both structure and function. When considering the uterine function in labor, the activity of the myometrium, endometrium (decidua), and cervix will be discussed.

Myometrium

Structurally, the myometrium protects the fetus during development and provides the expulsive

TABLE 16-1. Factors Involved in the Initiation of Labor

Factor	Research	Proposed Theory	Proposed Function in Human Labor
Progesterone (hormone produced primarily in the placenta)	Work done on animals, especially rabbits; not validated in humans (Csapo, 1959)	*Progesterone withdrawal or block theory*—Marked decline in production by placenta results in relative increase of estrogen level at site of the placenta, with an increase in myometrial activity and onset of labor	Inhibitory function on the transmission of electrical impulses through myometrium, thus preventing uterine contractions, is felt to be essential for maintenance of gestation
Oxytocin (hormone released from the posterior pituitary of the mother; also released by the fetus)	No increase before onset of labor in humans; as labor progresses there is a spurt release of oxytocin (Caldeyro-Barcia and Serino, 1961; Chard, 1973)	*Oxytocin stimulation theory*—Uterus is extremely sensitive to oxytocin at term. Long thought that oxytocin is released to stimulate myometrium and initiate labor	Oxytocin, from mother and fetus, is felt to be important in determining strength and duration of uterine contractions once labor is established; but that, by itself, does not start labor. Oxytocin is thought to facilitate contraction of uterus after delivery
Estrogens (hormones from both maternal and fetal sources—difficult to determine exact source of each compound)	In humans as well as animals the level of estrogen rises progressively until term	No theory has been proposed for the role of estrogens as initiators of labor, although estrogen is known to stimulate myometrial contractions and to oppose action of progesterone	Estrogens are important in the storage of arachidonic acid, precursor of prostaglandin in fetal membranes and possibly decidua. They may serve an essential role in bringing about synthesis of prostaglandin through release of phospholipase in fetal membranes or decidua
Cortisol (hormone produced by the fetal adrenal cortex)	Work done primarily on sheep; has not been documented in human pregnancies (Liggins, 1973)	*Fetal cortisol theory*—Experiments on fetal lambs demonstrated that hypophysectomies and more specifically adrenalectomies prevent onset of labor. Administration of ACTH or cortisol to the fetus triggers labor. Therefore, it appears that fetal adrenals in the lamb are responsible for labor and that this may occur in a similar way in humans. According to theory, cortisol acts on placenta to increase level of estrogen, decrease progesterone, and release prostaglandins to activate uterus	Fetal corticosteroids have role in indicating maturational changes in several organs. Cortisol has been shown to play a role in fetal lung maturity by encouraging development of surfactant production
Prostaglandins (substances found in almost every human tissue thus far examined; fetal membranes and uterine decidua are rich sources of prostaglandin precursors—E_2 and $F_2\alpha$)	Studies done on humans demonstrate six-fold increase in concentration of arachidonic acid in amniotic fluid of women in labor; high levels of prostaglandin found in women near term or in labor; studies show that aspirin and indomethacin block prostaglandin synthesis and delay labor	*Fetal membrane glycerophospholipid arachidonic acid–prostaglandin theory*—The obligator precursor of the two prostaglandins, E_2 and $F_2\alpha$, which are known to initiate myometrial contractions, is free form of arachidonic acid found incorporated in glycerophospholipids of fetal membranes	Prostaglandins are probably major hormone in activation of labor. They enhance labor by acting as cell messengers to stimulate smooth muscle of uterus to contractions, mediate oxytocin activity, and ripen cervix, particularly connective tissue
Uterine distention		*Uterine distention theory*—As pregnancy advances the uterus distends to point where pressure is exerted on muscles and nerve endings in cervix, initiating labor	Theory has gradually lost acceptance, although with multiple pregnancies and polyhydramnios there is tendency for premature labor to occur

forces during parturition. It is composed of long smooth cells, forming a network of intricately interwoven bundles. The cells in these bundles have few contacts until the end of pregnancy, when a number of gap junctions appear. These junctions are areas of specialized contact allowing synchronization of their contractile function. The formation of these gap junctions is facilitated by estrogens and prostaglandins, and inhibited by progesterone.

The action of the myometrium depends on the delicate balance between factors that keep the uterus at rest and those that facilitate contractions. The major role of estrogen is to maintain myometrial cellular structure and excitability. The actions of other hormones may be viewed as modifying or dependent on the properties of the estrogen-controlled myometrium. Progesterone has a negative influence on uterine activity in that it limits uterine contractions by stabilizing membrane-bound pools of calcium. This calcium must be released in order to interact with the proteins actin and myosin within the cell to eventually cause contractions. It is possible that oxytocin or the prostaglandins may act as calcium releasers.

During pregnancy, pacemaker activity appears to be randomly distributed, with bursts of action associated with contractions. Near labor, the pacemaker activity in the cornua seems to dominate and the contractions become regular and synchronous.

Endometrium (Decidua)

The endometrium, composed of connective tissue and epithelium, has been the main source of prostaglandin $F_2\alpha$ production in the nonpregnant human uterus. Physical damage to the decidua or fetal membranes is a potent stimulus for the release of prostaglandins and possibly for the initiation of labor.

Indeed, rupture of the membranes is associated with a marked increase in prostaglandin synthesis which may explain its accelerating effects on labor.

Cervix

The cervix functions to help protect the fetus by remaining closed during pregnancy to prevent ascending infection and by providing resistance to pressure from above caused by the upright position and by the Braxton-Hicks contractions. During labor it must, however, be able to efface and dilate to allow the birth of the fetus. The changes in the connective tissue of the cervix occur less noticeably than with the smooth muscle contractions in the myometrium and may precede delivery by days or weeks. *Effacement*, the obliteration or taking up of the cervix, is the shortening of the cervical canal from a structure about 2 cm in length to one in which only a circular orifice with paper-thin edges remains. It is assessed in percentages, from 0 to 100 percent. By the onset of labor in the primigravid woman, the cervix is usually about 50 percent effaced. The cervical canal is 1–1.5 cm long, and from 2 to 3 cm dilated, but still resistant as labor proceeds. *Dilation* refers to the opening of the cervical canal to a maximum of 10 cm diameter. When the dilation reaches 5–6 cm, the cervix is usually very thin and completely effaced. The cervix has been found to be a source for the synthesis of prostaglandin E_2, which may prove to have a role in cervical ripening.

Uterine Contractions

The uterus contracts throughout pregnancy. In early pregnancy the contractions are irregular and weak and are generally not noticed by the woman nor felt by abdominal palpation. As pregnancy progresses, contractions increase in intensity and frequency and by the third trimester are noticed by the woman. The contractions are usually painless until they become more rhythmic and stronger (see Fig. 16–1). The contractions that are palpable abdominally are known as Braxton-Hicks contractions. Late in pregnancy these contractions may cause some discomfort and are considered "false labor" contractions.

Uterine contractions occur when the muscle cells of the myometrium tighten and shorten. They are described in terms of frequency, duration, and intensity. Frequency refers to the time between the beginning of one contraction and the beginning of the next contraction. (It cannot be determined without subsequent contractions.) Duration is the length of contraction from the beginning of the tightening of the uterus until the relaxation. *Intensity* is the strength of contraction, measured by abdominal palpation as mild, moderate, or strong. When measured by external topography or intrauterine measures, intensity is the difference between the peak pressure during a contraction and zero pressure.

Uterine contractions are involuntary and generally independent of extrauterine control. They are known to start in the fundal, uppermost section of the uterus, causing the upper part of the uterus to contract and thicken during labor. As the upper

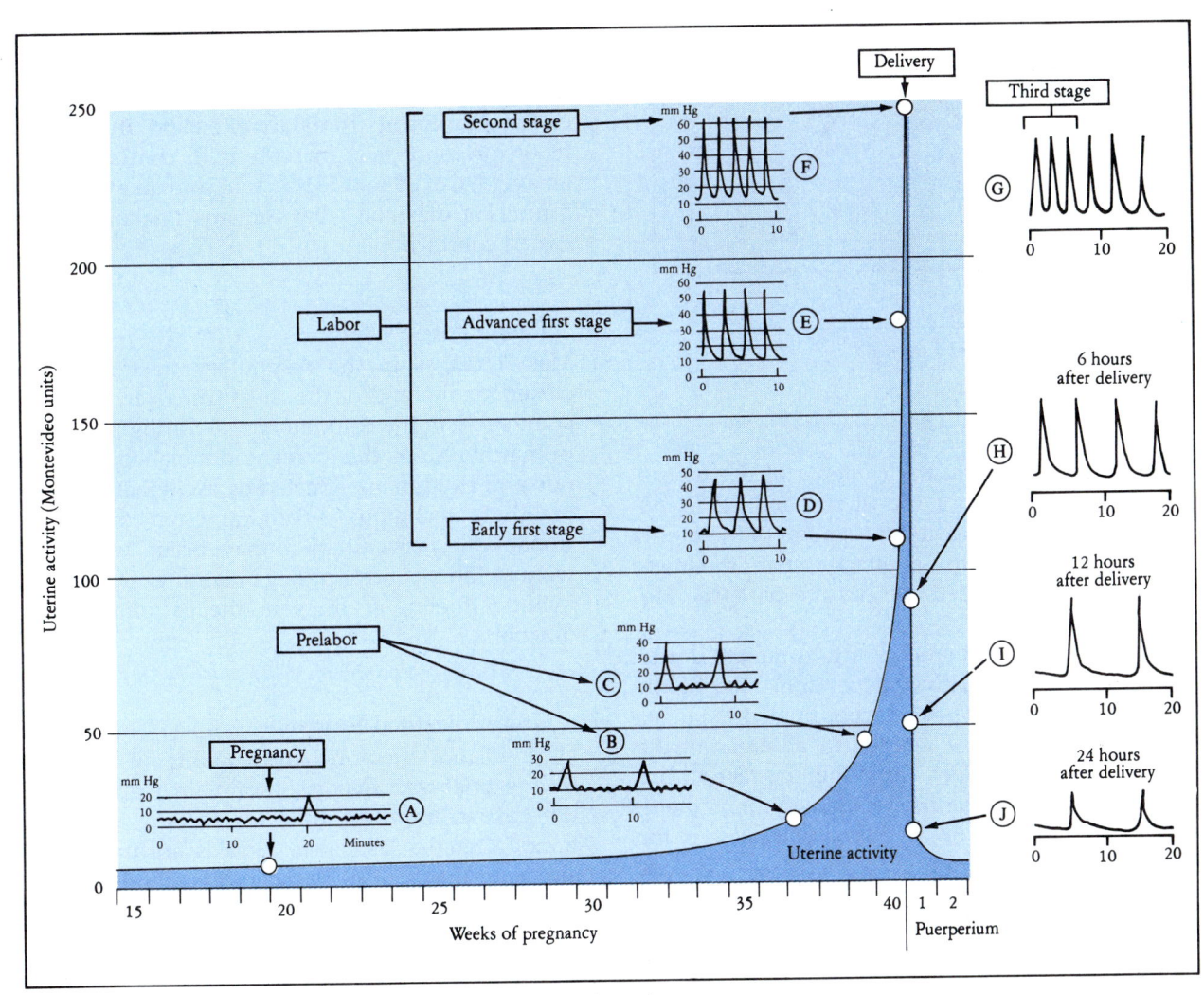

FIGURE 16-1. The evolution of spontaneous uterine activity throughout the cycle—illustrated by the shaded area and measured on the left-side scale. Typical tracings of uterine contractility at different stages of the cycle are shown.
SOURCE: Caldeyro-Barcia and Poseiro (1959).

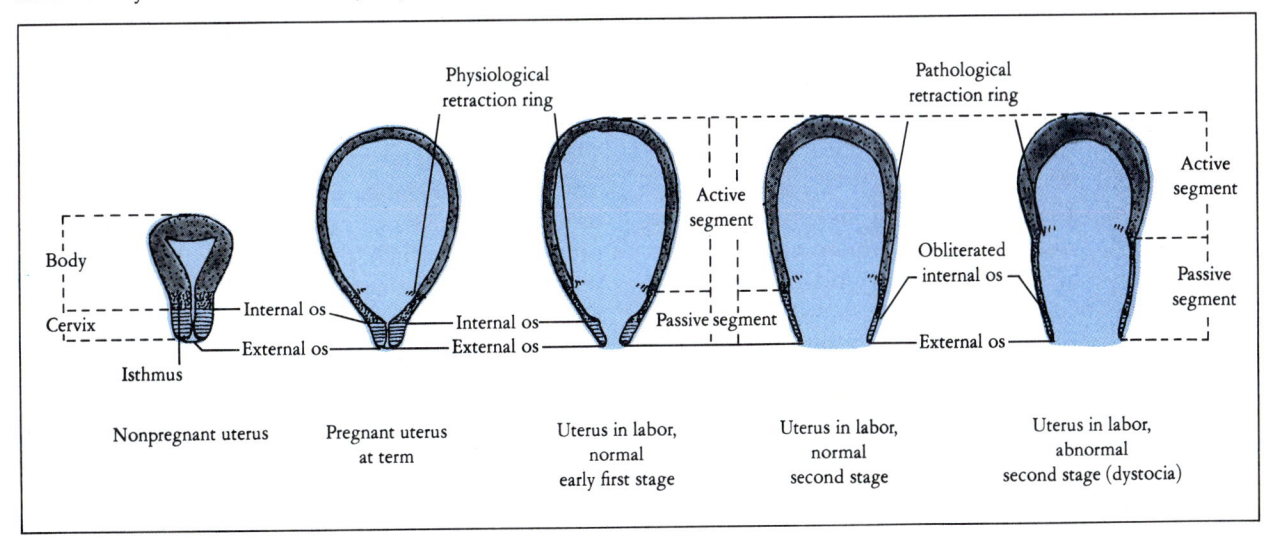

FIGURE 16-2. The progressive development of uterine segments: active upper segment, passive lower segment.
SOURCE: Pritchard, MacDonald, and Gant (1985).

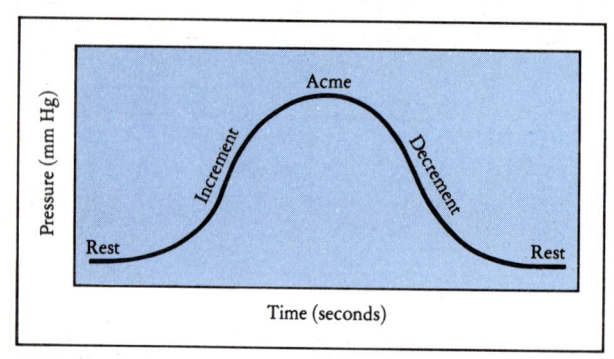

FIGURE 16-3. Phases of a normal contraction.

segment contracts on the contents of the uterus, the lower segment of the uterus and cervix expands and thins. The upper segment of the uterus is considered the active contracting part; the lower segment is considered the passive part (see Fig. 16-2).

Forces of the normal contraction radiate downward to the least active, dependent area of the uterus, the cervix. They are coordinated in such a way that the peak is reached in all areas of the uterus simultaneously. Thus, the contraction has three phases to describe its intensity: increment, acme, and decrement. The *increment phase* is the period in which the intensity increases, the *acme phase* is the point at which the contraction is at its strongest, and the *decrement phase* is the period of decreasing intensity (see Fig. 16-3). As the cervical resistance decreases, the forces from above form a thinned-out muscular and fibromuscular tube through which the fetus can pass.

Other Changes in Maternal Systems

Cardiovascular System

Changes that occur in maternal systems prepare the woman to cope with the events of labor. Pregnancy and labor require an increased cardiac work load, with moderately increased cardiac output at the beginning of labor and an appreciably greater increase during the expulsion stage. The pulse undergoes marked changes during contractions and remains slightly higher between contractions because of the increased metabolism that occurs with labor.

Toward the end of pregnancy, as the uterus becomes enlarged, the position of the woman's body affects circulation and blood pressure. The supine position compresses the venous system that returns blood from the lower half of the body, thereby reducing blood flow to the heart and decreasing cardiac output. Occasionally, this causes significant arterial hypotension. In general, blood pressure may increase with contractions—an average of 15 mm Hg systolic and an average of 5 mm Hg diastolic—but remains unchanged between contractions.

Respiratory System

Most changes in the respiratory tract have occurred by the end of the third trimester. There is an increase in the respiratory rate during labor that primarily reflects the increase in metabolism. Both rate and rhythm are affected by excitement, use of breathing techniques, pain, and tension. Occasionally, hyperventilation may occur when the woman loses control of her breathing. Symptoms include tingling feelings in the extremities and dizziness.

Gastrointestinal System

During labor the tone and motility of the gastrointestinal tract decrease noticeably, prolonging the gastric emptying time for as long as 12-36 hours after the last meal. Liquids are unaffected and leave the stomach in the usual amount of time. With the decrease in emptying time of gastric contents, there is an increase in the acidity of the contents. For women in labor who need to have general anesthesia, administration of an antacid will help to neutralize the gastric contents, thereby helping to prevent the complications involved in regurgitating and aspirating acidic contents. Nausea and vomiting are not uncommon in labor, particularly during the transition phase and after the administration of intravenous pain medication.

Musculoskeletal System

The musculoskeletal system provides for increased mobility of the sacroiliac, sacrococcygeal, and pubic joints, which promotes flexibility as labor progresses. The soft tissues in the perineum hypertrophy and blood supply to the area increases, providing for stretching during the birth process.

FETAL ATTRIBUTES

The way the fetus adapts to the trip down the birth canal is called the *mechanism of labor*. The maneuvers or adaptations that occur as the fetus descends depend on several factors, including fetal posture, lie, presentation, position, station, and engagement.

In the last months or weeks of pregnancy the fetus assumes a characteristic *posture* or *attitude* that conforms to the shape of the uterine cavity. The most common posture finds the fetus curved inward toward itself, with the back convex, head flexed toward the chest, legs bent at knees, thighs resting on abdomen, arms crossed over the chest, and umbilical cord in the space between arms and legs (see Fig. 16–4).

As noted in Chapter 15, the *lie* of the fetus is the relation of the longitudinal axis of the fetus to that of the mother. Longitudinal lies (see Fig. 16–5), present in over 95 percent of labors at term, occur when the maternal and fetal spines are parallel. Transverse lies occur when the maternal and fetal spines are at right angles. Oblique lies, with spines at 45-degree angles, are unstable and resolve into either the transverse or longitudinal lies during the course of labor.

Presentation of the fetus refers to that part which enters the birth canal first. Cephalic (head first) presentations are the most common, comprising approximately 96 percent of term presentations (see Fig. 16–4). Other presentations include breech, pelvis first, and shoulder. The presenting part is the area the finger first makes contact with during a vaginal or rectal exam. This may be the occiput (vertex), chin, or sacrum.

Position refers to the relation of an arbitrarily chosen position of the fetus to the right or left side of the mother's pelvis. The relationship is designated by capital letters. The first and last letters refer to the mother and the middle initial to the presenting part of the infant. Thus, ROA signifies that the fetal occiput is on the right side of the mother facing anteriorly (see Fig. 16–6 for examples of positions of the fetus).

Station is the term used to measure the descent of the presenting part through the birth canal. Station is recorded in terms of centimeters above or below the ischial spines, usually ranging from -5 through $+5$ (see Fig. 16–7). Engagement is said to occur when the widest diameter of the fetal head (the biparietal plane) has passed the pelvic inlet (see Fig. 16–8).

The anatomy, size, and pliability of the fetal skull must also be considered in understanding the mechanisms of labor. The important bones of the fetal head during labor are those that make up the skull: two frontal, two parietal, two temporal, and

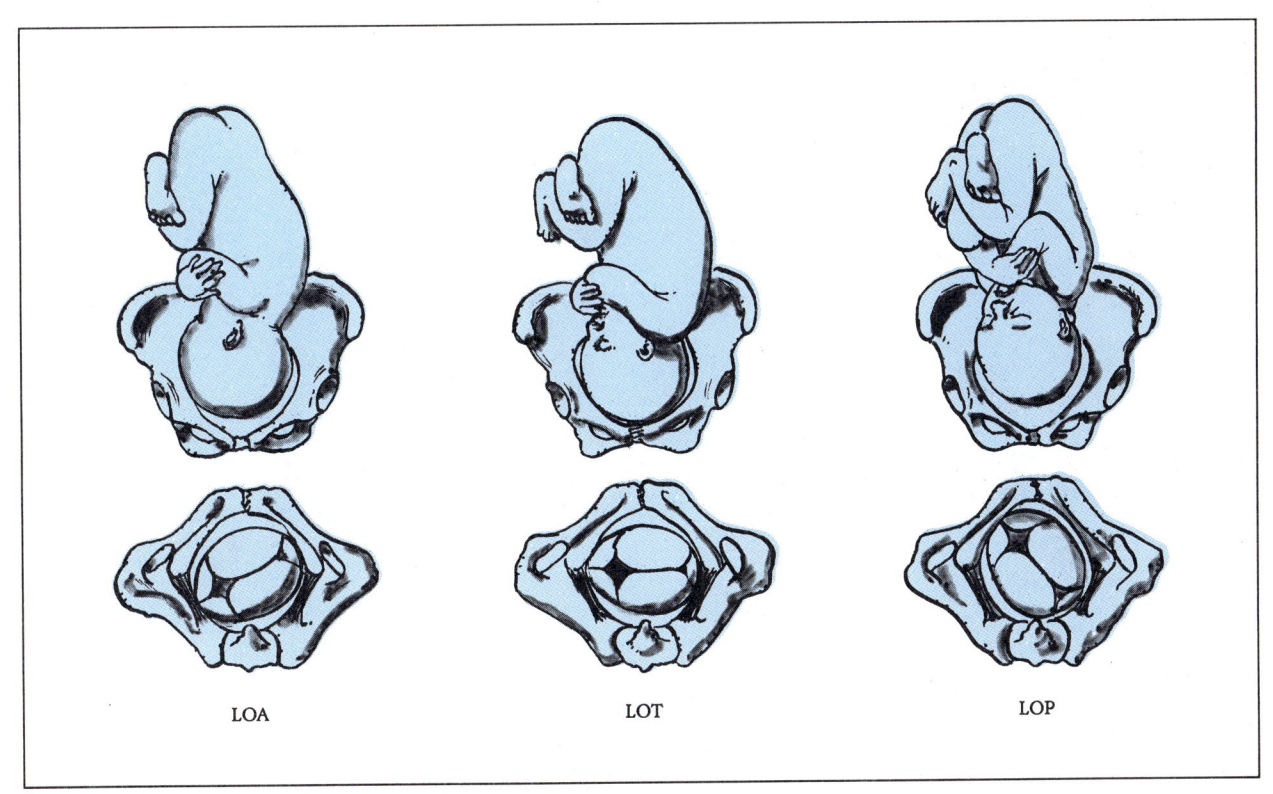

FIGURE 16–4. Common cephalic presentations showing flexed attitude, longitudinal lie, and three positions in the maternal pelvis.

346 CHANGE: THE INTRAPARTAL PERIOD

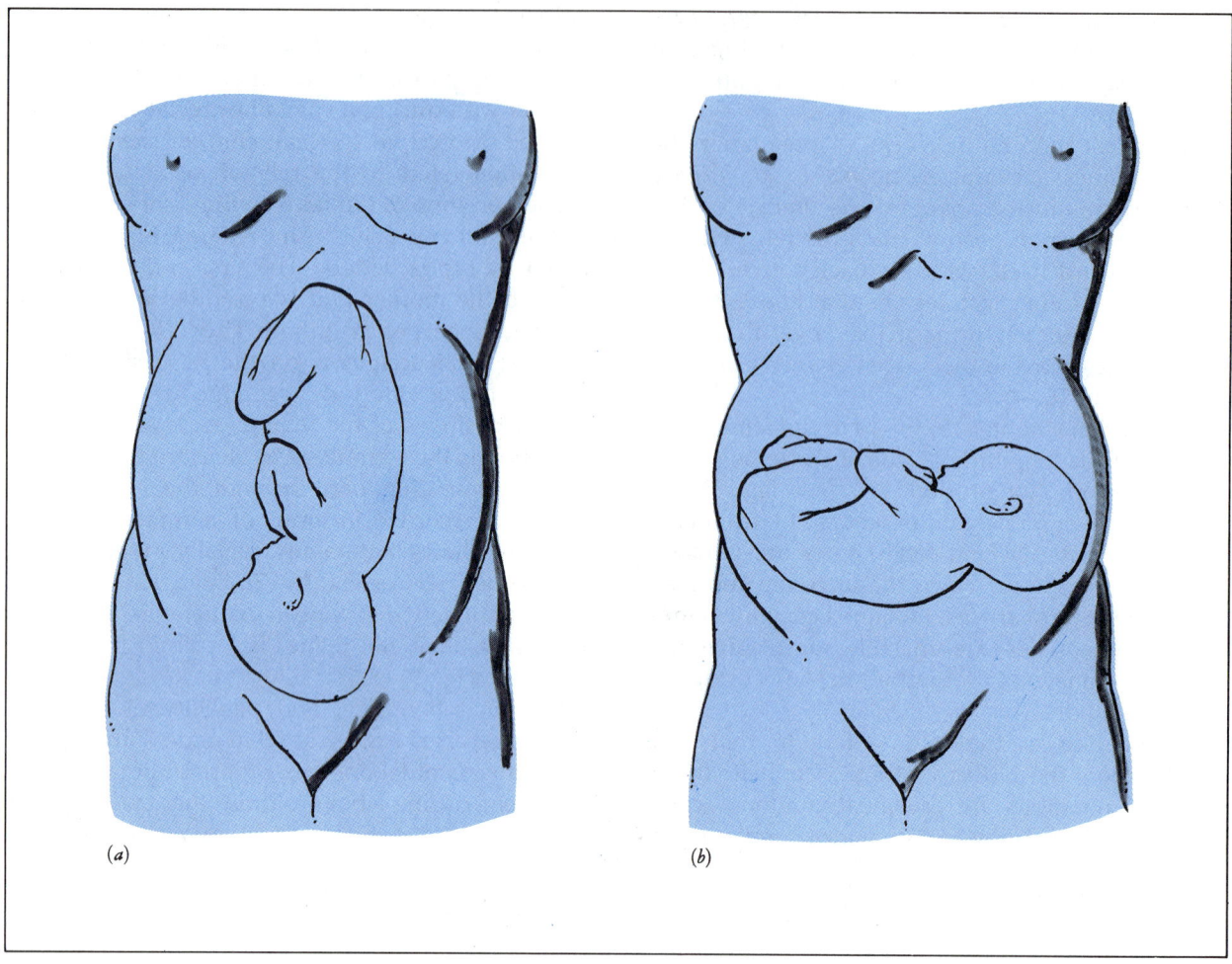

FIGURE 16–5. Types of lie. (*a*) Longitudinal lie; (*b*) transverse lie.
SOURCE: Oxorn and Foote (1980).

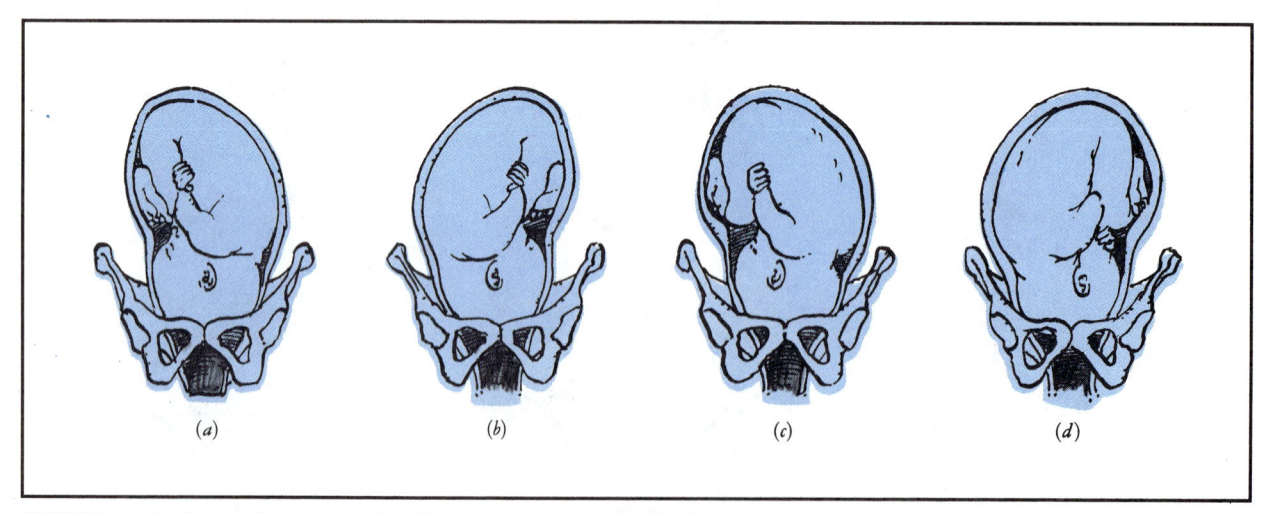

FIGURE 16–6. Types of positions. (*a*) Left occiput transverse (LOT), the most common position. (*b*) Right occiput transverse (ROT), the second most common position. (*c*) Left occiput anterior (LOA) position. (*d*) Right occiput anterior (ROA) position.

The Labor Process: Change in the Mother and Fetus 347

the occipital bone. As can be seen in Fig. 16-9, the bones are not rigidly fused but are separated by membranous space, the sutures. With vertex presentation these sutures, as well as the two fontanelles, can be palpated during vaginal examination and can give valuable information regarding the position and presentation of the fetus.

As the head maneuvers through the birth canal it accommodates to the various measurements of the maternal pelvis. This occurs through utilization of the mechanisms of labor and the process of molding. Molding involves the overlapping of one bone over another to adapt the diameter of the fetal head as it pushes downward.

PELVIC CHARACTERISTICS

The process by which the fetus must pass through the pelvis is basically one of accommodation. The

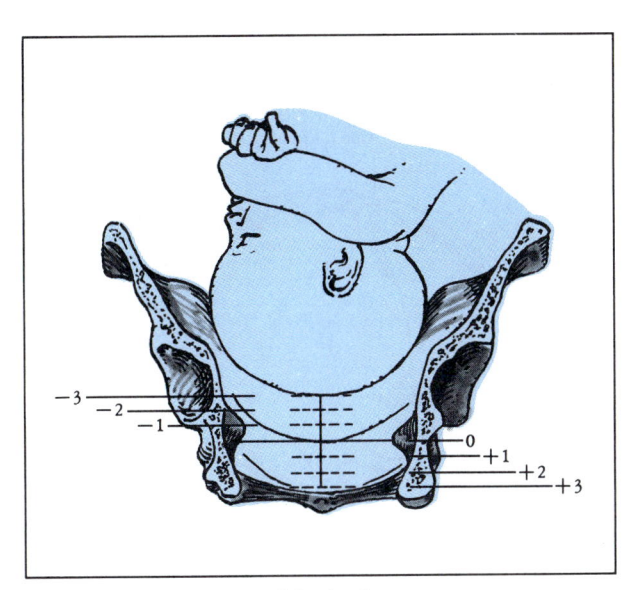

FIGURE 16-7. Stations of the fetal head.

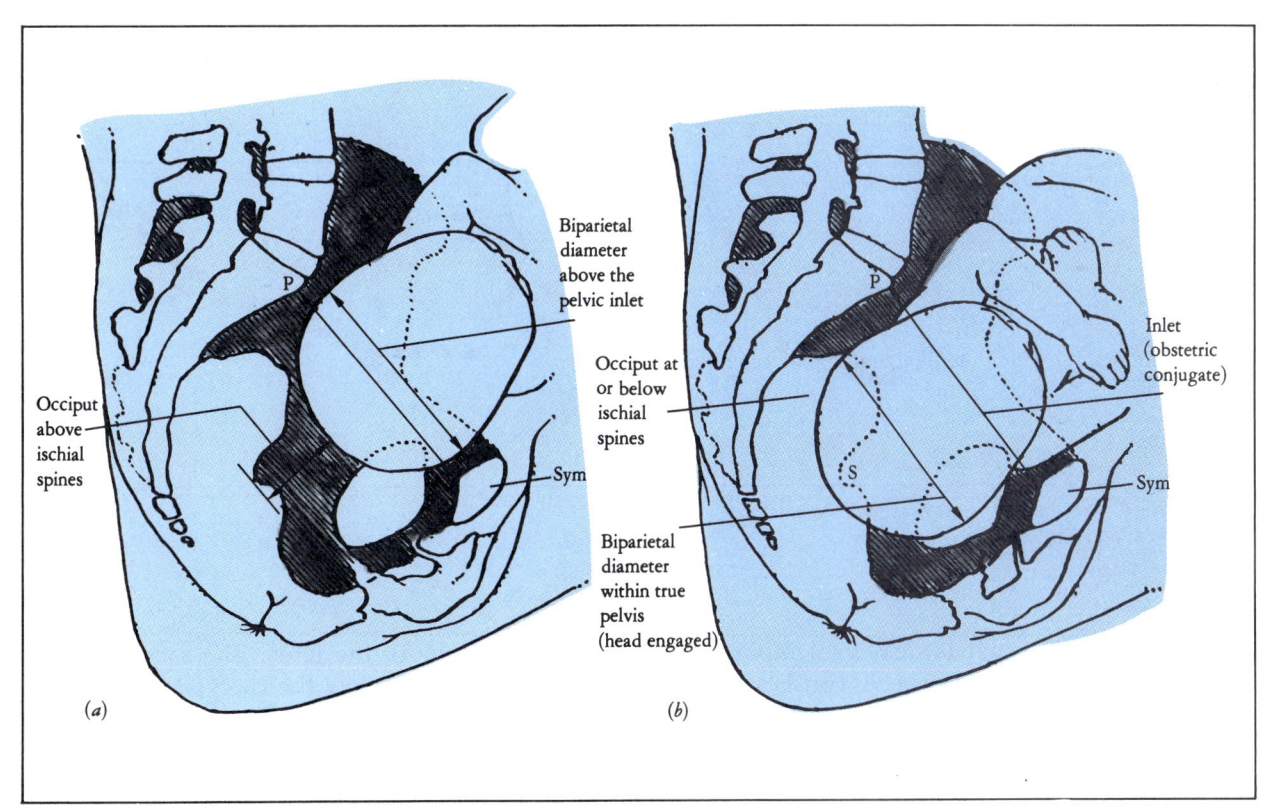

FIGURE 16-8. Engagement. (*a*) When the lowermost portion of the fetal head is above the ischial spines, the biparietal diameter of the head is not likely to have passed through the pelvic inlet and, therefore, is not engaged. (*b*) When the lowermost portion of the fetal head is at or below the ischial spines, it is usually engaged. Exceptions occur when there is considerable molding, caput formation, or both. P, sacral promontory; Sym, symphysis pubis; S, ischial spine.
SOURCE: Pritchard, MacDonald, and Gant (1985).

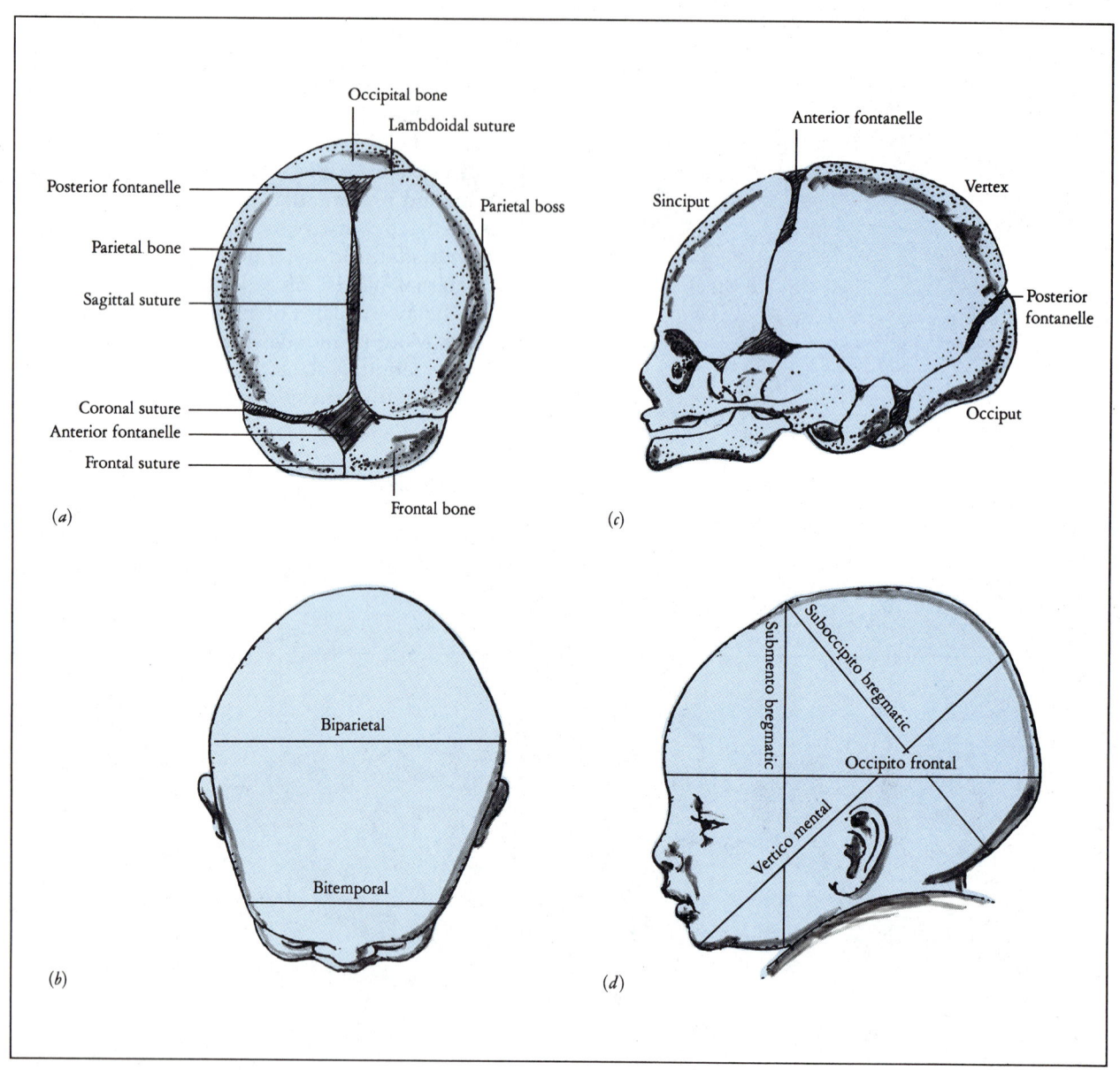

FIGURE 16–9. Fetal skull: landmarks and diameters.
SOURCE: Oxorn and Foote (1980).

size and shape of the pelvis are of vital importance in labor (see Fig. 16–10). The pelvis consists of four bones: the sacrum, the coccyx, and the two innominate bones. (The innominate bones are composed of the illium, ischium, and pubis). The pelvic bones are connected by four important joints: two sacroiliac joints, the sacrococcygeal joint, and the symphysis pubis. Whereas in the nonpregnant state there is little movement in these joints, during late pregnancy a certain amount of softening and stretching takes place, and during labor additional space provided by this "give" permits passage of the fetus. The sacrococcygeal joint may actually allow the coccyx to bend backward as the head is delivered.

The bony pelvis is divided into two parts, the false and the true. The *false pelvis* is the flaring part above the linea terminales and has no importance in labor. The *true pelvis* is the curved bony canal through which the fetus must pass. The pelvic *inlet* is bounded by the sacral promontory, the linea terminales, and the upper margin of the symphysis pubis. The anterior–posterior diameter (sometimes called the obstetric conjugate) is an impor-

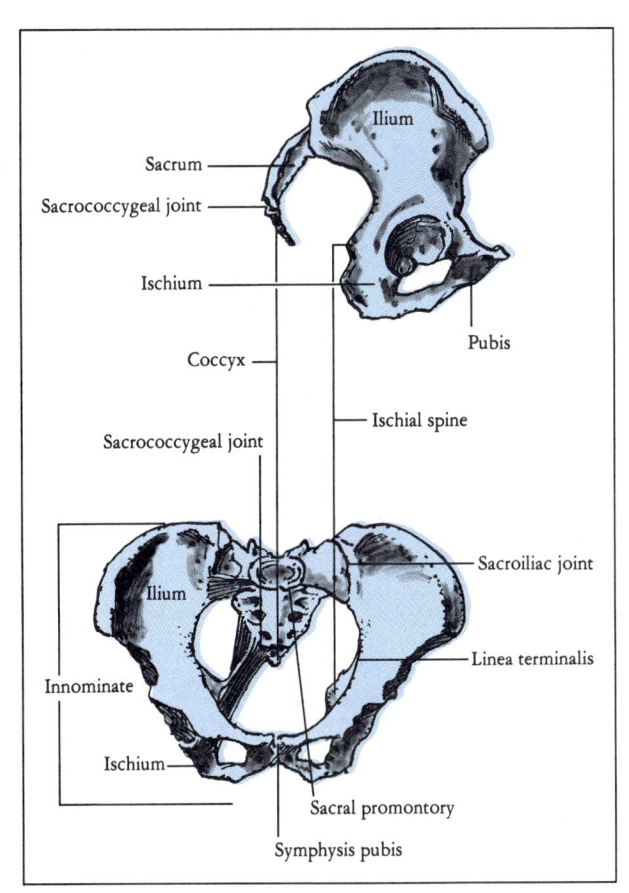

FIGURE 16–10. The joints of the pelvis. The sacrum, the coccyx, and the two innominate bones are linked together by four joints: the symphysis pubis, the sacrococcygeal, and the two sacroiliac joints.
SOURCE: Oxorn and Foote (1980).

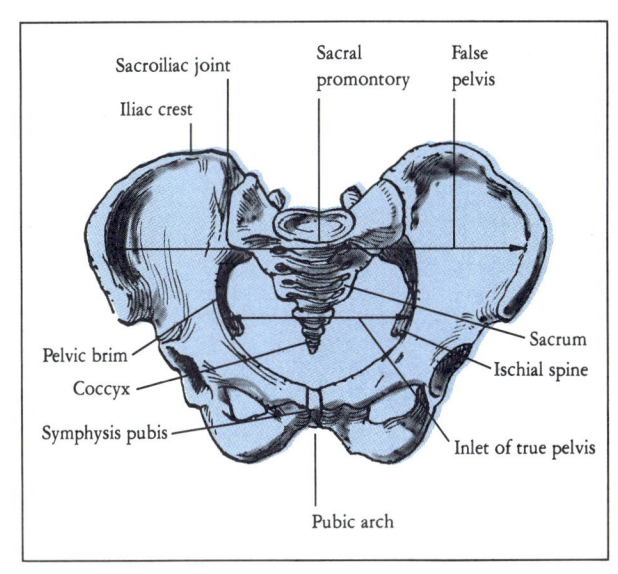

FIGURE 16–11. Female pelvis showing pelvic inlet.
SOURCE: Spence and Mason (1979).

tant measurement to approximate, to assure adequacy for vaginal delivery. Normally, this distance is 10 cm. Assessment can be done on vaginal examination by using the length of the examining finger to measure the distance between the lower margin of the symphysis pubis and the promontory of the sacrum and subtracting 1.5 cm. Thus, if the examiner measures 11.5 cm with the finger, 1.5 cm is subtracted to arrive at an estimation of 10 cm for the anterior–posterior diameter of the inlet.

The pelvic *outlet* can be visualized as two triangular areas with a joined common base. The anterior plane has the symphysis as the apex, and the base is a line drawn between the two ischial tuberosities. The apex of the posterior triangle is the tip of the coccyx (as is shown in Fig. 16–11).

In the female, four distinct types of pelves have been identified, using Caldwell-Moloy classifications (see Fig. 16–12). Quite often a mixture of two types rather than a pure form is found. Briefly, the types are:

1. *Gynecoid:* the normal female pelvis. The inlet is usually round, and the pubic arch is wide. This is a fairly easy pelvis for the fetus to navigate. It occurs in 40 percent of women.
2. *Android:* heart-shaped pelvis. The inlet is heart shaped, the pubic arch is narrow, and ischial spines are sharp and prominent. This is a difficult passageway for the fetus. It occurs in 30 percent of women.
3. *Anthropoid:* long, narrow pelvis. The inlet is oval shaped, ischial spines are prominent, and the pubic arch is narrow. This type occurs more in nonwhite women (40 percent) than in white women (22 percent).
4. *Platypelloid:* flat pelvis. The inlet is wide with a narrow anterior–posterior diameter. The ischial spines are wide apart, the sacrum is short, and the pubic arch is quite wide, creating a shallow pelvis. This type occurs in less than 3 percent of women.

The type of pelvis is an important factor in the process of labor. An initial evaluation of the pelvis can be made early in pregnancy. However, another assessment is usually made at the time of

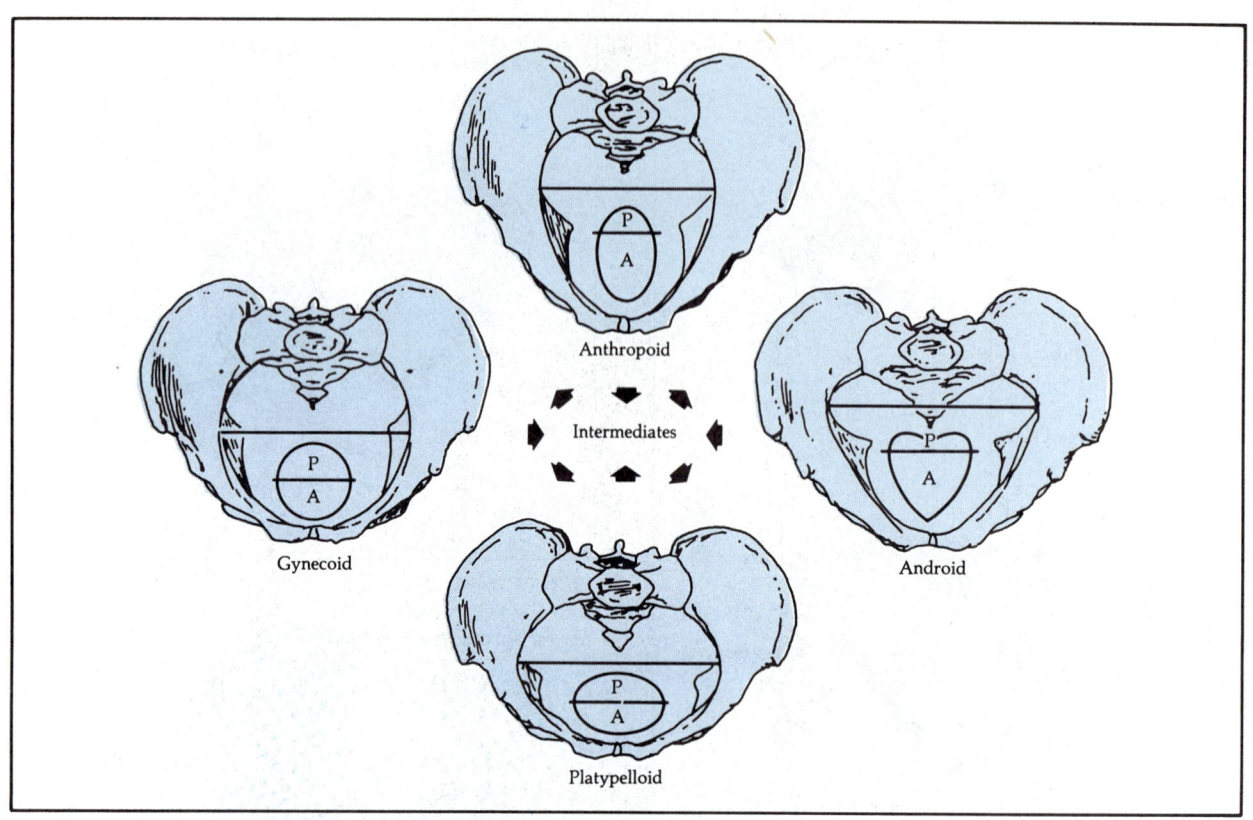

FIGURE 16–12. Four major pelvic types showing flexion of the fetal head.
SOURCE: Pritchard, MacDonald, and Gant (1985).

labor to compare pelvic measurements with the data obtained about the presentation, position, and size of the fetus.

PREMONITORY SIGNS OF LABOR

Certain maternal–fetal changes provide an anticipatory sign of the onset of labor. These include:

1. *Lightening:* the sensation of decreased abdominal distention or pressure on the diaphragm caused by the settling of the lowest part of the fetus in the uterus, or presenting part, into the pelvic cavity. In the primigravid woman, lightening often occurs as a sudden or gradual feeling 2–3 weeks before labor begins. For women who have had other children, lightening usually does not occur until after labor has begun.
2. *Braxton-Hicks contractions:* the irregular, mild contractions of the myometrium present throughout pregnancy that become more noticeable to the woman as the pregnancy nears its last weeks. They may become uncomfortable, even painful, and occur more frequently.
3. *Cervical changes:* the softening and shortening of the cervix (effacement) are documented by vaginal examination. These changes are a result of Braxton-Hicks contractions and increasing hormonal action. The hormonal changes increase the vascularity in the area and promote increased vaginal mucous secretions. Once a woman has had a vaginal delivery her cervix never returns to a nulliparous state.
4. *Bloody show:* blood and mucus found in vaginal secretions. This is due to the rupture of superficial blood vessels as the cervix dilates.
5. *Rupture of membranes (ROM):* a gush or trickle of amniotic fluid, normally clear in color, that occurs when amniotic membranes "tear" or "spring a leak" at some point during pregnancy or labor. As an early sign of labor, ROM usually occurs just before or after contractions begin. This leakage is uncontrollable and can be differ-

entiated from urine by testing with nitrazine paper. This paper will turn blue if the fluid is alkaline (pH 6.5–7.5), indicating amniotic fluid.

Premature rupture of membranes (PROM) may occur before the onset of labor and may not be followed by contractions. (Note: the abbreviation PROM may also be used to indicate *prolonged* rupture of membranes more than 12–24 hours before birth.) Premature rupture of membranes may also be associated with premature labor *at any time during the last half of pregnancy*. However, membranes may also remain intact until the time of delivery. When necessary (as for stimulation of labor or application of a fetal scalp electrode), the "bag of waters" or membranes may be punctured artificially (AROM) as opposed to the spontaneously occurring rupture (SROM).

A woman may encounter one or more of these premonitory signs at the end of pregnancy, but when she will go into labor cannot be accurately predicted. This is the case both for the woman who is having her first child and for the woman who has had several children. There are a number of signals that indicate labor is imminent but not immediate. Labor may not be ready to proceed into its predictable rhythmic stages for hours or days. Some signals or symptoms may be used to differentiate between "false" labor and "true" labor, as listed in Table 16–2.

Instructors in prenatal classes inform the couple about the differences between false labor and true labor. The physician and midwife also go into detail as to when to call them or when to go the hospital or birthing center. However, the diagnosis of true labor is not always clearcut, and the pregnant woman may need to seek professional advice and be observed in the hospital labor room for a period of time to confirm whether this is indeed the onset of labor. The pregnant woman should always notify her physician or midwife when (1) the membranes rupture, (2) she feels the contractions have become regular and remain so, and (3) there is vaginal bleeding or spotting.

STAGES OF LABOR

Traditionally, labor has been divided into three stages, encompassing the birth of the baby and the placenta. In recent years, a fourth stage has been identified as crucial to the childbirth experience:

1. The *first stage of labor* begins with regular contractions that efface and dilate the cervix. This stage ends with full dilation of the cervix.
2. The *second stage of labor* begins with full dilation of the cervix and ends with the delivery of the infant.
3. The *third stage of labor* begins after the delivery of the infant and ends with the delivery of the placenta.
4. The *fourth stage of labor* includes the first hour after delivery of the placenta.

First Stage of Labor

The first stage of labor is the longest and most variable stage and includes three phases (Fig. 16–13):

1. *Latent phase:* duration is sensitive to outside interference, such as heavy medication or stimulation (mean = 8.6 hours for primiparas, 5.3 hours for multiparas).

TABLE 16–2. Characteristics of Labor

False Labor (Braxton-Hicks Contractions)	True Labor (Labor Contractions)
No perceptible change in cervix	Cervical changes of effacement, dilation
Irregular pattern, often starting close together and then decreasing in frequency	Progressively closer frequency, stronger intensity, longer duration
Discomfort more in lower abdomen and groin	Discomfort noted in back, sometimes radiating toward front
Contractions often slacken with activity, disappear when asleep	Contractions intensify with activity, continue even when sleeping

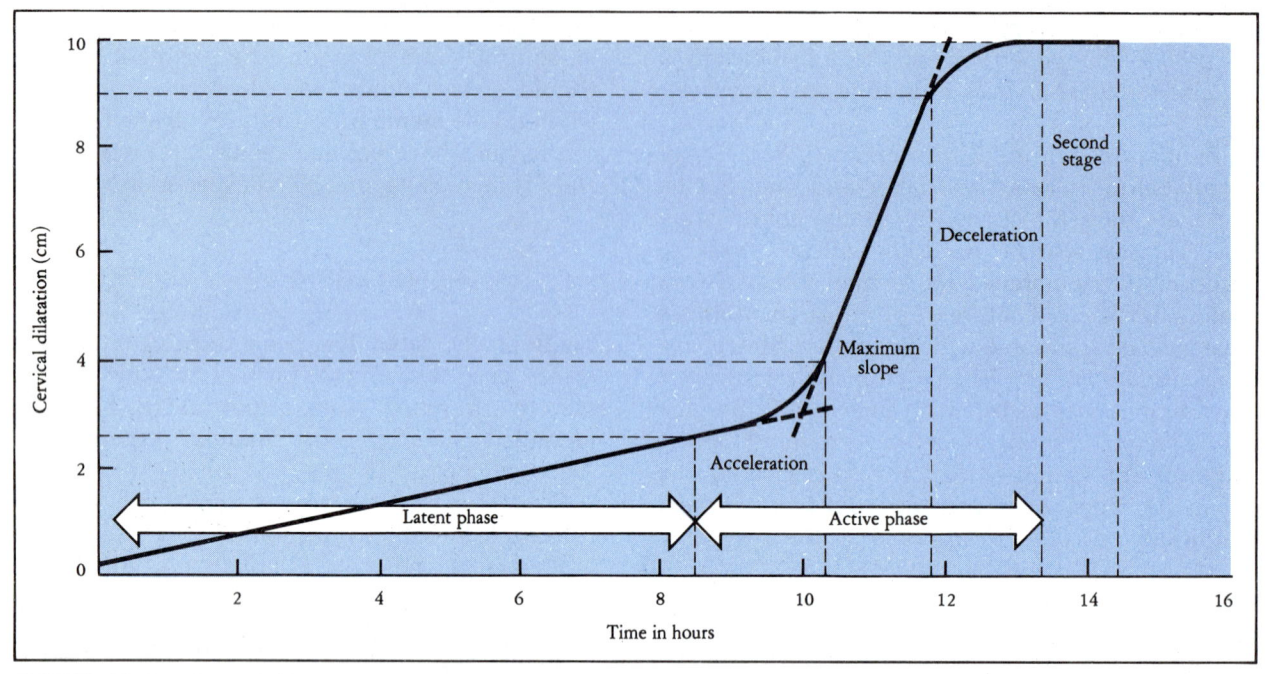

FIGURE. 16–13. Cervical dilation time in the three phases of the first stage of labor.
SOURCE: Friedman (1955).

2. *Active phase:* short and variable (mean = 4.9 hours for primiparas, 2.2 hours for multiparas).
3. *Transitional phase:* cervical retraction about the fetal head occurs (mean = 57 min for primiparas, 2 hours, 14 min for multiparas) (Friedman, 1955).

Frequently, these phases have been combined so that two major phases are discussed, latent and active. The active phase includes the accelerated phase, maximum slope, and the deceleration phase shown in Fig. 16–13.

The Phases of the First Stage

During the latent phase, contractions become stabilized as they increase in frequency, duration, and intensity. Beginning contractions are of mild intensity, occurring every 10–15 min and lasting 15–20 sec. These contractions progress to those of moderate intensity (about 40 mm Hg), occurring every 5–7 min and lasting 30–40 sec. There may be no appreciable change in cervical dilation, usually less than 2–2.5 cm. However, the cervix at this point is apparently being primed for the subsequent phases, and effacement may be completed. Since the fetus is passive during labor, it makes little effort to descend. The duration of this phase is quite variable and particularly sensitive to outside interference.

The woman during this phase is usually excited and happy to finally have the long waiting period over, yet somewhat anxious and apprehensive about what is to come. She is usually not too uncomfortable and is responsive to suggestions, information, and words of support.

The active phase is the period from the end of latency to full dilation. Acceleration characterizes this phase. Contractions are relatively short in duration and lead into the phase of maximum slope. This phase rapidly takes the cervix from 3 to 4 cm to about 8 cm, averaging about 3 cm/hour for primigravidas and 1.2 cm/hour for multiparas.

The transitional phase marks the slowing of cervical dilation from 8 to 10 cm as descent of the fetus reaches its maximum rate. Contractions during the active phase become increasingly more frequent, occurring every 1–2 min. These contractions last longer, approximately 50–60 sec and are of greater intensity, averaging 55–60 mm Hg. Membranes are usually ruptured by this time. Bloody show increases and low back pain occurs.

As labor progresses, the woman experiences more discomfort with contractions, becomes more apprehensive, and appears less interested in outside activities. She becomes more serious and intense with each contraction, needing support and constant attention (see Chapter 17).

Second Stage of Labor

The second stage of labor begins when the cervix is fully dilated (10 cm) and effaced 100 percent. At this time the woman may feel the urge to bear down. She may now use her abdominal muscles to assist the involuntary uterine contractions as a force in the descent of the fetus. She is able to participate actively at this stage, as she coordinates her breathing and abdominal muscles with the contractions. During this stage the fetus moves through the lower segment of the cervix and vagina to the perineal floor and out the introitus. The vaginal walls and perineal floor muscles must be stretched and thinned. Generally, this stage is considerably shorter than the first stage—from a few minutes in some cases to 1–2 hours in others. Mean times are 0.9 hour for primiparas and 0.3 hour for multiparas.

Uterine contractions during the second stage are forceful, occurring every 2–3 min and lasting 60–90 sec. They have an intensity of 70–80 mm Hg. There is an increase in bloody show, and more amniotic fluid may be released. As the fetal head descends, the perineum begins to bulge and the labia separate with contractions (see Fig. 16–14c). As the head reaches the perineal floor, it appears at the introitus, then crowns (Fig. 16–14d, e). If there is a need for an episiotomy, a midline or mediolateral one may be performed at this time. With the physician or midwife supporting, the head delivers and rotates, the mouth is suctioned, and then the shoulders appear (Fig. 16–14g, h, i). A quick check is made to assure that the mouth is clear and that there is no umbilical cord around the neck (Fig. 16–14j). First one shoulder, then the other is delivered under the symphysis pubis, and the body quickly follows (Fig. 16–14k). Again, the airway is immediately checked for obstructions and the placenta is delivered (Fig. 16–14l).

The Mechanisms of Labor

The mechanisms of labor consist of a series of sequential movements (also known as cardinal movements) that reflect changes in posture as the fetus passively conforms itself to the birth canal during descent and birth.

The six cardinal movements of the fetus in the vertex position are (1) descent and engagement, (2) flexion, (3) internal rotation, (4) extension, (5) restitution and external rotation, and (6) expulsion (see Fig. 16–15).

DESCENT AND ENGAGEMENT. As the head moves toward the pelvic inlet, it is described first as *floating*, then as *dipping* into the inlet. Once the biparietal diameter passes through the inlet, the head becomes *engaged*. This may occur before or after labor begins and is due to the pressure of contractions, amniotic fluid, and abdominal muscles.

FLEXION. During descent, the head flexes so that the chin rests on the chest. This *flexion* reduces the presenting fetal diameter, as the head enters the inlet and moves down through the birth canal.

INTERNAL ROTATION. In this maneuver the fetus gradually turns—first head, then shoulders and body—to fit the curving of the birth canal. The head accommodates itself to the space available, and then the shoulders turn to fit the widest diameter available.

EXTENSION. As the fetal head reaches the pelvic floor, it pivots under the symphysis pubis and pubic arch and advances through the introitus and over the perineum.

RESTITUTION AND EXTERNAL ROTATION. After the head is delivered, it immediately rotates to its original position, as the shoulders align themselves to the anterior–posterior plane of the outlet.

EXPULSION. The anterior shoulder moves under the pubic arch and the posterior shoulder moves forward and is usually delivered first, followed by the anterior shoulder. The rest of the infant is born in one movement.

Third Stage of Labor

Following the delivery of the infant, the umbilical cord is still attached. At this time the practitioner will check to see if the cord is around the neck. If so, she or he will slip the cord over the head to release it and then clear the mucus from the nose and mouth when possible. Many physicians now clamp the cord. The umbilical cord is clamped in two places and cut between the two clamps a few inches from the navel. Some practitioners, however, wait 5–10 min for the cord to stop pulsating before clamping in order to maximize blood flow to the infant. Right after birth the infant is evaluated with a 1-min Apgar score (from 1 to 10; see Chapter 25). As soon as possible the infant is placed on the mother's abdomen or in her arms (Fig. 16–16). The uterine contractions continue, forcing the uterus to contract on itself. The walls thicken, and the site of placental implantation shrinks, causing the placenta to buckle and separate. Separation occurs within a few minutes after birth, and its process is enhanced by a hematoma that forms behind the placenta. There may be a sudden trickle or gush of blood, and there is a noticeable lengthening of the umbilical cord visible at the vaginal introitus. If the woman is supine, the abdominal contour changes with a rise in the uterus as the placenta slides downward (see Fig. 16–17). Usually the placenta delivers itself, but sometimes it needs to be manually separated. The normal blood loss during the third stage is approximately 150–350 ml. The episiotomy, if one has been made, is repaired after the delivery of the placenta.

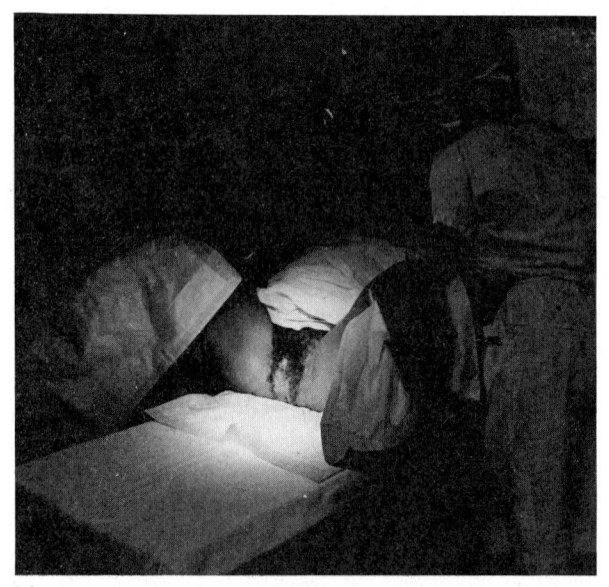

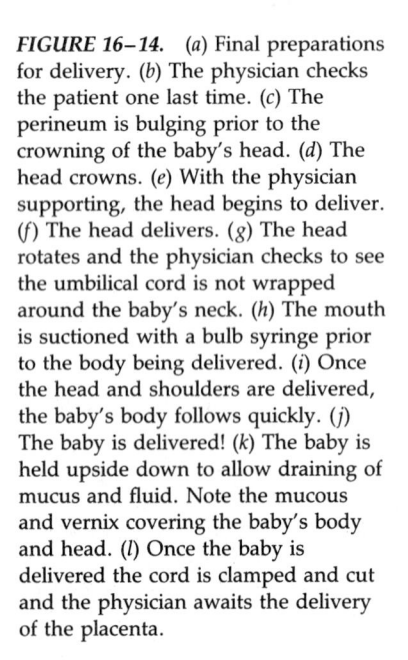

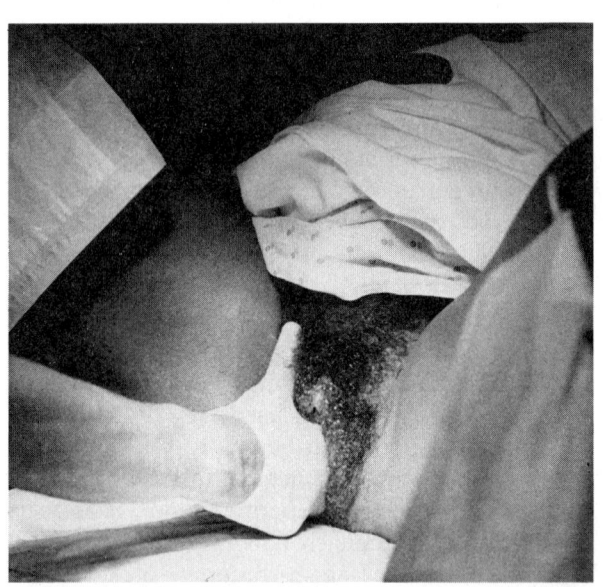

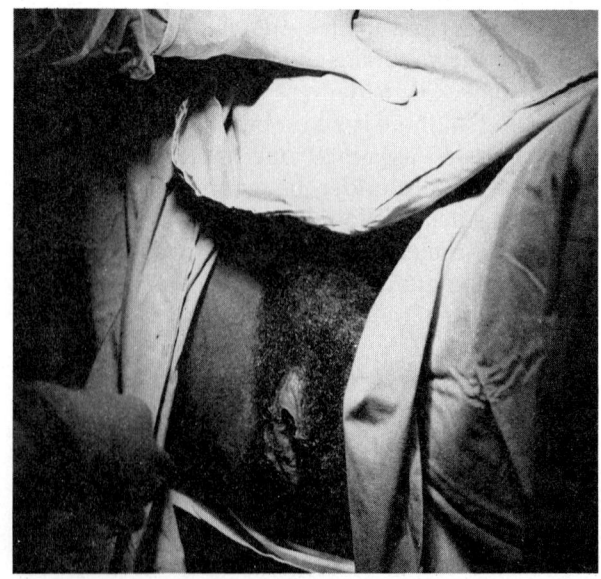

FIGURE 16–14. (a) Final preparations for delivery. (b) The physician checks the patient one last time. (c) The perineum is bulging prior to the crowning of the baby's head. (d) The head crowns. (e) With the physician supporting, the head begins to deliver. (f) The head delivers. (g) The head rotates and the physician checks to see the umbilical cord is not wrapped around the baby's neck. (h) The mouth is suctioned with a bulb syringe prior to the body being delivered. (i) Once the head and shoulders are delivered, the baby's body follows quickly. (j) The baby is delivered! (k) The baby is held upside down to allow draining of mucus and fluid. Note the mucous and vernix covering the baby's body and head. (l) Once the baby is delivered the cord is clamped and cut and the physician awaits the delivery of the placenta.

(d)

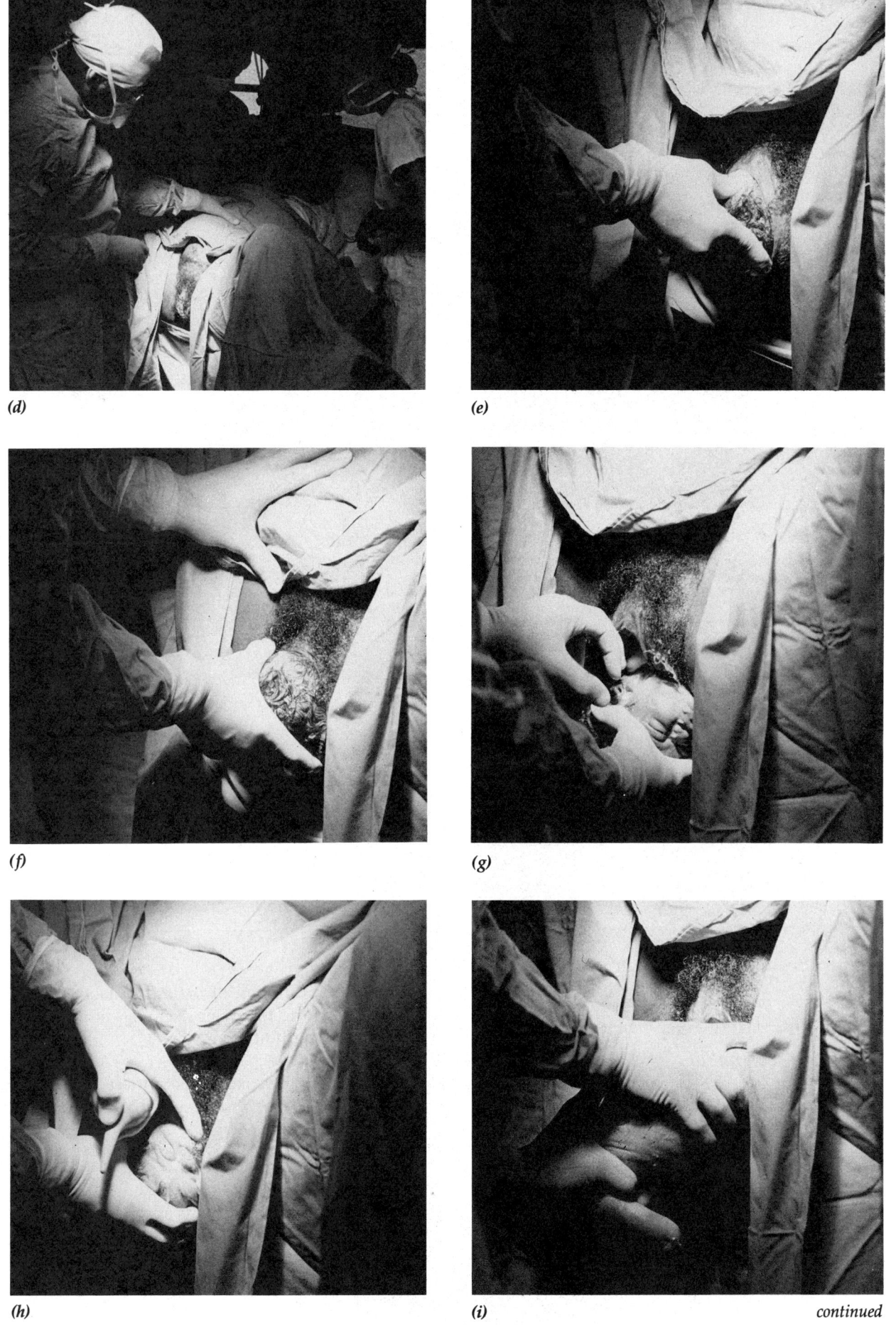

(e)

(f)

(g)

(h)

(i)

continued

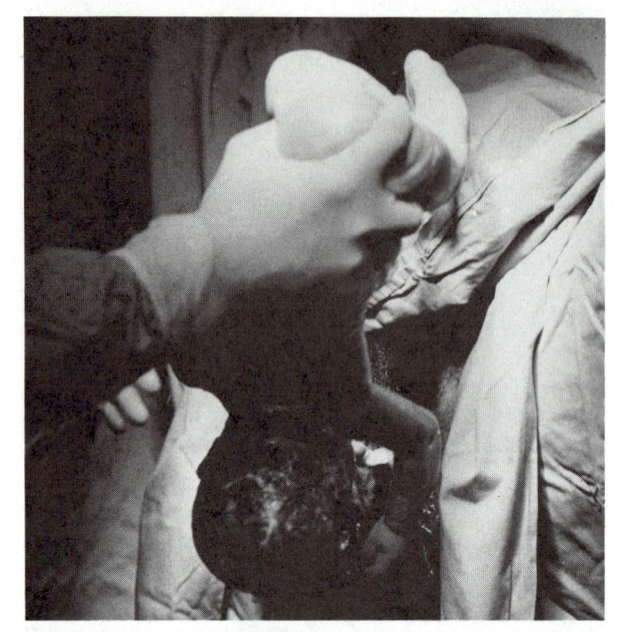

(j)

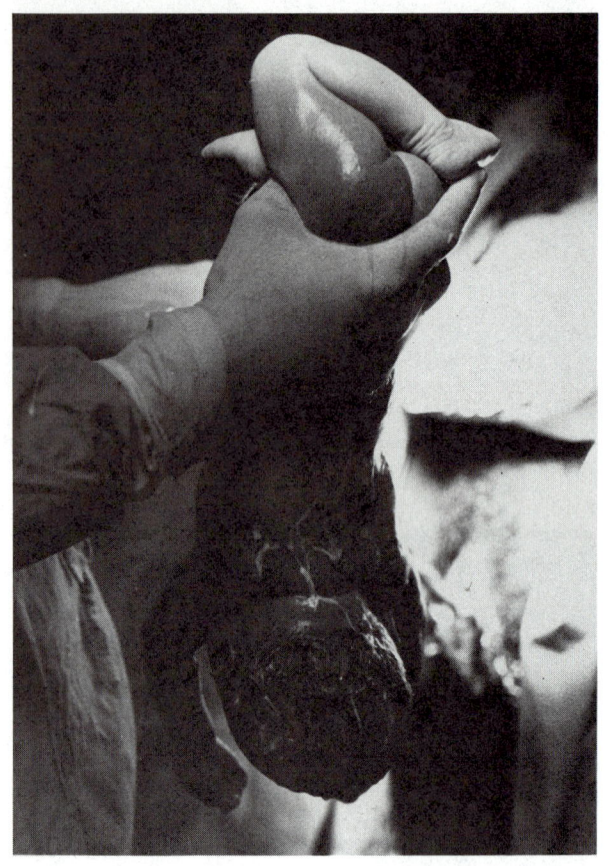

(k)

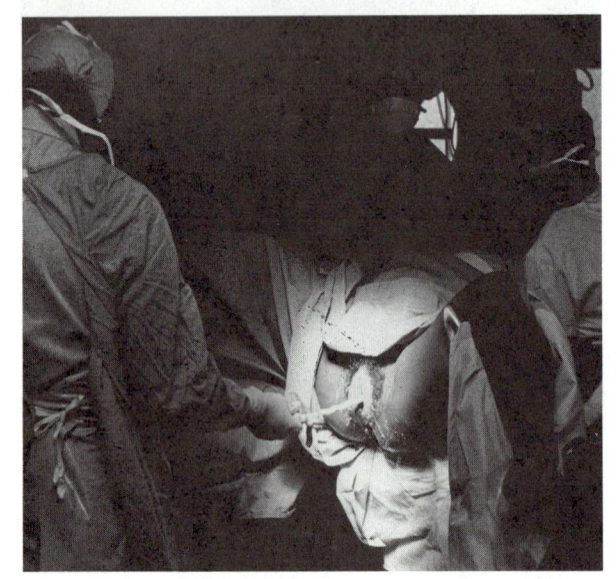

(l)

Fourth Stage of Labor

After delivery of the placenta, the uterine muscles continue to contract and relax as they compress the open blood vessels and sinuses at the placental site. Uterine tone can be increased by having the mother breastfeed her newborn. Breastfeeding releases oxytocin, which stimulates contractions. Preparations of oxytocin or ergotrate may also be administered. For the first hour after delivery, it is critical to observe the woman for physiologic reactions and readjustments to all the changes that have occurred during labor and birth, such as return of uterine tone, control of vaginal bleeding, and return of normal values for vital signs (see Chapter 20).

DURATION OF LABOR

Although the duration of individual labor cannot be predicted, the following factors will affect the course and length of labor:

1. *Parity.* With increasing parity there is shortening of total labor and of each of the separate phases of the first stage.
2. *Intervals between birth.* Women who have had an extended period between births may have longer labors than those who have more closely spaced pregnancies.
3. *Relationship between size of fetus and pelvic measurements.* Small fetuses with ample maternal pelvis will have shorter labors than large fe-

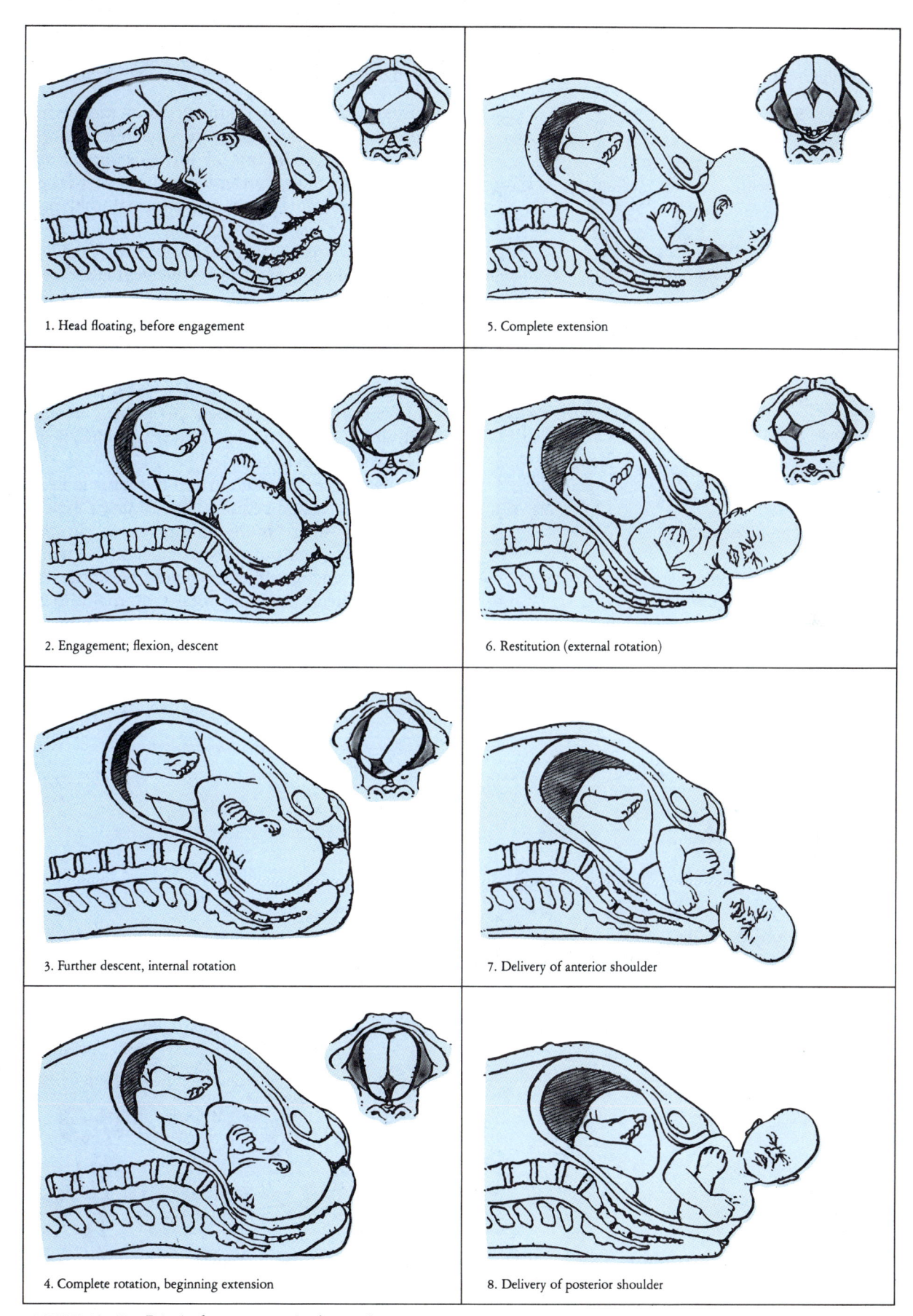

1. Head floating, before engagement
2. Engagement; flexion, descent
3. Further descent, internal rotation
4. Complete rotation, beginning extension
5. Complete extension
6. Restitution (external rotation)
7. Delivery of anterior shoulder
8. Delivery of posterior shoulder

FIGURE 16–15. Principal movements in the mechanism of labor and delivery, LOA position.

358 CHANGE: THE INTRAPARTAL PERIOD

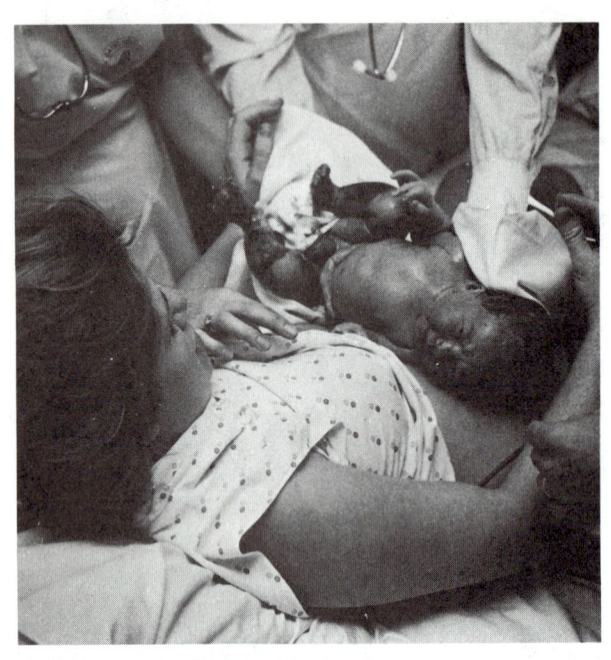

FIGURE 16–16. The infant is placed on the mother's abdomen immediately after delivery.

tuses, who will have difficulty in maneuvering through an average or narrow birth canal.
4. *Gestational age.* Infants of low gestational age will usually have shorter labors because of their greater ease in negotiating the maternal passageway.
5. *Nutritional status, fatigue.* Women in excellent nutritional state and those who start labor with adequate rest and do not become exhausted will have an easier and usually shorter labor.
6. *Medication.* Medication in the latent phase is known to prolong early labor. Sedatives, narcotics, as well as ethanol, magnesium sulfate, and ritodrine are known to reduce uterine activity. Certain types of regional anesthesia may also prolong labor.
7. *Position of the fetal head.* When the fetus is in an occiput posterior position, the woman experiences a longer, more painful labor. In this position the occiput presses against the woman's sacrum, resulting in severe backaches. If the fetal head does not rotate internally to an anterior position, the mechanisms of labor are

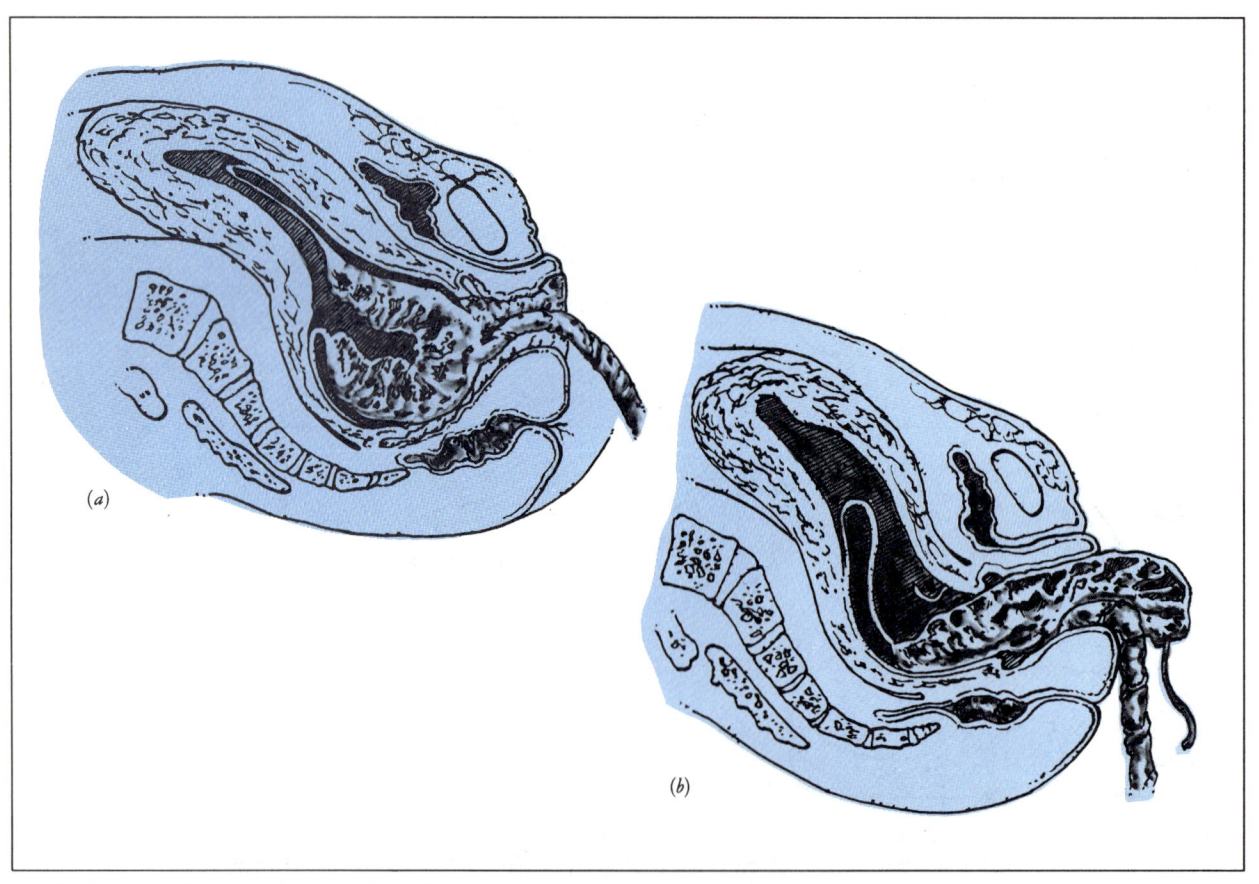

FIGURE 16–17. Usual mechanism of expulsion of placenta. (a) Separation of placenta from wall of uterus. (b) Movement of placenta through vagina.

slowed down and are more arduously maneuvered. As the fetal head extends under the symphysis and pubic arch, the face is turned upward rather than in the more usual face downward position.

8. *Maternal position during labor.* The maternal position has been found to have a definite effect on labor, particularly on both uterine activity and comfort. In the supine position, contractions occur more frequently but are lower in intensity and less efficient in dilating the cervix. In the lateral recumbent position the uterus is more effective in dilating the cervix, although frequency is decreased and the intensity is greater. In research by Roberts, Malasanos, and Mendez-Bauer (1981) women were found to be more comfortable sitting up in early labor and lying on their side in later labor. The standing position has also been found to be an efficient position for cervical dilation. Maternal position during the second stage will also influence the ability of the woman to work effectively with each contraction. The traditional lithotomy position recommended in order to visualize the perineum more clearly and deal with any complications is not necessarily the most comfortable or the most effective. The use of birthing beds permits flexibility of position during labor and delivery (see Chapter 42).

SUMMARY

Parturition or labor is a complex, intricate, and coordinated performance by the woman and her fetus. Their roles are still only partially understood—"as through a glass, darkly"—but a great deal of progress has been made in recognizing the supporting factors that influence the course and outcome of the childbearing experience.

These changes or increase in knowledge of the reproductive cycle will necessitate changes in the clinical practice of both obstetrics and maternity nursing. Procedures, protocols, and practice based on knowledge that is outdated or static become rigid, task-centered, and restricted. New knowledge and the prospect of more to come encourages a future-oriented, flexible practice that is goal-oriented and tolerant of individual expectations and alternatives. The goal for health care providers is a safe, healthy, and satisfying childbirth experience for mother and infant. Providing alternatives for the childbearing family will keep health care providers and their delivery system an open system with two-way open flow that encourages expanding knowledge yet assures a homeostatic relationship between client and provider.

SUGGESTED READINGS

Caldeyro-Barcia, R., and Serino, J. A. 1961. The response of the human uterus to oxytocin throughout pregnancy. In *Oxytocin,* eds. R. Caldeyro-Barcia and H. Heller. New York: Pergamon Press.

Chard, T. 1973. The role of the posterior pituitaries of the mother and fetus in spontaneous parturition. In *Fetal and neonatal physiology,* eds. K. S. Comline, K. W. Cross, and D. S. Dawes. Cambridge: Cambridge University Press.

Chard, T., and Richards, M. 1977. *Benefits and hazards of the new obstetrics.* Philadelphia: J. B. Lippincott.

Csapo, A. 1959. Function and regulation of the myometrium. *Ann. N. Y. Acad. Sci.* 75:790–808.

Friedmann, E. 1955. Primigravid labor: A graphico statistical analysis. *Obstet. Gynecol.* 6:570.

Friedman, E. 1956. Labor in multiparas: A graphico statistical analysis. *Obstet. Gynecol.* 8:691–703.

Friedman, E. 1971. The functional division of labor. *Am. J. Obstet. Gynecol.* 109:274–280.

Friedman, E. 1978. *Labor: Clinical evaluation and management.* 2nd ed. New York: Appleton-Century-Crofts.

LeBoyer, F. 1975. *Birth without violence.* New York: Knopf.

Liggins, G. C. 1973. Fetal influences on myometrial contractibility. *Clin. Obstet. Gynecol.* 16(3):148–165.

CURRENT REFERENCES

Danforth, D., and Scott, J. R. 1986. *Obstetrics and gynecology.* Philadelphia: J. B. Lippincott.

Fuchs, F. 1983. Endocrinology of parturition. In *Endocrinology of pregnancy,* 3rd ed, Eds. F. Fuchs and A. Klopper. Philadelphia: Harper and Row.

Mackey, M. C. 1984. *Women's views of the childbirth experience.* Doctoral dissertation, University of Illinois. Ann Arbor, Michigan. University Microfilms International.

Oxorn, H. 1980. *Oxorn-Foote human labor and birth.* 4th ed. New York: Appleton-Century-Crofts.

Pincus, J. 1984. Childbirth. In *The new our bodies, ourselves* by The Boston Women's Health Book Collective. New York: Simon and Schuster, Inc.

Pritchard, J. A.; MacDonald, P. C.; and Gant, N. F. 1985. *Williams obstetrics.* 17th ed. Norwalk, Conn.: Appleton-Century-Crofts.

Roberts, J.; Malasanos, L.; and Mendez-Bauer, C. 1981. Maternal positions in labor: Analysis in relation to comfort and efficiency. *Birth Defects: Original Article Series.* 17(6):97–128.

Roberts, J. E. 1979. *The effect of maternal position on labor.* Doctoral dissertation, University of Illinois. Ann Arbor, Michigan. University Microfilms International.

Summer, P. E., and Phillips, C. P. 1981. *Birthing rooms, concept and reality.* St. Louis: C. V. Mosby.

Trevathan, W. R. 1987. *Human birth: An evolutionary perspective.* New York: Aldine DeGruyter.

Varney, H. 1987. *Nurse-midwifery.* 2nd ed. Boston: Blackwell Scientific.

17

The Nurse's Role During the Intrapartal Period

BEHAVIORAL OBJECTIVES

Upon completion of this chapter, the reader should be able to:

- Identify and describe the nurse's role in assessment of the intrapartal family.

- Demonstrate the ability to assess fetal heart rate and uterine contraction patterns during labor.

- Identify and describe purposes, techniques, and applications for direct and indirect fetal monitoring.

- Identify emotional considerations and stressors of the intrapartal experience.

- Describe and discuss the nurse's role during clinical examinations throughout the intrapartal period.

- Identify and describe assessment of acute fetal distress, including interpretation of abnormal fetal monitor readings and fetal scalp sampling.

- Describe and discuss nursing actions in cases of acute fetal distress.

Never in the childbearing cycle is the nurse's role more important than in the intrapartal period. In the long, lonely hours of work and waiting, an emerging family depends on the nurse for help and reassurance during the labor and delivery process. The nurse is at the bedside throughout some of the most exciting and important hours in the lives of the new family. How the nurse administers to them and facilitates their adaptation to the new parenting role makes a difference in the family's ability to have a positive intrapartal experience. The purpose of this chapter is to enable the health care provider to offer supportive care to the client family during and immediately following labor and delivery. This chapter focuses on the role of the nurse in providing care and monitoring the progress of the client and family throughout the intrapartal period.

LABOR AND DELIVERY AS STRESSORS

Labor is a direct stressor to a mother and her baby. Also, significant others are indirectly stressed as they support their loved ones during the childbearing experience. Nursing care is directed toward identification and mediation of stressors, for all members of the emerging family—mother, father, and fetus. The goals of nursing care during the childbearing period are to assure (Clark and Affonso, 1979):

1. The safety and protection of the fetus.
2. The safety and protection of the mother.
3. Healthy outcomes for the fetus, mother, and family.

Professional nursing care promotes the safety, protection, and health of all members of the emerging family. Stressors are identified and mediated, and nursing care interventions are directed toward promoting optimal adaptation to the childbearing experience.

THE NURSE'S ROLE IN ASSESSMENT

One of the most frequently asked questions is "Will my baby be all right?" This question has been asked by mothers throughout the ages. Today, nurses have increased ability and responsibility to answer that question. Contemporary nursing involves using expanded assessment capabilities and offering nursing care to fetus, mother, and father throughout the childbearing experience.

Nursing Assessment of the Fetal Heart Rate: Periodic Auscultation

Nursing actions during the intrapartal period have traditionally included *periodic auscultation* of the fetal heart rate, because of the stress known to occur during labor and delivery. The fetal heart responds to stress during the intrapartum by accelerating or decelerating (Clark and Affonso, 1979; Krebs et al., 1982). The normal fetal heart rate ranges from 120 to 160 beats/min (bpm). The term *bradycardia* describes a fetal heart rate below 120 bpm; *tachycardia* describes a fetal heart rate above 160 bpm. Assessment of the fetal heart rate is a nursing responsibility throughout the intrapartal period.

Listening to the fetal heart with a fetoscope is a method of *intermittent auscultation* (see Fig. 17–1). The nurse places the fetoscope on each of the four quadrants of the maternal abdomen to find out the most audible fetal heart tones. The fetal heart rate is counted for 1 min, between contractions. The nurse also assesses the regularity of the rhythm and strength of the heart beat. This manual method of assessment of the fetal heart rate is common but is considered less reliable than electronic fetal monitoring for diagnosing fetal distress.

Electronically enhanced, portable fetal monitors (fetone, Doppler) are available in many labor and delivery rooms (see Fig. 17–2). These machines are used with a conductive gel. They electronically convert the movement of the fetal heart into an audible sound. The fetone is easy to use and makes it possible for everyone in the room to hear the fetal heart rate simultaneously.

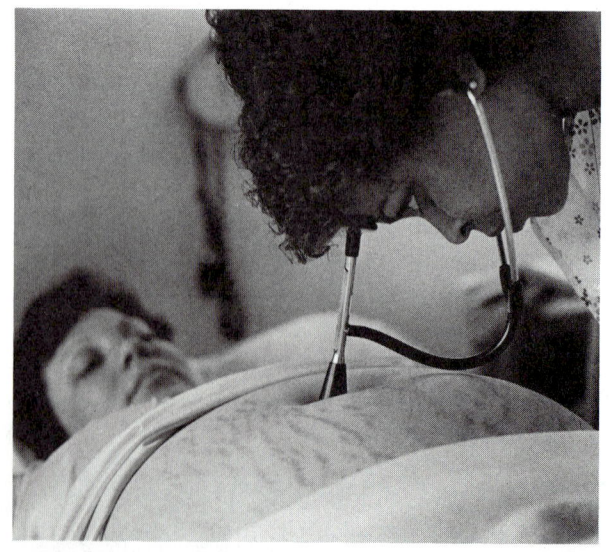

FIGURE 17–1. Auscultation of the fetal heartbeat using the fetoscope.

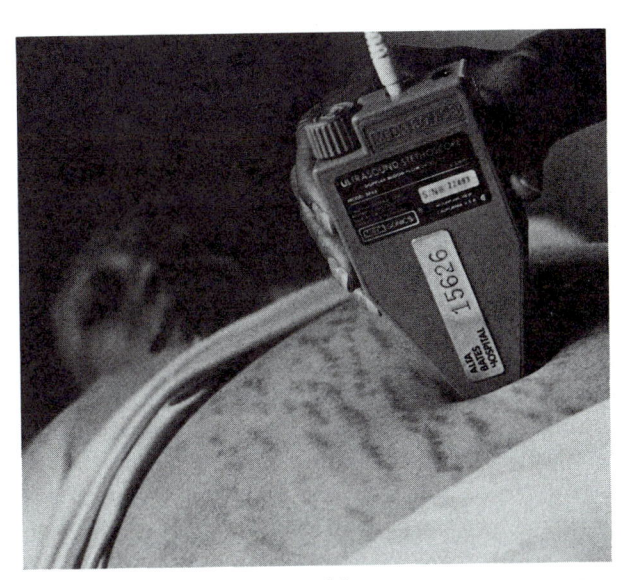

FIGURE 17-2. A Doppler used for fetal heart rate assessment.

Nursing Assessment of Uterine Contractions

Uterine contractions are stressful to both mother and fetus during labor. Adequate perfusion of the placenta during labor depends on normal patterns of contraction and relaxation of the uterus throughout the intrapartum. To assess the fetal–maternal response to labor, the nurse assesses the uterine contraction patterns.

The following four steps are suggested for the manual assessment of uterine contractions:

1. Gently place the fingertips of one hand on the uterine fundus.
2. Note the degree of uterine pressure under the fingertips as a contraction begins.
3. The intensity will increase. Note the peak in uterine hardness at the *acme* of the contraction. The hardness will then slowly diminish.
4. Contractions normally begin in the fundus; if they begin elsewhere (midabdomen or lower quadrant), it may indicate abnormalities and should be reported to the physician or midwife managing the labor and delivery.

A nurse is responsible for assessing the frequency, duration, and intensity of uterine contractions. *Frequency* is assessed by measuring the interval between the beginning of one contraction and the beginning of the next, in minutes. *Duration* is measured in seconds and describes the interval between the beginning and end of any one contraction. *Intensity* of the contraction is subjectively defined as mild, moderate, or strong, depending on the degree of uterine indentation possible during a contraction (see Chapter 16). The nurse's notes include a statement about the frequency, duration, and intensity of the uterine contractions at specified time intervals according to the standards specified by an institution.

Electronic Fetal Monitoring

Use of continuous electronic fetal monitoring during labor and delivery enables health care providers to make continuous, immediate assessments of the fetal–maternal unit throughout the intrapartal period. Interpretation of the assessment data allows caregivers to initiate prompt and specific treatment for episodes of fetal distress. Nurses are responsible for managing the continuous monitoring during the intrapartal period and assessment of the data gathered.

Use of electronic fetal monitoring in the perinatal period significantly decreases the infant mortality rate (Neutra, Rienberg, and Griedman, 1978; Reeder, Mastroianni, and Martin, 1983). Although some studies question the value of electronic fetal monitoring in normal labor, continuous monitoring has become commonplace in labor and delivery rooms across the country. With the widespread use of fetal monitoring, the nurse's role includes teaching the childbearing family about the procedures and equipment. The nurse teaches the family the purpose and techniques of monitoring, provides anticipatory guidance about application and management of the monitoring apparatus, and serves as the primary professional to screen and interpret data gathered. Thus, knowledge about electronic fetal monitoring, the equipment, underlying principles, basic interpretations, and data management have become important for intrapartal nursing.

Electronic fetal monitors use a strip graph to record the fetal heart rate (FHR) and the uterine contractions (UCs) on perforated accordion paper. The perforated paper is placed in a fetal monitoring system, with the output immediately available at the bedside. Some hospitals also have fetal monitor readouts at the central nurse's station. The strip graph display is recorded using two monitor channels. The lower channel represents the uterine contraction activity. Uterine contraction data are presented as pressure readings, in milimeters of mercury (mm Hg). Normal uterine pressure during labor ranges from 5 to 15 mm Hg between contractions, and 30 to 75 mm Hg during a contraction (Hon, 1976; Freeman and Garite, 1981; Krebs et al., 1982). Monitors have calibrating and zeroing devices to ensure accuracy of pressure readings. The upper channel of the strip graph displays fetal heart rates in beats/min. Some monitors are also equipped with digital readouts of FHR. The paper speed of the monitor can be adjusted by the nurse to correlate the uterine contraction and fetal heart rate channels for easy calculation of elapsed time; the paper speed is usually set at 3 cm/sec. The entire fetal monitor strip graph becomes part of the permanent patient record.

Types of Electronic Fetal Monitoring

Two types of electronic fetal monitoring are currently in use: indirect and direct (Hodnett, 1982). *Indirect fetal monitoring* is also called external pressure monitoring. In indirect monitoring, the uterine contractions are assessed using a *tocodynamometer*, or *pressure transducer*, placed on the abdomen above the uterine fundus. The external pressure transducer converts the uterine fundal pressure of the contractions into an electrical signal that is recorded on the lower channel of the strip graph. The tocodynamometer measures and records the frequency and duration of uterine contractions. Intensity of contractions is not measured during indirect monitoring.

During indirect monitoring, a second transducer reflects high-frequency sound waves from the fetal heart and valves. This is called an *ultrasound transducer*. The ultrasound transducer data are recorded as FHR on the upper channel of the strip graph. The indirect method is often used in early labor, prior to rupture of the fetal membranes. This method is also used in the antepartum period for perinatal screening purposes, the nonstress test (NST), or the oxytocin challenge test (OCT).

The nurse is responsible for initial and subsequent positioning of both external transducers during indirect fetal monitoring procedures (see Fig. 17–3). The equipment is easy to apply and is

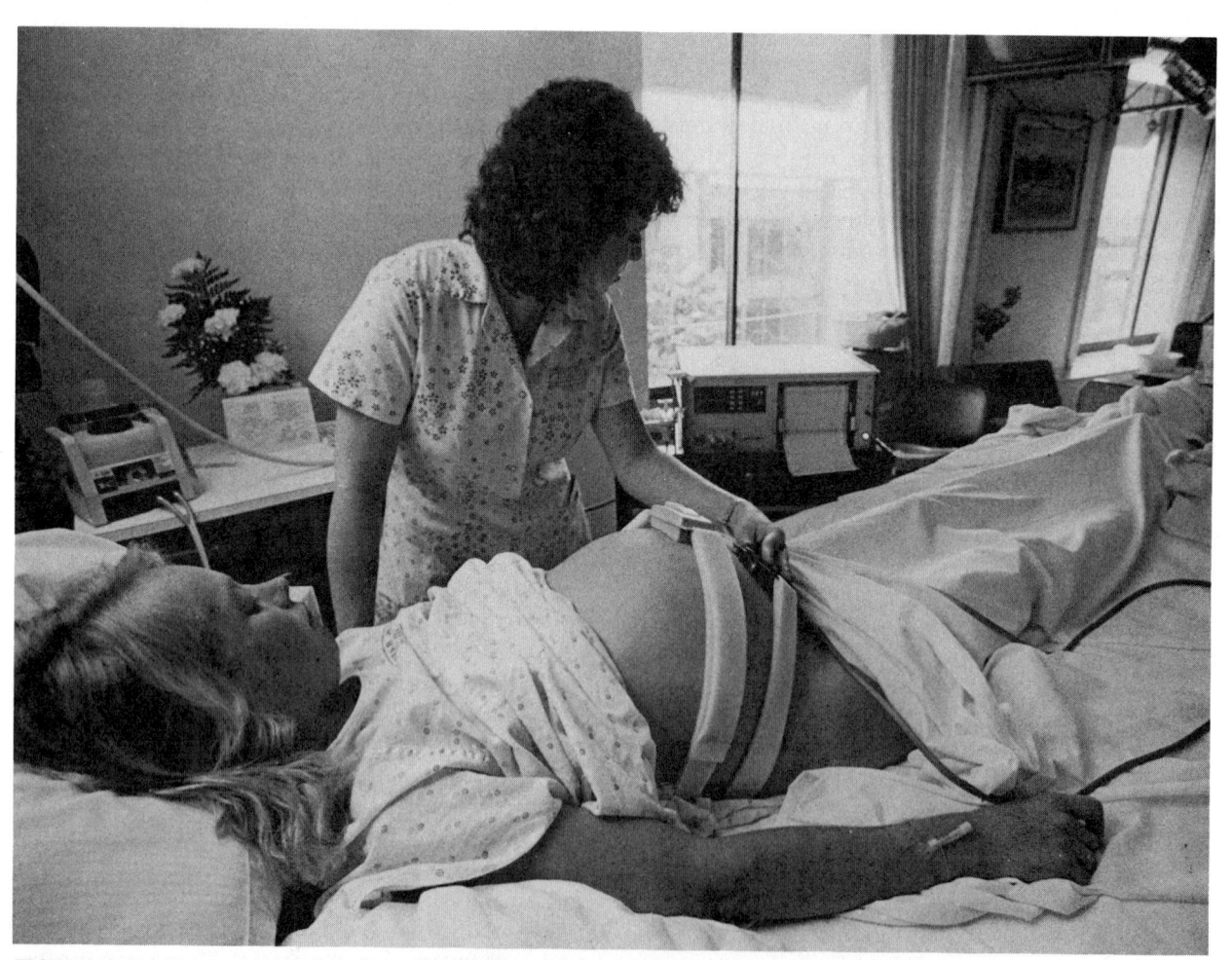

FIGURE 17–3. Patient with external fetal monitor applied. Note that the monitor function can be observed by the patient.

not invasive. The indirect monitor allows the patient substantial freedom of movement and does not cause discomfort during application. However, most manufacturers recommend its use in the supine position. With assistance, the patient can assume the side-lying or semi-sitting position. The patient can also be assisted to the bathroom. The nurse will find that it is necessary to reposition the external transducers frequently. These repositioning intervals can be used to wash application sites, provide comfort measures, give a back rub, or initiate other supportive actions.

Direct fetal monitoring is used more frequently than indirect monitoring in contemporary maternity settings. This type of monitoring is also called internal monitoring. The direct method uses an electrode transducer applied directly to the fetal scalp or presenting part (see Fig. 17–4). Application of the internal electrode transducer requires that the mother has ruptured membranes and a cervical dilation of 1–2 cm. The application procedure is usually carried out by a physician or a specially trained nurse. The scalp electrode is inserted using a flexible, soft plastic guide; it attaches to the presenting fetal part by a small wire, gently turned clockwise (Tucker, 1978; Jensen, Benson, and Bobak, 1981).

In direct fetal monitoring, uterine contractions are assessed using a soft, fluid-filled, transvaginal catheter. The catheter is filled with sterile water and positioned inside the uterine cavity. The fluid acts as a direct transmitter of intrauterine pressure. Pressure changes that occur with contractions are converted by the pressure transducer into readings in mm Hg. Both pressure and FHT readings are recorded on the appropriate channel of the strip graph. Because the procedure is invasive, the nurse is responsible for cleansing the vulva with an antiseptic solution before the procedure and for maintaining aseptic technique throughout fetal monitoring.

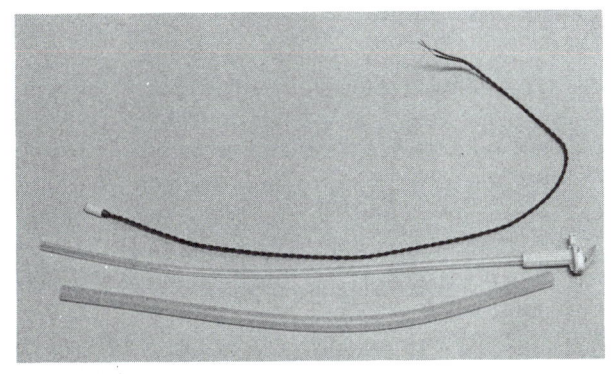

FIGURE 17–4. Scalp electrode and transducer for fetal heart monitoring.

Application of the Electronic Fetal Monitor

Although the primary decision to monitor a patient is the physician's, nurses often set priorities within the clinical setting (NAACOG, 1980; Perez, 1981; Reeder, Mastroianni, and Martin, 1983). Once the decision to monitor is made, the nurse is responsible for preparing the patient for the application procedure and for obtaining informed consent. In most cases the application of indirect monitoring (external) is done by the nurse. Patients can be told that indirect monitoring will not hurt them and will allow them a certain degree of freedom of movement after application. Direct monitoring (internal) is uncomfortable during initial application and restricts the patient's freedom of movement substantially. Nursing support and encouragement is appropriate throughout the procedure.

Most patients and their significant others are moderately anxious about, but also very interested in, the monitoring procedures and data tracings. The equipment should be fully explained to the family and kept in full view of all labor and delivery participants. A nurse's teaching should include an explanation of both the upper and lower channel strip graphs, fetal heart rate, uterine contraction, and normal variations in the strip graph data. Many couples find the monitor data helpful in using their prepared childbirth breathing techniques.

Evaluation of Interactions of Significant Others

Each laboring couple is unique and brings to the intrapartum experience personal hopes, dreams, expectations, abilities, and preparation. Nurses have the responsibility of helping others give support to women during labor and delivery. Nurses should be aware that angry behavior or hostile remarks from significant others may be expressions of fear and anxiety, or a plea for help. The desire to escape, outbursts of anger, and feelings of helplessness are often verbalized by significant others during the intrapartal period. Nurses should include significant others in their family assessment, plan appropriate helping interventions, and use continuous evaluations to enhance the experiences of all members of the childbearing family.

Fathers have proved helpful, comforting, and reassuring to their wives during labor and delivery (Campbell and Worthington, 1982). As supporting others, fathers are involved in the intrapartum period as:

1. Patient advocates.
2. Support givers, providing comfort measures such as pillows, ice chips, and back rubs.
3. Company during the labor process.
4. Coparticipants in a joyful life event.

These supportive behaviors of the father have been classified into three categories.

1. Physical care actions.
2. Nonverbal supportive actions (such as hand-holding, smiling, and kissing).
3. Verbal care (such as coaching, encouraging relaxation, and complimenting) (Jensen, Benson, and Bobak, 1981).

The nurse supports significant others as a member of the family unit. Support and care reinforces the value of the significant other's role and validates the supporting position. Regardless of the degree of involvement fathers or supporting others desire, their needs include adequate orientation to the labor and delivery area and procedures, respect as active participants in the intrapartum or as caring support persons, praise for helpful actions, and teaching of patient comfort measures throughout the labor and delivery. Supporting others should always be kept well informed about the progress of the labor and delivery.

The Oakland County Lamaze Association (1982) suggests that nurses can help significant others feel more comfortable and can plan nursing interventions to assist the entire family throughout the intrapartum by:

1. Introducing themselves to both patient and support person.
2. Adjusting the room environment to promote relaxation.
3. Encouraging reasonable decision making and self-care.
4. Praising the efforts of mother and coach.
5. Encouraging the coach to praise the mother.
6. Demonstrating comfort measures.
7. Allowing the coach to assume care according to his or her individual desires.

The nurse uses professional judgment to assess the supporting other's need for relief or nourishment. The nurse can facilitate the support person's separation from the laboring patient by replacing the significant other during the relief period and validating for the family the importance of meeting self-care needs during the intrapartal period.

Emotional and Psychologic Considerations

Along with physiologic assessment of the mother during labor, psychosocial care to the woman and her significant others is an important responsibility of the nurse. Assessment of the emotional stressors of the intrapartal period, for all the labor participants, and recognition of and attention to specific stressors are the appropriate concerns of the intrapartum nurse.

Clark and Affonso (1979) suggest the following important psychosocial concerns of maternity patients and families during the intrapartal experience:

1. *Concerns about self and identity.* Childbirth can be a positive or negative experience for any woman and her family. The perceived meaning of the event, expectations of the participants, and feedback received may vary and will contribute to the overall intrapartum experience. In perspective, the childbearing experience can strengthen or weaken the self-concept and ego strength of the participants.
2. *Role expectations.* Personal expectations of a woman and her significant others are defined by self, culture, and family. Conflict and stress result from discrepancies between role expectations and role performance, and are demonstrated as increased anxiety in the woman and her significant others.
3. *Anxiety and the wish for control over events.* These concerns are common throughout the intrapartal period. Concerns center around fear for self and for the child. These fears are exacerbated by strange environments, lack of knowledge, fear of the unknown, and the normal discomforts of the labor and delivery experiences.
4. *Sensory alteration.* Sensory overload is caused by the physiologic manifestations of labor and delivery and by environmental stressors. Sensory deprivation arises from the interruption of usual routines, the decrease in sensory stimulation in the environment, and the social isolation of the setting.
5. *Feelings of loss.* The woman and her significant others fear loss of the baby, of expectations,

of values, and of some aspects of the self (e.g. body image, self-esteem, and former roles).

6. *Perceptions of crisis.* Intrapartum is a period of increased stress, predisposing the emerging family to crisis.

Within this framework, the nurse interacts with the intrapartal family to mediate stress and facilitate optimal adaptation to the childbearing event. The nurse responds to the feelings and behaviors of the laboring patient during the different phases of labor and provides appropriate nursing interventions.

Latent Phase Labor
This part of labor can cause mild anxiety in the woman and her significant others. They are excited and ready to learn. The nurse's role is to assess client expectations and perceptions about labor and delivery, identify knowledge deficits and fears, and offer whatever anticipatory guidance is required. Nurses assess the support a woman wants and expects throughout the labor and delivery. Nurses use interviewing techniques and observation to assess needs and make nursing diagnoses during latent phase labor. Actions are planned and implemented that (1) facilitate trust, (2) promote relaxation, (3) provide support, (4) teach specific knowledge, (5) create a comfortable environment, and (6) meet hygiene needs of the client (Reeder, Mastroianni, and Martin, 1983). Nurses should be accepting and supportive in their approach. They should offer encouragement, be empathetic, and establish rapport and positive communication patterns during the latent phase to establish a basis for optimal care as the labor progresses.

Active Phase Labor
Active phase labor is characterized by increasing anxiety levels. Women need the nurse to help rationalize the stressors and the treatment, to reinforce previous teaching, and to offer continued anticipatory guidance as transition approaches (Clark and Affonso, 1979). The use of gentle touch and counterpressure techniques and selective positioning is helpful during active-phase labor (Saltenes, 1962; Jensen, Benson, and Bobak, 1981). But the most important of all interventions for most women is the assured presence of the nurse at the bedside. To stay with a woman during labor and offer support and reassurance to her and her family is an important nursing role.

Transitional Phase Labor
As transition approaches, client anxiety increases rapidly. Significant others experience fear and anxiety along with the laboring woman. Both the family and client experience narrowing of their perceptions. Nurses should teach in brief sessions during this transition phase, with emphasis on enhancing coping skills (Clark and Affonso, 1979). Nurses should try to convey empathy and understanding, respect and caring throughout this period. During transition women are tired, irritable, and uncomfortable. It is suggested that one nurse follow the woman through labor and delivery to minimize environmental changes and facilitate development of trust (Jensen, Benson, and Bobak, 1981). Decreasing anxiety, increasing relaxation, and facilitating coping are the primary nursing goals of the transition period.

Second Stage: Delivery
Nurses can offer support and comfort as delivery is completed. During this time the nurse encourages the patient to push or not to push, depending on the readiness of the cervix, and carefully monitors the condition of the mother and baby. Maximizing the patient's comfort by adjusting her position on the delivery table and providing an opportunity for the new family to interact together are major nursing priorities during the delivery period.

Third Stage: Delivery of the Placenta
During the delivery of the placenta, the nurse tells the woman and her significant others what is happening and encourages the patient to use her breathing techniques to cope with the discomforts of this stage. The nurse promotes opportunities for interaction with the infant during this stage, both for the value of the interaction itself and for purposes of diversion.

Fourth Stage: Postpartum
During the immediate postpartum period, many women express dramatic emotional release. This expression might appear as crying, anger, or feelings of helplessness (Reeder, Mastroianni, and Martin, 1983). A nurse reassures the woman that feelings and expressions of this sort are common in the immediate postpartum period and that she and the baby are being well cared for. Special attention to comfort measures meets the woman's dependency needs of this period and helps her to meet

the newborn's needs in the days to come. Some women demonstrate "sleep hunger" in the immediate postpartum period and can be assisted to rest and relax.

Most women review the events of the labor and delivery process during the immediate postpartum, to define the personal meaning of their experiences. The nurse helps by listening and filling in forgotten or missing pieces of information. Also, the woman and her family can be assisted to "claim the baby" during this period. If the status of the mother and child allow it, the nurse can facilitate opportunities for the new family to interact and begin the process of learning to love one another. Many women breastfeed for the first time during the immediate postpartum period.

A Summary of Behaviors and Interventions

Table 17–1 summarizes the feelings, behaviors, anxiety levels, pain experiences, and coping mechanisms of the patient as well as nursing interventions for the four stages of labor.

TABLE 17–1. *Impact and Coping During Human Labor and Birth: A Guide for Professional Nursing Care*

Stage		Nursing Interventions
First stage: **Latent phase of labor**	Onset of contractions to 4 cm Mean: Primipara—8.6 hours Multipara—5.3 hours	
Beginning: Onset of contractions to 3 cm		
Feelings of patient	High energy and activity. Happy with admission—eagerly waiting for labor. Contentment—relief that pregnancy is over. Generally tired of being pregnant.	1. Excellent time for assessment of expectations, attitudes, past experiences, what she's been told or heard, fears, and anxieties. 2. Set atmosphere positively. Explain routines, procedures.
Common behaviors	Smiling, talking, laughing, comfortable. Spontaneous expression of feelings. Focus on others besides self—e.g. mate, family. Healthy use of defenses.	3. Excellent time for teaching; patient alert and retains. Clarify misconceptions and what to expect, how to help self, use of breathing techniques. 4. Involve patient in care; give her decision-making power. 5. Manipulate environment; control stressors.
Impact of labor: 1. Anxiety level	Mild. Alert: sees, hears, attends, retains information well. Anxiety enhances learning: can observe, describe, analyze, make decisions, evaluate.	
2. Pain experience	Patient's pain tolerance (PPT) high; minimal physiologic effects of contractions. Factors to lower PPT: traumatic admission events; environmental factors creating stress; fears, attitudes, lack of significant support.	
3. Coping mechanisms	Laughing, crying, increased talking, sleep, increased activity, daydreaming, rocking, efforts to gain approval; exercises self-discipline; demonstrates pride; desires to make decisions.	

TABLE 17-1. Continued

Stage			Nursing Interventions
Ending: 4 cm			
Feelings of patient		Contractions are more threatening.	1. Explain purpose of contractions (why they are becoming more stressful and threatening).
		Compares feelings during contractions with past experiences of discomfort.	
		Increased preoccupation with threats, especially contractions.	2. Explain what feelings are expected and which bodily sensations will be experienced during contractions.
		Anxious and apprehensive about what is to come.	
Common behaviors		Verbalizes feelings of helplessness during contractions.	3. Use distraction to tackle pain.
		Can still relate to others, family.	4. Accept coping behaviors, even if patient is hostile.
		Autonomic stress responses: flush, increased respiration, nausea, vomiting, pallor, dry mouth, diaphoresis.	5. Offer anticipatory guidance regarding rupture of membranes; frequency, intensity, duration of contractions; increased pressure in perineum.
Impact of labor:			
1. Anxiety level		Anxiety increases to moderate.	
		Perceptual field narrows—hears, sees, grasps less.	
		Selective attention and inattention (especially to time and contractions).	
		Can focus when given direction.	
		Beginning fears of isolation if left alone.	
2. Pain experience		PPT lowered by physiologic effects of contractions; dilatation; effacement; descent.	
		Uses word *pain* to describe contractions.	
		Increased verbalizations of pain and discomfort.	
3. Coping mechanisms		Skeletal muscle responses to communicate plea for help—grimace, clenched fists, restlessness, rigidity, facial expressions.	
		Aggressive, hostile behaviors (means to maintain self-control).	
		May depreciate others to save control of self.	
		May not always give verbal cues for help.	
First stage:		3–4 cm to 8 cm	
Active phase of labor		Mean: Primipara—4.9 hours	
		Multipara—2.2 hours	
3–8 cm			
Feelings of patient		Serious, determined, weary.	1. Take measures to promote relaxation.
		Upset when routines involve restrictions (nothing by mouth, bedpan, bedrest).	2. Organize care for decreased disturbance to patient.
		May not want to be disturbed (vital signs, FHTs, vaginal exams).	3. Meet dependency needs.
			4. Provide comfort measures to

continued

TABLE 17–1. Continued

Stage			Nursing Interventions
Common behaviors		Less talking; dependency needs manifested. Breathing labored; hyperventilation. Preoccupation with self. Increased diaphoresis; sympathetic autonomic responses continue and increase discomforts. Restless; unable to assume comfortable position. Autonomic behaviors not requiring thought; regression.	relieve discomforts of sympathetic autonomic nervous system. 5. Speak in short sentences, phrases. 6. Decrease feeling of abandonment by increasing contact time with patient. 7. Provide pain relief measures; follow physician orders for pain medication; use less distraction. 8. Begin teaching of what to do for second stage, and practice.
Impact of labor			
	1. Anxiety level	Increases from moderate to severe. Rapid reduction of perceptual field—possibility of distortion; decreased attention span. Increased focus on scattered detail, especially contractions, pain, time. Difficulty with hearing, retaining, and making connections. Fear of abandonment. Anxiety—specific fears for self, baby, of unknown.	
	2. Pain experience	Increased factors to lower PPT: frequency, intensity, duration of contractions; descent, dilatation; pressure, asphyxia of muscles; fatigue; increased fears, anxiety. Increased attention to pain. Difficult to distract; desires immediate pain relief.	
	3. Coping mechanisms	Cannot rely on own resources to cope; cries for "wanting something." Behaviors oriented toward immediate pain relief. Behaviors range from hostility to depression to withdrawal to regression. Frequent demands or praise for others to sustain human contact. May complain of tremors during contractions. Beginning behaviors of losing self-control.	
First stage: **Transitional phase of labor**		Mean: Primipara—0.9 hours Multipara—0.2 hours	
8–10 cm			
Feelings of patient		Focus on self only. Exhausted; wants to give up; feels like she can't go on. Increased sensations in perineum.	1. Do less talking, explaining to patient. 2. Do not expect patient to respond to you as previously.

TABLE 17–1. Continued

Stage		Nursing Interventions
Common behaviors	Beads of perspiration on forehead. Shaking, chills, nausea, vomiting. Restless. Lowered response to environment, difficult to get her attention.	3. Stay with patient as much as possible. 4. Increase positive reinforcement for efforts. 5. Repeat instructions for managing contractions with *each* contraction.
Impact of labor: 1. Anxiety level	Severe to panic state. Details blown out of proportion—contractions, pain, death fears. Difficult to get attention; decreased attention span. Decreased ability to make decisions. Increasing fear.	
2. Pain experience	Increased stimuli for sensory overload, pain; sensations on perineum, increased vaginals, VS, FHT. Pain of contractions a big threat. Pain appears constant. Difficulty to differentiate intervals between contractions.	
3. Coping mechanisms	Conservation of energy for self-preservation; increased withdrawal from environment; amnesic between contractions; transitory episodes of unrealistic thinking (i.e. regarding time, person, place). May demoralize self or others to prevent panic.	
Second stage Mean:	Primipara—0.9 hours Multipara—0.3 hours	
Feelings of patient	Fatigue continues. Uncontrollable feelings regarding desire to defecate, fear of making mess.	
Common behaviors	Exhausted. Cannot safeguard self against injury. Minimal reactions between contractions. Restlessness during contractions. Amnesic episodes.	
Impact of labor: 1. Anxiety level	Moderate to severe panic. Difficulty to attend to commands to push or not to push; decreasing ability to work with labor process.	
2. Pain experience	Pain stimulus mainly operating on interpretation of pain and effects of fatigue. May desire to have infant removed or to die to escape pain experience.	

continued

TABLE 17–1. Continued

Stage		Nursing Interventions
3. Coping mechanisms	Verbal remarks reflect loss of coping—"I can't", "Take it out", "I want to die". Aggressive behaviors: clawing nurse, vulgar comments, may be last attempt to prevent ego dysfunction. Behaviors to conserve energy continue—withdrawal, etc.	
Third–Fourth stages	Median: 10 min 5–30 min	
Feelings of patient	Focus on others—baby, husband. Sense of relief, excitement.	
Common behaviors	Dozing, sleeping, talking, crying. Increased attention to environment.	
Impact of labor:		
1. Anxiety level	Decreased—mild to moderate. Alert—sees, hears, grasps well. Increased attention to environment. Factors that increase anxiety are: fears for baby and self, expectations unmet, guilt feelings about behaviors during labor.	
2. Pain experience	Physiologic pain source decreased. Pain experience augmented by increased anxiety: threats to ego during labor; punitive remarks received regarding behaviors; isolation, alienation during labor.	
3. Coping mechanisms	Talkative, laughing, crying. Healthy use of defenses again. Frequent questions—seeking pieces to find a meaningful whole. Data collection regarding own behaviors. Apologizing for behaviors. Focus on baby—wants to see; questions appearance; tests reality of event. Focus on family—husband and siblings, relative reactions.	

SOURCE: Modified from Clark and Affonso (1979).

The Use of Touch

Therapeutic touch has been recognized as a helpful, necessary element of health care since the nineteenth century. The "laying on of hands" helps patients maintain or achieve good health (Saltenes, 1962; Reeder, Mastroianni, and Martin, 1983). Most women respond positively to gentle touch during the intrapartal period (Jensen, Benson, and Bobak, 1981). Therapeutic touch can help establish rapport, enhance communication, and demonstrate concern or empathy when verbal communication is difficult or impossible (Reeder, Mastroianni, and Martin, 1983). Therapeutic touch nursing behaviors include back rubs, hand-holding, and brow-stroking.

Although there is little scientific data on the subject, a recent study showed that maternity patients could work with their contractions more effectively if they experienced extensive physical contact. This ability decreased as contact was withdrawn (Saltenes, 1962; Reeder, Mastroianni, and Martin, 1983).

Many techniques from prepared childbirth classes clearly depend on the use of gentle touch—for example, effleurage and counterpressure. However, these and other forms of gentle touch must be used with discrimination, especially as labor progresses. Some women express the desire *not* to be touched during the latter phases of active labor (Jensen, Benson, and Bobak, 1981).

THE NURSE'S ROLE IN EXAMINATIONS

General Role

Routine assessments of temperature, pulse, and respirations (TPR) are done every 2–4 hours during the intrapartal period. In cases of maternal fever, prolonged rupture of membranes, or long labors, TPR may be ordered as often as every hour. Blood pressure readings are ordered every 2–4 hours. A complete assessment including a history and a physical examination is done by the physician soon after the woman is admitted to the labor and delivery suite.

Assessment of the Uterus

Fetal size, position, attitude, and presentation are estimated by abdominal palpation using Leopold's maneuvers (see Chapter 15). Fetal heart rate and uterine contraction patterns are also assessed. The nurse offers the woman an opportunity to urinate prior to the abdominal assessment and offers anticipatory guidance about each part of the exam to mediate anxiety and fear.

Rectal and Vaginal Examinations

Nurses and physicians perform rectal and vaginal examinations during the intrapartal period to assess the dilatation and effacement of the cervix, as well as the position and station of the fetal presenting part. For either exam, the patient lies in a supine position, with her knees flexed. A drape is placed over her chest and abdomen and is wrapped around her legs to provide warmth and privacy. The examiner wears a sterile glove for the vaginal exam and then may also perform a rectal examination.

The vaginal exam has essentially replaced the rectal exam, since its safety has been substantiated (Jensen, Benson, and Bobak, 1981). For a vaginal exam, the vulvar area is cleansed using an antiseptic preparation. Sterile gloves are used, and two lubricated fingers are gently introduced into the vagina. Cervical effacement and dilatation and fetal fontaneles, station, and presentation can be directly assessed by palpation. After completion of the vaginal exam, the perianal area is cleansed and dried and the examiner disposes of the gloves and washes hands.

For a rectal exam, two lubricated gloved fingers are gently introduced into the rectum. The cervix and fetal presenting part can be palpated through the anterior rectal wall, and dilatation, effacement, presentation, and station can be inferred. After the procedure is completed, the woman's perianal area is washed and dried. The examiner disposes of the glove, and washes hands carefully.

Sterile water is often used as a lubricant in vaginal exams conducted prior to rupture of fetal membranes, because some lubricating gels may alter the response of nitrazine paper. Nitrazine paper is used to assess the vaginal pH, to determine whether fetal membranes have ruptured. Vaginal exams are contraindicated for women with unusual vaginal bleeding.

TECHNOLOGY

Maternity nursing has been dramatically affected by the advances of supporting technologies. Electronic fetal monitoring alone has changed the role of the maternity nurse.

Care of the Patient as Opposed to Care of the Machine

Early fears that fetal monitoring would cause a tendency to nurse the machine rather than the patient have not been borne out (McDonough, Sheriff, and Simmel, 1981; Reeder, Mastroianni, and Martin, 1983). A woman in labor needs to feel that she is being given attention as a person and not as an appendage of the monitoring equipment (Clark and Affonso, 1979).

In reality, fetal monitoring has freed the nurse

from repetitive tasks and given increased opportunity for individualized and comprehensive nursing care in maternity settings (Reeder, Mastroianni, and Martin, 1983). As a result of the widespread use of electronic fetal monitoring, maternity nurses:

1. Are functioning in expanded roles as primary caregivers to monitored patients.
2. Are offering increased parent education and counseling to families using monitors.
3. Have identified mother, fetus, and supporting others as the nursing clients.
4. Make independent assessments of fetal well-being and distress.
5. Initiate early treatment for abnormal monitor tracings.
6. Have become increasingly necessary (one on one) throughout the period of labor and delivery.

Special Patient Considerations

Electronic fetal monitoring is well received by husbands and significant others during labor and delivery. Frequently, the support person is fascinated with the monitor, a fact that is sometimes irritating to the laboring woman (Clark and Affonso, 1979; McDonough, Sheriff, and Simmel, 1981). The nurse demonstrates an ability to evaluate contractions from the patient's perspective, not only as they appear on the monitor; thus, the nurse assures the woman of continued supportive care throughout the labor and delivery.

Some women and their families are anxious about fetal monitoring procedures. When anxiety is identified, nursing interventions can be planned to mediate or modify the anxiety level. Patients should be taught what electronic fetal monitoring is, why it is being used for them, how it is applied, and what the data mean. Patients are less anxious if they understand the basic concepts of the monitoring procedure.

A second nursing concern for the monitored patient is pain relief and coping, which become more difficult for some monitored patients because of the anxiety, fear, and the loss of freedom of movement they experience (Clark and Affonso, 1979). Nurses can plan careful assessments of pain and coping, as well as measures to reduce the fear associated with the monitoring procedure (see Chapter 18).

ASSESSMENT OF FETAL DISTRESS

Acute fetal distress is compromised fetal well-being resulting from the recurring stress of uterine contractions during labor or from umbilical cord compression. The signs of fetal distress include persistent acceleration of the fetal heart rate, eventual deceleration of heart rate that continues between uterine contractions, or meconium in the amniotic fluid in a vertex presentation (Hon, 1976). Data from electronic fetal monitors is extremely helpful in diagnosing acute fetal distress.

A systematic approach must be used to assess and interpret electronic fetal monitor data and to correlate the data with clinical events (Hon, 1976; Reeder, Mastroianni, and Martin, 1983). Data about fetal heart rate are evaluated first for baseline rate, and then for beat-to-beat variability. Episodes of tachycardia or bradycardia are described relative to the baseline heart rate. The baseline fetal heart rate levels increase as the fetus matures, indicating maturation of the fetal autonomic nervous system. Accelerations of the baseline rate can result from maternal fever, fetal hypoxia, or early fetal acidosis. Decreases in baseline rate are most often associated with fetal congestive heart failure, congenital heart defects, or longstanding fetal hypoxia.

Beat-to-beat variability is seen as a fine, irregular line on the normal fetal heart tracing from an internal fetal monitor (see Fig. 17-5). Normal beat-to-beat variability (greater than 5 bpm) implies an intact fetal central nervous system. Lower levels (3-5 bpm) of variability suggest depressed CNS activity in the fetus. Variability of 0-2 bpm is considered ominous. Use of drugs to relieve the pain of labor causes diminished or absent beat-to-beat variability of the fetal heart rate (FHR) (Martin and Gingerich, 1976; Reeder, Mastroianni, and Martin, 1983).

Assessment of Uterine Contraction Tracings

In external monitoring procedures, the frequency and duration of uterine contractions can be determined from tracings by observing the increment, acme, and decrement of each uterine contraction. With internal monitoring procedures, exact uterine pressures may be calculated. *Baseline tonus* is measured as the height of the baseline between the contractions. Amplitude of the contractions is

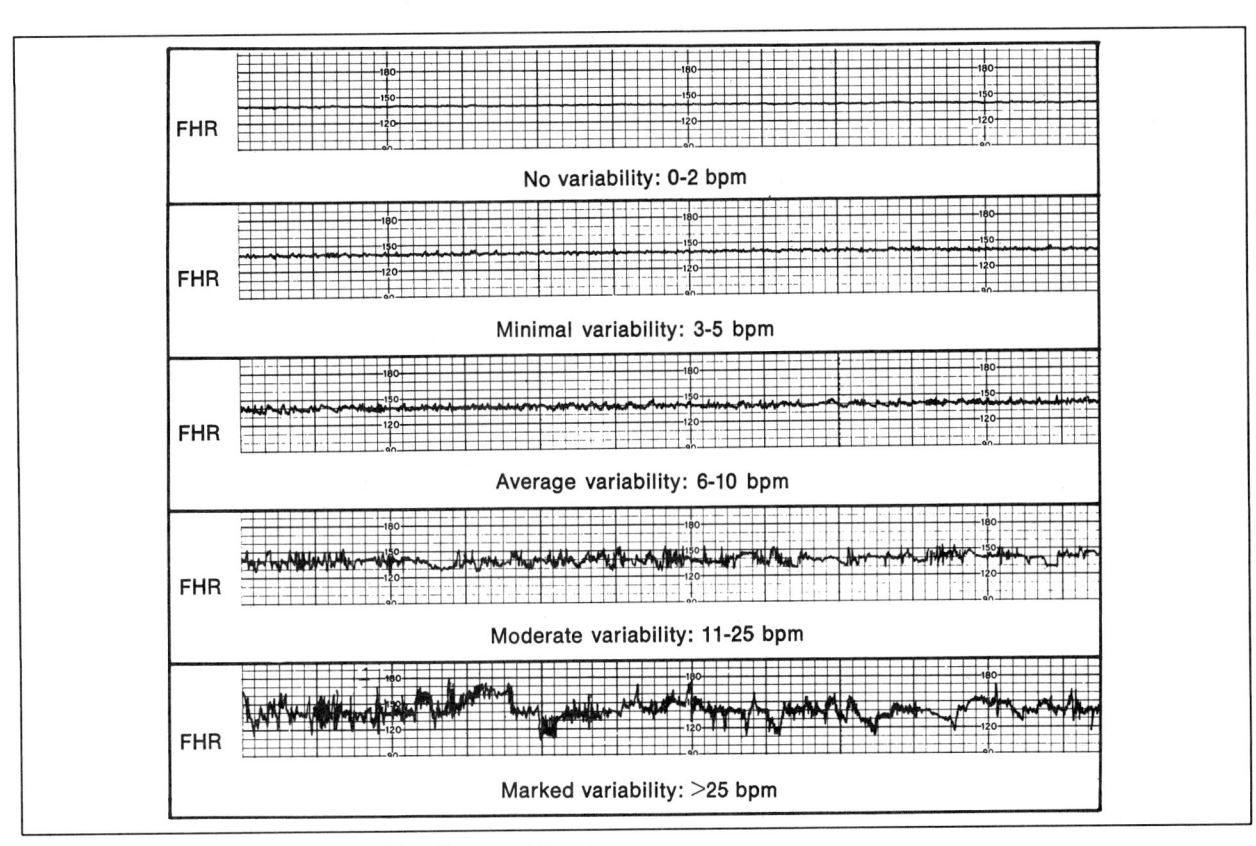

FIGURE 17-5. Fetal heart rate variability. Short- and long-term variability tend to increase and decrease together.
SOURCE: Tucker (1978).

measured at the acme and can range from 30 to 75 mm Hg. *Hypotonic labor* is the term used to describe low levels of uterine contractions. *Hypertonic labor* is indicated when the amplitude of the uterine pressure exceeds 75 mm Hg, when uterine contractions occur more often than every 2 min, or when contractions last for longer than 90 sec. Hypertonic labor can be the result of excessive amounts of oxytocin, placental abruption, or uterine dysfunction. Any deviations from normal should be reported promptly.

Fetal well-being during labor is assessed by correlating changes in the FHR with uterine contraction patterns to look for periodic changes. In normal labor, the FHR remains between 120 and 160, with normal variability, during the uterine contractions. Changes in the FHR that occur during uterine contractions are described as *accelerations* or *decelerations* of FHR. Accelerations can also be *nonperiodic*, occurring during periods of fetal movement.

Periodic accelerations of FHR occur during uterine contractions and are defined as increases in the FHR greater than 15 bpm for longer than 15 sec. Generally, periodic accelerations are considered within normal limits. The ability of a healthy fetus to accelerate the heart rate with movement is the basis of several prenatal tests of fetal well-being (see Chapter 13).

Periodic decelerations can be early, late, or variable in onset, when compared to the uterine contraction patterns. *Early decelerations* appear on the strip graph as a wave form that coincides with the uterine contraction wave. This type of deceleration pattern is most often associated with fetal head compression during contractions. The characteristic wave tracing shows a deceleration of uniform shape, short duration, and low amplitude (seldom dropping below 100 bpm) (Krebs et al., 1982). No nursing action is required for early periodic decelerations (see Fig. 17-6).

Late decelerations appear on the strip graph as a uniform wave with consistently late onset in relationship to the uterine contraction pattern. FHR recovery time is also delayed. This pattern may occur completely within the normal FHR

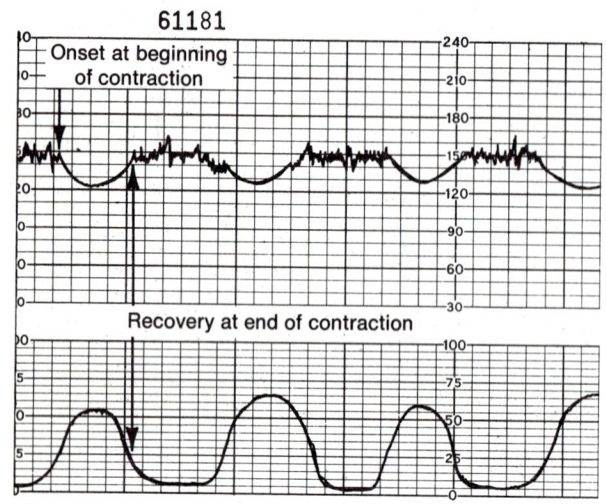

FIGURE 17–6. Early deceleration (head compression).
SOURCE: Tucker (1978).

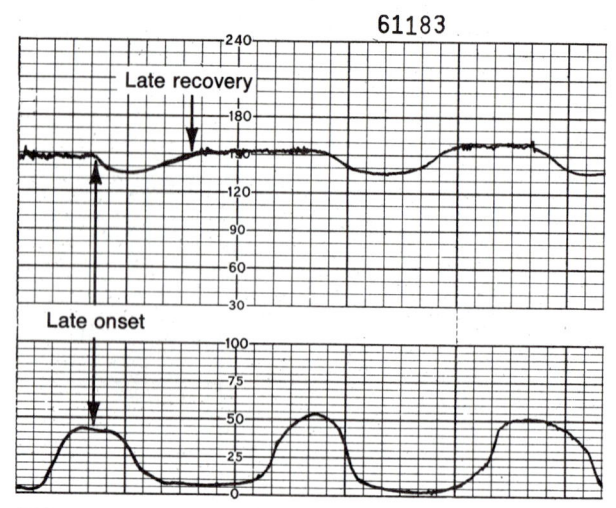

FIGURE 17–7. Late deceleration (uteroplacental insufficiency).
SOURCE: Tucker (1978).

range and yet be ominous (Hon, 1976). Etiology is direct fetal hypoxia due to reduced oxygen exchange from the placenta.

Transient decelerations may be associated with maternal hypotension. Correcting the maternal hypotension usually results in fetal recovery. Persistent patterns of late decelerations of fetal heart rate indicate fetal distress (see Fig. 17–7). Nursing indications in fetal distress include the following actions:

1. Discontinue all oxytocin stimulation of labor.
2. Change the maternal position from back to side-lying (preferably left lateral).
3. Administer oxygen by face mask at 10 liters.
4. Increase the flow rate of the primary intravenous solution (not oxytocin).
5. Continue to support the client and family at the bedside.
6. Report the situation promptly.

Variable decelerations appear on the strip graph as irregular wave forms that have an inconsistent relationship to the uterine contraction pattern. Variable decelerations are the most common FHR deviation in labor (Reeder, Mastroianni, and Martin, 1983). The etiology is thought to be a reflex response to compression of the umbilical cord during labor and delivery. Variable decelerations are labeled mild, moderate, or severe depending on the degree of deceleration of the FHR (see Fig. 17–8). Nursing actions for variable decelerations include:

1. Changing the mother's position to left side-lying, knee-chest, or right side-lying.
2. Administering oxygen by face mask at 10 liters.
3. Discontinuing oxytocin.
4. Continuing emotional support to the family.
5. Notifying the physician.

Periodic Fetal Scalp Blood Sampling

Periodic fetal scalp blood sampling measures fetal blood pH and is useful in determining the well-being of the fetus. The test is used to diagnose fetal distress. The normal pH of fetal blood is 7.25–7.35, with a mild progressive decline throughout labor. A pH of 7.20 or below indicates fetal hypoxia and acidosis. Two such readings suggest the need to deliver the infant immediately (Freeman and Garite, 1981; Reeder, Mastroianni, and Martin, 1983). Compromised fetal pH readings (below 7.15) correlate with abnormal FHR and low Apgar scores in newborns (Paul and Petrie, 1973; Clark and Affonso, 1979).

Fetal scalp blood sampling is an invasive procedure that requires ruptured fetal membranes and cervical dilatation of 3–4 cm. The fetal presenting part must also be fixed in the pelvis. The nurse assists the woman to lithotomy position in a well-lighted room. The patient is draped, and a sterile technique is maintained throughout the procedure. The physician uses a lighted amnioscope to visualize the fetal scalp. The scalp is cleansed with an antiseptic solution, dried, and

The Nurse's Role During the Intrapartal Period 377

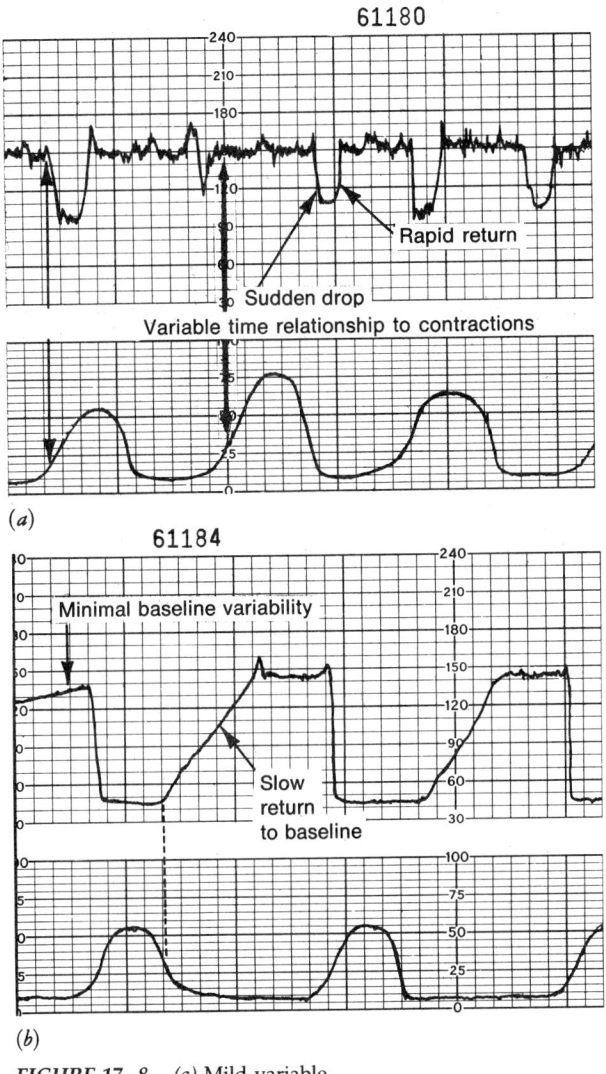

FIGURE 17-8. (a) Mild variable deceleration (cord compression). (b) Severe variable deceleration (cord compression).
SOURCE: Tucker (1978).

vaginal bleeding in the mother and FHR in the infant. A sustained increase in vaginal bleeding or persistent fetal tachycardia is ominous and must be reported promptly.

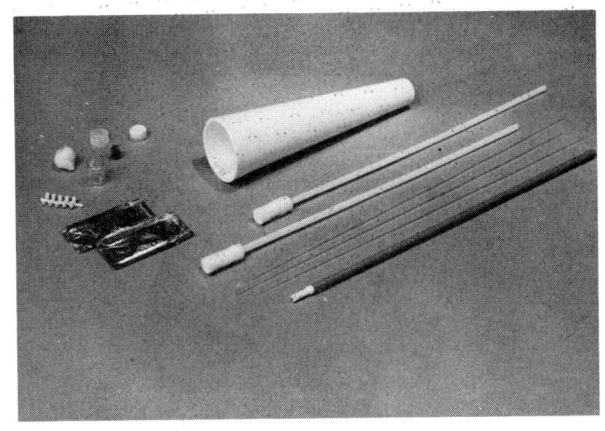

FIGURE 17-9. Fetal scalp kit. Contents include funnel, blade, capillary tubes, antiseptic, and silicon gel.

sprayed with a silicone preparation, to facilitate "beading" of the blood sample. The scalp puncture is made with a small metal blade. The sample is collected into a long capillary tube. The blood is mixed, sealed, and iced, and sent immediately to the laboratory for fetal pH. The test results are usually available within 20 min. A fetal scalp kit is shown in Fig. 17-9 and Fig. 17-10 shows fetal pH machine.

After the sampling procedure, the nurse plans care with consideration to known postprocedure risks to the fetus. Postprocedure risks include: (1) continued scalp bleeding, (2) ecchymosis, (3) hematoma, and (4) risk of infection at the wound site. The nurse should carefully assess postprocedural

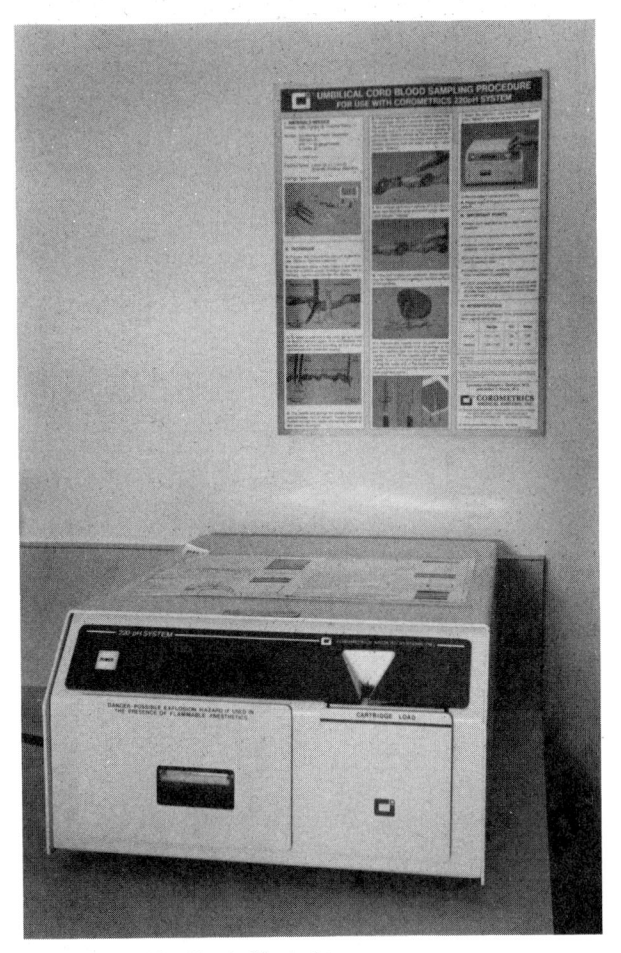

FIGURE 17-10. Fetal pH machine.

Occasionally, altered fetal blood pH is secondary to maternal pH changes. Simultaneous blood sampling for pH for mother and fetus will specify diagnosis and treatment.

SUMMARY

The nurse plays a primary role in the assessment of and support to the childbearing family throughout the intrapartal period. Nurses use both traditional and contemporary assessment methods to monitor the progress of labor and identify stressors to the mother, fetus, and significant others. In addition to noting the physiologic realities of labor and delivery, the nurse is aware of the emotional and psychologic stressors of the client family. Using positive communication techniques, gentle touch, and observation skills, the nurse assesses the client, makes appropriate nursing diagnoses, sets goals and criteria, plans interventions, acts to mediate stressors, and evaluates the care given. The nurse is careful to direct care to the patient and family, not to the many technical devices surrounding the emerging family in the modern labor and delivery suite. Special procedures to evaluate fetal distress are incorporated into the nursing care when appropriate. Attention is given to education and support to the family regarding all procedures and treatments. The overall goal of nursing care of the family during intrapartum is to facilitate optimum adaptation to the childbearing experience, an important goal for an important moment in time.

REFERENCES

Campbell, A., and Worthington, E. L. 1982. Teaching expectant fathers how to be better childbirth coaches. *MCN.* 7:28.

Clark, A. L., and Affonso, D. D. 1979. *Childbearing: A nursing perspective.* Philadelphia: F. A. Davis.

Freeman, R. K., and Garite, F. J. 1981. *Fetal heart rate monitoring.* Baltimore: Williams & Wilkins.

Hodnett, E. 1982. Patient control during labor. Effects of two types of fetal monitors. *J. Obstet. Gynecol. Neonatal Nurs.* 11:94.

Hon, E. H. 1976. *An introduction to fetal heart rate monitoring.* 2nd ed. Los Angeles, Calif.: University of Southern California School of Medicine.

Jensen, M. D.; Benson, R. C.; and Bobak, I. M. 1981. *Maternity care: The nurse and the family.* St. Louis: C. V. Mosby.

Krebs, H. B.; Petree, R. E.; Dunn, L. J.; and Smith, P. J. 1982. Intrapartum fetal heart rate monitoring. *Am. J. Obstet. Gynecol.* 142(3):297.

Martin, C. B., and Gingerich, B. 1976. Factors affecting the fetal heart rate: Genesis of FHR patterns. *J. Obstet. Gynecol. Neonatal Nurs.* 5(5):305.

McDonough, M.; Sheriff, D.; and Simmel, P. 1981. Parents' responses to fetal monitoring. *MCN.* 6:32.

NAACOG. 1980. The nurse's role in electronic fetal monitoring. Technical Bulletin No. 7.

Neutra, R. R.; Rienberg, S. E.; and Griedman, E. A. 1978. The effect of fetal monitoring on neonatal death rates. *New Engl. J. Med.* 299:324.

Oakland Country Lamaze Association. 1982. *Supporting laboring patients.* Oakland County, Mich.: Lamaze Association.

Paul, R. H., and Petrie, R. H. 1973. *Fetal intensive care: Current concepts.* Los Angeles, Calif.: University of Southern California School of Medicine.

Perez, R. H. 1981. Fetal monitoring. In *Protocols for perinatal nursing practice.* St. Louis: C. V. Mosby.

Reeder, S. J.; Mastroianni, L.; and Martin, L. L. 1983. *Maternity nursing.* 15th ed. Philadelphia: J. B. Lippincott.

Saltenes, S. J. 1962. *Physical touch and nursing support in labor.* Unpublished Master's Thesis, Yale University.

Tucker, S. M. 1978. *Fetal monitoring and fetal assessment in high-risk pregnancy.* St. Louis: C. V. Mosby.

18

Comfort Management During Labor and Delivery

BEHAVIORAL OBJECTIVES

Upon completion of this chapter, the reader should be able to:

- Discuss the significance of current theories of pain mechanisms and relationship to discomfort in childbirth.

- Identify factors that influence pain perception in labor.

- Describe physiologic causes of pain in labor.

- Describe three approaches to relief of discomfort in labor.

- Describe the various types of analgesia and anesthesia used during labor and delivery, their indications and contraindications.

- Develop a plan of care based on the assessment of the alterations in comfort experienced during labor.

"Labor," "travail," "confinement," and "pain" are words that have been associated with childbirth for hundreds of years and have conveyed the notions of hard work, discomfort, and even punishment. Although our many cultures have expressed their values of childbirth and the role of women and men in family life in different ways, all acknowledge in some manner, changes in emotion and behavior during the childbirth process. Generally, all recognize and/or demonstrate that women do go through varying degrees of discomfort that we call pain.

Pain may be as undefinable and unmeasurable for the individual experiencing it as for the scientist studying it and the health care practitioner trying to control it. Pain has been defined as bodily suffering or distress due to injury or illness, as mental or emotional suffering or torment, and as a sensation of discomfort or suffering resulting from provocation of sensory nerves.

Pain is a personal experience, involving feelings and sensations. Thus, individuals can respond differently to the same sensory stimulus, which explains why one person may react strongly to a stimulus while another may not react at all. Even though pain as a concept or as a neurophysiologic mediation may be difficult to describe for the individual who feels it, what remains is that pain hurts.

This chapter looks first at advances in pain research that provide a more thorough understanding of pain and at the factors that influence pain and pain control. Next it considers pain measurement, physiologic pain in labor, and the role of the health care provider, particularly the nurse, in the care of the woman during labor and delivery. Finally, it discusses the three approaches to relieve the discomfort of labor: pharmacologic, sensory modulation, and psychologic.

RESEARCH ON PAIN MECHANISMS

Early pain theories included the specificity theory and the theory of specific nerve energies. Both were based on the idea that specialized sensory receptors communicate specific senses (touch, cold, warmth, and pain) and that when these receptors are stimulated, messages are relayed to specific central areas in the brain. According to these theories, then, the experience of pain was determined by the receptor of the specific nerve innervated.

Each of these old concepts concerned a single isolated system of afferent signals and central cells which constituted *the* pain mechanism. The nervous system, however, is not recognized today as a series of separate compartments each designated to handle a single problem. The first new stage came, when in 1965, two Canadian scientists proposed a new theory for the mechanism of pain that has offered a new and broader insight into the nature of pain and has stimulated a surge of basic research and subsequent clinical applications. These scientists, Ronald Melzack, a psychiatrist, and Patrick Wall, a neurophysiologist, developed what is known as the gate control theory of pain.

Basically, their theory proposes that a neural mechanism in the dorsal horns of the spinal cord acts as a gate that may increase or decrease the flow of nerve impulses that come from peripheral fibers and travel through the central nervous system. Somatic input is subjected to the mediating influence of the gate before it evokes pain perception and response (Melzack and Wall, 1983). The degree to which the gate increases or decreases sensory transmission is determined by the activity of large-diameter or small-diameter fibers and by descending influences from the brain (see Figs. 18–1 and 18–2).

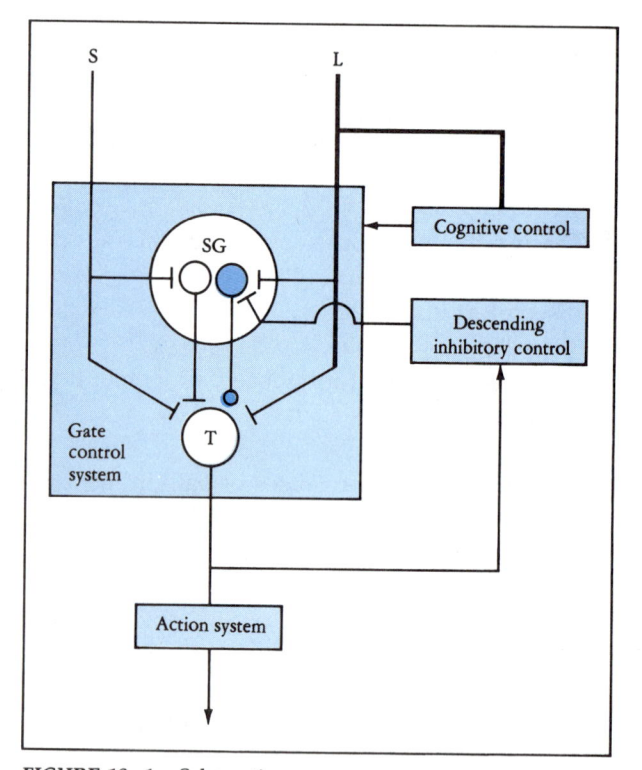

FIGURE 18–1. Schematic representation of the gate control theory. The large (L) and small (S) fibers project impulses to the substantia gelatinosa (SG) and first central transmission (T) cells in the spinal cord. The central control trigger is represented by a line running from the large-fiber system to central (cognitive) control mechanisms, which in turn project back to the gate control system. The gate tends to be closed by large-fiber stimuli, opened by small-fiber impulses, and modulated by descending fiber impulses.
SOURCE: Melzack and Wall (1983).

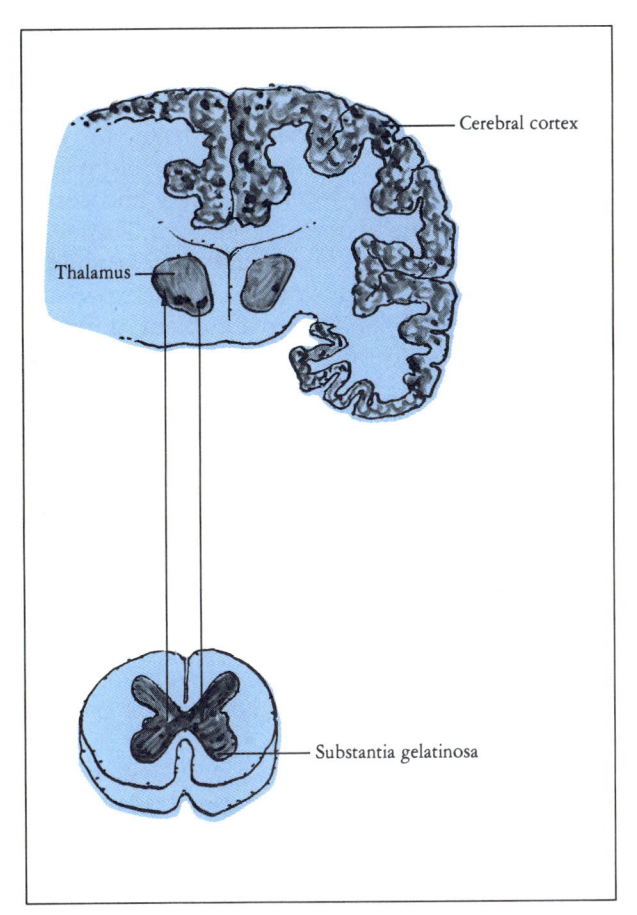

FIGURE 18–2. Simplified model of pain pathway in gate control theory. An unpleasant stimulus to the skin sends impulses to the gate in the substantia gelatinosa in the dorsal horn of the spinal cord. Impulses are then sent up the spinal cord to the brain. There, complex interactions between the thalamus and cerebral cortex take place, and a new message travels down the spinal cord. The "gate" is then opened or closed. The resulting action will then determine perception of pain.

Melzack and Wall proposed that pain phenomena are determined by interactions among the following three spinal cord systems:

1. The cells found in the substantia gelatinosa in the dorsal horn (the "gate").
2. The dorsal column fibers of the cord that project toward the brain (the central control trigger that activates brain processes).
3. The central transmission (T) cells in the dorsal horn (which activate the action system responsible for perception and response).

Although this theory has generated a great deal of excitement, controversy, and conflicting evidence, clinically it has been able to provide useful explanations for understanding and treating the person in pain.

One of the first effects of the gate control theory was to do away with the idea that pain is a simple sensation with a direct transmission line to a pain center. Instead, this new theory recognizes that pain is a complex phenomenon that is an integration of sensitivity-discriminative, affective-motivational, and cognitive dimensions. The spinal gating theory suggests that impulses travel along several pathways, both ascending and descending, carrying information that must be received, acted upon, and then processed at the "gate". Thus, lesions in any of the pathways, interference from additional sensory input such as pressure or temperature, and mental processes—including attentions, emotions, and expectations based on past experiences—may account for variations in the pain perception and response in the individual. A deep cut in the foot from a piece of glass may not be perceived as painful by an individual whose attention has been on the marathon race in which he is competing. Conversely, a gentle touch on the shoulder can trigger severe pain in someone who has neuralgia or who is very anxious.

This brief look at the pain research which has been done indicates that we still need new knowledge but, as practitioners, we must utilize the existing knowledge as effectively as possible. Pain remains to be what the patient tells us (s)he feels, and the test of our current pain theory, or framework, should result in a decrease or disappearance of this pain.

FACTORS INFLUENCING PAIN IN LABOR

Pain perception cannot be defined simply in terms of specific kinds of stimuli. In addition to the role played by such intrinsic factors as the physiologic and biochemical mechanisms influencing the intensity, duration, and pattern of contractions, the amount or degree of discomfort associated with childbirth is influenced by cultural, physical, psychological, and emotional factors.

Cultural Influences

From as far back as the Babylonians, early Egyptians, and Chinese, we have records of childbirth pain. The way an individual perceives, interprets, and responds to pain is intimately associated with cultural attitudes and values. Childbirth may be viewed as an illness or as a normal physiologic process, as an open sexual event or as an event calling for privacy or secrecy. It may represent achievement, something to be paid for in some way, or even the result of supernatural forces (Mead and Newton, 1967). The emotions and feelings aroused by these cultural attitudes influence the woman's pain perception and behavior in labor.

In some cultures, such as the Alor Islanders of Indonesia and the Jarara in South America, the labor process is viewed as a normal, painless experience (Newton and Newton, 1973). The Japanese, on the other hand, view birthing as uncomfortable and painful but bearable. No medication or herb is used, and the woman maintains a stoic, controlled manner throughout (Okamoto, 1978). The Filipino-American Woman, on the other hand, sees pain and labor as inseparable and childbirth as potentially life threatening (Affonso, 1978).

According to the gate control theory, cultural background affects both the pain perception threshold (the lowest stimulus value at which the person reports that the stimulus feels painful) and pain tolerance (the upper threshold at which the stimulus is tolerated). Thus, the cultural values that a person takes on and carries through life must be considered in any evaluation of pain.

Bonica (1984), in describing several extensive studies of women in labor conducted in six continents and over 40 years, reported that women, regardless of culture, varied with extent of discomfort perceived and exhibited. Even some of the women who did not show pain during childbirth, would afterwards describe the experience as painful. Statistically, the findings indicated that 15 percent of women studied had little or no pain, 35 percent had moderate pain, 30 percent had severe pain, and 20 percent had very severe pain.

Past Experience

Attitudes toward pain are acquired early in life. They are influenced first by the attitudes of parents and then by early experiences with pain itself, such as childhood accidents and illnesses or family and peer illnesses. The quality and quantity of these experiences, as well as the meaning of the situation associated with them, play an important role in pain perception and behavior in later years.

Psychologic Factors

Whether or not a person's attention is focused on a potentially painful experience will influence pain perception. The mere anticipation of pain may be sufficient to raise the level of anxiety and consequently the intensity of perceived pain. Dispelling anxiety or reassuring the person that he or she has control over the stimulus can cause the experience to be perceived as less painful. In addition, distracting attention away from pain or unpleasant stimuli, such as by talking, watching TV, or listening to music, may reduce the intensity of pain, particularly if the person can become interested or involved in the distracting activity.

Studies have demonstrated that persons who feel they have control over a pain-provoking situation, or at least certain aspects of the situation, report significantly less pain than those who do not know what to expect or how to cope with the pain (Jacox, 1977; Melzack and Wall, 1983). For example, it has been found that surgical patients who have been carefully prepared for and informed about the upcoming surgery and what to expect about postoperative routines request less medication and report less pain than patients who have not been so prepared.

The unique past history of the individual, the meaning he or she gives to the pain-producing situation, and his or her state of mind at the time, all influence the perceptual experience of pain. Other factors, such as age, sex, and socioeconomic status, have also been found in certain circumstances to influence pain perception. Depending on the situation, one or more factors may play a significant role in determining the actual pattern of nerve impulses that ascend from the spinal cord to the brain, are received there and acted upon by other input, and are then finally transmitted downward for final action.

MEASUREMENT OF PAIN

Measurement of pain has been approached in three ways: (1) subjectively, by asking the person to describe the pain; (2) objectively by observing the person's behavior; and (3) by using instruments to measure autonomic signs of pain, such as pulse or blood pressure. The person's subjective report is probably the best single indicator of pain. If someone says he is in pain, then he probably is. However, the intensity of pain reported by the individual may or may not be easily related to pathology or to the amount of tissue damage involved. The expression of pain is primarily the person's interpretation of what is happening.

In order to obtain some measure of this subjective and sometimes elusive phenomenon, a number of tools, verbal and written, have been developed. These tools range from simply asking the person to describe the location, intensity, and pattern of the pain to more elaborate rating scales and questionnaires. The person may even be asked to draw or color the pain.

One relatively new tool, the McGill Pain Questionnaire, has been used to study women in labor (Melzack et al., 1981). As shown in Fig. 18–3, this questionnaire consists of 20 sets of words describing: (1) the sensory qualities of the pain experience (pressure, thermal, spatial, etc.; items 1–10); (2)

McGill - Melzack Pain Questionnaire

Patient's Name______ Date______ Time_____ am/pm
Analgesic(s) ______ Dosage______ Time Given _____ am/pm
______ Dosage______ Time Given_____ am/pm

Analgesic Time Difference (hours): +4 +1 +2 +3
PRI: S____ (1-10) A____ (11-15) E____ (16) M(S)____ (17-19) M(AE)____ (20) M(T)____ (17-20) PRI(T)____ (1-20)

1 FLICKERING, QUIVERING, PULSING, THROBBING, BEATING, POUNDING
2 JUMPING, FLASHING, SHOOTING
3 PRICKING, BORING, DRILLING, STABBING, LANCINATING
4 SHARP, CUTTING, LACERATING
5 PINCHING, PRESSING, GNAWING, CRAMPING, CRUSHING
6 TUGGING, PULLING, WRENCHING
7 HOT, BURNING, SCALDING, SEARING
8 TINGLING, ITCHY, SMARTING, STINGING
9 DULL, SORE, HURTING, ACHING, HEAVY
10 TENDER, TAUT, RASPING, SPLITTING
11 TIRING, EXHAUSTING
12 SICKENING, SUFFOCATING
13 FEARFUL, FRIGHTFUL, TERRIFYING
14 PUNISHING, GRUELLING, CRUEL, VICIOUS, KILLING
15 WRETCHED, BLINDING
16 ANNOYING, TROUBLESOME, MISERABLE, INTENSE, UNBEARABLE
17 SPREADING, RADIATING, PENETRATING, PIERCING
18 TIGHT, NUMB, DRAWING, SQUEEZING, TEARING
19 COOL, COLD, FREEZING
20 NAGGING, NAUSEATING, AGONIZING, DREADFUL, TORTURING

PPI
0 No pain
1 MILD
2 DISCOMFORTING
3 DISTRESSING
4 HORRIBLE
5 EXCRUCIATING

PPI____ COMMENTS:

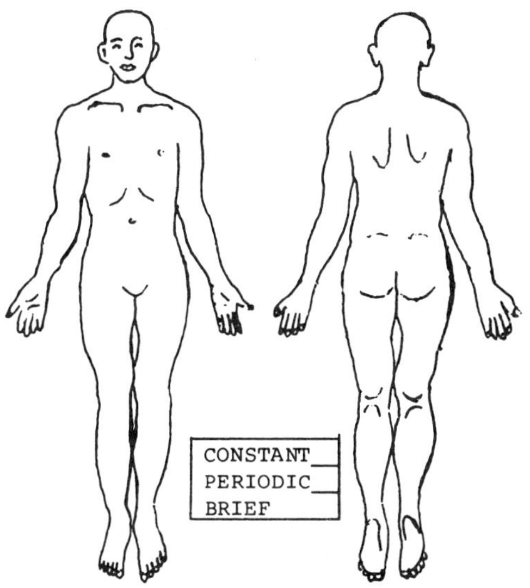

CONSTANT__ PERIODIC__ BRIEF__

ACCOMPANYING SYMPTOMS: NAUSEA, HEADACHE, DIZZINESS, DROWSINESS, CONSTIPATION, DIARRHEA
COMMENTS:

SLEEP: GOOD, FITFUL, CAN'T SLEEP
COMMENTS:

FOOD INTAKE: GOOD, SOME, LITTLE, NONE
COMMENTS:

ACTIVITY: GOOD, SOME, LITTLE, NONE
COMMENTS:

FIGURE 18–3. McGill-Melzack Pain Questionnaire.
SOURCE: Melzack et al. (1981).

the affective qualities (tension, fear, etc.; items 11–15); and, (3) the subjective overall intensity of the experience. The words in each item are rank-ordered and scored, and then totaled by subgroups to arrive at a total score, termed the Pain Rating Index (PRI). The last item on the questionnaire measures the present pain intensity (PPI) on a scale of 0–5.

PAIN IN LABOR

First and Second Stages

Most research supports the hypothesis that the pain of the first stage of labor is due primarily to the dilation of the cervix and lower uterine segment and, consequently, to the stretching and distention of these structures during contractions. Impulses from the cervix and uterus are transmitted by afferent nerves along the sympathetic pathways through the pelvic, inferior, middle, and superior hypogastric plexuses, the lumbar sympathetic chain, and the spinal nerves of T10, T11, T12, and L1. In early labor only the nerve roots of T11 and T12 are involved, but as labor progresses, T10 and L1 become involved (see Fig. 18–4).

During the second stage of labor, the cervix is now fully dilated with a decrease in the stimulation of its pain pathways. Continued distention of the lower uterine segments, however, causes pain in the same area. In addition, the descent of the presenting part of the fetus has a progressive impact on the pelvic structures. The distention of the outlet and perineum, and pressure on roots of the lumbosacral plexus, produce referred pain via nerve roots L2 and below. Pain may therefore be felt in the low back and in the thighs and legs.

Pain produced by stretching the perineum is transmitted via the pudendal nerve. This nerve is derived from the sacral nerves S2, S3, and S4 and passes posterior to the junction of the ischial spine and sacrospinous ligament.

Physiologic Effects of Pain in Labor

Major changes in respiratory, cardiovascular, and gastrointestinal systems during labor are summarized in Chapter 16. However, several physiologic and biochemical changes also occur as a result of the pain itself and should be considered. Knowledge of these changes will assist in assessing the woman's condition in labor and in managing her

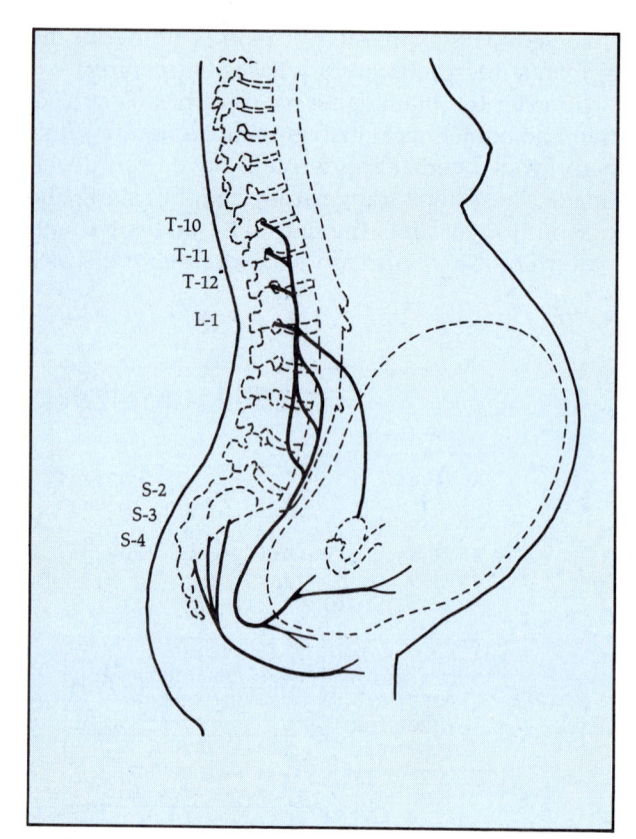

FIGURE 18–4. Neuroanatomy of pelvic and perineal structures.

nursing care. Pain, if unrelieved, causes a series of changes that will affect both mother and fetus (see Fig. 18–5). Contractions are the stimuli that initiate the pain experience. As they become strong enough to generate pressure on the pain receptors, many factors will influence pain perception and interpretation. As noted earlier, such factors as anxiety, fear, fatigue, intensity of contractions, past experiences, cultural norms, meaning of this event, preparation for childbirth, and support during labor, all have potential for altering the pain experience.

Without relief of unpleasant and negative interpretations of pain, increased autonomic responses will trigger further changes that affect labor, mother, and infant. These changes may include increases in cardiac output, peripheral resistance, blood pressure, hyperventilation, lactic acid production, oxygen consumption, and catecholamine release. At the same time, there may be a decrease in uterine contractile activity, uterine blood supply, and cerebral perfusion. During the first stage of labor, without relief of pain, a progressive maternal acidosis occurs (Brownridge, Taylor, and Ralston, 1980). Fetal hypoxia and fetal acidosis closely follow the change in the mother. Any or all

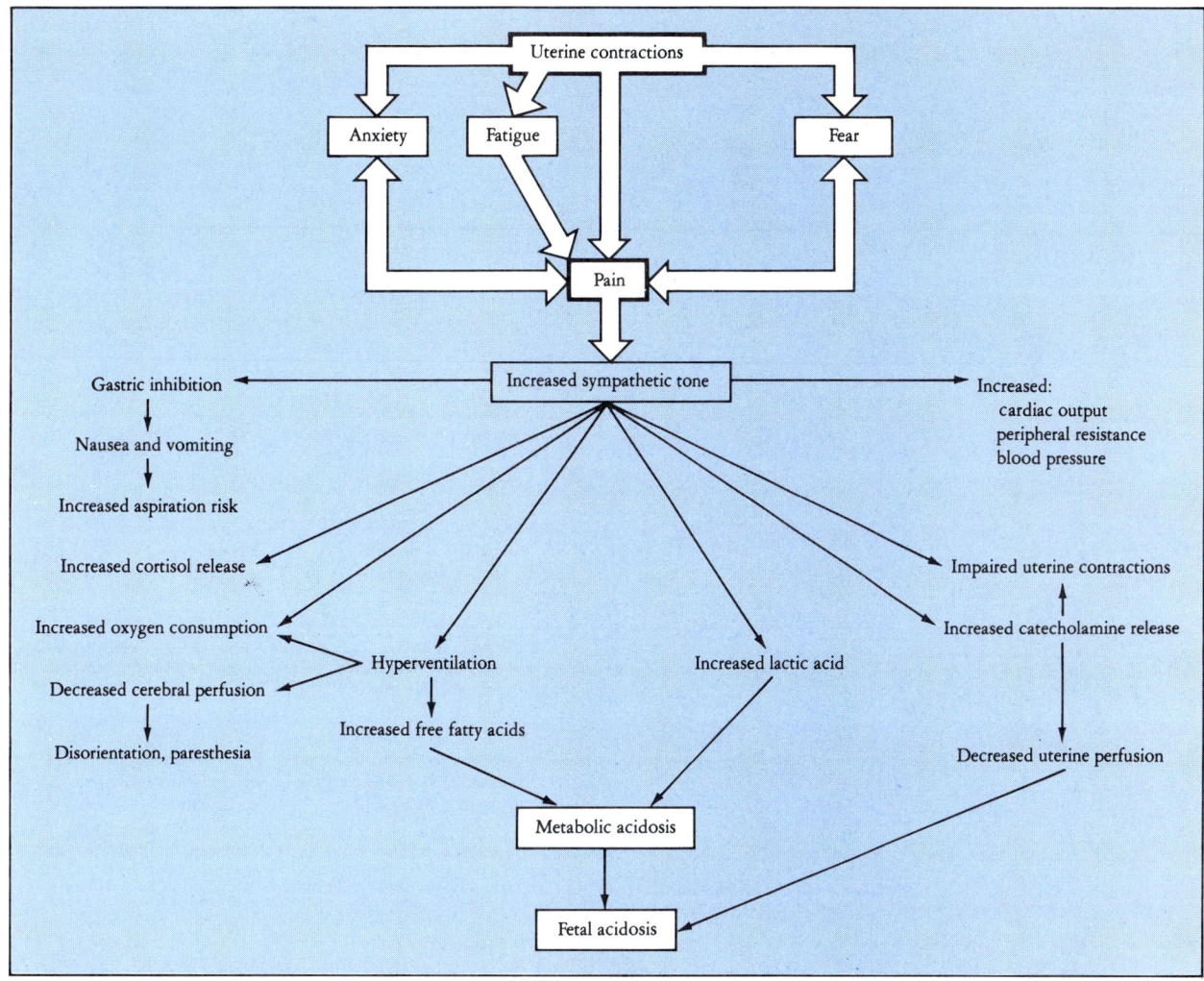

FIGURE 18–5. Physiologic consequences of unrelieved pain in labor.
SOURCE: Brownridge, Taylor, and Ralston (1980).

of these sequelae can be blocked by interventions at the appropriate levels.

ROLE OF THE NURSE IN PAIN ASSESSMENT

As the nurse begins care for the woman in labor (s)he needs to follow the steps of the nursing process as a guide for planning. Because the childbirth experience each woman wants and has prepared for is unique, the nurse should be prepared to individualize the care.

As pain appears and persists, the person's life becomes increasingly governed by the pain and new needs take precedence over all others. Melzack and Wall (1983), in their extensive research on pain, have identified three compelling needs during this time. First is a need to communicate something of the nature of the pain to others. Second is the need to seek a behavior that will reduce the pain, such as rest, sleep, and a general decrease in activity. Third is the need to search for treatment and relief. Although labor pain is a more finite phenomenon than chronic pain, these needs are still relevant.

A unique consideration in assessing and managing pain in labor is that at least two individuals are involved in the process. The woman's responses to pain and to pain-relief techniques pass over to the fetus. If the woman hyperventilates, the oxygen supply to the fetus is compromised. Medication administered to the mother also reaches the fetus.

Table 18–1 summarizes the nursing management of comfort during labor, using the nursing diagnosis, alteration in comfort related to the pain and/or progress in labor, and the needs identified by Melzack.

TABLE 18-1. *Management of Alterations in Comfort During Childbirth*

Assessment Diagnosis	Expected Outcome Criteria	Nursing Intervention	Rationale

Alteration in comfort related to the pain and/or progress of labor	A. Woman will feel free to communicate her feelings to her care	1. Observe patient's physiologic and behavioral signs of unrelieved pain
		  a. Increases in blood pressure and pulse.
		  b. Increases in respiration leading to hyperventilation.
		  c. Increase in muscle tension.
		  d. Nausea and vomiting
		  e. Increases in anxiety and fear.
		  f. Excessive perspiration
			1. To assess woman's physiologic responses to labor and/or pain

		2. Periodically ask patient how she is feeling and observe facial, body expressions of discomfort	2. To assess patient's perception and interpretation of pain
		3. Communicate to other caregivers, the patient's feelings and needs, verbally or in writing	3. To promote continuity and consistency of care, along with acceptance of her feelings
	B. Woman will identify and demonstrate behaviors that will increase her comfort during labor	1. In early labor, discuss with patient comfort measures and positions for various stages of labor	1. To provide the patient time to share her past experiences with pain, as well as her cultural values and beliefs relating to labor, pain and birth
		2. Provide attractive, clean, restful environment for patient	2. To promote relaxation, comfort and a positive feeling about the childbirth experience
		3. Include husband or support person in planning of an enjoyable, comfortable labor setting	3. To encourage input from patient's support system as early as possible for the comfort of both the patient and support person
		4. Discuss with patient upcoming options for relief of discomfort in regard to analgesia and/or anesthesia	4. To individualize comfort measures, and to plan ahead for consultation with other practitioners and arrange for other comfort measures as needed
	C. Woman will demonstrate and/or express feelings of increased comfort or no pain	1. Record specific nursing and/or medical interventions to relieve discomfort and the effectiveness of each intervention	1. To assure that medications and other comfort measures are effective, or if not, whether more or less of each measure would be helpful later. Also to look for untoward effects with any medication, anesthesia, ambulation, or other modality

It is essential for the nurse to be with the woman long enough to hear what she is saying or trying to communicate. This requirement may or may not imply constant attendance, depending on the phase of labor and other support persons present. The purpose of this communication is to assess the woman's perception and interpretation of pain. If possible, information seeking should be accomplished before the contractions intensify and the woman is decreasingly interested in long conversations. Early in labor the woman may be interested in sharing her past experiences with pain and how she handled it and discussing her cultural values and beliefs related to labor, pain, and birth. The nurse can also assess the woman's knowledge of childbirth and her preparation-for-childbirth training with this or a previous labor.

Words that the woman uses to describe pain indicate how she is responding to labor. Pain may be cramping, aching, tiring, sharp, shooting, or unbearable. As labor progresses, communication may take other forms. Facial expression, vocalization such as grunting or crying, use of single words and short phrases rather than full sentences, and body language provide important information the nurse can utilize in her assessment.

The nurse must assess pain response in terms of the progress being made in the labor process. What level of pain relief is the woman expecting, and what does she want? What phase of labor is she in? Can the nurse anticipate time of delivery? This information is particularly important if analgesia or anesthesia is to be used.

APPROACHES TO RELIEVING PAIN IN LABOR

Nursing intervention in pain control is based on the nurse's knowledge of the childbirth process, on assessment of the pain experienced by the woman, and on the nursing measures appropriate to the situation. Although several pain control approaches are available to the nurse, namely pharmacologic, sensory modulation, and psychologic, there are basic measures that should be considered first. They include:

1. Providing the woman and her family with information. A woman who is kept informed about what is happening to her is more likely to feel in control of herself and the situation. She is therefore more likely to recognize the pain of labor as a bearable experience.

2. Encouraging relaxation. Relaxation should be considered an essential component of all approaches to the relief of pain. The stress, anxiety, and fear associated with pain all produce muscle tension, increased epinephrine flow, and increased vital signs. Activities that can result in muscle relaxation will also help decrease blood pressure and respiratory rate. When analgesics and anesthesia are indicated, relaxation of the muscles will facilitate administrations and absorption of the pharmacologic agent.

3. Including the woman and her family in decision-making. From the time of admission the atmosphere should be warm and open. All the participants should be goal-oriented, with an easy flow of communication between the family and health care providers and encouragement of relevant participation by all those affected.

To be informed means to have the information necessary to give understanding consent to treatment and participate in decisions. Two important documents focus on the patient's right to know and be informed. The Patient's Bill of Rights was adopted by the American Hospital Association in 1972 and, more recently, The Pregnant Patient's Bill of Rights has been developed (see Appendix E). The nurse should review these rights as she plans the management of pain in labor.

PHARMACOLOGIC APPROACHES

The use of pharmacologic agents plays an important part in the relief of pain. In the management of care for the woman in labor, the selection of analgesia and anesthesia must be carefully determined. Analgesia ("no pain") refers to the absence or decreased awareness of a normal sensation of pain. It is usually brought about by the administration of drugs and is usually given in the first stage of labor.

Anesthesia ("without sensation") is the partial or complete loss of sensation with or without loss of consciousness; it results from the administration of an anesthetic agent, usually by injection or inhalation. Anesthesia may be employed during the active phase of the first stage, at the end of the first stage, or during the second and third stages. Both types of agents act to inhibit neural stimuli and to block pain pathways.

Keeping in mind the goal of providing as safe and satisfactory pain relief as possible for the mother during labor and delivery with the least harm to the fetus/infant, the following factors should be carefully examined in making the decision to use drugs:

1. The physical and chemical properties of the drug that may affect transfer across the placenta.
2. Optimal dose, therapeutic effect, time of peak activity, and duration of effect of the drug.
3. Possible side-effects of the drug on the woman, fetus/newborn, and labor.
4. Progress made in labor. If pain medication is given too early, it may interfere with uterine activity by slowing down the frequency, intensity, and duration of the contractions. If administered late in labor (within 30–60 min of delivery), it may lead to the delivery of a medicated newborn who may need resuscitative measures.
5. Gestational ages of the fetus. Immaturity of fetal systems such as the liver will interfere with metabolism of drugs that cross the placenta and may well affect the condition of the premature newborn.

Effects of Drugs on the Fetus

Almost all drugs used to produce anesthesia, analgesia, and sedation have properties that assure rapid crossing of the placenta from mother to fetus. Drug properties that favor rapid diffusion are: (1) low molecular weight (under 500); (2) low protein binding; (3) high lipid solubility; and, (4) low degree of ionization. Almost all of the pain relief drugs possess these qualities and therefore diffuse easily.

Other factors that influence transfer of a drug across the placenta include: (1) placental blood flow, whether obstructed or not, as by hypotension, aortal-caval obstruction, hypertonic uterine contractions, diabetes, or preeclampsia; and, (2) route of administration, with drugs that are given intravenously being the most rapidly absorbed and eliminated.

Drugs that do cross the placenta enter the umbilical vein. Most of the drug (85 percent) enters the fetal liver and then the vena cava, the rest bypasses the liver to enter the vena cava directly and be dispersed to the rest of the fetal circulation. The final amount of drug reaching a vital organ is related to the organ's blood supply. Because the central nervous system is the most highly vascularized fetal organ, it receives the greatest amount of drug. The threat of hypoxia or asphyxia to the fetus is known to increase uterine blood flow and consequently increase fetal drug intake (Avery, 1987).

The ability of the fetal liver to metabolize drugs is limited, particularly in the premature fetus. In addition, the immature functioning of the kidneys reduces the ability of the fetus to excrete drugs. Indeed, it is believed that some drugs excreted by fetal kidneys into the amniotic fluid are reabsorbed by the fetal intestines.

Although some is known about the circulation and absorption of drugs into fetal tissues, less is known of the fetal metabolism and excretion. In general, the most common effect on the fetus of drugs given in labor is depression of the central nervous system in varying degrees. Specific effects will be discussed as we examine each type of drug.

It is almost impossible to maintain expertise in the use of all the currently available techniques in obstetric analgesia and anesthesia. However, the major ones will be presented in this chapter with a general discussion of each category, and some indication of the scope and trends of each.

Systemic Medications

Three groups of medications are included in the category of systemic medications: (1) sedatives and tranquilizers, (2) analgesics (including narcotics), and (3) dissociative or amnesia-producing drugs (see Table 18–2).

Sedatives

Early in the first stage of labor, women, particularly primigravidas, may be anxious and fearful. To calm these feelings, barbiturates are given as sedatives, which act primarily by depressing activity of excitable tissues. They do not relieve pain and are not considered to be analgesics. Barbiturates readily cross the placental barrier, and within a few minutes after the injection of a short-acting barbiturate, such as Seconal, the concentration in the fetal blood approaches that in the maternal venous blood. Evaluation of the effects of such drug concentrations on fetus and neonate has been difficult, and results are still controversial.

Barbiturates are not commonly used today because the potential adverse effects on the newborn

TABLE 18-2. *Common Systemic Medications Used During Childbirth*

Drug	Usual Dosage and Action	Desired Effects	Effects on Mother and Fetus	Comments
Sedatives				
Barbiturates	100–200 mg, PO 100 mg IM	Promote relaxation, sleep, hypnosis in the presence of mild pain only	In presence of severe pain, tend to excite rather than calm; may depress fetal respirations at birth with large doses	Useful in early latent phase of labor, when delivery is not expected for 12–24 hours
Pentobarbital (Nembutal)	Intermediate acting			
Secobarbital (Seconal)	Short acting			
Tranquilizers				
Promethazine (Phenergan)	25–50 mg IM, PO	Relieve apprehension and anxiety; control nausea and vomiting; when given with narcotic, decrease amount of narcotic needed	May depress respirations of newborn	Used in early labor
Propiomazine (Largon)	10–20 mg IM, PO			
Promazine (Sparine)			Sparine and Thorazine tend to lower maternal blood pressure	
Chlorpromazine (Thorazine)				
Hydroxyzine (Vistaril)	25–100 mg IM, PO		Decreases fetal beat-to-beat variability; large doses may cause fetal hypotonia or hypothermia, or lethargic feeding of newborn	
Diazepam (Valium)	2–10 mg IV, IM			Used preoperatively for cesarean sections and with narcotics throughout labor
Analgesics				
Morphine	5–10 mg SC or IM Peak effect: 1–2 h IM Duration: 4–6 h IM	Reduce pain, spasms, and anxiety Used to relieve pain in patients with cardiac disease	Respiratory distress in newborns; respiratory depression in mothers	Not used as often as other analgesics because of delayed peak effect, longer duration, and depressant effect
Meperidine (Demerol)	50–100 mg IM Onset: 15 min Peak effect: 40–50 min Duration: 2–3 h 25–50 mg IV Onset: 30 sec Duration: 1½–2 h		In mother: nausea and vomiting; respiratory and circulatory depression; delayed gastrointestinal action In newborn: respiratory depression, decreased beat-to-beat variability	Used in active phase of first stage, and in second and third stages
Pentazocine (Talwin)	30 mg IM, IV Peak effect: 15–20 min IM 2–3 min IV 30 mg = 75–100 mg Demerol	Relieve moderate to severe pain	Respiratory depression May precipitate withdrawal reaction in addicts; delayed gastric emptying, drowsiness	Used with caution in women delivering premature infants
Butorphanol (Stadol)	2–4 mg IM 1 mg IV Onset: 10 min IM Peak effect: 30–60 min IM Duration: 3–4 h		In mother: nausea, increased perspiration (reversed by Narcan) In newborn: respiratory distress	2 mg Stadol depresses respirations to degree equal to 10 mg morphine or 75 Demerol
Dissociative (amnesia-producing) drugs				
Scopolamine (hyoscine)	0.2–0.6 mg IM, IV	Produce sedation, tranquilization, and amnesia	Side effects: excitement, restlessness with contractions, dry mouth	Best results when given with analgesic, rarely used today

are more widely recognized. In large doses, barbiturates depress respiration in both mother and the newborn. Since these drugs rapidly traverse the placenta, fetal levels may be high at birth (Dickason, 1978). Poor sucking behavior has been observed during the first 4 days of life in newborns whose mothers received Seconal during labor (Kron, Stein, and Goddard, 1966).

A variety of tranquilizing agents may also be given early in labor. Also known as ataratic (quieting) drugs, they are effective in relieving apprehension and anxiety and in controlling nausea and vomiting. Hydroxyzine (Atarax, Vistaril) and diazepam (Valium) are popular tranquilizer-amnesics. Valium is popular for use in the first stage of labor because it has a good tranquilizing effect and because it enables a reduction in the dosage of analgesic.

Valium, in addition to relieving anxiety and potentiating the effect of narcotics, can be used preoperatively for cesarean sections. It can also be administered as an anticonvulsant in the treatment of toxemia. Although Valium crosses the placenta rapidly, the fetus can metabolize small doses of it.

Analgesics

Narcotics are used in labor in dosages that are aimed at reducing pain, not eliminating it. Overdoses cause respiratory depression, decreased reflexes, and postural hypotension. They may be administered alone or with a tranquilizer or amnesic drug. Neonatal depression is related to dose and to the time interval between drug administration in the woman and delivery of the infant. Studies indicate that infants born within 1 hour or more than 4 hours after administration of 50–100 mg of Demerol (meperidine) are no more depressed than infants whose mothers had not received Demerol.

Naloxon hydrochloride (Narcan) is a narcotic antagonist capable of reversing respiratory depression induced by narcotics with opium derivations by displacing the narcotic from specific receptors in the central nervous system. When given to the woman in labor, however, it inhibits the analgesic effect produced by the narcotic. The suggested dose for the newborn infant is 10 µg/kg injected into the umbilical vein. When so injected, it usually acts within 2 min and lasts approximately 30 min. If depression persists, this dosage may be repeated.

The greatest amount of meperidine is found in the neonate when the drug is given 2–3 hours before delivery. Elimination of the half-life of meperidine has been reported to be within 13 and 23 hours. The neonate will continue to excrete the drug for 3–6 days (Schnider, 1987).

Dissociative or Amnesia-producing Drugs

Drugs in this category were used in labor and delivery a number of years ago to provide the woman with amnesia for the childbirth experience, but today they are seldom used for this purpose. One such drug is scopolamine, a belladonna alkaloid with many atropine-like properties. In labor it produces sedation and amnesia. When given alone in the presence of pain or severe anxiety, however, it may induce outbursts of uncontrolled behavior, during which it is almost impossible to communicate with the patient. Patients may experience delusions, hallucination, and hyperactivity. Thus, use of scopolamine requires constant nursing attention for the safety of the woman and fetus.

All of the systemic drugs used obstetrically are intended to have beneficial effects on the woman in labor—to make her more comfortable, relaxed, and pain free. Given in safe dosages and at the appropriate time in labor, they may indeed make the woman "feel" better. However, all of these drugs have noxious though short-term effects on the fetus/newborn. The nurse must therefore be alert to the timing and dosage of each medication and to the possible effect on the infant at birth. Although numerous studies have been done on the effect of these drugs on the infant and on mother–infant interactions, so far results are not conclusive.

Regional Anesthesia

Blocking or temporarily interrupting the conduction of sensory nerve impulses by the injection of an anesthetic substance into or very near a nerve trunk can be classified as local, regional, or conduction anesthesia. Regional and conduction anesthesia are terms that are used interchangeably. The types of nerve blocks used for regional anesthesia include local infiltration, pudendal block, paracervical block, spinal block, caudal block, and lumbar epidural block (see Fig. 18–6 and Table 18–3).

Local Anesthesia Infiltration

Local anesthesia in childbirth refers to the injection of an agent such as lidocaine 1 percent into the

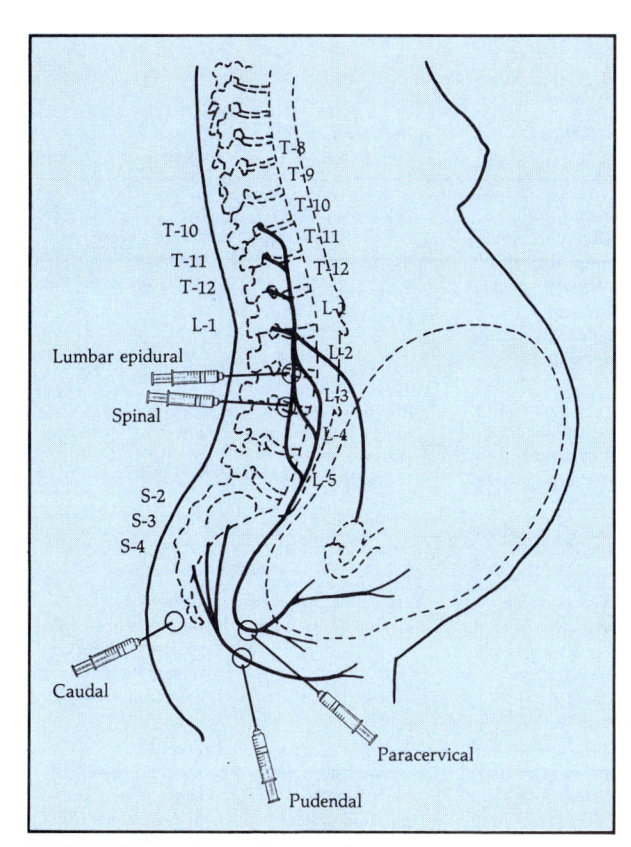

FIGURE 18-6. Types of regional blocks that may be used to provide analgesia during obstetric and gynecologic surgery.

after delivery into the site of lacerations to be repaired.

The episiotomy, or incision of the perineum, substitutes a straight, surgical incision for a ragged laceration that might otherwise result. It is felt to be easier to repair and heal than a tear.

Need for an episiotomy is based on one or more of the following considerations (Varney, 1980):

1. The stated preference by the woman.
2. Policy of the physician or midwife based on the concept of prophylactic gynecology.
3. Size of the infant.
4. Fetal malposition or malpresentation.
5. Probability of lacerating the perineum.

If episiotomy is indicated, pudendal anesthesia, which alleviates the sensation of stretching in the vaginal tract, will also alleviate feelings of being cut.

Paracervical Block

A paracervical block blocks nerve pathways from the uterus during labor. It is usually administered in active labor, lasts for approximately 1 hour, and then must be repeated throughout the first stage of labor. There is no perineal anesthesia, and another type of anesthesia must be added for the delivery. Because this method has been found to increase the incidence of fetal arrhythmias, it is no longer recommended for labor. If used, it requires careful monitoring of the fetus and mother.

Spinal Anesthesia (Saddle Block)

A saddle block is a type of anesthesia used primarily for delivery; it is given at the end of the first stage of labor. In this variation of spinal anesthesia, medication is administered with the woman in a sitting position at the side of the bed. She remains upright for 3–5 min to ensure a low level of anesthesia. The woman can still push when instructed. Frequent monitoring of vital signs is important before delivery. Postpartally, the woman should be watched carefully for any signs of complications (see Chapter 20).

Caudal and Lumbar Epidural Anesthesia

Caudal anesthesia was once quite popular for women in labor, but it has largely given way to lumbar epidural anesthesia. The lumbar epidural is easier, less painful, and more reliable to admin-

perineum. The procedure is simple and free from complications. It is used when other anesthesia has failed, when the labor has progressed too rapidly to give other anesthesia, or when a woman has elected to have no anesthesia but an episiotomy is needed at the last minute. It is often used for women who desire to have as natural a childbirth as possible.

Pudendal Block

The pudendal block is a relatively simple and safe procedure that has no effect on the uterus or its contractions. The block is administered just prior to delivery; the onset of action is immediate and may last from 30 to 90 min. The most common route is transvaginal insertion of a long (5–6 inch) needle in a guide through the sacrospinous ligament to a space just in front of the pudendal nerve plexus (see Fig. 18-7). This technique is particularly indicated for women who may choose minimal analgesia and anesthesia but are known ahead of time to need episiotomies. It may also be used

TABLE 18–3. Regional Anesthesia Used in Childbirth

Type of Block	Procedure	Areas Affected	Indication for Use	Untoward or Side-Effects	Comments
Local infiltration	Injection of drug, up to 10 ml, into perineum; short-acting; may be repeated several times	Perineum	Given prior to delivery to prepare for episiotomy; given after delivery to repair episiotomy or lacerations	None when agent remains in perineal tissues	May be administered by physician or nurse-midwife
Pudendal	Two injections of up to 19 ml transvaginally into space in front of pudendal nerve plexus	Perineum, vulva, rectal area	Gives immediate anesthesia for 30–90 min; given in second stage after presenting part is through cervix	Minimal effect on mother and infant if administered properly	May be given by physician or nurse-midwife
Paracervical	Two injections transvaginally into lateral fornix, on each side of cervix; may be repeated	Lower uterine segment and cervix, as well as upper third of vagina	Used in active labor (when cervix is at least 4–5 cm dilated); lasts about 1 hour	Increased incidence of fetal bradycardia	There is no perineal anesthesia; requires skillful administration and careful monitoring
Spinal (saddle block)	Injection of agent through dura into subarachnoid space containing spinal fluid, below spinal cord, usually between L3–L4 or L4–L5	Perineum, lower pelvic area, upper thigh	Given at end of first stage of labor; effective for 1–2 hours; larger dose raises level up to T8–T10, may be used for cesarean	Maternal hypotension; possible infection of spinal fluid; loss of spinal fluid causing severe headaches; increased tendency for uterine and bladder atony	Frequent monitoring of vital signs of woman and fetus before delivery; woman needs to be instructed to push; skillful administration needed
Caudal	Injection of agent into sacral foramen and caudal space below dura; "one shot" or continuous administration available	Pelvic area	Used in the active phase of the first stage and during delivery; woman needs direction to push in second stage	Maternal hypotension; in late labor risk of puncturing rectum and fetal head	Careful monitoring of blood pressure and progress in labor since woman is unaware of contractions; forceps usually needed for delivery
Lumbar epidural	Injection of agent into epidural space, in lumbar area, L2–L3 or anywhere between L2 and S1	Affects all nerves from T10–T12 to S4, level of umbilicus to the thighs, and sometimes down to toes	Primary indication is woman's desire for complete pain relief; started in active labor relieves pain and anxiety and reduces: cardiac output, B.P., hyperventilation, endocrines ACTH, cortisol, and catecholamines	Possible puncture of dural membrane; hypotension; bladder dysfunction	Special training needed to administer; forceps needed to deliver; contraindicated with clotting defects, sepsis; used with obstetric emergencies needing immediate delivery

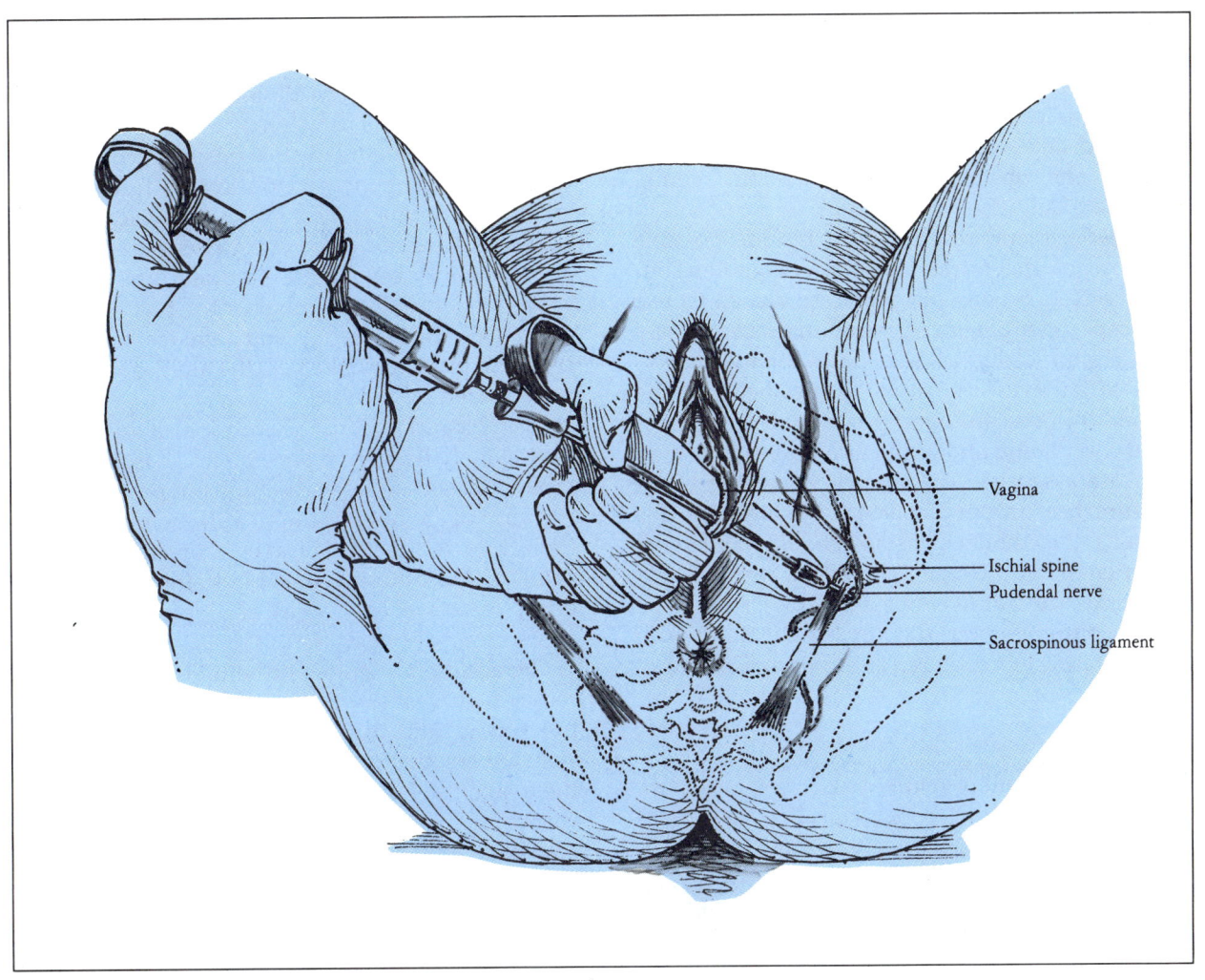

FIGURE 18-7. Local infiltration of the pudendal nerve using the transvaginal technique. Note needle passing through the sacrospinous ligament. A needle guard is usually used
SOURCE: Pritchard and MacDonald (1980).

ister than the caudal. Both types require special training and expertise to administer, as well as careful observation by the administrator, whether obstetrician or anesthesiologist, and by the nurse caring for the woman. The woman is usually placed on her side and the needle, or catheter if continuous, can be inserted in any of the lumbar spaces.

The blood pressure should be taken every 5 min and the woman should be carefully observed to ensure that spinal anesthesia has not been given inadvertently. Constant nursing observations and support are necessary. The woman's legs may be placed on a pillow to facilitate venous drainage, and the head may be elevated slightly. Once anesthesia has occurred, the woman may be positioned on her right side to relieve uterine pressure on the inferior vena cava. The success rate for analgesia is approximately 85 percent, with readjustments necessary 18 percent of the time because of the woman changing position or movement of the catheter.

There is disagreement over the use of epidural anesthesia in the presence of hypertension and preeclampsia. Some advocate regional anesthesia to lower blood pressure while others prefer local anesthesia, such as a pudendal block.

The primary indication for using lumbar epidural should be the woman's desire for this kind of pain relief. Anesthesia may be instituted at any time in active labor, but labor may be slowed significantly for up to 30 min after a dose is injected. During the second stage the woman cannot push effectively. Therefore, forceps delivery is almost always required.

Contraindications to the lumbar epidural are patient dislike, clotting defects, sepsis in the mother, and obstetric emergencies that require immediate delivery.

Side-effects and complications include possible puncture of the dural membrane, hypotension, bladder dysfunction, and problems caused by use of forceps. Neurologic complications are extremely rare. The procedure is safe for the fetus, unless there is an overdose of local anesthetic or the mother's blood pressure becomes hypotensive. Close observation and frequent monitoring of vital signs are essential. The first clue that the blood pressure has dropped is sudden nausea. If this happens, the woman's position should be changed to left lateral and oxygen should be administered by mask. The intravenous fluid rate should be increased (intravenous therapy is initiated prior to administering any required anesthesia) (Gorvine et al., 1982).

Local Anesthetic Agents

Regional anesthesia has been used in labor and delivery since the beginning of the twentieth century. The drugs used are alkaloids that belong to the "caine" family, related to cocaine. They act on the cell membrane to block both generation and conduction of the nerve impulse.

Local agents may be divided into two groups, *esters* and *amides*. The esters (procaine, chloroprocaine, tetracaine) have a slow onset of action, short duration, and poor penetration of tissues. The amides (lidocaine, mepivacaine, bupivacaine, and prilocaine) are the group most commonly used in regional anesthesia because of their rapid onset of action and prolonged duration of pharmacologic effect (see Table 18–4). Both amides and esters cross the placenta; however, the amides are poorly metabolized by the fetus.

Lidocaine hydrochloride (Xylocaine) is one of the most widely used local anesthetics. It is an amide, rapidly absorbed after administration. It has a half-life of 3 hours; thus, although it crosses rapidly to the fetus, it leaves more rapidly than some of the other agents. Lidocaine has a rapid onset of action (2–3 min) and reaches its peak action in 15–30 min.

The addition of epinephrine to local anesthetics reduces drug absorption and therefore enhances the spread and quality of the neural blocks. It also lowers the peak blood levels of the anesthetic agents. However, because epinephrine is a vasoconstrictor and acts to decrease uterine tone and contractility, it must be used carefully in labor.

Toxic effects of local anesthetics on the fetus are

TABLE 18–4. Local Anesthetic Agents

Drugs	Characteristics	Actions	Effect on Fetus
Alkaloids of "caine" family		Act on cell membranes of nerve fibers to block both generation and conduction of the nerve impulse; action completely reversible	May affect central nervous system, cardiovascular system; effects disappear within 12 hours
Ester group Procaine (Novocain) Chloroprocaine (Nesacaine) Tetracaine (Pontocaine)	Slow action Short duration Penetrate poorly into tissues		
Amide group Lidocaine (Xylocaine) Mepivacaine (Carboncaine) Bupivacaine (Marcaine) Prilocaine (Citanest)	Rapid action Prolonged duration Rapidly absorbed into tissues		

found in the central nervous system and the cardiovascular system. Such depressant effects, if mild, disappear within 12 hours (Brownridge, 1980).

Inhalation Analgesics, Inhalation Anesthesia, and General Anesthesia

Although the use of inhalation analgesia and anesthesia is declining in the United States, there will continue to be a need for alternate methods of pain relief during labor to meet varying situations and conditions.

Inhalation analgesia is the administration of subanesthetic concentrations of inhalation anesthetic agents to provide analgesia for labor or delivery with or without supplemental narcotics or regional anesthesia. The woman is awake and cooperative. The agent is usually administered by mask or a special mouthpiece (inhaler) either by the woman or by an anesthesiologist. The degree of pain relief can be regulated by the woman and is a good alternative for the woman who refuses needles or fears the headache that can accompany spinal block. Also, in some hospitals or other settings, there may not be expert personnel to administer regional anesthesia.

Commonly used inhalants include nitrous oxide and methoxyflurane. Nitrous oxide may be self-administered in a blender device that delivers various percentages of nitrous oxide and mixed with oxygen. Methoxyflurane (Penthrane) may be self-administered in low concentrations with an inhaler. Other agents include halothane (Fluothane) and trichloroethylene (Trilene).

All these agents may be inhaled intermittently (during contractions only) or continuously (during and between contractions), although the former is more common. The dose should be regulated according to the woman's response. That is, if she becomes confused, drowsy, or excited, the concentration should be lowered at once or stopped. The major risk of this technique is inadvertent overdose.

The nurse has an important role in explaining the use of the inhaler if the woman is to use it herself and in observing the woman as labor progresses, to see that there are no side-effects and no overdose.

Inhalation analgesics cross the placenta rapidly; however, there has been no incidence of neonatal depression when awake-inhalers using nitrous oxide or methoxyflurane have been employed, particularly when they are used intermittently.

Inhalation anesthesia is the practice of administering inhalation drugs with the intent of producing unconsciousness. By itself, there is little use for this type of anesthesia for normal vaginal deliveries today. It is, however, used as part of a general anesthetics routine used for cesarean section or a difficult delivery. This routine includes intravenous anesthetic induction agents, muscle relaxants, and endotracheal intubation.

General anesthesia historically was produced with the inhalation of a gaseous anesthetic such as ether or cyclopropane. However, ether is unpleasant for the mother, depresses the fetus, causes the uterus to relax, and is explosive. Cyclopropane is also highly explosive and depresses the fetus. Today general anesthesia is a combined technique that includes an intravenous induction agent, muscle relaxants, various mixes of nitrous oxide and oxygen, endotracheal intubation, and maintenance anesthesia with narcotics or inhalation agents.

Thiopental sodium (Pentothal) is an ultrashort-acting barbiturate, injected intravenously, used as an induction agent. A dose of 3–4 mg/kg given intravenously will produce a loss of consciousness and a loss of sensation within 30 sec. The induction is smooth and pleasant, and so is the emergence. There is little nausea or vomiting. Given alone, Pentothal causes a drop in blood pressure, occasional laryngospasm, apnea, and other respiratory difficulties. Within a few minutes after injection into the woman, the concentration of the drug in the fetus equals that in the woman. The effect of Pentothal is transient, and by 30 min over 90 percent of the drug has left the brain and viscera to enter lean tissues and fat deposits. The plasma half-life in the brain is 3 min; for the rest of the body, the half-life is 3–8 hours (Goodman, 1985).

Pentothal is rarely used alone because of the severe respiratory distress possible. It is used for induction and as an adjunct to other anesthetics. The muscle relaxant administered is succinyl choline (Anectine). Administered intravenously, this neuromuscular blocking agent is given to obtain relaxation of skeletal muscle and abdominal muscle. It also facilitates the introduction of the endotracheal tube. Given in a drip, it can be monitored moment to moment for response of the patient.

General anesthesia may be used for elective or emergency cesarean section. For an elective section, regional anesthesia is usually preferred, although if regional anesthesia is not available or if the mother strongly prefers, general anesthesisa may be administered safely. For emergency cesarean section, when either mother or fetus is in immediate jeopardy, general anesthesia is preferred. Such cases would include prolapsed cord, massive bleeding, and ruptured uterus.

Complications of general anesthesia may include: (1) fetal depression if anesthesia has been long or deep; (2) uterine relaxation, which may lead to uterine atony; and, (3) vomiting and aspiration. If there is not a real emergency, the administration of 30 ml of a cold antacid (such as Maalox) given 30 min before induction will help neutralize stomach contents and avoid the complication of aspirating acidic contents.

The long-term effect of fetal depression has not been determined. Studies have shown that immediately postdelivery and up to 8 hours after delivery infants delivered under general anesthesia are more depressed neurobehaviorally than those delivered with spinal anesthesia.

Sensory Modulation Approaches

Sensory modulation methods include such simple techniques as relaxation, effleurage, superficial heat (dry or wet) and cold, which all produce sensory input. That is, they generate nerve impulses that enter the spinal cord and brain, where, it is believed, they ultimately inhibit pain signals and close the "gate". The gate control theory also indicates that cognitive activities such as distraction and suggestion can influence pain by interacting with afferent noxious stimuli.

PSYCHOLOGIC APPROACHES

A number of different methods of psychologic approaches have been used with varying degrees of success, which include (1) hypnosis, (2) natural childbirth, (3) psychoprophylaxis, (4) acupuncture, (5) LeBoyer techniques, and (6) transcutaneous electric nerve stimulation (TENS). They have been used independently, in combination and with modification, depending on the requirements of the woman and the situation. Table 18–5 summarizes alternate approaches to comfort in childbirth, with advantages and disadvantages of each. Natural childbirth and psychoprophylaxis

TABLE 18–5. Alternate Approaches to Comfort in Childbirth

Approach	Description or Definition	Anticipated Effect or Advantage	Negative Effect or Disadvantages	Comments
Hypnosis	Through a series of conditioning sessions, increasing degrees of trance are induced until a level of analgesia is achieved. May be able to function in labor without hypnotist present	Achieves maternal analgesia with no obstruction of airway, depressed reflexes, or hypotension, and no drug depression of neonate. May shorten labor. May be indicated for women for whom other methods are not indicated	Time consuming to prepare subject. Contraindicated in women with history of psychosis or psychoneurotic hysterical conversion reactions, or ambivalence toward birth or motherhood	Not always effective, depends on level of susceptibility
Natural childbirth, "childbirth without fear"	Introduced by Dr. Grantly Dick-Read. Based on the concept that fear and tension increase pain during labor. Provides for education and exercise prenatally. Decreasing fear and tension minimizes pain	Increased personal attention. Increased relaxation. Increased understanding of childbirth experience	Too much technical knowledge may increase tension or expectations. Presentation too emotional or spiritual for some practitioners	Raised awareness and consciousness of consumers and practitioners

TABLE 18–5. Continued

Approach	Description or Definition	Anticipated Effect or Advantage	Negative Effect or Disadvantages	Comments
Psychoprophylaxis, "childbirth without pain"	Introduced to Western World by Dr. Lamaze. Combines positive conditioning of mother with education on process of childbirth	Reduces amount of chemical anesthesia required by mother. Woman is well prepared for birth process. She and husband may participate in delivery	Possibly hyperventilation with breathing techniques. Need to maintain control thoroughly labor. Woman may be reluctant to ask for medication. May feel a failure if medication is needed	This movement led by consumers has continued to grow and evolve
Acupuncture	Manual or elective acupuncture in sites traditionally used for vaginal hysterectomy and dysmenorrhea	Safe for mother and infant	Dependent on motivation and cultural conditioning. Not found to be adequate thus far	Technique practiced in China, but not used traditionally by Chinese woman in labor. So far, not judged to be adequate analgesia for labor pains
LeBoyer, "birth without violence"	Promotes concept of childbirth without violence. Decreases noise, lights and other noxious stimuli during delivery. Provides warm bath to infant right after birth	Appealiing and attractive to many couples who are anticipating a normal delivery	Delivery room may be too dark to see adequately. Music may be distracting. Placing neonate on mother's abdomen may cause depletion of blood volume into placenta	Emphasis on sensations fetus may feel during birth process.
TENS	Skin electrodes placed symmetrically on either side of T10–T11 region of spine. Electric current may be controlled by mother or staff. Thought to stimulate nerve fibers which close "pain gate"	Safe for mother and baby. Can be controlled by mother, increased as needed. Instantly reversible. Decreases use of chemicals. Easily applied	Possibly unsatisfactory analgesia	So far, use has been limited. Mechanism of action not confirmed

have already been discussed in detail in Chapter 14, but are briefly mentioned here as comparative approaches to pain control.

SUMMARY

Labor pains exist for only a limited number of hours. However, within those hours the pain progresses from an infrequent twinge to intense, seemingly unbearable sensations that come one atop the other. To the woman in labor, pain may indeed seem endless, with time going on forever; simultaneously, it may appear as though time is standing still.

To the nurse, pain is a challenge. With knowledge of labor, the causes of pain, pain pathways, and pain interventions, the nurse is prepared to assess the pregnant woman's pain experience, design a plan of care, and see that the plan is carried out effectively. The challenge is there, waiting with each woman who goes into labor. Working with the physician, nurse-midwife, and family, the nurse can respond to this challenge and make each delivery a safe and satisfying family-centered birth experience.

REFERENCES

Affonso, D. D. 1978. The Filipino American. In *Culture, childbearing, health professionals*, ed. A. L. Clark. Philadelphia: F. A. Davis.

Albright, G.; Ferguson, J.; Joyce, T.; and Stevenson, D. 1986. *Anesthesia in obstetrics—Maternal, fetal, and neonatal aspects*, 2nd ed. Boston: Butterworths.

Avery, G. B. 1987. *Neonatology, pathophysiology and management of the newborn*, 3rd ed. Philadelphia: J. B. Lippincott.

Bonica, J. J. 1984. Labor pain. In *Textbook of Pain*, eds. P. D. Wall and R. Melzack. New York: Churchill Livingston.

Brownridge, P. R.; Taylor, G.; and Ralston, D. H. 1980. Neural blockade for obstetrics and gynecology. In *Neural blockade in clinical anesthesia and management of pain*, eds. M. J. Cousins and P. O. Bridenbaugh. Philadelphia: J. B. Lippincott.

Clark, A. L. 1981. *Culture and childbearing*. Philadelphia: F. A. Davis.

Coote, J. H., and Crawford, J. A. 1986. Neuroanatomy and neurophysiology of the female genitalia. In *Scientific foundation of obstetrics and gynecology*, 3rd ed, eds. E. Philipp, J. Barnes, and M. Newton. Chicago: William Heineman.

Dickason, E. J. 1978. Drugs used during labor and delivery. In *Maternal and infant drugs and nursing intervention*, eds. E. J. Dickason, M. O. Schult, and E. M. Morris. San Francisco: McGraw-Hill.

Gilman, A. G.; Goodman, L. S.; Wall, T. W.; and Murad, F. 1985. *Goodman and Gilman's the pharmocological basis of therapeutics*, 7th ed. New York: MacMillan.

Giuffre, M. 1983. *Validation of a visual analogue scale for pain measurement in childbirth*. University of Rochester, Ann Arbor: University of Microfilms International.

Horsely, J. A.; Drane, J.; and Reynolds, M. A. (1982). *Pain: Deliberative nursing intervention*. San Diego: Grune and Stratton.

Jacox, A. 1977. *Pain: A source book for nurses and other health professionals*. Boston: Little, Brown.

Kron, R. E.; Stein, M. S.; and Goddard, K. E. 1966. Newborn sucking behavior affected by obstetrical sedation. *Pediatrics*. 37:1012–1016.

Meade, M., and Newton, N. 1967. Cultural patterning of perinatal behavior. In *Childbearing: Its social and psychological aspects*, eds. S. A. Richardson and A. A. Guttmacher. Baltimore, Md.: Williams and Wilkins.

Melzack, R. 1975. The McGill Pain Questionnaire: Major properties and scoring methods. *Pain*. 1:277–299.

Melzack, R., ed. 1983. *Pain measurement and assessment*. New York: Raven Press.

Melzack, R., and Wall, P. D. 1983. *The challenge of pain*. New York: Basic Books.

Melzack, R.; Taenzer, P.; Feldman, P.; and Kinch, R. 1981. Labour is still painful after prepared childbirth training. *Canad. Med. Assoc. J.* 125:357–363.

Morse, J. M. 1981. *Descriptive analysis of cultural coping mechanisms utilized for the reduction of parturition pain and anxiety in Figi*. University of Utah, Ann Arbor: University Microfilms International.

Newton, N., and Newton, M. 1973. Childbirth in cross-cultural perspective. In *Modern perspectives in psychoobstetrics*, ed. J. C. Howells. New York: Brunner/Mazel.

Okamoto, N. I. 1978. The Japanese American. In *Culture, childbearing, health professionals*, ed. A. L. Clark. Philadelphia: F. A. Davis.

Sandelowski, M. 1984. *Pain, pleasure and American childbirth*. Westport, Conn.: Greenwood Press

Shnider, S. M., and Gershon, L. 1987. *Anesthesia for obstetrics*, 2nd ed. Baltimore: Williams and Wilkins.

Varney, H. 1980. *Nurse-midwifery*. Boston: Blackwell Scientific.

Winsberg, B., and Greenlick, M. 1967. Pain response in Negro and white obstetrical patients. *J. Health Soc. Behav.* 8:222–228.

19
Care of the Newborn Immediately Following Birth

BEHAVIORAL OBJECTIVES

Upon completion of this chapter, the reader should be able to:

- Identify the high-priority needs of the infant immediately after birth.

- Discuss assessment of hypoxia and asphyxia and nursing care measures for prevention of both.

- Explain the Apgar scoring system and the scoring of each item.

- List basic resuscitation equipment that should be available in the delivery room and describe possible uses of each item.

- Demonstrate the basic technique for infant resuscitation.

- Discuss the prevention of hypothermia and cold stress.

- Explain how complications of hypercarbia, hypoglycemia, and hypotension may result from hypothermia or hypoxia.

- Compare hospital routines for prevention of infection, prevention of hypoprothrombinemia, assessment for anomalies, and identification.

- Discuss the rationale for promoting attachment of infant and family and identify safe methods the nurse can use to facilitate the attachment.

CHANGE: THE INTRAPARTAL PERIOD

- Identify interventions the nurse can provide for spiritual care of the family.

- Establish a nursing intervention plan to care for both infant and parents immediately after birth.

The cry of a newborn infant is thrilling. The change, long awaited and planned for, has finally occurred. The infant is delivered to the outside world by the doctor or midwife and the mother or father may hold the infant for a few seconds. The physician then usually focuses attention on the care of the mother by delivering the placenta and repairing the episiotomy. If the infant is not cared for by a pediatrician, the nurse assumes responsibility for immediate assessment and care of that newborn.

Immediately after birth the infant is very vulnerable. The care the nurse gives is important, as successful adaptation to changes in the outside world can make a difference in the infant's potential for physical and mental development. The nursing strategies implemented can also affect the parents and their attitudes toward the birth process and parenting. This chapter discusses the priorities and the routine procedures used in assessment and care of the infant immediately after birth, focusing on the first-priority nursing goals for prevention of complications.

PREVENTING ASPHYXIA

The biggest threat to the newborn is *asphyxia*. Avery (1987) lists four basic mechanisms that cause asphyxia in the newborn:

1. Interruption of the umbilical blood flow as a result of cord compression during labor.
2. Failure of oxygen exchange across the placenta because of placental separation, as in abruptio placentae.
3. Inadequate perfusion of the maternal side of the placenta, as in maternal hypertension (PIH).
4. Failure of the lungs to inflate and complete the change in the fetal circulatory systems, because of obstruction, fluid, or weak respiratory effort.

Asphyxia is potentially a problem for all newborns because of the need for change from the fetal to newborn respiratory and circulatory systems.

Prevention of asphyxia in the newborn begins before birth. As the nurse is caring for the labor client, she needs to be aware of conditions that may cause asphyxia (see Table 19–1).

The maternity nurse caring for the client during labor should communicate information regarding any of these high-risk conditions to the physicians or nurses who will be responsible for the care of the infant immediately after birth so that preparations can be made for emergency care. Equipment that should be present in the delivery room for immediate care of the infant is listed in Table 19–2.

The first priority in care of the newborn is to establish a clear airway and initiate respirations. Respirations are usually spontaneously initiated in the first 30 secs of life, and when the infant is 90 secs of age respirations are normally regular, as indicated in Fig. 19–1 (Berman and Saunders 1980).

Initial breathing in the infant is the result of a reflex triggered by chemical changes in the aortic blood flow due to the occlusion of the umbilical cord. As the O_2 falls from 80 to 15 mm Hg, arterial pCO_2 rises from 40 to 70 mm Hg and arterial pH falls below 7.35, the respiratory center is stimulated to initiate respirations (Butnarescu and Tillotson, 1983). Other sensory changes of the birth process such as pressure changes, chilling, noise,

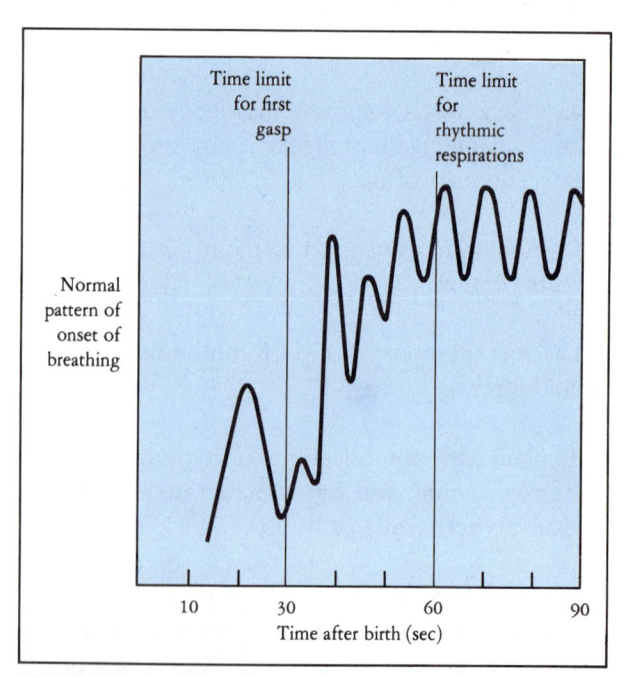

FIGURE 19–1. Time after birth needed to establish respirations.
SOURCE: Clark, Affonso, and Harris (1979).

TABLE 19-1. *Some Factors That Place the Newborn Infant at High Risk for Asphyxia*

Maternal Conditions

Age: under 15 or over 35
Parity: primigravida or greater than gravida 5
Single parent
Nutrition: obesity, underweight, inadequate caloric or protein intake
Drug usage: nicotine, alcohol, other habituating or addictive drugs, aspirin, caffeine, prescription and over-the-counter drugs
Unusual stress or anxiety
Environment and occupation
Family history of inheritable disorder
Previous infant with congenital anomalies
Consanguinity
Stature (height below 60 in, small pelvis)
Diabetes mellitus
Cardiac disease
Endocrine dysfunction
Positive serology for syphilis
Hypertension
Renal disease
Malignancy

Anemia
Epilepsy
Acute viral infections, hepatitis
Urinary tract infections
Psychiatric disorders
History of previous high-risk pregnancy:
    Premature labor
    Small-for-gestational-age or large-for-gestational-age infants
    Cesarean section or other operative delivery
    Abortion or stillbirth
    Neonatal morbidity
Present pregnancy:
    Exposure to teratogens (radiation, chemicals, accident)
    Hyperemesis gravidarum, dehydration, ketosis, acidosis
    Vaginal bleeding, placenta previa, abruptio placentae
    Isoimmune disease
    Prolonged rupture of membranes
    Premature labor

Fetal Conditions

Premature delivery
Multiple births
Acidosis (fetal scalp capillary blood)
Abnormal heart rate or rhythm
Meconium-stained amniotic fluid
Forceps delivery other than low-elective or vacuum-extraction
Breech or other abnormal presentation and delivery
Cesarean section
Prolonged labor (1st stage 24 hours; 2nd stage 2 hours)
Prolapsed umbilical cord

Polyhydramnios
Decreased rate of growth (uterine size or fetal size by ultrasound)
Immaturity of pulmonary surfactant system
Fetal malformations (by ultrasound)
Cord compression (nuchal cord, cord knot, compression by after-coming head in breech delivery)
Maternal hypotension
Sedative or analgesic drugs given i.v. within 1 hour of delivery or i.m. within 2 hours of delivery
Prolonged rupture of membranes
Premature labor

SOURCE: Avery (1987).

---

and light are also believed to stimulate respirations.

Before the birth process begins, the term infant has approximately 80–110 ml of fluid in the respiratory passages. Between 7 and 42 ml of this fluid is squeezed out during vaginal delivery, and the rest is either swallowed, aspirated, or absorbed rapidly. A large amount of mucus, amniotic fluid, blood, and possibly meconium is present in the nasopharynx at birth and should be removed as soon as the infant's head is delivered by the clinician. A bulb syringe or a DeLee catheter may be used to suction first the mouth and then the nose. (Suctioning the nose first would cause the infant to gasp and aspirate the large amount of fluid in the mouth.) Suctioning prior to the first respirations prevents aspiration of the mucoid fluid from the oropharynx into the bronchi with the first breaths. This is especially important if meconium has been present in amniotic fluid,

TABLE 19–2.	Equipment Required for Adequate Neonatal Resuscitation

Radiantly heated resuscitation platform with sterile drapes
Sterile bulb suction and vacuum suction with sterile catheters
Thermometer and thermal control for radiant heater
Laryngoscope and blades (at least 2 sizes), spare parts, batteries
Oropharyngeal airways
DeLee suction catheter
Endotracheal tubes, with stylets
Source of oxygen and air with an oxygen–air proportioner and heated nebulizer
Face masks—preterm and term sizes
Connectors from endotracheal tube or mask to soft 500 ml anesthesia bag and air–oxygen source
Sterile umbilical vessel catheterization tray, including small iris scissors, cord tie, and 3½ and 5F umbilical vessel catheters with 3-way stopcocks
Sterile syringes, needles, straight and sterile 1 ml heparinized syringes for blood gas sampling
Good light (a procedure spotlight may be helpful)
Pressure transducers and monitor for vascular pressures
ECG electrodes and heart-rate monitor
Blood gas and pH electrodes
Clock with sweep second hand
Infant stethoscope
Fresh bottle of glucose reagent sticks for heelstick glucose estimator
Scissors, tape, tape measures
Medications
#8 feeding tubes
Apgar timer

SOURCE: Moore (1983).

against too much nasopharyngeal stimulation with a catheter since reflex bradycardia or laryngospasm may occur (10 sec is adequate) (Hazinsky, 1987).

Keeping the infant in a semi-Trendelenberg's position, with head down, immediately after delivery will promote drainage of mucus from respiratory passages. This position is contraindicated when the infant may have suffered cerebral trauma or intracranial hemorrhage. Holding the infant by its heels or spanking is not recommended to stimulate respirations. Rubbing the back and the rest of the body while quickly drying the infant is usually sufficient stimulus for respirations. Additional suctioning with a bulb syringe or a DeLee catheter may be necessary (see Fig. 19–2). When a bulb syringe is used for suctioning, it should be collapsed before it is inserted. Otherwise, the material in the nose or oropharynx will be forced into the bronchi and lungs when the bulb is collapsed. When suctioning with a catheter, the nurse should take care not to traumatize the tissues of the oropharynx with the tip of the catheter or with forceful suction. If wall suction is used, it should be set on low or at a range of 0–80 mm Hg. Oversuctioning should be avoided because it deprives the infant of oxygen and irritates the mucous membranes. If deep suctioning is provided, the infant should receive supplemental oxygen therapy; adequate ventilation should be ensured before and following any suctioning.

INITIAL ASSESSMENT: THE APGAR SCORE

Once an infant has initiated respirations and the airway is patent, an initial assessment of the infant should be carried out. The first assessment done in the delivery room by the nurse, nurse anesthetist, or doctor is known as the *Apgar score*.

The Apgar scoring system was introduced by Virginia Apgar (1953) as a simple system for evaluating the physical condition of the infant. The newborn is rated at 1 min after birth and again at 5 min. A total score ranging from 0 to 10 is assigned, with the more vigorous infant receiving a high score. The following criteria are used for scoring (see also Table 19–3):

1. *A—appearance, or color.* Color evaluation is for cyanosis and pallor. Frequently, the infant is completely blue and pale at birth, receiving a

because aspiration of the meconium will keep alveoli from expanding with air. If meconium staining is present during delivery, the neonate's oropharynx must be suctioned immediately in an attempt to prevent aspiration of the meconium. If the neonate does aspirate thick meconium, intubation should be performed immediately, and the meconium should be suctioned from the trachea using direct application of the suction to the endotracheal tube. The neonate should then be reintubated with a new endotracheal tube, and additional suctioning should be performed as needed. Berman and Saunders (1980) cautions

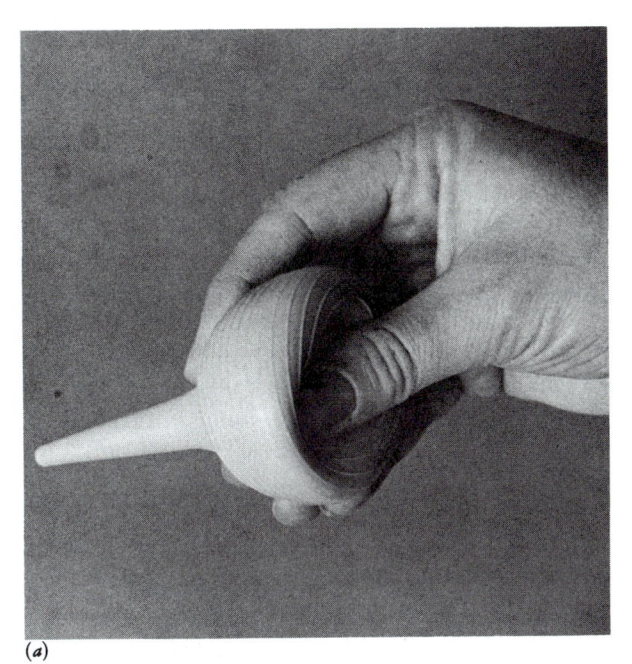

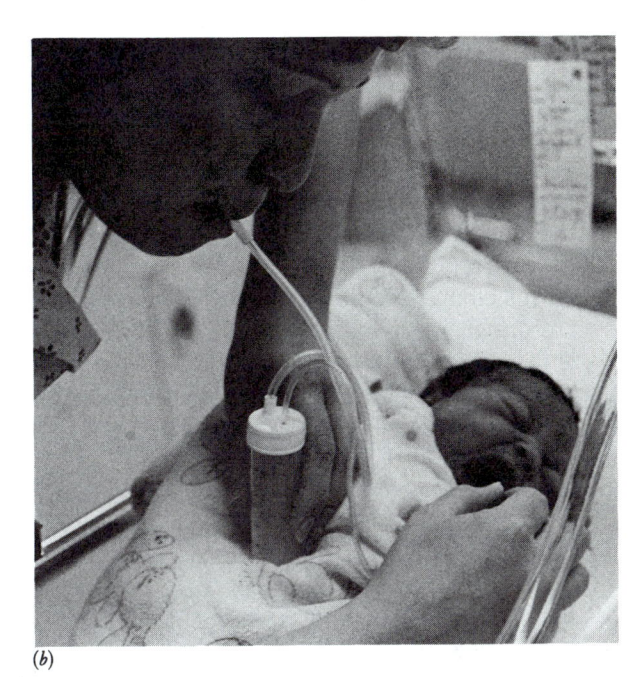

FIGURE 19-2. (a) Bulb syringe for suctioning the nose and mouth. (b) De Lee trap for suctioning the nose, mouth, and nearby areas.

score of 0. At 1 or 5 min after birth many infants have become pink but continue to have blue extremities (acrocyanosis) and receive a score of 1. Only a few infants become completely pink by 5 min after birth and are rated 2 (Korones, 1986).

2. *P—pulse, or heart rate.* The heart rate is the most important diagnostic and prognostic item to assess in measuring asphyxia. The heart rate is auscultated for at least 30 sec, or the pulse may be palpated at the junction of the umbilical cord and the skin. A heart rate of over 100 beats/min rates a 2. If the rate is less than 100 beats/min, the rating is 1, severe asphyxia is present, and the infant must be immediately resuscitated. No heart rate equals a score of 0.

3. *G—grimace, or reflex irritability.* Reflex irritability is evaluated by noting the infant's response to stimuli. A catheter may be touched to the nostril (after the oropharynx is clear). In the healthy infant a cough or sneeze is elicited. Only a grimace rates a 1, and no response is a 0.

TABLE 19-3. Apgar Scoring Chart

Sign	0	1	2
Appearance or color	Blue, pale	Body pink, extremities blue	Completely pink
Pulse or heart rate	Absent	Slow (below 100)	Over 100
Grimace or reflex response	No response	Grimace	Cough or sneeze
1. Response to catheter in nostril (tested after oropharynx is clear)			
or			
2. Tangential foot slap	No response	Grimace	Cry and withdrawal of foot
Activity or muscle tone	Limp	Some flexion of extremities	Well flexed
Respirations or respiratory effort	Absent	Weak cry, hypoventilation	Good strong cry

SOURCE: Apgar (1958).

Reflex irritability can also be tested by flicking the sole of the foot; if the infant cries, a score of 2 is given. If he only grimaces or cries feebly, a score of 1 is given. No response is a sign of severe neurologic depression and rates a 0.

4. *A—activity, or muscle tone.* Muscle tone refers to the degree of flexion and the resistance offered to straightening the extremities. A normal newborn's elbows are flexed, and thighs and knees are drawn up toward the abdomen. When the leg is straightened, some resistance is felt. The asphyxiated infant (0) is limp with no flexion or resistance. An intermediate state is given 1 point.

5. *R—respirations, or respiratory effort.* Respiratory effort refers to the infant's ability to initiate respirations. Regular respirations and a vigorous cry merit a score of 2. If the respirations are shallow, irregular, or gasping, a score of 1 is appropriate. Zero (0) denotes complete absence of respiratory effort, or apnea.

The 5-min Apgar score has been shown to have a close relationship to neurologic status at 1 year of age. The Apgar scoring will be lowered by depression due to maternal analgesia and anesthesia, low birth weight, or neonatal asphyxia. Most infants score 6–7 at 1 min and 8–10 by 5 min after birth. If the score is 7 or less at 5 min, the rating should be repeated in 10 min (Korones, 1986).

The total 1-min Apgar score indicates whether there is need for resuscitation. A score of 8, 9, or 10 indicates an infant in good condition who requires only nasal and oral suctioning, drying, and warming.

The infant with a score of 5, 6, or 7 is a slightly depressed infant. These infants may have a heart rate of over 100, but are cyanotic or pale, and may be dyspneic and less reactive to stimuli. After nasopharyngeal suctioning, moist oxygen may be given directly by blowing oxygen over the face while cupping one's hand over the infant's nose and mouth to form a funnel (Shaffer, 1980). Stimulating the infant by rubbing the back vigorously will also encourage crying and adequate respirations. When the newborn is in distress, resuscitative efforts are begun before the 1-min Apgar is officially completed.

An infant with an Apgar of 3 or 4 is moderately depressed and will require more aggressive oxygen therapy with a resuscitation bag and oxygen mask. The mouth, nose, and pharynx should be thoroughly suctioned. Endotracheal intubation and suctioning may be necessary and will make respiratory assistance more effective. The infant resuscitation bag can administer 100 percent oxygen to the infant. (For this short time, 100 percent oxygen will not harm the eyes, but will give adequate oxygen to the bloodstream to overcome the effects of severe asphyxia.) Hyperventilate at 40–50 breaths/min.

If the Apgar score is 0 to 2, the infant is severely depressed. The infant is blue and limp with no reflex irritability, and heart rate is below 100/min. Immediate endotracheal intubation with a laryngoscope and suctioning, and ventilating are the only procedures that can save this infant. Frequently, the delivery of oxygen to the lungs brings about a quick response, the heartbeat returns, and the baby becomes pink.

If there is no audible heart rate, or if it remains below 100 after 1 min of assisted ventilation, cardiac massage should be initiated. This should be coordinated with the ventilation in a 5:1 ratio (5 heartbeats, pause for 1 breath, 5 heartbeats, pause for 1 breath). As with an adult, cardiac massage is best accomplished over a hard surface.

There are two acceptable techniques of chest compression. Both thumbs may be placed in the middle of the infant's sternum, just below the nipple line, with both hands encircling the infant's torso. The sternum may also be compressed using two fingers (the ring and middle finger), placed one finger-breadth below the nipple line.

Chest compression should be smooth, and the thumbs or fingers should not leave the infant's sternum between compressions. Care should be taken to avoid compression of the lower portion of the infant's sternum since this may result in damage to abdominal organs. Compressions may be discontinued if the infant's spontaneous heart rate reaches or exceeds 80/min (Avery, 1987; Hazinsky, 1987) (see Fig. 19–3).

Positioning the infant with neck hyperextended with a towel roll will stretch the trachea and the floor of the mouth, providing a more patent airway. As the face mask is placed over the infant's mouth and nose, care should be taken not to compress the eyes but to obtain an air-tight seal around the face mask (Sheldon and Dominiak 1980) (see Fig. 19–4).

When the bag and mask are used, there is a tendency to inflate the stomach with air. Insertion of a nasogastric tube will keep the stomach decompressed to give more room for pulmonary expansion.

Massage can be discontinued for a few seconds periodically to evaluate spontaneous rate. If lengthy resuscitation and massage are necessary, connection to an ECG monitor will show heart

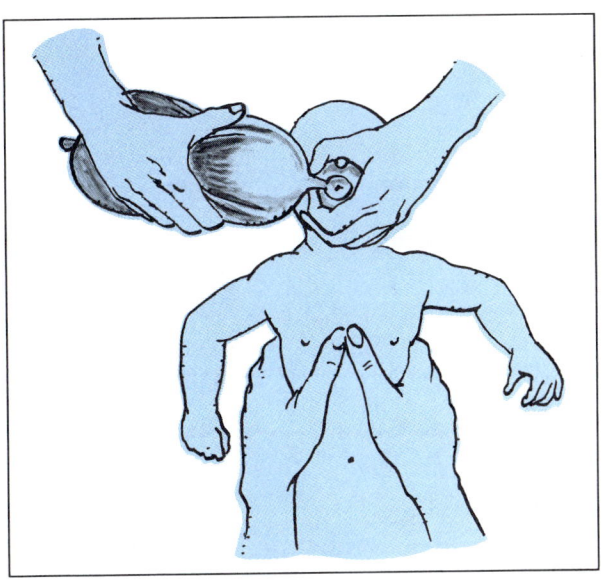

FIGURE 19-3. Cardiopulmonary resuscitation, with bag and mask technique for ventilation and external cardiac massage with the thumbs of the second resuscitator applied at the midsternum.
SOURCE: Hodson and Truog (1983).

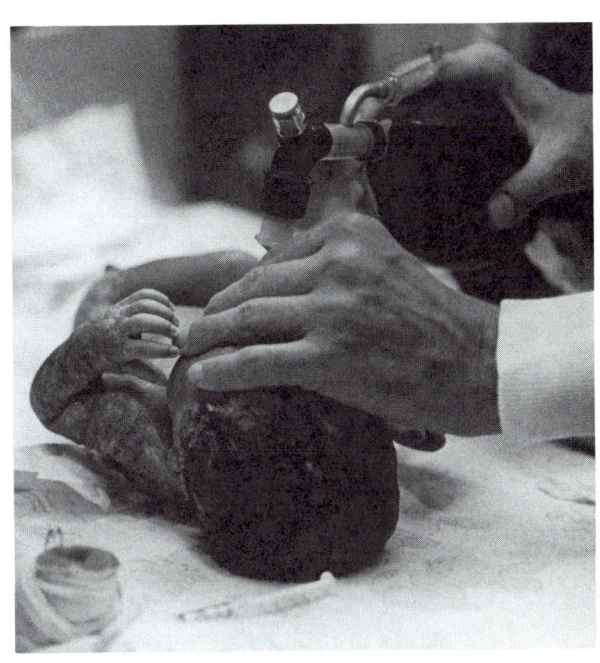

FIGURE 19-4. Position of infant with face mask for resuscitation.

action. Intermittent positive pressure breathing (IPPB) may be utilized to provide an initial inflating pressure that will aid in expansion of the lungs and in preventing atelectasis (collapse of lung alveoli) as the infant exhales.

When artificial ventilation with 100 percent oxygen and cardiac massage are not effective, administration of medications may be necessary. Table 19-4 lists the drugs most commonly used in resuscitation, indications for use, routes and concentrations for administration, usual dosages, side-effects, and nursing implications.

Intravenous medications are frequently administered to a newborn through an umbilical catheter, which the physician inserts shortly after birth. The nurse must ensure that a sterile tray with all necessary equipment is available in the delivery room for this procedure. She may assist the physician by restraining the infant or by handling equipment. Assisting with maintenance of sterile technique during this procedure is an important nursing intervention.

HYPOTHERMIA

The human organism is homeothermic. This means that it can and must maintain its body temperature within narrow limits in spite of gross changes in the atmosphere. The newborn infant has several disadvantages in this process of adaptation to changes in surrounding temperatures because it has (1) a relatively large surface area, (2) inadequate thermal insulation, (3) a small body mass to retain heat, and (4) limited metabolic capabilities for heat production (see Chapter 25).

Thermal Control in the Infant

The control of body temperature is accomplished primarily by the central nervous system. The hypothalamus receives data from skin and central sensory receptors that note minute changes in the environment. The functioning of this sending (affector) arc can be affected by drugs, intracranial hemorrhage, cerebral abnormalities, asphyxia, trauma, cerebral edema, and infection (Perez, 1981).

The receiving (effector) arc is the responding component of the sensory temperature control system. Four primary factors limit or potentiate the infant's ability to produce and retain heat. These include vasomotor control, thermal insulation, muscular activity and body movement, and metabolism of brown fat.

Vasomotor control—vasoconstriction in particular—allows the newborn to control loss of heat

TABLE 19-4. *Drugs Most Commonly Used in Resuscitation of Infant*

Medication	Indications	Suggested Dosage	Usual Concentration	Side-Effects and Nursing Implications
Atropine	Neonatal bradycardia	0.01–0.08 mg/kg IV	0.4 mg/ml	Tachycardia; decreased cardiac output
Calcium chloride	Low cardiac output	25 mg/kg IV; may repeat every 10 min; 0.5–1.0 mg/kg/24 h IV	1 g/10 ml (100 mg/ml) 10% solution	Toxic to tissues if it infiltrates; hypotension
Dopamine	Low cardiac output	100 mg/100 ml D_5W (1000 μg/ml) IV; small infant: 50 mg/100 ml D_5W (500 μg/ml); range: 2–20 μg/kg/min IV	200 mg/5 ml	Cardiac arrhythmias; protect from light; discard discolored solution
Dextrose	Hypoglycemia	6–7 mg/kg/min IV	10%	Monitor blood sugar frequently to prevent diabetes acidosis
Calcium gluconate	Low cardiac output, hypocalcemia, hypermagnesemia	100 (1 ml) mg/kg IV over 5–10 min	10%	Monitor ECG for arrhythmias
Epinephrine 1:10,000	Cardiac arrest; given while performing cardiac massage	0.1 ml/kg (0.01 mg/kg) IV; drip: 1 mg/100 ml D_5W (5 μg/ml) IV; small infant: 0.5 mg/100 ml D_5W (5 μg/ml) start at 0.1 μg/kg/min; IV or intracardiac injector	1:1000 (1 mg/ml) (0.1 mg/ml or 100 μg/ml) 1:10,000 = 1 ml + 9 ml normal saline	Hypertension; ventricular fibrillation
Isuprel (isoproterenol)	Bradycardia, hypotension	1 mg/100 ml D_5W (1000 μg/ml) IV; small infant: 0.5 mg/100 ml D_5W (5 μg/ml); start with 0.1 μg/kg/min IV	0.2 mg/ml or 1 mg/5 ml (200 μg/ml)	Arrhythmias; tachycardia; if pulse above 160/min, lower rate
Narcan	Narcotic antagonist	0.01 mg/kg IV or i.m.	0.02 mg/ml	Do not administer to infants of addicted mothers as it may precipitate withdrawal
Sodium bicarbonate	Acidosis	1–3 meq/kg IV over 5 min IV; every 10 min × 2, then arterial blood gases	44.6 meq/50 ml (1 meq/ml)	May cause further decrease in pH acidemia without adequate pulmonary exchange
CNS stimulants—caffeine, Dexaprin, Coremine	Harmful and should not be given to neonates			

through the skin surface. This mechanism is limited by the fact that the infant has a large ratio of body surface to body weight. At birth, the full-term infant is only 5 percent of adult body weight. However, its body surface is 15 percent of that of the adult. A larger surface area provides more extensive exposure to the environment, thus promoting more heat loss. Loss of heat is four times greater in the full-term newborn than in the adult. This rapid loss of heat is the principal source of the neonate's difficulty in maintaining thermal balance (Korones, 1986).

Thermal insulation depends on the thin layer of white subcutaneous fat on the neonate. Deep-body core temperature is generally higher than skin or surface temperature. Since a gradient exists between the core and the surface, heat is constantly transferred to the surface. This transfer is impeded by a layer of subcutaneous fat (Korones, 1986). Substantial amounts of fat do not accumulate until after 32 weeks' gestation. Therefore, a preterm infant or one weighing less than 2000 g lacks adequate insulation to prevent rapid heat loss or to permit the body core mass to act as a heat reservoir (Perez, 1981).

Muscular activity and *body movement* contribute to chemical thermogenesis. Shivering is an important mechanism of heat production in the adult. However, it is very limited in the neonate and occurs only in the presence of extreme cold stress.

Metabolism of brown fat is the most important mechanism of heat production. Brown fat is located between the scapulae; behind the sternum; around the neck, head, heart, great vessels, kidneys, and adrenal glands; and in the axilla. It comprises 2–6 percent of the neonate's body weight. Brown fat cells first appear at 26–30 weeks of gestation and continue to enlarge during the neonatal period. The brown color is due to a copious blood supply, a dense cellular content, and a profusion of sympathetic nerve endings. When cooling occurs, these sympathetic nerve endings are stimulated to secrete norepinephrine, which then stimulates fat metabolism in the brown tissue with the end result of heat production and oxygen depletion. Prolonged cold stress seems to deplete brown fat stores and may even eliminate this nonshivering thermogenesis mechanism (Korones, 1986).

Although the most common problem in thermal regulation of the neonate is cold stress, the infant can also become stressed if it is too warm. The neonate's sweating mechanism is not mature; therefore, the overheated neonate must seek to eliminate heat through increased respiratory and metabolic rates, thus compromising the homeostatic capacities of the infant.

Maintaining a Neutral Thermal Environment

The goal for nursing care is to maintain a neutral thermal environment. Measurement of temperature by axillary or skin electrodes is recommended. Rectal or "core" temperature changes more slowly and shows differences only when cold stress is already occurring. Rectal temperatures require more exposure to room air and cooling besides the danger of bowel perforation. The newborn infant loses heat through four processes: evaporation, conduction, convection, and radiation (see Chapter 25).

Evaporation

Immediately after delivery, heat loss may occur by evaporation of the amniotic fluid covering the body or through the lungs via normal breathing. Nursing interventions that lessen evaporative heat loss are:

1. Drying the baby off as rapidly as possible after birth with a warm blanket. Dry the hair and head carefully, as this is a large surface area and loses heat rapidly.
2. Replacing the wet blanket with a warm, dry one. Do not leave infant in a wet blanket.
3. Bathing the infant only after its temperature is stabilized at 98–99°F (axilla). This occurs at about 4–6 hours of age in most infants.
4. Allowing the vernix to be absorbed or to wear off rather than vigorously scrubbing or soaking it.

Conduction

Conductive heat loss at the time of birth frequently occurs through contact with cold blankets, cold clothing, and cold surfaces such as exam tables and scales. Conductive heat loss can be prevented by:

1. Placing the infant under a prewarmed (98°F) radiant warmer immediately after birth for unwrapped observation or any needed treatments.
2. Warming blankets and clothing before using them on the infant.

Convection

Heat loss by convection is caused by air currents passing over the baby. This can result from: (1) air conditioning of the delivery room; (2) administration of cold oxygen; or, (3) transportation of the infant through cold or drafty corridors or elevators. Heat loss by convection may be prevented by:

1. Planning for control of the environment of the delivery room, recovery room, and nursery so that cooling vents are not near an infant warmer or crib.
2. Wrapping the infant in a thick blanket for holding or transporting.
3. Utilizing a covered crib or transport isolette for transportation in halls and elevators.

Radiation

Heat loss by radiation can occur through cold window panes, cold walls, or cold isolette walls close to an air conditioner vent. Radiation heat loss is prevented by:

1. Placing the infant in a radiant warmer or warmed isolette away from cold windows or walls (32–35°C or 90–95°F). *Note:* The infant's temperature should be carefully monitored if a servo-controlled overhead warmer is used. The infant can become overheated, which will cause a heat stress problem. The rectal probe is not recommended for monitoring because of the danger of rectal perforation. A skin monitor will be sufficient to note overheating that might occur in the delivery room. Insensible water loss may occur if the infant is left under the warmer for a long period of time (see Chapter 25).
2. Leaving the infant unwrapped under the warmer, since the radiant heat does not go through the blanket.
3. Using an overhead radiant warmer over both mother and baby (see Fig. 19–5). This is safe even for a premature baby weighing 1.0–1.5 kg (Behrman, 1983).
4. Laying the infant skin to skin with the mother with a layered blanket covering the baby's back. This has been found to keep the infant 1 degree warmer than a heated crib (Gardner, 1979; Korones, 1986).
5. Dressing the infant in long-sleeved gown and cap and wrapping in a warm blanket (if the infant is not under the warmer or next to mother's skin) (see Fig. 19–6). The recom-

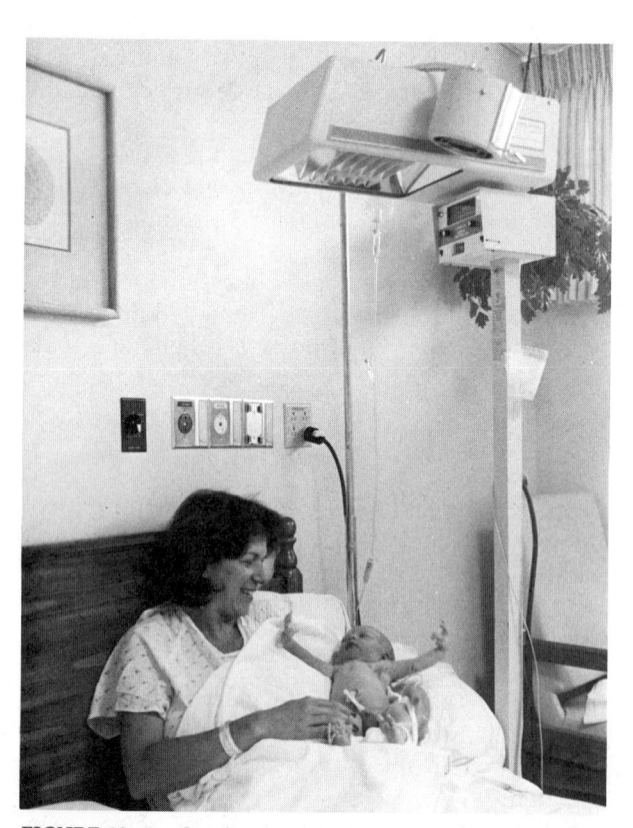

FIGURE 19–5. Overhead warmer with mother and baby.

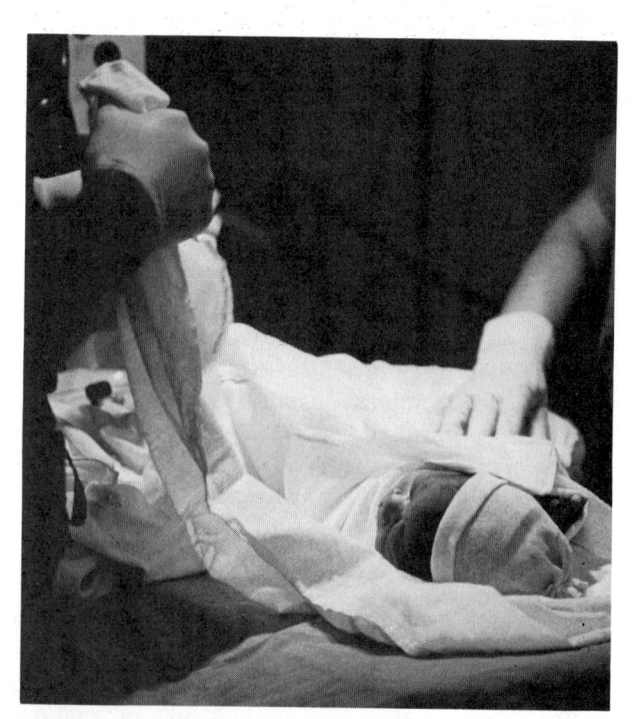

FIGURE 19–6. Newborn being wrapped in a warm blanket with a stocking cap.

mended temperature for nurseries/delivery rooms is 78°F (25.5°C) (Korones, 1986).

HYPOGLYCEMIA

Hypoglycemia can be expected in the severely cold-stressed newborn infant. The infant responds to chilling by increasing the metabolic rate, which increases oxygen needs. Breakdown of glycogen to glucose then occurs under hypoxic conditions. This anaerobic glycolysis metabolizes glucose at 20 times the normal aerobic rate and will quickly induce hypoglycemia (Steele, 1981). Since normal brain function depends on an adequate level of glucose being available in the blood, the potential for brain damage exists with severe hypoglycemia.

During pregnancy the fetal glucose level is 70–80 percent of that of the mother. During the last trimester of pregnancy, the fetus stores glucose as glycogen. These glycogen stores can be utilized during the birth process and immediately after birth before feeding begins. Diabetes, toxemia, multiple fetuses, and any maternal condition that may cause intrauterine growth retardation or prematurity may predispose the infant to hypoglycemia (Steele, 1981). In the normal newborn, the blood glucose reaches its lowest level between 1.5 and 3 hours of age. In the absence of high-risk conditions, there is a gradual return of the glucose level to normal, and stabilization is reached by 4–6 hours of age.

Screening is the most effective way of preventing hypoglycemia. A Dextrostix test at 1 hour of age will identify those infants already hypoglycemic. Glucose levels for the newborn are normally 70–80 mg/100 ml. If the glucose is under 40 mg/100 ml, blood sugar level should be determined by the laboratory. If desired, the Dextrostix test may be repeated at 2- or 4-hour intervals if the infant is small or at special risk for hypoglycemia.

If the Dextrostix shows the glucose level to be below 40 mg/100 ml, an early feeding of 5–10 percent glucose water may be given. In some hospitals, a physician's order may be required prior to feeding. If the glucose level is below 25 mg/100 ml, the physician may order the administration of dextrose intravenously.

HYPERCARBIA

Anaerobic glycolysis generates excess lactic acid. The metabolism of brown fat also releases fatty acids into the bloodstream. These excess acids cause a metabolic acidosis in the cold-stressed newborn (Steele, 1981).

The hypoxic infant cannot maintain an adequate oxygen supply. Vasoconstriction results, which reduces pulmonary perfusion and results in further decreased oxygen and increased carbon dioxide in the bloodstream. Thus, respiratory acidosis is induced in the newborn.

Measurement of acidosis is done by obtaining pH and blood-gas values. If the arterial pH level is below 7.0 or the pCO_2 is over 70 mm Hg, sodium bicarbonate will usually be given (see Table 19-4). Resuscitation of the infant should also be continued.

HYPOTENSION

Newborns can be in shock due to hypoxic conditions or loss of blood. The moderately depressed neonate's blood pressure should be obtained shortly after birth. This can be obtained with a Doppler or by other monitoring devices. Normal newborn blood pressure values are 46/20 to 96/69.

BLOOD TESTS

A hematocrit and hemoglobin may be routinely obtained within 1 hour after birth. Blood can be drawn at the same time the Dextrostix test is done, if the heel is adequately warmed to ease filling of the tubes. Normal range for the hematocrit is 50–70 percent. If it is below 40 percent, the physician may order a transfusion.

The procedure for heel-stick to obtain capillary blood for Dextrostix or hematocrit is as follows:

1. Warm the infant's foot by applying a moist warm pack for at least 5 min.
2. Cleanse the heel by rubbing with 70 percent alcohol.
3. Wipe alcohol off with a sterile cotton ball or 2" × 2" gauze pad.
4. Using a lancet, puncture the outer edge of the heel deeply enough to get a free flow of blood.
5. Cover the reagent area of the Dextrostix completely with blood.
6. After 60 sec, rinse the Dextrostix and read it by comparing it with the chart or by using a glucometer.
7. While waiting for 60 sec to elapse, you may begin filling capillary tubes with blood for the hematocrit.

The most important actions the nurse can take to prevent hypoglycemia, hypercarbia, and hypotension are to establish a clear airway and adequate respirations and to prevent hypothermia. These are the highest priorities of care for the infant immediately after birth. Other care may vary according to hospital routines and physicians' orders. Explanations to the parents of procedures being performed lessens their emotional distress and facilitates attachment later.

PREVENTING INFECTION

Adequate handwashing is the one best method for prevention of infection. A 3-min vigorous scrubbing of hands and arms to elbows with antibacterial soap or betadine solution should be done by all personnel each day before working on the obstetric unit. Parents and other family members who may be holding the infant should also be taught proper handwashing techniques. Careful 1-min handwashing should also be performed before handling each infant, after diaper changes, and before and after caring for the mother. Center for Disease Control (CDC) guidelines specify gloving to prevent spread of infectious diseases from moist secretions. Since the infant is usually wet with amniotic fluid, it is recommended that those caring for the infant before it is bathed wear gloves to protect themselves. Protective gown, goggles, and mask should be worn in delivery rooms to prevent contamination with amniotic fluid or while suctioning. Careful cleaning and/or disposal of all blankets and articles contacted by amniotic or other body fluids is also important (CDC, 1987). Gloving is recommended before procedures such as laryngoscopy or endotracheal suctioning.

Bathing is not recommended until the temperature of the infant is stabilized. A mild baby soap can be used to remove blood or meconium from face, head, and perianal area. Hexachlorophene (HCP) derivatives have been found to be neurotoxic to infants and should not be used (Feigin and Callanan, 1983). Vernix, a white cheesy substance frequently covering the newborn skin, especially in the folds, is a lubricating substance and does not need to be removed. However, removing blood or meconium-stained amniotic fluid helps the infant's appearance and aids bonding.

Cord Care

After the baby is delivered and the cord has ceased pulsating, the physician will clamp the cord in two places and cut between. If the physician does not place a small disposable clamp on the umbilical cord near to the infant's umbilicus, it may be the nurse's responsibility to do so. The nurse should also examine the cord for the presence of three vessels—two arteries and one vein—and record their presence on the delivery room record. The cord is clamped 0.5–1 inch from the abdomen to allow air space between the abdomen and the clamp to aid drying of the cord. The clamp must not catch any abdominal skin because this will cause necrosis of the tissue. The clamp is removed in the newborn nursery approximately 24 hours after the cord has dried (Olds et al., 1980). The cord should be inspected along with the placenta for abnormalities such as the absence of an artery, knots, strictures, hematomas, torsion, extremes of cord length, and unusual patterns of placental insertion. The nurse should check the cord frequently for bleeding or oozing, because 30 ml of a baby's total blood volume is the equivalent of 600 ml in an adult. Such bleeding is usually due to an ineffectively applied cord clamp but might also be indicative of a bleeding disorder or infection (Perry, 1982).

If the mother of the infant is Rh negative, or if the infant is considered to be high risk, the cord may be left 8–10 inches long so that umbilical catheterization will be possible if necessary. The cord may be kept in a sterile, moist saline gauze until blood type, Coombs' test, and other test results are obtained.

Topical applications of several medications are currently used to dry the cord and prevent infection. These include alcohol, triple dye, bismuth subgallate powder and antimicrobial agents such as bacitracin, or silver sulfadiazine cream. All are found to be equally effective (Arad, Eyal, and Fainmesser, 1981). Often a combination is used, with a moist antimicrobial ointment such as bacitracin being used once daily and antiseptic solutions such as alcohol or triple dye being applied with diaper changes. The umbilical area should be kept clean and uncovered to promote healing and drying.

Preventing Eye Infection

The use of an antibacterial agent as prophylaxis against ophthalmia neonatorum is mandatory by law in all states. Ophthalmia neonatorum is a gonococcal infection of the eye contracted during labor and delivery through a cervix and vagina infected with gonococcal organisms. Prior to this practice of prophylaxis of all infants, ophthalmia neonatorum had reached epidemic proportions. Because gonococcal infections can be present asymptomatically, prophylaxis of all infants is necessary.

Acceptable prophylactic agents that prevent gonococcal ophthalmia neonatorum include:

1. Silver nitrate solution (1 percent) in single-dose ampules.
2. Erythromycin (0.5 percent ophthalmic ointment or drops in single-use tubes or ampules)
3. Tetracycline (1 percent) ophthalmic ointment or drops in single-use tubes or ampules.

Erythromycin and tetracycline ointment and drops have also been found to prevent chlamydial ophthalmia neonatorum, which has become a common problem in recent years. Silver nitrate drops do not prevent this chlamydial infection. Therefore, the Committee on Ophthalmia Neonatorum of the National Society to Prevent Blindness (1981) and the American Academy of Pediatrics (1983) currently recommend installation of erythromycin or tetracycline ointment or drops shortly after birth in all infants.

The recommended method for administration of eye prophylaxis medications follows. Use of individual-dose wax ampules or tubes that will be discarded after use on one infant is recommended.

Silver Nitrate

1. Carefully clean the eyelids and surrounding skin with sterile cotton, which may be moistened with sterile water.
2. Gently open the baby's eyelid, particularly pulling down the lower eyelid, and install two drops of silver nitrate on the conjunctival sac. Allow the silver nitrate to run across the whole conjunctival sac. Carefully manipulate lids to ensure spread of the drops. Repeat in the other eye. Use two ampules, one for each eye.
3. After 1 min, gently wipe excess silver nitrate from eyelids and surrounding skin with sterile water. Do not irrigate the eyes.

Ophthalmic Ointment (Erythromycin or Tetracycline)

1. Carefully clean the eyelids and surrounding skin with sterile cotton, which may be moistened with sterile water. Do not irrigate the eyes.
2. Gently open the baby's eyelid, particularly pulling down the lower eyelid, and place a thin line of ointment, at least 0.5 inches (1–2 cm), along the junction of the bulbar and palpebral conjunctiva of the lower lid. Try to cover the whole lower conjunctival area. Carefully manipulate the lids to ensure spread of the ointment. Be careful not to touch the eyelid or eyeball with the tip of the tube. Repeat in the other eye. Use one tube per baby.
3. After 1 min, gently wipe excess ointment from the eyelids and surrounding skin with sterile water. Do not irrigate the eyes (National Society to Prevent Blindness, 1981).

Cautions in Instillation

The instillation must be carefully performed so that the agent reaches all parts of the conjunctival surface. Careful manipulation of the lids with fingers to ensure spreading of the medication is recommended. If the medication strikes only the eyelids and lid margins but fails to reach the cornea, the instillation should be repeated (National Society to Prevent Blindness, 1981).

Although a temporary chemical conjunctivitis may occasionally occur as a result of instillation, irrigation or rinsing of the eye after instillation is not recommended, because it may reduce the efficacy of the prophylaxis.

The instillation of eye drops or ointment appears to blur the infant's vision temporarily and is felt by many sources to be a hindrance to bonding. Delay of prophylactic eye instillation for 1 to 2 hours after birth gives the infant time to interact with the parents and has not increased the incidence of ophthalmic infections (Klaus and Kennell, 1981). The American Academy of Pediatrics (1983) states that prophylaxis can be delayed for 1 hour after birth, but a check should be set up to ensure that the medication is not omitted.

Other Prophylaxis

Other recommendations of the American Academy of Pediatrics (AAP) regarding the prophylaxis of ophthalmia neonatorum include:

1. Infants born by cesarean section should also receive prophylaxis against gonococcal ophthalmia. Although gonococcal infection is usually transmitted during passage through the birth canal, ascending infections also occur.

2. Most infants born to mothers with clinically apparent gonorrhea are prevented from developing gonococcal ophthalmia with the recommended modes of prophylaxis. However, an occasional case of gonococcal ophthalmia may occur in such infants. Intravenous or intramuscular aqueous crystalline penicillin G should be administered to these infants. A single dose of 50,000 units for term infants or 20,000 units for low-birth-weight infants is recommended.
3. Infants with clinical evidence of ophthalmia or complicated disseminated gonococcal infection should be hospitalized under isolation and treated appropriately.
4. Screening for gonococcal infections should be part of prenatal care, because they are associated with fetal wastage, early and prolonged rupture of membranes, premature labor, and delivery of low-birth-weight infants. They also may result in sepsis or scalp abscess if intrauterine fetal monitoring is used. Failure to treat an infected mother before or at the time of delivery may result in transmission of gonococcal infection postnatally to infants who escape infection at delivery (American Academy of Pediatrics, 1983).

PREVENTING HYPOPROTHROMBINEMIA

The Committee on Nutrition of the American Academy of Pediatrics recommends that vitamin K_1 be given to newborns. A routine physician's order in many hospitals is Aquamephyton 1 mg (0.5 ml) intramuscularly. This is a clear, yellow-tinged solution of phytonadione (vitamin K_1) given for prophylaxis of hemorrhagic disease of the newborn. Vitamin K is synthesized by normal flora of the human intestine. The fetus has a sterile gut and does not synthesize vitamin K until after birth. A small store is present within the liver, but if the newborn is premature, is breastfed, or fasts for more than 12 hours, there may be a deficiency of vitamin K–dependent factors, a prolonged prothrombin time, and an increased risk of significant bleeding (Avery, 1987).

Some sources (Brewer and Greene, 1981; Mendelsohn, 1981; Cohen and Estner, 1983) state that newborn hemorrhagic disease is so rare that it would not be necessary to use prophylaxis except in high-risk cases. Others (Shearer et al., 1982; McNinch, Ormes, and Tripp, 1983) have found an increase in incidence of hemorrhagic disease when vitamin K is not given to newborns routinely.

Possible side-effects of intramuscular Aquamephyton include pain, swelling, and tenderness at the site, anaphylactic reactions, and hyperbilirubinemia. However, no evidence of these effects is reported with the 1 mg dosage (Avery, 1987). The nurse should check carefully to ascertain that the dosage in the vial is the 1.0 mg (0.5 ml) neonatal concentration. An adult dosage vial of 10 mg could be fatal for the infant. The vitamin K injection is administered to the infant intramuscularly in the lateral thigh area with a $\frac{5}{8}$-inch needle.

EXAMINING FOR CONGENITAL ANOMALIES

Congenital anomalies occur in 1–7 percent of all live-born infants. Approximately 2–3 percent of all live-born infants show one or more significant congenital malformations that may require medical attention soon after birth (James, 1983). The professional nurse can perform a brief assessment to discover gross anomalies that may require medical attention soon after birth. This can be done as a head-to-toe assessment:

1. Beginning with the head, note the fontanelles, which should be soft. A bulging anterior fontanelle may indicate intracranial pressure resulting from hydrocephalus or intracranial hemorrhage. A depressed fontanelle may indicate dehydration. Although the posterior fontanelle may be closed because of molding, a closed anterior fontanelle may indicate microcephaly. Rarely, a cranial bone may be absent or forms of anencephaly may occur.
2. Check the nose for obstruction and suction it. Occlusion of each side for a few seconds will cause respiratory difficulty if choanal atresia is present.
3. Examine the mouth for cleft palate by feeling along the inner roof with a finger.
4. Inspect neck for webbing or anomalies.
5. Move the shoulders while placing a finger over the clavicle. A crepitus indicates a fracture.
6. Auscultate the chest for heart rate, proper position of heart, and normal air exchange.
7. Palpate the abdomen for masses, distention, or enlargement of the liver, spleen, or kidneys.
8. Examine the cord for the normal number of vessels (two arteries, one vein).
9. Examine the genitals for normal sexuality and the anus for patency. Record elimination of urine or stool.
10. Examine the back and sacral region for pig-

mentation and abnormal hair, which may be associated with occult spina bifida and meningocele and myelomeningocele.
11. Check the extremities for normal number of digits.
12. Inspect the skin for scaling, lesions, bruises, and jaundice.
13. Note any asymmetry of face, extremities, or body movement.

Several sources recommend that a screening examination be done on all infants for hidden congenital anomalies (Van Leeuwen and Glenn, 1968; Shaffer, 1980; Pillitteri, 1981). This procedure and the rationale for using it are detailed in Table 19-5.

A variation in the procedure for assessing choanal atresia (item 2) requires that a nasogastric tube be passed only if respiratory difficulty persists after pharyngeal suctioning. Since infants are obligatory nose breathers, choanal atresia usually results in complete respiratory obstruction (James, 1983). Once breathing is established, it is recommended to check for choanal atresia by occluding the mouth and the right or left nostril. A catheter may be inserted into each nostril and should pass for 3-4 cm. A small infant airway will allow ventilation if choanal atresia is present. If a tube is to be inserted into the nasopharynx, it must be done with care. The catheter is directed toward the middle of the nose and down, rather than directing it upward and back as in an adult. Color should be observed carefully. Nasogastric stimulation and suctioning have been demonstrated to induce laryngospasm, bradycardia, and apnea (Fanaroff and Klaus, 1979; Behrman, 1983). There is also a danger that a catheter passed through the nasal canals may cause edema and may result in partial or complete airway obstruction.

Introducing a tiny, flexible catheter into the mouth on the left or right side of the tongue and advancing it down into the esophagus and stomach is suggested. The tip of the catheter may be felt in the left half of the abdomen as it is gently advanced, or a minute amount of air can be pushed by syringe into the stomach and heard with a stethoscope held over the stomach (James, 1983).

There is some question as to whether gastric aspiration is as desirable as allowing amniotic fluid to remain in the stomach, for caloric content and nutritional value. Infants at risk for hypoglycemia, such as premature infants, infants of diabetic mothers, and those small for gestational age or subjected to perinatal stress, need this fluid containing significant amounts of glucose and protein. It is suggested that gastric suctioning be reserved for those infants known to have swallowed meconium or blood, for infants whose mothers have polyhydramnios, and for the ill infant with abdominal distention (Brown, 1982).

It is important that a brief assessment of the infant be performed immediately after delivery. If the head-to-toe assessment does not detect problems needing immediate intervention, this more invasive hidden anomaly check could be delayed until after the initial bonding period.

FACILITATION OF ATTACHMENT

Hugs, Holding, and Bonding

The parents have waited for months to hold and look at their baby. During the first hour after birth the healthy infant is very alert and responds to stimulation. That first hour is a sensitive, critical period during which close contact between infant and parents can facilitate the attachment process (Klaus and Kennell, 1981). Erickson (1963) has defined the first developmental task of the infant as "trust versus mistrust." The infant is sometimes placed on the mother's abdomen for a few brief moments while the cord is cut. Most hospital routines then stipulate that the infant must be placed under the radiant warmer while various procedures, including injections and administration of eye ointments, are performed. Finally, the infant is given to the mother to hold for a few brief moments on the way to the nursery. They are then taken to separate rooms for close observation and nursing care.

Placing the infant skin to skin with the mother, covering the infant, and drying it will keep the infant's temperature within normal limits (Gardner, 1979; Broadribb, 1983). This may be more soothing to the infant and may lessen the stress of adaptation to the changes of birth. It was found that at 1, 3, 6, 9, and 12 months of age, babies who had spent more time with their mothers immediately after birth gained more weight and had fewer infections. Their mothers were more affectionate toward them. At 5 years after birth, these children were found to have higher IQs and superior scores on language tests (Phillips and Anzalone, 1978).

The nurse can perform a brief suctioning, drying, and Apgar assessment under the radiant warmer. During this time, the mother has a few seconds to rest while she is being cleansed and

TABLE 19-5. Assessment to Determine Anomalies

Assessment	Procedure	Abnormalities Considered
Inquire for hydramnios	Polyhydramnios: This information is obtained from the obstetrician. This is a clinical diagnosis based on the observation of the obstetrician that more than 2500 ml of amniotic fluid was present. We are not able to obtain information concerning the actual measurement of amniotic fluid	Presence of hydramnios suggests congenital gastrointestinal or genitourinary obstruction or extreme prematurity
Appearance of abdomen	Observation of abdomen: Careful observation of the convexity or concavity of the abdomen is made. This may suggest presence of abdominal mass or diaphragmatic hernia	Distended abdomen suggests ascites or tumor. Empty abdomen suggests diaphragmatic hernia
Passage of nasogastric tube (No. 5 feeding catheter)	Nasogastric tube: A feeding tube is passed through each nasal orifice into the nasopharynx. If this is impossible and a $3\frac{1}{2}$ French catheter can be passed with difficulty, the diagnosis of choanal stenosis is made. The catheter is then advanced into the stomach and 5 ml of air is injected while the examiner listens over the abdomen to ensure actual presence of the catheter in the stomach	Failure to pass nasogastric tube through naris on either side establishes choanal atresia. Failure to pass it into the stomach confirms presence of esophageal atresia
Aspiration of stomach with recording of color and amount of fluid	Aspiration of stomach: The ability to obtain 1–2 ml of aspirate is not proof that the tip is in the stomach, because the "gastric aspirate" obtained may be mucus and saliva from the blind pouch of an esophageal atresia. Therefore, one must previously have ascertained presence of the catheter in the stomach as described. Note the volume and character of fluid. Suction should be maintained on the catheter as it is withdrawn to prevent leakage of contents into the pharynx and resultant aspiration	With excess of 20 ml of fluid, or yellow fluid, duodenal or ileal atresia is suspected
Insertion of rectal catheter	Rectal catheter: The same catheter used previously is inserted into the rectum as far as it can be easily passed. If meconium is not present on the tip of the catheter after withdrawal, a digital examination is performed. If no meconium is produced by this means, careful observation of the infant for gastrointestinal abnormality is indicated	Failure to obtain meconium suggests imperforate anus or higher obstruction
Counting of umbilical arteries	Umbilical arteries: The umbilical stump is examined at the point of entry into the infant. Unless both arteries are easily identified, they are examined under magnification with a hand lens and probed. One artery suggests the need for genitourinary evaluation	The presence of one artery suggests possible congenital urinary anomalies or chromosomal trisomy (if other portions of examination are consistent)

SOURCE: Van Leeuwen and Glenn (1968).

while any necessary suturing of the episiotomy is being done. If there is no respiratory distress, the infant should then be wrapped in a warm blanket and handed to the father, or it should be placed skin to skin with the mother and both should be covered with a heavy blanket. Radiant warmers are available that extend over mother and infant. The mother may wish to nurse the infant soon after birth.

Routines such as eye prophylaxis, vitamin K injection, and screening for hidden anomalies could be delayed until after the first hour. At this time, the infant usually becomes sleepy and the mother is more relaxed and ready for a rest.

During the first hour both the mother and infant must be observed closely, vital signs must be assessed every 15 min, and other physical assessments must be made. One nurse can perform these assessments for one mother–infant pair, whereas two nurses are required to observe them closely in separate rooms.

The parents may wish a few minutes of privacy during this time. If no complications seem to have occurred during the first 30 min, some private intervals may be allowed. The nurse should instruct the parents in suctioning with the bulb syringe and in signs or symptoms that will require immediate nursing or medical intervention. Ideally, she will remain close enough to hear distress signals and intervene immediately.

Cultural Customs and Individual Preferences

The parents may want to observe numerous cultural customs. Assessment of preferences regarding birthing and bonding is best accomplished before labor has even begun. The health care provider should discuss alternate birthing practices and allow the parents to make choices within safe limits. This helps the couple to feel they have control over the changes that are occurring.

The process of birth in most U.S. hospitals has been described as a "violent tidal wave of sensations" resulting in confusion, pain, suffering, abandonment, fear, and despair (Leboyer, 1974). The many sensory changes the infant must cope with after birth, such as bright lights, loud noise, rough handling, invasive procedures, and cold air, all contribute to these sensations. Dimming the delivery room lights, using gentle stimulation to help the newborn to breathe, speaking quietly, and immersing the newborn in a tub of warm water shortly after birth may help to minimize these sensations. If couples desire this approach, it can be carried out safely if care is taken not to chill the infant during the bath. Some hospitals are using a modification of this procedure by using only a spotlight over the perineum and a light on the baby's warmer. The atmosphere is kept quiet, and the number of observers is limited. This atmosphere has been noted to calm the client during delivery and to facilitate attachment of infants and parents (see Chapter 37).

SPIRITUAL CARE

During the labor process assessment should be made of the parents' religious affiliation and belief in infant baptism. Immediate infant baptism may be desired if a high-risk situation is present and there is any probability the infant will not live. Many people in the Catholic church, the Episcopal church, and the Lutheran church believe that baptism is essential to spiritual salvation and ask that in case of emergency any baptized Christian present baptize the infant. The nurse may assume this responsibility by pouring or sprinkling water on the head of the child while saying, "I baptize thee in the name of the Father, and of the Son, and of the Holy Ghost. Amen." A short prayer such as the Lord's Prayer may also be said (Lutheran Church, 1943).

The Catholic church prefers the water be pure and made to flow when poured on the infant's head. If there is any doubt the infant is alive or dead, it should be baptized, but conditionally, "If thou art alive, I baptize thee" (Reeder, Mastroianni, and Martin, 1983).

If possible, the nurse should try to contact the priest or pastor before a high-risk delivery, so that he can be present to administer this sacrament and comfort the parents. If the nurse has not been baptized or does not believe in baptism, she should ascertain that someone else will be present to assume this responsibility.

IDENTIFICATION

The footprinting of newborn infants and fingerprinting of the mother has been a hospital routine for years. Today, this practice is in question as studies have shown that only about 10–20 percent of newborn footprints are identifiable and most of these will not withstand legal scrutiny in the courts (Shepard, Erickson, and Fromm, 1966; Thompson et al., 1981). Although some hospitals have discontinued routine footprinting, Lohnes (1986) describes several cases in which flexure creases have been important in identifying kidnapped newborns. If footprinting is desired, it is recommended to wait until the feet have been bathed or vernix has been absorbed or removed and then the following procedure should be utilized:

1. Use a disposable footprinter ink plate and smooth, high-gloss paper.
2. Wipe the baby's foot immediately after birth so that the vernix will not dry on it. This will make the foot easier to clean when the footprint is made.
3. Before making the print, be sure the baby's foot is clean and dry. Cleaning should be gentle, so that the skin of the baby's foot will not peel.

4. Be sure that there is not too much ink on the pad.
5. Flex the baby's knee so that the leg is close to the body; grasp the ankle between the thumb and middle finger, with the index finger pressing on the upper surface of the foot just behind the baby's toes to prevent the toes from curling.
6. Press the footprinter firmly to the baby's foot.
7. Touch the baby's foot gently to the footprint chart, which should be attached to a hard surface such as a clipboard. Place the heel on the paper first and "walk" the foot gently onto the chart with a heel-to-toe motion. Then lift the foot off the chart; do not slide it off. The foot should not be rolled back and forth, either on the inking pad or on the footprint chart.
8. If the footprint is to be used for identification, it is particularly important to get a good impression of the ball of the foot, and the great toe. The flexure creases are unique to the individual foot and remain relatively stable during the first weeks and even through the first years of life. Check the print for legible flexure creases, preferably with a magnifying glass. If the creases are not clear, take another print. The mother's fingerprints of the thumb or third finger, are commonly placed on the same sheet as the baby's footprint.
9. After a satisfactory print is made, the excess ink is wiped from the baby's foot. Vaseline on clean gauze pads can be used to cleanse the feet without irritating the skin. As in every other aspect of newborn care, it is most important that the baby not be chilled during the process (Moore, 1983).

The most common method of identification is banding (see Fig. 19–7). Three plastic bands with identical numbers and information detailing sex, mother's name, room number, hospital number, date and time of birth, and physician's name are utilized. Two bands are placed on the infant's extremities and one on the mother's wrist. Because the infant will lose 5–10 percent of birth weight shortly after birth, the band should be applied snugly, but not so tightly as to obstruct circulation. When the infant is taken to the mother, the bands should be checked for matching identification. If a band falls off the baby, it should be replaced, not just taped on the crib.

An alternate method of identification might be to write a number or a name on the infant's chest with a silver nitrate treated pencil. The silver nitrate leaves an indelible tatoo that lasts 3–4 weeks, eventually disappearing completely (Shepard, Erickson, and Fromm, 1966). Still another method is to utilize ear photos, as it has been found that infants' ears have differential markings that can be used for identification (Ziegel and Cranley, 1978).

CHARTING

An example of a form for recording care of the newborn immediately after birth is shown in Fig. 19–8. The infant's chart should document assessment and care of the infant, e.g.:

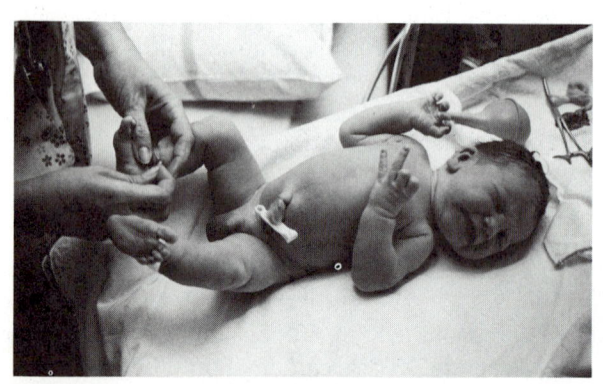

FIGURE 19–7. Banding a newborn.

FIGURE 19–8. Sample of newborn record.
SOURCE: Good Samaritan Hospital, Kearney, Nebraska.

NURSING CARE PLAN: The Newborn

Nursing Diagnosis	Nursing Expected Outcome	Interventions	Rationale
1. Potential for impaired gas exchange	1. Vigorous respirations and crying; color pinking with only some acrocyanosis	1a. Suction mouth, with bulb syringe b. 1- and 5-min Apgars c. Stimulate by rubbing back vigorously d. Use O_2 as needed, blow over nose e. If 1-min Apgar is below 6, intubate and suction tracheally f. CPR as necessary	1. To maintain patent airway; establish adequate respirations
2. Potential alteration in body temperature, R/T ineffective thermoregulation	2. Maintenance of neutral thermal environment; prevention of cold stress; body temp. 97.4–98.4 °F by skin or axillary; color pink.	2a. Place infant on radiant warmer or skin to skin with mother b. Dry quickly with warm blanket, especially head and hair c. Replace wet blanket with dry blanket d. Do not bathe infant until temperature is stable e. Avoid drafts in delivery room and during transport f. Place stockinette cap on head	2. To maintain infant's temperature stable
3. Potential for infection related to immune system	3. Prevention of infections; no drainage or odor to umbilical cord, skin lesions	3a. Gloves, goggles, mask in delivery room b. Wash hands before and after all cares c. Use sterile supplies: blankets, syringes d. Perform eye infection prophylaxis e. Perform cord care f. Encourage early and frequent nursing (colostrum contains antibodies)	3. To prevent spread of infections and to protect caretaker and infant; to allow transmission of antibodies by mother's colostrum
4. Potential for alterations in tissue perfusion	4. Prevention/detection of complications such as anemia, hypoglycemia	4a. Administer vitamin K_1 b. Take hemoglobin and hematocrit c. Check for blood type and Rh d. Check Dextrostix	4. To prevent any bleeding disorders and note anomalies; prevent system damage
5. Potential for alteration in parent-infant attachment	5. Facilitation of early bonding of parents and infant; parents focus eye contact on infant, stroke and touch infant	5a. Dry and suction infant, establish respirations; take any emergency measures b. Delay prophylaxis and other assessments 1-2 hours c. May lay infant skin to skin on mother's abdomen or allow father to hold well-swaddled infant d. Do recovery care of mother and infant together	5. To allow mother (parents) to remain with infant and to provide minimal stress to infant to facilitate early bonding

1. Time of birth.
2. Initiation of respirations—time, spontaneity, resuscitation utilized.
3. Medications administered:
    a. Vitamin K,
    b. Eye prophylaxis.
4. Apgar score at 1 and 5 min.
5. Assessment or anomaly check.
6. Voidings or stooling.
7. General condition of infant.
8. Identification—band number or footprints.

The form might also contain information about the maternal labor and delivery such as analgesia, anesthesia, maternal Rh and blood type, and any complication of pregnancy or delivery. This information might be helpful to the health care team caring for the infant during the neonatal period.

CERTIFICATES

All states require the registration of births with the Bureau of Vital Statistics. Information required may vary but will include the infant's name, parents' names, and date, time, and place of birth. Other information may be included such as birthplaces and birthdates of parents, prenatal care, past obstetric history, and abnormalities of the birth process. The hospital usually provides for the collection of this information. Sometimes an unofficial birth certificate is given to the parents as a keepsake for the baby book.

SUMMARY

The newborn infant requires quick assessment and care of the six h's: hypoxia, hypothermia, heart rate, hypercarbia, hypoglycemia, and hypotension (Shaffer, 1980a). The nurse functions as a member of the health team in providing for these needs.

Hospital routines such as prevention of infection, administration of vitamin K, assessment for anomalies, and identification of the infant are usually part of the nurse's responsibility. Besides providing skillful physical care, the nurse has an important role in facilitation of attachment. She may function as a client advocate by helping to meet individual preferences for bonding. The nursing interventions discussed in this chapter are summarized in the accompanying nursing care plan for newborns. Some of these practices are continually changing.

The nurse caring for the newborn must contribute insight and skill, yet remain flexible to respond to frequent changes in knowledge and the need for research in this area. Only a short time has elapsed since newborn infants were believed to be sightless, without feelings, and helpless. We now know them to be alert to their new world, taking in and studying those around them and possibly heavily influenced by the treatment they receive. This is a time of transition and change.

REFERENCES

American Academy of Pediatrics and American College of Obstetricians and Gynecologists. 1983. *Guidelines for perinatal care.* Evanston, Ill.: AAP, and Washington, D.C.: ACOG.

Apgar, V. 1953. A proposal for a new method of evaluation of the newborn infant. *Curr. Res. Anesthes. Analges.* 32(260):260–262.

Apgar, V. 1958. Evaluation of the newborn infant—second report. *JAMA.* 168:1985–1988.

Arad, I.; Eyal, F.; and Fainmesser, P. 1981. Umbilical care and cord separation. *Arch. Dis. Childhood* 56(11):887–888.

Avery, B. 1987. *Neonatology.* Philadelphia: J. B. Lippincott.

Behrman, R., ed. 1983. *Neonatal and perinatal medicine.* St. Louis: C. V. Mosby.

Berman, L., and Saunders, B. 1980. Newborn resuscitation. *Perinatology–Neonatology.* 14(1):22–30.

Brewer, G., and Greene, J. 1981. *Right from the start.* Emmaus, Pa.: Rodale Press.

Broadribb, V. 1983. *Introduction to pediatric nursing.* Philadelphia: J. B. Lippincott.

Brown, J. 1982. Effects of suctioning newborn stomach contents during resuscitation. *New Engl. J. Med.* 306(22):1366.

Butnarescu, G., and Tillotson, D. 1983. *Maternity nursing: Theory to practice.* New York: John Wiley & Sons.

Center for Disease Control. 1987. Morbidity and mortality weekly report. Vol. 36, No. 19, 25.

Clark, A. L.; Affonso, D. D.; and Harris, T. B. 1979. *Childbearing: A nursing perspective.* Philadelphia: F. A. Davis.

Cohen, N., and Estner, L. 1983. *Silent knife.* South Halley, Mass.: Bergin & Garvey.

Erickson, E. 1963. *Childhood and society.* New York: Norton.

Fanaroff, A., and Klaus, M. 1979. *Care of the high risk neonate.* Philadelphia: W. B. Saunders.

Feigin, R. D., and Callanan, D. L. 1983. Postnatally acquired infections. In *Behrman's neonatal-perinatal medicine,* 3rd ed., eds. A. A. Fanaroff, R. J. Martin, and I. R. Merkatz. St. Louis: C. V. Mosby.

Gardner, S. 1979. The mother as incubator after delivery. *J. Obstet. Gynecol. Neonatal Nurs.* 8(3):174–176.

Good Samaritan Hospital. 1983. *Nursery forms. Procedure book.* Kearney, Neb.: Good Samaritan Hospital.

Hazinsky, M. F. 1987. New guidelines for pediatric and neonatal resuscitation and Advanced Life Support. *Pediatric Nursing.* 13:1.

Hodson, W., and Truog, W. 1983. *Critical care of the Newborn.* Philadelphia: W. B. Saunders.

James, L. S. 1983. Emergencies in the delivery room. In *Behrman's neonatal-perinatal medicine,* 3rd ed., eds. A. A. Fanaroff, R. J. Martin, and I. R. Merkatz. St. Louis: C. V. Mosby.

Klaus, M., and Kennell, J. 1981. *Maternal–infant bonding.* St. Louis: C. V. Mosby.

Korones, S. 1986. *The high risk newborn infant,* 4th ed. St. Louis: C. V. Mosby.

Leboyer, F. 1974. *Childbirth without violence.* New York: Knopf.

Lohnes, R. C. 1986. Reading the fine print. *Am. J. Nurs.* 9.

Lutheran Church. 1943. *Dr. Martin Luther's small catechism.* St. Louis: Concordia.

McNinch, A. W.; Ormes, R. L.; and Tripp, J. H. 1983. Haemorrhagic disease of the newborn returns. *Lancet.* 2(8301):770.

Mendelsohn, R. 1981. *Mal(e) practice.* Chicago: Contemporary.

Moore, M. L. 1983. *Realities in childbearing.* 2nd ed. Philadelphia: W. B. Saunders.

National Society to Prevent Blindness. 1981. *Prevention and treatment of ophthalmia neonatorum.* New York: NSPB.

Olds, S. B.; Landon, M. L.; Ladewig, P. A.; and Davidson, S. V. 1980. *Obstetric nursing.* Menlo Park, Calif.: Addison-Wesley.

Perez, R. H. 1981. *Protocols for perinatal nursing practice.* St. Louis: C. V. Mosby.

Perry, D. 1982. The umbilical cord, transcultural care and customs, *J. Nurse-Midwifery.* 27(4):25–30.

Phillips, C. R., and Anzalone, J. T. 1978. *Fathering.* St. Louis: C. V. Mosby.

Pillitteri, A. 1981. *Maternal–newborn nursing.* 2nd ed. Boston: Little, Brown.

Reeder, S. J.; Mastroianni, L.; and Martin, L. L. 1983. *Maternity nursing.* 15th ed. Philadelphia: J. B. Lippincott.

Shaffer, K. 1980a. Neonatal resuscitation, Part I. *Nebraska Med. J.* 65(4):122.

Shaffer, K. 1980b. Neonatal resuscitation, Part II. *Nebraska Med. J.* 65(5):122.

Shearer, M. J.; Rahim, S.; Barkhan, P.; and Stimmler, K. 1982. Plasma vitamin K in mothers and their newborn babies. *Lancet.* 2(8296):1090.

Sheldon, R., and Dominiak, P. 1980. *The expanding role of the nurse in neonatal intensive care.* San Diego: Grune & Stratton.

Shepard, K.; Erickson, T.; and Fromm, H. 1966. Limitations of footprinting as a means of infant identification. *Pediatrics.* 37(1):107–108.

Steele, S. 1981. *Child health and the family.* New York: Mason.

Thompson, J. E.; Clark, D. A.; Salisbury, B.; and Cahill, J. 1981. Footprinting the infant, not cost effective, *J. Pediatrics.* 5(99):797–798.

Van Leeuwen, G., and Glenn, L. 1968. Screening for hidden congenital anomalies. *Pediatrics.* 41:147.

Ziegel, E., and Cranley, M. 1978. *Obstetric nursing.* New York: Macmillan.

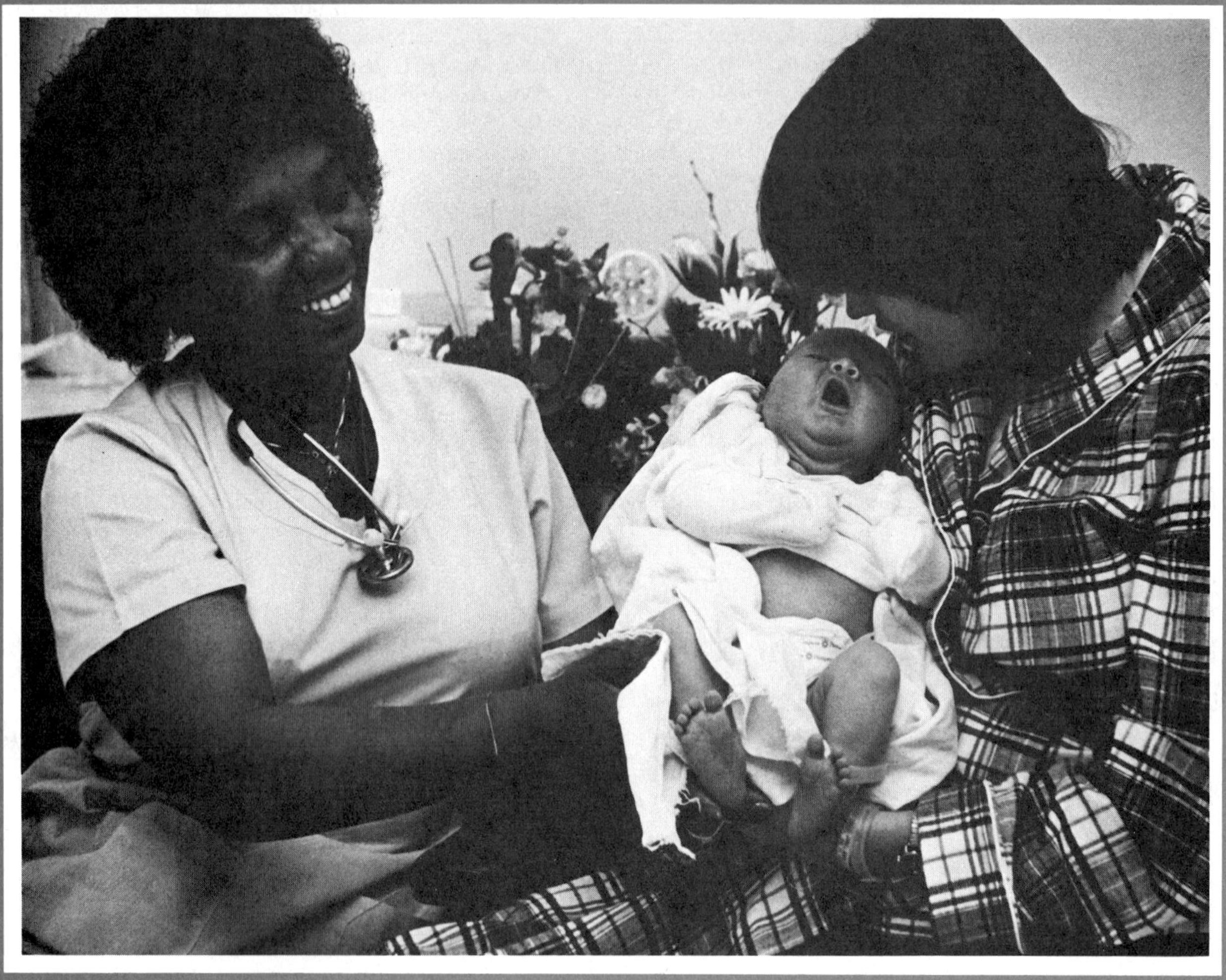

UNIT FOUR

CHANGE: THE POST-PARTAL PERIOD

20

Maternal Physiologic Adaptation

BEHAVIORAL OBJECTIVES

Upon completion of this chapter, the reader should be able to:

- Describe the physiologic adaptations that occur in each of the following body parts during the postpartal period: uterus, cervix, vagina, and breasts.

- Define *involution* and its role in the postpartum period.

- Briefly outline the time frame for the return to menstrual cycling.

- Explain the physiologic basis for postpartal fainting, postpartal diuresis, "afterpains," and the need for sleep.

- List the benefits of early ambulation in the postpartal period.

- Describe the factors that influence a woman's self-image after delivery.

- List the signs, symptoms, and nursing interventions for spinal headaches, hemorrhoids, hematomas, and trauma to the bladder.

- Identify warning signals that indicate an abnormal course of healing for episiotomy or laceration.

- Identify key features of assessment for the postpartal bladder.

- Describe nursing interventions to promote optimal postpartal bladder function.

The physical and physiologic changes that accompany pregnancy are many. Most of these changes occur over a 40-week period. The postpartal period (also referred to as the *puerperium*) lasts one-sixth as long as pregnancy. It is during this short 6- to 8-week period that all of the changes of pregnancy are reversed. The challenge of nursing care for a patient during such a dynamic period requires rigorous application of the nursing process. To provide the knowledge base on which this process depends, this chapter explores maternal physiologic adaptation, the characteristics of the return to the steady state, and special problems that may arise during this period.

THE REPRODUCTIVE SYSTEM

Two types of changes occur in the postpartal period: *involution*, the retrogressive process of the uterus and genital organs, and the progressive processes, i.e. beginning lactation and the return to menstrual cycling. The reproductive organs do not regain their prepregnant character once a pregnancy has taken place. At the end of the postpartal period, the woman is said to have reached a nonpregnant, *parous* state.

Involution

Immediately after delivery of the placenta, the uterus weighs about 1000 g, is firmly contracted, and rests about 12 cm above the symphysis pubis. About 1 hour later, the uterine fundus has risen to the level of the umbilicus, and it remains there for the next 24 hours (see Fig. 20-1). This first hour is a critical one; should the uterus relax, the woman could lose a very large amount of blood from vessels at the placental site.

During the first postpartal week the weight of the uterus is decreased by 500 g, reaching about 60 g after 6 weeks. This is due to a decrease in the size of each uterine muscle cell, which occurs as the result of uterine muscle contraction and autolysis (breakdown of uterine cell material).

Beginning on the second postpartal day, the

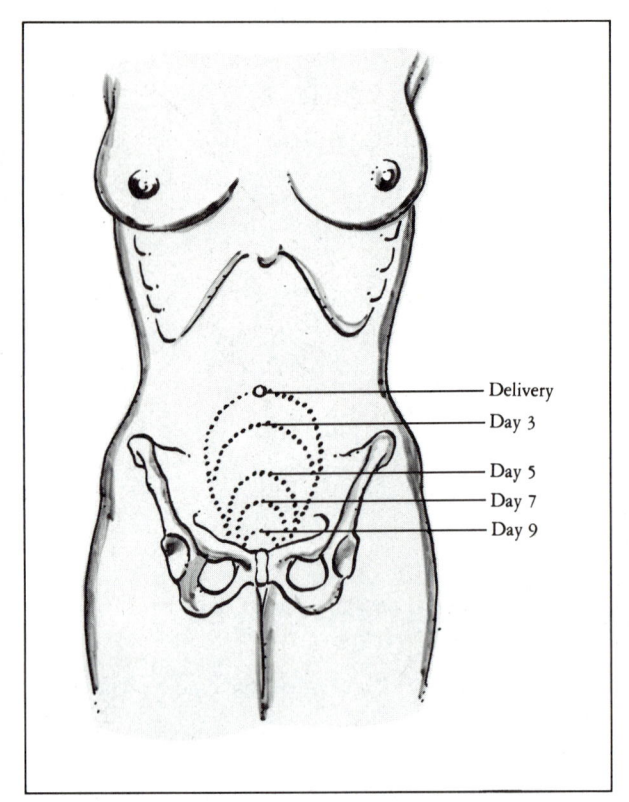

FIGURE 20-1. Involution of the uterus.
SOURCE: Reeder, Mastroianni, and Martin (1983).

fundus descends 1 cm further below the umbilicus each day. Ligaments that hold the uterus in place do not regain tone as rapidly as the uterus itself, so the uterus is easily moved about in the abdomen during the first few days after delivery. Before palpating the fundus, the nurse should have the woman empty her bladder, because a full bladder can cause the fundus to rise in the abdomen and deviate to one side.

By the tenth day, the fundus should no longer be palpable abdominally. If the fundus does not continue to descend, if it climbs higher in the abdomen, or if it is frequently found to be relaxed (boggy), the uterus may contain clots. Massage can express clots; if it does not, the physician should expect subinvolution (see Chapter 30). Anytime a uterus is found to be relaxed or boggy, it should be massaged until it becomes firmly contracted. However, massage or manipulation of the contracted uterus should be kept to a minimum, as it may cause muscle fatigue. The uterine atony and subsequent hemorrhage that results from muscle fatigue is difficult to control, because the muscle no longer responds to massage. While massage of the uterus may be mildly painful for the vaginally delivered woman, for the woman delivered by cesarean section, massage, or even palpation, can be very painful.

The endometrial lining of the uterus separates into two layers during the 3 days after delivery. The upper layer becomes necrotic and is sloughed off as *lochia*, which is seen as a vaginal discharge. The lower layer is the basis of the new endometrium, which is generated by the third week except at the placental site.

At separation, the placental site is about 6 cm in diameter, and the vessels in the area quickly thrombose. Scar formation does not occur, because the new endometrium is generated from glands and stroma that remain in the basalis layer of the decidua after placental separation. Endometrium at the placental site is completely restored in 6 weeks.

The lochia that flows from the vagina consists of the necrotic upper layer of the endometrium combined with blood and lymph tissue that ooze from the placental site. Lochial flow progresses through three distinct phases (see Table 20-1):

1. *Rubra lochia* is red, has the odor of fresh blood, and continues to flow for 1-3 days. It is composed of blood, decidual cells, and fetal debris.
2. *Serosa lochia* is brownish and indicates that healing of the placental site is taking place. Serosa lochia contains red and white blood cells, uterine debris, bacteria, and mucus. Serosa is thicker than rubra and lasts up to 10 days.
3. *Alba lochia* is composed of degenerating decidual cells, white blood cells, epithelial cells, debris from healing wounds, mucus, bacteria, and cholesterin crystals (composed of cholesterol). The duration of alba lochia is usually 10-15 days, although it may sometimes last until 6 weeks after delivery.

The flow of lochia peaks on the third or fourth day and is often more profuse in multiparas. Increasing parity has been found to result in a shorter duration of lochia. However, the larger the size of the infant, the longer the duration of lochia. After the peak, the amount rapidly decreases. There may be occasional gushes of lochia when the woman first gets out of bed or increases activity. However, the reappearance of rubra lochia and a steady flow of red lochia with no decrease or with frequent soaking of perineal pads are abnormal signs and require medical attention. Any pungent or foul odors should also be considered abnormal. There is evidence that approximately one-third of women will cease lochia flow after serosa lochia. (Oppenheimer *et al.*, 1986). The lack of alba lochia should not be considered a cause for concern.

The progress of lochial flow is followed by examining the amount, color, and odor of the lochia on the perineal pads. After being educated, most women cooperate with this assessment by reporting abnormalities of their lochia.

After vaginal delivery, the cervix is edematous, relaxed, and very congested with blood. It often has several lacerations of various sizes due to trauma from the birth. However, in only 18 hours, the cervix regains much of its prelabor form. By the seventh day, the external cervical os is only dilated 1 cm. However, once a vaginal delivery has been accomplished, the cervix never recovers its nulliparous character. The internal os will close, but the external os remains slightly dilated.

Birth greatly stretches the vagina, which is often swollen and bruised as well. Healing progresses rapidly because of the high vascularity of the perineum. Perineal tone also returns rapidly. The vaginal mucosa regains rugae by 3 weeks postpartum. These rugae are not as prominent as those of the nullipara. The hymen is torn by delivery, resulting in tissue tags referred to as *myrtiform caruncles* (Monheit, Cousins, and Resnik, 1980). Complications such as infection or unrecognized lacerations can retard this healing, just as they can

TABLE 20-1. Characteristics of Lochia

Type of Lochia	Color	Duration	Composition
Rubra	Red	1-3 days	Blood, fragments of decidua and mucus
Serosa	Pink or brown-tinged	3-10 days	Blood, mucus, and invading leukocytes
Alba	White	10-14 days May last for 6 weeks	Largely mucus; leukocyte count high

SOURCE: Pillitteri (1981).

retard the entire involutional process (see Chapter 30).

The Progressive Process

Beginning Lactation

Breast changes that result in lactation begin during pregnancy. These early changes are mediated by estrogen and progesterone. The changes of the postpartal period are mediated by prolactin and become more evident between the second and fourth days. The breasts have a bluish cast because of increased vascularity. They become fuller and swollen as the veins and lymph vessels become enlarged. Pigmentation of the areola increases, and many women report tenderness.

Internally, there is an increase in the number and size of the alveoli. Usually on the third day, milk production begins, and the alveoli and ducts dilate markedly. This process is more gradual in the multipara and less likely to be uncomfortable.

Examination of the breasts is incorporated into each physical assessment. Breasts are visually examined for areas of redness, and nipples are checked for cracks and fissures. Next, the breasts are palpated to detect fullness and hardened or hot areas indicative of mastitis (an infection of the breast) or congested milk ducts. The assessment period is an excellent time to discuss breastfeeding and breast self-examination (see Chapter 21).

The Return of Menstrual Cycling

While a great deal of information about the neuroendocrinology of the postpartum period is yet to be learned, the presence or absence of lactation appears to be the major factor in the timing of the first postpartal ovulation and menstruation.

The prolactin level stimulated by breastfeeding suppresses luteinizing hormone (LH) and estrogen. These substances are necessary to induce ovulation.

Women who continue to breastfeed for at least 1 hour at night and delay supplementation will have longer periods of amenorrhea. These periods of amenorrhea may last as long as 18 months. It is thought that the contraceptive effect of breastfeeding is a result of the high output of prolactin during lactation. Prolactin inhibits the secretion of LH and may also have a direct inhibitory effect on the ovaries, thereby suppressing ovulation (Short, 1984).

THE CARDIOVASCULAR SYSTEM

During pregnancy there is a 30–50 percent increase in blood volume. Beginning with the 500–600 ml of blood usually lost at vaginal delivery (twice that amount at cesarean section), the blood volume rapidly decreases.

Obstruction of the vena cava is relieved, and the veins of the broad ligament contract as the uterus is emptied. There is an increased venous return to the heart and decreased volume in the uteroplacental vascular bed.

In the first 2–3 days postpartum a 15–30 percent increase in circulating blood volume results from the elimination of the placental circulation, an increase in venous return, and a shift of extracellular fluids into the systemic circulation. This increase in blood volume accounts for the hemodilution fall in hematocrit and promotes profound diuresis. The cardiac output increases by 35 percent. Patients with limited cardiac reserve are most vulnerable for heart failure at this time (Iffy and Kaminetzky, 1981).

The Coagulation and Fibrinolytic Systems

The coagulation and fibrinolytic systems exist in a dynamic balance to maintain the patency of the vascular system. The failure of one system results in hemorrhage; the failure of the other in thrombosis. Both of these disorders are significant complications of the postpartal period.

There are four mechanisms that prevent hemorrhage: (1) muscle contraction, (2) tissue pressure, (3) platelet activity, and (4) the coagulation system. They are called upon at delivery to meet the challenges of placental separation, episiotomy, and lacerations (Bonnar, 1975).

The blood flow to the placenta is 600–700 ml/min and must be rapidly decreased at separation to prevent exsanguination. Activation of the clotting system is particularly evident during placental separation, as thromboplastin is released locally. This assists the contracting myometrium in slowing blood loss. After 1 hour, the vessels at the site are thrombosed. Rapidly, a fibrin mesh develops that covers the site, and platelets are consumed in large numbers. Consumption of platelets and fibrinogen continues during the entire postpartal period.

During pregnancy, the plasma fibrinogen (necessary for coagulation) has increased to a greater extent than the plasminogen (necessary for fibrinolysis), so that the newly delivered woman has a greater ability to produce fibrin clots and a decreased ability to remove them. Therefore, clots are very likely to form in the uterus. This tendency should decrease after the first 1–2 hours, and subsequent clots greater than 1 cm in diameter should be considered abnormal. Refer to Table 20–2 for coagulation factors and inhibitors during normal pregnancy.

This increased coagulation activity is even greater in the presence of exogenous estrogen sources such as medications. It also contributes to the thrombophlebitis that sometimes complicates this period. Early ambulation lowers the likelihood of blood stasis and subsequent thrombus formation.

By 3–4 weeks postpartum, the coagulation and fibrinolytic systems have returned to prepregnancy status (Hathaway and Bonnar, 1978). Some women may continue to have thromboembolic complications during the third postpartum week. Therefore, thrombosis prophylaxis in a woman with a history of thromboses may last for at least 6 weeks after delivery (Dahlman, Hellgren, and Blomback, 1985).

Vital Signs

Blood pressure decreases during the first two trimesters of pregnancy, only to return to prepregnant levels during the final trimester. During labor, although blood pressure rises during a uterine contraction, the blood pressure between contractions will be the same as third-trimester values. After delivery, blood pressure readings are an indication of vascular stabilization and should remain unchanged from those recorded during labor. A lower blood pressure may indicate blood loss exceeding normal limits, while an increasing blood pressure could be the first indication of preeclampsia.

The woman's temperature may show a slight elevation after delivery because of dehydration, fatigue, and hormonal changes. A temperature greater than 100.4°F (38°C) that occurs in any 2 of the first 10 days postpartum, exclusive of the first 24 hours, is defined by the U.S. Joint Committee on Maternal Welfare as puerperal morbidity (Iffy and Kaminetzky, 1981). Any elevation after 24 hours usually indicates an infection.

As mentioned earlier, a bradycardic pulse may

TABLE 20–2. *Coagulation Factors and Inhibitors During Normal Pregnancy*

Factor	Non-pregnant	Late Pregnancy
Fibrinogen	2–4.5 g/liter	4.0–6.5 g/liter
Factor II	75–125%	100–125%
Factor V	75–125%	100–150%
Factor VII	75–125%	150–250%
Factor VIII	75–150%	200–500%
Factor IX	75–125%	100–150%
Factor X	75–125%	150–250%
Factor XI	75–125%	50–100%
Factor XII	75–125%	100–200%
Factor XIII	75–125%	35–75%
Antithrombin III	85–110%	75–100%
Antifactor Xa	85–110%	75–100%

SOURCE: Hathaway and Bonnar (1978).

be found in the early postpartal period. While the usual range is 68–80, a pulse of 40–50 is not unusual (Greenhill and Friedman, 1974). Tachycardia may be indicative of anemia or hypotension. However, the pulse rate fluctuates with pain and emotional highs and lows. The pulse returns to the prepregnant rate about 10 days after delivery.

THE ENDOCRINE SYSTEM

As discussed earlier, many of the endocrine changes of pregnancy result from hormone production in the placenta or from the influence of these hormones on other glands. The endocrine functions of the nonlactating woman nearly reach prepregnancy activity by the end of the 6th postpartal week, resulting in a decrease in circulating hormones. The placental hormones are affected first. After delivery, human placental lactogen (HPL) can no longer be detected. At the end of 2 weeks, human chorionic gonadotropin (HCG) and corticosteroid binding globulin (an adrenal hormone) have disappeared. Prolactin disappears in 1–2 weeks. Within 4–6 weeks after delivery, the pituitary begins its monthly cycling with follicle simulating hormone (FSH) release preceding the release of LH.

Failure of the pituitary gland (Sheehan's syndrome) may follow an episode of hypovolemic shock caused by intrapartum or postpartum hemorrhage. The decreased blood supply leads to necrosis of the anterior pituitary. Since pituitary function influences the normal functioning of the thyroid, adrenal glands, and ovaries, multiple symptoms and signs appear. The first symptom of this conditon is the lack of lactation in a woman attempting to breastfeed. Later signs include decreased breast size, a regression of secondary sexual characteristics, lack of menses, and the signs of thyroid deficiency. Treatment of this condition consists of hormone replacement.

Finally, by 6 weeks postpartum, adrenal hormones have also returned to prepregnant levels. The levels of prolactin are, of course, different in the lactating woman (see Chapter 21).

THE GASTROINTESTINAL SYSTEM

Within 2 weeks after vaginal delivery, the gastrointestinal tract tone and motility return to normal. The woman may be thirsty for the first 2–3 days, and constipation is common (Pritchard, MacDonald, and Gant, 1985). A mild laxative, stool softeners, or enema may be necessary prior to the return of normal bowel function. The decreased fluid intake during labor, possibly a predelivery enema, decreased abdominal tone, decreased intraabdominal pressure, and fear of pain from the episiotomy or hemorrhoids contribute to the delay of the first stool.

The day after a cesarean delivery the women can usually tolerate liquids unless there was excessive manipulation or infection of the bowel. Bowel action begins to recover from the trauma of surgery by the second day as evidenced by audible bowel sounds.

At first, bowel action is not well coordinated and results in gas pains. Activity, fluids, and resumption of a normal diet will help resolve this problem. If these are ineffective, a rectal suppository may be ordered to provide relief (Pritchard, MacDonald, and Gant, 1985).

THE RENAL SYSTEM

The immediate effect of delivery on the renal system is a decrease of intraabdominal pressure. The stretched and relaxed abdominal muscles exert less pressure on the bladder, increasing bladder capacity. Bladder tone can be diminished as a result of length of labor, analgesia, and anesthesia. Soon after the delivery of the baby, diuresis of the retained fluid and sodium begins. This diuresis may continue for up to 21 days or until the woman's fluid and sodium balance is restored.

During the postpartal period the woman may void up to 3000 ml/day for the first 4–5 days. This is a larger amount (by as much as 2–3 times) than is usual for the adult. Volumes of urine over 500 ml predispose a bladder to atony, so women should be encouraged to void frequently.

By the end of the first postpartal week, the bladder achieves its prepregnant tone. Dilatation of the ureters and renal pelvis returns to normal after 3–6 weeks but may persist for up to 3 months. The functional activities of the kidneys, plasma flow, glomerular filtration rate (GFR), plasma creatinine, and nitrogen return to prepregnant levels by 6 weeks postpartum. Many newly delivered women have lactose in their urine, and increased nitrogen results from uterine involution (Pillitteri, 1981).

THE MUSCULOSKELETAL SYSTEM

The neck and arm muscles may ache as a result of the vigorous use of these muscles during pushing. Any malpositions of the legs in stirrups during delivery will lead to soreness in the lower back and legs.

The abdominal wall muscles have poor tone after their "big stretch." Sometimes, the growth of the abdomen has been so great that the muscles actually separate. This is known as a *diastasis recti*. Exercises to restore muscle tone may begin immediately after vaginal delivery and after soreness has decreased in the cesarean section patient (see Chapter 22).

THE IMMUNE SYSTEM

Blood-type Incompatibilities

Labor and delivery are times of risk for fetal–maternal transfusion. This situation has great significance for the Rh^- mother who receives cells from an Rh^+ fetus. The mother's system responds to the foreign (+) antigens by producing antibodies that may complicate future pregnancies. During the early postpartal period, the immune system can be manipulated to prevent antibody formation by the administration of anti-Rh$_O$ (D) immune globulin.

The antibodies in the immune globulin destroy fetal antigens before they are able to stimulate production of permanent maternal antibodies. The immune globulin must be given within 72 hours after delivery to be effective, and it is only helpful in those women who have not developed Rh$^+$ antibodies. The single dose of immune globulin should be sufficient to destroy the antigens in a moderate fetal–maternal transfusion. If a large transfusion is suspected, a Kleihauer Betke blood test is ordered. This test will detect 20 ml or more of fetal blood cells in the mother's bloodstream. If the test is positive, an additional dose of immune globulin is given.

Rh$_O$ (D) immune globulin should also be given after each miscarriage or abortion. In recent years, it has also been given at 28 weeks' gestation, to prevent antibody formation that may result from any bleeding complications of the last trimester of pregnancy.

Maternal–fetal blood group incompatibility may occur with other blood groupings in addition to Rh. In 20 percent of pregnancies the mother is type O while her fetus is A, B, or AB (Pritchard, MacDonald, and Gant, 1985). In 5 percent of these infants this incompatibility leads to a mild to moderate hemolytic disease. These infants may become jaundiced within the first 24 hours and require phototherapy. Very rarely a blood transfusion will be required to lower bilirubin levels and correct anemia. Because the ABO antigens are common in the intrauterine environment, the primigravida may be sensitized and have an infant with hemolytic disease.

Other blood groups (for example, Kell, Duffy, and Kidd) also produce incompatibilities and hemolytic disease in the infant. Although the occurrence of these blood types is rare, the resulting neonatal disease may be severe.

Early detection of blood type incompatibilities is vital to reduce neonatal morbidity. Early in pregnancy each woman's blood type is determined, and a screening test for antibodies is carried out. If the screening test is positive, further tests are used to discover the identity of the specific antibody. The father of the baby may also have blood typing performed to determine whether the potential exists for a maternal–fetal incompatibility. For example, an Rh$^-$ mother and an Rh$^+$ father might produce an Rh$^+$ fetus and maternal–fetal incompatibility. However, if the father is Rh$^-$ or the mother is Rh$^+$, no maternal–fetal Rh incompatibility can result.

At birth, the infant's cord blood is sent to the laboratory for blood typing and a direct Coombs' test, which detects antibodies from the mother that are coating the infant's cells. This test is always positive in all cases of incompatibility sensitization except ABO. Thus, blood typing of the infant is done to determine whether the newborn is at risk for hemolytic disease.

Rubella

Women who have been found during pregnancy to have no immunity to rubella should receive rubella vaccine in the postpartal period to prevent them from acquiring the disease during some future pregnancy.

The live, attenuated virus used in the vaccine is not communicable, so the woman may breastfeed and may visit with pregnant women. However, the virus in the vaccine is teratogenic. The woman must be made aware of this fact and must practice contraception for at least 2 months to avoid conception and possible injury to the fetus. While data suggest that rubella vaccine virus is less teratogenic than the wild virus, the risk to the fetus has not been precisely defined (American Academy of Pediatrics and American College of Obstetricians and Gynecologists, 1983).

The side-effects to the woman include a rash, mild arthralgia, and an elevated temperature. The vaccine is usually given on the day of discharge so that any appearance of the side-effects does not prolong hospitalization.

OTHER CHANGES

The anabolic protein metabolism of pregnancy returns to normal 6 weeks after delivery. Carbohydrate metabolism returns to normal quite slowly, as does the reversal of the hyperlipidemia of pregnancy.

In the early postpartal period, a hyperaminoacidemia is due to uterine autolysis. By 2–3 months postpartum the plasma proteins rise to normal levels.

After delivery, the diaphragm descends. This allows the woman to revert to abdominal costal breathing rather than the costal breathing of late pregnancy. This leads to the end of the respiratory alkalosis of pregnancy by improving CO_2 exchange.

RETURN TO THE STEADY STATE

The physiologic adaptation required in the postpartal period is so great that the transition to the nonpregnant state is not always a smooth one. "Afterpains" and the woman's body image are two aspects of the return to the steady state that are problematic for many women. They are both intimately related to the involution process.

"Afterpains"

Afterpains are spasmodic uterine contractions that occur during the first few days after delivery to keep the uterus firmly contracted. They are not usually noticed by primiparous women, who have good uterine tone and whose uteri are more likely to stay firmly contracted. The pains increase in severity with each delivery, as the uterus becomes more distended, so the multipara feels them more intensely than the primipara. They can usually be relieved by an analgesic or by activity. The woman can also be reassured that afterpains seldom last more than 3 days.

Afterpains are aggravated by breastfeeding, as oxytocin release is stimulated. Medications used to stimulate contractions—oxytocin (Pitocin), ergonovine (Ergotrate), or methylergonovine maleate (Methergine)—also aggravate them. Increasing or prolonged afterpains may indicate that the uterus is attempting to expel clots. In this instance, uterine size and abdominal position are assessed, and this information is relayed to the birth attendant. The women may be experiencing subinvolution.

Body Image

During pregnancy, women usually dream of the return to their former selves that will follow delivery. After delivery, the uterus sitting at the umbilicus, the numbers on the scales, and the striae can be very disappointing. A quick review of the process of involution by the nurse, however, can be reassuring. This is also a good opportunity to teach the woman to examine and know her own body.

The usual weight loss after delivery is 12 lb. An additional 5–8 lb is soon lost as a result of diuresis and involution. However, further weight loss will depend on the woman's diet and her exercise schedule.

Striae may be found on the skin of the breasts, abdomen, buttocks, and thighs. These reddish lines that most women refer to as "stretch marks" have been caused by adrenal cortical stimulation and mechanical overdistention of the skin, which lead to tearing of the elastic fibers under the epidermis. While striae do not disappear, they do fade, becoming a silvery white.

The increased skin pigmentations that appear with pregnancy (chloasma) usually disappear during the postpartal period.

Armed with this information, the woman can begin to adjust her image to the expected course of physiologic changes and make decisions regarding how to achieve her goal image.

Rest and Ambulation

Labor is exhausting work. At the end of labor, women have often been without sleep for many hours. While the new mother is excited about her accomplishment and relieved that her discomfort is decreased, within an hour or two she will just want to sleep. Also contributing to this fatigue are blood loss and the continuing effects of medications. The fatigue must be relieved to promote healing and to promote milk production in the lactating mother.

In the past the baby was sequestered from the mother in order to promote rest. However, because of the sleep–wake cycles of the neonate, the rooming-in baby will most likely sleep right along with his or her mother. It is more likely that health care activities such as abdominal examinations and vital signs determinations will interrupt the woman's rest. These activities should be carried out as quickly and gently as possible to allow the woman to rest, and schedules should be bent to allow for sleep. Women do not learn well when exhausted, so little teaching should be done until after an initial sleep period.

The woman is encouraged to continue to nap when the baby is asleep. Activity should be increased gradually when the woman returns home. She must be reminded to avoid fatigue.

Early ambulation is encouraged. The woman who has had an unmedicated delivery may be up taking a shower within 1 hour. This short trip may actually promote a longer sleep. The cesarean patient is ambulated with the first 24 hours. This early ambulation encourages elimination and decreases pooling of blood in the legs, which can lead to thrombophlebitis. Early ambulation also decreases the discomforts noted after delivery. However, because of the possibility of fainting, this ambulation must be supervised.

Disequilibrium

Three factors contribute to the dizziness and fainting frequently experienced during the early postpartal period: (1) the dilation of vessels caused by continued estrogen influence; (2) decreased intraabdominal pressure causing splanchnic engorgement (pooling of blood in the vessel of the gut); and, (3) larger than normal blood losses leading to hypovolemia (Bearg, personal communication). Even in cases of normal blood loss, it may be a few hours before the woman's blood volume equilibrates. While most women no longer experience fainting after 48 hours, they should be treated on an individual basis. Each woman should be accompanied on her first 2–3 ambulations to ensure safety. If signs of dizziness and fainting persist, they should be reported as they may indicate hypovolemia.

Hypothermic Reactions

Postpartum chilling, which often occurs after delivery, is accompanied by uncontrollable shaking in the early postpartal period. The chilling usually lasts no longer than 15 min but is often frightening for the patient. The etiology of this chilling is not known, but it is not considered an ominous sign. Several explanations have been offered, including the following: sudden release of intraabdominal pressure after delivery, nervous and exhaustion responses related to the stress of childbirth, disequilibrium in the internal and external body temperature resulting from the waste products of muscular exertion, and previous maternal sensitization to elements of fetal blood (Reeder, Mastroianni, and Martin, 1983). Nursing interventions to help prevent and control this chilling can include dry and warm blankets, an environment free of drafts, and warm fluids by mouth.

Diuresis and Diaphoresis

Within 24–48 hours after delivery, the woman begins to mobilize and excrete the 2–3 liters of fluid she has retained during pregnancy. With the loss of placental progesterone, there is no longer increased propensity to retain sodium. The excretion of fluid is most evident as a diuresis, reaching as much as 3000 ml/day. Women also experience diaphoresis, often soaking their gowns and bed linens. Linen change and frequent showers will provide comfort and rest. Also, the woman should be reassured that this is a normal process.

PROBLEMS AND SPECIAL CONSIDERATIONS

Special problems and considerations may arise after delivery because of postpartal physiology or as a result of procedures performed in association with delivery. Nursing assessment and interventions can minimize discomfort and lead to the early detection of deviations from the expected recuperative course.

Spinal Headache

When the spinal canal is penetrated, either to inject anesthesia medication or inadvertently during the effort to place an epidural catheter, a spinal headache may result. The puncture allows fluid to leak out. With bearing-down efforts during the second stage, leakage can be as much as 10 ml/hour. Escape of cerebrospinal fluid causes depletion of fluid volume, especially in the cisterna around the base of the brain, resulting in a loss of its cushioning effect. When the patient sits up, pain is caused by traction on the structures that support and anchor the brain, particularly the dura mater and the tentorium (Iffy and Kaminetzky, 1981).

The patient should be encouraged to lie flat for at least 6 hours after delivery, to avoid straining and coughing, and to increase fluid intake. For mild cases of spinal headache, maintaining the supine position, hydration, analysis, and reassurance are sufficient nursing measures.

The location of the headache may vary, but it is commonly felt in the occipital area and back of the neck. The headache varies in intensity but is precipitated by standing or sitting and is relieved by lying flat. The headache usually begins by the second day and may last for 2–3 days.

In some women, the headaches are severe and persist. For these women, a blood patch procedure is performed. The anesthesiologist withdraws 20 ml of the patient's blood and injects it into the epidural space. The blood then clots, sealing the puncture site. Blood patches have been known to provide effective and dynamic relief. The only side-effect or complication of the blood patch procedure is a sensation of bruising in the area of the procedure.

Morphine Epidurals

An injection of 5–7.5 mg morphine through the epidural catheter during a cesarean section provides the patient with relief of visceral pain during the first hours, when she is most likely to require pain medication. The onset of pain relief is prolonged, and so the morphine is injected after the umbilical cord is cut to insure that relief begins as the surgical anesthetic decreases. The pain relief may last for 12–36 hours, with most women being comfortable for approximately 24 hours. Women who have received epidural morphine may ambulate and care for themselves and their new baby.

The most disturbing side-effect of this medication is delayed respiratory depression. About 4–8 hours after injection is the most likely period for depression, although it may occur as late as 12 hours. The onset of respiratory depression is gradual with a slow decrease in respiratory rate. This decrease is detected by careful nursing assessment. The current recommendation for evaluation of respiratory function is every 30 min for 12 hours, and then every 60 min for the second 12 hours (Hughes, 1987). Other narcotics also potentiate respiratory depression, so the anesthesiologist will leave orders to be called if the woman requests further pain medication during the first 24 hours after delivery.

Other side-effects of epidural morphine include pruritis, nausea, vomiting, and urinary retention, and usually last as long as the analgesic effect. For itching, Narcan (0.2 mg intramuscularly or 0.08 mg intravenously) may be given every 2 hours as needed. This small dose of Narcan will frequently relieve the itching without reversing analgesia.

Episiotomies and Lacerations

Some trauma to the cervix and birth canal is inevitable during vaginal delivery. The trauma ranges from small tears to major lacerations requiring extensive repair. Most physicians prefer the controlled episiotomy wound to the possibility of an uncontrolled laceration.

Episiotomies first became popular in the U.S. at the end of WW II. Besides minimizing trauma to the maternal perineum, the episiotomy relieves pressure to the fetal head and shortens the second stage of labor.

Timing of the episiotomy is important. If it is cut too soon, the woman may lose a great deal of blood. If it is cut too late, it does not relieve pressure on the fetal head or shorten the second stage. The ideal time is when 3–4 cm of the fetal scalp is visible.

There are two types of incisions made, median and mediolateral (see Fig. 20–2). The *median* episiotomy is cut down the midline of the perineum. The major disadvantage of the median episiotomy is the risk that it will be extended down through the anal sphincter as the fetal head is delivered. The *mediolateral* episiotomy is cut at a 30-degree angle from the midline of the perineum. It has the advantage of being less likely to extend into the anal sphincter but is less easily repaired and more susceptible to complications of healing. Both types of episiotomies are repaired after delivery of the placenta and after the cervix and vagina have been explored for lacerations.

Lacerations can occur to the vagina and cervix, around the urethra, into the uterus, and to the perineum. They are graded as to the amount of tissue involvement. First-degree lacerations involve only the skin or mucosa; second-degree involve the underlying muscle; third-degree in-

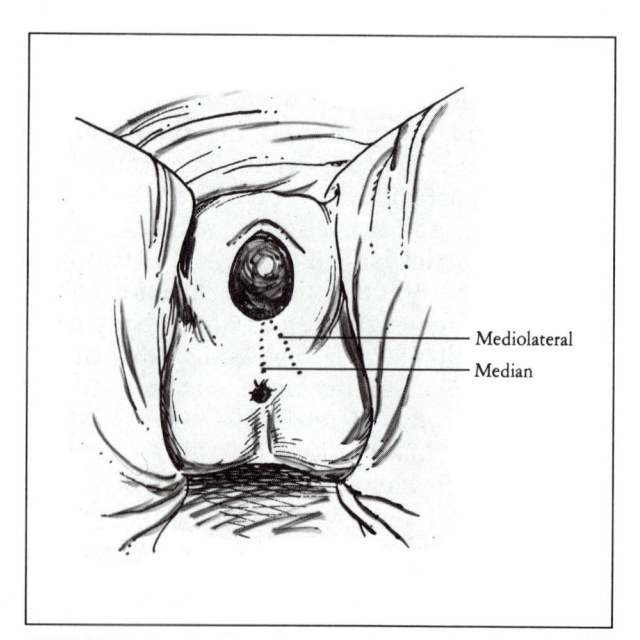

FIGURE 20–2. Types of episiotomies.
SOURCE: Reeder, Mastroianni, and Martin (1983).

volve the anal sphincter; fourth-degree involve the rectal mucosa. The degree of the laceration directly influences the plan of care for the wound.

Rapid labors, uncontrolled deliveries, large babies, abnormal presentations, rigid tissues, and instrumental deliveries predispose to lacerations or extensions of episiotomies by lacerations. Immediately after delivery, the entire genital area is inspected by the physician, as lacerations can lead to significant blood loss and hematoma formation.

Perineal and vaginal wounds heal rapidly because of the abundant blood supply to the region. Within 3–4 weeks an episiotomy site is usually so well healed there is no discomfort during intercourse. The perineum is checked for healing every 8 hours. The woman either lies in the lithotomy position or rolls on to her side with the superior leg pulled up toward her chest for the examination. The nurse chooses the position in which the repaired episiotomy or laceration can be most completely visualized. The nurse looks for a discolored mass indicative of a hematoma, reddened areas indicative of infections, or discharges from the wound. These abnormalities usually require medical management. There is evidence that the most important factor in the eventual strengthening of the perineal muscle is exercise, i.e. Kegel's exercise (Gordon and Logue, 1985). This exercise appears to be more important than the route of delivery or the presence or absence of an episiotomy.

To relieve the discomfort and edema from perineal wounds, an ice-pack is applied as soon as the repair is completed. The ice-pack is replaced often and used for 12–24 hours. After 24 hours a warm sitz bath given 3–4 times each day is encouraged. If the woman has a third- or fourth-degree laceration, sitz baths with an iodophor preparation may be ordered to prevent infection.

Hemorrhoids

Hemorrhoids are venous channels that drain the rectum and anus. External hemorrhoids drain the lower anal canal and perineal area while internal hemorrhoids drain the upper anal canal and the lower rectum.

Treatment of hemorrhoids is not indicated unless they become symptomatic, develop external thromboses, or prolapse and develop internal bleeding. Hemorrhoids often develop during pregnancy as the enlarging uterus exerts pressure on the perineal veins. Also during pregnancy, there is a likelihood of constipation and straining, and the hormones of pregnancy cause the pelvic tissue to relax.

Labor often exacerbates hemorrhoids and leads to increased pain, especially during the first few days after delivery. Treatment is at first conservative. Hydrophilic agents such as Metamucil or wetting agents such as Colace will soften stools. Increased fluid and a high-fiber diet will decrease the chance of constipation. Anesthetic sprays and ointments, witch hazel pads (tucks), and warm sitz baths also provide relief in the postpartum period. The woman should be taught to examine herself with a mirror for signs of discoloration, indicative of thrombosis. In some cases of continued pain, a clot may need to be removed surgically.

Usually after a delivery, the symptoms resolve within 1–3 weeks, although large skin tags may remain. The hemorrhoids that appear during pregnancy recede appreciably after delivery, often reappearing with the next pregnancy.

Hematomas

Damage to underlying vessels can occur during delivery without injury to the skin or mucosa. This damage results from pressure of the fetal head (especially at the point of the prominent ischial spines), the use of forceps, or the puncture of a vessel during the insertion of a needle for anesthesia or suturing. The blood loss from the vessel is often gradual, and a great deal of blood can be lost before the hematoma is discovered.

The sites of hematomas are the vulva, the vagina, and the subperitoneal space. The hematoma may first be noted as a discolored (bluish or reddish) mass during a physical examination of the perineum, or the woman may complain of intense pain in the area of perineum. All complaints must be examined, because a large, growing hematoma not only results in significant blood loss but may also become infected.

Large hematomas are incised and evacuated, and bleeding vessels are ligated. Small hematomas usually require no treatment and are reabsorbed spontaneously.

Bladder Trauma and Urine Retention

The passage of the fetal head through the birth canal causes edema, tenderness, and hyperemia of the vulva and perineum. The tenderness is even greater after a rapid delivery, long periods of pushing, the use of forceps, or episiotomies and lacerations.

Trauma to the bladder or urethra may lead to nerve damage that decreases bladder tone. Anesthesia used for delivery also decreases bladder tone as well as the new mother's perception of bladder fullness. These circumstances place the woman at risk of an overdistended bladder.

The distended bladder can be palpated just above the symphysis pubis. It displaces the uterus higher in the abdomen and causes it to deviate to one side. Percussion of the bladder elicits the distinct sound of fluid. The woman may void in small amounts (less than 100 ml). Small overflow amounts of urine are passed when the detrusor muscle has lost its tone and cannot empty the bladder. When a woman has reached this state, an indwelling catheter is inserted to keep the bladder empty for 48–72 hours to enable the detrusor to retain its tone.

The need for an indwelling catheter may be avoided by careful nursing management of the woman's bladder. This begins with frequent encouragement to void. Treatments to promote urination should be used, including relief of pain and warm fluids to the perineum. If, after 6 hours, these treatments have failed and fluid can be palpated in the bladder, the physician should be notified of the woman's inability to void. A straight catheterization at this point may prevent the need for an indwelling catheter later.

The key point in preventing a distended bladder is remembering that the woman will often have no perception of bladder fullness. She will depend on the nurse to let her know when she should void.

SUMMARY

For 40 weeks every system in a woman's body undergoes alterations to meet the needs of the fetus and to ensure the successful outcome of the pregnancy. At delivery an abrupt return to the nonpregnant state begins. Alterations occur in most body systems, contributing to special problems and considerations unique to the puerperium. The woman's body is vulnerable to complications after delivery because of the abruptness of the changes that are occurring, and she depends on the assessment skills of the nurse to promote safe passage through the postpartal period. If nurses understand the physiology of the postpartum adaptation, they are better able to assess the patient and to provide her with the information she needs.

REFERENCES

Albright, G. A.; Ferguson, J. E.; Joyce, T. H.; and Stevenson, D. K. 1986. *Anesthesia in obstetrics: Maternal, fetal, and neonatal aspects.* 2nd ed. Boston: Butterworth.

American Academy of Pediatrics and American College of Obstetricians and Gynecologists. 1983. *Guidelines for perinatal care.* Evanston, Ill.: AAP, and Washington, D.C.: ACOG.

Bonnar, J. 1975. The blood coagulation and fibronolytic systems during pregnancy. *Clinics in Obstet. Gynecol.* 2:321–344.

Chestnut, D. H.; Choi, W. W.; and Isbell, T. J. 1986. Epidural hydromorthone for postcesarean analgesia. *Obstet. Gynecol.* 68:65–69.

Crawford, J. S. 1985. Epidural blood patch. *Anesthesia.* 40:381.

Dahlman, T.; Hellgren, M.; and Blomback, M. 1985. Changes in blood coagulation and fibrinolysis in the normal puerperium. *Gynecol. Obstet. Invest.* 20:37–44.

Elias, M. F.; Teas, J.; Johnston, J.; and Bora, C. 1986. Nursing practices and lactation amenorrhoea. *J. Biosocial Sci.* 18:1–10.

Gordon, H., and Logue, M. 1985. Perineal muscle function after childbirth. *Lancet.* 2:123–125.

Greenhill, J. P., and Friedman, E. A. 1974. *Biological principles and modern practice of obstetrics.* Philadelphia: W. B. Saunders.

Hathaway, W. E., and Bonnar, J. 1978. *Perinatal coagulation.* San Diego: Grune and Stratton.

Hawkins, J. W., and Higgins, L. P. 1981. *Maternity and gynecological nursing, women's health care.* Philadelphia: J. B. Lippincott.

Herbert, W. N. P. 1982. Complications of the immediate puerperium. *Clin. Obstet. Gynecol.* 25:219–232.

Hughes, S. C. 1987. Intraspinal opiates in obstetrics. In *Anesthesia for obstetrics,* 2nd ed., eds. S. M. Shnider and G. Levinson. Baltimore: Williams and Wilkins.

Iffy, L., and Kaminetzky, H. A., eds. 1981. *Principles and practice of obstetrics and perinatology.* New York: John Wiley.

Jaffe, D. J. 1985. Postpartum evaluation of renal function. *Clin. Obstet. Gynecol.* 28:298–309.

Jennings, B., and Edmundson, M. 1980. The postpartum period: After confinement: The fourth trimester. *Clin. Obstet. Gynecol.* 23:1093–1103.

Liu, J.; Rebar, R. W.; and Yen, S. S. C. 1983. Neuroendocrine control of the postpartum period. *Clinics in Perinatology.* 10:723–736.

Malinowski, J. 1978. Bladder assessment in the postpartum patient. *J. Obstet. Gynecol. Neonatal Nurs.* 7(4):14–16.

McKenzie, C. A.; Canaday, M. E.; and Carroll, E. 1982. Comprehensive care during the postpartum period. *Nurs. Clin. N. Amer.* 17(1):23–48.

Metcalfe, J.; McAnulty, J. H.; and Ueland, K. 1981. Cardiovascular physiology. *Clin. Obstet. Gynecol.* 24:693–708.

Monheit, A. G.; Cousins, L.; and Resnik, R. 1980. The puerperium–anatomic and physiologic readjustments. *Clin. Obstet. Gynecol.* 23:973–984.

Oppenheimer, L. W.; Sherriff, E. A.; Goodman, J. D. S.; Shah, D.; and James, C. E. 1986. The duration of lochia. *Br. J. Obstet. Gynecol.* 93:754–757.

Osathanondh, R. 1980. Endocrine tests in obstetrics and gynecology. *Curr. Prob. Obstet. Gynecol.* 3(10):5–20.

Pillitteri, A. 1981. *Maternal–newborn nursing, care of the growing family.* 2nd ed. Boston: Little, Brown.

Pritchard, J. A.; McDonald, P. C.; and Gant, N. F. 1985. *Williams Obstetrics.* 17th ed. Norwalk, Conn.: Appleton-Century-Crofts.

Reeder, S. J.; Mastroianni, L.; and Martin, L. 1983. *Maternity nursing.* 15th ed. Philadelphia: J. B. Lippincott.

Russell, T. R. 1983. Managing hemorrhoids during and after pregnancy. *Contemp. Ob./Gyn. Special Issue: Update on General Surgery.* 21(S.I.):75–79.

Scott, D. B., and Sinclair, C. 1982. Advances in regional anesthesia and analgesia. *Clinics in Obstet. Gynecol.* 9:273–289.

Short, R. V. 1984. Breastfeeding. *Sci. Amer.* 250(4):35–41.

Wiggins, J. 1979. *Childbearing, physiology, experiences, needs.* St. Louis: C. V. Mosby.

Williams, W. J.; Bentler, E.; Erslev, A.; and Lichtman, M. A. 1983. *Hematology.* 3rd ed. New York: McGraw-Hill.

21

Breastfeeding: Physiology and Management

BEHAVIORAL OBJECTIVES

Upon completion of this chapter, the reader should be able to:

- Evaluate the importance of nursing care to breastfeeding women and identify counseling information that is based on sound rationale.

- Apply the principles of the anatomy and physiology of lactation to the nursing care of breastfeeding women.

- Apply the nursing process in meeting the needs of breastfeeding women for support and information.

- Identify common problems with breastfeeding and possible solutions.

- Analyze how mothers can adapt breastfeeding to special situations.

Health care professionals can help mothers to understand the benefits of breastfeeding and to achieve success in implementing this method of feeding their infants. Recently, breastfeeding has been definitively shown to have particular advantages over bottle feeding, for both mother and baby.

HISTORY AND TRENDS

History

For thousands of years in all cultures breastfeeding was the only acceptable method of feeding an infant. Women of hunting and gathering and agrarian societies—societies that have dominated the span of human history—breastfed their infants. As these women walked, gathering food or farming, they carried their children, ever ready to feed when the child needed them. During the day nursing tended to be infrequent, for the walking motion of the mother rocked the baby to sleep. In the evening and during the night the infant awakened and fed more frequently, often nestled against the sleeping mother.

Despite the commonness of the practice of breastfeeding, evidence exists that artificial feeding was attempted quite early in our history. Various types of feeding implements such as cups, spoons, and bottles were used to feed infants mixtures of milk, water, and grain (see Figs. 21–1 and 21–2). Feeding vessels have been found in Egyptian graves dating from as long ago as 2500 B.C. (Riordan, 1983), and throughout Europe spouted feeding cups have been found in infants' graves dating from 2000 B.C. (Lawrence, 1985). In addition, there is sound evidence that direct suckling from animals was attempted.

However, the dangers of early artificial feeding are well documented. Without the immunologic protection of breast milk, many infants died from infections, especially gastrointestinal infections. Foundling hospitals in the late 1700s had a mortality rate of 80 percent or higher in artificially fed infants (Riordan, 1983).

To avoid the dangers of artificial feeding, affluent mothers employed wet nurses. Wet nurses became so popular in England that illegitimacy among young girls became common. In France, wet nursing became so prevalent that laws were established to control its practice (Garrison, 1929).

The value of a mother's nursing her own infant was also well known. Wet nurses were often cruel and neglectful. If the wet nurse was loving and nursed the child until weaning, usually 18 months, separation from the mother substitute and return to the natural mother was traumatic. Spartan royal lawmakers in 4 B.C. dictated that all mothers should breastfeed, even the kings's wife. Plutarch reported that a second son of King Themestes inherited the kingdom of Sparta only because he had been been nursed with his mother's milk and his brother had not. The eldest son had been nursed by a stranger and was therefore rejected (Lawrence, 1985). In 1762 in *Emile*, Jean-Jacques Rousseau protested the decline of breastfeeding in France as a "source of weakness to the nation" (Garrison, 1929).

Trends

The scientific discoveries and changing social and cultural patterns of the late nineteenth and early twentieth centuries brought a decline in breastfeeding. Pasteurization, refrigeration, and the manufacture of canned milk made bottle feeding less hazardous. The scientific community began to place great value in preciseness and measurement. Thus, bottle feeding seemed superior, because the exact amounts fed could be calculated. Concurrently, changing social practices were not supportive of successful breastfeeding. The move from urban areas to the city forced many women to go

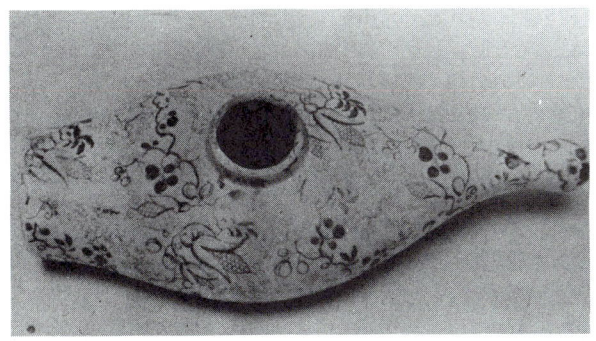

FIGURE 21–1. Staffordshire nursing bottle.
SOURCE: Courtesy of the Maxwell Museum of Anthropology, University of New Mexico.

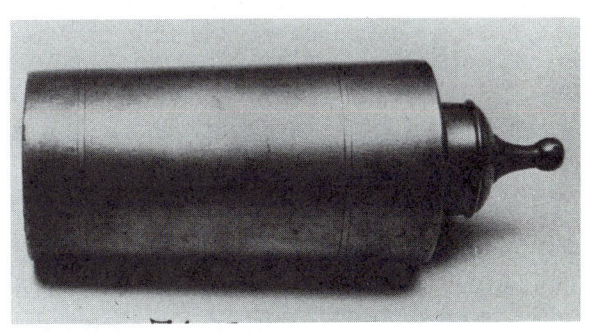

FIGURE 21–2. Pewter nursing bottle–German, late eighteenth or early nineteenth century.
SOURCE: Courtesy of the Maxwell Museum of Anthropology, University of New Mexico.

to work in environments such as factories, which were not suitable for an infant. Thus, mothers became separated from their infants. Childrearing practices also changed. In America, childrearing was influenced by the dogmatic teaching of Luther Emmet Holt and his pamphlet, "The Care and Feeding Of Children," first published in 1894 (Montague, 1978). In this work he recommended abolishing the cradle, not picking up the crying baby, not handling the baby too much, and feeding the baby by the clock. Separation and such infant care practices made breastfeeding difficult. In addition, Western culture began promoting the female breast as an object of sex, excluding its primary nutritive function. Consequently, many women became inhibited and embarrassed at the thought of breastfeeding. Many thought it uncivilized and not "modern." Thus, the modern woman of the 1920s was "symbolized by short hair, short skirts, contraceptives, cigarettes, and bottle feeding" (Lawrence, 1985).

The decline in breastfeeding was dramatic. What had been a common practice for thousands of years became uncommon. In the United States in the 1930s over 70 percent of infants were breastfed, but by the late 1960s breastfeeding had dropped to an all-time low of 18 percent (Riordan, 1983). However, as dramatically as the trend toward bottle feeding arose, a reverse trend toward breastfeeding appeared. By the late 1970s, studies were reporting that over 50 percent of babies were being breastfed (Cole, 1977; Stanway and Stanway, 1980; Houston, 1981; Yeung et al., 1981). Reports by scientists on the benefits of breastfeeding were emerging. Women were now choosing breastfeeding not because of cultural influences but because of knowledge of the benefits for both the mother and the infant (Stanway and Stanway, 1980; Yeung et al., 1981; Eckhardt and Hendershot, 1984). In one study, 9 out of 12 reasons why women chose breastfeeding were comments related to the positive benefits for the mother or infant (Yeung et al., 1981). The largest percentage of women stated that they were breastfeeding because breast milk was better for the baby.

However, these statistics are deceiving. First, they reflect trends in only certain populations. In lower socioeconomic groups and black populations, lower percentages of women breastfeed (Arafat et al., 1981; Riordan, 1983; Eckhardt and Hendershot, 1984). There has also been a steady decline in breastfeeding in Third World countries, where formula companies have promoted bottle feeding as the "modern way" to feed babies. Also, even though many women are choosing breastfeeding, many are discontinuing breastfeeding within a few weeks following delivery. One study reported that 97 percent of the mothers who left a certain hospital breastfeeding were totally bottle feeding at the end of the first week (Frantz, 1982). Other studies also report that many women stop breastfeeding (Stanway and Stanway, 1980; Houston, 1981; Houston, Howie, and McNeilly, 1983). In one study, 64 percent of women who breastfed said they would not breastfeed a second child or were not certain they would (Arafat et al., 1981).

The reasons women give for discontinuing breastfeeding do not indicate that this is an independent decision. One study reports that over 50 percent of women discontinued breastfeeding before they intended (Ellis and Hewat, 1984). The reasons indicate that the mothers were having difficulties breastfeeding. A lack of confidence in the ability to breastfeed, not having enough milk, painful or sore breasts or nipples, the baby not nursing well, and maternal discomforts are common reasons given by mothers for terminating breastfeeding (Evans, Thigpen, and Hamrick, 1969; Wallace, 1980; Houston, 1981; Yeung et al., 1981; Houston, Howie, and McNeilly, 1983; Loughlin et al., 1985). All of these are situations that can be prevented or resolved with good counseling from the nurse.

Women need accurate and complete information about breastfeeding so that they can prevent or resolve problems and thus continue breastfeeding as long as they desire. Studies show that health professionals often give conflicting information to breastfeeding mothers and that some of this information is not based on sound rationale (Estok, 1973; Maclean, 1977; Crowder, 1981; Hayes, 1981). Counseling is often based on opinion and personal experience. One author has remarked that the advice given to breastfeeding mothers is not lacking in quantity, but in some areas to say that it excels in diversity would not be exaggerating (Maclean, 1977). Nurses need to develop a good knowledge base regarding breastfeeding before they can adequately counsel breastfeeding mothers.

ANATOMY AND PHYSIOLOGY OF THE BREAST

To begin counseling breastfeeding women, the nurse must have a thorough knowledge of the anatomy and physiology of the breast. This enables the nurse to help the mother establish and maintain practices that are in synchrony with the natural process of lactation.

Anatomy of the Breast

Glandular tissue

The breast is composed of glandular tissue, surrounded by nutritive, supportive, and protective tissue and structures, including connective, fat, and lymphatic tissue and blood vessels (see Fig. 21–3). The glandular tissue can be visualized as a tree-like structure. Arising from the nipple are 10–20 large branch-like structures called *lobes*. Branching off from each lobe are 20–40 *lobules*, which each branches further into 10–100 sac-like structures called *alveoli*. It is in the alveoli that milk is produced. These sac-like structures are lined with secretory cells called *acini*, which produce and secrete the milk. Surrounding each cluster of cells of each alveolus are contractile cells called *myoepithelial cells*, which contract the alveolus and eject milk from the sac through small *ductules* into the larger *lactiferous ducts*. As the lactiferous ducts approach the nipple they widen into milk-collecting areas called the *lactiferous sinuses*. From these sinuses the infant extracts the milk through openings in the *mammary papilla*, or nipple.

Some mammary glandular tissue projects into the axillary region. This tissue, known as the *tail of Spence*, is more prominent during lactation and its enlargement may cause maternal discomfort if the breasts become engorged.

A few mother have accessory mammary glands. Glandular tissue that developed when the mother was a fetus (from a line of tissue called the *milk line*, which extends from the lavicular to the inguinal regions) can develop accessory mammary glands. This is called *hypermastia* and occurs in 2–6 percent of women (Lawrence, 1985). If there is breast tissue in these accessory breasts, enlargement and secretion may occur during pregnancy and lactation.

Fat and Connective Tissue

Connective tissue supports the milk ducts. Fat tissue surrounds the glandular tissue, giving the breast its round shape. Much of the size variation of the breast is due to the amount of fat and connective tissue present and not the amount of glandular tissue. The human is the only mammal that has protuberant breasts. Thus, it is not the size of the breasts that is significant in lactation.

Innervation and Blood Supply

The breast is well supplied with blood and nerves. The blood supply arises from branches of the intercostal arteries and the internal thoracic artery, the major portion coming from the internal mammary and the lateral thoracic arteries. Nerves of the breast are from the branches of the fourth, fifth, and sixth intercostal nerves and consist of sensory fibers and sympathetic fibers innervating smooth muscles in the nipple and blood vessels. The sensory innervation of the nipple and areola is extensive.

Skin

The outer covering of the breast includes the nipple, areola, and surrounding skin. The skin, an elastic cover of the breast tissue, adheres to the fatty subcutaneous tissue. The *nipple* is a darkly pigmented, sometimes erect structure located slightly below the middle of the breast. It contains the opening of the milk ducts. Surrounding the nipple is a darkly pigmented area called the *areola*, which is variable in size. Behind this area lie the lactiferous sinuses. The areola contains the *Montgomery glands*, sebaceous glands that secrete a substance for nipple lubrication and antisepsis.

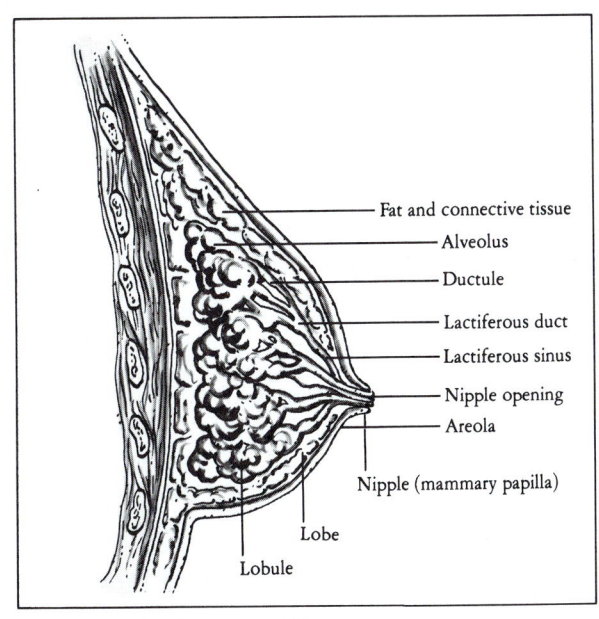

FIGURE 21–3. Anatomy of the breast.

Physiology of Lactation

During Pregnancy

During pregnancy circulating hormones cause changes in the breast tissue. There is rapid growth of the alveoli, lobes, and ducts. Estrogen stimulates ductal growth, and progesterone stimulates lobular and alveolar increases. Prolactin levels increase and influence the development of the secretory alveolar cells. As pregnancy progresses, this prolactin response stimulates the production of colostrum in the breast. Colostrum can be found in the breast as early as the third month of gestation (Lawrence, 1985).

Postpartum

At delivery, with the expulsion of the placenta there is an abrupt decline in estrogen and progesterone. Estrogen inhibits milk secretion. Thus, after delivery, prolactin is free to stimulate milk production. Infant suckling provides for continued release of prolactin from the anterior pituitary (see Fig. 21–4). A reduction of suckling results in a decrease in prolactin and, therefore, a decrease in milk synthesis.

Infant stimulation of the breast also effects the release of oxytocin from the posterior pituitary. Oxytocin stimulates contraction of the myoepithelial cells that cause ejection of milk from the alveoli into the ductal system, making it available for the infant. This mechanism is called the *let-down reflex*. This reflex, though stimulated by infant suckling, can also be initiated by the mother's thoughts, usually positive thoughts about her baby. Conversely, it can be inhibited by thoughts. Feelings of anxiety and insecurity can inhibit the let-down reflex (see Fig. 21–5). When milk does not let down, the infant becomes frustrated at the breast. The mother interprets this as rejection, which reinforces her insecure feelings. In addition, when milk is not removed from the alveoli, pressure on capillary blood flow inhibits lactation. Thus, unless these feelings are minimized by reassurance and support, a cycle begins that leads to lactation failure.

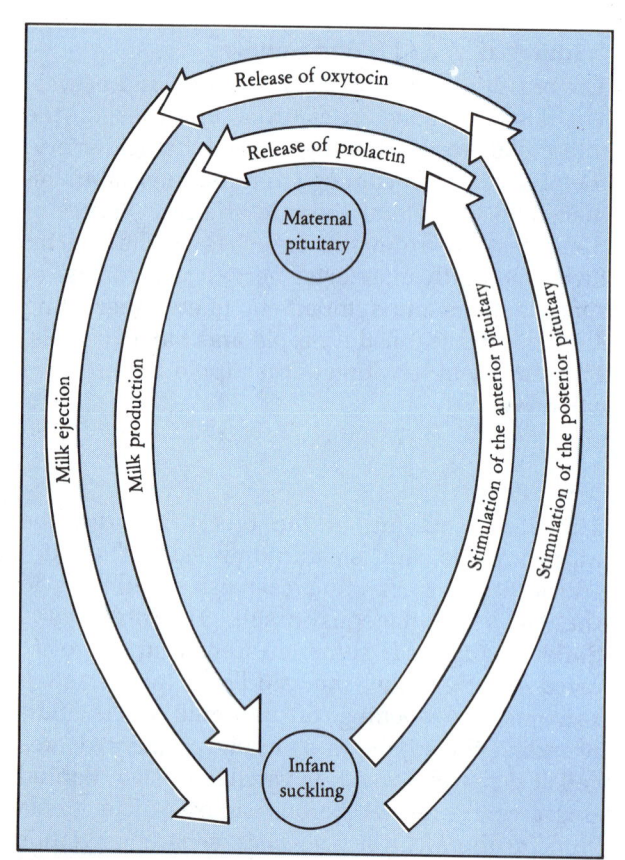

FIGURE 21–4. Milk production and ejection.

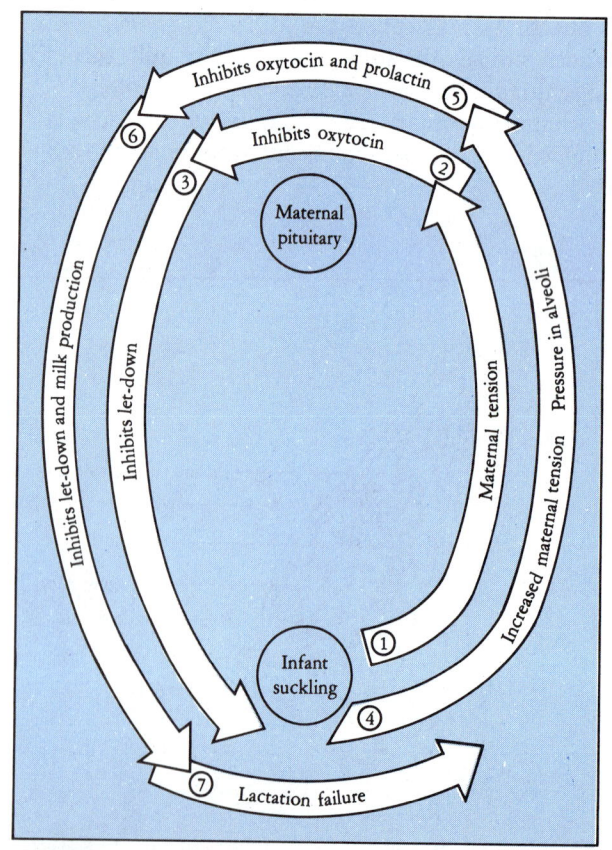

FIGURE 21–5. The effect of maternal tension on milk production and ejection.

Sensory receptors that trigger both oxytocin and prolactin release are located in the nipple. These receptors respond somewhat to the negative pressures of suckling. However, it is the tactile stimulation of the nipple that is most important for milk ejection (Lawrence, 1985). This need for tactile stimulation has implications for the mother who is using a breast shield or who is pumping her breast with a mechanical or electric pump. Tactile stimulation by these devices is not the same as that from an infant suckling. Additional support may be needed to ensure milk production and ejection.

NURSING MANAGEMENT OF SUCCESSFUL BREASTFEEDING

Nursing management of breastfeeding in the postpartum period involves application of the nursing process to facilitate successful breastfeeding. Success in breastfeeding is defined as follows: (1) the mother has breastfed as long as she and the baby desired, (2) the baby's nutritional needs have been met, and (3) the mother verbalizes satisfaction with the experience. How is this outcome achieved? Many authors report that it is important that health care personnel provide support and information to the breastfeeding mother (Sloper, McKean, and Baum, 1975; Meara, 1976; Cole, 1977; Berger, 1978; Beske and Garvis, 1982). Two studies report that successful breastfeeding occurs when both support and information are provided to the breastfeeding woman (Ladas, 1970; Hall, 1978). These kinds of support are important because women have not had breastfeeding role models. They have not learned the art of breastfeeding from a family member, nor are these members nearby for support. Thus, nursing management of postpartum breastfeeding women involves assessing their support and informational needs, planning for and meeting those needs, and evaluating the effectiveness of the support provided (see Fig. 21–6).

Support Needs

Support needs are physical and psychologic needs that, if met by the nurse, enhance the natural functioning of breastfeeding, prevent problems, facilitate skill development, and increase maternal confidence. These needs include (1) early initiation of breastfeeding, (2) correct positioning of the baby at the breast, (3) encouragement of a demand feeding schedule, (4) offering no supplementary feedings unless medically indicated, (5) enhancement of the let-down reflex, and (6) psychologic support.

Early Initiation of Breastfeeding

It is important that the mother and infant have the opportunity to breastfeed as soon after delivery as possible. Mothers who feed during the first hour of life breastfeed longer and have more positive comments about their experience than women who first breastfeed at 16 or more hours after birth. The initial satisfying breastfeeding experience acts as a reinforcer for subsequent feedings (Johnson, 1976). This early breastfeeding has an imprinting effect (Riordan and Countryman, 1980). It reinforces not only the infant's sucking reflex and pattern but also the mother's self-esteem.

There are few contraindications to early initiation of breastfeeding. Concern for hypothermia should not prohibit this practice. Studies indicate that the temperature of infants placed skin to skin with the mother or in a warm blanket next to the mother are similar to those of infants heated in an isolette or with an overhead heater (Gardner, 1979; Hill and Shronk, 1979). Breastfeeding may be delayed if (1) a mother is heavily medicated, (2) an infant has a 5-min Apgar score under 6, or (3) an infant is under 36 weeks' gestation (Lawrence, 1985). Occasionally, a mother will express extreme fatigue and will not desire to breastfeed immediately after delivery. She may wish merely to observe and hold her infant. In this situation, encouraging her to breastfeed may have a negative rather than a positive effect. The mother should have the opportunity to breastfeed as soon as she and the infant are ready and able.

Frequently, the infant does not latch onto the nipple as soon as he or she is put to the breast after delivery. The infant may lick and nuzzle the breast but not attach and suck. However, the benefit of this close contact is important to the establishment of the mother–infant relationship. Also, tactile stimulation from licking will stimulate the mother's hormonal response.

Positioning the Infant on the Breast

Helping the mother position the infant on the breast the first few times the baby feeds is important in initiating and maintaining a milk supply and in preventing nipple problems. Incorrect positioning of the infant on the breast prevents the

Breastfeeding Assessment Tool

Needs or problems	Need or problem active	Need met or problem resolved
Supportive needs		
1. Early initiation of breastfeeding (note when baby first breastfed).		
2. Correct position is being used (observed twice).		
3. Baby is feeding on a demand schedule.		
4. Baby is receiving no supplements. (If so, state reason.)		
5. Let-down reflex is present.		
6. Mother makes positive statements about her feeding skills.		
7. Support is present after mother goes home.		
Teaching needs		
1. Advantages and disadvantages of breastfeeding (usually done prenatally).		
2. Knowledge of breasts and their function.		
3. Breast care.		
Wash once daily with no soap.		
Air dry for 10–15 minutes after feedings.		
Knowledge of lubricants and their use.		
Use of both breasts at each feeding.		
Knowledge of how to take baby off the breast.		
Inverted or retracted nipples—use of breast cups (may have been done prenatally).		
4. Diet for breastfeeding.		
5. How to tell if baby is getting enough.		
6. Growth spurts.		
7. Infant feeding behavior.		
8. Normal stool patterns.		
9. Additional reading sources.		
Breastfeeding problems (hospital/home/well-baby visit)		
Possible hospital problems		
1. Engorgement		
2. Sore nipples		
3. Difficult attachment		
Later problems		
4. Colicky baby		
5. Mastitis		
6. Slow weight gain		
7. Other		

FIGURE 21–6. A breastfeeding assessment tool.

infant from properly stimulating and milking the breast. As a result, milk production diminishes. Incorrect positioning also creates excessive pressure on breast tissue, and nipple soreness results.

To position the mother correctly, the nurse should first help her to an upright, comfortable position. If she has discomfort from a perineal or abdominal incision or from "after birth" pains, medical and nonmedical means should be instituted to relieve that discomfort. Her arms may need to be supported by pillows if they are not supported by the arms of a chair. A pillow on the abdomen may be held in place by the bent knees of the mother who has had a cesarean birth, to give support to the baby and to lift the infant off the incision (see Fig. 21–7). If the mother needs privacy, it should be provided.

Next, the mother should place the infant across her abdomen with the head at her antecubital fossa, or the crook of her holding arm (Frantz, 1980). With this holding arm she then turns the infant's body so that it entirely faces her (see Fig. 21–8). The infant's face, chest, genitals, and knees should be facing the mother's body. Then the mother holds her breast not in the cigarette hold as frequently recommended but with the thumb and fingers spread. The thumb is placed on the upper breast and the remaining fingers and hand under the breast (see Fig. 21–9). This keeps the fingers away from areola and gives good support to the breast. A common mistake mothers make is to grasp the areola behind the nipple and by doing so inadvertently offer the nipple to the baby's waiting jaws (see Fig. 21–10). In a properly suckling infant, the jaws should fit behind the nipple and the breast should stretch so that the nipple is positioned deep within the infant's mouth (see Fig. 21–11). This places the nipple far away from the pressing jaws that milk the sinuses under areola.

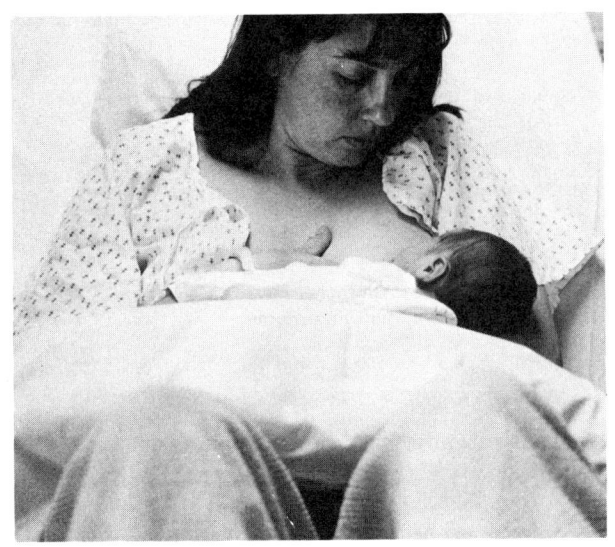

FIGURE 21–7. A comfortable breastfeeding position with pillows placed between the bent knees of the mother and the baby.

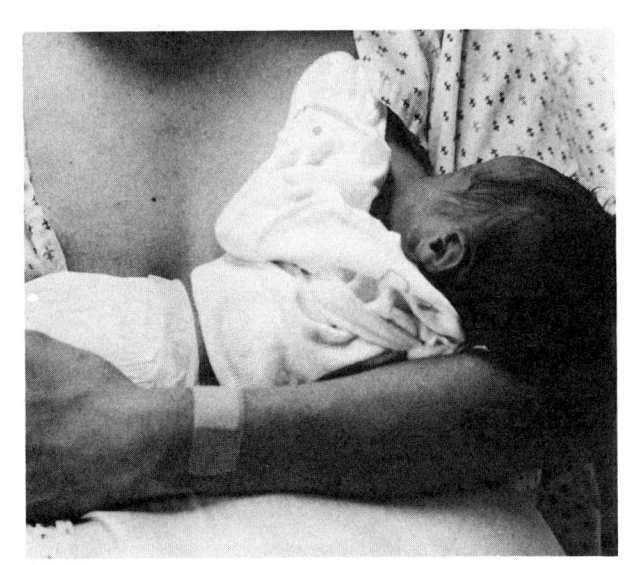

FIGURE 21–8. Infant placed across abdomen with head in mother's antecubital fossa. Infant entirely faces the mother.

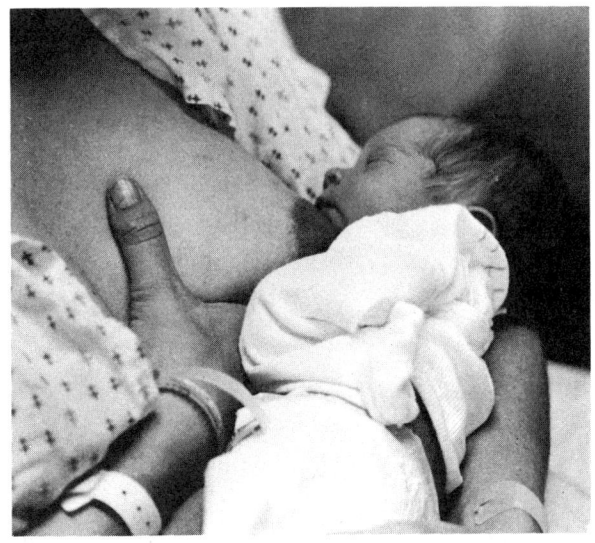

FIGURE 21–9. The thumb is placed on the upper breast and the fingers and hand under the breast to give the breast good support.

444 CHANGE: THE POSTPARTAL PERIOD

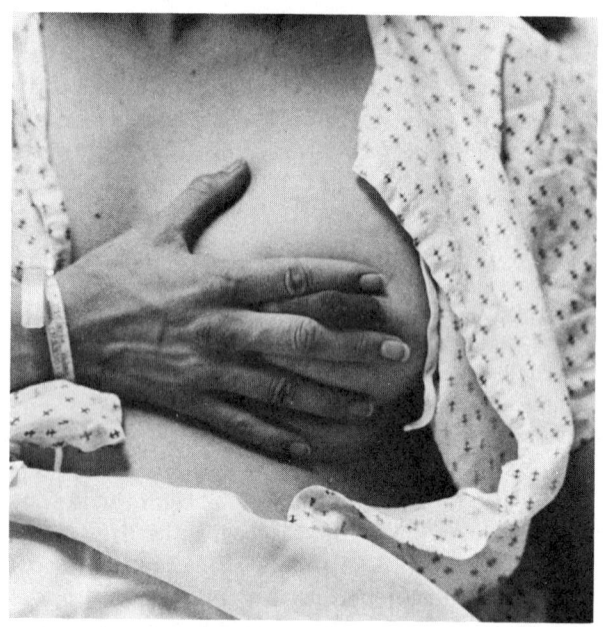

FIGURE 21–10. The cigarette hold is frequently recommended; however, having the thumb and fingers spread is more effective.

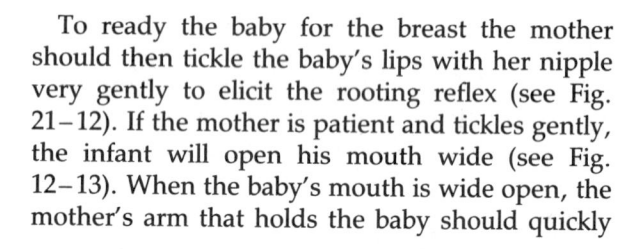

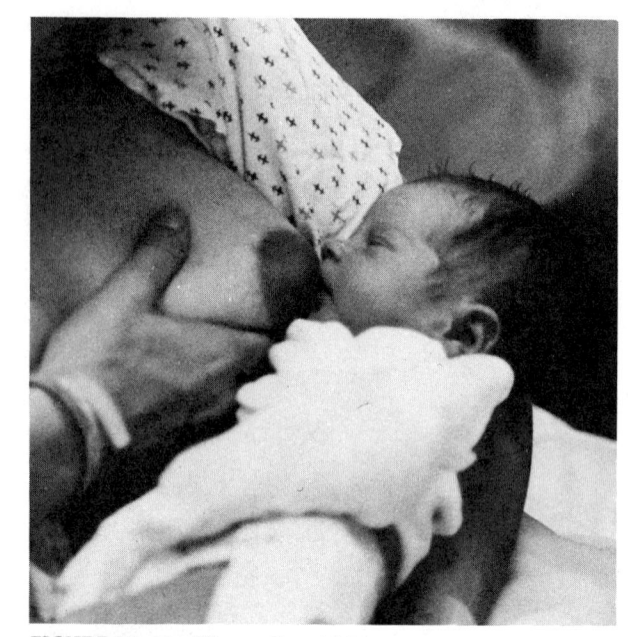

FIGURE 21–11. The mother tickles the infant's lower lip with her nipple.

To ready the baby for the breast the mother should then tickle the baby's lips with her nipple very gently to elicit the rooting reflex (see Fig. 21–12). If the mother is patient and tickles gently, the infant will open his mouth wide (see Fig. 12–13). When the baby's mouth is wide open, the mother's arm that holds the baby should quickly pull the infant toward her as close as as she can so that the baby's nose just barely touches the breast. The buttocks should be pulled in toward the mother as much as the baby's upper torso. In this position the infant uses the minimum amount of suction on the breast.

Holding the infant supine across the mother's

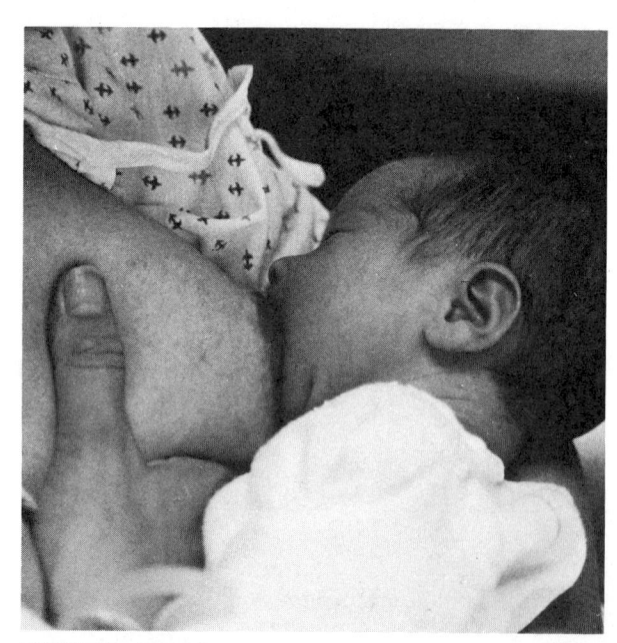

FIGURE 21–12. If the mother waits patiently, the infant will open his mouth wide.

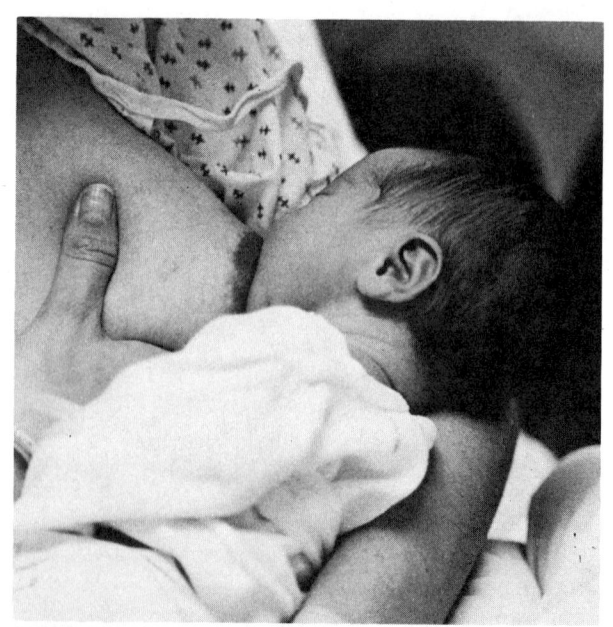

FIGURE 21–13. The infant's buttocks should be pulled in toward the mother's torso.

abdomen will increase suction on the breast, because the baby's shoulder will prevent him from getting close to the breast and the weight of his body will tend to pull him away from the breast. If the baby is not close enough to the breast to fit his mouth well back onto the areola, he will only grasp the nipple. Pressure by the jaws on the nipple will cause trauma. Also, trauma to the jaws may occur if the mother presses her finger against the breast as is often recommended to ensure that the infant can breathe. Keeping the baby's body straight and even, with the nose tip touching the breast, should provide enough of an airway. If more of an airway is needed, it is better to have the mother lift the baby off the breast slightly rather than depress the thumb. Some mothers depress the thumb too vigorously, inadvertently pulling the breast up and out of the posterior part of the infant's mouth.

During a 4-year period when this technique for positioning the infant was used at the Natural Childbirth Institute in Los Angeles, there was not one case of sore nipples (Frantz, 1980). In addition, another study reports that most of the cases of sore nipples detected at 1 or 2 weeks postpartum at the University of Southern California Breastfeeding clinic were eliminated when this method was used (Herbin, 1981). Clinically, when this position is used, women report immediate relief of soreness or pain accompanying breastfeeding.

Once the infant is nursing, it is important for the nurse to continue to observe a feeding periodically to assess for proper positioning. This is particularly true if the mother is complaining of any nipple soreness and especially if pain occurs throughout the feeding. Treatment for nipple soreness should not be initiated without observing the mother to determine the cause.

ENCOURAGING DEMAND FEEDING

It is important that the mother nurse her infant whenever the infant is hungry and for as long as the infant wants to nurse. During the first month, most breastfed infants nurse about 8–10 times in a 24-hour period. One study reported that the mean frequency of feedings during the first 2 weeks of life was 9.8 in 24 hours; at 1 month it was 7.2 (De Carvalho et al., 1982a). The length of a feeding will vary between infants; one study reported a range of 7–30 min (Howie et al., 1981), and 70–80 percent of milk volume was taken in the first 5 min. Thus, when infants nurse for short periods, it may be inappropriate to force the infant to feed longer. In contrast, other infants may need to nurse longer. De Carvalho et al. (1982a) found that heavier newborns nursed longer and more frequently. Although the nutritive time may be only 10 min. or less, the value of non-nutritive sucking is not known. The caloric content of hind milk is higher because of the higher fat content and, therefore, small amounts at the end of the feeding may be important to some infants (Howie et al., 1981). Therefore, it is important to teach the mother to "read" her infant's signs of hunger and satiation.

Demand feedings offer benefits to the mother and infant. Demand feedings help to establish a good milk supply and prevent engorgement and sore nipples. Frequent feedings help clear the lactiferous ducts of colostrum and allow milk to flow freely. Thus, the conditions that lead to engorgement are lessened or even prevented. The amount of milk produced is directly related to the number of feedings. The greater the number of feedings, the greater the quantity of milk produced (Newton, 1971; Egli, Egli, and Newton, 1961).

Allowing suckling and active nursing for as long as the infant desires, provides additional breast stimulation and satisfaction of sucking. In many hospitals it is routine to limit the time the infant nurses during early feedings to 3–5 min at the first feeding and to gradually increase the length of the feedings. Contrary to common belief, this does not prevent nipple soreness (Whitley, 1978; L'Esperance, 1980; Slaven, 1981; Ramirez, 1982; L'Esperance and Frantz, 1985; De Carvalho, Robertson, and Klaus, 1984). Limiting nursing time merely delays nipple irritation (Newton, 1952; Whitley, 1978). In actuality, it is excessive pressure unrelieved by sucking that causes nipple damage (Gunther, 1945). A sleepy infant creates more pressure than a baby who is actively sucking. Thus, it is important to allow the infant to nurse when he is awake and hungry rather than to wake a sleeping infant to feed.

The Importance of Avoiding Supplementation with Early Feedings

Offering supplemental bottles of water or formula is not necessary and, to the contrary, can be detrimental to breastfeeding (Cohen, 1980; La Cerva, 1981; Frantz, 1983; Lawrence, 1985). Studies have demonstrated that supplementary feedings are not necessary to prevent jaundice, elevated bilirubin levels, or weight loss (Dahms et al., 1973; De Carvalho, Hall, and Harvey, 1981; Nicoll, Ginsburg, and Tripp, 1982; De Carvalho, Klaus, and Merkatz, 1982b; Maisel and Gifford, 1983; Lawrence, 1985). In addition, frequent nursing significantly reduces serum bilirubin levels (De Carvalho, Klaus, and Merkatz, 1982b). However, supplementary feedings do negatively affect the establishment of breastfeeding. Offering early water or formula supplements undermines a woman's confidence. This action by health professionals may indicate to her that her breasts will not produce enough milk. Providing complimentary formula packs when the mother leaves hospital tells her that the nurse thinks she may not have enough milk either. One study found less mothers breastfeeding at 1 month if they received these samples. This was especially significant among the less well educated, primiparas, and mothers who were ill postpartum (Bergevin, Dougherty, and Kramer, 1983). One young mother who was given a case of glucose water from the hospital was still giving water supplements after every feeding at the second postpartum week, despite full, dripping breasts. The mother and father stated that these feedings were against their better judgment but that they had continued because they thought it was what they were supposed to do.

Giving the infant a supplement can also cause what is termed *nipple confusion*. The sucking action required of the infant for a rubber nipple is totally different from that required for the breast. With the rubber nipple the infant thrusts the tongue forward and presses upward at varying intervals to stop the easy flow of milk. With breastfeeding the infant thrusts the tongue under the areola, pulling the breast so that the nipple is in the back of the mouth and the jaws are on the areola. He then curves the tongue and thrusts it back to create a suction to milk the breast. Trying to learn these two different actions after birth can be confusing to some infants. Usually, they discover that it is easier to suck on a rubber nipple and refuse the breast. Or they merely become confused and fuss and cry whenever they feed on the breast, which is a more difficult procedure. The mother then interprets this as the baby's not liking the breast, her breast milk, or sometimes even her.

Enhancement of the Let-down Reflex

Initially, the nurse assesses whether let-down is occurring. If let-down is present, infant swallowing noises will be heard. The mother may feel a tingling sensation in her breasts, or leaking of the breasts may be noted before or during a feeding. Uterine cramping caused by the effect of oxytocin on the uterus is also a sign that the let-down reflex is being stimulated. Knowing this is often consoling to a mother who is experiencing the discomfort of cramping.

The nurse can enhance the let-down reflex response by creating a relaxed physical and psychologic atmosphere. Ensuring a comfortable position, offering warm liquids, offering methods of pain relief, and teaching relaxation techniques help the mother relax physically. To help the mother relax mentally the nurse needs to make sincere positive comments that increase the mother's confidence about breastfeeding. Pleasant conversation is also helpful and relaxing during breastfeeding.

Psychologic Support

The behavior of a woman in the postpartum period has been characterized as "taking-in" and "taking-hold" (Rubin, 1961). During the taking-hold period, a woman is eager to learn about breastfeeding. However, her self-esteem in this new role is fragile. Comments by nurses can have a significant impact. This is particularly true of breastfeeding. Feeding is an important part of the mothering role, and breastfeeding is viewed by the mother as dependent solely upon her functioning. Therefore, it is extremely important that the nurse support any and all efforts a mother makes in her breastfeeding attempts. Remarks should, as much as possible, be positive without being artificial. Negative situations can be turned from negative to positive. For example, if a sleepy baby does not want to nurse the first day, the nurse can remark that the infant seems very happy and content just being near the mother. When the mother has cramping from breastfeeding, the nurse can remark that this is a positive sign that her milk is letting down. Remarks, such as "Oh, your breasts are so small" or "Your nipples are too flat" are devastating to a new mother, can inhibit her let-down, and can eat away at her confidence in her ability to produce breast milk and to breastfeed.

Even if the nurse does not make a negative comment, his or her attitude may transmit negativism to the new mother. One mother reports that the hospital was no help at all. The staff's attitude was: "It's natural, so get on with it!" An introductory statement in a journal article stated that breastfeeding has long been a bane to nursing supervisors and in-service educators (Jarkowsky, 1980). Even though the article was an honest effort to help the breastfeeding mother, it reflects an attitude prevalent among many nurses—that these mothers are a bother. In such a situation the woman feels that she is inadequate as a mother and a woman. If there is a problem, it must be her fault. In reality, when there is a problem with breastfeeding, it is because management of breastfeeding is faulty or because the infant is not feeding properly. Mothers should be approached in a nonjudgmental manner and should be treated as intelligent adults. They should be given information about breastfeeding based on sound rationale. The nurse, then, does not give directives and advice but merely helps the mother to identify a problematic situation and to determine a solution.

In addition, mothers need support after they go home if they are to be successful (Raphael, 1976; Hall, 1978). Mothers who are enthusiastically committed to breastfeeding fail as often as those who are not. The factor that distinguishes those who succeed is the amount and type of help they receive after they return home. Mothers without help or with help that is insufficient, hostile, or coercive are quick to lose their milk. They often suffer a longlasting sense of failure (Raphael, 1976). Nurses should help mothers plan so that they have positive, nonjudgmental support for breastfeeding once they go home. The nurse can provide support by giving the postpartum or nursery phone number. Mothers who have questions in the middle of the night generally feel comfortable in calling the nurse. If the mother is having difficulty with early breastfeeding, a referral to a community health nurse or to a Certified Lactation Consultant can be initiated. Assessment of the family situation is important. Are the patient's husband and mother supportive? Beske and Garvis (1982) see the support of both as being necessary. If the nurse determines that they are not supportive, he or she should assess why they are not. If they are misinformed, the nurse can correct this by providing them with information about breastfeeding. If they have negative attitudes, the nurse can provide understanding while emphasizing the mother's desire to breastfeed and the importance of their support. The nurse can also encourage the mother to call on friends who have successfully breastfed their infants.

Breastfeeding support groups can also provide help. There are various self-help groups of breastfeeding mothers who offer their time to provide new mothers with support for, and information about, breastfeeding. The La Leche League is one of these organizations. It began in 1956 and now services women internationally. The nurse can provide the mother with the telephone number of the La Leche League representative in her area. The mother can utilize the group to answer questions about breastfeeding or can become a member of the organization (see Appendix F).

Questions regarding matters that may affect the health of the infant, such as medications or symptoms of the mother or her infant, should be referred to the mother's or infant's physician.

Information Needs

Information needs are the teaching and learning needs of the mother and her family that, if met, help the mother to care for herself and her infant and to prevent or resolve breastfeeding problems. These needs include information regarding:

1. General knowledge about the breasts and the benefits of breastfeeding.
2. Care of the mother, including breast care and diet.
3. Knowledge of the infant, including how to determine whether the infant is getting enough milk, understanding infant feeding behavior, recognizing growth spurts and normal stool patterns.
4. References that will provide additional information for the breastfeeding mother.

Each mother should be assessed for learning readiness, educational background, prior knowledge and experience, and culture, so that an individual teaching plan can be developed to present this information.

General Knowledge

The breastfeeding mother needs to have a basic understanding of the breasts and how they function. She also needs information about the advantages and disadvantages of breastfeeding so that she can make an informed decision about how she will feed her infant.

Breastfeeding provides many advantages for a mother and her newborn infant. For the mother, it accelerates involution of the uterus through the effects of oxytocin. For the infant, breastfeeding provides a food composed of over 100 elements different in proportions and chemical composition from equally complex milks of other mammals. It supplies nutrition perfectly suited for the infant, and it is difficult to replicate (Jeliffe and Jeliffe, 1971, 1977; Applebaum, 1975). Antibodies and other resistant factors in human milk also offer protection from infection for the newborn (Gunther, 1963; Grams, 1978; Campbell, 1981;

Pittard, 1981). Infants fed breast milk have lower incidences of infant colic, allergy, eczema, obesity, colitis, dental caries, and orthodontic problems (Applebaum, 1970, 1975; Jelliffe and Jelliffe, 1971, 1977; Sugarman, 1977). Affirming these advantages for the infant in 1978, the American Academy of Pediatrics stated that all full-term newborns should be breastfed (American Academy of Pediatrics, Committee on Nutrition, 1978).

Breastfeeding also provides emotional advantages for the mother and infant. For the mother, breastfeeding can offer pleasure comparable to that experienced in coitus. Breastfeeding, like coitus, was necessary for the survival of the human species; therefore, it had to be sufficiently pleasurable to ensure its frequent occurrence (Newton and Newton, 1967; Riordan and Rapp, 1980). In addition, the mother experiences other sensations in response to circulating hormones. Pleasurable to many women are the uterine contractions, the sensation of the let-down, and the relief of breast tension produced in response to the hormone oxytocin. Circulating prolactin appears to have a psychologic effect that is euphoric and tranquilizing and may be important in diminishing the "baby blues" caused by a reduction in certain circulating hormones after birth (Newton, 1971; Sugarman, 1977).

For the infant, breastfeeding provides obligatory and frequent close body contact with the mother. It provides for a variety of sensory stimuli, such as skin-to-skin contact, the special smells of the mother, and the taste and texture of the mother's nipples. The position for breastfeeding itself provides an opportunity for close and frequent eye-to-eye contact. These factors are felt to be essential to the beginning of the maternal–infant bonding process (Klaus and Kennell, 1982; see Chapter 29). Studies investigating the long-term benefits of breastfeeding on personality reveal that although there seems to be no difference between children bottle fed and children breastfed for a short time, children breastfed for 6 months or more have fewer undesirable behavior characteristics, are less anxious, and are more secure (Childers and Hamil, 1932; Maslow and Szilagyi-Kessler, 1946; Hughes and Bushnell, 1977). To clearly determine the long-range psychologic advantages of breastfeeding, many factors affecting the development of the child must be explored. However, pleasure experienced by the mother and infant in breastfeeding tends to attract the mother and infant together and enhance the potential for maternal–infant attachment during the early years (Bowlby, 1958; Sugarman, 1977).

Women also need to be prepared for what is required of them during breastfeeding, especially during the first few weeks. Many are wooed by pamphlets that discuss the "natural" method of feeding; they expect the infant to attach to their breast immediately, and they expect to feel confident and comfortable immediately. Before the infant is born, the mother should be informed that initiation of breastfeeding takes at least 2 weeks, during which time the mother is feeding her infant at least every 2–3 hours to build up her milk supply. The infant may also have difficulty attaching to the breast, and the mother may feel awkward in holding the infant at the breast. Often the infant is sleepy the first few days and does not nurse well. Some women experience breast and nipple discomfort. Providing a woman with accurate information prenatally not only helps her make a knowledgeable choice but also helps her to form realistic expectations about feeding in the postpartum period.

Breast Care and Diet

Breast care involves proper hygiene and measures to keep the skin in good condition. The breasts should be cleansed once a day during the daily shower or bath. Only water should be used on the breasts because soap tends to dry and irritate the skin (Newton, 1952). The breasts should *not* be washed before or after each feeding as is sometimes recommended. Cleansing with every feeding washes off natural lubricants and antiseptic secretions and can be irritating to the skin of the nipple and areola. The mother should be taught to air dry her breasts and nipples for 10–15 min after each feeding. Breast pads without plastic can be used in between feedings to keep the breasts dry (see Fig. 21–14). Moisture will macerate breast tissue.

After drying, a lubricating cream or ointment can be applied to soothe the nipples and prevent excessive dryness. Lubricants should be pure and free of additives such as alcohol, dyes, and perfumes, which are irritating to the skin and distasteful to the infant. Mothers should be taught to read the labels of breast preparations to detect these substances. If instructions on the label recommend washing off the lubricant before each feeding, it should *not* be used on the nipples. Examples of pure lubricants include pure lanolin (mothers allergic to wool should not use this product), pure cocoa butter, vegetable oil, and olive oil. If the mother desires, these lubricants can be applied prenatally to help condition the skin.

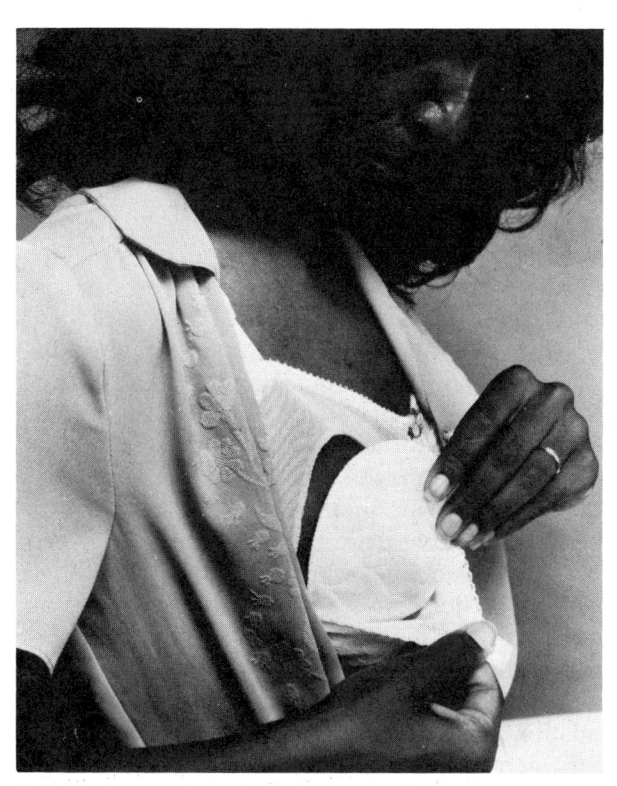

FIGURE 21-14. Comfy Care nursing pad.
SOURCE: Reproduced with the permission of Happy Family Products, Inc.

Traditional methods of preparing the nipples for breastfeeding have included variations of rubbing, rolling, massaging, and scrubbing in order to toughen the nipples. Most studies demonstrate that these methods are not effective (Brown and Hurlock, 1975; Hall, 1978; Whitley, 1978). One study reported that the amount of extreme pain was reduced when the mother implemented a regime of gentle friction with a terry towel, nipple rolling twice a day for 2 minutes, and airing the nipples for 2 hours a day (Atkinson, 1979). However, more research is needed before this can be recommended to women. Friction removes the natural oils provided for the breast and nipples, and can also cause blisters and abrasions (Levit, 1977; Akers, 1985). Cleansing the breasts and nipples with clear water during the daily bath or shower and applying a natural lubricant is sufficient prenatal care.

The mother should also be taught the techniques of putting the baby on and off the breast. Both breasts should be used at each feeding so that both receive adequate stimulation. The mother should start on the breast that she ended the last feeding on. This will even stimulation to both breasts. Mothers often place a safety pin on the bra strap of the breast that the baby last suckled to remind them which one should be used to start the next feeding. When taking the baby off the breast, the mother should be taught to insert her little finger into the infant's mouth to break suction; this minimizes trauma to the nipple from the infant's sucking action.

Mothers with inverted nipples should be taught to use corrective breast cups. Inverted nipples can be detected by using the "pinch test". In this test the nipple is pulled gently between the thumb and forefinger. Then, with the fingers placed on the areola at the nipple base, light compression is applied to make the nipple protrude farther. If the nipple and the areola flatten and move forward, the infant should not have difficulty grasping the breast. This is true even if the nipple is flat. If the nipple retracts or inverts, it indicates that the adhesions within the underlying connective tissue will prevent the infant from being able to compress the breast easily and draw it into the mouth. This condition can be corrected with the use of the Woolrich breast shield or a similar type of breast cup (Cadwell, 1981; Riordan, 1983; see Fig. 21-15). If inverted or retracted nipples are detected prenatally, the mother is taught to wear the cups inside the bra during the last two trimesters, starting with an hour or two each day and gradually increasing the length of wearing time (Riordan, 1983). While the woman is wearing this breast cup, the nipple is

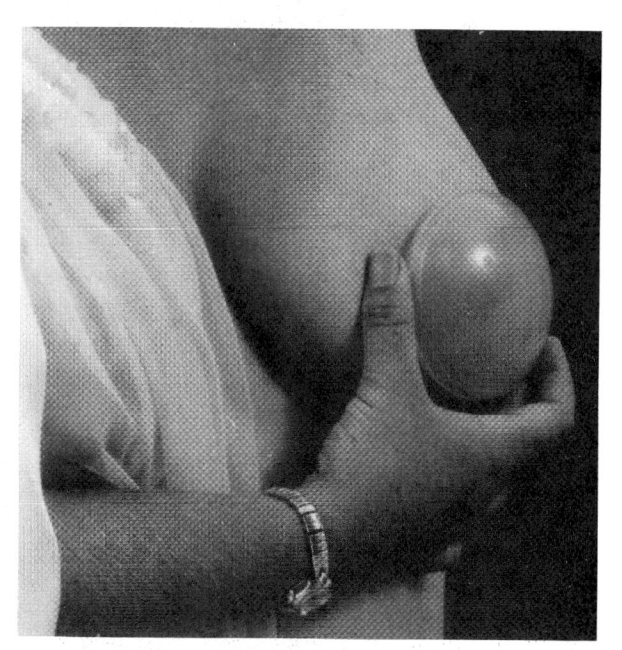

FIGURE 21-15. Comfy Care breast shields.
SOURCE: Reproduced with the permission of Happy Family Products, Inc.

gently pushed through the central opening of the concave portion, and thus the adhesions are slowly released and the nipple is everted. If inverted or retracted nipples are not assessed until the postpartum period, the use of these breast cups can be initiated then. The infant may initially have some difficulty attaching; however, this should not prevent the infant from nursing. Eventually, the sucking action of the infant will break the nipple adhesions.

The diet of a woman who is breastfeeding should be assessed, and a plan for dietary teaching should be established. Breastfeeding women need 300 additional calories over the requirements for pregnant women and 4–6 pints of liquids per day (see Chapter 12). They should be encouraged not to begin a weight-loss program. The fat deposited during pregnancy will be utilized in the lactation process, as breastfeeding results in a gradual loss of the weight gained during pregnancy.

Knowledge of the Infant

ADEQUATE MILK SUPPLY The question most frequently asked by breastfeeding mothers is: "How will I know if my baby is getting enough?" The nurse can assure the mother verbally that she will produce enough milk to feed her infant. Often the mother interprets the frequency of feedings as "I don't have enough milk." The mother needs to know that frequent feedings are normal because of the easy digestibility of breast milk. Also, the mother needs to know that if her infant is wetting diapers 6–8 times a day, going 2 hours between feedings, and seems content after a feeding, the baby is getting enough nourishment. Sometimes babies are fussy not because they are hungry but because they need additional sucking. The mother can provide this by allowing the infant to nurse longer or by occasionally using a pacifier.

GROWTH SPURTS The infant will experience periods in which he needs more nutrition to meet the demands of growth. These are called *growth spurts*. They are characterized by changes in the baby's feeding behavior. Behavior changes include fussiness and wanting to nurse more frequently. They can occur at 2 weeks, 6 weeks, 2–3 months, and 4–6 months. At each of these growth spurts, frequent nursing for 24–48 hours will increase milk supply to meet the new requirements.

INFANT FEEDING BEHAVIOR Feeding during the first few days is infrequent and feeding behavior is sometimes erratic. The mother needs to know that the baby will sleep much of the first day and may not be too interested in nursing. As the days progress, the infant will assume a pattern of frequent, active feedings. This will not be a rigidly predictable pattern but an individual one in which a 24-hour period will include periods of fussiness and frequent nursing and periods of less frequent feedings. The nurse should help the mother discover her infant's individual pattern. A simple tool (see Fig. 21–16) on which the mother records infant feedings for 24 hours can be useful. When the mother has finished filling in the information, the nurse and the mother can look at the feedings and identify a pattern. Women enjoy this exercise and are often surprised to learn that their baby really does have a schedule. The nurse can also teach the mother how to identify and predict infant sleep–wake states as well as behavior cues that signify hunger and those that signify satiation. It is more beneficial for the mother to learn about her baby than to learn to watch the clock.

NORMAL STOOL PATTERNS Mothers are often concerned about their breastfed infant's stools, since they are different from the stools of bottle-fed infants. Mothers need to know that breast milk is almost completely digested; therefore, if there is residue, it is excess fluid. Bowel movements, then, can be frequent, occurring with every feeding, or they can be infrequent, occurring every few days. Frequent stools are liquid in consistency and bright yellow in color. Infrequent stools are similar but may have a soft, more solid consistency. They should not be hard or difficult to pass. Mothers are often concerned that their breastfed infants have diarrhea or constipation. This knowledge of normal stools of breastfed babies will prepare and reassure them.

Other Resources

Mothers can receive additional information from excellent reading sources. There are many books and pamphlets on breastfeeding. Some are good; some are inaccurate and misleading. The nurse should carefully read any book or pamphlet before giving or suggesting it to a mother. Excellent reading resources include Pryor (1973), Higgins (1986), and the La Leche League (1987).

Date	Feeding Time			Comments and Questions
	Began	Ended	Time/breast	Feeding behavior—signs of hunger, signs baby has finished feeding, behavior during feeding

MOTHER'S INFANT FEEDING RECORD

FIGURE 21–16. A tool for recording infant feeding patterns.

BREASTFEEDING PROBLEMS

Despite nursing support and information, problems with breastfeeding can occur. These include engorgement, sore nipples, difficult attachment, colicky baby, mastitis, and slow weight gain for the infant.

Engorgement

Engorgement is a condition in which the breasts become very full and firm. This condition is due to the combination of filling of the breasts with milk and breast tissue edema. It can occur when the milk first comes in at about 48–72 hours postpartum or anytime a mother lengthens the time between feedings once milk supply has been established. The later commonly occurs, for example, on the morning after the baby sleeps all night for the first time.

Encouraging the mother to feed on a demand schedule often prevents or minimizes this condition in the early postpartum period. If it does occur, it is extremely important to ensure that the infant attaches to the breast and nurses well. Build-up of pressure inside the breast will inhibit lactation and decrease milk supply. Hot, moist towels or a paper diaper soaked with warm water can be applied to the breast before each feeding. A hot shower also helps. This stimulates letdown and dilates the lactiferous ducts to help milk flow. If the areola is firm, the mother may have to express milk until this area is soft enough for the infant to grasp. The mother should be encouraged to nurse the infant as often as he/she is hungry. If the infant is unable to nurse, the mother should pump her breast every 3 hours. After 24–48 hours, the engorgement lessens. By the end of 1 week, the mother will feel full before a feeding and soft after a feeding. She needs to know that the decrease in size of her breast is a decrease in tissue edema *not* a decrease in milk supply.

Engorgement can also occur when the plan is to wean or skip feedings. This can be avoided if the mother begins eliminating one feeding at a time over a period of several weeks.

Sore Nipples

As noted, sore nipples can be avoided much of the time by proper placement of the infant on the breast. Thus, if a woman is complaining of sore nipples, the nurse should observe a feeding and determine whether the infant is positioned properly. If placement is found not to be the cause of soreness, other causes should be explored.

Occasionally, sore nipples are caused by an infant who does not have his tongue under the breast. The infant sucks the roof of his mouth, creating constant suction against the mother's breast without relief of pressure provided by swallowing. The nurse can observe this by opening the baby's mouth slightly. The tongue will be seen on the breast rather than under it. To correct this gently remove the baby from the breast; when the baby opens his mouth wide, help the mother to get the baby on the breast quickly, before the tongue reaches the roof of the mouth. Gently pressing down on the baby's chin will keep the tongue down until the infant attaches to the breast. Because the infant probably sucked his tongue *in utero*, it may take several feedings to reverse this habit.

Some babies draw in their lower lip with the breast when sucking, causing an abrasion to the nipple. To correct this, gently remove the baby from the breast and reattach when the baby's mouth is wide open. When the baby is fixed to the breast, pull out the lower lip (Frantz, 1982).

Other possible causes of sore nipples include reaction from a nipple cream, too much washing of the nipples, infrequent nursing, and breast pads that adhere to the nipples or that contain plastic. Prolonged soreness or soreness of sudden onset may be caused by *Candida albicans*. Typically, women with a monilia infection have severe burning, stinging nipple pain which radiates throughout the breast, and persists long after feedings. This symptom is usually accompanied by a history of prenatal or postpartum monilial vaginitis, a recent history of antibiotic therapy, or evidence of thrush in the infant (Neville and Neifert, 1983). If monilial infection is suspected, a physician should be contacted so that both the mother and infant can be treated concurrently.

Once the cause of the soreness is eliminated, then the sore nipples can be treated. Breast cups such as the Woolrich cups worn inside the bra protect the nipples from the chafing of clothes. Wearing tea strainers inside the bra has also served this purpose. Dry heat to breast tissue increases circulation and helps heal sore nipples. This can be accomplished by exposing the breasts to the sun from an open window for 10–15 min after daytime feedings. During cloudy days the use of an ultraviolet lamp is recommended as a substitute (Riordan, 1983). In using this light the mother needs to be careful to protect herself and others from the burns. The mother should sit 4 feet away from the light and should expose the nipples gradually, starting with 30 seconds the first day, then 1 minute twice a day on the second and third days. If ultraviolet lamp treatment is needed for more than 3 days, it should never be used for more than 3 minutes per treatment. Using a blow dryer on a low setting for 1–2 minutes after each feeding is also soothing to sore nipples.

When breastfeeding with sore nipples, the mother should start the infant on the least sore side. This prevents the infant from applying the strong suction used to induce let-down to the sore breast. Also, varying the position of the baby on the breast from the elbow to the football hold from feeding to feeding, will vary the pressure exerted by the hard palate on certain areas of the breast.

Rubber or plastic nipple shields that cover the breast during a feeding should never be used to help sore nipples. If shields are used, the cause of the sore nipples may be ignored. When the shields are removed, the mother will again develop sore nipples. Also, infants become accustomed to them and may refuse the unshielded breast. The most important reasons for not using them are that when they are used, the breasts do not receive adequate tactile stimulation and the infant cannot extract milk adequately. A study measuring infant intake with two types of breast shields revealed that the shields reduced milk intake by 22–58 percent (Woolridge, Baum, and Drewitt, 1980). Thus, with inadequate milk intake and a decreasing milk supply, an infant may not thrive.

Difficult Attachment

Occasionally, babies have difficulty attaching to the breast. This usually resolves itself as the baby becomes accustomed to the particular configuration of the mother's breast and learns the sucking motion needed for breastfeeding. Sometimes, an infant refuses one breast in preference to the other. Engorgement makes the areola difficult to flatten; therefore, before putting the baby to the breast, the mother should express enough milk to soften the areola. Inverted or retracted nipples sometimes make attachment difficult. This can be corrected with breast cups, as noted previously.

In all these situations patience is the key. When the nurse brings the infant to the mother, the mother should be informed that it may take some time, but the baby will eventually attach. The nurse can set a relaxed atmosphere by sitting rather than standing at the bedside. The baby should be placed in the proper position for attachment. If the baby becomes frustrated, he can be cuddled for a time and then put back to the breast. Sometimes the football hold places the infant in a position that makes attachment easier.

If the infant is unable to attach in the first 3 days postpartum, the mother should pump her breast milk and feed it to her baby by bottle syringe, or eye dropper. A referral should be made to a lactation consultant who specializes in attachment problems. The baby should also be evaluated by the baby's physician for transient neurological problems that can often be treated with physical therapy.

Rubber nipple shields should *not* be used because of the dangers previously discussed.

Slow Weight Gain

When an infant is slow to gain weight with breastfeeding, formula supplements or discontinuation of breastfeeding are frequently recommended. Both infant and the mother should be examined to determine what problems may be affecting breastfeeding. Maternal or infant illness, poor infant sucking, poor breastfeeding technique, or the use of supplements or breast shields can prevent the mother from building a good milk supply and adequately nourishing her infant. There is almost always a solution for these problems that allows the mother to continue breastfeeding (Frantz, 1983). The infant should be seen by the infant's physician and a lactation consultant for a full evaluation.

Colicky Baby

Although colic is less frequent in breastfed infants, it does occur. The exact cause is unknown; therefore, treatment is not specific, and it varies. Jakobsson and Lindberg (1978, 1983) have studied the relationship of colic in breastfed infants to ingestion of cow's milk by the mother, and they recommend a diet free of cow's milk as the first method of treatment for colic in breastfed infants. The mother should eliminate dairy products for 1 week. If she sees no improvement in the baby, she can resume eating these foods. If there is an improvement in the symptoms, she can start taking calcium supplements. Some women can eat some dairy products such as cheese and yogurt. Other foods when ingested by the mother can also cause colic. However, because sensitivity to foods by the baby is very individual, the mother should not be given an arbitrary list of foods "not to eat." The specific food causing the problem can only be assessed through a dietary history.

Other techniques attempt to relieve the symptoms of colic. Small, frequent feedings may be easier on a digestive system that is immature. Warmth applied to the abdomen may help relieve the pain of abdominal cramping. The baby may receive warmth by lying prone on the mother or father's abdomen or by immersion in a warm bath. Parents of colicky infants need to be reassured that they are not "bad" parents, and they should be given reinforcement for their parenting. Comforting to some parents is the fact that colic will disappear in about 3 months.

All crying and fussiness is not colic. Some babies have a time of the day in which they are more awake and fussy. These times are frustrating for new parents. However, like colic, as the child gets older, these outbursts will disappear.

Mastitis

Mastitis is an infection involving inflammation of either the connective tissue of the breast or the mammary ducts. It is characterized by symptoms which include fever of 38.5°C or more, extreme fatigue, and a hot, red, swollen area on the breast. Some mothers feel as though they have the flu. Mastitis is thought to be caused by factors that restrict milk flow, allow bacteria to be introduced into the breast, or decrease maternal resistance. Restriction of milk flow can be caused by engorgement, by a decrease in the number of feedings, or by a restrictive bra. A cracked and fissured nipple can be an avenue for bacterial entry. Poor maternal nutrition, fatigue, and stress lower a mother's resistance to infection. Thus, the best management of mastitis involves prevention by proper breastfeeding counseling. Mastitis can be treated as any other infection—with rest, fluids, heat to the site, and antibiotics. It is especially important that the mother nurse frequently and adequately on the affected breast to allow milk to flow, preventing further stasis and infection. Continuing to breastfeed has not been found to be harmful to the mother or the infant. In fact, mothers who continue to breastfeed have a better outcome and a shorter duration of symptoms (Neville and Neifert, 1983; Thomsen, Espersen, and Maigaard, 1984; Lawrence, 1985).

Plugged ducts are hard, warm, swollen areas on the breast without the flu-like symptoms. They can be treated with warm, moist heat to the area, gentle massage of the area toward the nipple, and nursing or pumping until the area becomes soft. If the lump-like area remains above 24°C, or if other symptoms develop, a physician should be notified.

ADAPTING BREASTFEEDING TO SPECIAL SITUATIONS

Breastfeeding is most easily established and maintained when the mother and the infant are together and in good health. However, in certain instances, the mother and the infant must be separated or breastfeeding must be adapted to a special condition of the mother or the infant.

Mother–Infant Separation

Milk Expression and Storage

If a mother is to breastfeed her infant successfully during periods of separation, she must learn the art of milk expression and storage. Breast milk can be expressed manually, with a hand pump, or with an electric breast pump.

For many mothers, hand expression is the most convenient and efficient method of expression. To hand express, the mother should be instructed to cup her hand around the breast with the fingers around the areola. With the thumb on top and the fingers underneath, the fingers should be squeezed together rhythmically, at the same time pushing toward the chest wall (see Fig. 21–17). The fingers should not slide along the skin, because this can cause irritation and soreness. The hands should then be rotated around the areola to express milk from all the lactiferous sinuses. Milk can be expressed into a wide-mouthed container or directly into a bottle using a hand expression funnel (see Fig. 21–18).

Some mothers feel uncomfortable or embarrassed about using hand expression, whereas others find it tiring. Thus, a hand or electric pump may be more suitable (Fig. 21–19). Hand pumps

1. Position the thumb and first two fingers about 1 to 1½ in. behind the nipple.

2. Push straight into the chest wall. Avoid spreading the fingers apart. For large breasts, first lift and then push into the chest wall.

3. Roll thumb and fingers forward as if making thumb and fingerprints at the same time. The rolling motion of the thumb and fingers compresses and empties the milk reservoirs without hurting sensitive breast tissue. Note the changing position of the thumbnail and fingernails in illustration.

4. Repeat rhythmically to drain the reservoirs. Position, push, roll; position, push, roll.

5. Rotate the thumb and finger position to milk the other reservoirs. Use both hands on each breast. These pictures show hand positions on the right breast.

FIGURE 21–17. Marmet technique for manual expression of breast milk.
SOURCE: Reproduced with the permission of the Lactation Institute.

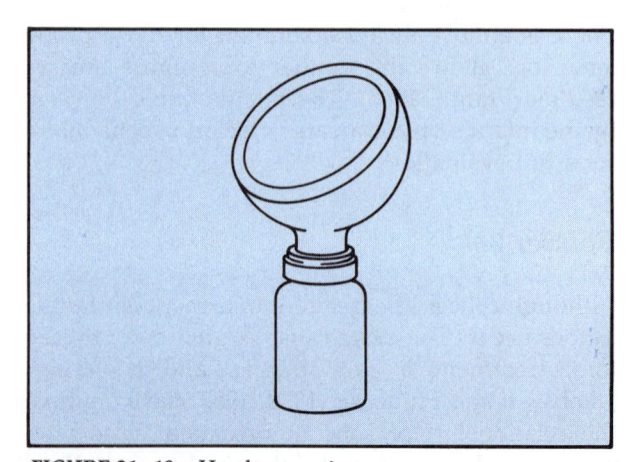

FIGURE 21–18. Hand expression funnel.

Breastfeeding: Physiology and Management 455

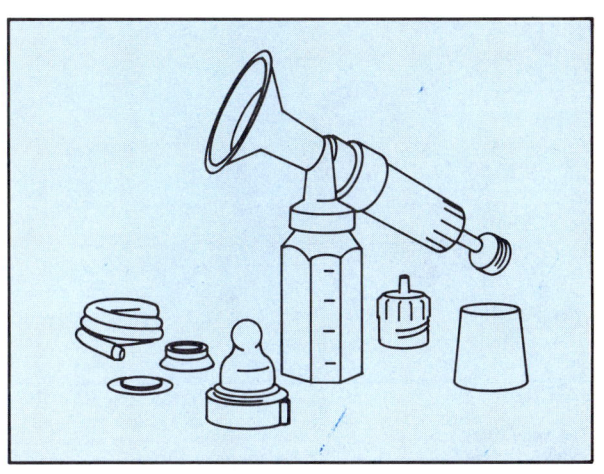

FIGURE 21–19A. Medela breast pump attachment.

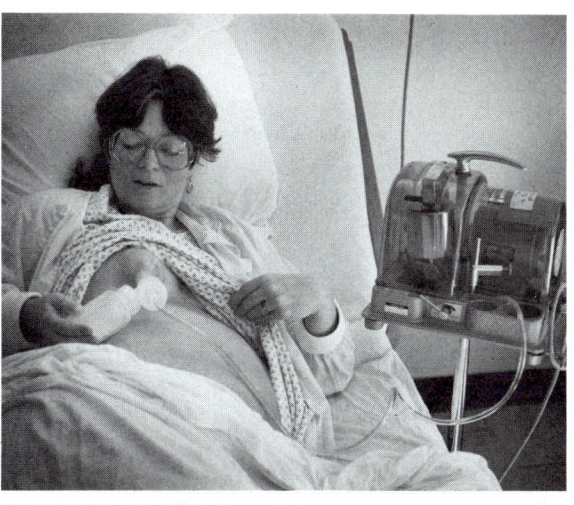

FIGURE 21–19B. Mother using Egnell electric pump.

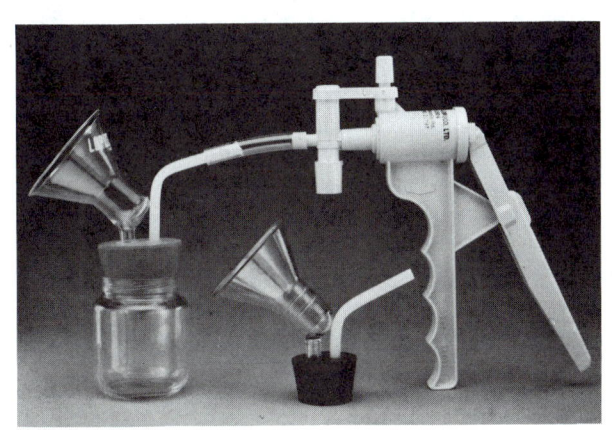

FIGURE 21–20. Loyd-B hand-operated breast pump.
SOURCE: Courtesy of Lopuco, Ltd

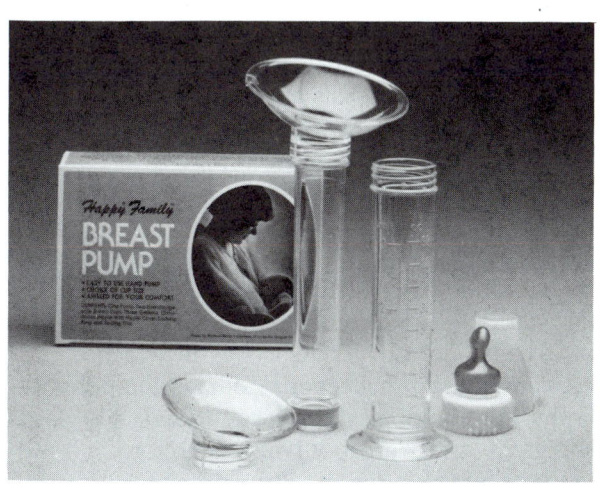

FIGURE 21–21. Happy Family breast pump.
SOURCE: Reproduced with the permission of Happy Family Products, Inc.

include the cycling, pump and hold, and diaphragm types. The Medela cycling pump exerts pressure for 1 second and then releases. Pump and hold types include the cylinder-type pumps, such as the Loyd-B (Fig. 21–20) and the Happy Family (Fig. 21–21). Diaphragm pumps are either electrically- or battery-operated, such as the Gentle Expression, a battery pump, and the Gerber electric pump. It is difficult to recommend the best hand pump, because some pumps work better for some women than others. However, all the above are good hand pumps and do work. Pumping is a skill each woman learns (Fig. 21–22). It takes time and patience in the beginning. For working women, however, the electrically- or battery-operated pumps are often preferred. Regarding the former, women need to know that they last only 6–9 months. Also, for battery pumps, the batteries need to be changed frequently, unless they are rechargeable.

Hand pumps (bicycle-horn type) that include a suction bulb should not be used. Bacterial growth that can occur in the bulb makes these pumps unsafe for expressing milk that is to be stored (Tibbetts and Cadwell, 1981). In addition, the suction cannot be controlled and, therefore, breast tissue can be traumatized. Electric pumps such as the Egnel (Fig. 21–23) are easy for mothers to use, especially if they must pump for long periods of time. They can be rented for home use through local hospital supply companies or through a La Leche League representative. Both have attachments that convert to hand pumps for continued use when the electric pump is no longer needed. The Medela also has a double attachment for

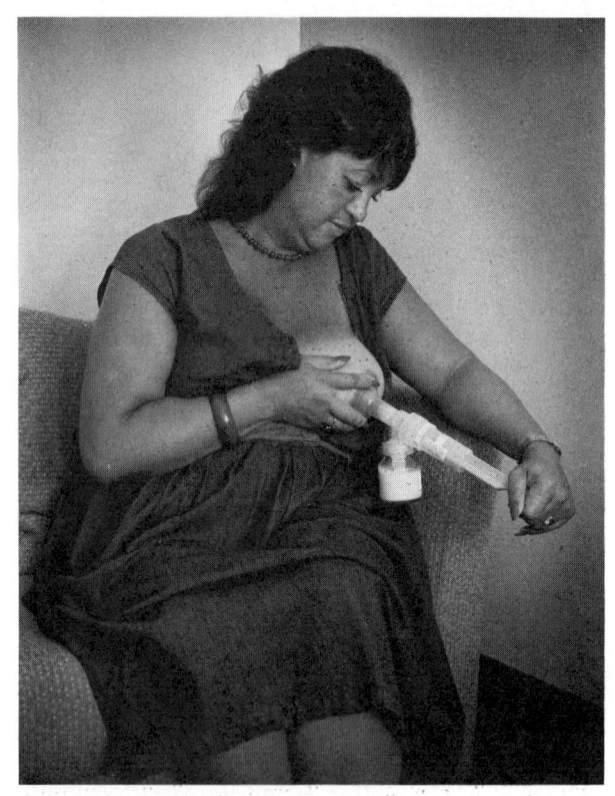

FIGURE 21-22. Mother using piston-type (Medela) hand pump.

pumping both breasts at the same time. This reduces pumping time and increases milk supply.

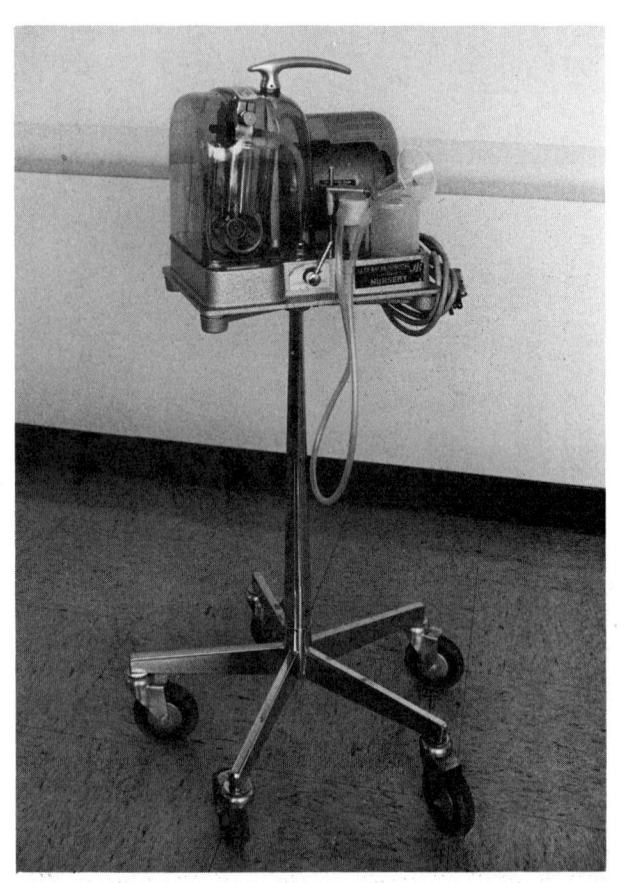

FIGURE 21-23. Egnel electric breast pump.
SOURCE: Reproduced with the permission of Egnel, Inc.

Milk Expression Procedure

The mother should be taught to wash her hands thoroughly before beginning collection. Refrigeration and freezing retard bacterial growth, but they do not destroy bacteria. All pump parts should be thoroughly washed with hot soap and water before each pumping. If the milk is being collected for a premature infant, the parts of the pump should be sterilized twice a day in boiling water or in a dishwasher (Meier and Riordan, 1983). To pump, the mother should:

1. Find a comfortable, relaxing place to sit.
2. Stimulate let down by:
   - massaging the breasts, starting at the chest wall and working toward the nipple;
   - stimulating the nipple by gently stroking or rolling;
   - thinking about her baby, looking at a picture of the baby, or reading a baby magazine;
   - using stress relaxation techniques;
   - listening to relaxing music.
3. Express milk from one breast until the milk flow slows (5–7 min), and then switch to the opposite breast.
4. Massage the breasts again.
5. Express milk from both breasts again until the milk flow slows (2–5 min).
6. Massage the breasts again.
7. Express milk from both breasts again until the milk flow slows (2–3 min).

Milk Storage

Milk can then be collected in sterile glass containers, sterile plastic containers, or sterile plastic bottle bags. Controversy exists as to which is the best container for collection. Cellular components of the immunologic response adhere to glass (Shepherd and Yarrow, 1982); therefore, plastic may be preferable for the ill or premature infant. However, Shepherd and Yarrow (1982) suggest that the slightly acidic human milk may draw out plasticizers from the plastic. Breaks can occur in plastic bags. To minimize problems with plastic bags, use only nurser bags (designed to hold milk) and use double bags to prevent breakages. In addition, the bags must be tied securely to prevent any spillage, and the section above the tie needs to be folded down to prevent the collection of bacteria. At this time there is not enough data to disqualify any of these collection containers. Therefore, the mother and family's individual situation should be the primary consideration when a container is selected for milk collection.

After the milk is collected, it should be cooled immediately by placing it in a refrigerator or on ice in a cooler. Whenever possible, breast milk should be given fresh so that the infant receives all its benefits. However, if it is not to be given to the baby within 48 hours, it should be frozen. Breast milk can be frozen in the freezer compartment for 2 weeks and for 6 months in a freezer maintained at 0°F. The milk should be frozen in amounts equal to or slightly more than one feeding. It is also helpful to store some in smaller amounts for smaller feedings for when the infant wants more, because once defrosted it cannot be refrozen. If small amounts of fresh milk are added to milk already frozen to complete a feeding bottle, the fresh milk should be cooled first.

Breast milk should be defrosted by placing the jar or bag under cool water and increasing the temperature until the milk is at room temperature. Boiling or defrosting the milk with hot water will alter its nutritional and anti-infective properties. Milk should not be microwaved until the safety of this process has been determined. All frozen milk should be labeled, marked with tape indicating the date and time collected. If the milk is stored at the hospital for a sick or premature infant, the infant's name should also be included on the tape.

The Working Mother

Today many women are choosing to work after they have a baby. Many must return to work because of economic necessity. If a woman wants to breastfeed, going back to work presents a dilemma. How will she manage breastfeeding and working? For most of human history this situation was not a problem. Women worked and breastfed their infants. The difficulty today is not that women work, but that to work, a woman must be separated from her infant. Thus, the nurse's goal in supporting the woman who plans to return to work is to help her maintain breastfeeding during periods of mother–infant separation

Initially, the nurse should inform the mother that, if she desires, she *can* breastfeed and work.

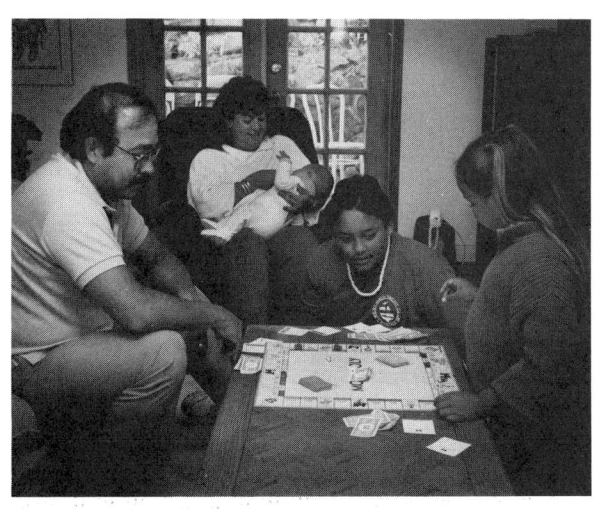

FIGURE 21–24. Mother going home to breast feed during work day.

Also, she needs to know that she has various ways she can accomplish this. Some mothers can continue exclusive breastfeeding because they can take their infants to work with them. Others can breastfeed during the day because they can go home for feedings or the childcare provider can bring the baby to work (Fig. 21–24). But in many instances the mother cannot feed during the day. She can instead have the childcare provider feed supplements of formula or breast milk. To supplement with breast milk, the mother will need to pump her breasts during the day and save her milk. Some recommend pumping on a regular schedule during the workday; others recommend that the breasts be pumped whenever they become full or uncomfortable.

To help the mother maintain breastfeeding while working, the nurse should emphasize several important points (Mack, 1983):

1. The mother must establish a good milk supply. It is especially important for the nurse to meet the mother's supportive and educational needs so that she can facilitate breastfeeding in those early days. The mother should be encouraged to spend time with the baby once she goes home from the hospital, to continue building a milk supply.
2. The mother should plan how and where she will pump at work if she is going to supplement with breast milk. At least 2 weeks before going back to work, the mother should begin eliminating one feeding at a time until her body has become adjusted to not feeding during the time she will be at work. She should select a

childcare provider who will be supportive not only of her beliefs about childcare but also about breastfeeding.
3. Once back to work, she should breastfeed as much as possible while with the infant.
4. The mother should rest as much as possible. Stress, fatigue, and spacing of feedings are all factors that predispose a working mother to mastitis.
5. The mother should be able to adapt breastfeeding and working to whatever works for her and the baby. In most instances the mother finds that even breastfeeding a few times a day is rewarding. One mother states: "For those moments at least, it's reassuring to know that there is one thing that no babysitter, no matter how wonderful, can give your baby."

The nurse as a client advocate should support and encourage work policies that support breastfeeding. Many electric breast pump companies will supply electric pumps free if their manual–electric pumps are purchased. Break times for pumping should be permitted. Employers should be encouraged to offer extended leave policies to new mothers and fathers.

The Premature or Ill Infant

The benefits of human milk for the premature infant, especially the mother's preterm milk, are now well known. The immunologic properties of the milk protect the vulnerable premature infant from infection. Fresh breast milk, particularly, contains leukocytes that are thought to protect the premature infant from necrotizing enterocolitis. Preterm breast milk has a higher protein and lipid content; lower lactose concentrations; higher sodium, chloride, magnesium, and iron concentrations; and a lower lactose concentration—all helpful for the rapid growth and special developmental needs of the premature infant (Gross et al., 1980; Schanler and Oh, 1980). In addition, both preterm and full-term human milk have long-chain fatty acids thought to be essential for neurologic development (Oakland Perinatal Health Project, 1983).

Nursing care for the mother of a premature infant who has decided to breastfeed involves supporting the decision, helping her initiate a milk supply, initiating breastfeeding with the infant, and supporting her when she goes home.

If a mother has decided to breastfeed and she delivers a premature infant, she should be supported in continuing in that decision. The mother who decided to bottle feed should have information about the benefits of breast milk for premature babies. Then she should be supported in whatever decision she makes.

For the mother who plans to breastfeed her premature infant, the nurse needs to ensure that all the normal supportive and educational needs are met. Pumping of the breasts will substitute for the infant's stimulation of the breast. Pumping should occur as early as possible and as frequently as possible, preferably every 3–4 hours. This scheduling should be adapted to the mother's individual situation. The stress of having a premature infant utilizes much energy. Thus, the benefits of the rest provided by sleeping through one night, for example, may outweigh the benefits of pumping during that night.

When the infant is ready to begin breastfeeding, the nurse should provide much help and support. Boggs and Rau (1983) recommend that breastfeeding be initiated before a bottle is introduced. If a nipple is introduced first, the baby will become accustomed to the nipple. Nipple–bottle confusion is an even greater problem. The premature nipple is so soft that the infant does not have to open its mouth wide. Thus when the baby is put to breast, its mouth is not opened in response to stimulation and, therefore, the infant does not attach to the breast. If the infant must have feedings from a bottle, the Nuk® brand nipple is recommended (Meier and Riordan, 1983; see Fig. 21–25). Attempts to initiate breastfeeding early have been reported to have no untoward effect on

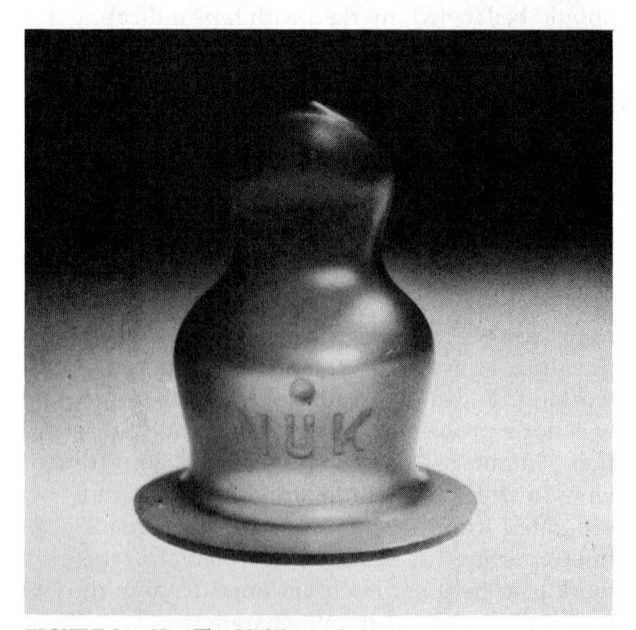

FIGURE 21–25. The Nuk® nipple.
SOURCE: Courtesy of Gerber Products Co.

the infant (Boggs and Rau, 1983; Meier and Riordan, 1983). Criteria for determining when a premature infant is ready to breastfeed include the infant's ability to suck and swallow (Boggs and Rau, 1983; Meier and Riordan, 1983). In addition, it is recommended that the premature infant weigh 1500 g, experience short wakeful periods, tolerate gavage feedings, and no longer require oxygen therapy (Boggs and Rau, 1983).

Initial breastfeeding should take place at a time during the day when the infant is awake and alert. The position of the infant at the breast should be varied for a premature infant. The football hold (Boggs and Rau, 1983) or holding the infant's head with the hand opposite the breast (Meier and Riordan, 1983) gives more support to the infant's head and neck, allowing the infant to use most of the available energy for sucking. During early sessions, the infant may merely nuzzle the breast or suck once or twice and fall asleep. Switching from breast to breast with frequent burping may help keep the infant awake. Feedings should not be long at first, and the infant should be observed for temperature, heart and respiratory rate, and color. Until the infant is nursing steadily on the breast for 10–15 minutes per feeding, supplementary gavage feedings should follow each feeding and should also be given when the mother cannot be present (Boggs and Rau, 1983). Gavage feedings following breastfeeding should be done at least 20–30 minutes after the infant nurses.

Before the infant is discharged, it is important for the mother to spend several days at the hospital if possible. There should be at least one 24-hour period when the mother can assume responsibility not only for feedings but for other care as well. After discharge the mother should be encouraged to feed the infant frequently to build up her milk supply and to help the infant continue to gain weight. When being fed on demand, a premature infant should not go longer than 4 hours between feedings. Continued support by the nurse and the physician by phone or home visit is necessary to answer questions and to relieve parental anxiety.

Breastfeeding Twins

A mother of twins can breastfeed both her infants. The mother needs to be assured that she will produce enough milk to nourish two infants. A sibling of nursing twins understood the logic of this phenomenon when she saw her aunt breastfeeding a single child. She exclaimed: "Aunt Linda, why do you have two nipples when you have only one baby?" (Speight, 1980).

With twins it is particularly important to help the mother build a good milk supply. This may take longer than for the mother with one child. Often mothers of twins do not realize this and interpret it as the inability to produce enough milk. Also, since the mother is producing twice as much milk, diet is especially important. The Recommended Dietary Allowance for a mother breastfeeding twins is an extra 1000 kcal/day. It takes 1500 kcal/day to produce enough breast milk for twins; therefore, when the mother regains her normal weight or desired weight she should add another 500 calories to her diet (Leonard, 1982).

The logistics of feeding the infants is also an important issue. Usually, in the beginning, it is advisable to feed them separately, each on a demand schedule. This offers several advantages: the mother's breasts are stimulated frequently; the infants are wide awake for feedings, which facilitates their learning the skill of attaching to the breast and feeding; and the mother gets to know and bond with each twin. After the milk supply is established, it becomes important to allow the mother time and rest. The mother also needs more time to play with the babies rather than spending all her time feeding. The mother can slowly get the babies on the same schedule and feed them together. Simultaneous feedings are most easily accomplished with both babies in the football hold with pillows supporting the infants. With the infants in this position the mother has both hands free to burp or care for an infant when it is necessary. Because there is more care in general for a mother with twins, support from family and friends to help with cooking and housework is essential

Infant with a Cleft Lip or Palate

The mother of a baby with a cleft lip or palate can breastfeed her baby. In fact breast milk provides some important advantages for a baby with this condition. Nutritional and anti-infective properties help prevent middle-ear and upper-respiratory infections common to these children (Styer and Freeh, 1981). Breast milk is less irritating to body tissues; therefore, the choking–coughing reaction often experienced by a child with a cleft lip or palate while eating does not occur (Grady, 1980). The action of breastfeeding creates less pressure in the middle ear and helps promote facial development.

The infant is usually able to attach onto the breast when it is the fullest. The mother needs to shape and hold the breast, because the infant cannot create suction in the oral cavity. The baby will then "milk" the breast with the gums and the tongue (Grady, 1980). Sometimes the infant does learn to create suction by placing the tongue over the cleft (Styer and Freeh, 1981). Support from the nurse is needed. Referral to another mother who has breastfed a child with this condition is also very helpful.

Cesarean Birth

Mothers who have had a cesarean birth have the same supportive and educational needs as mothers who deliver vaginally. However, support and education will have to be adapted to the individual needs of a woman who has had surgery. Basically, adjusting the pace at which a woman assumes breastfeeding skills is important. Because the mother has had surgery, her physical needs are greater and the "taking-in" period may be extended. Also, the nurse needs to assess the length of labor if the woman labored before the surgery, the type of anesthesia used, the mother's general health, and the mother's normal response to stress. If a mother did not labor, is in good health, had an epidural anesthetic, and responds well to stress, she may be ready to breastfeed in the recovery room soon after delivery. Some mothers may want to see and hold their infants but may be too tired to nurse. For other mothers the desire to nurse is stronger than the need for rest. The nurse should also help the woman who has had a cesarean birth find a comfortable nursing position. The side-lying position is most frequently used. Sitting up with a pillow supporting the infant is also a comfortable position.

Induced Lactation and Relactation

Knowledgeable of the benefits of breastfeeding, some women are attempting to breastfeed their adopted infants. Also, some women are breastfeeding after they have stopped breastfeeding because of maternal or infant illness. Other women try breastfeeding after they have received a lactation suppressant or have bottle fed for a time and then decide that they want to breastfeed. When the mother has never given birth, the process is called *induced lactation;* when the mother has given birth, it is called *relactation.* In either case the success of breastfeeding is variable.

Drugs have been used to stimulate lactation in these situations. Phenothiazines increase prolactin levels by reducing the prolactin inhibiting factor. Some drugs, such as theophylline, directly influence prolactin secretion. Oxytocin nasal spray can be used temporarily to help the let-down reflex (Lawrence, 1985). However, breast stimulation is the most important factor in influencing milk production. With induced lactation, when possible the mother should begin breast stimulation at least 2 months before the arrival of the infant. A mother who is relactating can put the infant directly to breast. In both situations the mother will need to supplement with formula. Supplements can be given by dropper or cup, depending on the age of the infant. In addition, the Lact-Aid® Nursing Trainer System (Fig. 21–26) and the Medela SNS (Supplemental Nutritional System) have been found to be very effective for supplementing without using a bottle. Both systems incorporate a plastic bag attached to the body/nursing tube (or tubes). They are hung from the mother's neck. The nursing tube(s) are placed along the mother's

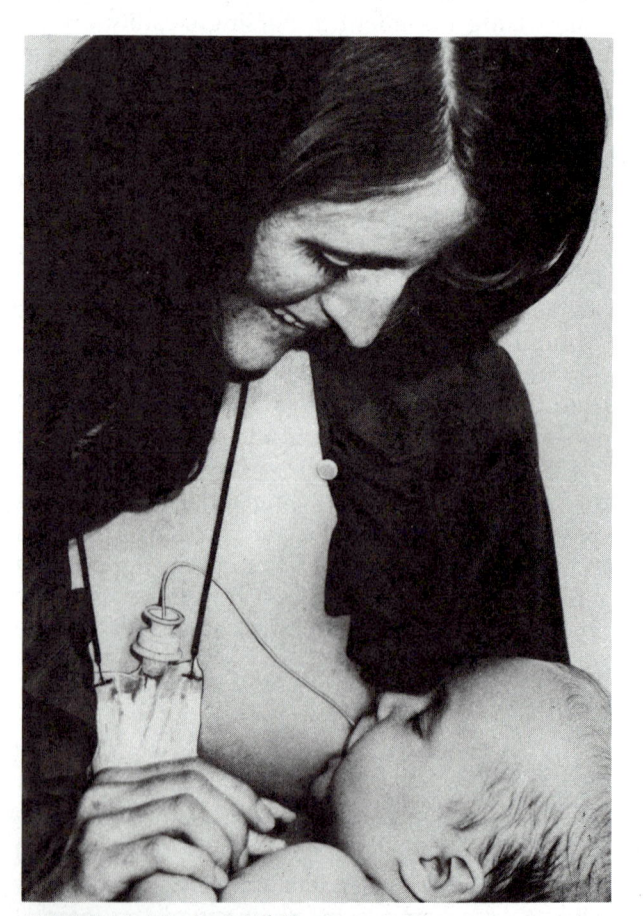

FIGURE 21–26. Lact-Aid Nurser.
SOURCE: Couresty of Lact-Aid® International, Inc.

nipple. The infant can provide breast stimulation and receive supplements of milk at the same time. Mothers can start by filling the container with the amount of milk required for an infant of comparable age. As lactation increases, the infant will gradually self-decrease the amount of supplement taken.

Mothers who attempt to induce lactation or to relactate need to be highly motivated and persistent in their efforts. They need to understand that their success cannot be measured in the amount of milk they are producing. In induced lactation/relactation, most babies are supplemented, with the supplements supplying about 50 percent of their needs (Zimmerman, 1981; Avery, 1983). With relactation, one study reports that out of seven mothers who had not breastfed for at least 2 weeks, three mothers were able to breastfeed completely, two breastfed partially, and two never produced significant amounts of milk (Bose et al., 1981). Thus, women who desire to breastfeed in these situations need to measure their success in relation to the degree of enjoyment experienced by mother and infant. Most women felt they were successful in the relationship that developed with their infant. One mother commented: "I never did get to go without some supplements, but what did I care: That was such a small nuisance compared to such great joy" (Raphael, 1983, p. 44).

Drugs and Breastfeeding

Current studies suggest that most drugs can be administered to nursing mothers without producing adverse effects on nursing infants (Rivera-Calim, 1987). Many drugs have been mentioned as being contraindicated during breastfeeding; however, some recommendations have been made on the basis of a single-dose reaction in an infant, theoretical concerns only, or reports from pharmacologic assays that lacked precision, sensitivity, and specificity (Reisner et al., 1983). When there is a concern, the benefits of breastfeeding need to be weighed against the possible side-effects in the infant receiving the drug. Also, when possible, an alternate drug that is excreted into the breast milk in lower proportion and that provides a similar therapeutic effect for the mother should be prescribed.

The Committee on Drugs of the American Academy of Pediatrics (1983) has listed the following drugs as contraindicated during breastfeeding: amethopterin, bromocriptine, cimetidine, clemastine, cyclophosphamide, ergotamine, cold salts, methimazole, phedindione, and thiouracil (no contraindication with propylthiouracil). In addition, Reisner et al. (1983) recommend that breastfeeding women be advised against the use of marijuana while nursing. Studies indicate that marijuana and its metabolites are found in breast milk and are absorbed and utilized by the infant. Although no study demonstrates the effects of marijuana on infants, rodents were shown to have endocrinologic and behavioral changes after absorption of this drug.

Other drugs, although not absolutely contraindicated, need special consideration (American Academy of Pediatrics, Committee on Drugs, 1983). When a mother receives a radiopharmaceutical drug, she should pump her breasts and discard the milk until all of the drug is excreted. Infants of mothers who ingested alcohol were found to be drowsy and weak and to show an abnormal weight gain. In some mothers, alcohol has been found to decrease milk ejection. In contrast, small amounts of alcohol in tense mothers are known to enhance let-down of milk. Sulfa drugs should be used with caution if the infant has jaundice or is prone to jaundice. Contraceptives may cause breast enlargement and decrease milk production and are usually not recommended during lactation if another method of contraception is acceptable. Eating or drinking too many foods that have large amounts of caffeine can cause irritability in the infant. Lawrence (1985) suggests that a mother should not receive tetracycline or kanamycin for longer than 10 days. The former can cause staining of first and second teeth; the latter may be toxic to the auditory nerve and the kidneys.

Much knowledge and research are needed in the area of drugs and breastfeeding. Data are needed on drug excretion in breast milk and on infant response to drugs. Methods must be developed to determine the optimum time for a mother to take certain drugs. A mother who is breastfeeding should be taught to consult her physician before taking any medication.

SUMMARY

The nurse plays a significant role in helping the mother breastfeed successfully by assessing the mother's needs for support and information, planning for individualized care to meet those needs, and evaluating whether the methods chosen are effective. Despite this nursing care, problems with breastfeeding can occur. Early and efficient intervention can help resolve those problems. In addition, some mothers encounter special situations that make breastfeeding more challenging and to which the nurse must help them adapt.

REFERENCES

Akers, W. 1985. Measurement of friction injuries in man. *Am. J. Industrial Med.* 8:473–481.

American Academy of Pediatrics, Committee on Drugs. 1983. The transfer of drugs and other chemicals into human breast milk. *Pediatrics.* 72(3):375–383.

American Academy of Pediatrics, Committee on Nutrition. 1978. *Pediatrics.* 62:591–599.

Applebaum, R. M. 1970. The modern management of breastfeeding. *Pediatr. Clin. N. Amer.* 17(1):203–225.

Applebaum, R. M. 1975. The obstetrician's approach to breast and breastfeeding. *J. Reproductive Med.* 14(3):98–112.

Arafat, T.; Allen, D.; and Fox, E. 1981. Maternal practices and attitudes toward breastfeeding. *J. Obstet. Gynecol. Neonatal Nurs.* 10(2):91–95.

Atkinson, L. 1979. Prenatal nipple conditioning for breastfeeding. *Nurs. Res.* 23(5):267–271.

Avery, J. L. 1983. Relactation and induced lactation. In *A practical guide to breastfeeding*, ed. J. Riordan. St. Louis: C. V. Mosby.

Berger, L. 1978. Factors influencing breastfeeding. *J. Cont. Ed. Pediatrics.* 13–29.

Bergevin, Y.; Dougherty, C.; and Kramer, M. 1983. Do infant formula samples shorten the duration of breast feeding? *Lancet.* May:21.

Beske, E. J., and Garvis, N. S. 1982. Important factors in breastfeeding success. *MCN.* 7(3):174–179.

Boggs, K., and Rau, P. 1983. Breastfeeding the premature infant. *Am. J. Nurs.* 83(10):1437–1439.

Bose, C.; D'Ercole, A. J.; Lester, A. G.; Hunter, R. S.; and Barrett, J. R. 1981. Relactation by mothers of sick and premature infants. *Pediatrics.* 67(4):565.

Bowlby, J. 1958. The nature of the child's tie to his mother. *Int. J. Psychoanal.* 39:350–373.

Brown, J. S., and Hurlock, J. T. 1975. Preparation of the breast for breastfeeding. *Nurs. Research.* 24(6):448–451.

Cadwell, K. 1981. Improving nipple graspability for success at breastfeeding. *J. Obstet. Gynecol. Neonatal Nurs.* 10(1):277–279.

Campbell, N. 1981. The nutritional and immunological benefits of breast milk. *Austral. Nurses' J.* 10(11):40–47.

Childers, A. T., and Hamil, B. M. 1932. Emotional problems in children as related to the duration of breast-feeding in infancy. *Am. J. Orthopsychiatry.* 2:134–142.

Cohen, S. A. 1980. Postpartum teaching and the subsequent use of milk supplements. *Birth Fam. J.* 7(3):163–167.

Cole, J. 1977. Breastfeeding in the Boston suburbs in relation to personal-social factors. *Clin. Pediatrics.* 16:352–356.

Crowder, D. S. 1981. Maternity nurse's knowledge of factors promoting successful breastfeeding. *J. Obstet. Gynecol. Neonatal Nurs.* 10(1):28–30.

Dahms, B. B.; Krauss, A. N.; Gartner, L. M.; Klain, D. B.; Soodalter, B. A.; and Auld, P. A. M. 1973. Breastfeeding and serum bilirubin values during the first 4 days of life. *J. Pediatrics.* 83:1049–1054.

De Carvalho, M.; Hall, M.; and Harvey, D. 1981. Effects of water supplementation on physiological jaundice in breastfed babies. *Arch. Dis. Children.* 57(7):568–569.

De Carvalho, M.; Robertson, S.; Merkatz, R.; and Klaus, M. 1982a. Milk intake and frequency of feeding in breast-fed infants. *Early Human Development.* 7:155–163.

De Carvalho, M.; Klaus, M.; and Merkatz, R. 1982b. Frequency of breastfeeding and serum bilirubin concentration. *Arch. J. Dis. Child.* 136:737–738.

De Carvalho, M.; Robertson, S.; and Klaus, M. 1984. Does the duration and frequency of early breastfeeding affect nipple pain? *Birth.* 11(2):81–84.

Eckhardt, K., and Hendershot, G. 1984. Analysis of the reversal in breastfeeding trends in the early 1970's. *Public Health Reports.* 9(4):410–415.

Egli, G. E.; Egli, N. S.; and Newton, N. 1961. The influence of the number of breastfeedings on the milk production. *Pediatrics.* 27:314.

Ellis, D., and Hewat, R. 1984. Breast-feeding: Motivation and outcome. *J. Nosoc. Sci.* 16:81–88.

Estok, P. 1973. What do nurses know about breastfeeding problems? *J. Obstet. Gynecol. Neonatal Nurs.* 2(6):36–39.

Evans, R.; Thigpen, L.; and Hamrick, M. 1969. Exploration of factors involved in maternal physiologic adaptation to breastfeeding. *Nurs. Research.* 18(1):28–33.

Frantz, K. 1980. Techniques for successfully managing nipple problems and the reluctant nurser in the early postpartum period. In *Human milk: Its biological and social value*, eds. S. E. Frier and A. I. Eidelman. New York: Elsevier Science.

Frantz, K. 1982. *Managing nipple problems.* Franklin Park, Ill.: La Leche League International Reprint No. 11.

Frantz, K. 1983. Slow weight gain. In *A practical guide to breastfeeding*, ed. J. Riordan. St. Louis: C. V. Mosby.

Gardner, S. 1979. The mother as incubator—after delivery. *J. Obstet. Gynecol. Neonatal Nurs.* 8(3):174–176.

Garrison, F. H. 1929. *An introduction to the history of medicine.* 4th ed. Philadelphia: W. B. Saunders.

Grady, E. 1980. *Breastfeeding the baby with a cleft of the soft palate.* Franklin Park, Ill.: La Leche League Reprint No. 82.

Grams, K. E. 1978. Breastfeeding as a means of imparting immunity? *MCN.* 3(6):340–344.

Gross, S. J.; David, R.; Bauman, L.; and Tomarelli, R. M. 1980. Nutritional composition of milk produced by mothers delivering preterm. *J. Pediatrics.* 96(4):640–644.

Gunther, M. 1945. Sore nipples, causes, and prevention. *Lancet.* 2:290–293.

Gunther, M. 1963. Comparative merits of breast and bottle feeding. *Proc. Nutr. Soc.* 22:134–139.

Hall, J. M. 1978. Influencing breastfeeding success. *J. Obstet. Gynecol. Neonatal Nurs.* 7(6):28–32.

Hayes, B. 1981. Inconsistencies among nurses in breastfeeding knowledge and counseling. *J. Obstet. Gynecol. Neonatal Nurs.* 10(6):430–433.

Herbin, B. 1981. Avoid sore nipples—position the baby properly. *La Leche League News.* March–April:29.

Hill, S. T., and Shronk, L. K. 1979. The effect of early parent–infant contact on newborn body temperature. *J. Obstet. Gynecol. Neonatal Nurs.* 8(5):287–290.

Houston, J. J. 1981. Breastfeeding: Success or failure. *J. Adv. Nurs.* 6:447–454.

Houston, M. J.; Howie, P.; and McNeilly, A. 1983. Midwife forum, 2. Breastfeeding. *Nurs. Mirror.* 156(6):1–8.

Howie, P. W.; Houston, M. J.; Cook, A.; Smart, L.; McArdle, T.; and McNeilly, A. S. 1981. How long should a breast feed last? *Early Human Development.* 5:71–77.

Huggins, K. 1986. *The nursing mother's companion.* Boston: Harvard Common Press.

Hughes, R. N., and Bushnell, J. A. 1978. Further relationships between IPAT anxiety scale performance and infantile feeding experiences. *J. Clin. Psychol.* 33(3):698–700.

Jakobsson, I., and Lindberg, T. 1978. Cow's milk as a cause of infantile colic in breastfed infants. *Lancet.* 2:437.

Jakobsson, I., and Lindberg, T. 1983. Cow's milk proteins cause infantile colic in breastfed infants: A double-blind crossover study. *Pediatrics.* 71(2):268–271.

Jarkowsky, M. J. 1980. How to prevent breastfeeding problems. *Supervisor Nurse.* 11(1):43–44.

Jelliffe, D. B., and Jelliffe, E. F. P. 1971. An overview. *Am. J. Clin. Nutr.* 24:1013–1024.

Johnson, N. W. 1976. Breastfeeding at one hour of age. *MCN.* 1(1):12–16.

Klaus, M., and Kennell, J. 1982. *Parent–infant bonding.* 2nd ed. St. Louis: C. V. Mosby.

La Cerva, V. 1981. *Breastfeeding: A manual for health professionals.* New York: Medical Examination Publishing.

Ladas, A. 1970. How to help mothers breastfeed. *Clin. Pediatr.* 9(12):702–705.

La Leche League. 1987. *The womanly art of breastfeeding,* 3rd ed. Franklin Park, Ill.: La Leche League International.

Lawrence, R. A. 1985. *Breastfeeding: A guide for the medical profession.* St. Louis: C. V. Mosby.

Leonard, L. G. 1982. Breastfeeding twins: Maternal–infant nutrition. *J. Obstet. Gynecol. Neonatal Nurs.* 11:148–153.

L'Esperance, C. 1980. Pain or pleasure—the dilemma of early breastfeeding. *Birth Fam. J.* 7(1):21–25.

L'Esperance, C., and Frantz, K. 1985. A case against time limitation for early breastfeeding and nursing implications. *J. Obstet. Gynecol. Neonatal Nurs.* (14)2.

Levit, F. 1977. Joggers' nipples. *NEJM.* 297:1127.

Loughlin, H.; Clapp-Channing, N.; Gehlbach, S.; Pollard, J.; and McCutchen, T. 1985. Early termination of breastfeeding: Identifying those at risk. *Pediatrics.* 75(3):508–513.

Mack, E. 1983. One mother's story. *Baby Talk.* January:26–28.

Maclean, G. 1977. An appraisal of the concepts of infant feeding and their application in practice. *J. Adv. Nurs.* 2:111–125.

Maisel, M., and Gifford, K. 1983. Breast-feeding, weight loss and jaundice. *Clin. Lab. Observations.* 102(1):117–118.

Maslow, A. H., and Szilagyi-Kessler, I. 1946. Security and breastfeeding. *J. Ab. Soc. Psych.* 1(4):302–311.

McDonald, L. 1978. *The joy of breastfeeding.* Pasadena, Calif.: Oaklawn Press.

Meara, H. 1976. A key to successful breastfeeding in a nonsupportive culture. *Keeping Abreast J.* 1(4):302–311.

Meier, P., and Riordan, J. 1983. Breastfeeding support in the high risk nursery and at home. In *A practical guide to breastfeeding,* ed. J. Riordan. St. Louis: C. V. Mosby.

Montague, A. 1978. *Touching.* 2nd ed. New York: Harper & Row.

Neville, M., and Neifert, M. 1983. *Lactation: Physiology, nutrition, and breastfeeding.* New York and London: Plenum Press.

Newton, N. 1952. Nipple pain and damage. *J. Pediatrics.* 41:411–423.

Newton, N. 1971. Psychologic differences between breast and bottle feeding. *Am. J. Clin. Nutr.* 24:993–1004.

Newton, N., and Newton, M. 1967. Psychologic aspects at lactation. *New Engl. J. Med.* 277:1179–1187.

Nicoll, A.; Ginsburg, R.; and Tripp, J. 1982. Supplementary feeding and jaundice in newborns. *Acta. Paediatr. Scand.* 71:759–761.

Oakland Perinatal Health Project. Summer 1983. *Nutrition Newsletter.* Oakland, Calif.: Alameda County Health Care Services Agency.

Pittard, W. B. 1981. Special properties of human milk. *Birth Fam. J.* 8(4):229–235.

Pryor, K. 1973. *Nursing your baby.* New York: Pocket Books.

Ramirez, N. 1982. *The relationship between selected predisposing factors and nipple pain in breastfeeding mothers.* Unpublished master's thesis. California State University, Fresno.

Raphael, D. 1976. *The tender gift of breastfeeding.* New York: Schocken Books.

Raphael, D. 1983. Nursing the adopted baby. *Childbirth Educator.* 2(4):43–44.

Reisner, S.; Eisenberg, N.; Stahl, B.; and Hauser, G.

1983. Maternal medications and breastfeeding. *Dev. Pharmacol. Ther.* 6:285–304.

Riordan, J. 1983. *A practical guide to breastfeeding.* St. Louis: C. V. Mosby.

Riordan, J., and Countryman, B. A. 1980. Preparation for breastfeeding and early optimal functioning. *J. Obstet. Gynecol. Neonatal Nurs.* 9(5):277–283.

Riordan, J., and Rapp, E. T. 1980. Pleasure and purpose: The sensuousness of breastfeeding. *J. Obstet. Gynecol. Neonatal Nurs.* 9(2)109–112.

Rivera-Calim, L. 1987. The significance of drugs in breast milk. *Clinics in Perinatology.* 14(1):51–70.

Rubin, R. 1961. Puerperal change. *Nurs. Outlook.* 9:753–755.

Schanler, R., and Oh, W. 1980. Composition of breast milk obtained from mothers of premature infants as compared to breast milk obtained from donors. *J. Pediatrics.* 9(4):679–681.

Shepherd, S. C., and Yarrow, R. E. 1982. Breastfeeding and the working mother. *J. Nurse-Midwifery.* 27(6):16–20.

Slaven, S. 1981. Unlimited sucking time improves breastfeeding. *Lancet.* 8216:392–393.

Sloper, K.; McKean, L.; and Baum, J. D. 1975. Factors influencing breastfeeding. *Arch. Dis. Childhood.* 50:165–170.

Speight, L. 1980. Nursing twins? I double dare you. *Mothering.* Summer: 24–28.

Stanway, P., and Stanway, A. 1978. *Breast is best.* London: Pan Books.

Styer, G. W., and Freeh, K. 1981. Feeding infants with cleft lip and/or palate. *J. Obstet. Gynecol. Neonatal Nurs.* 10(5):329–331.

Sugarman, M. 1977. Perinatal influences on maternal-infant attachment. *Am. J. Orthopsych.* 47(3):407.

Thomsen, A. C.; Espersen, T.; and Maigaard, S. 1984. Course and treatment of milk stasis, noninfectious inflammation of the breast and infectious mastitis in nursing women. *Am. J. Obstet. Gynecol.* 149(5): 492–495.

Tibbetts, E., and Cadwell, K. 1981. Selecting the right breast pump. *MCN.* 5(4):262–264.

Wallace, A. 1980. Nursing mothers then and now. *Canad. Nurs.* 44–47.

Whitley, N. 1978. Preparation for breastfeeding—one year follow-up of 34 nursing mothers. *J. Obstet. Gynecol. Neonatal Nurs.* 7(3):44–48.

Woolridge, M. W.; Baum, J. D.; and Drewett, R. F. 1980. Effect of a traditional and of a new nipple shield on sucking patterns and milk flow. *Early Human Development.* 4:357–364.

Yeung, D.; Pennell, M. D.; Leung, M.; and Hall, J. 1981. Breastfeeding: Prevalence and influencing factors. *Canad. J. Public Health.* 72:323–329.

Zimmerman, J. A. 1981. Breastfeeding the adopted newborn. *Pediatric Nurs.* 7(1):9–12.

22

Postpartum Exercises

BEHAVIORAL OBJECTIVES

Upon completion of this chapter, the reader should be able to:

- Provide a rationale for beginning an early exercise and relaxation program for a postpartum mother.

- Provide instruction for the new postpartum mother in comfort measures, proper posture, proper body mechanics, appropriate early exercises, and relaxation techniques.

- Provide the new postpartum mother with instruction in progressive exercises appropriate to the individual and to the length of her hospital stay.

- Provide the postcesarean mother with an appropriate physical restoration program.

Women in this country are becoming more aware of the need for being in good physical condition during the childbearing years. The United States is several decades behind other countries, however, in providing well-defined exercise programs for the postpartum mother, and even further behind in incorporating a physical therapist into the postpartum routine at the hospital. The nurse is placed in the new and challenging position of filling this gap. She has an opportunity to develop new skills and introduce change in traditional postpartum care.

The current national trend toward early discharge presents an additional challenge. Women are often discharged 12–24 hours following a normal vaginal delivery and within 3–4 days following a cesarean section delivery. Such short inpatient care for the new mother makes the educational role of the nurse even more important. A summary chart of recommended exercises is included at the end of this chapter to facilitate discharge planning and follow-up (Fig. 22–34).

Postpartum restorative exercises are significant in preventing or minimizing potential discomforts and dysfunctions and in aiding the new mother to resume a fully functional routine. The primary aims of the postpartum exercise program are to restore alignment of the pelvic girdle, to restore function of the abdominal and pelvic floor muscle groups, and to restore placement of the pelvic organs. Proper body mechanics and posture ensure longer-term protection. Relaxation exercises facilitate comfort and stress management.

Pelvic floor weakness results in poor urinary control, prolonged discomfort, hemorrhoids, possible prolapse of pelvic organs, a weakened low back, and can detract from normal sexual responses. Weak abdominal muscles lead to poor posture and eventually to low-back syndrome. Poor postural habits in the upper body can contribute to cervical and shoulder problems, improper breathing, and poor digestion. These problems are common after both vaginal and cesarean births.

The cesarean birth rate has increased significantly in the past 5 years. The exercise program for the cesarean patient must be modified, and additional comfort measures must be considered.

Physical exercise "feels good." One's sense of well-being, self-esteem, and positive body image are fortified by a balanced program of exercise and relaxation. A woman can manage fatigue, tension, and emotional stresses more easily when she gains in physical strength and stamina; this aids in her acceptance of her new and demanding role. A woman must be encouraged to take some time to nurture herself so that she will feel more fulfilled. Experience has shown that "stress-resistant" parents are less prone to the anger and frustrations that can trigger patterns of child abuse.

Women are frequently overwhelmed by their new responsibilities as mothers and need practical hints on how to incorporate exercise and relaxation techniques into their daily routines. The husband/father may be able to play a proactive role in the mother's postpartum restoration. If the couple participated in childbirth education classes, the cooperative effort established before delivery provides a natural bridge to the postpartum recovery the mother now faces. The husband/father can encourage her to exercise, assist her, or have a "special time" with the baby, thereby freeing her mentally and physically to focus on her own restoration. In addition, any new program must reflect the needs of the individual mother and must incorporate or relate to her cultural practices and attitudes, or she may reject the program in favor of family or cultural advice (Marecki, 1979).

EARLY POSTPARTUM RESTORATION: DAY 1

Postpartum restoration begins in the first hour following delivery. Early exercises initiate the important process of pelvic realignment and muscle rebalancing. In addition, the first day's program is designed to facilitate healing, increase comfort and promote safe body mechanics.

Initial Comfort Measures

Ideally, immediately following delivery and any necessary perineal repair, an ice pack should be applied to the woman's perineum for 30 minutes to minimize edema, stiffness, and soreness and to reduce hemorrhoids. When the ice pack is removed, encourage the woman to begin pelvic floor contractions, also known as *Kegel exercises*.

Pelvic Floor (Kegel) Exercises

Pelvic floor contractions stimulate circulation to promote healing; alleviate pain, stiffness, and edema; encourage return of bladder control; aid in shrinkage of hemorrhoids; and reestablish support of the pelvic organs. Micturation difficulties may be related to reflex muscle spasms of the pelvic floor, which can occur as a response to pain. Awareness and conscious relaxation of the muscles will help remedy the problem (Blankfield, 1967).

For this exercise, the woman should be in a supine or side-lying position with head and knees supported on pillows (see Figs. 22–1 and 22–2). Ask the woman to gently contract the pelvic floor muscles, tightening the sphincters, especially around the vagina. She may need to tighten the buttocks muscles to initiate the action. The contraction should be brief, held for only 1–3 seconds, and should be followed by complete muscle release. Repeat five times each hour. Often, a woman cannot feel the results of her action. Feedback from the nurse viewing the pelvic floor is helpful and encouraging. A firmer contraction can be achieved during exhalation, and more complete relaxation during inhalation.

Positions of Comfort

Spinal and pelvic alignment in resting positions must be considered so that the low back will be protected. Comfort will facilitate the rest of the entire body. Pelvic floor contractions can be performed in all of the following positions (breast-feeding and cuddling an infant are easier in the first two positions):

1. *Supine.* A woman may lie supine with head and knees supported by pillows or by adjusting the bed (see Fig. 22–1).
2. *Side lying.* Alternatively, she might lie on her side with head, upper leg, and low back supported with pillows (see Fig. 22–2). This position is preferable if hemorrhoids are uncomfortable.
3. *Three-quarter position.* The woman may prefer to lie turned farther over and to use an extra pillow under the abdomen to avoid low-back strain (see Fig. 22–3).
4. *Prone lying.* A woman may eagerly request a prone lying position for resting. It is essential to put a pillow under the woman's hips to place her pelvis in proper alignment and prevent excessive lumbar lordosis (see Fig. 22–4). This relieves strain on her low back, relaxes and avoids stretching of the weakened abdominal wall, and encourages repositioning of the pelvic organs. Additional pillows under her head and shoulders will reduce pressure on tender breasts (see Fig. 22–5). The woman should not be allowed to prop herself on her elbows, as this will stretch the abdominal muscles and compress the low back. The prone lying position can be maintained for 30–60 minutes twice daily. It is a safer alternative to the knee–chest position, which must be avoided in the early postpartum period, especially during the first 11 days, when retained amniotic membranes, clots, or placental fragments can keep the uterine sinuses open and vulnerable to air entry. In the past the knee–chest position was linked to air embolism (Forbes, 1944), but this has not been documented as a problem.

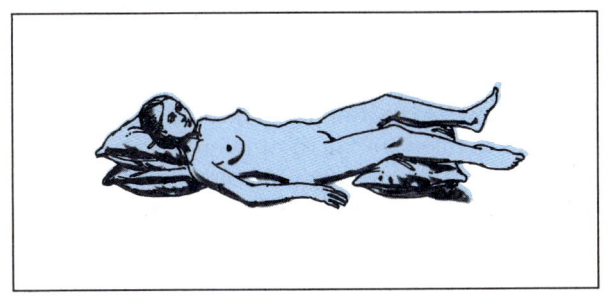

FIGURE 22–1. Supine position.

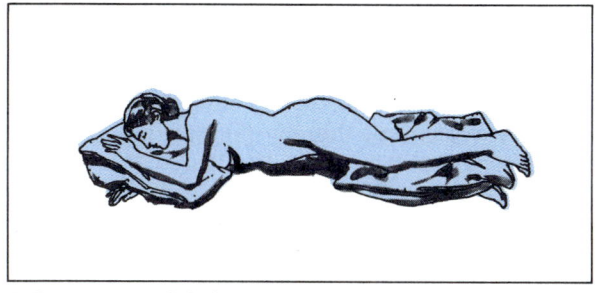

FIGURE 22–2. Side-lying position. Place a pillow between the legs.

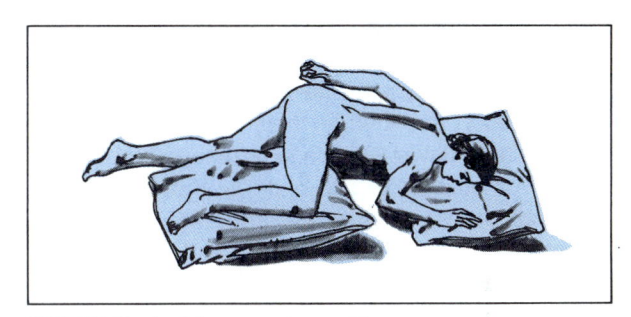

FIGURE 22–3. Three-quarter position with pillow support.

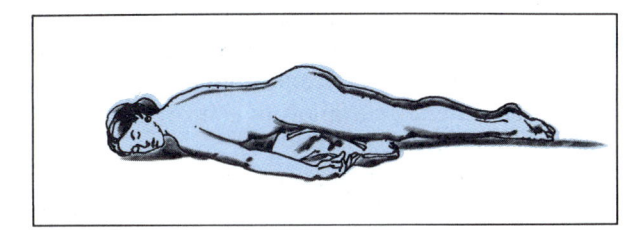

FIGURE 22–4. Prone position.

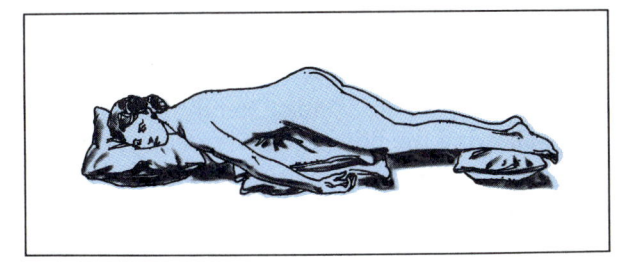

FIGURE 22–5. Pillow support protects the low back and tender breasts.

Basic Diaphragmatic Breathing Exercise

Diaphragmatic breathing enhances a state of well-being. It is the foundation of many relaxation and meditation techniques and should be incorporated into exercise programs to improve efficiency and reduce fatigue.

Proper diaphragmatic breathing has been found to improve ventilation. Blood distribution and gas exchange is more concentrated in the lower half of the lungs. Thoracic breathing brings air primarily into the upper two-thirds of the lungs. In diaphragmatic breathing, the diaphragm contracts during inhalation and moves downward, creating more of a vacuum, thereby pulling the air down into the lower, blood-rich lobes. Thoracic breathers may take 16–20 breaths/min (22,000–25,000 in a 24-hour period), whereas diaphragmatic breathers may need to take only 6–8 breaths/min (10,000–12,000 in a 24-hour period) for adequate oxygen intake. In diaphragmatic breathing, the workload of the lungs and heart may be reduced by 35–50 percent (Nuernberger, 1981).

The downward action of the diaphragm during inhalation has a gentle massaging effect on abdominal organs, improving their circulation. Blood flow in the inferior vena cava returning blood from the lower portion of the body is enhanced. Peristaltic activity of the intestines is stimulated. Movement of the thoracic cavity and the pressure within it have a stimulating effect on the vagus nerve and so affect the balance of the sympathetic and parasympathetic nervous systems. Inspiration is linked to an increase in sympathetic (arousal) activity, and exhalation to parasympathetic (inhibitory) activity. Respiration is the autonomic body function most easily controlled and is primary in achieving general relaxation to combat the stress response (Nuernberger, 1981).

To perform the diaphragmatic breathing exercise, the woman should lie supine with knees bent, left hand on the abdomen below the rib cage, right hand over the sternum (see Fig. 22–6). The head and knees can be supported with pillows. A side-lying position can be used if the supine position is uncomfortable.

The woman should inhale gently through the nose, allowing the breath to move deeply into the lower lungs. The diaphragm will descend, and the abdomen will rise under the left hand. The chest should remain relaxed and quiet under the right hand, with little or no movement. Breaths should be exhaled through the nose. The abdomen will flatten under the left hand. The breathing pattern

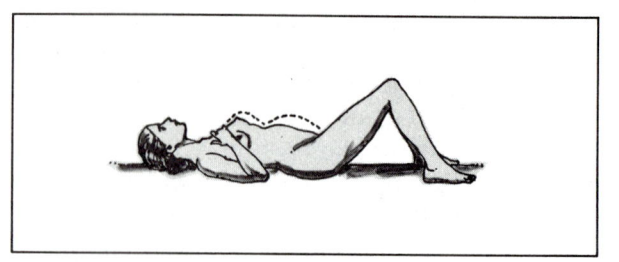

FIGURE 22–6. Diaphragmatic breathing.

should be smooth, slow, and regular, without holding or pausing. Exhalation through the mouth will help control hyperventilation if needed. A woman with nasal congestion may breathe entirely through her mouth.

Once the postpartum woman has reviewed or learned diaphragmatic breathing, she can go on to the relaxation technique or exercise program she needs. Building upon her skill in diaphragmatic breathing allows an exercise regimen to flow naturally, minimizing physical strain and emotional resistance.

Pelvic Realignment Exercise

The primary function of early postpartum exercises is to coax the muscles that realign the pelvis back into use. These exercises should begin as soon as the mother has been settled and has had time to rest. Fatigue and soreness may make the woman resist beginning this program. The nurse should assure the woman that the exercises will improve her comfort and that if she waits, healing and recovery may be delayed. Prolonged delay can lead to muscle atrophy and tissue degeneration (Noble, 1976).

For the following exercises, the woman can be side-lying or supine with head and knees supported on low pillows (see Figs. 22–2 through 22–5; Noble, 1976).

1. ABDOMINAL TIGHTENING. Instruct the woman to inhale deeply. She should exhale slowly while contracting (tightening or pulling in) the abdominal muscles. She should then gently build up and release the contraction over a 5–10 seconds period. She will be able to feel the muscles working by placing her hands on the abdominal wall (see Fig. 22–7). Have her repeat this exercise five times. The abdominal muscles have been stretched an inch or so and this simple exercise will begin to shorten them.

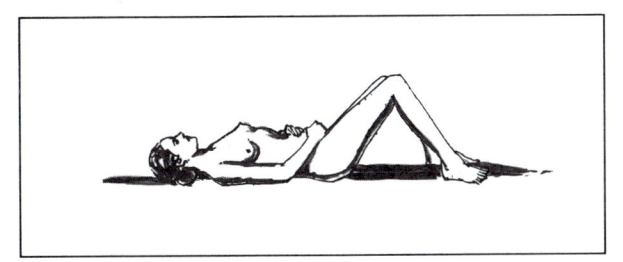

FIGURE 22–7. Abdominal tightening. Tighten the abdominal muscles on the outward breath.

2. ABDOMINAL AND PELVIC FLOOR TIGHTENING. As the woman exhales and tightens her abdominal muscles, she should tighten the pelvic floor, squeezing the sphincters and gradually tightening the vagina, holding from 3 to 5 seconds and then releasing slowly. This sensation is the same as shutting off the desire to urinate. Have her repeat the exercise five times.

3. ABDOMINAL, PELVIC FLOOR, AND GLUTEAL TIGHTENING. As she performs exercise 2, she should add tightening (pinching together) of her buttocks muscles. If she does this properly, she can hold her buttocks and feel them contract. Have her repeat this exercise five times.

4. LUMBO-PELVIC REALIGNMENT–FINDING NEUTRAL SPINE. Exercise 3 is performed more strongly, and the woman feels her low back flattening into the bed. She can increase her awareness of this movement by placing one hand at the small of her back and the other on her abdomen. She should become aware of action in the three muscle groups that move the pelvis, rather than pushing down on her legs to accomplish this movement. The back arches during inhalation as the muscles relax, and it flattens during exhalation as the muscles contract (see Fig. 22–8). Have her repeat this exercise 5–10 times, oscillating in progressively smaller arcs until her neutral position is found. This position should be pain-free and the amount of lumbar curve will be approximately equal to her normal (prepregnancy) standing lumbar curve. Over-arching or over-flattening of the lumbar curve are avoided in this "neutral" alignment (Johnson et al., 1987).

Lower Extremity Exercises

Prior to getting out of bed, a woman will "find her legs" again and will feel more secure on her feet if she follows a few simple exercises. The following

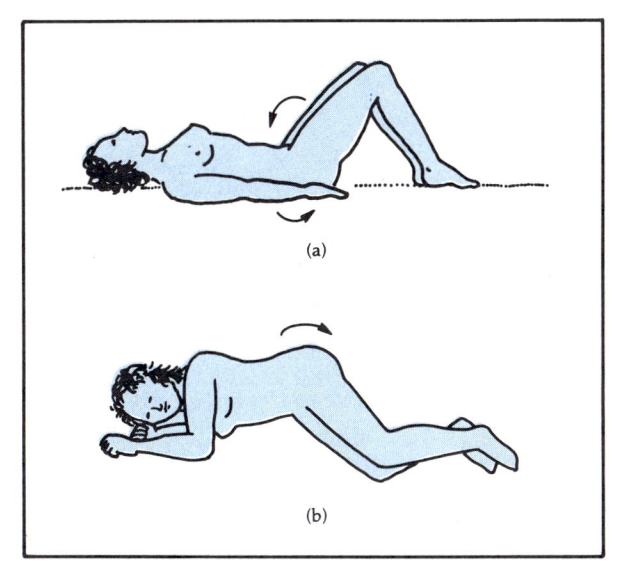

FIGURE 22–8. Lumbo-pelvic realignment. (*a*) Supine. (*b*) Side-lying.

exercises are performed in the supine position with the head slightly elevated and the legs straight.

1. ANKLE FLEXION AND EXTENSION. Instruct the woman to dorsiflex her foot strongly, with a sense of stretching down through the heel, and then to plantar-flex the foot strongly, keeping the toes extended (see Fig. 22–9). (Flexing or pointing the toes may initiate a cramp and should be avoided for this reason.) She should repeat this exercise 10 times.

2. ANKLE CIRCLES. Have her draw circles with the great toe in clockwise and counterclockwise directions. She should repeat this exercise five times in each direction (see Fig. 22–9).

3. QUADRICEPS EXERCISES. Instruct the woman to perform an isometric contraction of the quadriceps muscle group, holding for 5–10 seconds, then releasing. This exercise should be repeated 10

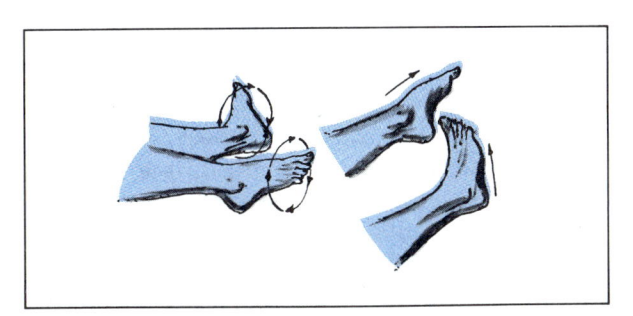

FIGURE 22–9. Ankle exercises.

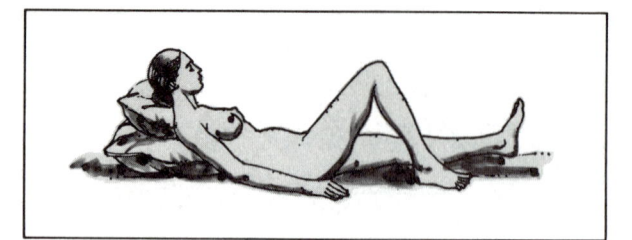

FIGURE 22–10. Alternate leg flexion and extension.

times. These muscles keep the knees strong when the woman is standing.

4. ALTERNATE LEG FLEXION AND EXTENSION. Have the woman bend one knee, keeping the foot flat on the bed. She should gently draw the other heel up toward the buttock while inhaling, and then slide the leg out straight while exhaling and maintaining a pelvic tilt (see Fig. 22–10). This exercise should be alternated with each leg and should be repeated five times.

The sequence of exercises for pelvic realignment and lower extremities should be as follows: Kegel exercises for the pelvic floor should be done each hour; diaphragmatic breathing should gradually become a normal breathing pattern (practice during feeding times), and the remaining exercises should be done before each meal and at bedtime.

Body Mechanics: First Transfers, Posture, and Early Ambulation

Pelvic joint instability and overstretched muscles put the low back at risk and contribute to a feeling of pelvic looseness when the patient first moves and gets up. The woman must be encouraged to move slowly and safely. After she has performed the preparatory exercises described previously, she should be encouraged to hold the pelvic floor, buttocks, and abdominal muscles tight in order to stabilize the pelvis as she moves.

1. GETTING OUT OF BED. To get out of bed safely, without putting any strain on the lower back, she should move close to the edge of the bed, roll on to her side with her hips and knees flexed to a 90-degree angle, and then push up into a sitting position, using her arms while allowing her legs to dangle over the edge of the bed (see Fig. 22–11). Once sitting, she should slowly release the muscles around the pelvis, swing her legs several times, and then perform several more pelvic

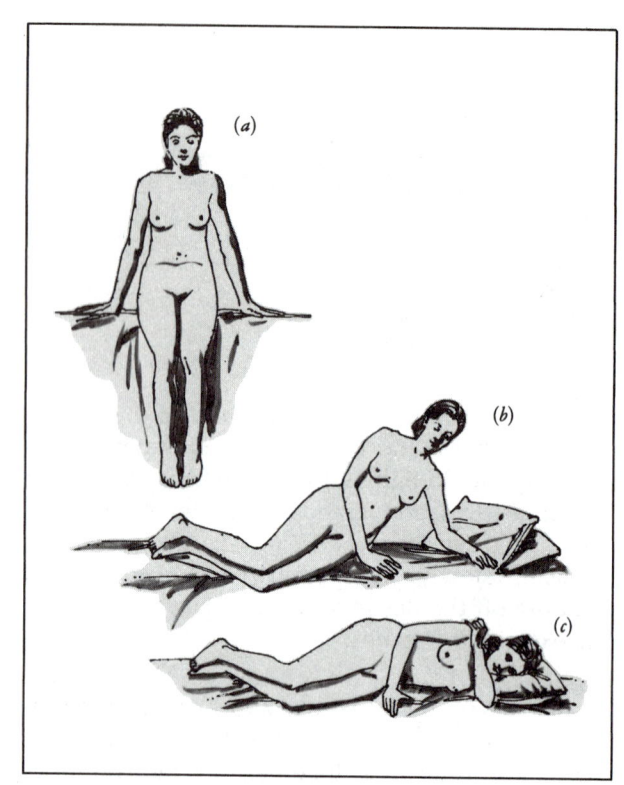

FIGURE 22–11. Procedures for getting in and out of bed. Getting in: (*a*) Sit on the edge of the bed. (*b*) Bring both arms to one side; lower the side of the body to the bed, keeping the knees bent at an angle of 45 degrees. Put the feet into bed. Remain on the side or roll on to the back. Getting out: (*c*) Roll to the side; push with the hands to a sitting position; keep the knees bent and swing the legs over the edge of the bed.

realignment contractions to establish the neutral spine position, holding it as she stands up. Once standing, she should repeat the contractions oscillating her pelvis several more times, paying particular attention to realigning the pelvis into a neutral spine position (see Fig. 22–12). Since the woman's weakened muscles generally allow too much lordosis after childbirth, she will be moving into a partial posterior pelvic tilt position.

2. STANDING. She should stand as erect as possible. Her weight should be equal on both feet and should be balanced between the heels and balls of her feet. Her toes should be relaxed, not gripping the floor. Her knees should be flexible, not locked. The pelvis will move posteriorly into the neutral spine position. The nurse should check the woman's shoulders to see that they are released away from her ears and not raised or rounded forward.

Her chest should feel open. The top of her head should stretch up and her chin should tuck slightly. Her breathing should be free and even.

3. WALKING. After delivery, most women tend to ambulate with legs wide apart and shoulders slouched forward over their protruding abdomens. They frequently look down at their feet. Performing the preparatory exercises and achieving proper posture will help to counter the development of poor gait habits. The legs should swing straight forward with each step, and normal heel-to-toe foot placement should be achieved. Maintaining the neutral position of the pelvis while ambulating is important in reestablishing proper placement of the pelvic and abdominal organs and in protecting the low back. This will be difficult to achieve initially. The nurse should persist in encouraging proper posture and the return of the woman's normal gait pattern.

4. GETTING INTO BED. The postpartum mother can protect her low back when transferring back into bed by first sitting on the edge and then lowering on to one side with the knees flexed. After putting her feet into bed with the knees still flexed, she should roll on to her back and then straighten her legs one at a time. Pelvic stability will be enhanced if the pelvic muscles are held tight during these maneuvers and a few pelvic realignment contractions are performed once the woman is in the resting position. When in bed, she should roll to one side by bending the knees and pushing on the legs, keeping the trunk straight and the pelvic muscles tight. Turning by twisting can strain the low back, and it relies more on abdominal muscle action (see Fig. 22–11).

Relaxation

Following delivery, many women experience a surge of energy and euphoria and are unable to rest effectively. Other women are overcome with feelings of fatigue, exhaustion, sadness, depression, or detachment. Performing a relaxation technique soon after delivery can aid in reestablishing a sense of balance and harmony between mind, body, and emotions. A woman can regain her sense of centeredness and can deal more effectively with the crisis of bearing an infant. When deep muscular relaxation is achieved, superficial thoughts and emotions quiet (Shealy, 1980). As the "static" subsides, a woman can experience deeper emotions more openly which often reside in the memories of her muscles. Past experiences and emotions are often internalized and become "natural" or familiar levels of increased muscle tension or armor. Just as a particular sound or smell may trigger a memory and its emotions, a state of mental and physical relaxation may also serve as a direct path to a deeper emotion. Her feelings can be dealt with more completely, and her growth can be enhanced. Deep relaxation soon after delivery may lead to a positive integration of the mother's birthing experience and prevent unnecessary armoring or muscle tension from developing. Physically, she will benefit by resting more completely and comfortably.

Once the woman has performed the *diaphragmatic breathing* exercise, the nurse can easily guide her into relaxation. Be certain she is comfortable before beginning the exercise.

1. BEGINNING RELAXATION. The nurse should speak to the woman slowly, in a calm, controlled voice. For example, she might say, "As you inhale the next time, say to yourself, 'I breathe in', and as you exhale say, 'I breathe out.'" Allow her to do this silently for several breaths. Then proceed: "With the next inhalation, repeat the phrase 'I am', and

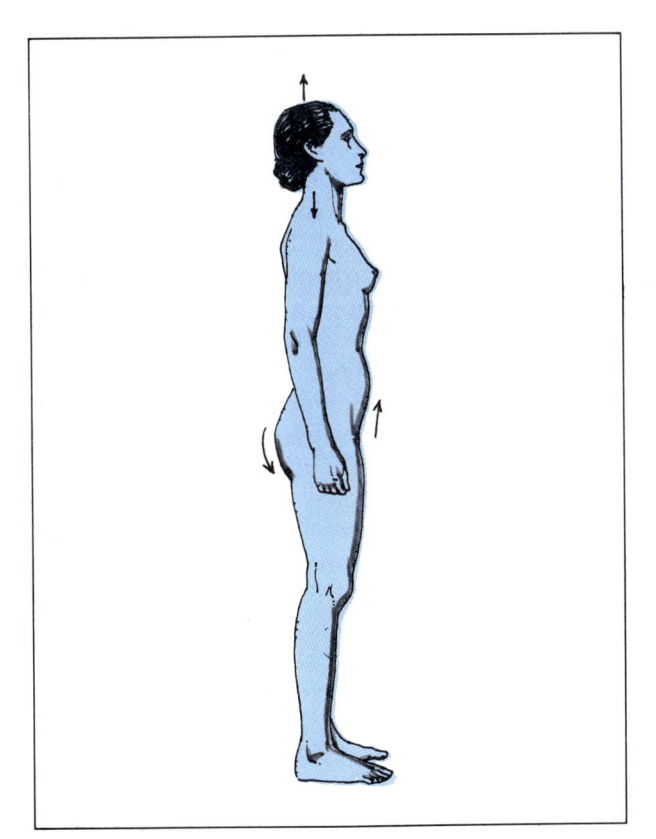

FIGURE 22–12. Proper posture.

as you exhale, repeat 'relaxing'." After several more breaths, the nurse might say, "With each exhalation allow your body to soften, to release gently and comfortably into the bed. Allow your body to feel completely supported and at ease." The nurse can then call attention to parts of the woman's body, moving from head to foot or foot to head, suggesting that each part "release," "soften," "open," become "heavy" or "light." To simply tell a woman to relax is to no avail; she must be instructed and encouraged.

2. PROGRESSIVE RELAXATION. If the nurse observes that the woman is having difficulty controlling her muscles or that an area of her body (such as forehead, eyes, jaws, shoulders, hands, or toes) is especially tense, progressive relaxation techniques can be utilized. The following is a sample of instruction for progressive relaxation: "Gradually tighten your right hand, making a fist. Make it tighter and tighter. Hold it. Feel the sensations of tension, and compare it to your left hand. Now gradually release your fist, allowing your hand to soften and open and feel at ease on the bed. Feel the sensations of relaxation as they unfold in your right hand. Compare it to your left hand."

This method teaches that a muscle can be contracted strongly and held contracted. By doing the exercise, the woman can carefully learn the feeling of tension. Then the muscle is allowed to relax and the contrasting sensations are observed. This technique can be applied to the entire body or to a specific trouble area only. As the patient's ability to relax improves, more subtle movements or contractions can be performed and, finally, they can be imagined rather than carried out (Jacobson, 1965).

3. TOUCH-RELEASE TECHNIQUES. The nurse can gently touch the region of the woman's body that is to be relaxed. This helps the body–mind connection to become clearer and the release to be more complete.

4. POSITIVE AFFIRMATIONS. Once physical relaxation is apparent, the woman can be redirected to observe her diaphragmatic breathing pattern and then to appreciate and enjoy the state of "serenity, peace, balance, and harmony" she has achieved.

This is an ideal time for the nurse to encourage positive affirmations. She can guide the woman in open-ended or specific, goal-oriented images. If the woman has had an opportunity to express her personal concerns, fears, or problems, the nurse can use that information in developing an image.

The following is a suggested list of positive affirmations:

1. My body is healthy and strong. I will regain more of my normal strength and stamina each day.
2. My baby is unique, and I enjoy getting to know my baby.
3. My baby is strong and healthy and suckles well.
4. Breastfeeding is progressing normally.
5. I am experiencing strong emotions. I will flow with them, allowing them to finish, knowing I can return to my center and feel at peace.

Massage

A woman works hard in labor and exerts much effort during delivery. Her muscles may ache with fatigue. She may have pain. Massage is an appropriate treatment after delivery to enhance relaxation and comfort for the new mother. In reality, few nurses have time to perform massage on their patients, beyond the uterine massage; but they can suggest it to the woman's partner or significant others. Areas to emphasize include the neck and shoulders, low back, and legs. Massage strokes should begin lightly, then build in strength and depth, but remain comfortable. Kneading of tight muscle masses and gentle pressure over trigger points can be incorporated into the massage. Pressure during the massage strokes should be heavier when going toward the heart and lighter when moving distally. One or both of the nurse's hands should remain in contact with the patient's body at all times to avoid startling her. The hands should be kept open to avoid pinching and should mold to her body for greater comfort. Avoid scratching the patient with fingernails, rings, or bracelets. Massage lotion will reduce friction and increase comfort. In addition to increasing physical comfort, massage can help to soothe, comfort, and relax the new mother. Touch is nurturing and can give a woman additional emotional strength in beginning her new mothering role (Downing, 1972). Massage can become a vehicle for opening lines of communication between partners or between patient and nurse.

POSTPARTUM RESTORATION: DAY 2

The focus of the second day's restoration program is to further strengthen the abdominal wall and pelvic floor muscles, to alleviate discomfort in the woman's body, and to instruct her in proper body mechanics for moving about and handling her infant.

Comfort Measures

Encourage the new mother to wear her nursing bra. This will help to protect her ligamentous breast tissue from overstretching and will also help to redistribute a portion of the carrying load from her back to her shoulders. Some women can wear a bra day and night. Others cannot tolerate it at night. Minimally, a bra should be worn whenever the woman is out of bed.

Pelvic floor comfort will be enhanced if the woman alternately takes warm sitz baths and exposes the pelvic floor to dry heat (the peri-lamp). The woman should allow the pelvic floor muscles to warm up and relax for 5 minutes during each treatment and should then start pelvic floor exercises. The intensity and duration of each contraction will be dictated by the woman's sensitivity and the condition of her pelvic floor but, ideally, contractions will be stronger and longer than those performed on the first day.

Overall comfort will be improved by periods of activity, exercise, and ambulation, continued use of diaphragmatic breathing, and relaxation techniques.

Positions of Comfort

Continue to encourage the woman to lie prone (as shown in Fig. 22–4) for 30–60 minutes twice daily. While supine and side-lying positions remain appropriate, many women are feeling more energetic by the second postpartum day and request more upright positions. Assist the woman to use the following proper sitting positions.

Correct Position for Sitting Up in Bed

When sitting up in bed, the woman must support the lumbar spine properly with an extra pillow or rolled towel (approximately 4 inches in diameter; see Fig. 22–13a). The entire back, neck, and head should be supported with two pillows, and the knees should be comfortably flexed and supported, the hips and feet should be relaxed, or the legs should be crossed in tailor fashion. This position maintains the normal lordotic curve of the low back and prevents overstretching

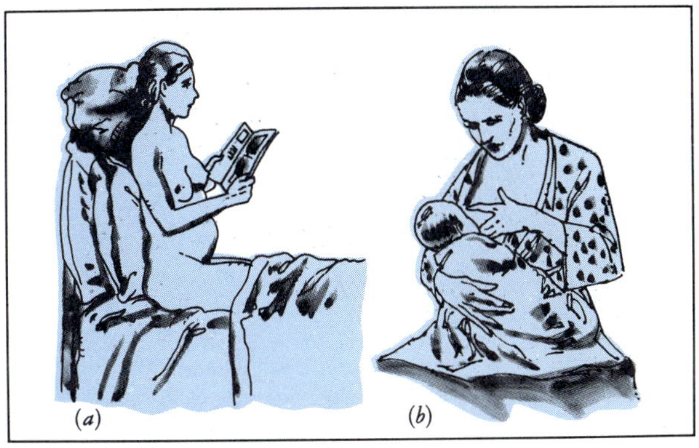

FIGURE 22–13. Correct position for sitting up in bed. (a) Reading, (b) nursing. Use pillows to support the spine.

of the spinal ligaments. Overstretching will occur if the spine is allowed to round excessively (slouch) or arch excessively (sway) for prolonged periods. Overstretching will cause pain and, possibly, joint instability with persistent or recurring low-back pain. The back must be carefully protected until the softening hormones are no longer present in the woman's body, approximately 6–8 weeks postpartum (Danforth, 1967). This position is ideal for reading, writing, or chatting with friends.

If the new mother wishes to nurse the baby while sitting up in bed, place the baby in her lap elevated by a pillow or two for easy access to the breast. The mother should not lean forward but should have her back against the supporting pillows, bringing the baby in close to her body (see Fig. 22–13b). The baby can lie across the front of her body or can be tucked under her arm "football" style, with the baby's body curving around her side and the baby's head supported by her hand. Twins can be nursed in any combination of these two positions (see Fig. 22–14).

Proper position and support of the infant are essential in preventing upper-back tension and arm fatigue. The mother should not hold the baby up while nursing but should cradle the baby while it rests in her lap. Her shoulders must remain relaxed to avoid tension. A gentle touch and verbal remainder from the nurse can be helpful (see Chapter 21).

Correct Position for Sitting in a Chair

When the woman is sitting in a chair (see Fig. 22–15), support her lumbar spine with a pillow or rolled towel, elevate the baby, and maximize support of the mother by using armrests and a

474 CHANGE: THE POSTPARTAL PERIOD

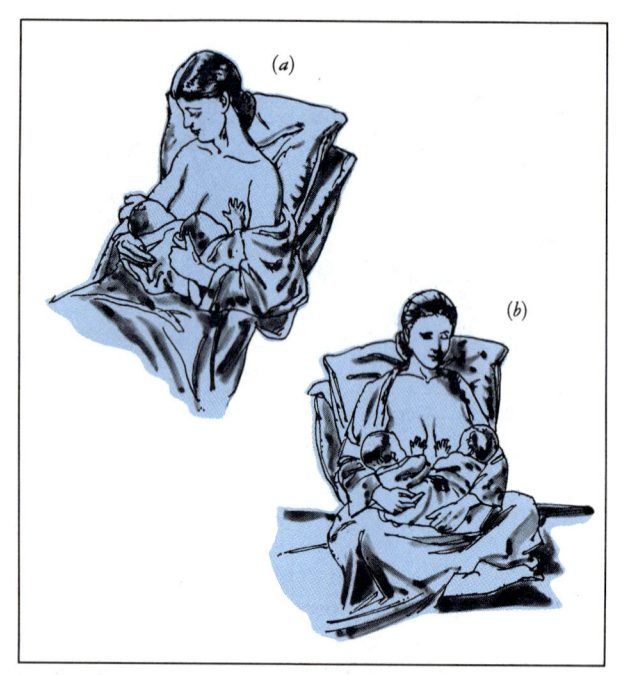

FIGURE 22–14. Nursing twins. (*a*) The "football" style; (*b*) babies lying across the front of the body.

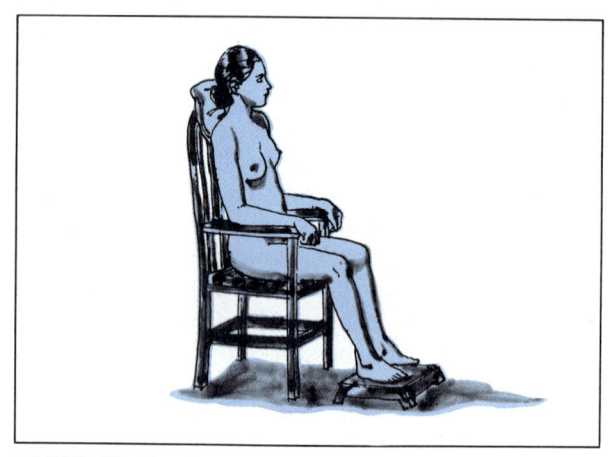

FIGURE 22–15. Correct position for sitting in a chair.

The mother should be cautioned against leaning or bending forward when caring for her infant in order to prevent low-back strain (see Fig. 22–17). Her infant should be raised approximately to countertop level for easy bathing, diapering, and dressing. The mother should be instructed to place one foot forward with the toes in the recessed toe space beneath the cupboard doors and the knee slightly bent. Her pelvis should remain properly aligned (neutral position), her shoulders should be relaxed, and her breathing should be diaphragmatic.

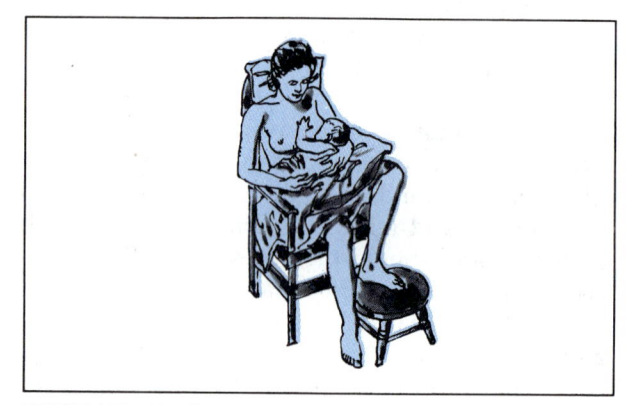

FIGURE 22–16. Proper support when breastfeeding reduces strain.

footstool on the side from which the baby is nursing (see Fig. 22–16).

Body Mechanics: Caring for the Infant

The woman becomes more active on the second postpartum day and begins to spend more time out of bed caring for her newborn infant. She should observe the proper transfer and ambulation techniques described for the first day postpartum.

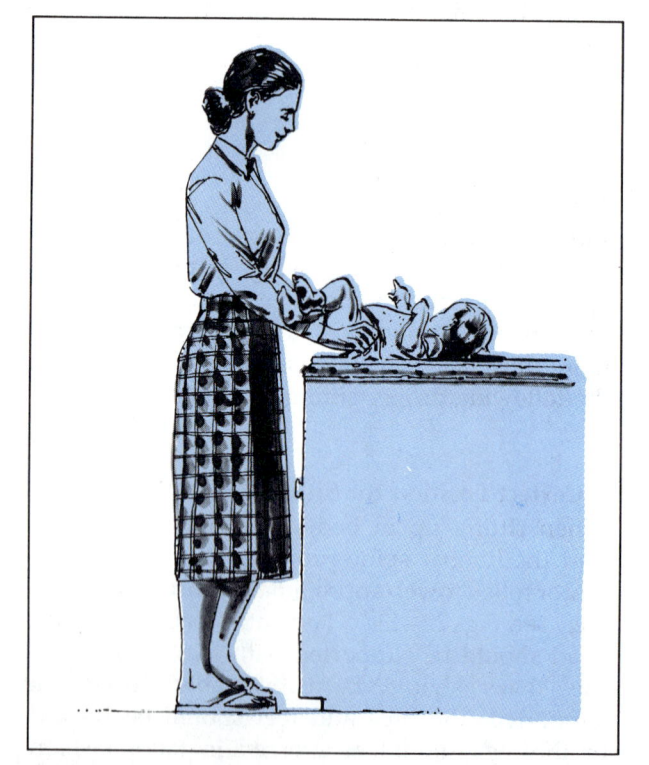

FIGURE 22–17. Correct working posture.

The mother should always be instructed to bend her knees when picking up an object and to keep her spine straight. She will not be able to lift heavy objects and older children safely until her pelvic floor and abdominal muscles begin to regain their normal position and strength. Older siblings should be encouraged to crawl up into their mother's lap or to sit beside her for attention and cuddling.

Pelvic alignment is easiest to maintain when the mother carries her infant across the front of her body with one or both arms, or with the infant lying prone over one arm, her hand supporting its head. Pelvic alignment is most difficult to maintain when the mother holds her infant upright over her shoulder. To do this, most women lean backward, overarching the low back and locking the knees, which creates stress and overstretches the ligaments. To hold or carry an infant correctly over her shoulder, the new mother must emphasize proper neutral alignment of her lumbar spine and pelvis, keeping her abdominal, buttocks, and perineal muscles firm. To facilitate maintenance of lumbopelvic alignment when standing, she must keep one foot forward with the knees slightly bent.

Abdominal Exercises

Abdominal strengthening exercises can progress only when the pelvic floor is able to withstand increased intraabdominal pressure (Noble, 1976).

The following pretest allows the nurse to determine whether the new mother's pelvic floor is of sufficient strength.

1. PELVIC FLOOR ASSESSMENT. Have the woman sit on the toilet with legs separated and feet flat. After she begins to urinate, have her attempt to stop and restart the urinary flow several times. If she has good control, it means that the strength of the pelvic floor has improved and the next set of exercises can be tolerated. If control is poor, or if the woman reports pelvic floor strain, she should not progress.

Progressive Abdominal Exercises

1. HIP HIKING. This exercise activates the lateral portions of the abdominal muscle and is performed in a supine position with head slightly elevated and legs straight. The woman should bring one hip up toward the shoulder during exhalation, pushing down with the other leg. Both legs should be kept straight. The first leg will feel as if it is becoming shorter, the other leg longer. She should alternate legs, repeating the exercise five times on each leg.

2. SUPINE BICYCLE. Having the patient move her legs will activate the lower portions of the abdominal muscles. This exercise is performed in the same position as hip hiking. The woman slides one heel up toward the buttocks and then returns it to the straight starting position while bringing up the opposite leg (see Fig. 22–18). She should be instructed to maintain the pelvis in a neutral position and to breathe smoothly. She should alternate legs, repeating the exercise five times.

Exercises in the Supine Position

The following exercises are performed in the supine position with the head flat, knees bent, and feet flat. A hand can be placed over the abdomen.

1. BUTTOCKS LIFT. Have the woman inhale and then exhale while stabilizing the pelvis in neutral and lifting the buttocks very slightly off the bed (Moore et al., 1987). The woman should then inhale again while holding the buttocks up, and then the buttocks should be lowered slowly during the next exhalation (see Fig. 22–19). This exercise is repeated five times. The buttocks should be kept low to prevent air from entering the vagina. Overstretching of the abdominal muscles and overarching of the lumbar spine should also be avoided (Shrock, Simpkin, and Shearer, 1981).

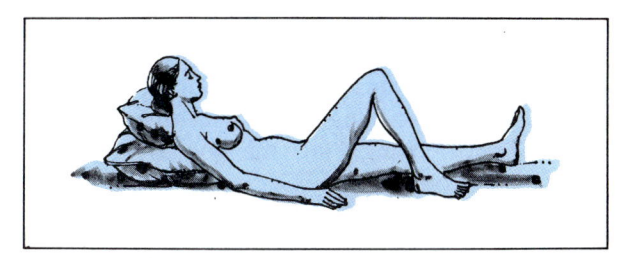

FIGURE 22–18. Supine bicycle.

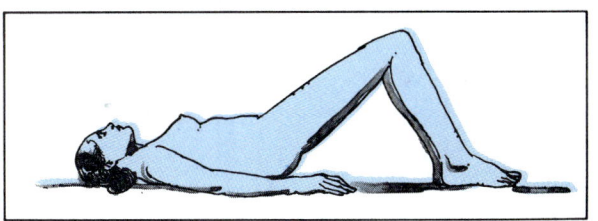

FIGURE 22–19. Buttocks lift.

476 CHANGE: THE POSTPARTAL PERIOD

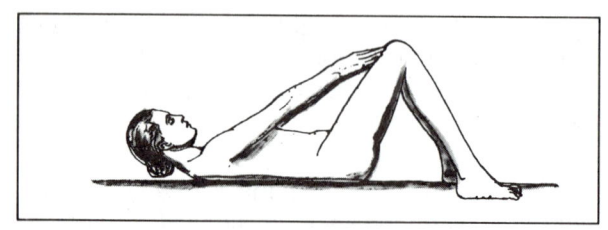

FIGURE 22–20. Head lift.

Head Lift

Position the woman with her knees bent, spine in neutral, and arms crossed on her chest, looking straight up at the ceiling (Moore et al., 1987). The exercise begins with an inhalation. The woman should exhale while lifting her head and neck straight up toward the ceiling (see Fig. 22–20). She should then slowly lower her head during inhalation. Lifting the head activates the upper regions of the abdominal muscles. Have her repeat this exercise five times.

Cervical and Thoracic Exercises

Heavy breasts and various nursing positions can create tension in the neck and upper back. The following exercises will aid relaxation in these areas.

For all but the flying exercise, the woman sits tailor fashion in the middle of the bed or on the edge of the bed with the feet on a stool.

1. POKE AND TUCK. Have the woman poke (jut) her chin forward and then tuck it back, as if to create a double chin. This exercise stretches the posterior cervical muscle group, which becomes tense if the head is allowed to hang forward, as often happens during breastfeeding. Have the woman repeat this exercise five times.

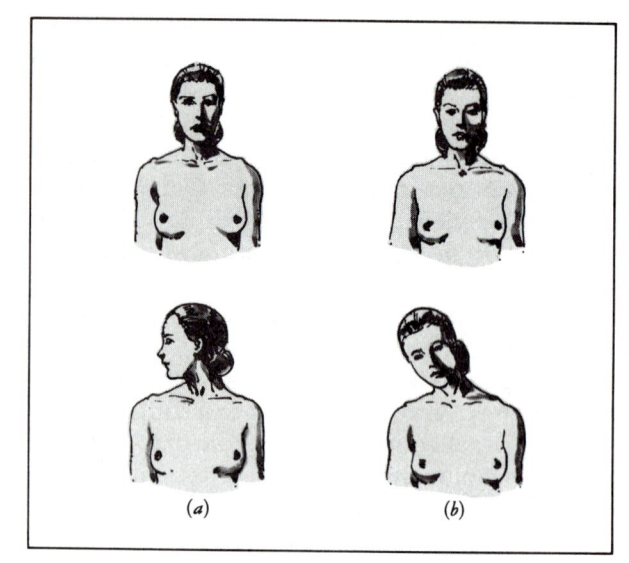

FIGURE 22–21. Neck exercises. (*a*) Rotation; (*b*) lateral flexion.

2. GENERAL CERVICAL RANGE OF MOTION. These exercises help to relieve tension in the neck.

   a. *Rotation.* Have the woman turn her head from side to side, looking over each shoulder. She should repeat this motion five times on each side (see Fig. 22–21*a*).
   b. *Lateral flexion.* The woman tilts her head from side to side bringing her ear close to the shoulder (see Fig. 22–21*b*). The shoulders remain level. Have her repeat the exercise five times on each side.

3. SCAPULAR ROTATION. The shoulders should be rotated forward and up during inhalation, back and down during exhalation (see Fig. 22–22). Have the woman repeat the exercise five times.

4. ELBOW CIRCLES. Place the woman's fingertips on her shoulders, and then have her rotate her elbows forward and up during inhalation, back

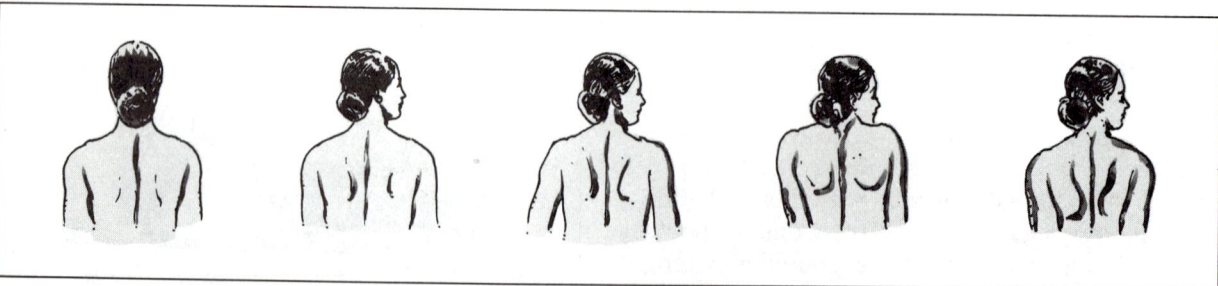

FIGURE 22–22. Scapular rotation.

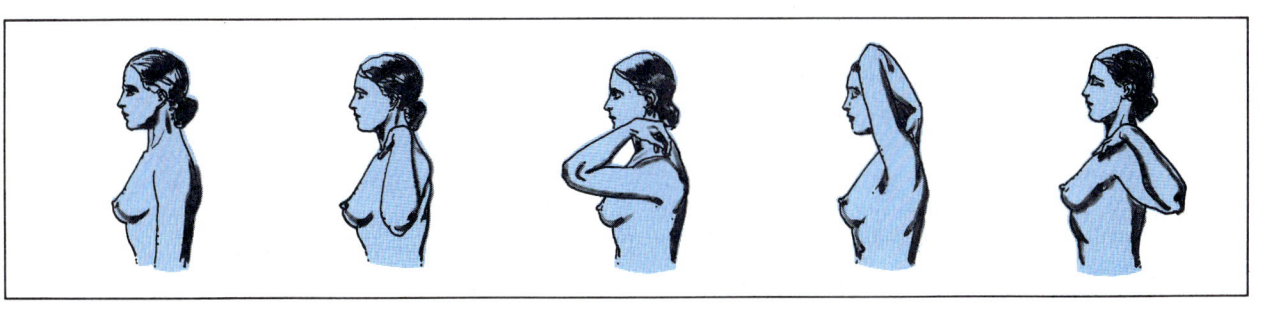

FIGURE 22–23. Elbow circles.

and down during exhalation (see Fig. 22–23). Have her repeat this exercise five times.

5. SCAPULAR RETRACTION AND PROTRACTION. The arms are abducted and the elbows are bent, each to 90 degrees. Have the woman retract the scapulae strongly during inhalation, bringing the elbows toward each other. Instruct the patient to protract the scapulae strongly and stretch the arms forward during exhalation, repeating this exercise five times (see Fig. 22–24). This action stretches the intrascapular muscle group, which frequently becomes tense in new mothers.

6. FLYING EXERCISE. Have the woman stretch her arms straight forward, over her head, and then down and back (see Fig. 22–25). Instruct her to push backward five times. Repeat the sequence five times. This movement encourages the chest to remain open and stimulates circulation around the breasts.

Visualizations

The nurse can suggest visualizations that may be helpful in achieving relaxation and in helping the woman to maintain a sense of herself as an individual.

As many sensual characteristics as possible should be incorporated when she views a scene – sights, sounds, colors, textures, tastes, smells, temperature, movements. Some suggested visualizations may include:

1. A perfect place – mountains, beach, home, forest.
2. An ideal room – study, nursery, bedroom.
3. Floating on water – lake, ocean, pool, hot tub.
4. Standing under a waterfall.
5. A favorite activity.
6. Her most successful job or most enjoyable work.
7. A prepregnancy time that was most satisfying.
8. A pleasant experience shared with her partner.
9. A pleasant experience shared with her new baby.

The visualization technique can also be used to help solve problems, reach goals, and break habits (Shealy, 1980). A picture of the desired improve-

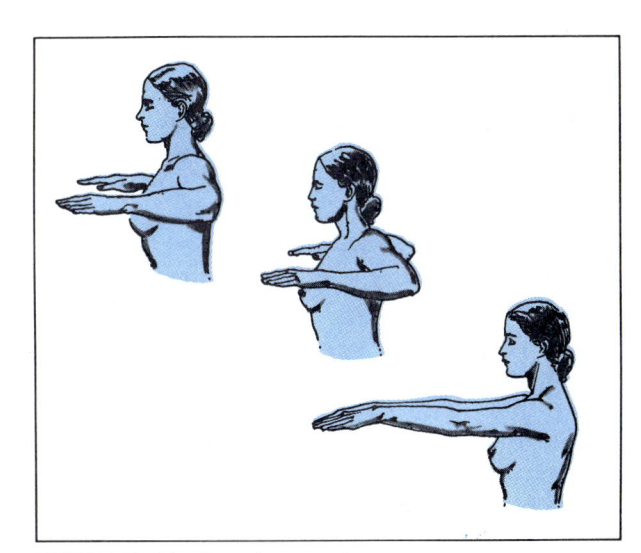

FIGURE 22–24. Scapular retraction and protraction.

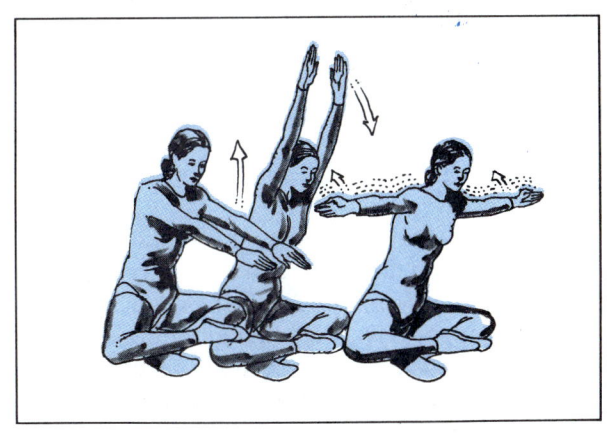

FIGURE 22–25. Flying exercise.

ment or result can be created in the mind. Emil Coué, a French pharmacist who lived in the early 1900s, proposed that the imagination is more powerful than the will. He referred to guiding the imagination as "conscious autosuggestion" (Shealy, 1980).

As the new mother becomes more active and busy with the care of her newborn, it is helpful for her to develop relaxation "cues" or ways of incorporating short relaxation exercises into her normal activities. Tension-producing situations can be recognized and can become cues for a relaxation response rather than a stress response. For a new mother, the newborn's cry is a useful cue. When she hears crying, the mother can inhale deeply and then consciously release tension as she exhales, allowing a wave of relaxation to flow over her face, jaw, neck, shoulders, body, and limbs. The entire response consumes only 6 seconds. One hundred repetitions per day would take only 10 minutes (Stroebel, 1982).

As the nurse performs routine nursing activities in the woman's room, she or he can teach the woman this technique. The nurse may also benefit from performing these relaxation exercises. Autogenic training phrases can be introduced to aid in achieving self-regulation and reducing stress.

The woman must be in a comfortable position prior to being asked to respond to the following phrases:

1. My arms and legs are heavy.
2. My arms and legs are warm.
3. My heartbeat is calm and regular.
4. It breathes me.
5. My solar plexus is warm.
6. My forehead is cool.

Each phrase is repeated silently, six times, and the entire sequence is repeated three times (Luthe, 1969).

POSTPARTUM RESTORATION: DAY 3

On the third postpartum day the abdominal muscles are evaluated to determine whether strengthening exercises can progress. If the muscles are strong enough, advanced strengthening exercises are introduced. Posture and body mechanics are reviewed. Relaxation is reinforced, and an additional technique is introduced.

Progressive Abdominal Exercises

The standing pelvic tilt exercise may be done on day 3. More advanced abdominal exercises should not be initiated if diastasis (separation) of the rectus muscles of the abdomen is greater than 1 inch. Special diagnostic tests and special abdominal exercises may be needed (Noble, 1976).

1. STANDING PELVIC REALIGNMENT EXERCISE. The patient should stand on a firm surface, keeping in mind all the points for good posture. To begin the exercise the nurse should instruct the patient to inhale and to release the abdominal, buttocks, and pelvic floor muscles, allowing the pelvis to tip anteriorly. This increases lordosis of the lumbar spine. While exhaling, the patient should perform a posterior pelvic tilt, consciously activating all of the abdominal muscles (see Fig. 22–26). The knees should be flexed slightly, and the buttocks should be tucked under. Instruct the patient to inhale, release, exhale, contract. Have her repeat the exercise 10 times. If the patient palpates the abdominal wall during this exercise, awareness of muscle action will be increased. She should palpate in the central abdominal region, inside the iliac crests, above the pubic bone and below the

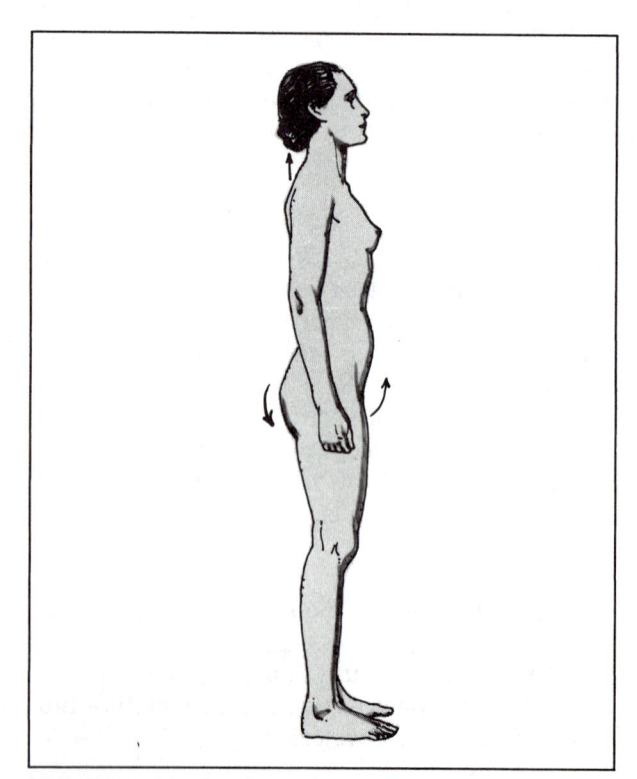

FIGURE 22–26. Standing pelvic realignment.

lower ribs. This exercise should end with progressively smaller oscillations until the lumbar spine and pelvis are in a "neutral" position (Johnson et al., 1987).

2. ABDOMINAL WALL CHECK. To test for separation of the rectus muscles the patient should be in the supine position, knees flexed, feet flat. The nurse should place fingers of one hand firmly into the abdominal wall near the navel. During an exhalation the woman is instructed to flatten her low back and raise her head and shoulders off the bed. The rectus muscles should contract and pull toward the midline. The soft separation between the tensed muscles is then measured by fingerbreadths. A small separation, one or two fingers wide, represents normally stretched tissues and exercises can progress (see Fig. 22–27a). A larger gap, three or four fingers wide, represents muscle weakness and mis-alignment (see Fig. 22–27b). A special exercise to protect and strengthen this area must then be performed until the muscles become normal (Noble, 1976).

3. ABDOMINAL EXERCISE FOR DIASTASIS. The patient should be in a supine position, knees bent, feet flat, hands crossed over the abdominal wall, positioned so that the muscles can be pulled toward the midline. Begin the exercise by having the patient inhale. Have her support the abdominal muscles firmly. While exhaling, she should hold the pelvis in neutral and pull the abdominal muscles together as she raises her head and upper scapulae up toward the ceiling (see Fig. 22–28). The buttocks and muscles of the pelvic floor are firmly contracted to help stabilize the pelvis. After several days she can lift both scapulae from the bed several inches. Have her repeat this exercise 10 times.

When abdominal strengthening exercises are

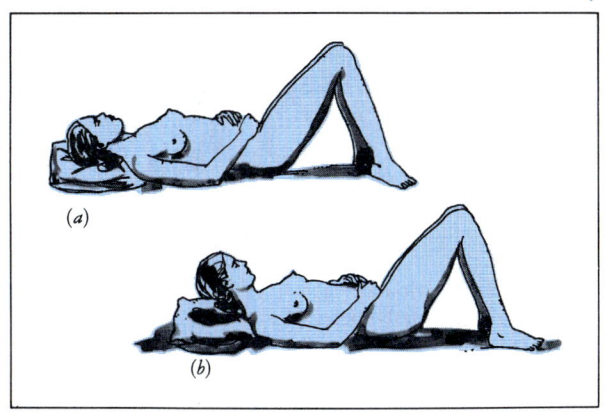

FIGURE 22–28. Abdominal exercise for diastasis. The rectus muscles must be supported. (*a*) Relaxation occurs during inhalation. (*b*) During exhalation, the woman performs a pelvic realignment and lifts her head.

designed, all four layers of abdominal muscles must be considered. The transverse abdominal muscle acts as a circular girdle (see Fig. 22–29). It is strongly activated when an exercise is performed during exhalation. The rectus abdominis muscle is more active during midline lift-ups. The internal and external oblique muscles are most active in diagonal lifts. The upper portions of these muscles work hardest when the woman lifts her head and upper body, the lower portions when she stabilizes the pelvis during leg lifts.

The nurse should help the patient coordinate the breath with each exercise. Exhaling reduces intraabdominal pressure during exercise, thereby minimizing strain on the pelvic floor, on the lumbar spine, and especially on the abdominal wall itself.

4. DOUBLE LEG SLIDING. Instruct the patient to assume a supine position, knees bent, feet flat. Have her inhale. While exhaling she should

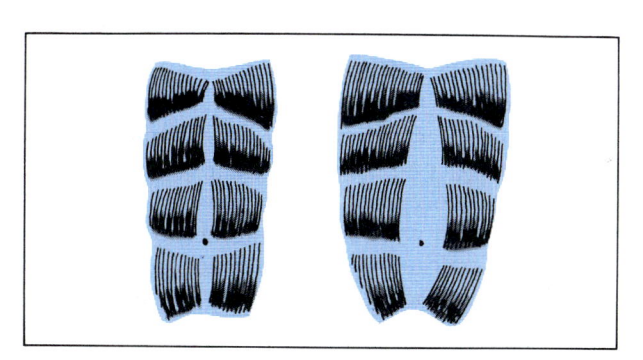

FIGURE 22–27. Diastasis. The rectus muscles of the abdomen can separate.

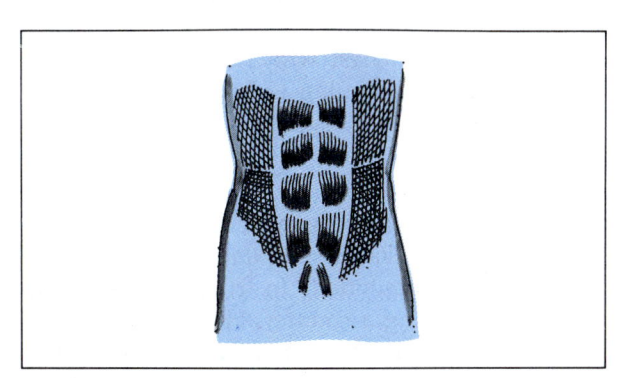

FIGURE 22–29. The muscles of the abdominal wall.

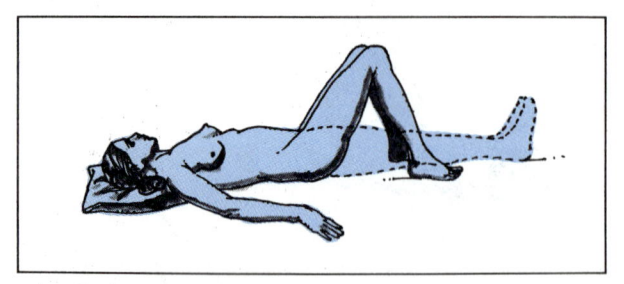

FIGURE 22-30. Double leg sliding. Maintain neutral lumbo-pelvic alignment.

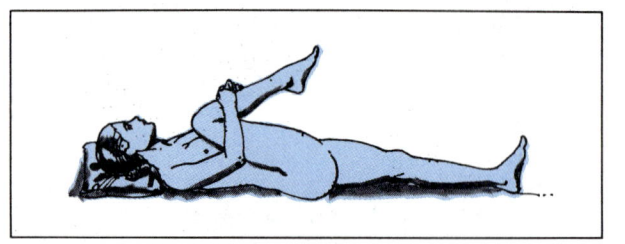

FIGURE 22-31. Single knee-to-chest stretch.

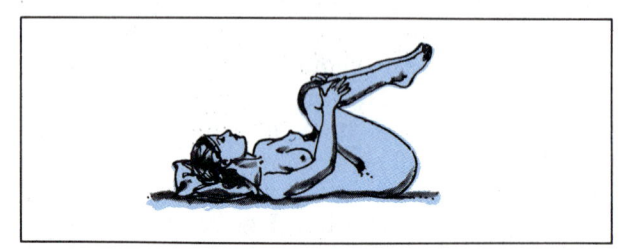

FIGURE 22-32. Double knee-to-chest stretch.

strongly stabilize her pelvis in neutral, slowly sliding her legs out straight until her back begins to arch (see Fig. 22-30). This indicates the limit of adequate abdominal wall function. She should then slide her heels back up to the starting position during inhalation. As her strength improves, pelvic stability will be maintained through the complete range of lower extremity extension. This exercise should be repeated 10 times.

Low Back Exercises

If low-back discomfort is present, emphasize proper posture and the pelvic realignment exercise, and encourage the following stretching exercises, to be done in a supine position, with knees bent and feet flat.

1. SINGLE KNEE-TO-CHEST STRETCH. Have the patient inhale. While she is exhaling, have her lift one knee toward the chest and then gently pull it up as far as possible with the hands (see Fig. 22-31). As the stretch is released, she should inhale but continue to hold the knee. The stretch should be repeated 5-10 times for each leg.

2. DOUBLE KNEE-TO-CHEST STRETCH. Have the patient inhale. While she is exhaling, have her lift one knee, then the other. She should stretch them both toward her chest with her hands (see Fig. 22-32). While continuing to hold her knees, she releases the stretch. This exercise is repeated 5-10 times.

3. SUPPORTED FORWARD BENDING STRETCH. To prevent general backache and fatigue, a standing stretch is recommended. Instruct the patient to stand erect, facing a counter. Have her place her hands on the counter and walk backward while bending at the hips until her arms and spine are straight (see Fig. 22-33). Ideally, her back should be flat, with the hips flexed 90 degrees. Have her complete five slow, full breaths, lengthening the spine and stretching the legs and shoulders more with each breath. Then instruct her to walk toward the counter when finished, relaxing her arms to her sides and slowly coming to an erect position.

POSTCESAREAN SECTION RESTORATION

The postcesarean new mother presents a dual problem. She has undergone surgery as well as childbirth. Both conditions must be considered in her postpartum exercise program. Several important points typically distinguish the mother who gives birth by cesarean section:

1. Her hospital stay will be longer.
2. She becomes fatigued more easily.
3. She has more pain.
4. Her period of dependency may be prolonged and intense (Rubin, 1961).
5. She may need closer emotional support or counseling, particularly if complications or an emergency occurred during her labor.
6. Her postpartum program will incorporate postsurgical precautionary breathing and exercise techniques, special comfort measures and relaxation.
7. Her restoration exercises are nearly identical to

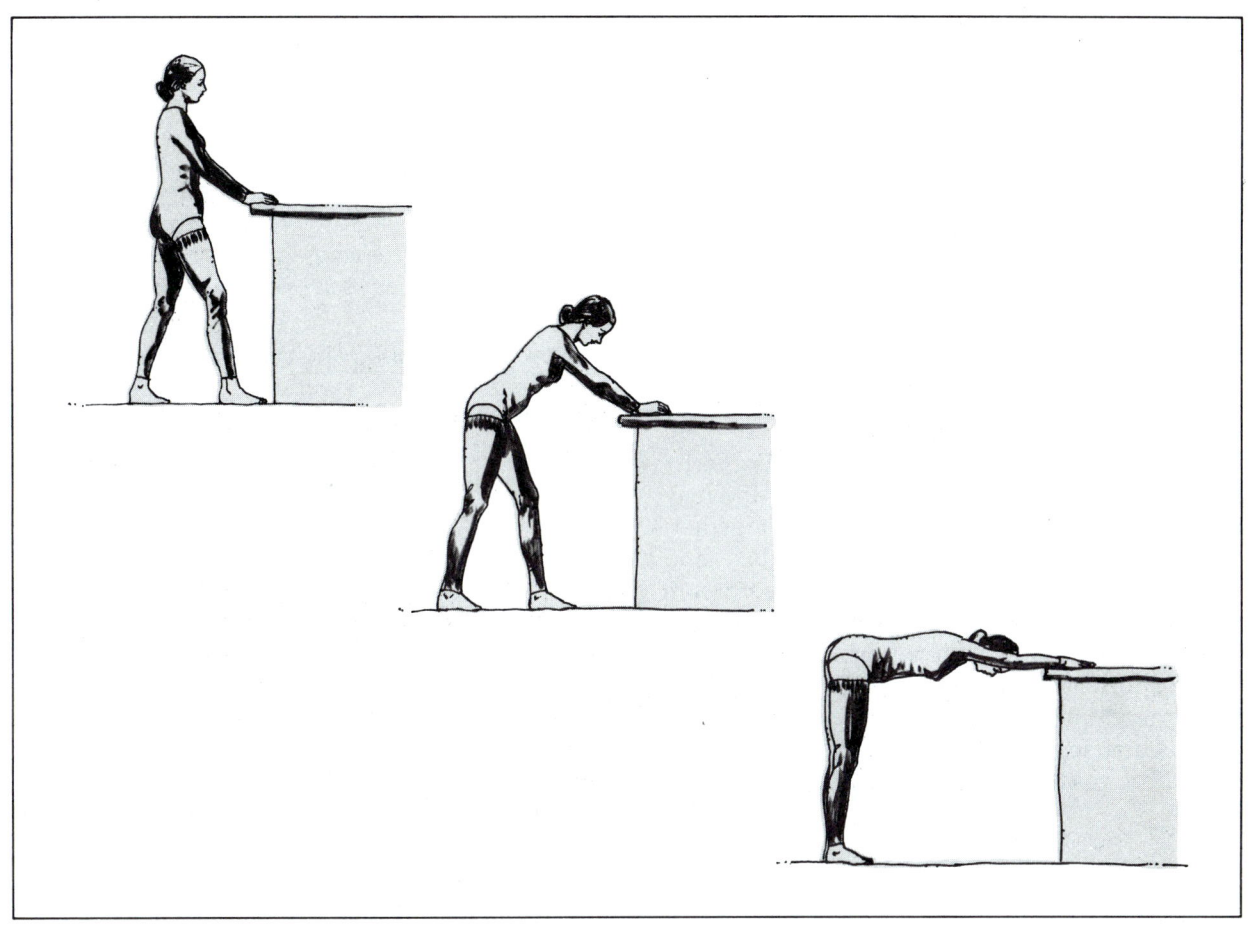

FIGURE 22–33. Supported forward-bending stretch.

the program for mothers who delivered vaginally, but they progress at a different rate.

Comfort Measures and Body Mechanics

Although these new mothers experience pain postpartally, they are eager to care for their infants as soon as possible. When the nurse observes the level of discomfort and intervenes effectively with exercise techniques, the need for pain medication may be reduced considerably.

Maintaining the abdominal muscles in a relaxed state with the head and shoulders supported on pillows will improve comfort of the abdominal wall immediately after surgery. The side-lying position is also comfortable initially. Later, when comfort permits, the prone position with pillow support under the lower abdomen can be used (see Figs. 22–1 through 22–3). The woman's abdominal muscles can be protected further if she avoids actively lifting her head. During the first few hours, the nurse should provide the woman with a flexible straw for drinking fluids, or should ensure that someone assists the patient to lift her head.

When the mother is ready to breastfeed, the nurse can recommend the side-lying position or the football hold, or place a pillow over the incision to support and protect it.

For the first 1–2 days, moving in bed or getting out of bed should be done slowly to avoid strain and discomfort, and the woman should support the incisional area with her hands or a pillow. Mothers who have had cesarean sections may need to have the head of the bed fully raised before getting up. They can also use an overhead trapeze to improve mobility in bed and to assist in transfers. When the mother stands up, she will tend to lean forward excessively to protect her sore and distended abdomen. She will need firm encouragement to perform her restorative exercise program. She will also need assurance from the nurse that her comfort and posture will improve with gentle activity and early ambulation.

Early ambulation is the key to postcesarean

comfort and recovery. Gentle, slow ambulation will:

1. Stimulate circulation, thus reducing stiffness and pain.
2. Encourage kidney, bladder and intestinal activity.
3. Facilitate healing.
4. Eliminate anesthetic agents from her system more quickly.

If the patient can begin to move before she becomes too stiff, her need for pain medication may be reduced. Conversely, medication often leads to lethargy and prolonged inactivity. Early, gentle activity is the preferred alternative and may eliminate the need for pain medication altogether.

Ideally, women should be out of bed and ambulating in their rooms and to the bathroom within 12–18 hours after delivery. Ambulating in the corridors should begin within 24 hours.

Flatus formation is increased following abdominal surgery, particularly if general anesthesia was used, because anesthesia slows bowel action. Relief from gas discomfort can be gained in several ways:

1. Lying on the left side with the right knee drawn up and supported will aid in opening the bowel passage.
2. Massaging the abdomen will stimulate peristaltic action.
3. Diaphragmatic breathing, pelvic realignment exercises, and early ambulation will stimulate bowel activity.
4. A light enema or flush will clear the bowels (Harris, 1980).

Postsurgical Exercises: Day 1

The two primary postsurgical conditions that can be prevented by proper early exercises include collection of mucus in the lungs and thrombosis formation (Jesscoate and Tindall, 1965). The first can aggravate existing respiratory conditions or end in pneumonia. The second can have more serious consequences.

Respiratory Exercises
A thorough breathing regimen activates all regions of the lungs and ensures complete ventilation and mobilization of secretions. The following exercises are conducted when the patient is in a supine or side-lying position with head, shoulders, and knees supported.

1. DIAPHRAGMATIC BREATHING. Encourage gentle movement of the abdominal wall. The postcesarean mother may tend to splint the region because of its sensitivity. As the woman's pain subsides, the nurse should encourage stronger contraction of the abdominal muscles during exhalation.

2. LOW RIB EXPANSION. Instruct the patient to place her hands over the inverted "V" formed by the low ribs. Have her apply gentle pressure during inhalation. At the end of exhalation firmer pressure may be applied to facilitate emptying of the lungs.

3. MIDDLE RIB EXPANSION. The patient should place the backs of her hands over the sides of the ribs about 3 inches below the axillae. During the inhalation, have her apply gentle pressure while expanding the ribs. Firmer pressure should be applied during exhalation.

4. UPPER CHEST EXPANSION. Have the patient place one hand over the mid-sternum and apply gentle pressure while she tries to raise the sternum during inhalation. She should apply only slightly firmer pressure at the end of the exhalation.

5. HUFFING. This exercise should replace coughing for several reasons. It is easier to perform, it is less painful, it does not strain the incision and, most important, it does not stress the muscles of the pelvic floor or abdominal wall. Coughing requires closure of the glottis and tensing of the abdominal muscles, with an increase in intraabdominal pressure. Huffing is performed during exhalation, with the diaphragm moving up, the abdominal muscles contracting inward, and the intraabdominal pressure decreasing. Thus, strain on the incision and the pelvic floor is avoided. To instruct the patient in this exercise, have her inhale deeply. She should then open her mouth, keeping the jaw relaxed. The patient should say "huff" or "ha" quickly and briskly while exhaling, forcefully contracting the abdominal muscles and diaphragm to dislodge any mucus. She should then spit out the mucus. This exercise should be repeated three times each waking hour. If chest secretions are present, have her repeat the breathing and huffing sequence two or three times each time she does it. Respiratory therapy is available to treat more serious chest conditions (Noble, 1976).

Lower-Extremity Exercises

Ankle exercises are important in preventing thrombosis following surgery. Lower-extremity exercises will help prepare the woman for early ambulation, particularly following regional anesthesia.

Beginning Restoration Exercises: Days 2 Through 4

Before the woman begins walking, introduce pelvic realignment exercises and a more active lower-extremity exercise. These exercises will improve comfort, facilitate mobility, and encourage good posture. They will also help to stimulate gastrointestinal activity and bladder function that have been suppressed by the anesthesia. Early, gentle exercises will reassure the mother that her muscles can work and that her incision is secure.

Most postcesarean mothers can begin ambulating in the halls on day 2. The woman should support her incision with her hands while getting up. Once she is standing erect, her tightened abdominal wall can begin to take over the supportive function of her hands.

1. MODIFIED HEAD LIFT. The patient assumes a semireclining position with knees bent and arms crossed on her chest. Have the patient inhale. While exhaling, the woman should lift her head and neck slowly toward the ceiling. She should again inhale, while slowly returning to the starting position. This exercise should be repeated five times. The new mother should support her incision with her hands for comfort if needed.

2. STANDING PELVIC REALIGNMENT. By the third day the postcesarean mother's comfort should be improved adequately to allow her to perform this exercise. Her posture should begin to show improvement (see Fig. 22–26).

Progressive Restoration Exercises: Day 5

Women with low transverse incisions may be able to progress to abdominal exercises by the fifth day, particularly if they have exercised prenatally. Each woman must be assessed carefully by the nurse before, during, and after performing the exercises.

Women who have a classical midline incision should not increase abdominal exercises beyond the head lift and supine, side-lying and standing pelvic realignment exercises for 2 weeks.

Relaxation

The postcesarean mother will experience more fatigue as a result of the surgical procedure. Her emotions may be quite labile and may include negative feelings toward herself, the baby, and possibly the medical staff (Harris, 1980). This array of feelings might include disappointment, sadness or grief, anger, resentment, feelings of failure, and a sense of being invaded. Because her hospital stay is longer and her care more intensive, the nurse will have a greater opportunity to counsel and guide her in relaxation techniques. These will improve her physical comfort and the efficiency of her rest. There are psychologic and emotional benefits as well. Regular relaxation periods will help her accept reality, help create a sense of inner peace, enhance closure of past events, and heighten interest in meeting life's next challenges.

DISCHARGE PLANNING

Prior to discharge, the nurse should review the following with the new mother:

1. Diaphragmatic breathing.
2. Correct posture – neutral lumbo-pelvic alignment.
3. Pelvic floor exercises, including comfort measures and evaluation.
4. Abdominal strengthening exercises, including evaluation.
5. Comfortable positions for resting and feeding, giving several alternatives.
6. Body mechanics for transferring, standing, bending, lifting, and working.
7. Relaxation techniques.
8. Safety precaution:
   - no heavy lifting;
   - no full sit-ups;
   - no supine double leg lifts.

The summary chart (Fig. 22–34) can be given to the new mother upon discharge. The trend toward early discharge allows for less educational time in the hospital. The chart is a useful reminder and guide to a medically approved postpartum return to health.

Once the new mother is at home, she will gradually return to her normal activities. House-

Comfort Measures Day 1	Perineum: Ice pack, Kegel exercise Positions: Supine, Side-lying, 3/4, prone; all with pillow supports at head, knees and at pelvis for prone only
Day 2	Use nursing bra, take warm sitz baths, continue Kegel exercise, lie in prone position (twice/day for 30–60 minutes), ambulate
Breathing	Diaphragmatic preferred to thoracic

Exercises		Duration	Reps	Freq
Day 1 Begin	**Pelvic Realignment** 1. Tighten pelvic floor (Kegel) 2. Tighten abdominals 3. Tighten abdominals and pelvic floor 4. Tighten abdominals, pelvic floor, and gluteals 5. *Find neutral spine*	1–3–5 secs 5–10 secs 3–5–10 secs 3–5–10 secs	5 5 5 5	Hourly 2Xday 2Xday 2Xday
	Lower Extremities 6. Flex/extend ankle 7. Circle ankle 8. Activate quadriceps (thighs)	 5–10 secs	10 10 10	Hourly Hourly Hourly
Day 2 Add	**Abdominals/Pelvis** 1. Assess pelvic floor (control urinating w/hold-release) 2. Hip-hiking 3. Supine bicycle 4. Buttocks lift 5. Head lift	 5 secs Continuous 5 secs 5 secs	 1 5 5 5 5	 Daily 2Xday 2Xday 2Xday 2Xday
	Cervical/Thoracic Spine 6. Poke and tuck chin 7. Rotate/laterally flex neck 8. Rotate scapulae (shldr blades) 9. Circle elbows 10. Retract and protract scapulae	 All slow Continuous	5 5 5 5 5	2Xday 2Xday 2Xday 2Xday 2Xday
Day 3 Add	**Abdominals/Lumbar Spine** 1. Standing pelvic realignment 2. Assess abdominal wall 3. Abdominal exercise for diastasis (muscle separation) 4. Double leg sliding 5. Single knee-to-chest stretch 6. Double knee-to-chest stretch 7. Supported forward-bending stretch	 5 secs Continuous 5–10 secs 5–10 secs 5 breaths	 when up 1 10 10 5–10 5–10 1	Daily Daily 2Xday 2Xday 2Xday 2Xday 3Xday

Body Mechanics	Getting out of bed, standing, walking, getting into bed, sitting up in bed, sitting in chair, nursing; maintain *neutral spine*, use lumbar pillow support
Relaxation Techniques	Progressive Relaxation, Touch-Release Response, Positive Affirmation, Massage, Visualization (15 min 2Xday)

FIGURE 22–34. Recommended postpartum restoration summary.

work will help to prevent general muscle wasting but will not strengthen weakened muscles (Blankfield, 1967). When helping the patient to choose an exercise program or activity, the nurse should remind her that the musculoskeletal changes will take 6–8 weeks to return to a normal, nonpregnant state (Danforth, 1967). During this period, the ligaments will remain soft and the joints loose. Therefore, exercises that include excessive stretching and jarring (such as vigorous gymnastics, running, and certain types of aerobic dancing) should be avoided during this period to prevent strain. Safe activities include walking, swimming, and cycling. A woman can begin an exercise or yoga class 2 weeks after a vaginal delivery and 4–6 weeks after a cesarean delivery. Ideally, she should seek an instructor with experience in dealing with postnatal women. With or without such a class, the mother must be responsible for observing proper body mechanics and avoiding overstretching and strain.

Mothers usually have difficulty finding time to exercise or practice relaxation techniques at home. The nurse must encourage the woman to rest when the baby sleeps and not try to accomplish her work during that time.

Women are usually impatient to return to their usual body shape. The nurse should remind the new mother that when she is breastfeeding she will need to carry some extra fat on her body, and that, while good nutrition is important, excessive dieting is not appropriate. The nurse can reassure the mother that the time needed for a woman to return to her normal figure after delivery is quite variable and the process may require 6–12 months.

SUMMARY

A complete postpartum restoration program for the hospitalized new mother includes exercises, posture, body mechanics, positions of comfort, and relaxation techniques. The nurse should be able to plan and safely guide a new postpartum mother in an appropriate restorative program.

REFERENCES

Blankfield, A. 1967. Is exercise necessary for the obstetric patient? *Med. J. Australia.* 1:163–165.

Cherry, L. 1978. Interview with Hans Selye. Eustress. *Psych. Today.* 12(2):60–69.

Danforth, D. N. 1967. Pregnancy and labor. *Am. J. Phys. Med.* 46:653–658.

Downing, G. 1972. *The massage book.* New York: Random House, The Book Works.

Forbes, G. 1944. Air embolism as a complication of vaginal douching in pregnancy. *Brit. Med. J.* 2:529–531.

Harris, J. K. 1980. Self-care is possible after cesarean delivery. *Nurs. Clin. N. Amer.* 15(1):191–204.

Helfer, R., and Kemp, H. 1974. *The battered child.* 2nd ed. Chicago: University of Chicago Press.

Jacobson, E. 1965. *Progressive relaxation.* Chicago: University of Chicago Press.

Jesscoate, T. N. A., and Tindall, V. R. 1965. Venous thrombosis and embolism in obstetrics and gynecology. *Australia-New Zealand J. Obstet. Gynecol.* 5:119.

Jesscoate, T. N. A., and Tindall, V. R. 1973. Knee-chest exercises and maternal death. *Med. J. Australia.* 1:1127.

Johnson, G. S., et al. 1987. Institute of Physical Art, class notes.

Luthe, W. 1969. *Autogenic therapy. Vol. I: Autogenic methods.* San Diego: Grune & Stratton.

Marecki, M. P. 1979. Postpartum follow-up: Goals and assessment. *J. Obstet. Gynecol. Neonatal Nurs.* 8(4):214–218.

Moore, M., et al. 1987. "Training the patient with low back dysfunction," class notes.

Noble, E. 1976. *Essential exercises for the childbearing year.* Boston: Houghton Mifflin.

Nuernberger, P. 1981. *Freedom from stress, a holistic approach.* Honesdale, Pa.: Himalayan International Institute of Yoga, Science and Philosophy.

Rubin, R. 1961. Puerperal changes. *Nurs. Outlook.* 9:753.

Shealy, C. N. 1980. *90 days to self-health.* New York: Bantam Books.

Shrock, P.; Simpkin, P.; and Shearer, M. 1981. Teaching prenatal exercise. Part II: Exercises to think twice about. *Birth Fam. J.* 8(2):167–175.

Stroebel, C. 1982. *QR: The quieting reflex.* New York: Putnam.

23

The Nurse's Role in the Postpartum Period

BEHAVIORAL OBJECTIVES

Upon completion of this chapter, the reader should be able to:

- Assess the physiologic behaviors of a postpartum patient.

- Plan nursing interventions that promote postpartal adaptation.

- Identify mothering behaviors in terms of Rubin's phases of maternal development, Ludington-Hoe's concept of maternicity, and Mercer's criteria for mother–infant bonding.

- Assess the readiness of the patient to assume the maternal role.

- Implement nursing interventions to foster mothering behaviors.

- Discuss the process of transition to motherhood.

- Identify situations that hinder role transition to motherhood.

- List criteria for early hospital discharge.

The period following delivery is exciting yet stressful for the postpartal patient. The physiologic and psychologic changes that occur during the puerperium are stimuli for the maternal adaptation process and the development of new coping mechanisms. The pregnant woman is changing both physically, as her body undergoes the process of involution, and emotionally, as the process of maternal role transition begins. The ease with which she progresses through these changes is determined in part by her level of knowledge and by the availability of support systems. Nurses serve as invaluable resource personnel, since they are able to provide information, offer support, and function as role models.

This chapter focuses on the physical assessment of the postpartal patient, along with nursing care related to the promotion of postpartal physical well-being. The chapter also presents several frameworks for the identification of mothering behaviors and emphasizes the nurse's role in assisting the woman to assume the maternal role and in encouraging adaptive mothering behaviors.

PHYSICAL ASSESSMENT

Physical assessments should be performed routinely on every maternity patient. The frequency of postpartum checks after transfer to the maternity unit from the recovery room varies with each hospital. As a guideline, the nurse should palpate the fundus and observe the lochia every 4 hours during the first 24 hours if the results are within normal limits. Following that, assessments are done at the beginning of each shift, or every 8 hours.

To perform a postpartum physical assessment, the practitioner proceeds in a logical and systematic sequence starting with the vital signs and then working from the breasts downward. Prior to the examination the patient is encouraged to void, since a full bladder can displace the uterus and can also be a source of discomfort during the procedure. The nurse should check the mother's perineal pad before it is discarded in the bathroom.

Vital Signs

The temperature may be slightly elevated following delivery because of dehydration in the first 24 hours (see Chapter 20). An infection should be suspected, however, if the temperature exceeds 38°C (100.4°F) after the first 24 hours. If the temperature is elevated, the nurse should assess the patient for signs and symptoms of infection, such as complaints of discomfort, localized pain, or tenderness. The patient's pulse rate should be checked, since an increase is significant if it occurs in conjunction with a rising temperature.

During the early puerperium, the pulse rate normally decreases, usually to about 60–70 beats/min. The pulse may be as low as 40–50 beats/min on postpartal days one and two but returns to the patient's baseline by the tenth day following delivery. A pulse rate above 100 beats/min indicates a possible problem, and the physician should be notified. An elevated pulse could be a sign of infection, blood loss, cardiac abnormalities, or anxiety.

The blood pressure and respiratory rate should remain fairly constant and within the range of the woman's baseline values.

Lungs

The chest assessment should include palpation, percussion, and auscultation. During palpation, the chest can be observed for symmetrical lung expansion. On percussion healthy lung tissue will be resonant. Breathing sounds should be assessed posteriorly, laterally, and anteriorly. The patient should be instructed to breathe more deeply through her mouth as the nurse listens to the lung areas. Any abnormal or adventitious sounds (such as rales and rhonchi) should be noted.

Breasts

Breasts should be observed for color, secretions, nipple shape (erect or inverted), and nipple condition (intact, cracked, or fissured), and should be palpated to determine fullness, firmness, and warmth. The mother should be asked whether she feels any tingling or tenderness upon palpation. Breasts that are red and warm may indicate an infection, especially when these conditions are accompanied by an increased temperature. Breasts that are tender, lumpy, hard, and feel tense indicate the problem of engorgement. In this condition, the skin covering the breasts appears to be shiny and tight (see Chapter 21).

Abdomen

The abdomen should be auscultated with a stethoscope. Bowel sounds should be assessed in all four quadrants and described in the patient's record. The nurse should observe for the presence of diastasis recti, which is the separation of the rectus muscles of the abdominal wall. The width of the diastasis recti can be measured by palpating the separation below the umbilicus and the length can be measured by ascertaining the distance from the symphysis pubis to the xiphoid process. If the diastasis is difficult to locate, the patient should raise her head without assistance, since this action helps to define the rectus muscle through contraction. Nursing interventions for this condition would focus on exercises to increase the muscle tone of the abdominal area (see Chapter 22).

Palpating the fundus is one of the most important methods for determining the progress of involution. Firmness of the fundus indicates whether the uterus is contracting properly. The nurse should place one hand at the symphysis pubis and the other hand above the umbilicus. The fundus should be palpable at the level of the umbilicus. The fundus should feel firm, with a size and consistency similar to that of a grapefruit. If the fundus feels boggy or flabby, the nurse can intervene by massaging it until it becomes firm. Caution should be exercised to avoid overmassaging since the uterus can be overstimulated, contributing to muscle fatigue.

The rate of uterine involution is determined by measuring the height of the fundus in relation to the umbilicus (see Fig. 23–1). Decreasing fundal height indicates that involution is progressing satisfactorily. The nurse should also note the location of the fundus in relation to the midline position. If the fundus is elevated or deviated from the midline to the right side of the abdomen, the nurse can suspect a full bladder. Because a full bladder obstructs the uterus from contracting, nursing interventions are directed toward urinary elimination (see Chapter 20).

The mother who has had a cesarean section requires slightly different nursing management. Assessment is similar to that required for a surgical patient. The woman's bowel sounds should be checked to determine whether peristalsis has returned, since general anesthesia may have been administered. The abdominal dressing should be assessed for drainage and the surgical incision evaluated for signs of infection. Palpation of the fundus must be done gently. Flatus is a concern of many cesarean section patients. Nursing interventions for this problem include promoting ambulation, assessing for bowel elimination, and providing effervescent beverages.

A common discomfort experienced by postpartal patients of both types is "afterpains." When the fundus is palpated, many patients will comment on the discomfort and pain caused by the contract-

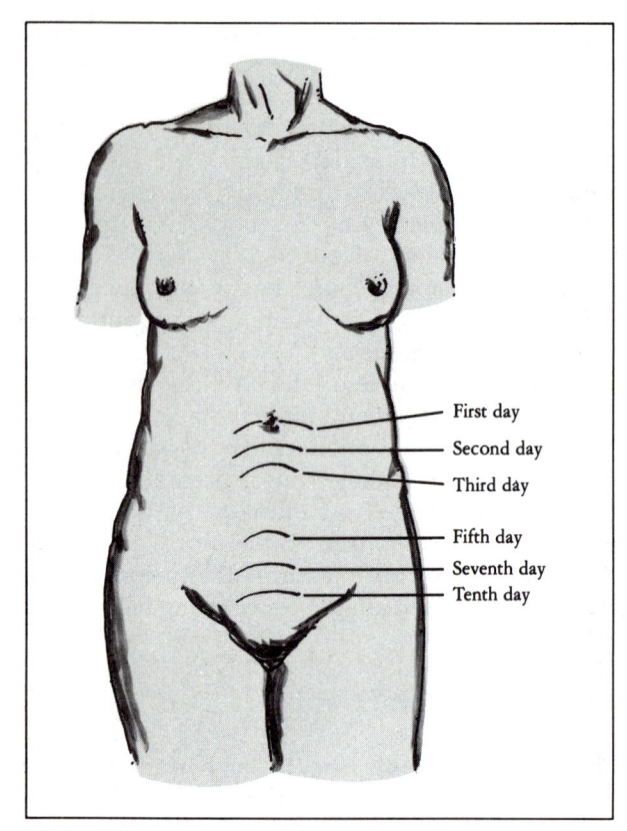

FIGURE 23–1. Descent of the fundus.

ing uterus. The nurse can intervene by discussing the prevalence and etiology of afterpains and suggesting ways to decrease the discomfort. Several options are available, including taking an analgesic, practicing breathing and relaxation techniques utilized in labor, and lying flat on the abdomen (see Chapter 22 for relaxation techniques).

Suprapubic Area

The nurse should assess the bladder for fullness and determine the frequency and amount of voidings. A distended bladder will rise above the symphysis pubis; if it is markedly distended, it can be seen as a bulge between the symphysis pubis and the umbilicus (see Fig. 23–2). Upon palpation, a distended bladder feels like a fluid-filled sac, whereas the uterus has a firmer consistency and feels solid. Within 4 hours following delivery, a bedpan should be offered to the mother, as the urge to void may be diminished from overdistention of the bladder resulting in loss of bladder tone. An important nursing intervention is to record fluid intake and output for the first 24 hours

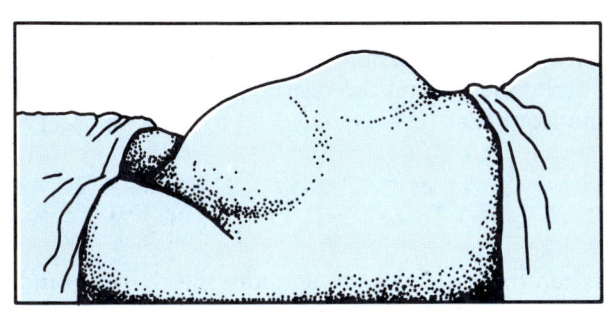

FIGURE 23-2. The uterus pushed up by a full bladder.

to ensure appropriate elimination. The first voiding should be at least 500 ml.

If the mother has difficulty voiding, the nurse can implement a care plan used for all patients who have problems with urination. Common interventions include having the woman pour warm water over the vulva, listen to the sound of running water, and drink a warm beverage. If the woman has to use a bedpan, have her sit upright, which places pressure on the urethra and facilitates urination. To increase the patient's comfort, a thoughtful nurse will provide privacy and offer a warmed bedpan.

If the woman is unable to urinate within 6-8 hours after delivery or if her voidings are frequent and less than 100 ml, catheterization must be considered. To avoid having the patient acquire a nosocomial (hospital-acquired) infection, the conscientious nurse is encouraged to be creative and persistent when attempting to promote adequate urinary elimination.

Vaginal and Perineal Area

The mother should be placed in a supine position so the nurse can observe the lochial discharge. Assessment of the lochia includes type of discharge (rubra, serosa, or alba), odor, and amount (see Chapter 20). The odor of lochia varies among patients; however, it should not be offensive. Foul-smelling discharge is indicative of an infection or the presence of decomposing blood clots and further assessment is required. The quantity of lochia can be ascertained by determining the number of pads soaked in 1 hour; pads should also be checked for large clots or pieces of tissue. A postpartal patient can be expected to use two pads during the first hour following delivery, then one pad every 2-4 hours for the next 8 hours. After 8 hours, the quantity of discharge should resemble the woman's normal menstrual flow. When assessing the quantity of lochia, the nurse can use the following standard: (1) scant is defined as blood only on tissue when wiped or less than one-inch stain on a peripad; (2) light is defined as less than four-inch stain on a peripad; (3) moderate as less than six-inch stain on a peripad; and (4) heavy as saturated peripad within one hour (Jacobson, 1985).

From the supine position, the mother should turn on her side, with the top leg flexed forward, to allow visualization of the perineum and anal area. Good lighting is essential when inspecting for hematomas, swelling, proper healing of episiotomy, and hemorrhoids. Complaints of severe perineal pain accompanied by a tumor or mass of varying size and by discolored skin indicate the possible development of a hematoma. Small hematomas are allowed to reabsorb; large hematomas require medical intervention. Hemorrhoids are usually more painful during the early puerperium and will gradually decrease in size. Nursing management of this common postpartal problem involves teaching various techniques for reducing the discomfort. The mother can be taught to reinsert the hemorrhoid using a glove or finger cot while maintaining digital pressure for 1-2 minutes, to utilize Sims's position to relieve some of the congestion from the rectal veins, and to remove or loosen the perineal pad to minimize irritating the area. In addition to these measures, sitz baths, local anesthetic sprays, and cool, medicated compresses can provide soothing relief to the patient.

While the nurse is assessing the vaginal and perineal area, it seems logical to question the mother about her bowel patterns, since many women experience postdelivery constipation. To promote natural bowel elimination, the nurse can encourage the patient to increase her roughage and fluid intake and to ambulate soon after delivery. Many physicians prescribe stool softeners as a prophylactic measure; however, if the mother has not had a bowel movement by the time of discharge, a laxative, suppository, or enema is usually ordered. Suppositories and enemas are contraindicated for patients with third- or fourth-degree lacerations because the hard suppository or enema tubing may rupture the suture.

Generalized perineal discomfort is a major source of concern to most mothers and becomes a priority for nursing care. Immediately after delivery, ice packs may be applied to the perineum at 15-minute intervals for a 24-hour period to reduce swelling in the area. Commercial ice packs can be used, or the nurse can use a rubber glove filled with ice and wrapped in gauze. After the first 24 hours, localized heat is effective in promoting circulation, comfort, and healing of the episiotomy. Warm sitz baths in plain water can be taken three to four times a day for 10–15 minutes at a time. A recent study, however, has indicated that cold sitz baths produced greater immediate pain relief than warm sitz baths (Ramler and Roberts, 1986). Therefore, a nurse can vary the temperature of the sitz bath water depending upon the patient's individual comfort level. Most hospitals have portable sitz baths that are disposable and that fit over the toilet. Following the sitz bath, a heat lamp placed 10–12 inches from the perineum offers the woman another source of comfort (see Fig. 23–3). The patient lies in a dorsal recumbent position using the top sheet as a drape for 15–20 minutes; the treatment can be repeated two to three times. Other measures to promote comfort include sitting on a pillow or rubber donut, tightening the buttocks before sitting to avoid pressure on the area, taking a mild analgesic, and using a local anesthetic spray.

Teaching good perineal care is an important intervention to promote healing, cleanliness, and comfort of the area. At first the nurse administers and demonstrates the procedure; the woman is then instructed to repeat the technique after each voiding or bowel movement. Because pelvic infections that begin during the postpartum period usually come from the patient's own intestinal flora and are ascending in nature, clean technique is very important. The patient should wash her hands before beginning. After removing the perineal pad, the mother sits on the toilet and pours warm water over the perineum using a plastic squeeze bottle. To dry the area, gauze pads may be used in a single stroke downward from the pubis. To replace the perineal pad, the mother should handle the pad on the outside surface and secure the front first.

Back

When the patient is on her side, the nurse should assess for acute back pain or tenderness in the flank area, which may indicate a kidney infection. Acute pyelonephritis has an abrupt onset, with unilateral or bilateral pain in the lumbar region. Further assessment will reveal a temperature greater than 100.4°F accompanied by chills, loss of appetite, nausea, and vomiting.

Lower Extremities

With the patient in a dorsal recumbent position, the nurse should examine the legs for color, edema, warmth, symmetry, and varicosities.

Thrombophlebitis can be assessed by checking for Homans' sign. Homans' sign, which is elicited by extending the leg and dorsiflexing the foot, may be an early indicator of deep-vein thrombosis. A positive response is when the patient complains of leg pain. Other signs that may accompany this condition include fever, swelling, and absence of a pulse in an extremity. The incidence of thrombophlebitis is increased when bedrest is prolonged, as in recovery from a cesarean section. Nursing management focuses on preventive care; therefore, early ambulation or leg exercises in bed are encouraged. While in bed, the patient can flex and extend her legs and feet and also rotate her feet.

The legs should be inspected for superficial varicosities. The mother should be advised of the following interventions that are helpful in treating varicose veins: avoid clothing that restricts the return of blood flow from the lower extremities, wear supportive elastic stockings, and elevate the legs. The legs should not be elevated above the pelvis when the head is also elevated, since this position causes blood to pool in the pelvic region.

Other Considerations

A thorough nursing care plan also includes assessment of rest and sleep, ambulation, diaphoresis, and nutrition.

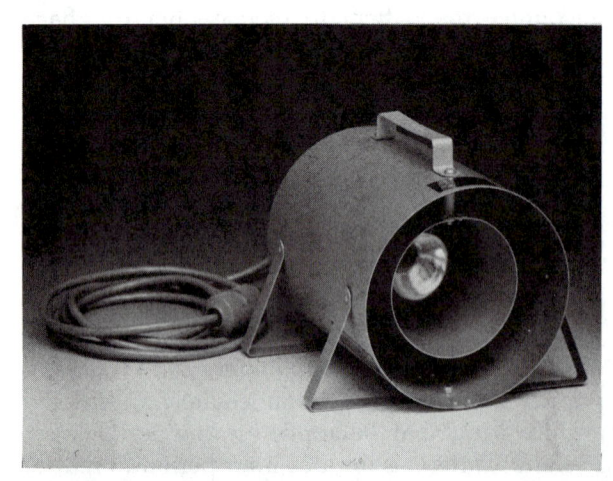

FIGURE 23–3. Perineal heat lamp.

Rest and Sleep

The mother needs enough rest and sleep to feel relaxed and comfortable so she can enjoy her infant during the postpartal period. Factors influencing the need for rest include length and difficulty of labor, type of delivery, and kind of anesthesia or analgesia used.

The woman should be allowed to sleep for several hours following normal delivery, longer for cesarean section. Uninterrupted rest periods of 1–2 hours during the day and 4 hours of continuous sleep at night is the minimal requirement. If the mother appears tired, the number of visitors and length of stay should be limited and the baby can be returned to the nursery. The father can also be enlisted to help care for the infant if the nurse determines this behavior to be culturally acceptable.

Ambulation

Ambulation within 4–8 hours after delivery is encouraged because it promotes circulation and the functioning of bowel and bladder elimination. An exception to early ambulation is made for women receiving spinal anesthesia. Many physicians request that these patients remain flat in bed for 8–12 hours postdelivery to avoid leakage of fluid from the puncture site. Spinal headache is also thought to be less likely to occur if the head is kept flat until the puncture site has healed.

The mother should be told to ask for assistance before attempting to ambulate for the first time. Because she may feel faint and weak following delivery, rapid elevation to a walking position is discouraged (see Chapter 22). The patient should initially dangle her legs at the bedside and then walk from the bed to a chair, gradually increasing the distance. She should be told the location of the call bell and taught to sit down, even on the floor, if she feels faint. On the first postpartum day, a nurse should remain close by when the mother is in the bathroom or walking. The patient's response should be recorded on the chart (such as "tolerated ambulation well").

Diaphoresis

Profuse diuresis and diaphoresis, evidenced by beads of perspiration on the upper lip and brow, is prominent for several days, especially during the night, subsiding in about 1 week. The nurse should remind the patient that this process is a normal physiologic response following childbirth.

The mother should be encouraged to wear a hospital gown at night to keep her own garments from becoming soaked and to change her damp clothing frequently to avoid becoming chilled. Nylon and polyester materials tend to be very warm and may aggravate the problem; therefore, the nurse should suggest cotton gowns. The nurse may also suggest frequent showers and offer cool washcloths during the day.

Nutrition

Good nutrition is as important during the puerperium as it is in the prenatal period. Nourishing foods help to promote a sense of well-being and speed the recovery phase. The mother who eats well is better able to resist infection and can produce more milk of greater quality. Women are usually very hungry after delivery and can receive a meal tray unless they were administered a general anesthetic.

ASSESSMENT OF MOTHERING BEHAVIORS

The behavior of *mothering* requires the individual to demonstrate those skills and attitudes that are essential to adaptive role performance as a mother (Perdue, Andrews-Horowitz, and Herz, 1977). The goal of nursing is to promote mastery within the psychomotor, cognitive, and affective domains of the maternal role. Neonatal and maternity nurses can have a significant impact on the developing mother–infant relationship because they are present during the periods of early interaction. Nurses can utilize teaching plans, role playing, group discussions, and active participation as ways to encourage the growth of adaptive mothering behavior.

In assessing mothering behaviors, nurses must identify those factors that can influence a woman's readiness for role transition. Among possible stimuli that can contribute to ineffective behaviors are:

1. Physical condition of the patient, such as long and difficult labor, chronic illness, and use of certain medications, such as narcotics.
2. Limited knowledge of infant care, increasing the woman's anxiety level regarding the basic skills essential to mothering.
3. Lack of adequate support systems available to offer physical and emotional security to the woman and her baby. Psychologic support is

necessary because it conveys feelings of importance and worth to the patient and helps raise her confidence as a mother. Women who have a limited support network display fewer attachment behaviors (Cropley, Lester, and Pennington, 1976).

It is difficult to rely on only one framework as a basis for the assessment of mothering behavior since it is such a complex phenomenon. As a result, we present three perspectives here: Rubin's phases of maternal behavior, Ludington-Hoe's concept of maternicity, and Mercer's criteria for mother-infant bonding.

Phases of Maternal Behavior

Rubin (1961b, 1967a,b) has identified three phases of maternal behavior demonstrated by hospitalized women during the puerperium: the *taking-in phase*, the *taking-hold phase*, and the *going-home phase*. The process is completed by about 10 days postpartum, although it may be more rapid with multiparas. A time frame for each phase is suggested; however, variation is normal. Mothers may also move back and forth between phases during the early puerperium.

Rubin's three phases of maternal behavior have been questioned in a study conducted by Martell and Mitchell (1984). These investigators did not find a strong "taking-in" phase and noted that the "taking-hold" phase seemed to peak on the second postpartum day. The following section will continue to describe Rubin's three phases; however, the nurse needs to consider the current socioeconomic and cultural influences on the woman such as the desire for early discharge and self-care and its resulting implications.

The Taking-In Phase

The taking-in phase occurs during the first few days after delivery. The woman's physical and emotional energy is centered on herself and on the experience of childbirth. She has an intense desire to discuss her labor experience in order to give meaning to it. Recreating the event helps the mother to accept the reality of the situation and to begin the process of interaction with her new baby. Discussion of her labor with an informed nurse helps to clarify details of the experience. Nursing staff on the postpartum unit can serve as good listeners and share the excitement of the woman who wants to discuss her experience.

During this phase, the mother appears passive and dependent. She does not initiate self-care or assume responsibility for the infant. Her attention is focused primarily on meeting her own needs. At this time, the role of the nurse is to provide physical care for the woman and assist her with any tasks that she may initiate. The mother's physical and emotional needs must be fulfilled before she can meet the needs of her child.

The desire for rest and food is strong during the taking-in phase. Women frequently mention how tired and hungry they are. Uninterrupted periods of rest are necessary to prevent the problem of "sleep hunger," which can be disruptive to the mother. Food becomes a preoccupation. Nurses can be supportive by recognizing the mother's need for food and providing nourishing meals and snacks.

The Taking-hold Phase

The taking-hold phase usually occurs sometime during the third day and lasts about 10 days. Unlike the taking-in phase, in which the mother's attention is centered on past events, her focus now centers on the immediate present and the reality of today. The woman seeks to assert her independence and autonomy by initiating self-care activities and meeting infant needs. Regaining control of her bodily functions, such as bowel and bladder elimination, becomes paramount, and the woman feels anxious if she cannot gain immediate control. The mother may be receptive to learning infant care and personal hygiene skills during this time. Anticipatory guidance about possible problems in the future, such as what to expect immediately after discharge from the hospital, and a discussion of coping methods should be included in the nursing care plan.

The mother has an intense desire to carry out infant care activities perfectly, and when she is unable to meet her high self-expectations, she experiences feelings of inadequacy and frustration. In addition to concern for caretaking skills, the mother shows great interest in her infant's bodily functions and physical characteristics (Fig. 23–4). She can benefit from assistance in trying to understand her baby's unique behavior and responses. In order to increase her self-confidence, the mother should be given opportunities to make decisions about the infant's needs. Nursery nurses are also in a good position to share their observations of the newborn, thus helping to identify the baby as a separate individual (see Chapter 29). Because psychomotor skills are considered to be

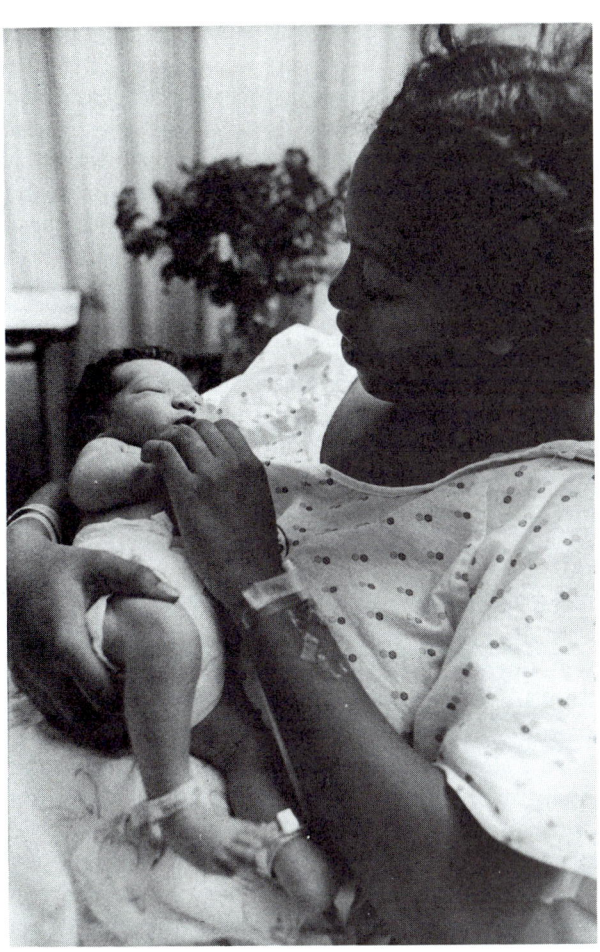

FIGURE 23-4. Mother identifying her newborn through fingering.

the foundation for mothering, the critical goal of nursing is to assess the woman's ability and teach necessary infant care tasks. An effective teaching method is role modeling while assisting the mother (see Chapter 24).

Since the taking-hold phase is marked by intense activity, frequent mood changes occur until equilibrium is achieved. Increased responsibility creates feelings of anxiety, and exhaustion from overexertion can be expected. Realistic expectations and limits should be set in collaboration with the patient.

The Going-Home Phase

The final phase occurs on the day of departure from the hospital. Characteristically, the mother is organized and ready to leave early. She is at a maximum for new learning during this phase, even though her intentions are set on "going home."

Maternicity

According to Ludington-Hoe (1977), the maternal role is divided into two components: maternicity and mothering: *Maternicity* represents the emotional factors involved; *mothering* focuses on the physical caretaking skills. The concept of maternicity refers to the mother's long-term feelings of affection, concern, and devotion for the infant. Mothering behaviors revolve around such psychomotor tasks of childcare as feeding, diapering, and bathing. Therefore, a woman can display the qualities of mothering without experiencing the emotional feelings of maternicity. Women who develop maternicity have a high probability of developing a successful and healthy relationship with their children (Ludington-Hoe, 1977).

An adaptive mother–infant relationship does not automatically appear with the child's birth; rather, it has to develop and grow. Rubin (1961a) defines maternal behavior as learned behavior. Both mother and infant need to learn appropriate ways of responding to each other. Until the newborn can actively participate in the relationship, there is little reward in caring for someone who is totally dependent and acts indifferently. Changing attitudes, added responsibilities, and altered relationships are incorporated into the new mother's lifestyle as she begins to develop mothering and maternicity behaviors.

The mother–infant relationship is initially established through the process of identification, which has its beginnings in the prenatal period. After delivery, the woman continues to identify her baby by inquiring about its sex, size, and condition (Fig. 23-5). The actual infant is compared to the mother's fantasy child and the degree to which the two are similar is a factor that facilitates the identification. Rubin (1961a) has studied the process of identifying the newborn and considers association and differentiation to be the mother's major tasks. According to Rubin, the infant's sex is the foremost differentiating factor. The mother looks for traits that represent maleness (a strong, rugged chin, for example) or femaleness (dainty fingers, a soft cry) (Fig. 23-5).

The act of *reaching* is another indicator of the identification process and the development of maternicity. The mother needs to hold her baby to realize the reality of the birth. At first, she holds the infant passively and then progresses to *actively reaching*. The mother's trunk and arms move forward with extended fingers to seek out the child (Ludington-Hoe, 1977).

Nurses can foster the identification process by

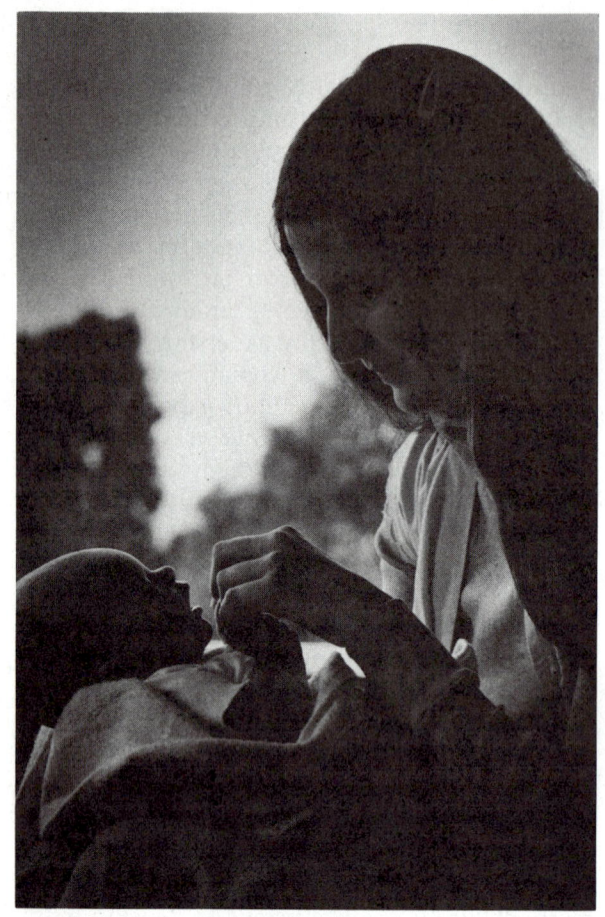

FIGURE 23–5. A mother identifies her newborn by visually taking in physical characteristics.

calling the infant by name and writing the baby's first name on the crib card. Sharing observations of the child's unique traits and mannerisms can also help to separate the infant as an individual person.

Verbal identifying behaviors follow a pronounced progression and indicate the development of maternicity. The mother initially refers to her child with such remarks as: "It looks funny because the head is so long," and "This boy is always hungry." Later, the pronoun changes to "he," and finally the first name is used. Ludington-Hoe (1977) and Rubin (1961a) have observed the identification of family features in the newborn as part of the differentiation process. Associating physical characteristics of the infant with various relatives also helps to incorporate the child into the family.

Chest positioning is another measure of maternicity. Most mothers hold their infants close to the left side of their chest, where the familiar heartbeat can be heard by the newborn (Fig. 23–6). Women who experience infant contact within 1–2 hours following delivery demonstrate a higher likelihood of chest positioning on the left side than those mothers who do not have such early interaction (Salk, 1970). To facilitate touch progression if the mother is receiving intravenous therapy, the nurse should place the baby on the same side as the arm with the IV infusion so the mother can stroke the infant with her free hand.

Eye-to-eye contact between the mother and infant is the primary indicator in assessing maternicity. The *en face position*, in which the woman rotates her face so the infant's eyes meet hers in the same vertical plane, is the preferred way to secure the baby's attention (Klaus et al., 1970). Making eye contact is critical to the evolution of the emotional feeling that constitutes maternicity (see Chapter 29).

Mothers who have some amount of maternicity will unconsciously demonstrate speech patterns that are soothing to their infants. A quiet voice pattern with many inflections can capture a newborn's attention, since it is the quality and not the quantity of verbalization that is appealing (Condon and Sander, 1974). Using the infant's name or the pronoun "you" in short sentences is also effective. Nurses can help mothers in developing maternicity by pointing out the newborn's response to the various speech patterns and noting which ones are successful.

The development of maternicity becomes more evident as time passes, allowing the mother and infant to share experiences together in daily life. As maternicity grows, the woman's desire for continued contact with her child increases in intensity. Failure to display most of the behaviors described here is a potential nursing problem that can lead to a disruptive relationship.

Mother–Infant Bond

Mercer (1981) has identified six tasks of the postpartal period that are necessary to mother–infant bonding:

Integrating Process
The woman relives the experience of childbirth and evaluates her own performance. She compares the actual delivery to the expected one. To promote integration between the real and the fantasy, nurses can listen to the mother express

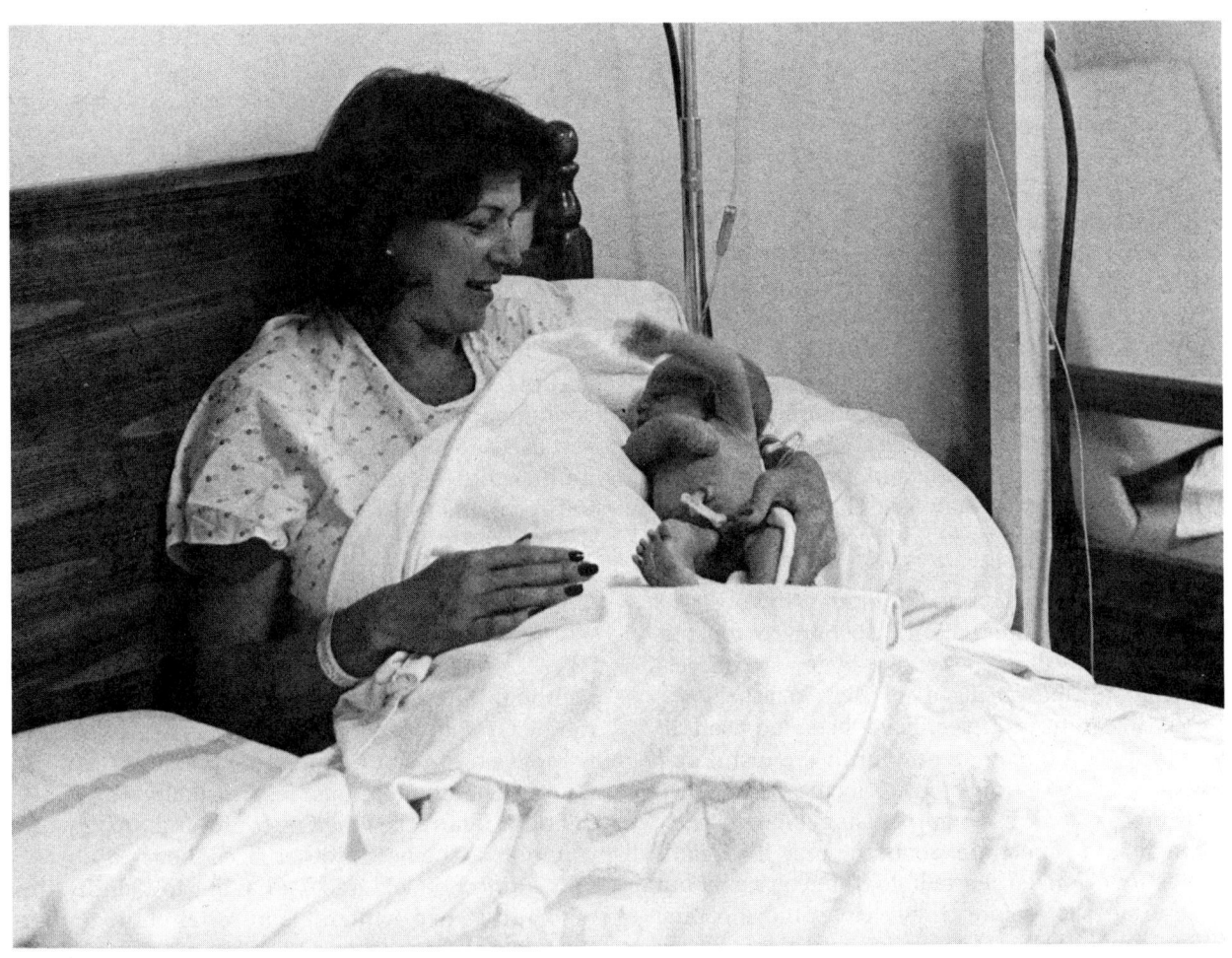

FIGURE 23-6. Most mothers hold their infants to the left side of their chest.

her concerns and can clarify any events that are unclear.

Grief Work

The mother must reconcile her expectations regarding the fantasy baby with the realities of the actual child. In this phase the woman must also accept her postpartum body instead of a preconceived "ideal" body image. Allowing the mother an opportunity to vent her anxieties brings forth possible topics for discussion. If she is unhappy about the baby's characteristics or sex, the nurse should explain the reasons for the child's appearance and encourage the woman to express her disappointment. The nurse can also describe the physical restoration of the mother's body during the puerperium and its accompanying changes. A teaching plan incorporating an exercise schedule with diet counseling can help the mother to achieve her desired appearance. Acceptance of the infant and of the woman's postpartum body by her significant others may be instrumental in the resolution phase of grief work.

Concern About the Infant's Performance

The mother compares her baby's behaviors to those of other infants as a measure of wellness. Activities such as feeding, crying, and burping become important indicators to the woman that her baby is whole. As an intervention, nurses can point out the individual variations exhibited by newborns and reassure the mother of her infant's normalcy.

Mothering Skills

This task is of greater significance to primiparas. They spend much time and effort on learning mothering behaviors in an attempt to perform them perfectly. Multiparas are more concerned with the integration of this infant into the family and with how mothering will differ for this child.

Redefining Roles

This task centers on building a relationship with the infant's father and on incorporating the life changes brought about by the birth. The mother studies her mate's responses and actions closely to observe any differences. Her efforts are directed toward the maintenance of an adaptive, healthy relationship. The father can be educated regarding the process of involution and the resulting expected physiologic behaviors. The nurse emphasizes the mother's need for rest to avoid sleep deprivation and its effects.

Coitus is best postponed until after the postpartum visit and examination. Abstinence for this period is considered excessive by most couples, but it should be practiced for 2–3 weeks (Novy, 1982). Recently, couples have been advised to refrain from intercourse only until the lochia has changed to the straw-colored lochia alba. Since men are as anxious about causing pain to their partner as women are about having it. Health professionals need to talk to the couple about postpartal sex before they leave the hospital (Weinberg, 1982). The episiotomy site will be completely healed by 7 days postdelivery, so infection of, or injury to, this area is not probable. The couple should be advised to use positions that keep pressure off the episiotomy site. Although the cervix is essentially closed 24 hours after delivery, the couple should be told of the possibility of infection, and proper hygiene of the area should be stressed. Adequate lubrication of the penis may also make the initial experience of postdelivery intercourse more comfortable (Anderson, Clancy, and Quirk, 1978).

Resuming Other Responsibilities

The final task is to make the transition from the dependent role of patient to the busy and complex world waiting for the mother at home. Primiparas can benefit from a discussion of what it is like to have the responsibility for an infant for 24 hours a day. The nurse can plan interventions that include:

1. Exploring the availability of support systems to assist the parents in caring for the home.
2. Helping the mother and father decide on a plan for division of labor.
3. Encouraging the couple to set aside time for their own activities.
4. Providing the phone number of the postpartum or nursery unit.

ROLE TRANSITION TO MOTHERHOOD

The transition to motherhood is sudden and abrupt, necessitating the development of new coping mechanisms (Le Masters, 1965). In this section the actual transition to motherhood, factors influencing the process, and supportive nursing interventions to facilitate role change will be described.

The Process of Transition

Although most women have prepared for the mother role throughout pregnancy, the transition is rapid and is accompanied by a sudden realization of the tremendous responsibility for a dependent infant. Feelings of fright and anxiety are common as the new mother faces the tasks ahead. She is often bewildered by having to identify the newborn as her own and is uncertain how to play the new role of mother. Quite often, the woman is concerned because she lacks the expected maternal feelings for the infant and does not associate herself as the mother.

For purposes of analysis, the transition process can be separated into three stages: (1) immediate postpartal feelings; (2) the first 3 months of actual coping; and, (3) the year of long-term adjustments (Boston Women's Health Book Collective, 1976). During this time, the mother experiences a series of highs and lows as she progresses through role transition.

Immediate Postpartal Feelings

At first the mother feels exhilarated about the birth and is relieved that everything went well. As she approaches the second postpartal day, the excitement dissipates as she tries to recover from the generalized discomfort of delivery. By the third day, she may feel tearful and alarmed by her lack of emotion for the child. The feelings of maternicity begin to develop as she spends more time with the infant and as the caring aspect is nurtured. During this stage, nursing interventions include providing a nonthreatening environment of acceptance and allowing the mother an opportunity to share her fears and anxiety.

First 3 Months

The second stage of transition is characterized by coping and living with the new baby. At this time, the woman discovers the disillusioning reality of sharing her life with an infant. The home often becomes the site of chaos and fragmentation, leaving the mother with a sense of being out of control. Because of her attempts to meet the baby's needs for physical care, the mother has less time for housework, activities, and others in the family. Her amount of work also increases. Since her sleep is interrupted, she is more fatigued during the day time. Stress is evident as the baby becomes integrated into the family constellation.

There will be times when the mother feels she is unable to cope and wishes that the baby would disappear. She experiences difficulty understanding the baby's responses and may even scream out in sheer frustration. Ambivalent feelings toward motherhood, and its resulting loss of independence, can give the mother a sense of being trapped for a lifetime.

The mother may also feel jealous, as the attention of others shifts from concern for her welfare to interest in the baby. Feelings of abandonment are prominent, as well-meaning friends and relatives swoop in to admire the newborn, neglecting to fuss over the mother. The nurse can provide some anticipatory guidance by encouraging the new mother's support systems to demonstrate affection toward her and not just the baby. The support systems should be encouraged to focus on the new mother's needs and concerns. Besides a gift for the baby, a personal item for the mother expresses interest and conveys concern. Discussion of jealousy with the mother as a normal and natural response should be included as part of the nursing care plan.

The issue of jealousy may also surface between parents as they both spend increasing amounts of time focused on the baby. The relationship between mates is stressful during this period of readjustment to changing roles. The father may unconsciously feel sexual jealousy when the infant is breastfeeding and may complain of emotional neglect.

Year of Long-Term Adjustment

During the first year, new mothers may be unhappy because of the changes in their lifestyle. First-time mothers should be helped to understand that their life will never be the same as it was. At times, social isolation and a desire for independence may arouse feelings of resentment. The new mother may feel that she is unable to live up to her image of the "ideal" mother. These feelings of inadequacy need a buffer, and yet American society lacks an adequate support network built into the system to help women through the transition to motherhood.

Factors Influencing Transition

The transition to motherhood is a complex behavioral process that is learned, not instinctive. Most parents are ill-prepared for the changes in relationships, lifestyle, and roles associated with the integration of the child into the family. Many factors are known to affect these role changes.

The ease of transition is affected by the parents' level of maturity and by their acceptance of each other as separate individuals holding particular values. Role change is facilitated when parents allow for mutual growth and development.

Past experience with childcare also affects the transition process. Many adults have had minimal exposure to infants, and the basic educational system has not offered adequate training in childcare. During pregnancy, women anticipate motherhood without gaining actual practice in developing mothering skills.

The transition to motherhood is facilitated by the availability of a strong support system. Unfortunately, life in America is characterized by increasing mobility, thus isolating new families from their extended kinship network and from helpful female relatives. As a result, women are forced to assume the mothering role with little guidance from others. Professional support is often minimal and can occur at an inopportune time, since follow-up visits are not usually scheduled until 4–6 weeks postpartum.

Supportive Interventions

One major task of the nurse is to provide supportive assistance to the mother and family as they begin the transition process. This need for guidance is particularly pressing in a highly mobile society where there is little stability for traditional role models.

During the assessment, it is important for the nurse to present a nonthreatening environment by avoiding a judgmental attitude. Areas of discussion can be introduced through statements indicating the normality of feelings: "Many mothers express a concern" or "Most women feel . . ." Open-ended questions are also helpful, because they allow the woman to share her thoughts and fears.

Because time during hospitalization is limited, nurses should identify priority areas for teaching and offer supportive interventions. Even if new mothers stay only 1 or 2 days, they are receptive to information. The best time to reinforce the teaching of infant-care and self-care skills is when the nurse has a captive audience, as during infant feedings, heat lamp treatments, and postpartum assessments. Written instructions such as brochures and pamphlets can be given to the mother in the hope that she will read them after being discharged.

Role modeling is an effective method of teaching since the mother can observe the caregiver–infant interaction and copy the psychomotor and affective behaviors (Fig. 23–7). The nurse can demonstrate ways of communicating with the newborn, serving as a role model for the mother by using the baby's first name and talking to the baby. By praising the woman for her efforts, the nurse helps to increase the mother's confidence, feelings of security, and self-esteem (see Chapter 24).

Organizing a support group on the postpartum floor will offer women an opportunity to share their feelings regarding childbirth and mothering. From the discussions, women can be reassured that many of their guilty feelings and fears of inadequacy are also experienced by others. Topics of discussion can include maintaining a relationship with one's mate, absence of maternal feelings, and the need to spend time away from the baby.

Other important nursing interventions include providing anticipatory guidance about what the new mother can expect at home and engaging her in the process of problem solving. The nurse can assist the woman in identifying changes in routine that will be necessitated by the baby's demands and altered interaction styles that may occur between other family members. This preparation is particularly important when there are other children.

The mother should be encouraged to keep her housework at a minimum by arranging for outside help or for assistance from her mate, relatives, or friends. Other time-savers include the use of paper plates, frozen foods, and take-out food. Nurses should encourage supplementing such a convenience-food diet with fresh fruits and vegetables, whole grain bread, and cheese.

Lack of rest and sleep becomes a critical problem when a newborn is added to the family. Allowing the father to be responsible for the late night or early morning feeding is helpful. If the mother is breastfeeding, the father can still assume responsibility for the baby by changing the diaper and bringing the baby to the mother for the feeding. Taking short naps while the infant is sleeping works out well and gives the mother extra energy.

The mother needs support as she resumes her interests and hobbies. The transition can be eased by adjusting her schedule and by avoiding an overload of insignificant tasks. The mother can be encouraged to seek out experienced parents who can help her sort out important and less important responsibilities. A search for a babysitter to be used in the future should begin early. The nurse should emphasize the importance of maintaining an open line of communication between parents by setting aside specific times for sharing. Mutual reassurance about the parenting role is vital in increasing their confidence as mother and father.

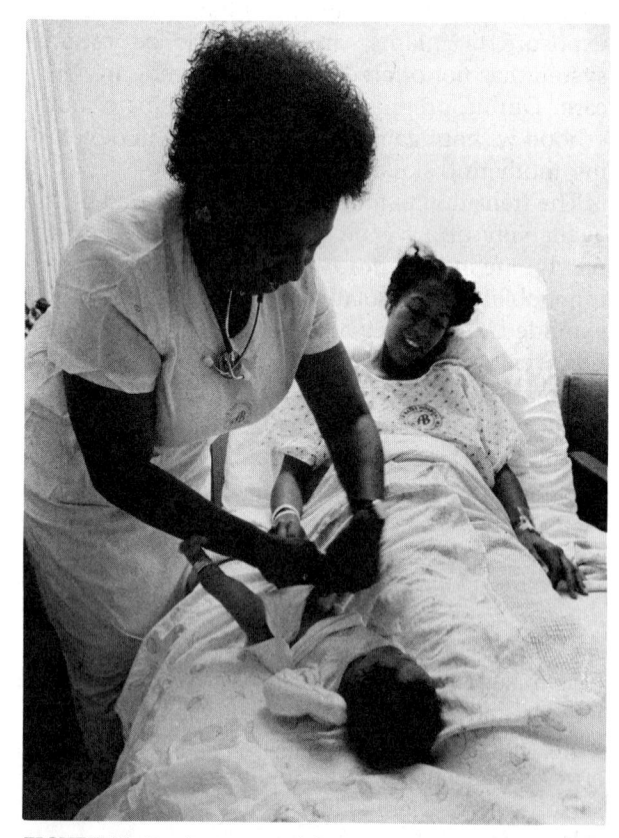

FIGURE 23–7. A nurse modeling care to a mother in a relaxed environment.

EARLY HOSPITAL DISCHARGE

Many mothers desire to return home within 24 hours after delivery – some as early as 6–12 hours. There are many reasons for preferring early discharge, including (1) facilitation of parent–infant attachment, (2) participation of family and friends in the baby's care, and (3) reduction of costs of medical care. The primary goal of the health care team in early discharge is to promote a safe and smooth transition from the hospital to the home environment for both mother and baby.

Careful planning during the prenatal period is essential to the preparation of parents for the tasks involved in early postpartum and newborn care (Avery et al., 1982). Expectant parents should be encouraged to attend parent education classes. Topics for discussion should include identification of potential problems of both mother and newborn, problem solving, nutrition, and baby care. Classes should offer:

1. Self-care instruction.
2. Assistance to parents in understanding the importance of having help at home and information on how to obtain help from either significant others or private duty nurses.
3. Information about possible equipment that might be needed (such as breast pumps, portable sitz baths, thermometers), where to obtain it, and how to use it.

Parents should secure a pediatrician early in the prenatal period. This physician should share a similar philosophy and should be available for consultation during the immediate neonatal period (the first 3–5 days of the newborn's life; Carr and Walton, 1982).

The American Academy of Pediatrics and the American College of Obstetricians and Gynecologists (1983) have developed guidelines for the early discharge of mother and newborn. The following criteria should be met:

1. The course of pregnancy (antepartum, intrapartum, and early postpartum) has been uncomplicated and should be expected to remain so.
2. Parents have attended classes regarding care of mother and newborn, including discussions of problems that might occur during the first days of life.
3. The mother had a vaginal delivery with no evidence of hemorrhage or infection.
4. The newborn is at term (38–42 weeks), is of normal weight (2500–4500 g), and is found to be normal by a physician at the discharge examination.
5. Hospitalization has been a minimum of 6 hours, preferably 12 hours, during which time the newborn has maintained stable temperature and demonstrated the ability to suck and swallow.
6. Laboratory data obtained were (a) serology on maternal or cord blood, (b) type and Coombs' test on cord blood or newborn blood if mother is Rh negative or type O, and (c) hemoglobin and blood sugar determinations, if indicated clinically.
7. The mother demonstrates ability to care for herself and the baby; she demonstrates skill in assessing the newborn's needs, feeding, and skin care.
8. She understands the need for continuing care by an obstetrician, pediatrician, and other health care professionals. Arrangements for examination of the newborn should be made at 1–3 days of age.
9. Support systems at home have been identified, and adequate help has been obtained.

The role of the nurse during the immediate postpartal period is to monitor the mother's physical condition. She may also monitor the newborn, particularly in a family-centered setting.

The infant's vital signs, ability to feed, eliminative patterns, and color should be assessed. Prior to discharge, the nurse is responsible for ascertaining whether the baby has been examined by a physician or pediatric nurse practitioner. Hospitalization for at least 6–21 hours is preferable, to allow the newborn's temperature to stabilize. During this time the nurse has an opportunity to watch the baby feed and to provide the mother with instruction in newborn care as needed: temperature taking, positioning, using the bulb syringe, cord care, diapering, and bathing. The mother's skill and comfort level as she performs the various infant care tasks should be assessed.

After the mother has rested and has spent time with her baby, the nurse can continue to evaluate her knowledge regarding self-care and newborn care. Individualized instruction can be provided, utilizing return demonstrations if needed. The patient and her support systems should be encouraged to participate in the activities. The nurse should suggest that they keep a record of the baby's routines, including both feedings (times and amounts) and elimination (number of stools and voidings). The nurse should emphasize that the infant be reexamined in 2–3 days and clarify with the parents the date, time, and place of the appointment. Resources in the community that offer additional guidance, such as the La Leche League and parent groups, should be discussed.

Many hospitals have a follow-up program in which the nurse contacts the patient by phone within 24 hours and makes a home visit by the second postpartal day. At the time of the follow-up visit the nurse assesses the well-being of mother and baby and answers any questions. Potential problems or areas of concern that the nurse identifies are then referred to the appropriate community agencies. Some common maternal problems encountered during home visits have centered on breastfeeding concerns, transitory depression, fatigue, and episiotomy pain. Concerns relating to the infant have included jaundice, breastfeeding, and excessive crying (Jansson, 1985). When making a referral, the nurse can inform the agency about the mother's ability, available support systems, and pertinent socioeconomic and cultural factors.

SUMMARY

The postpartal period is one of many changes. The woman's body begins the process of involution, during which physical restoration takes place. She practices and begins to perfect various infant care skills as she takes on the mothering role. With time, the emotional feelings of warmth and attachment toward the baby evolve and maternity is attained.

The transition to motherhood is a complex process requiring supportive care. Because of the mobility of the American family and its subsequent lack of support systems, the nurse may be the one who is most instrumental in obtaining support for the new mother and her family.

REFERENCES

American Academy of Pediatrics and the American College of Obstetricians and Gynecologists. 1983. *Guidelines for Perinatal Care.*

Anderson, C.; Clancy, B.; and Quirk, B. 1978. Sexuality during pregnancy. In *Human sexuality for health professionals*, eds. M. U. Barnard, B. J. Clancy, and K. E. Krantz. Philadelphia: W. B. Saunders.

Avery, M. D.; Fournier, L. C.; Jones, P. L.; and Sipovic, C. P. 1982. An early postpartum hospital discharge program. *J. Obstet. Gynecol. Neonatal. Nurs.* 11:233–235.

Boston Women's Health Book Collective. 1976. *Our bodies, ourselves.* 2nd ed. New York: Simon & Schuster.

Carr, K. C., and Walton, V. E. 1982. Early postpartum discharge. *J. Obstet. Gynecol. Neonatal. Nurs.* 11:29–30.

Condon, W. S., and Sander, L. W. 1974. Neonate movement is synchronized with adult speech: Interactional participation and language acquisition. *Science.* 183:99–101.

Cropley, C.; Lester, P.; and Pennington, S. 1976. Assessment tool for measuring maternal attachment behaviors. In *Current practice in obstetric and gynecologic nursing*, eds. L. K. McNall and J. T. Galeener. St. Louis: C. V. Mosby.

Jacobson, H. 1985. A standard for assessing lochia volume. *MCN.* 10:174–175.

Jansson, P. 1985. Early postpartum discharge. *Am. J. Nurs.* 85:547–550.

Klaus, M. H.; Kennell, J. H.; Plumb, N.; and Zuehlke, S. 1970. Human maternal behavior at first contact with her young. *Pediatrics.* 46:187–192.

Le Masters, E. 1965. Parenthood as crisis. In *Crisis intervention: Selected readings*, ed. H. J. Parad. New York: Family Service Association of America.

Ludington-Hoe, S. 1977. Postpartum: Development of maternicity. *Am. J. Nurs.* 77:1170–1174.

Martell, L. and Mitchell, S. 1984. Rubin's puerperal change reconsidered. *J. Obstet. Gynecol. Neonatal Nurs.* 13:145–149.

Mercer, R. 1981. The nurse and maternal tasks of early postpartum. *MCN.* 6:341–345.

Novy, M. J. 1982. The puerperium. In *Current obstetric and gynecologic diagnosis and treatment*, ed. R. C. Benson. Los Altos, Calif.: Lange Medical.

Perdue, B.; Andrews-Horowitz, J.; and Herz, F. 1977. Mothering. *Nurs. Clin. N. Amer.* 12:491–502.

Ramler, D., and Roberts, J. 1986. A comparison of cold and warm sitz baths for relief of postpartum perineal pain. *J. Obstet. Gynecol. Neonatal Nurs.* 15:471–474.

Rubin, R. 1961a. Basic maternal behavior. *Nurs. Outlook.* 9:603–608.

Rubin, R. 1961b. Puerperal change. *Nurs. Outlook.* 9:753–755.

Rubin, R. 1967a. Attainment of the maternal role, part I: Processes. *Nurs. Research.* 16(3):237–245.

Rubin, R. 1967b. Attainment of the maternal role, part II: Models and referrants. *Nurs. Research.* 16(4):342–346.

Salk, L. 1970. The critical nature of the postpartum period in the human for the establishment of the mother–infant bond: A controlled study. *Dis. Nerv. Sys.* 31(Suppl.):110–116.

Weinberg, J. S. 1982. *Sexuality: Human needs and nursing practice.* Philadelphia: W. B. Saunders.

24

Parent Education: Teaching/ Learning

BEHAVIORAL OBJECTIVES

Upon completion of this chapter, the reader should be able to:

- Discuss the role and importance of education in the nursing care of mothers, their infants and families.

- Compare and contrast major learning theories and resulting principles for instruction.

- Cite the major categories of influences that affect learning.

- Describe the curriculum planning and implementation process and its relationship to the nursing process.

- Discuss the curriculum for maternal and infant care and its individualization for a nursing client.

- Discuss evaluation of teaching as part of the nursing process and as part of the parent education and postpartal education programs

Education in general is a process of providing and acquiring knowledge, skill, or competence and, consequently, it is a teaching–learning process. Numerous definitions of learning have been put forth by authors in the social sciences (especially psychology) and by the helping professions of education and nursing. A composite definition of *learning* is: the relatively permanent change in behavior or potential behavior of an individual that reflects changes in insights, outlooks, and thought patterns and is a result of practice with reinforcement, such that the person becomes able to do something of a cognitive, affective, or psychomotor nature that was not possible before. The definition also allows for future behavior that reflects learning. By emphasizing relative permanence, the definition excludes the transitory effects on learning of such things as drugs, fatigue, and altered motives. In like manner, the changes in behavior associated with physiologic development, aging, and brain damage are excluded from this definition because they are not a result of practice and reinforcement. Finally, this definition acknowledges that the behavioral change need not be an improvement.

The definition of teaching seems to be less complex but no less broad: *teaching* is a combination of activities by which a teacher assists the student to learn (Redman, 1980). This definition incorporates the notion of the student's active participation. The teaching–learning process is a dynamic interaction between the teacher (in this context the nurse) and the learner (the client).

Education during the postpartal period is the process of learning self-care by the newly delivered mother, of learning infant care by the mother and her family, and of teaching such self-care and infant care by the nurse. Postpartal education and parent education are aspects of the overall nursing activity called *patient teaching in health education*, which itself is a process of helping people to learn how to reach their optimal level of physical and mental health for a longer and fuller life. Specific goals in patient teaching focus on health promotion, illness prevention, coping facilitation, health education, cost containment, and self-care. Inasmuch as this education deals primarily with adults as learners, it has received growing consumer acceptance as adult development and learning have become an important part of the whole educational process (Knox, 1977).

THE ROLE OF THE NURSE IN EDUCATION DURING POSTPARTUM

In the past attention given to growth and development tended to focus on childhood and adolescence, with adulthood considered a period of stability. Thus, education surrounding the childbearing process centered primarily on the process of childcare rather than on personal growth for the mother and father as individuals and as a family. However, it is now realized that adulthood involves a mix of outward adaptation, internal change, and established patterns of interests and activities. Childbearing is certainly a time of adaptation, giving the nurse an opportunity to facilitate the mix of stability and change. In this teaching role the nurse deals with the functioning person whose performance reflects his or her aspirations and limitations as well as the demands of his or her societal context.

The role of the nurse in postpartal education is important, since the first aim of maternal and child health nursing practice is to promote and maintain the optimal health of each individual and the family unit (American Nurses' Association, 1973a). Teaching is an integral part of nursing practice, as is reflected in the *Standards of nursing practice* (American Nurses' Association, 1973b). Teaching–learning principles are specifically noted as part of the criteria of Standard IV. Teaching–learning principles are to be incorporated into the plan of care, with objectives for learning stated in behavioral terms.

Nurses have an unparalleled opportunity to participate in postpartal education, since they are working with the mother and her family after delivery to meet physical needs and childcare needs, whether in a hospital maternity unit, the family's home, or a clinic setting. The nurse can be the most significant teacher on the health care team because of the nature of the nurse–client relationship in both one-to-one and group situations.

Much of learning involves changes in tasks or roles that a person performs in the course of daily life. Such changes occur when a woman assumes the client or patient role. The woman in this new role has some specific rights. She has both the need and the right to know about her condition in appropriate language and terminology. Like any client, she needs to know the related anatomy and physiology of her condition as well as the diagnosis, prognosis, therapy, and predictable events. She needs to know about the health care delivery system with which she is dealing–the personnel, the organizational structure, the routines, the norms, and the expectations. She also needs to know about the immediate environment in which she is placed when receiving care outside her own home. She also needs to develop the skills to do what needs to be done for herself, or to know that the staff has the skills to do what is necessary (Narrow, 1979).

Developmental changes are a strong impetus for learning. Having a baby represents a significant life event in an individual's and a family's development. Some of these changes specific to childbearing include becoming and functioning as a parent, becoming independent in self-care, accepting changes in relationships, and finding satisfaction in aging or in physical changes. Because of these major changes, some learning will occur whether or not the nurse assists. It is the nurse's unique opportunity to capitalize on developmental changes so that he or she can enhance the depth and breadth of learning.

LEARNING THEORIES

There are two major families of contemporary learning theories: behavioristic theories and Gestalt-field theories (Bigge, 1981). A primary area of commonality for these two scientific approaches to the study of human behavior is that neither assumes humans to be innately bad or innately good. Table 24–1 outlines the main differences between these two approaches. It lists six different learning theories divided equally between the behavioristic family and the Gestalt-field family, notes the concepts that characterize these theories, and identifies some theorists associated with each.

Under the category of "Conception of human nature in terms of activity" the table presents each theory's assumptions about the basic nature of humankind. Are humans basically passive in relationship to the environment, so that an individual is a product of environmental influences? Or are humans active, so that the environment is only a place where innate characteristics unfold? Or are humans interactive, meaning that individuals' psychologic characteristics develop from trying to make sense of their respective physical and social environments? The category "Basis for transfer of learning" indicates the relationship between the learning process and use of this learning in future learning situations. The category "Emphasis in teaching" pulls out the essential teaching concept for each theory.

It is useful for nurses to understand the assumptions within these major learning theories so that they can be applied in congruence with the assumptions of nursing practice. For example, it would be difficult to apply a learning theory that assumes humans are basically passive to a nursing practice where the client is viewed as an active participant in decisions about and provision of health care.

Behavioristic Theories

The behavioristic family of learning theories encompasses three main stimulus–response conditioning theories. Within these theories, *behavior* is defined as the actions, or *responses*, that result from forces, or *stimuli*, on an organism. Therefore, *learning* is seen as a change in behavior through formation of relationships of some sort between stimuli and responses.

Stimulus–Response Bond

The oldest and still fairly dominant behavioristic theory is that of *connectionism*, or *stimulus–response bond* (Thorndike, 1932; Bugelski, 1978). The basis of learning is the association—the bond or connection—between sense impressions and the impulses to act. The first part of this theory is the *law of effect*. When a connection between a stimulus and a response is made and followed by a satisfying state of affairs, the connection is strengthened. If the connection is followed by an annoying state of affairs, the connection is weakened. The next tenet of the theory is the *law of exercise*, which states that connections are strengthened with use and weakened with disuse; connections must result in success or the practice has no significance. The third basic tenet is the *law of readiness:* the learner has a preparedness, or *set*, for making the next response in a sequence. Fulfillment of the preparation is considered satisfying, while unfulfillment is annoying.

Other principles included in connectionism are (1) belongingness, in which a connection can be quickly learned if the stimulus and response belong together; (2) vividness, in which those elements of a stimulus situation that stand out are more quickly incorporated into behavior than those that are less vivid; and (3) associative shifting, in which some learning involves stimulus substitution.

Conditioning Without Reinforcement

Another learning theory in this family is that of *behaviorism*, also called *classical conditioning*, or conditioning without reinforcement. According to

TABLE 24-1. Two Families of Learning Theories

Theory of Learning (Related Psychologic System)	Conception of Human Nature in Terms of Activity	Basis for Transfer of Learning	Emphasis in Teaching
Behaviorist Family Stimulus-response S-R bond (connectionism)	Passive or reactive organism with many potential S-R connections	Identical elements in S-R connections	Enabling acquisition of desired S-R connections
Conditioning without reinforcement (behaviorism; classical conditioning)	Passive or reactive organism with many innate reflexive drives and emotions	Conditioned responses or reflexes	Promoting attachment of desired responses to appropriate stimuli
Conditioning through reinforcement (operant conditioning)	Passive organism with innate reflexes and needs with the drive stimuli	Reinforced or conditioned responses	Changing the organism's environment successively and systematically to increase the probability of desired responses
Gestalt-Field Family Insight (Gestalt psychology)	Active person whose activity follows psychologic laws of organization	Transposition of insights	Promoting insightful learning
Goal-insight (configurationalism)	Interactive, purposeful individual in sequential relationships with environment	Tested insights	Helping learners in developing high-quality insights
Cognitive-field (field psychology/positive relativism)	Interactive, purposive person in simultaneous mutual interaction with psychologic environment, including other persons	Continuity of life spaces, experiences, or insights	Helping learners restructure their life spaces and gain new insights into their contemporaneous situations

SOURCE: Bigge (1981).

this approach, a human being is born with a certain set of physical and emotional responses, and learning is a process of attaching different stimuli to these basic innate responses. Responses to any given stimuli can be conditioned. Conditioning is merely some sort of stimulus-response sequence that results in either an enduring change in behavior or an increase in the likelihood of a response. A response, in the form of some kind of movement or action, is immediately learned or conditioned to the stimuli that are present at the time. The strength of the response patterns is not determined by reward but by the frequency of contiguous association with stimuli.

Behaviorism includes the principles of extinction, generalization, discrimination, and postremity. In *extinction*, the omission of an unconditioned stimulus will result over time in the decrease and eventual disappearance of the conditioned response. In some cases, an extinguished response may reappear after a rest—a phenomenon known as spontaneous recovery. In *generalization*, once a response has been conditioned a similar stimulus can elicit it. The more similar the stimulus, the greater the amount of response. In *discrimination*, the response is made to one stimulus only and not to similar ones. According to the principle of *postremity*, individuals always learn the last thing that they do in response to any given stimulus situation.

Conditioning Through Reinforcement

The third theory in the behavioristic family is that emphasizing *instrumental* or *operant conditioning* (reinforcement) as the crucial event in learning (Skinner, 1953; Hilgard and Bower, 1974). *Reinforcement* is a special type of conditioning in which the drive stimulus increases the probability of the desired behavior, or response, in subsequent situations.

Reinforcement may be primary or secondary. With *primary reinforcement*, a response that is closely followed by a decrease of a drive or drive stimulus is likely to be repeated. There are three key assumptions underlying primary reinforcement. First, no learning occurs unless some physiologic need or drive is reduced; second, this drive does not need to be eliminated; and third, learning will proceed in increments. In *secondary reinforcement*, any stimulus that is present with and immediately preceded by a primary reinforcer takes on the characteristics of the primary reinforcer. Similarly, there are secondary drives: any stimulus that is present at the time a primary drive is activated and rapidly reduced can take on the properties of the basic drive and serve as a basis for future learning.

Use of reinforcement is more effective and desirable than punishment. Punishment is only a temporary suppression of a response, so no permanent weakening of the punished behavior occurs. The phenomenon of extinction is also seen in operant conditioning. If reinforcement is withheld for previously reinforced responses, the response will decrease in probability and will eventually be extinguished.

In operant conditioning it is important to control and manipulate the response rates of learners. Deprivation of some sort, but not necessarily of an organic need or drive, works as a reinforcer. Such a deprivation can be in the form of a secondary drive. The pattern or *schedule of reinforcement* controls the rate of responses. With a *ratio* schedule reinforcement is provided after a certain number of correct responses. With an *interval* schedule reinforcement is given after a set time has elapsed.

There are a number of other concepts within operant conditioning theory. The *continuity hypothesis* postulates that learning is continuous and cumulative so that every reinforcement adds strength to the learning. The *goal-gradient hypothesis* states that the closer the learner comes to the goal, the more active he or she becomes. The *fractional-antedating response* indicates that someone has learned something when he or she responds in a certain way before being required to give the response. The *habit-family hierarchy* recognizes that organisms are likely to vary their responses to any single stimulus with a hierarchy of probable responses. Since a given response or goal can be arrived at in a variety of ways, there are patterns of alternate routes of probable responses. Thus, different sequences in learning can follow the same initial stimulus and reach the same goal but vary in the process. A final concept to note is *reactive inhibition*. Every action or behavior generates some negative after-effect that is analogous to fatigue. Reactive inhibition is presumably dissipated with rest.

Gestalt or Cognitive-Field Theories

Cognitive-field theories of learning describe how individuals gain understanding of themselves and their world in the situation in which the self and environment make up a whole of mutually interdependent, coexisting events. In field psychology, the person is conceived of broadly in comparison to the narrower biologic concepts of organisms seen in behavioristic theories; the person is what an individual makes of himself or herself. Unique features of cognitive-field theories of learning are (1) a relativistic approach to perception and reality, (2) emphasis on purposiveness of behavior, (3) emphasis on psychologic function, (4) emphasis on the situation as a whole, (5) the principle of contemporaneity, and (6) the definition of learning (Lewin, 1951; Bruner, 1966; Bigge, 1981).

Principle of Relativism of Interactions

Everything is perceived or conceived of in relation to other things, so that reality consists of what one makes of information gained through the senses or other processes. How a given individual perceives his or her environment depends on maturity, knowledge level, and goals. The term *life space* is used to denote the series of unique overlapping situations in a person's existence that contribute and relate to the continuity of the person's life. A person's life space is his or her psychologic or contemporaneous situation of functional and symbolic relationships; it is not a physical entity. This relativism is incompatible with behavioristic approaches, which take a more mechanistic view. The behaviorist views a person as an organism that is a product of a unique history of stimulus–

response patterns and the environment is part of these patterns.

Purposiveness of Behavior

An individual acts to achieve personal goals or to satisfy personal wants or desires in the quickest and easiest way that he or she comprehends as possible under the existing conditions. A person moves forward toward a goal by a process of constantly searching out the conditions of the next step. The term *topology* is used to show the position of a person in relation to his or her functional goals and the barriers to their achievement. The concept of *vector* indicates the force influencing psychologic movement toward or away from a goal. Stimulus–response conditioning theories tend to ignore completely goal or purpose or to consider it as peripheral and incidental.

Emphasis on Psychologic Function

Individual behavior is looked at from the perspective of the learner. This psychologic orientation is systematized into constructs: a *construct* is a generalized idea not directly observable but formed from observed data. The meanings of all constructs are mutually interdependent. This emphasis on psychologic function is reflected in the concept of life space, which includes the person–a purposive behaving self–and his or her psychologic environment–perceived objects and events. Behavioristic learning theories tend to describe the character of an activity or behavior in terms of its physical aspects, to the exclusion of the influence of the psychologic situation.

Emphasis on Whole of the Situation

The situation as a whole, in terms of the psychologic field or life space, is considered as well as the detailed aspects of a given situation. Even though a given construct of a life space might be under consideration, it cannot be separated from other constructs or concepts; everything is to some degree dependent upon everything else. This further contrasts with behaviorist theories, which consider activity or behavior to have an independent physical existence.

Principle of Contemporaneity

The psychologic field or life space contains everything psychologic that is taking place in relation to a specific person at a given time; everything is going on at once. Psychologic events are determined by conditions at the time the behavior occurs rather than in the past or in the future. Through the continuity of life spaces, past psychologic fields do have some residue or trace in a present field and thus can influence behavior. This principle differs from behavioristic theories, where present behavior is seen as being determined by past events.

Definition of Learning

Learning is a dynamic process with interactive experiences where insights or cognitive structures of life spaces are changed so they are more useful in future guidance. Changes in the cognitive structure of life spaces are accomplished through differentiation, generalization, and restructurization. *Differentiation* is a process by which relatively vague and unstructured regions of a life space are made more specific and are cognitively structured. The individual is discerning more and more specific aspects of his or her environment and self. Differentiation proceeds at different rates at different times in one's life. Cognitive *generalization* is a process of formulating a concept or general ideas through discerning some common characteristics of a number of individual cases and then identifying these cases as a class. Cognitive *restructurization* is a process of redefining oneself and one's world–of changing the meanings of respective regions of one's life space in relationship to self and others. This definition of learning differs markedly from that of behaviorist theories, in which learning is a mechanistic change in behavior through formation of relationships between series of stimuli and responses.

The meaning of cognitive-field theories of learning can be applied to teaching situations. Briefly, the teacher tries to understand the learner as a person and his or her psychologic environment in order to facilitate change. In analyzing a psychologic situation, the teacher ascertains the relationships between regions of the learner's life space, establishes the nature of respective factors within, at, and outside its boundary, and assesses the permeability of regional boundariers for susceptibility to change. For teaching and learning to occur, the teacher's and learner's life spaces must intersect so they have regions in common. A person's peripheral regions are quite accessible; it is more difficult to reach more central regions where a teacher can have greater impact.

Theories as Guides for Teaching–Learning Principles

From the various theories, some general principles of learning can be distilled for use in improving instruction. The following grouping by theories provides a series of principles that most learning theorists agree upon (Bigge, 1981; Hilgard and Bower, 1974). Learning theories and these resulting principles are not recipes for direct application in postpartal education. Translating general conceptions about learning into workable instruction is difficult for even the most thoroughly trained educator (Anderson and Faust, 1973). However, these principles can serve as guides for structuring learning tasks so that teaching can be more effective and efficient and the knowledge base in the teaching–learning process can be expanded.

Principles emphasized within stimulus–response theories include:

1. The learner should be an active participant in the educational process rather than a passive listener or viewer. Genuine participation increases motivation, adaptability, and speed of learning.
2. Frequency of repetition of a skill develops that skill and provides for overlearning the skill to ensure retention.
3. Behaviors that are reinforced or rewarded are more likely to recur. Generally, the use of positive reinforcement and success is preferred over punishment and failure. Reinforcement, to be most effective, must follow almost immediately after the desired behavior and must be associated with the behavior in the mind of the learner.
4. The learning task should be repeated or practiced in varied contexts so the learning will be appropriate to a wide range of stimuli.
5. Repetition per se – doing the same thing over and over again – does not teach. Spaced practice instead of massed practice is more efficient because fatigue and boredom set in with concentrated practice.
6. Novelty in behavior can be enhanced through imitation of role models, through cuing, and through structured influence.
7. Drive conditions are important in learning. Personal-social motives operate in the same way as physiologic drives.
8. Because conflicts and frustrations arise and can impede learning, they need to be recognized and then resolved or accommodated.

Principles emphasized within cognitive theories include:

1. Presentation of the perceptual features of the learning problem facilitates learning. The problem or task should be so structured and presented that the essential features are open to inspection by the learner.
2. The organization of material to be learned contributes to learning when progression is from simplified wholes to more complex wholes. The developmental level of the learner seems to make a difference in the appropriate organization of material.
3. Learning with understanding is more permanent and transferable than rote learning or learning by formula.
4. Cognitive feedback corrects faulty learning and confirms accurate knowledge. Learning is enhanced by the learner's hypothesis testing.
5. Goal setting by the learner serves as motivation for learning, with the successes and failures in the learning tasks influencing future goal setting.
6. Both divergent thinking and convergent thinking contribute to the learning task and are to be nurtured. Divergent thinking leads to novel solutions, while convergent thinking leads to logically correct answers. Divergent thinking needs appropriate support so that the person may perceive himself or herself as potentially creative.

Principles drawn from theories of motivation, personality, and social psychology include:

1. The abilities of the learner influence the learning process, so provision must be made for differences, such as rapid or slow learning.
2. Inherent maturational factors as well as developmental influences make a difference in the ability and desire to learn.
3. Learning is culturally relative.
4. The anxiety level of the individual learner influences whether certain kinds of encouragement to learn have beneficial or detrimental effects. With some kinds of tasks, high-anxiety learners progress better if not reminded of how well or poorly they are doing, whereas low-anxiety learners do better if they are interrupted with progress reports.
5. The same situation may tap appropriate motives for one learner but not for another.

6. Learning is facilitated when the organization of motives and values within the individual learner is consistent over time. For example, short-range activities are considered relevant to long-range goals. The best time to learn is when the learning can be useful.
7. People tend to forget content with which they disagree, especially if it is controversial, and they tend to remember content with which they do agree. People also tend to forget unpleasant and painful experiences or to reconstruct the memory to be less disturbing.
8. Intrinsic motivation for learning tends to produce longer-term effects in learning than extrinsic motivation, where the learner tends to forget what he or she learned as soon as the extrinsic purpose is met.
9. Self-esteem and its related manifestations influence the learning process for teacher and learner.
10. The group atmosphere of learning will affect satisfaction in learning as well as the products of learning.

These principles are incorporated into postpartal education for self-care and infant care in several ways. For example, the mother actually does the procedures, such as perineal care, bathing her infant, or changing diapers, rather than relying upon the nurse or allowing the nurse to take over automatically. Demonstrations of activities are spaced throughout the day with return demonstrations completed the following day. This provides for purposeful, sequenced repetition. Praise is readily given as parents master steps in the various activities of infant care. Information is provided in several formats and situations. For example, the infant bath is presented in a group setting or via videotape. Printed directions with pictures and options about the bath are given to parents. The mother and father, when it's possible to have the father's participation, give their infant a bath in the mother's room. The nurse always includes some one-to-one teaching even if there are group classes on breastfeeding, bottlefeeding, and bathing. This provides for the rapid or slow learner, the learner of a different background than the dominant culture, and the anxious learner. These principles are to be integrated into the individual nurse's repertory of interventions but also can be part of a nursing unit's quality control by structuring standard practices and documentation.

INFLUENCES ON LEARNING

The activities we call learning take place in a whole organism. Thus, the physical and intellectual capacities of the individual have a relationship to learning. During the postpartal period, the mother's physical comfort, diet, metabolic balance, stamina, agility, sensory levels, psychologic concerns, and cognitive abilities can all influence learning. In addition, the woman's needs, motives, interests, and attitudes influence learning.

Psychologic Factors

Certain psychologic conditions must be met for effective learning to take place. Both security and stimulus are necessary. The learner needs to feel comfortable with herself and sufficiently confident that she can meet the learning challenge successfully. And the learning task itself must be challenging enough to create the change in behavior required for learning.

The woman during the postpartal period is in a period of disequilibrium because of the dependency needs created by her situation. She must balance the opposing needs of dependence and independence—she wants the hard things to be done by someone else but also wants to assert herself. The learner who understands that she has these opposing drives is in a better position to bring them into equilibrium.

Another factor that influences learning is previous experience. The experiences of the client may be limited and narrow, or extensive and varied. It is best not to assume background knowledge on the basis of age but instead to assess reproductive, self-care knowledge and attitudes, and infant care.

Learning also depends on the relevance of subject matter. Adults are generally unwilling to accept learning challenges without clear relevance. They expect to find relevance in both the objectives for learning and the methods employed for teaching. Thus, the postpartal client may clearly see the relevance of learning infant care because of the immediacy of the newborn's needs but may be reluctant to learn self-breast examination because it does not have a direct, immediate consequence.

Continued learning depends upon the achievement of satisfaction. This satisfaction must be felt not only in terms of the learner's own expectations but also in relation to the teacher and the subject matter. Thus, the nurse jointly sets objectives with the client so that completing them meets the client's satisfaction needs and not the nurse's. The nurse has a generalized curriculum of self-care and infant care to teach, but it is geared to the individual mother through contracting. In *contracting*, a therapeutic relationship is established to facilitate effective learning and to raise the level of client satisfaction. Effective learning occurs when interests and attitudes are focused and expressed. Interests and attitudes are closely linked to occupation, class, and culture but can still be created and changed if this is done with care.

The nurse should convey the idea that both parent and newborn are new to the situation and will be engaged in a process of learning about the other. By viewing infant care in this way, parents can recognize that a variety of approaches can be used without undue concern that everything be done "just right." Because they perceive each encounter with their infant as a pass or fail situation, parents may express, behaviorally or verbally, a fear that they are failures or that they are not "good" parents. By pointing out that both newborns and parents are learning about each other, the nurse positively influences the parents' perceptions of themselves. The nurse also needs to explain that there are a number of ways to provide infant care and that parents must experiment in order to find what works best for them. For example, the nurse can suggest different positions for burping the baby and then assist the parents in trying each position. The ultimate choice of what is "best" can then be decided by the parents.

The nurse, as an expert, shares vital information that can assist parents in adapting successfully to their parenting role. Take, for example, the baby bath. By demonstrating a bath with a real infant rather than a doll, the nurse can demonstrate necessary coping techniques that can be effectively utilized by new parents. Knowing how the baby will respond to tactile stimuli, the nurse can demonstrate how the baby will cry when uncovered but quit crying when covered with a blanket. In addition, the nurse who talks to the baby during the bath can, through modeling, demonstrate a method that parents can use to calm their baby in this new experience.

Environmental Factors

Environmental and organizational factors must also be considered in the teaching–learning process. Although these factors, such as the setting, the emotional climate, and the way learners are organized, are often viewed as discrete, they should be fitted together into a total learning environment over which the teacher has control.

The emotional climate in which learning is to take place needs to be intellectually stimulating but also supportive. The approach to the learner must be balanced between support and stimulus, dependence and independence. Thus, rules are made and administered for the welfare of clients rather than for the convenience and comfort of agency personnel. Instead of presenting the mother with a summary of self-care procedures on the morning of her discharge, the nurse begins discussion of self-care procedures upon the mother's admission to the unit and provides printed and audiovisual reinforcement up to the time of discharge. Furthermore, the procedures are discussed in terms of the mother's situation and concerns.

Physical factors favoring, supporting, and reinforcing the individual learner include such things as good illumination; absence of distracting sounds, odors, and glare; appropriate temperatures; and fresh air.

The physical environment may be a patient's room or a conference room, depending on the number of individuals to be addressed. The learners may wish to stand or sit for a specific session. Comfortable chairs should be available for women with episiotomies or cesarean sections. To ensure that the session not be interrupted, the nurse may request that visitors and telephone calls be restricted during the session, if the participants agree. Hospital rooms are generally suitable physical environments for individualized teaching, but few hospital units have facilities for group instruction. The size and shape of facilities have an impact on learning in a group setting. Participants benefit most from the face-to-face communication they can achieve in circular or U-shaped chair arrangements that place all participants within conversational distance of each other. Individuals who have previously had a baby may assist new parents by offering certain adaptations of infant care that they have been found to be helpful. Additionally, parents who already have children will have concerns unique to their situation, such as how to introduce the new child into the family and how to deal with sibling rivalry. Discussion of such topics is useful even to first-time parents. It is therefore recommended that when group teaching sessions are offered, the invitation be extended to all parents, whether first time or experienced. By structuring group classes in this manner, the nurse will attract a variety of individuals who can assist each other in the learning process.

Organizational Factors

The environment for learning consists of more than an emotional climate and furnishings. It also includes organizational forms, methods and techniques, and devices. The various organizational forms include the one learner–one teacher dyad, two or more learners with one teacher, and a group of learners with more than one teacher. Methods and techniques of instruction include lectures, discussion, demonstration, and skill and process practice. Instructional devices comprise all the various teaching aids, from chalkboards to electronic audiovisual machines. In making decisions regarding organizational forms, methods, and devices, the nurse should consider what is to be accomplished, what sort of instruction is necessary, what kinds of groupings are appropriate, what presentation methods will work best, and how to get the clients involved.

With the organizational form of one learner to one teacher (the familiar nurse–client relationship), the learning situation has two significant relationships for the learner: learner–teacher and learner–subject matter. When there is more than one learner, there are three significant relationships in the learning situation: learner–teacher, learner–subject matter, and learner-with-fellow-learners. This additional relationship adds complexity to the teaching but also provides valuable opportunities for reinforcement.

TEACHING–LEARNING TRANSACTIONS

As previously mentioned, the teaching–learning process is a transaction between teacher and learner that deals with a particular subject matter in a specific setting or situation. In postpartal education the process or transaction occurs between the nurse and the postpartal mother (and father) and involves teaching and learning about postpartal self-care, infant care, and family adjustments in the setting of a maternity unit of a hospital, a birthing center, a maternity clinic, or a family home. A given teaching–learning transaction could be Nurse A with Client B teaching and learning about toning exercises in Client B's hospital room. It is important to recognize all these elements, since each contributes to the process and influences the learning outcomes.

Nurses, as teachers, have control over some of the elements of the learning situation, so that desired outcomes can be optimized. Learners and teachers each bring something to the transaction, but teachers have most control over the subject matter and the setting. As a teacher, the nurse can examine what he or she contributes, such as skills and knowledge of postpartal mothers and families, attitudes toward clients and self as a teacher, and perceptions about the hospital or home situation. The nurse/teacher assumes the responsibility of sending a clear message to the client/learner. Thus, for example, the nurse communicates lack of understanding by asking for a repeat of a question or making comments such as, "I don't think I understand your question. Ask again." Also, the nurse rephrases explanations when it becomes clear that the learner is not understanding. Finally, the learner is not a passive individual in the transaction, she contributes, too.

With the therapeutic relationship between nurse and client, the nurse as teacher tries to adapt the other elements of the teaching–learning transaction to the client rather than expecting the client to fit into a rigid routine system of postpartal instruction. Such adaptation does not negate the need for and use of a curriculum of postpartal education; rather, the nurse adapts that curriculum to the learner.

Malcolm Knowles (1980), who has done extensive work in adult education, has identified several characteristics of a good teacher. The good teacher understands the goals of the course, lesson, or learning task and sees that the learner participates in setting such goals; accepts and respects the personality of self and the learner; plans for the environment; facilitates full participation of the learner; chooses a variety of presentation methods and media; and shows awareness that learning should be satisfying and free of compulsion.

POSTPARTUM CURRICULUM

A practical instructional strategy for postpartal education is to develop a curriculum for mothers and their families. A *postpartal curriculum* encompasses all the experiences that individual mothers and families are likely to have during the postpartal period. The purpose of this program of education is to achieve broad health promotion and self-care/infant care goals and specific client objectives within a framework of theory and research and past and present nursing practices.

For each individual mother or family, the actual curriculum is that mother's or family's experiences while participating in the learning opportunities. Specific objectives are developed with the mother or family to tailor instruction to individual needs.

The curriculum planning and implementation process is similar to the steps of the nursing process: assessment, planning, intervention, and evaluation. In curriculum planning, the nurse assesses the group of learners and plans the learning experiences and the evaluation process. The planned learning experiences are then offered and are evaluated as part of implementation, with planning beginning again based on the learners' outcomes. Such general curriculum planning applies primarily to groups of postpartal mothers and families for whom the nurse usually cares. When only one nurse and one mother are involved, the process would be far more specific to that one mother, allowing creation of a unique postpartal curriculum from the broader plan. Figure 24–1 depicts the curriculum process (Anderson and Faust, 1973), which will be examined in detail.

Defining Objectives

The first step in a successful instructional strategy for creating a postpartal curriculum is to identify clear, detailed statements of *objectives* for postpartal education. These objectives are best stated in behavioral terms, not in vague words such as "to understand," "to know," and "to appreciate." At this point individual clients are not the prime consideration but rather postpartal women and their families as a group. In the process of initiating a postpartal curriculum, the nurse needs to collect data about the characteristics of the population served, such as age, educational level, socioeconomic status, and predominant lifestyle; to survey the facilities and resources that are available; and to ascertain the support available from people influential in the organization (Bille, 1981).

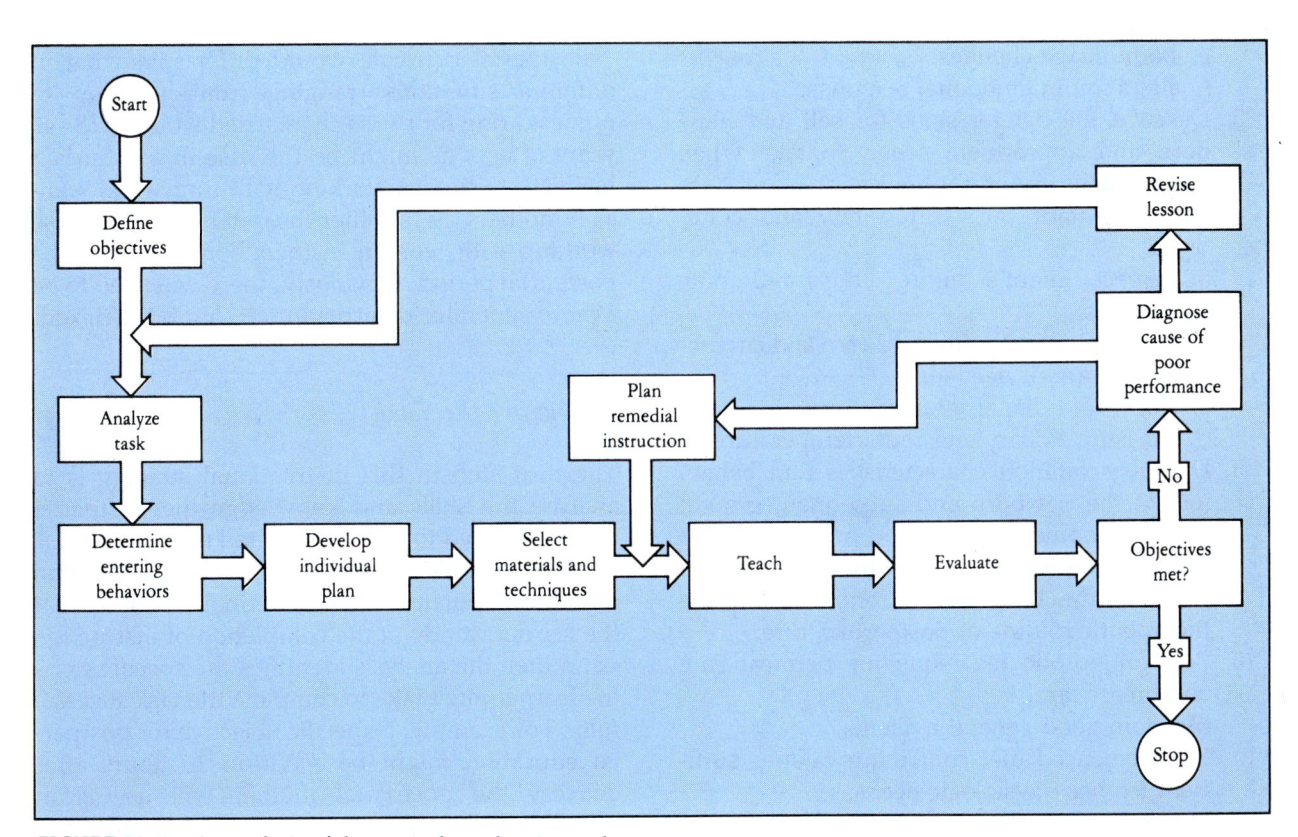

FIGURE 24–1. An analysis of the curriculum planning and implementation process.
SOURCE: Based on Anderson and Faust (1973).

The following is a sample set of objectives for postpartal education. These objectives are weighted most heavily toward meeting the client's knowledge needs. The practicing nurse converts these objectives into a postpartal curriculum for the client served, the postpartal mother:

The postpartal mother should be able to:

1. Explain physiologic adjustment during the puerperium:
   a. uterine involution;
   b. lochia changes;
   c. cervical and perineal healing;
   d. breast changes and lactation;
   e. return of menses and ovulation;
   f. muscle tone of abdominal wall;
   g. bowel and bladder functions;
   h. nutritional changes;
   i. rest and activity needs.
2. Discuss psychosocial adjustments during the puerperium:
   a. transition to parenthood;
   b. alteration in the marital relationship;
   c. temporary curtailment of social roles;
   d. transition of relationship with other children;
   e. body-image changes;
   f. alteration in emotional response.
3. Describe the danger signs for self and newborn and appropriate action to take when danger signs are present.
4. Perform infant care with safety and confidence:
   a. inspect infant's entire body and note changes;
   b. bath infant including cord care and circumcision care, if needed;
   c. clothe and diaper infant;
   d. measure axillary and rectal temperatures.
5. Describe common characteristics and behaviors of the newborn and subsequent growth and development.
6. Discuss measures to comfort the crying infant.
7. Describe the hospital environment and the therapeutic routine of postpartum care.
8. Perform aseptic technique for perineal care and breast care.
9. Maintain good general hygiene.
10. Eat a balanced diet containing calories sufficient for her physiologic needs.
11. Explain contraceptive needs and plans and intended resumption of sexual relations.
12. Establish infant feeding method.
13. Perform breast self-examination procedure.
14. Demonstrate postpartum exercises for muscle toning according to physical recovery.
15. Discuss self-health care measures and resources for healthy lifestyle.
16. Explain safety measures in use at home and plan for necessary changes.
17. Express confidence about ability to care for infant and to manage at home.
18. Discuss ways to utilize community resources.

Each objective can be made more specific and thus more functional by stipulating when and how the given behavior is to occur, e.g. "By the third postpartal day, when asked by the nurse, the postpartal mother will explain her future pregnancy plans and the steps she has planned to meet them." Such objectives are written with four steps or parts in mind. First, the objective describes the expected behavior of the learner with an action verb; in the example it is "explain." Next, the evaluation criteria are indicated; in the example they are the woman's future pregnancy plans. Then, the conditions for the performance evaluation are given; in the example, "when asked by the nurse." Finally, the acceptable performance level is indicated. The example does not specifically state a performance level but implies 100 percent.

Postpartal curricula would differ somewhat in different situations, ranging from a group of nurses caring for primarily married women, 18–40 years of age, as might be the case in a suburban hospital, to nurses working with unmarried teenage mothers in another hospital, to the nurse working with women in their homes during the postpartal period. Obviously, there will need to be a more generalized curriculum if clients are mixed.

Analyzing the Task

The next step in this instructional strategy is to analyze the skills and knowledge the postpartal client will need to attain the stated objectives. This process is called *task analysis*. The behavioral objective stipulates a task—a definable activity that the learner can do at the completion of instruction—and then the analysis identifies the specific steps the learner must take to complete the task successfully. For example, a specific objective for postpartal education might be: "Within 20 hours after delivery the postpartal mother will use clean technique in perineal care after voiding and pad changes." In the task analysis for this objective, the nurse identifies the steps necessary to achieving clean technique: washing the hands; assembling equipment (soap, water, basin, washcloth, gauze or cotton balls); removing the perineal pad; washing and rinsing the perineum from front to back; using washcloth, gauze, or cotton balls only once in a front-to-back wipe; replacing the clean perineal pad by grasping it on the outside and applying it in a front-to-back motion over the perineum; cleaning the equipment. From this task analysis, it becomes clear that an important subskill in this task is handling the perineal pad. Because it is a critical aspect of the procedure, it requires more specificity in description than, say, the subskill of assembling equipment. The concept that the nurse is trying to convey is prevention of infection by keeping the perineal area as clean as possible.

The relationship between components in a complex skill can be complicated, especially if all the details are specified. The nurse may be better able to focus on the whole if he or she conceives of the learning task as a set of chains and discriminations arranged in a pattern. A task analysis is detailed enough when the identified component skills and concepts are part of the clients' entering behavior. The subskill of handling the perineal pad, for example, would tend not to be a usual pattern in most women, and should be broken down into a series of usual patterns.

The task analysis serves several important functions in instructional planning. It obviously guides the selection and development of materials and techniques to be used in teaching the learning task. It also indicates the complexity of the task so that unnecessary steps can be eliminated. In addition, it guides the problem identification process if learning is poor: the nurse can look for deficiencies in the learner's mastery of subskills, in the task analysis itself, and in the resulting teaching.

Determining Entering Behaviors

The next step in the strategy for developing effective instruction is to determine the skills and knowledge the clients already have. These *entering behaviors* include information, capacities, and skills related to the postpartal curriculum objectives. In terms of perineal care, for example, the nursing assessment must include some way of determining what the client already knows about perineal care. Most often the mother is simply asked; other ways include having her demonstrate the skill or giving her a written test. If the nurse is going to meet individual needs and optimize nursing time, it is best to avoid simply assuming that all postpartum mothers are ignorant or that the multipara knows everything because she already has children.

Many agencies have developed tools to assess parents' current knowledge in infant care. Figure 24–2 is a tool which may be given to the parents to complete or could be read to the parents in situations of illiteracy in English, physical or mental handicaps, or high-anxiety.

Another aspect of entering behaviors is the readiness and willingness to learn, or motivation. Motivation comprises the learner's interest, alertness, attention, concentration, and persistence. For example, if a client being taught about contraception has little interest in the nurse's discussion, is drowsy, is more attentive to a TV program running at the same time, or lacks comprehension and has little willingness to listen to the nurse's presentation, she will learn little about contraception.

Assessment

It is in the step of determining entering behaviors that the individual postpartal mother is assessed. The client's readiness to learn can be assessed by dividing it into four components: comfort, energy, motivation, and capability (Narrow, 1979). These components reflect the variety of capacities of the learner that affect learning outcomes.

COMFORT. Physical and psychologic comfort affects readiness to learn in that an uncomfortable person is not ready to learn and thus does not profit from instruction. Physical discomfort is fairly straightforward to identify if the postpartal mother is willing to share her symptoms. The primary physical discomforts are from uterine contractions, breast congestion, and perineal tenderness. In a study done by Petrowski (1981), nurses generally saw mothers as being slightly more comfortable than the mothers rated themselves. Psychologic discomfort associated with fear, anxiety, worry, grief, and anger may be more difficult to identify, but nonverbal behavior may provide clues for making tentative judgments. Because the postpartal period is an emotionally satisfying, happy time for most mothers, it can be easy for the nurse to overlook or ignore other emotional aspects.

The mother's psychological comfort and thus readiness to learn is connected with where she is in her maternal role development. As originally described by Rubin, the mother is in a taking-in phase during the first 2 days postpartum when she

Questionnaire for Parents
in the Care-by-Parent Unit

PART I

INSTRUCTIONS: Please circle the answer that best describes your skills now.

1. **Feeding**
   A. Forms
      1. Nippling
         a. Can do without assistance
         b. Haven't done—need help
         c. Have tried but need help
         d. Never done—feel nervous
      2. Spoon
         a. Can do without assistance
         b. Haven't done—need help
         c. Have tried but need help
         d. Never done—feel nervous
      3. Breast
         a. Can do without assistance
         b. Haven't done—need help
         c. Have tried but need help
         d. Never done—feel nervous
   B. Preparations
      1. Concentrated
         a. Can do without assistance
         b. Haven't done—need help
         c. Have tried but need help
         d. Never done—feel nervous
      2. Ready-to-feed
         a. Can do without assistance
         b. Haven't done—need help
         c. Have tried but need help
         d. Never done—feel nervous
      3. Bottle preparation
         a. Can do without assistance
         b. Haven't done—need help
         c. Have tried but need help
         d. Never done—feel nervous

2. **Clothing**
   A. Diapers
      1. Choosing a kind
         a. Can do without assistance
         b. Haven't done—need help
         c. Have tried but need help
         d. Never done—feel nervous
      2. Washing
         a. Can do without assistance
         b. Haven't done—need help
         c. Have tried but need help
         d. Never done—feel nervous
   B. Clothes
      1. Choosing appropriate dress
         a. Can do without assistance
         b. Haven't done—need help
         c. Have tried but need help
         d. Never done—feel nervous
      2. Washing
         a. Can do without assistance
         b. Haven't done—need help
         c. Have tried but need help
         d. Never done—feel nervous

3. **Bathing**
   1. Daily bath
      a. Can do without assistance
      b. Haven't done—need help
      c. Have tried but need help
      d. Never done—feel nervous
   2. Shampoo
      a. Can do without assistance
      b. Haven't done—need help
      c. Have tried but need help
      d. Never done—feel nervous

4. **Medications**
   A. How to administer
      1. Dropper
         a. Can do without assistance
         b. Haven't done—need help
         c. Have tried but need help
         d. Never done—feel nervous
      2. Medication syringe
         a. Can do without assistance
         b. Haven't done—need help
         c. Have tried but need help
         d. Never done—feel nervous

5. **Health care maintenance**
   1. Temperature taking
      a. Can do without assistance
      b. Haven't done—need help
      c. Have tried but need help
      d. Never done—feel nervous

PART II

INSTRUCTIONS: Multiple choice (you may circle more than one).

1. **Changing diapers**
   When baby voids, what steps do you take?
   a. Take diaper off and replace it.
   b. Give baby a bath.
   c. Apply Vaseline.
   d. Rinse area with warm water.

2. **Throwing up**
   When baby throws up, you should:
   a. Lean baby forward or turn on side.
   b. If it is small amount of undigested formula shortly after feeding, clean baby and continue normal feeding schedule.
   c. If it is large amount and infant acts normal, continue normal feeding schedule at next feeding.
   d. If large or small amount and infant acts irritable, call the nurse or doctor.
   e. If small amount after each feeding, discontinue feedings.

3. You should call for help when baby displays:
   a. Forceful vomiting.
   b. Frequent watery loose stools.
   c. Spitting up after feeding.
   d. Fussing in bathtub.
   e. Crying and unable to be comforted.
   f. Lower than 97F or higher than 100F axillary temperature.

4. When baby has a loose stool, you should:
   a. Call the doctor.
   b. Change diaper and cleanse diaper area.
   c. Observe color, and if a water ring or blood is present, hold the next feeding.
   d. Change the formula.

5. When the baby has a rash in the diaper area, you should:
   a. Leave the diaper off and expose area to air for several periods during day.
   b. Call doctor for prescription.
   c. Use Vaseline.
   d. Stop using rubber pants or plastic diaper liners.
   e. Use Desitin (zinc oxide) or cornstarch in small amounts.

FIGURE 24–2. Questionnaire to determine parents' current knowledge.
SOURCE: Women's Hospital of Texas, Houston.

PART III

INSTRUCTIONS: Please answer in several short phrases.

1. What makes you most happy about taking your baby home?

2. What worries you about your ability to care for your baby?

3. Are there any special things about your baby that make you nervous?

4. Who will help you when you have problems with your baby?

FIGURE 24–2. Continued.

is focused on herself and her own physical restoration, especially through food and rest. Subsequently, she moves from dependent behaviors to the taking-hold phase where she widens her interests to include the infant, infant care, and self-care. By the end of the first week, she has moved to independence in her new role as indicated in the letting-go phase. The most "teachable" period is during the taking-hold phase when the mother is very open to acquiring information and skills in the mothering role, even though she is easily discouraged about her skills. Today it seems mothers move through the taking-in phase during the first day postpartum, especially in situations where limited drugs and anesthetics are used during labor and delivery. Within hours of delivery many mothers are ready to assimilate self-care skills and many are ready to learn infant care after 24 hours. The nurse can facilitate the mother's restorative process through good nursing care during the immediate postpartal period by providing sufficient time for family bonding, providing a tasty meal that meets personal preferences, and then controlling the environment for rest/sleep with interruptions only for physiologic monitoring. In this way, the nurse can facilitate the mother's readiness to learn.

ENERGY. The amount of energy available to the learner also affects her readiness to learn. This energy is closely related to the postpartal mother's physical condition; her reaction to the labor, delivery, and postpartal periods; the current number of stressors in her life; and the degree of situational or maturational crises.

The person's biorhythms can affect the amount of energy available at various times of the day. Thus, the nurse should not only assess the client's overall energy status but also try to determine her body rhythms. Possible questions for assessment include: "Do you have enough energy for what you need to do?" "What do you want to do that you can't?" "Do you seem to have more energy in the morning or in the evening?"

MOTIVATION. Unfortunately, it is not usually possible to determine a client's motivation from her behavior; in fact, she may not be aware of her own motivation. In addition, she may not want to share it with the nurse if she is aware of it. The nurse should resist the tendency to assume knowledge of what motivates a particular mother to learn; instead, the nurse should start at the client's own level of willingness to learn and should be glad if there is strong motivation, for whatever reason.

Some of the needs or desires that motivate a postpartal mother to learn are knowledge and understanding; pleasing others, especially professional staff; management of her own care; accommodation as a "good patient"; a higher level of wellness; avoidance of complications; avoidance of criticism; and concern for others, especially her infant and other family members.

CAPABILITY. The final component in readiness to learn is capability. Assessment of a client's capability to learn includes physical ability, intellectual ability, knowledge, attitudes, and skill.

In assessing a postpartal mother's physical capacity to learn a psychomotor skill, the nurse would assess her size, strength, coordination and dexterity, and senses. For most postpartal mothers, physical capacity is adequate because new mothers as a group comprise a basically healthy, normal segment of the population. Furthermore, even those with underlying problematic physical conditions can often master the learning tasks.

Intellectual ability is assessed in terms of basic mathematical skills, reading skills, verbal skills, problem-solving skills, and the ability to comprehend and follow instructions. For the postpartal mother, specific assessment questions or observations would include:

1. At what level can she do arithmetic calculations and read numbers?
2. At what level does she read directions and instructions?
3. Can she communicate successfully with others?
4. How well does she express herself?
5. Is she able to assess situations and know when and how to obtain help?
6. Can she apply instructions to her home situation?

Assessment of knowledge focuses on what the mother already knows about the material to be learned. For example, what basic concepts and facts has she learned about microorganisms, nutrition, contraception, and family relations? Assessment of attitudes entails talking to the mother about her beliefs and values regarding self-care, wellness, family life, and so forth. Among questions that could be asked are "What are the most important things you do to stay healthy?" and "What are some of the changes in yourself and family, and what can you do about them?" Assessment of skill involves looking at any psychomotor skills the mother has related to the learning topics. The nurse can either observe the skills or ask about them. For example, the nurse remains with the mother while the mother bathes the baby, or the father changes the diaper, or the mother breastfeeds, or the parents try to calm their infant during a crying spell.

Diagnosis

From the individualized nursing assessment, nursing diagnoses related to teaching for specific postpartal mothers and their families are formulated. These diagnoses direct intervention. The following diagnostic categories cover actual and potential problem areas as identified by Carpenito (1987).

1. *Alterations in family processes.* This diagnosis describes a usually supportive family being challenged by a stressor that has altered or may alter the family's functioning. The most common situational factor contributing to an alteration in family processes is the addition of a new family member.
2. *Alterations in health maintenance.* This diagnosis is made when an individual is experiencing disruption in her level of wellness, or is at risk to do so, because of an unhealthy lifestyle or inadequate preventive measures. Carpenito (1987) specifically defines a nursing goal of educating the individual and the family about health maintenance measures. The general interventions include first reviewing the daily health practices of dental and personal hygiene, food and fluid intake, exercise and rest patterns, leisure activities, use of tobacco, alcohol, and other drugs, safety practices, and interpersonal relations and then initiating health teaching and referrals as appropriate.
3. *Potential impaired home maintenance management.* This diagnosis is made when an individual or family may have difficulty in maintaining a home environment that is safe in terms of household hygiene, repairs, and finances. The addition of a new family member is a factor contributing to this situation. Again Carpenito (1987) suggests educating the individual and the family regarding home health practices. An example would be potential impaired home maintenance management related to poor time management with a newborn and two preschool children.
4. *Anxiety.* This diagnosis describes a state where the individual experiences feelings of uneasiness or apprehension and activation of the autonomic nervous system in response to a nonspecific threat. An example

of a specific diagnosis is: anxiety related to parenting first-born child, breastfeeding, and career development. The first-time mother is faced with several maturational factors that contribute to her anxiety. She is new to infant care and the parent role; with breastfeeding, she is establishing a whole new physiologic process for her body within all the psychosocial views our culture attaches to this natural process; and she is combining these activities within her career since she has been in, and plans to continue, employment outside the home. Anxiety interferes with learning because the person has an inability to concentrate, tends toward forgetfulness, and has an orientation to the past rather than to the present or the future. It is important to reduce the level of anxiety and assist the person to recognize her anxiety in order to initiate learning.

5. *Knowledge deficit.* This diagnosis is applied to individuals who have a deficiency in cognitive knowledge or psychomotor skills that actually or potentially affects health maintenance. Examples of specific diagnoses include: knowledge deficit related to contraception options while breastfeeding; knowledge deficit related to nutrition and an exercise program for weight reduction after having a baby; knowledge deficit related to the emotional changes commonly occurring in new mothers and fathers.

6. *Alteration in nutrition: more than body requirements.* This diagnosis is made when an individual is overweight. A specific example would be a 50-lb weight gain during pregnancy and a postpartum weight of 180 lb with a height of 5'5".

7. *Sexual dysfunction.* This diagnosis is applied when an individual experiences or is at risk for a change in sexual health or function leading the client to view sex as unrewarding or inadequate. During the postpartum, the woman must make a number of sexual adjustments. One source of sexual dysfunction is difficulty in coping with changes in lifestyle that result from the addition of a newborn to the family. Other sources of sexual dysfunction include lack of knowledge about and negative reactions to changes in body parts.

Nursing diagnoses for wellness emphasize strengths within an individual or family that can be identified and enhanced to attain the highest level of wellness or functioning possible for the client (Houldin, Salstein, and Ganley, 1987). Diagnoses reflecting wellness are as follows:

1. *Appropriate home maintenance.* This diagnosis refers to a situation in which the woman experiences or has the potential to experience a state of wellness because of adequate preventive measures or a healthy lifestyle. Childbearing is a normal maturational process, so wellness-oriented diagnoses are appropriate. The woman who has maintained a healthy lifestyle will need anticipatory guidance in stress management, parenting skills, and family relationships as she develops her mothering role. She would have already successfully managed a healthy satisfying pregnancy.

2. *Adequate accident prevention practices to support personal and family safety.* This diagnosis describes the approach to daily activities which minimizes potential and actual threats of bodily harm as manifested by lack of injury, consistent auto seat-belt use, effective time management, appropriate use of over-the-counter drugs, prescription medicines and alcohol, and a general safety awareness. Nursing interventions would reinforce her current practices and infant/child safety. The teaching plan would include demonstration of how to use an infant car seat, discussion of child growth and development, and how to childproof the home while maintaining an acceptable environment for other family members.

3. *Effective family coping.* This diagnosis is applied in a situation in which a family demonstrates constructive behaviors associated with the ability to manage internal and external stressors due to adequate physical, psychosocial, and cognitive resources. The family manifests open communication patterns, consensual decision making, role flexibility, constructive discipline practices, sensitivity to family members' needs, positive identification of child's (children's) individual characteristics, ability to meet responsibility, and request for and acceptance of help when needed.

Developing an Individual Plan

Part of the process of individualizing the postpartum curriculum is mutually setting specific learning goals with the postpartal mother and her family. A self-care framework is useful in maternity nursing, as clients are eager to accept responsibility for their own health through self-care activities. Using the self-care framework, participants in a parent education program set their own health goals, which usually include a healthy mother and infant, a comfortable pregnancy and birth, and a nurturing family relationship. The nurse functions in a teaching role, primarily leading discussions (Woolery, 1983).

Postpartal mothers and families are better able to participate in the goal-setting process if some kind of tool or guide is used. Schmidt (1978) describes a specific form that lists the categories of information about care of baby and mother necessary for new parents. A form of this type should be kept in the client's room and reviewed with the client. It should also provide space for documentation of teaching and learning.

Selecting Materials and Techniques

The next step in the strategy for developing effective instruction is to select instructional materials and techniques to teach the concepts and skills identified in the task analysis. A variety of well-developed methods and techniques are available, including lectures, explanation, group discussions, demonstrations, role modeling, role playing, case studies, and audiovisual materials.

Lectures

Lectures are primarily one-way transmissions of information from the teacher to the learner. This method can also take the form of a symposium or panel. It is well suited to sharing factual material but is poorly suited for handling attitudes. When the nurse sits down with a client and gives directions for self-care, he or she is using the lecture method. Even if aids such as slides are used, there is still only a one-way transmission of information.

If learning from lecture activities is to be effective, several criteria must be met: the motivation of the learner should already be high or must be stimulated by the talk; the content must be clearly relevant to the learner; provision should be made for some learner satisfaction by clarifying otherwise confusing concepts; and a learning dialogue should be established by engaging the learner's mind even though the learner is not participating verbally.

Explanation

A variation on the lecture is explanation. An explanation is a response to a real or potential learner need, so it may be initiated by either the learner through a question or the teacher through judgment of a knowledge deficit. If the nurse initiates the explanation, he or she must be sure to engage the client's attention, give as complete an explanation as possible, and assess the client's comprehension of the content (Narrow, 1979). If the client has asked a question, the nurse has the advantage of already having the client's attention. The nurse should then take enough time to answer, initially giving only the information requested in order to avoid overloading the client, and again assessing comprehension. A good way to conduct assessment is to ask for specific feedback, such as "Is that clear? Is there anything else I can cover?" and to observe for nonverbal cues, such as nods of agreement or puzzled looks.

Group Discussions

Another technique is small-group discussions. This form allows for considerable flexibility, depending on the objective of the discussion. The subject matter of the discussion group is contributed by participants, who share their experiences, ideas, and feelings. Such discussions should, however, be focused on a particular issue or question.

A postpartal discussion group should have a particular topic if learning is the objective rather than socialization or support. The success of group discussion depends on the effectiveness of the leadership. Thus, the nurse must not only have a thorough knowledge and clear understanding of the particular subject or problem but must also convey that knowledge to the group and provide adequate time for issues to be explored. It is not a group discussion if the nurse does most of the talking and group members only ask questions.

Demonstrations

The technique of demonstration is well suited to skill and process learning. A demonstration can be perceived by a variety of the senses and, if well planned, can provide the learner with opportunity for practice. In planning for skill learning, the nurse as teacher must ensure that the elements for practice and reinforcement are immediately available. Skill learning is enhanced if the learner is given some understanding of the reasons or principles for the skill, if the steps are clearly and sequentially outlined, and if the demonstration and practice are carried out under actual conditions and in the actual setting. Thus, the nurse who is demonstrating perineal self-care to a postpartal mother should have the woman in the bathroom with the supplies that unit uses and should demonstrate the procedure on the woman while explaining the steps and the reasons for perineal care. Female anatomy and physiology should also be reviewed, or specifically taught for those needing it, through use of the correct anatomical terms and functions. Such terms as "bottom," "butt," and "private parts" are appropriate only for introducing correct terms if learners lack the correct vocabulary.

Role Modeling

For the technique of role modeling to be effective, the learner must realize that the behavior is necessary or desirable, and she must be capable of copying the behavior and observing or identifying its essential characteristics. The role model must be seen as a person of influence and prestige by the learner; at times this can be a problem for nursing students. And, the learner must receive positive reinforcement when initiating modeling behavior (copying). For example, in postpartal education the nurse models good handwashing techniques by thoroughly washing her hands after handling soiled articles and when going from one mother or baby to the next. Mothers easily observe these behaviors in their rooms and in nurseries when they are viewing babies. They understand the importance of handwashing because it has been explained to them at some point and they have been given positive reinforcement for this behavior.

Role Playing

In the technique of role playing, members of the learning group act out a problem situation without a script. The purpose is to simulate reality for the purpose of gaining personal understanding and insight. Role playing is best suited for developing human relations skills, for sensitivity training, and for stimulating discussion. The nurse as teacher must consider the total environment of the learning setting in order to simulate a real setting as closely as possible. The nurse also needs to be prepared for the expression of genuine feelings in the role playing. In postpartal education, role playing could be a useful tool for stimulating discussion among couples about adaptations in their relationships as a result of the new infant or for having mothers go through what they would do with a baby who keeps crying as they go through comfort measures.

Case Studies

Another technique is the case study, which presents a thorough description of one individual's situation. The usefulness of this method depends on the case's reality, relevance to the learner's problems, completeness, and significance. It has tended not to be used in postpartal education, probably because of the preparation time needed. The case study method could be used in postpartal education for showing how a couple deals with the changes in their household when a newborn is brought home, how a couple considers their options for contraception, or how a postpartal woman deals with her body changes and her resulting body image. Nurses should scan popular books and magazines on childbearing and childrearing for first-person accounts that can help in developing case studies that meet set objectives.

Audiovisual Materials

All of the techniques mentioned here could incorporate audiovisual aids. Formats for audiovisual aids include:

chalkboard	radio
flannel board	telelecture
posters, charts	computers
scale models	textbooks
transparencies	printed programs
slides	magazines
filmstrips	pamphlets
film loops	photographs
16 mm films	diagrams
audiotapes	phonograph records
videotapes	duplicated "handouts"
live television	actual equipment/objects

Audiovisual materials are available from various sources—some for free, others for fees ranging from nominal to substantial. Sources include commerical audiovisual companies, publishers, pharmaceutical houses, state health departments, the National Institutes of Health, government extension agencies, the Government Printing Office, voluntary health organizations of consumers and professionals, the Public Health Service, libraries, colleges and universities, and individual creators.

Audiovisual materials can be used for a variety of purposes in postpartal education, such as providing information, showing skills and processes, raising questions, providing background for group discussion, and motivating reflection and change. Use of any audiovisual aid should not be an end in itself but rather part of an overall plan. Thus, a mother should receive an introduction to a given slide show, film, or whatever in terms of the learner's objectives and the relevance of the presentation to her. After viewing or listening, the nurse should clarify the major points and discuss their application with the mother. An advantage of audiovisual aids is that they can be easily repeated if the intended learning does not occur with the first presentation (see Fig. 24–3).

The nurse should not use audiovisual materials out of habit or in an effort to appear modern. Rather, their selection and use should be based on consideration of the learning objectives (What will be accomplished by using audiovisual materials?), the subject matter or topic (Is there an abstract concept, a motor skill, or a knowledge base to be learned? What audiovisual material can best cover the topic?), and the setting or situation in terms of staff, space, maintenance, schedule, and cost (What are the attitudes and skills of the nurse for using AV materials? What space is available for storage and use of the AV material? What is the upkeep for the materials and who will do it? How will accessibility be managed? What is the initial cost of hardware and software and the cost of upkeep and replacement?).

Printed materials should be reviewed according to their relevance as health education literature, readability, motivational appeal, legibility, learnability, and usability. A printed checklist to score possible materials and to guide development makes it feasible to fully and effectively use this medium (Allensworth and Luther, 1986).

Combining Techniques

The nurse needs to utilize a variety of teaching techniques in postpartal education, particularly demonstration, discussion, and role modeling, that are more supportive to the mother than are lectures and nurse-initiated explanations. Mothers need guidance in childcare, encouragement in their efforts, and discussion of expectations, perceptions, and concerns (Sheehan, 1981). Group discussion can be one way of helping primigravidas reconcile their expectations and actual experiences during the postpartal period (Pellegrom and Swartz, 1980). Austin (1980) has described one successful approach to group discussion for discharge planning. A congenial environment should be created for a group of mothers and families. A film on the postpartum experience can be introduced, viewed, and discussed with a nurse leader. Topics to be covered include infant care, feeding, sleep, illness, and resources; sibling rivalry; normal postpartal involution and activity levels; dieting; exercise; sexuality; couple self-nurturing; family planning; and baby blues. Sessions should last for 35–60 minutes. Participants have been found to be ready to learn because the discussion covers the situations they will soon be dealing with at home.

The mother who is illiterate in English especially benefits from teaching that combines techniques and incorporates learning principles. It is important to remember that the illiterate are not necessarily slow learners, economically or racially disadvantaged, nor without schooling. Doak, Doak, and Roat (1985) recommend some specific techniques for teaching clients with low literacy skills: struc-

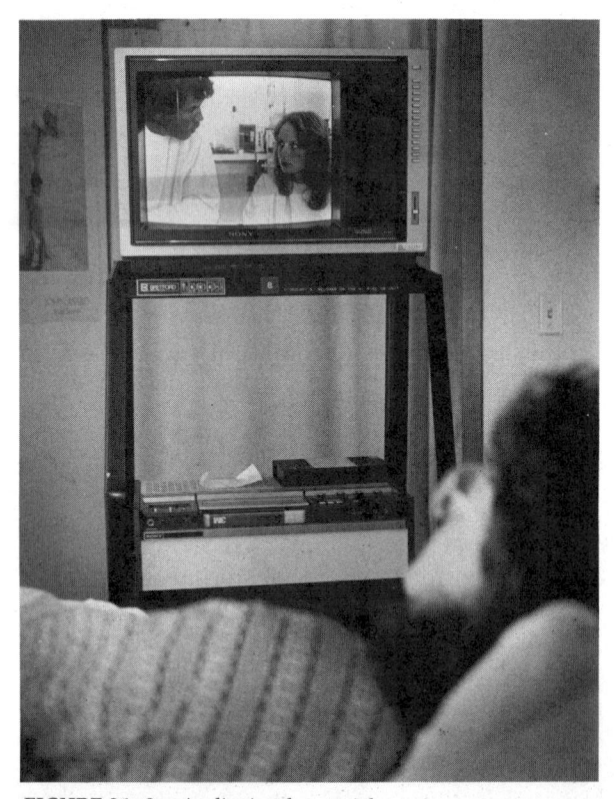

FIGURE 24–3. Audiovisual materials are useful for a variety of purposes.

ture content so the client needs to learn the smallest amount possible to accomplish the objectives; make points vivid and explicit; teach just one step of a process at a time; have the client restate and demonstrate content and skills; review information repeatedly; keep visual aids simple; and utilize taped resources instead of printed materials.

Teaching

The next step in the instructional plan is to actually *teach* the information, skills, or attitudes defined in the objectives. The nurse tries to carry out the plan. Even though it may not work perfectly, the plan should be followed until client feedback indicates that it is not working.

Some common barriers to teaching need to be kept in mind. Often nurses plead lack of time as an excuse to cover other reasons for lack of success. Perhaps they lack the knowledge of how to teach or fail to see the importance of the teaching. Or they may use inappropriate sources for objectives or attempt to teach too much. Another barrier is communication problems, whether because of language barriers or coordination difficulties of the physician, client, and nurse. Documentation becomes a barrier when nurses think they are too busy to write everything. Another barrier is limited involvement by the family. A final barrier is lack of continuity through planning.

SPECIAL TEACHING CONSIDERATIONS

Multiple Births

Parents experiencing a multiple birth will require special instruction in methods of scheduling care for each infant. Based on assessment of data concerning the resources and particular needs of the parents and infants, the nurse may suggest an alternate feeding schedule for infants who will be bottle-fed by only one caregiver or simultaneous feedings for infants who will be breastfeeding. The nurse may also arrange a visit with other parents of multiple births to ensure that a continuing source of support will be available for the new parents. There are several organizations that provide parent-to-parent support, including the National Organization of Mothers of Twins Club, Inc. (see Appendix G).

Premature Births

The problems of premature infants often necessitate a long hospitalization period following the birth. During the course of the hospitalization, parents need support and education regarding premature infants and their needs (see Chapter 32). The nurse should help the parents to recognize the appropriate amount for each feeding according to the infant's ability to consume and retain it; the need for more frequent, smaller feedings; the common need to awaken the infant for feedings; and appropriate stimulation methods that do not tire the infant. Because parents are usually concerned about the long-term effects of prematurity, the nurse will need to discuss the common delays in developmental milestones that occur with premature infants. This information can alleviate future anxiety when the parents compare their infant's abilities with those of full-term infants of the same chronologic age.

It is becoming more common for parents to be allowed a lot of contact time with their infant while he or she remains in the intermediate or high-risk hospital nursery. This time can be utilized by the nurse to instruct and assist the parents as they give some physical care (changing diapers, feeding) to their infant. It is useful to have a formal method of determining the specific content that has been covered with each set of parents. An example of one such record-keeping tool is provided in Fig. 24–3.

Another method of ensuring that the parents feel comfortable in assuming care of their baby is to entrust parents with total care of the infant for a period of 24–48 hours prior to the baby's discharge from the hospital. In many hospitals, parents stay in the hospital and provide care to their infant under the supervision of a nurse. This transition time is useful for instilling confidence in the parents' capabilities while ensuring that their understanding of pertinent knowledge is correct. To facilitate this process a questionnaire such as that presented in Fig. 24–3 may be completed by the parents at the beginning of the hospital stay. The answers then serve as data for the nurse to develop a nursing care plan specific for each set of parents.

Evaluating

The final step on a linear progression through the instructional strategy is evaluation; however, the evaluation process should permeate the whole teaching strategy. Evaluation entails measuring behaviors and interpreting the results in terms of the objectives – the desired behavioral changes. Evaluation within postpartal education occurs at both the individual client level and the level of the program of which the individual teacher–learner transactions are a part. The purpose of educational evaluation is to facilitate learning, to judge learners' progress, and to critique instructional methods and materials.

Setting clear, detailed behavioral objectives provides evaluation criteria for judging the teaching–learning outcomes. Once the teaching has begun, the learners' feedback can be used to modify content, approach, pace, and materials of instruction, so that progress is being made toward the learning objectives. This system of evaluation is based on learner outcomes rather than teacher inputs. The teacher does not assume the client has acquired knowledge just because information has been presented to her.

On the program level the evaluation process takes into account individual client outcomes as well as overall results. Evaluation of care is part of the standards of many accrediting organizations. For example, the Joint Commission on Accreditation of Hospitals requires evidence that patient and family teaching has been done and provides guidelines for evaluation. A flexible operational definition of teaching quality includes six elements:

1. Optimal achievable client results;
2. No harm done;
3. Client and family understanding;
4. Cost effectiveness;
5. Reasonable documentation, and
6. Appropriate utilization of resources (Bille, 1981).

A composite program evaluation strategy includes five steps (Bille, 1981):

1. The identification of problems in the delivery of quality postpartal education.
2. The selection of appropriate objective assessment strategies.
3. The assessment of the problem against established criteria to determine the extent of the problem and identify probable causes.

TABLE 24–2. *Postpartal Education Evaluation Planning Guide*

Components to Evaluate	What Do I Want to Know	Why Do I Need to Know?	Whom Will Be My Data Source?	What Will I Look For as Evidence?
Input				
Staff	Did the staff communicate?	To develop an inservice	Parents in the program	Favorable comments
Content	Is the content accurate?	To make program revisions	Medical and nursing staff	Opinions
Clients	Was knowledge gained?	To develop an instructional strategy	Mother and father on postpartal unit	Three-point gain in knowledge scores
Process/program	Were techniques appropriate?	To choose tactics to facilitate learning	Parents in the program	Satisfaction with techniques
Outcome	Do parents understand transition to parenthood?	To revise instruction, conduct more classes	Parents, hospital staff	75 percent of parents list adjustments to parenthood accurately

4. The identification of appropriate methods aimed at solving the problem.
5. The reassessment of the problem to ascertain resolution or reduction to an acceptable level.

Del Bueno (1978) has proposed a systems approach for evaluating programs. Such a systems approach would highlight problems and provide an assessment strategy. The nurse, then, would consider the inputs, process, and outcomes:

1. *Inputs:* the designed content, any audiovisual materials, the nurse, the client, and the setting or facilities.
2. *Process:* teaching activities, nurse and client attitudes, direct contacts, and time expended.
3. *Outcomes:* the specific client behaviors that resulted, staff attitudes, and cost per client. Costs must be considered in terms of personal costs (time spent), equipment costs, materials costs, and facility costs.

Table 24–2 pulls these concepts together into a completed postpartal education planning guide.

Evaluation as a process with the individual client consists of three sequential steps (Carnevali, 1983). The first is selecting criteria or standards that are logically related to the diagnosis and goals. Within the nursing process this step occurs as part of planning. Within the curriculum development process this step occurs as part of defining objectives and developing an individualized plan of instruction. The second step involves collecting data during the teaching–learning transaction as prescribed by the observational guide. Within the nursing process this step occurs during implementation but also becomes part of assessment because it is adding to the database. Within the teaching–learning process this step coincides with the actual teaching. The third step in the evaluation process is comparing the collected evidence to the criterion standards and any available baseline and then making judgments about the nature of the response. This step coincides with that of evaluation in both the nursing process and the curriculum planning/implementing process.

The first step of evaluation, setting criterion standards, has already been discussed in terms of defining clear behavioral objectives. The measurement process is greatly facilitated when criteria are

TABLE 24–2. continued

How Will I Collect the Data/Evidence?	When Will I Collect the Data/Evidence?	How Will I Analyze the Data/Evidence?	To Whom Will I Report the Data/Evidence?	How Will the Information Be Used?
Administer satisfaction tool	At end of program	Instructors should receive	Instructors	To improve communication ability
Review literature, interview staff	Prior to program	Content analysis	Medical, nursing consultants	To develop lesson plans, revise program
Administer short multiple-choice questionnaire	Prior to program	Compare pretest and post-test scores	Teaching staff	To determine effectiveness of teaching programs
Administer satisfaction tool	At end of each session	Number of individuals responding positively to techniques	Teaching staff	To modify teaching approach
Interview staff, observe parents	Within-hospital questionnaire, after discharge	Comparison of those attending class and those who do not	Director of nursing, education staff	To compute costs per client and allocate funds

SOURCE: Bille (1981).

specific because it is clear what behaviors the nurse should be looking for. Postpartal education has the advantage of having a similar group of clients needing generally the same kinds of information, so that validated criterion measures can be developed to test client retention (Petrowski, 1981).

Data collection for evaluation involves observation and measurement of behavior. Collection methods are more direct if the behavior is observed as it occurs, as in a demonstration, and less direct if the behavior is a response to a substitute situation, as in a verbal question. Some types of learning are not directly observable. Because a learner's "knowing" something cannot be observed, indirect evidence is given by explaining or discussing the "something."

Measurement involves obtaining a record of the behavior being evaluated (Redman, 1980). Because it is difficult and unnecessary to record all the behaviors that occur, key characteristics or critical activities are noted. Direct observation can take the form of anecdotal notes, a rating scale, or a checklist. A rating scale is a precise description of the pertinent behavior at several levels of achievement. A checklist summarizes crucial steps in the behavior without the levels. Even if the nurse does not have a written rating scale for evaluating a client's skills, he or she can use mental tools when teaching and when revising strategies. A major advantage of a written scale is that it can be used consistently and it allows careful discrimination of essential steps.

Oral questioning is a primary form of measurement in postpartal education and is often used in combination with direct observation. This form of measurement attempts to get at behaviors that are difficult to observe directly. In order to test the learning objective accurately and avoid misunderstanding, the nurse must phrase questions carefully. Wording must be tactful to prevent imposing an atmosphere of interrogation, and it must be well thought out to avoid telegraphing the right answer. Even though oral questioning may appear easy and quick, it is not; neither is it the most economical method when it comes to planning and replication.

Written measurement is a form of indirect observation that overcomes some of the drawbacks of oral questioning. It is not as time-consuming and provides greater consistency. However, it does require some reading and test-taking skills in the client. Tests are available from commercial sources or can be constructed for the specific teaching situation. Whether purchased or teacher-made, a test must be carefully reviewed to check whether it is really testing what is intended and whether it can do so consistently. A poorly constructed test is not worth the paper it is printed on. However, careful wording of questions, equal distribution of the subject matter in the questions, and thorough pretesting can avoid the worst problems.

Documenting

Documentation is not a direct part of the nursing or teaching–learning process but is important to the delivery of coordinated nursing care or education, depending on the system. Documentation entails recording client achievements and reactions to the teaching. It serves as a communication tool among coworkers, indicating what teaching has been done and what the mother's response to that teaching was. Documentation also fulfills the requirements of the Joint Commission for Accreditation of Hospitals and the standards of individual states. In addition, documentation can serve a research function by showing trends in instructional practices and in learners' responses to various practices.

The documentation tool should be designed to show what was taught and when, who did the teaching, the learner's response, and the setting if it was outside the usual clinical situation (see Fig. 24–4). For example, the documentation might note that perineal care was taught in the bathroom with the mother giving an accurate return demonstration, plus time, date, and nurse's signature. Figure 24–5 is a sample tool to be used for patient teaching documentation specific to postpartal and parent education.

Flowsheets are particularly useful for efficiently documenting the teaching–learning process. They fit well into the overall curriculum by showing the postpartal curriculum objectives and the times and dates when the objectives were met. Flowsheets can be open-ended, with the nurse describing the variables to be observed for each client. However, in postpartal education there is enough similarity of needs among clients to avoid the completely open-ended format. A checklist is a variation of the flowsheet. It is somewhat easier to complete but does not convey as much information about individual client responses as a flowsheet.

Another method of documentation is the progress report, which is an anecdotal record. Progress reports fit easily into the pattern of usual

INFANT TEACHING AND DISCHARGE CHECKLIST

MOTHER'S COMMENTS I have a good understanding of this subject	TOPIC LIST INFANT CARE	NURSE'S COMMENTS Comments/Initials (Handouts/Classes/Videos/etc.)	REVIEWED— Appears to understand Date/Initials
	1. Normal characteristics & behavior	1	
	2. Bathing/skin care *	2	
	3. Diapering *	3	
	4. Dressing *	4	
	5. Care of umbilical cord *	5	
	6. Care of male/female genitalia *	6	
	7. Care of circumcision *	7	
	8. Bowel & bladder patterns	8	
	9. Temperature taking	9	
	a. axillary	a	
	b. rectal *	b	
	10. Sleeping positions	10	
	11. Bulb syringe	11	
	12. Car safety *	12	
	13. Jaundice	13	
	14. When to call Dr. *	14	
	FEEDING ___ Breast ___ Bottle		
	1. Positioning *	1	
	2. Frequency	2	
	3. Duration/amount	3	
	4. Burping	4	
	5. Breaking suction *	5	
	6. Avoidance of supplementation	6	
	7. Formula preparation *	7	

*Subject can be found in *A Guide for New Parents*

Baby's Discharge Checklist
___ Discharge order
___ 48 hour assessment
___ Newborn screen
___ D/C record signed/identiband attached
___ Teaching checklist completed
___ Return appointment
___ Condition of infant & D/C charted
___ Notify desk of discharge

IDENTIFICATION SIGNATURE
1. _____
2. _____
3. _____
4. _____
5. _____
6. _____

FIGURE 24–4. Infant teaching and discharge checklist.
SOURCE: Alta Bates Hospital.

526 CHANGE: THE POSTPARTAL PERIOD

☐ EARLY DISCHARGE   _____ TUBAL LIGATION   _____ CESAREAN BIRTH
☐ ROUTINE STAY   DATE   DATE
_____ VAGINAL DELIVERY
         DATE

ASSESSMENT OF LEARNING NEEDS:
Previous baby care experience_____ Classes/Programs:_____
☐ Baby Care Booklet given   ☐ Informed regarding educational programs/films
Special Needs: _____

DISCHARGE PLANS:
Assistance available at home: _____   Referrals needed/made: _____
Educational films viewed: _____   Baby Care booklet read: _____

	Understands	Demo Returned	Family Included	COMMENTS	Date	Initial
A. SELF CARE						
Demonstrates good personal hygiene						
Demonstrates perineal care/care of hemorrhoids						
Verbalizes understanding of take home medications including peri meds/creams						
Verbalizes understanding of breast/nipple care (per standardized teaching plan)						
Swedish milk cups						
Hot/cold application						
Use of pump/manual expression						
Care of incision						
Signs/symptoms of infection						
B. PHYSICAL CHANGES						
Verbalizes understanding of physical change occurring post partum						
Involution/after contractions						
Lochial changes						
Bowel patterns						
Bladder patterns						
C. Rubella/Rhogam instruction (if applicable)						
D. DIET INSTRUCTION GIVEN						
E. OTHER: (HBIG) etc., if appropriate						

Identification signature
1   3
2   4

ALTA BATES HOSPITAL   A NON-PROFIT HEALTH CENTER
3001 COLBY STREET • BERKELEY, CA 94705

MATERNITY TEACHING CHECKLIST

SEQ. 1061 • NUR-093 (9/87)

FIGURE 24–5. Maternity teaching checklist.
SOURCE: Alta Bates Hospital.

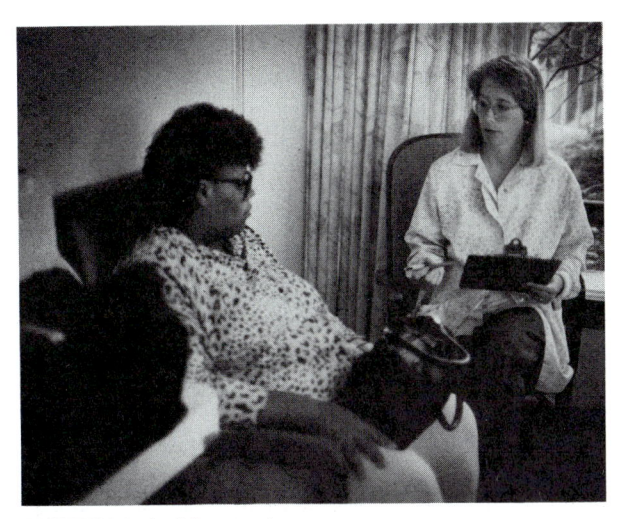

FIGURE 24–6. Nurse going over discharge teaching flow sheet (postpartum) with patient.

nursing notes or charting. However, in postpartal education, such written progress notes are far more time-consuming than the flowsheet or checklist and are really only necessary to document dramatic or untoward responses to teaching.

Whatever the form of documentation, it remains part of the client's legal medical record. As such, the client would have access to it. It is helpful to provide the postpartal mother and her family with a copy of the teaching–learning documentation tool as a way to highlight important points and to provide a review outline (Figure 24–6).

SUMMARY

The teaching-learning process is essential to the process of nursing. Through the process of education, the nurse serves as teacher and the new mother as active learner.

The behavioral sciences provide many learning theories that can be tested and integrated into nursing practice. Behavioristic and Gestalt-field theories are two major contemporary learning theories from which specific teaching-learning principles related to the adult learner can be derived.

Influences on learning include: 1. the learner's comfort level, energy level, motivation to learn, and physical, intellectual, and attitudinal capacities to learn; 2. the environment, and 3. the teacher.

Learning is a dynamic process with interactive experiences. Learning cannot be separated from teaching. The teaching-learning process is a transaction between teacher and learner.

The role of teaching includes curriculum planning and implementation. This process begins with defining objectives and moves to analyzing learning tasks, identifying entering behaviors, developing individualized plans, selecting appropriate methods, engaging in teaching, and thorough evaluation. In order to document teaching that has been done, recording is important. Teaching is one of many tools available to nurses for planned intervention through which they are active catalysts for change.

REFERENCES

Allensworth, D. D., and Luther, C. R. 1986. Evaluating printed materials. *Nurse Educator.* 11:18–22.

American Academy of Pediatrics. 1977. *You and your pediatrician: Common childhood problems.* Evanston, Ill.: The Academy.

American Nurses' Association. 1973a. *Standards of maternal and child health nursing practice.* Kansas City: The Association.

American Nurses' Association. 1973b. *Standards of nursing practice.* Kansas City: The Association.

Anderson, R. C., and Faust, G. W. 1973. *Educational psychology: The science of instruction and learning.* New York: Dodd, Mead.

Austin, S. J. 1980. Family-centered discharge planning classes. *MCN.* 5:96–97.

Barron, S. 1987. Documentation of patient education. *Patient Education and Counseling.* 9:81–85.

Bigge, M. L. 1981. *Learning theories for teachers.* 4th ed. New York: Harper & Row.

Bille, D. A. ed. 1981. *Practical approaches to patient teaching.* Boston: Little, Brown.

Boston Women's Health Book Collective. 1976. *Our bodies, ourselves: A book by and for women.* Rev. 2nd ed. New York: Simon & Schuster.

Brown, B. 1982. Maternity patient teaching – a nursing priority. *J. Obstet. Gynecol. Neonatal Nurs.* 11:11–14.

Bruner, J. S. 1966. *Toward a theory of instruction.* Cambridge, Mass.: Belknap Press of Harvard University Press.

Bugelski, B. R. 1978. *The psychology of learning applied to teaching.* Indianapolis: Bobbs-Merrill.

Bull, M., and Lawrence, D. 1985. Mothers' use of knowledge during first postpartum week. *J. Obstet. Gynecol. Neonatal Nurs.* 14:315–320.

Carnevali, D. L. 1983. *Nursing care planning: Diagnosis and management.* 3rd ed. Philadelphia: Lippincott.

Carpenito, L. J. 1983. *Nursing diagnoses: Application to clinical practice.* Philadelphia: Lippincott.

Consolvo, C. Questionnaire for parents in the Care by Parents Unit, Hermann Hospital, Houston, Texas.

Dean, P. G.; Morgan, P.; and Towle, J. M. 1982. Making baby's acquaintance: A unique attachment strategy. *MCN.* 7(Jan./Feb.):37–41.

del Bueno, D. J. 1978. Patient education: Planning for success. *J. Nurs. Admin.* 8:3–7.

Diagram Group. 1977. *Woman's body: An owner's manual.* New York: Paddington Press.

DiFlorio, I. A., and Duncan, P. A. 1986. Design for successful patient teaching. *Am. J. Nurs.* 11:246–249.

Doak, C.; Doak, L. R.; and Roat, J. H. 1985. *Teaching patients with literacy skills.* Philadelphia: J. B. Lippincott.

Duke University Hospital Nursing Services. 1983. *Guidelines for nursing care: Process and outcome.* Philadelphia: Lippincott.

Erickson, M. P. 1978. Trends in assessing the newborn and his parents. *MCN.* 3(March/April):99–103.

Giloth, B. 1985. Incentives for planned patient education. *Quart. Rev. Bull.* 11:295–301.

Gordon, M. 1982. *Nursing diagnosis: Process and application.* New York: McGraw-Hill.

Haber, J.; Leach, A. M.; Schudy, S. M.; and Sideleau, B. F. 1978. *Comprehensive psychiatric nursing.* San Francisco: McGraw-Hill.

Hilgard, E. R., and Bower, G. H. 1974. *Theories of learning.* 4th ed. New York: Appleton-Century-Crofts.

Hiser, P. L. 1987. Concerns of multiparas during the second postpartum week. *J. Obstet. Gynecol. Neonatal Nurs.* 16:195–203.

Hoff, L. A. 1978. *People in crisis.* Boston: Addison-Wesley.

Houldin, A. D.; Salstein, S. W.; and Ganley, K. M. 1987. *Nursing diagnoses for wellness: Supporting strengths.* Philadelphia: J. B. Lippincott.

Joint Commission on Accreditation of Hospitals. 1982. *Accreditation manual for hospitals.* Chicago: The Commission.

Klaus, M. H., and Kennell, J. H. 1976. *Maternal infant bonding.* St. Louis: C. V. Mosby.

Knowles, M. S. 1980. *The modern practice of androgogy versus pedragogy.* Rev. ed. Chicago: Follett.

Knox, A. B. 1977. *Adult development and learning.* San Francisco: Jossey-Bass.

Lewin, K. 1951. *Field theory in social science.* New York: Harper & Row.

Narrow, B. W. 1979. *Patient teaching in nursing practice: A patient and family-centered approach.* New York: John Wiley & Sons.

Pellegrom, P., and Swartz, L. 1980. Primigravidas' perceptions of early postpartum. *Pediatric Nurs.* 6:25–27.

Petrowski, D. D. 1981. Effectiveness of prenatal and postnatal instruction in postpartum care. *J. Obstet. Gynecol. Neonatal Nurs.* 10:386–389.

Price, J. P., and Cordell, B. 1984. Patient education evaluation: Beyond intuition. *Nurs. Forum.* 21:117–122.

Redman, B. K. 1980. *The process of patient teaching in nursing.* 4th ed. St. Louis: C. V. Mosby.

Redman, B. K.; Levine, D.; and Howard, D. 1987. Organizational resources in support of patient education programs: Relationship to reported delivery of instruction. *Patient Education and Counseling.* 9:177–197.

Rehm, R. 1983. Teaching cardiopulmonary resuscitation to parents. *MCN.* 8(Nov.):411–414.

Rubin, R. 1961. Puerperal change. *Nurs. Outlook.* 9:753–755.

Rutledge, D. L., and Pridham, K. F. 1987. Postpartum mothers' perceptions of competence for infant care. *J. Obstet. Gynecol. Neonatal Nurs.* 16:185–193.

Schmidt, J. 1978. Using a teaching guide for better postpartum and infant care. *J. Obstet. Gynecol. Neonatal Nurs.* 7:23–26.

Sheehan, F. 1981. Assessing postpartal adjustment. *J. Obstet. Gynecol. Neonatal Nurs.* 10:19–22.

Skinner, B. F. 1953. *Science and human behavior.* New York: Macmillan.

Smith, L. F. 1986. New parent teaching in the ambulatory care setting. *J. Obstet. Gynecol. Neonatal Nurs.* 11:256–258.

Summer, G., and Fritsch, J. 1987. Postnatal parental concerns: The first six weeks of life. *J. Obstet. Gynecol. Neonatal Nurs.* 6:27–32.

Thorndike, E. L. 1932. *The fundamentals of learning.* New York: Teachers College, Columbia University.

Tilley, J. D.; Gregor, F. M.; and Thiessen, V. 1987. The nurse's role in patient education: Incongruent perceptions among nurses and patients. *J. Advanced Nurs.* 12:291–301.

Wilson, H. S., and Kneisel, C. R. 1979. *Psychiatric nursing.* Menlo Park, Calif.: Addison-Wesley.

Woolery, L. F. 1983. Self-care for obstetrical patient: A nursing framework. *J. Obstet. Gynecol. Neonatal Nurs.* 12:33–37.

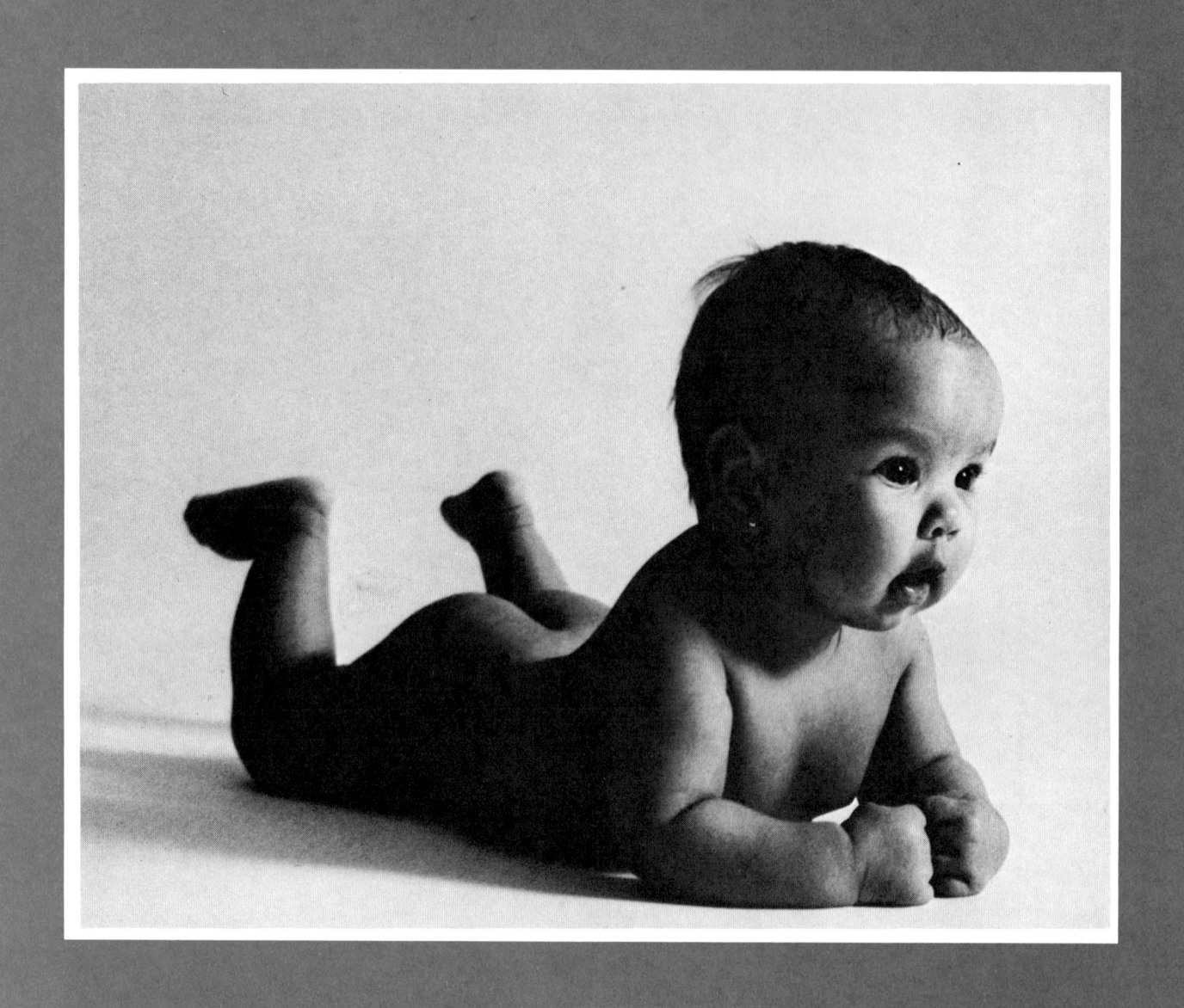

UNIT FIVE

CHANGE: THE NEONATAL PERIOD

25

Extrauterine Life Adaptation

BEHAVIORAL OBJECTIVES

Upon completion of this chapter, the reader should be able to:

- Compare and contrast fetal circulation and newborn circulation.

- Identify three structures essential to fetal circulation.

- Identify the stimuli that are important in the establishment of respirations.

- Explain mechanisms of heat loss common to the newborn.

- Define a neutral thermal environment.

- Describe mechanisms of heat production and conservation in the newborn.

- Identify the periods of reactivity of the newborn and describe the physiologic functions of each.

The delivery period and the first hours following birth are time spans in which phenomenal changes occur as the newborn adapts to a new environment. The warm, dark, fluid-filled environment that has provided security for the fetus is replaced by a cooler, light-filled environment of air. Adaptation to extrauterine life is one of the most dramatic adjustments that humans must make. It has been said that the journey from the womb to the outside world is the longest and most difficult human journey. In the intrauterine environment, the fetus is dependent on the mother for oxygenation, nutrition, excretion, thermoregulation, and fluid balance. Within seconds of delivery, the newborn must perform these functions independently. The essential event that must occur at birth is the shifting of respiration from the placenta to the infant's lungs (Ziai, Clarke, and Merritt, 1984).

Most newborns adjust to the stressors of the extrauterine environment and assume these functions without obvious difficulty. Less frequently, the adjustments are not made so smoothly, and external assistance is required for the newborn to make these transitions (Table 25–1).

The importance of the nursing role during this period of phenomenal physiologic adaptation cannot be overemphasized. Recognition of normal as well as abnormal physiologic responses to stressors is essential in providing accurate nursing assessment and appropriate nursing intervention.

INTRAUTERINE LIFE

Pulmonary Function

The fetus initiates respiratory movements as early as 13 weeks' gestation. These respiratory movements become more frequent, more organized, and more vigorous as term approaches. However, there is evidence that at approximately 3 days prior to birth the incidence of fetal breathing movements is greatly reduced.

Fetal breathing movements apparently have little to do with meeting the oxygen needs of the fetus. Prior to birth the oxygen needs are met by the placenta. It has been hypothesized that the fetal respiratory movements may aid in the development of alveolar and bronchial structures or may have some relationship to the synthesis, release, and distribution of surfactant (Reeder, Mastroianni, and Martin, 1983).

Just as it is known that fetal breathing movements occur *in utero*, it is also known that the fetal lungs do not remain collapsed *in utero*. The lungs produce fluid that keeps them inflated. By the time of birth, the lungs contain lung fluid similar in volume to the functional residual capacity in the neonatal period—30–35 ml/kg of body weight. Increasing amounts of surfactant are added to the

TABLE 25–1. Factors That Can Disturb the Normal Transition at Birth

Site	Factor
Maternal	Amnionitis
	Anemia
	Diabetes
	Hypertension
	Heart disease
	Hypotension
	Respiratory
	Maternal genetic
	Drugs
	Infection
	Maternal deformities
Uterine	Preterm labor
	Multiple pregnancies
	Abnormal fetal presentations
Placental	Placenta previa
	Abruptio
	Acretia
	Placental insufficiency
	Postterm pregnancy
Umbilical	Cord prolapse
	Entanglement
	Compression
Fetal	Cephalopelvic disproportion
	Erythroblastosis fetalis
Newborn	Hypothermia
	Meconium aspiration
	Respiratory distress syndrome
	Congenital pneumonia
	Maternal medication
	Mechanical trauma
	Increased lung water
	Congenital defects

SOURCE: Ziai, Clarke, and Merritt (1984).

lung fluid during the last weeks of pregnancy. The presence of surfactant is important in maintaining lung stability and in decreasing the surface tension of the lung and thereby allowing expansion and the establishment of a functional residual capacity.

Fetal lung fluid takes on additional significance for births involving certain presentations and for cesarean births (Milner and Vyas, 1982). The infant delivered by cesarean section does not benefit from the thoracic squeeze of vaginal pressure or from the effect of gravity on fluid drainage. It is postulated that the vaginal squeeze as well as the effect of gravity in the vertex position assists the newborn in evacuation of fetal lung fluid and preparation for aeration of the lung at birth (see Fig. 25–1). The small amount of lung fluid that is

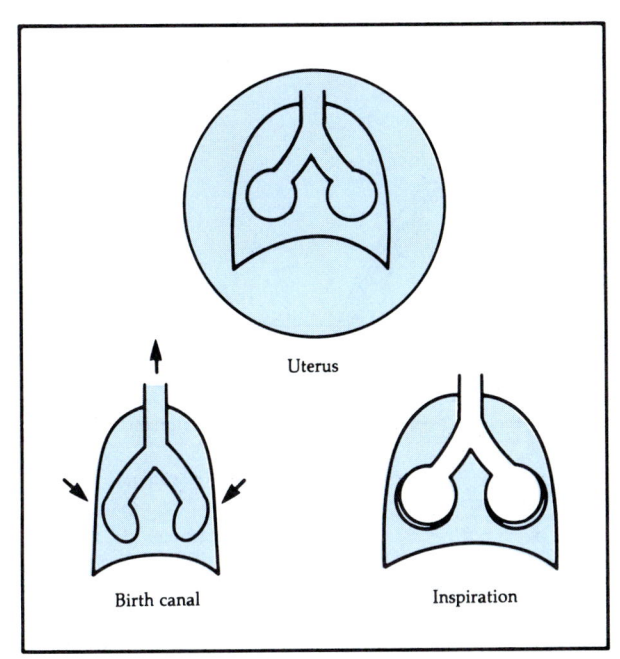

FIGURE 25–1. Fluid distribution in the lung.
SOURCE: Ziai, Clarke, and Merritt (1984).

not "squeezed" out or drained by gravity during a vaginal birth is reabsorbed through the lymphatic system. Thus the newborn delivered by cesarean section is more at risk for the development of respiratory problems, and so is the newborn delivered in a presentation other than vertex due to the relatively low functioning of the fetal lungs.

Fetal Circulation

Just as there are intrauterine pulmonary factors that influence the transition of the newborn to extrauterine life, there are also significant intrauterine circulatory factors. Because the placenta acts as an organ of transfer between mother and fetus, fetal circulation differs significantly from extrauterine circulation. Three unique circulatory structures are especially efficient in meeting the needs of the fetus *in utero:* (1) the ductus venosus, (2) the foramen ovale, and (3) the ductus arteriosus. The *ductus arteriosus* and the *foramen ovale* serve to shunt most of the blood to bypass the lungs. Only enough blood is circulated to the lungs to provide nourishment to maintain tissue integrity. The *ductus venosus* provides freshly oxygenated blood (from the placenta) more directly to the inferior vena cava.

To understand the adaptation that takes place shortly after birth, it seems useful to trace the entire route of fetal circulation. From the placenta the oxygenated blood flows to the fetus through the umbilical vein. Approximately half of the blood flows to the liver (see Fig. 25–2). The rest of the blood bypasses the liver through the special fetal structure, the ductus venosus. Blood from the ductus venosus enters the inferior vena cava, where it mixes with blood from the lower portion of the fetus's body and then enters the right atrium. The blood from the right atrium flows directly to the left atrium through the special fetal structure, the foramen ovale. It then flows to the left ventricle and to the head and neck by way of the ascending aorta. Note that this route ensures a well-oxygenated blood supply to these areas.

The blood that circulates to the upper extremities and head returns through the superior vena cava to the right atrium. Instead of passing through the foramen ovale, it is directed downward into the right ventricle. From the right ventricle the blood enters the pulmonary arteries, where a small amount of the blood goes to the lungs as the rest is shunted to the great aorta through the ductus arteriosus. This blood supplies oxygen and nutrients to the trunk and lower extremities. Most of it then finds its way back through the internal iliac arteries, through the umbilical cord, to the placenta, where it is reoxygenated. A small amount of this blood from the lower extremities passes back into the ascending vena cava, where it mingles with fresh blood from the umbilical vein and again travels the route of the entire body (Moore, 1983). Fetal circulation differs significantly from normal newborn circulation. Fetal circulation *in utero* is uniquely suited to the maintenance of a well-oxygenated blood supply to the vital organs.

PULMONARY EXTRAUTERINE LIFE ADAPTATION

First Breath

The phenomenon of the first breath has been studied for many years (Milner and Vyas, 1982). Yet many questions remain unanswered. The first breath heralds the beginning of an independent life–the newborn is capable of existence outside the intrauterine environment. It is hypothesized that several factors are responsible for the initiation of the first breath. Mechanical, sensory, and

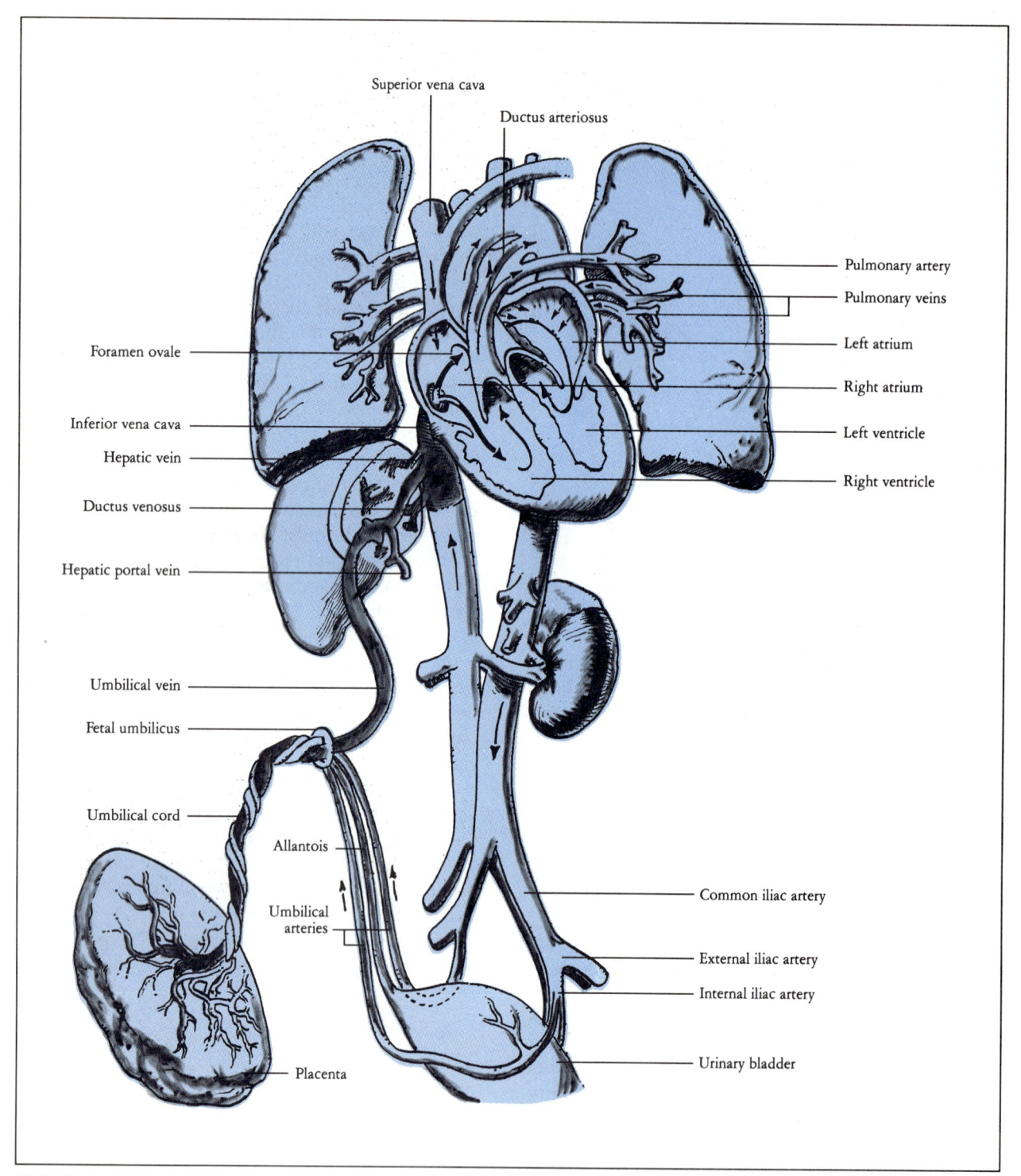

FIGURE 25–2. Fetal circulation.

chemical factors all seem to be involved (see Table 25–2).

The birth canal squeeze and the change from intrauterine pressure to extrauterine pressure are mechanical forces applied to the fetus secondary to muscular contractions from labor. As noted earlier, when the newborn is delivered in a presentation other than vertex, this fluid is not as easily expelled from the lungs. For this reason newborns delivered in other presentations should be closely

TABLE 25–2. *Factors Influencing the Respiratory Center and Respirations in the Fetus and Newborn*

Stimulate Respirations	Depress Respirations
Cord clamping	Maternal narcotics, sedatives
Hypoxemia (low P_{O_2})	Profound hypoxemia (P_{O_2} < 15 mm Hg)
Hypercarbia (high P_{CO_2})	Severe hypercarbia (P_{CO_2} > 70 mm Hg)
Acidosis (pH between 7.30 and 7.05)	Profound acidosis (pH < 7.00) or alkalosis (pH > 7.50)
	Heating (rapid or overheating)
Cooling	Severe cold stress
Stretching of lung tissue (Head's paradoxical reflex)	Overstretching of alveoli (Hering-Breuer reflex)
Deflation (Hering-Breuer reflex)	
Focal atelectasis	Massive atelectasis
Proprioceptive motion: change in position of body or individual joints	Floating
Tactile: touch, pain	Darkness
Auditory: noise	
Visual: light	

SOURCE: Clark, Affonso, and Harris (1979).

observed for the development of respiratory symptoms (Moore, 1983), secondary to retained amniotic fluid. It is thought that the intrauterine squeeze not only assists in expelling some of the fetal lung fluid but also creates a negative intrathoracic pressure that assists the "recoil" that occurs with the first breath. When the uterus is not contracting, the intrauterine pressure is 15 cm H_2O. While the membranes remain intact, the pressure is distributed equally and cannot influence the amount of pressure in the lungs. When the membranes are ruptured and the fetus descends into the lower uterine segment, the contractions create pressures of up to 75 cm H_2O that result in the squeezing of the fetus's thorax and the expulsion of lung fluid. Higher pressures have been recorded during the second stage of labor (Milner and Vyas, 1982).

The sensory stimuli that are thought to be associated with the initiation of respiration include cold, pain, touch, light, sound, and gravity (Reeder, Mastroianni, and Martin, 1983). This does not mean that cold stress should not be a concern to the nurse. On the contrary, it remains a prime concern, and care should be taken to minimize newborn heat loss. Excessive cooling of the newborn will interfere with breathing by increasing the need for oxygen and producing acidosis that affects blood flow through the lungs (Clark, Affonso, and Harris, 1979).

Delivery does result in a change of environmental temperature for the newborn. The normal intrauterine temperature is about 37°C, while the delivery room temperature may be as low as 22°C. This obviously represents a major environmental change.

Other changes that occur during the initiation of respiration may be categorized as chemical. Surfactant production increases as the fetus nears term. Surfactant is necessary to prevent alveolar collapse after birth. A great respiratory effort, as high as 40–80 cm H_2O pressure, is required to expand the newborn lungs even in the presence of sufficient surfactant. The relationship between the pressure necessary to inflate the lungs and the volume of gas brought into the lungs during the first few breaths after birth is shown in Fig. 25–3. Subsequent breaths require less effort than the first breath, because the airways are already open. This can be compared with blowing up a partially inflated balloon and one which is totally collapsed.

Chemical change due to a transient asphyxia also seems to be of prime importance (*asphyxia* is a condition in which oxygen is decreased and carbon dioxide is increased). Asphyxia-associated changes that tend to stimulate breathing include a decreased oxygen level, an increased carbon dioxide level, and a lowered pH level in the blood. However, if these chemical changes are prolonged, the respiratory center becomes depressed

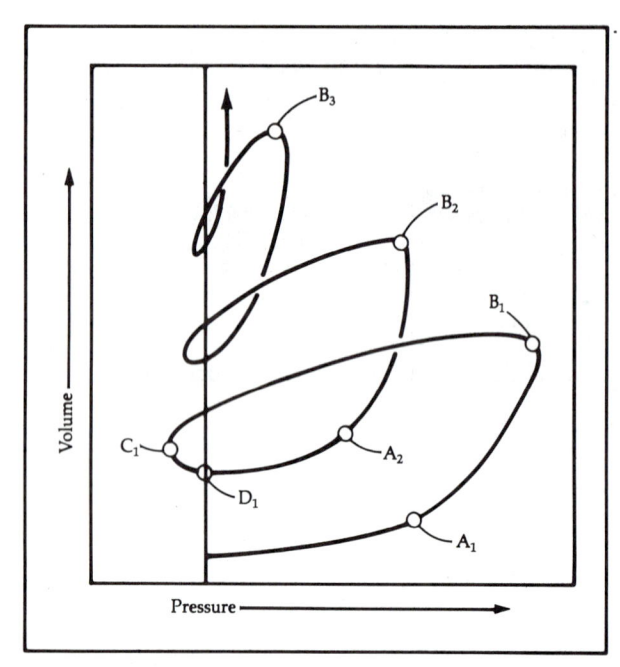

FIGURE 25-3. Pressure-volume loops during the first few breaths.
SOURCE: Clark, Affonso, and Harris (1979).

rather than stimulated. Drugs administered to the mother too close to the time of delivery may also serve to depress the respiratory center in the newborn. If all goes well, the infant usually takes his/her first breath within 30 sec and is breathing rhythmically after 90 sec (Ziai, Clarke, and Merritt, 1984).

Mechanical, Sensory, and Chemical Factors as Negative Stressors

While mechanical, sensory, and chemical stressors may combine to form a positive stimulus to the initiation of respiration, these stressors may also be associated with a negative adaptation to extrauterine life.

Mechanical Stressors

The intrauterine pressure secondary to uterine contractions may negatively influence the adaptation of the neonate. The pressure on the fetal skull may decrease the cerebral blood flow, which may activate the central vagus nerve and result in a decreased heart rate and decreased cardiac output (Tucker, 1978). During normal labor each uterine contraction decreases blood flow in the placental intervillous space to some degree. If placental reserve is adequate, the normal fetus will not be stressed significantly. However, if placental blood flow is compromised in the resting state, decreased blood flow in the intervillous space during uterine contractions will significantly diminish fetal oxygen supply. When the amount of oxygen needed by the fetus is decreased, fetal tissues begin to use the anaerobic metabolic pathway to meet energy requirements, and metabolic and respiratory acidosis occurs.

The newborn adjusts to the mechanical pressure of contractions if it is not prolonged. Intrauterine electronic monitoring as well as traditional labor monitoring techniques are necessary to assess the duration of contractions and the response of the fetus (see Chapter 16).

Localized pressure to the fetal head may also cause a mechanical injury to the fetus. The fetal skull tolerates molding and some localized pressure. The mildly convex plates of the head (occipital, frontal, and parietal) are connected by elastic connective tissue. Although the head of the newborn is able to mold, differential pressure (pressure of one area against the other) results in a shift of mass from the point of lesser pressure to the point of greater pressure (see Fig. 25-4). This pressure may cause a *caput succedaneum*, localized edema of the fetal head, which may cross the suture lines. This edema is present at birth but generally subsides within a few days after birth. If the pressure exerted upon the head is exception-

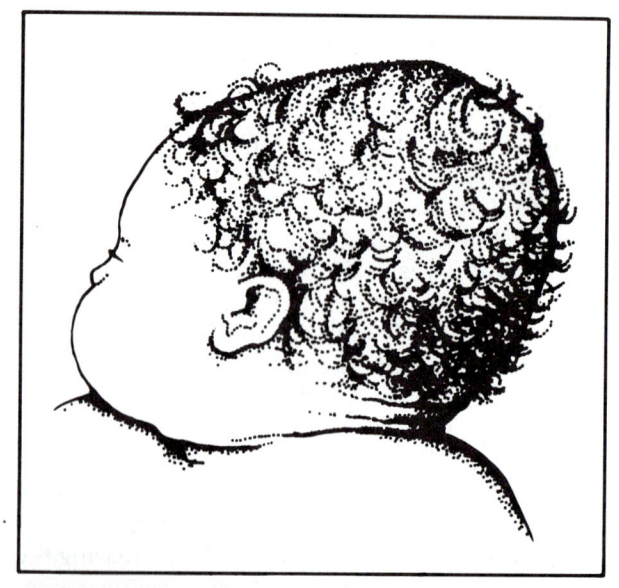

FIGURE 25-4. Vertex presentation molding.
SOURCE: Korones (1981).

ally hard and long, a *cephalhematoma* may result. A cephalhematoma is a collection of blood between the skull bone or bones and the periosteum. Because the bleeding occurs between the bone and the periosteum, the cephalhematoma does not cross the suture lines. The cephalhematoma may be further differentiated from the caput in that it is usually not present at birth but develops afterward, and it may take longer than 1 month to be reabsorbed (see Fig. 25–4). The nurse needs to provide information and support for the parents about either occurrence in order to alleviate anxiety. Other mechanical injuries to the fetus are listed in Table 25–3.

Sensory Stressors

Harsh sensory stimuli may also have negative effects upon the extrauterine adaptation of the newborn. Frederick Leboyer (1976) suggests that exposing the newborn to the abrupt change from the warm, dark, fluid-filled, and relatively quiet intrauterine environment to the cooler, air-filled, light, and noise-filled extrauterine environment may have negative psychologic effects on later development. He suggests that the sensory stimuli be reduced as much as possible in order to simulate the intrauterine environment. (The negative effects of cold stress are discussed later in this chapter.) Essentially, a cold environment negatively affects extrauterine adaptation by making cardiorespiratory adaptation more difficult. It also contributes to hypoglycemia and the development of hyperbilirubinemia.

Chemical Stressors

Transient and minor decreases in pO_2 and pH accompanied by minor increases in pCO_2 serve to stimulate the respiratory center. However, severe asphyxia poses a major threat to the fetus. With severe asphyxia the heart rate falls, cardiac output decreases, superior vena cava blood crosses the foramen ovale, meconium may be passed, and deep inspiratory gasping may occur. If severe fetal asphyxia occurs *in utero*, it may be followed by inhibition of respiration at birth, cyanosis from persistent fetal circulation, a heart rate below 100, and intense peripheral vasoconstriction.

The fetus is at greatest risk of severe asphyxia during labor and delivery. Most fetal asphyxia is caused by a reduction of oxygen transfer across the placenta. Among maternal factors associated with

TABLE 25–3. Mechanical Injuries to the Fetus

1. *Skin, subcutaneous tissue*
   a. Caput succedaneum
   b. Cyanosis and edema of buttocks, upper or lower extremities
   c. Diffuse scalp hemorrhage
   d. Subcutaneous fat necrosis (pressure necrosis)
   e. Abrasion of the skin
   f. Petechiae and ecchymoses of the skin
2. *Skull*
   a. Molding
   b. Fracture (linear or depressed)
   c. Cephalhematoma
3. *Long bone fractures*
   a. Clavicle
   b. Humerus
   c. Femur
4. *Central nervous system*
   a. Hemorrhage into brain substance
   b. Subdural hematoma
   c. Spinal cord injury
5. *Ocular*
   a. Subconjunctival (scleral) hemorrhage
   b. Retinal hemorrhage
   c. Rupture of inner membrane of cornea (Descemet's)
6. *Peripheral nerves*
   a. Brachial plexus injury
   b. Diaphragmatic paralysis (phrenic nerve injury)
   c. Facial paralysis
7. *Hemorrhage into abdominal organs*
   a. Liver
   b. Spleen
   c. Kidney
   d. Adrenals
8. *Rib fracture*

SOURCE: Korones (1981).

reduction of oxygen transfer are (1) maternal hypoxia, (2) maternal hypotension, (3) maternal hypertension, and (4) maternal blood loss.

Establishment of Rhythmic Respirations

Respiratory control in the immediate newborn period is relatively stable, although the chemoreceptor mechanism is probably sluggish (Milner and Vyas, 1982). In the term infant a respiratory pattern may not be established until about 20 sec after birth, but never later than 30 sec. After three to five gasplike efforts, sustained rhythmic respirations should be established by no later than 60 sec after birth. A premature infant may take 15–20 sec longer than the healthy term infant to achieve each of these goals.

Once ventilation and normal respirations are established, there are many factors that sustain ventilation. These factors include some degree of pain, cold, touch, noise, acidosis, hypoxia, and CO_2 retention, and to some extent cord clamping. In order for infants to move air in and out of the lungs, they must have (1) a functioning respiratory center to regulate the rate of breathing, (2) intact nerves from the brain to the breathing muscles in the chest (these nerves carry messages of how often the muscles of breathing should contract or relax), (3) enough energy to supply the respiratory muscles with the strength needed to do the work of breathing, and (4) a free and clear airway to allow passage of air into and out of the lungs.

A respiratory rate as high as 80 breaths/min may be noted during the first 15–30 min after delivery. This period is one of intense activity for the healthy newborn. The newborn normally sleeps after this first period of reactivity and then initiates a second period of reactivity upon awakening. (Periods of reactivity are discussed in greater detail later in this chapter.) After the second period of reactivity the newborn generally assumes an average respiratory rate of about 40 breaths/min (Klaus and Fanaroff, 1979). During the intermediate period, between the ages of 48 hours and 3 months, the control system is rapid but relatively unstable. It is only at age 4–6 months that the mature response, combining stability with speed, is consistently observed (Milner and Vyas, 1982).

CIRCULATORY EXTRAUTERINE LIFE ADAPTATION

Fetal circulation ends when the umbilical cord is clamped. Concurrent with the cessation of umbilical–placental flow, there is a marked increase in systemic vascular resistance, a rapid reduction in pulmonary vascular resistance, and a marked increase in pulmonary blood flow associated with expansion of the lungs with air. The pulmonary vasodilation is largely related to the effects of the increased pO_2 to which the pulmonary vessels are exposed. With the closure of the fetal shunts, the right ventricle now ejects all its blood into the pulmonary circulation.

Cord Clamping

There seem to be both advantages and disadvantages to early as well as later cord clamping. Many studies have been done to help decide the issue, but it remains unclear whether later cord clamping is advantageous. As much as 50–100 ml of blood may be added to newborn circulation if cord clamping is delayed several minutes and the infant is placed below the level of the placenta. However, it has been reported that rapid increases in blood volume may stress the newborn heart and the pulmonary vasculature, adding to the likelihood of respiratory distress, bleeding problems, and clotting in vessels with very slow flow, i.e. renal veins. While it has been reported that this additional blood assists in maintaining higher levels of iron stores, there is additional evidence that this extra blood may contribute to hyperbilirubinemia during the first week of life (Reeder, Mastroianni, and Martin, 1983). Regardless of when cord clamping occurs, it begins a period of circulatory adaptation for the newborn.

Closing of Shunts

With the initial respiration of the newborn, many circulatory changes occur simultaneously. Many of the structures and vessels that were necessary for fetal circulation now become useless. With the first breath and the clamping and cutting of the umbilical cord, a large amount of blood is returned to the fetal heart and lungs. Due to this increase in the amount of blood in the lungs and heart, a larger amount of blood under higher pressure enters the left atrium. The resulting increased pressure in the left atrium is responsible for the closing of the foramen ovale (Sacksteder, 1978).

As the oxygen concentration increases following the changes in pulmonary circulation, the ductus arteriosus is stimulated to constrict. Normally, functional closure is complete by 15 hours of age, while anatomic closure *(fibrosis)* is usually not complete until 3 weeks of age (Korones, 1981).

The mechanism of closure of the ductus venosus, the vessel that connects the fetal portal circulation with the inferior vena cava, remains unknown. With the ligation of the umbilical cord, the ductus venosus no longer transports blood. Fibrosis of the ductus venosus is usually completed in 3–7 days (Korones, 1981). After birth the umbilical vein and arteries no longer transport blood. These structures are obliterated except for the proximal portions of the umbilical arteries, which remain open (Sacksteder, 1978).

ADAPTATION OF OTHER SYSTEMS

Thermoregulation

The regulation of body temperature is essentially a balance of heat production and heat loss. In the newborn, the maintenance of a stable body temperature, where the amount of heat lost is about equal to that being produced, is possible only within a narrow range of environmental temperature fluctuation.

The newborn has a capacity for reasonably effective heat production, but the tendency for heat loss is excessive. The newborn's increased tendency to lose body heat is related to several factors: (1) large surface area in relation to mass; (2) limited metabolic capabilities; and (3) decreased thermal insulation because of limited fat deposits. Hypothermia is therefore the principal problem of heat regulation in the newborn. The tendency to lose heat rapidly at ordinary room temperature may be a threat to the survival of the newborn (Alistair, 1977; Korones, 1981).

Mechanisms of Heat Conservation and Production

The primary mechanisms by which the newborn is able to respond to heat loss include (1) vasomotor control, (2) thermal insulation, (3) shivering and muscular activity, and (4) nonshivering thermogenesis.

VASOMOTOR CONTROL. Newborns are able to conserve heat through constricting blood vessels in the skin and by increasing production of heat. On the other hand, the newborn is able to dissipate heat through vasodilation if exposed to excessive warmth (Perez, 1981). Essential to the newborn's ability to adapt to changes in environmental temperature is the ability to respond to peripheral stimulation. Peripheral stimulation activates vasomotor and metabolic processes to control the balance of heat.

THERMAL INSULATION. Thermal insulation varies directly with the amount of white fat in the body, since fat is a heat-retaining tissue. At birth about 11–17 percent of body weight is white fat. Substantial amounts of fat do not accumulate until after 32 weeks' gestation. Therefore, the premature or the intrauterine growth–retarded infant lacks adequate body insulation to prevent rapid heat loss or to permit the body mass to act as a heat reservoir (Perez, 1981; see Chapter 32).

SHIVERING AND MUSCULAR ACTIVITY. Muscular activity and body movement contribute to heat production in the newborn. Restlessness and hyperactivity are noted when the infant is first exposed to cold. Although this activity contributes somewhat to heat production, it is not considered a significant heat source. The newborn may also conserve heat by assuming a position similar to the *in utero* position. Flexion of the extremities reduces the surface area of the skin exposed to the environment (Korones, 1981).

Although shivering is an important mechanism of heat production in adults, its function appears to be limited in the newborn. Some report that the newborn does not shiver (Korones, 1981), whereas others report that the newborn shivers only in the presence of extreme cold stress (Perez, 1981). At any rate, shivering does not appear to be a significant mechanism of heat production in the newborn.

NONSHIVERING THERMOGENESIS. Nonshivering thermogenesis refers to the heat that is produced by a metabolic rate (and therefore an oxygen consumption) that is minimal in a neutral thermal environment, or increased in a cold one (Korones, 1981). Nonshivering thermogenesis appears to be the most important and consistent mechanism of heat production in the newborn (Alistair, 1977; Korones, 1981; Perez, 1981; Moore, 1983). The newborn's brain, liver, and possibly skeletal muscle are important thermogenic organs.

A major source of heat produced in the newborn by nonshivering thermogenesis appears to be *brown fat* (Korones, 1981), which makes up about 1.5 percent of total body weight. It is located between the scapulae; behind the sternum; around the neck, head, heart, great vessels, kidneys, and adrenal glands; and in the axilla. Note that the distribution is such that it forms a vest around the thorax and a collar around the neck. Brown fat provides local as well as central heat. It warms the blood as it enters and leaves the heart. Brown fat is easily distinguished from white fat: it has a copious blood supply, a dense cellular content, and a profusion of nerve endings. It seems that sympathetic nerves furnish the stimulus for the release of norepinephrine, which is thought to be the principal mediator of nonshivering thermogenesis (Perez, 1981). Norepinephrine stimulates fat metabolism in brown adipose tissue. The result of this increased chemical activity is an increased amount of heat, which perfuses the tissue mass. Skin temperatures recorded over subcutaneous deposits of brown fat are warmer during periods of cold stress than during nonstress periods (Korones, 1981).

Mechanisms of Heat Loss

Mechanisms of heat loss in the newborn include (1) radiation, (2) conduction, (3) convection, and (4) evaporation.

RADIATION. Radiant heat loss occurs when heat is lost to a cooler, solid environmental surface that is not in direct contact with the newborn. Environmental surfaces that may typically be cool include nursery walls and isolette walls. Radiant heat loss occurs independent of the surrounding temperature of the air. Radiant heat loss is suggested as the major mechanism of heat transfer in the newborn. It is important that the newborn be placed away from cool objects and walls. Also, it cannot be assumed that because the air temperature of an isolette is appropriately warmed, the walls of the isolette are also warm. The inside wall of an isolette acts as a radiant receiving surface (Perez, 1981).

CONDUCTION. Conduction is the heat loss that occurs during direct contact of the skin with a cooler solid object. Both the thermal conductivity of the surface and the surface temperature affect the amount of heat transferred. Placement of an infant on a cold table or cold scale promotes conductive heat loss (Korones, 1981).

EVAPORATION. Evaporative heat loss occurs when moisture on the skin of the newborn turns to vapor in the presence of dry air. Heat is lost by evaporation of insensible water, visible sweat, and moisture released from the respiratory tract during exhalation (Korones, 1981). Evaporative heat loss is minimal in the presence of high humidity and is maximal in dry environments. Nursing consideration should be given to evaporative heat loss at the time of delivery, because the newborn is covered with amniotic fluid. Heat loss from evaporation of amniotic fluid can be minimized if the newborn is dried immediately with a warm towel.

CONVECTION. Convective heat loss involves the transfer of body heat from the body surface to cooler surrounding air. This mechanism depends on the temperature and velocity of the surrounding air. Drafts should be minimized to prevent this type of heat loss (Perez, 1981).

Maintaining a Neutral Thermal Environment

A neutral thermal environment is an environment that provides optimal conditions for the maintenance of a normal core temperature with minimal caloric and oxygen consumption. The metabolic needs of a newborn increase as soon as the newborn leaves a neutral thermal environment and decrease as soon as the neutral thermal environment is restored (Scharping, 1983). The average newborn who is left wet and uncovered after birth will lose about 100 cal of heat/kg per min, leading to an increase in oxygen consumption and the development of progressive metabolic acidosis (Ziai, Clarke, and Merritt, 1984).

The abdominal skin temperature is indicative of a neutral thermal environment and should be maintained between 36 and 36.5°C, or 96.8 and 97.7°F (Perez, 1981). Axillary temperatures should also be maintained in this range.

Of all the vital signs, temperature is probably the most significant for successful extrauterine adaptation of the newborn. The detrimental effects of hypothermia in the normal newborn can be prevented by adequately monitoring environmental and body temperatures and assisting the newborn in conservation of body heat.

Endocrine System

While the endocrine system is ordinarily adequately developed in the term newborn, some of its functions are immature. For example, the newborn is particularly susceptible to dehydration because of the limited quantities of antidiuretic hormone (ADH) produced by the posterior pituitary gland (Whaley and Wong, 1983).

High levels of maternal estrogen and progesterone tend to cause a transient "miniature puberty." The breasts of the newborn may be engorged and may secrete milk during the first few days of life because of the abrupt decrease in hormonal transfer from the mother. Female newborns sometimes have hypertrophied labia as well as pseudomenstruation due to maternal hormonal effects. These occurrences sometimes cause concern on the part of the parents. Nurses should explain to parents that these occurrences are normal and transient.

Metabolic Changes

The abrupt termination of a continuous intrauterine supply of glucose and calcium requires profound changes in metabolism for the newborn in the extrauterine environment. There are rapid changes in plasma glucose and calcium during the first days of life. Blood glucose at birth is normally 60–70 percent of the maternal level. The blood glucose then falls over the next 1–2 hours and stabilizes at a minimum of 35–40 mg/100 ml. By 6 hours after birth the blood glucose generally rises to 60 mg/100 ml in normal unstressed newborns (Klaus and Fanaroff, 1979).

Like the blood glucose, serum calcium normally falls after birth. In the normal newborn it continues to fall for about 24–48 hours and then stabilizes. Hypocalcemia is defined by a serum calcium of less than 7 mg/100 ml in the normal newborn. Hypocalcemia is most likely to occur during the first 2 days of life or at 6–10 days of life. The later-onset hypocalcemia is most often attributed to milk preparations that contain an inappropriate calcium-to-phosphorus ratio (Korones, 1981).

Hypoglycemia and hypocalcemia are the principal metabolic disorders that produce seizures in the newborn. Additional symptoms of both disorders are similar and may include irritability, "jitteriness," cyanosis, apnea, listlessness, poor feeding, hypothermia, and hypotonia. Early observation for the development of hypoglycemia and hypocalcemia is essential in the management of these disorders and in the prevention of long-term problems (Alistair, 1977).

Gastrointestinal System

The gastrointestinal system of the fetus is not responsible for meeting nutritional needs *in utero*. While the fetus is *in utero*, the placenta provides nutrients to meet its nutritional needs. Once the infant is delivered, nutrition must be provided through other means. The normal newborn is able to digest, absorb, and metabolize food.

While the fetus drinks amniotic fluid and excretes it by way of the kidneys, no stool is normally passed while the fetus is *in utero*. (Meconium in the amniotic fluid of fetuses in positions other than breech is considered a sign of fetal distress.) The newborn passes meconium stool within 24–48 hours following delivery (Phillips, 1980). The first meconium stool is dark greenish-black, tarry, and odorless. Bowel sounds should be present a few hours after delivery.

The gastrointestinal tract is usually sterile at birth. Normal flora must accumulate before vitamin K can be synthesized and, as a result, vitamin K (acquamephyton) is routinely given to newborns within the first few hours after birth in most hospitals.

The normal newborn is equipped with reflexes that enable the baby to begin feeding competently. The full-term newborn has coordinated sucking and swallowing reflexes as well as the rooting reflex that causes the infant to turn toward a stimulus with its mouth open.

Oral feedings are usually started within about 6 hours of birth. Long periods of "starvation" are not recommended, because the newborn's glycogen stores are limited. However, the nurse should exercise careful clinical judgment before initiating oral feeding. The infant should be relatively physiologically stable before feeding begins. Sucking and swallowing reflexes should be present, and there should be an absence of respiratory distress prior to oral feeding. Occasionally, a newborn swallows some maternal blood during delivery and may vomit fresh blood. Maternal blood may be differentiated from fetal blood by an Apt test.

In spite of early feeding, a weight loss of 5–10 percent of the birth weight is typical. By about 10 days of age the newborn regains the birth weight. Weekly gains of 5–7 ounces are expected thereafter. The birth weight is generally doubled by 5 months and tripled by 1 year. The birth weight of bottle-fed babies may be doubled in 3–4 months.

The newborn needs water, protein, carbohydrates, fat, vitamins, and minerals for adequate nutrition. The nutritional and fluid requirements are in proportion to body weight. The newborn requires approximately 100 ml of water/kg per day and approximately 100–120 calories/kg per day (see Chapter 28). Enzymes are sufficient to handle proteins and simple carbohydrates, but deficient production of pancreatic amylase impairs the newborn's ability to digest complex carbohydrates. In addition, a deficiency of pancreatic lipase limits the absorption of fats.

The successful initiation of the feeding process is not only essential for the newborn but closely associated with feelings of self-esteem of the mother. If the newborn regurgitates feedings or rejects the mother's breast, the mother may interpret this as a "mothering failure." Support is required from nursing staff to bolster the mother's feelings of self-esteem.

Hepatic System

A major function of the liver after birth is the excretion and breakdown of bilirubin. Prior to birth the placenta was essentially responsible for this function. While the liver takes on a new function after birth, it also gives up a major function of the fetal period. The liver functioned as the chief organ of blood formation from the third to the sixth month of gestation. After birth, a significant increase in blood flow to the liver is noted as the fetal ductus venosus closes and blood is no longer shunted around the liver. The bone marrow becomes the chief site of blood formation in extrauterine life, although the liver continues to produce a limited number of cells into the first postnatal week (Moore, 1983).

Several stressors may prevent the liver from adequately performing the new function of bilirubin breakdown and excretion. Stressors that may prevent adequate liver functioning include infection, hemolysis, hypoglycemia, hypothermia, and prematurity. It is also hypothesized that without exceptional stressors the newborn liver produces insufficient quantities of glucuronyl transferase, an enzyme necessary for the conversion of indirect bilirubin to the water-soluble and thus excretable direct bilirubin. Consequently, with normal newborn hemolysis, it is not uncommon to find elevated levels of indirect bilirubin.

Bilirubin Levels and Liver Function

It is necessary for the nurse to understand the relationship of increased bilirubin levels and liver function in the neonate in order to provide predictive care. Bilirubin is the end-product of red blood cell breakdown. The normal lifespan of the neonatal red blood cell is approximately 80–100 days (adult RBC lifespan is 120 days). As the red cell ages, it becomes fragile, and hemoglobin is split into two fragments, heme and globin. Unconjugated (indirect) bilirubin is formed from the heme fraction (Korones, 1977).

Indirect bilirubin is fat soluble and cannot be excreted by the kidneys. Because it is fat soluble, it has a high affinity for fat tissue and brain tissue. Staining of fat tissues in the body causes the yellow, or *icteric*, appearance in the skin. About 50 percent of all newborns become visibly jaundiced by 48 hours of age. This frequently occurring jaundice may be termed "physiologic jaundice." Physiologic jaundice does not appear before 24 hours of age and disappears by the time the baby is 1 week old. The newborn with physiologic jaundice is otherwise well, and the bilirubin level generally does not exceed 12 mg/100 ml.

Bilirubin staining of brain tissue is called *kernicterus*. Serum bilirubin concentrations in excess of 20 mg/100 ml in term infants, 15 mg/100 ml in preterm infants, and 10–20 mg/100 ml in the smallest premature infants are generally accepted as the levels at which kernicterus is likely to occur (Korones, 1981). Through early observation and initiation of treatment, health professionals attempt to prevent bilirubin levels from rising to dangerous levels.

If bilirubin is albumin-bound, or conjugated, by liver enzymes (making it direct), it cannot stain extravascular or brain tissue. Thus, infants with either decreased albumin levels or particularly immature liver function may be more prone to jaundice (see Table 25–4).

Assessing Insufficient Liver Function

While in most newborns the function of the liver is adequate to meet physiologic needs, this discussion has included those times when liver function may be insufficient to meet those demands. The nurse must differentiate between physiologic and pathologic jaundice. The nurse must also be able to identify risk factors that may predict the development of pathologic jaundice. Through prediction the nurse is able to initiate care that may prevent bilirubin accumulation from reaching levels that could cause permanent brain damage.

PERIODS OF REACTIVITY

Two periods of reactivity, interrupted by a period of sleep, have been identified during the immediate newborn period (see Fig. 25–5).

First Period of Reactivity

The first period of reactivity is characterized by heightened responsivity and intense activity. Ap-

TABLE 25–4. *Factors Contributing to Jaundice in the Newborn*

Factors Contributing to Physiologic Jaundice	Factors Contribution to Pathologic Jaundice

Shorter red blood cell lifespan
Decreased production of liver enzymes
Increase in numbers of red blood cells
	Hemolysis from any cause
	  RH or ABO incompatibility
	  Hematomas
	  Ecchymosis, petechiae
	Decreases in albumin-binding sites
	Infection
	Metabolic factors
	  Hypoglycemia
	  Diabetic mother

proximately 40 min of the first hour of life are spent in this quiet, alert state (see Chapter 26). The infant is active and the eyes may be open. This is an appropriate time to initiate a relationship between newborn and parents. The nurse should be active in assisting the establishment of this relationship by placing the newborn where the parents can watch while initial care is given. After drying the newborn and providing initial care, the nurse may enhance the establishment of the mother–infant relationship by placing the infant in the mother's arms. It is suggested that administration of prophylactic eye drops or ointment be delayed so that early parent–newborn eye contact can be initiated. Care should be exercised throughout this early period to prevent cold stress to the

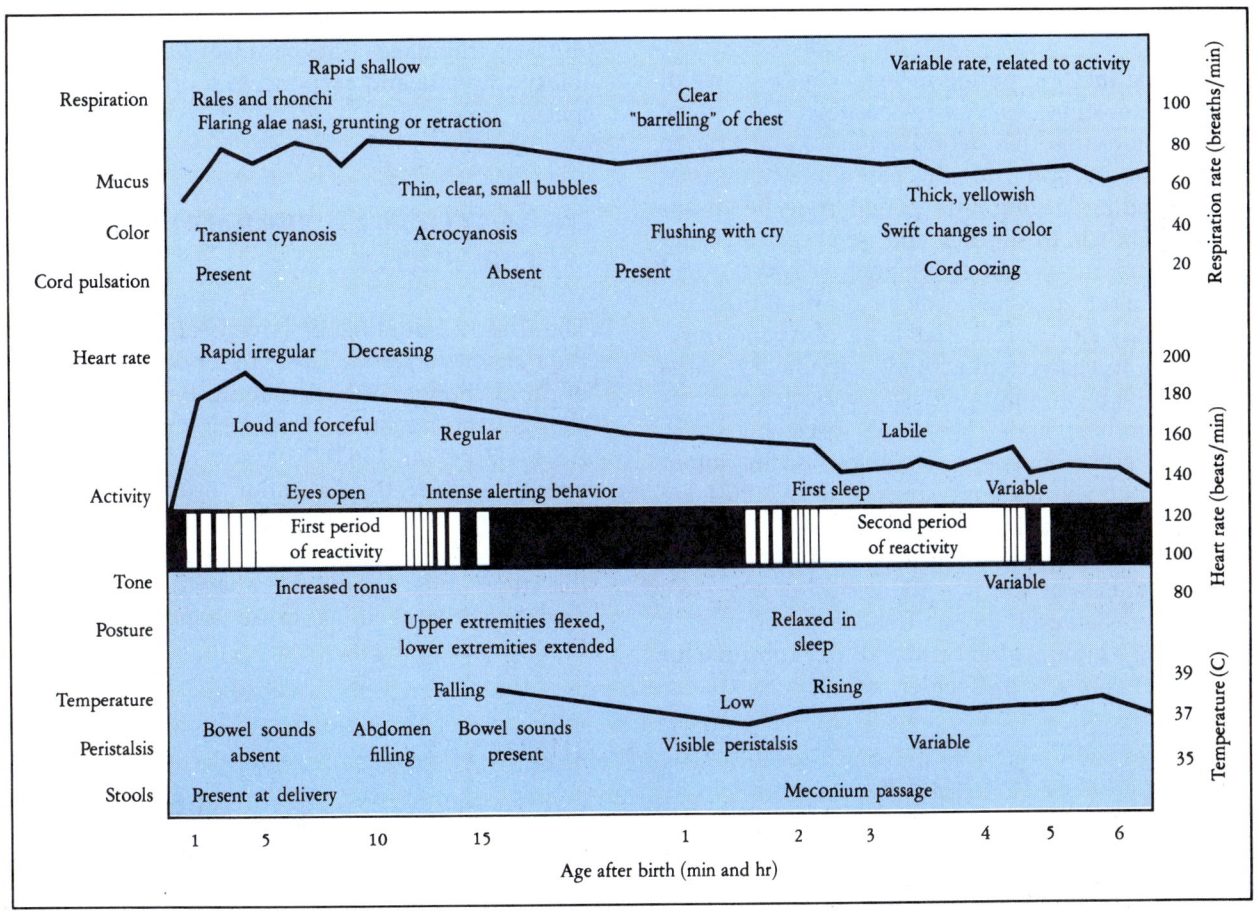

FIGURE 25–5. Periods of reactivity.
SOURCE: Arnold (1965).

newborn and to assist in extrauterine adaptation. Characteristic reactions and responses with alert exploratory behavior include nasal flaring or "sniffing" unrelated to respiratory difficulty; movements of the head from side to side; spontaneous startles and the Moro reflex; grimacing; sucking; swallowing; pursing and smacking of the lips; tremors of the extremities and mandible; opening and closing of the eyelids; short, rapid, jerky movements of the eyeball; sudden outcries; and abrupt cessations of crying (Desmond et al., 1963; Klaus and Fanaroff, 1979).

During the first period of reactivity, the newborn exhibits changes that are predominately sympathetic. It is not uncommon for the heart rate to reach 180 beats/min during the first minutes following delivery. Rapid and irregular respirations may be noted as well as transient rales, grunting, and flaring of the nares. *(Note: these respiratory symptoms are indicative of respiratory distress during periods other than reactivity.)* The body temperature decreases, while there is an increase in activity and muscle tone during this time.

Sleep Period

Following the first period of reactivity, a phase of unresponsiveness or sleep ensues. The nurse should note that this period is not a good time to initiate interaction with the parents. Attempts at breastfeeding during this period may be disappointing for both mother and newborn. A rapid respiratory rate without dyspnea may be noted during this sleep period. The heart rate at this time is generally slower (120–140 beats/min) and unresponsive to changes in activity. Circulatory status is reflected by an improved acrocyanosis (cyanosis of extremities) and a generally excellent color. General responsiveness decreases as the infant sleeps, but spontaneous jerks and twitches are common. Abdominal peristaltic waves may be observed during sleep, as well as small amounts of watery mucus at the lips (Desmond et al., 1963; Klaus and Fanaroff, 1979). This sleep period may begin at 1–3 hours after birth and may continue for 3–6 hours after birth (Oehler, 1981).

Second Period of Reactivity

Following this sleep period, the second period of reactivity occurs. An exaggerated responsiveness is exhibited, with marked swings in the intensity of activity. This second period of reactivity may be brief or it may continue over several hours. It begins when the infant is 3–6 hours of age. During this period the heart rate is very labile, with episodes of tachycardia as well as bradycardia. The skin color reflects improved vasomotor tone, as it remains pink. Respirations are again irregular at a rate of 30–60 breaths/min, and apneic pauses may occur. Oral secretions are now thick and yellow, and gagging and vomiting are common. During this period nursing care must include not only the monitoring of vital signs but continued monitoring of airway patency, as secretions may interfere with airway maintenance. Transitional nurseries should have suctioning equipment and oxygen readily accessible.

The bowel is generally cleared of meconium during this second period of reactivity. It is thought that as this second period of reactivity diminishes, a relative stability is reached and the newborn is ready to begin feedings.

These periods of reactivity and sleep occur in all infants, but the length of each period can be affected by maternal medication, anesthesia, length and difficulty of labor, and amount of stress to the fetus during labor. These are important periods to know about—not only because of the physical changes, but because of the infant's ability to relate and respond to its parents during specific times.

TRANSITIONAL PERIOD AFTER BIRTH

The first 12 hours of life have been designated as the *transitional period*. These first hours are periods of rapid change and adaptation. Because of rapid change, the newborn must be monitored closely (Desmond et al., 1963). Vital signs should be taken every 15 min in the first hour, every 60 min for 4 hours, and then every 4 hours until stable. The nurse should focus on physical assessment during this time. She should be able to detect subtle deviations as well as gross abnormalities (see Chapters 19 and 26).

SUMMARY

Birth is a "new beginning" that requires major physiologic and psychologic adjustments. The infant must adjust from an intrauterine, acquatic environment to an extrauterine, atmospheric environment. With the clamping of the cord the infant's body systems must assume all of the functions previously met by the placenta.

One of the biggest changes will be the closure of the three shunts which were vital for fetal circulation: the ductus venosus, the foramen ovale, and the ductus arteriosus. Mechanical, sensory, and chemical factors are involved in the initiation of the infant's first breath and heralds the beginning of an independent life.

In addition to respiratory and circulatory stabilization, temperature maintenance is extremely important for successful extrauterine adaptation. In the newborn, the maintenance of a stable body temperature is possible within a narrow range of environmental temperature fluctuations. The detrimental effects of hypothermia in the normal newborn can be prevented by adequately monitoring environmental and body temperatures and assisting the newborn in conservation of body heat. During the immediate period after birth, two periods of reactivity, interrupted by a period of sleep, also occur.

In addition to providing physiologic support, the nurse is in a unique position to foster early positive parent–infant interaction. As soon after delivery as possible, the nurse should allow the parents to see and hold their infant. The newborn should be placed in such a position that visual contact can be initiated. Early contact contributes to the earlier formation of attachment and a healthier parent–infant bond (see Chapter 37). The newborn is capable of responding to its parents within minutes after birth.

REFERENCES

Alistair, G. S. P. 1977. *Neonatology: A practical guide*. Flushing, N. Y.: Medical Examination Publishing.

Arnold, H. W.; Putnam, N. J.: Barnard, B. L.; Desmond, M. M.; and Rudolph, A. J. 1965. Transition to extrauterine life. *Am. J. Nurs.* 65(10):77–84.

Clark, A.; Affonso, D.; and Harris, T. 1979. *Childbearing: A nursing perspective*. 2nd ed. Philadelphia: F. A. Davis.

Desmond, M. M.; Franklin, R. R.; Vellvona, C.; Hill, R. M.; Plumb, R.; Arnold, H.; and Watts, J. 1963. The clinical behavior of the newly born. *J. Pediatrics*. 62:307–318.

Klaus, M. H., and Fanaroff, A. A. 1979. *Care of the high-risk neonate*. 2nd ed. Philadelphia: W. B. Saunders.

Korones, S. B. 1981. *High-risk newborn infants: The basis for intensive nursing care*. 3rd ed. St. Louis: C. V. Mosby.

Leboyer, F. 1976. *Birth without violence*. New York: A. A. Knopf.

Milner, A. D., and Vyas, H. 1982. Lung expansion at birth. *J. Pediatrics*. 101:879–886.

Moore, M. L. 1977. *Newborn, family, and nurse*. Philadelphia: W. B. Saunders.

Moore, M. L. 1983. *Realities in childbearing*. Philadelphia: W. B. Saunders.

Oehler, J. M. 1981. *Family-centered neonatal nursing care*. Philadelphia: J. B. Lippincott.

Perez, R. H. 1981. *Protocols for perinatal nursing practice*. St. Louis: C. V. Mosby.

Phillips, C. R. 1980. *Family-centered maternity and newborn care: A basic text*. St. Louis: C. V. Mosby.

Reeder, S. J.; Mastroianni, L.; and Martin, L. L. 1983. *Maternity nursing*. 15th ed. Philadelphia: J. B. Lippincott.

Sacksteder, S. 1978. Embryology and fetal circulation. *Am. J. Nurs.* 78:262–264.

Scharping, E. M. 1983. Physiologic measurements of the neonate. *MCN*. 8(Jan./Feb.):70–75.

Spence, A. P., and Mason, E. B. 1979. *Human anatomy and physiology*. Menlo Park, Calif.: Benjamin Cummings.

Tucker, S. M. 1978. *Fetal monitoring and assessment in high-risk pregnancy*. St. Louis: C. V. Mosby.

Whaley, L. F., and Wong, D. L. 1983. *Nursing care of infants and children*. 2nd ed. St. Louis: C. V. Mosby.

Ziai, M.; Clarke, T.; and Merritt, T. 1984. *Assessment of the newborn: A guide for the practitioner*. Boston: Little, Brown.

26

Assessment of the Normal Newborn

BEHAVIORAL OBJECTIVES

Upon completion of this chapter, the reader should be able to:

- Discuss the importance of assessment in the care of the normal newborn infant.

- Define gestational age and discuss various methods for determining it.

- List the steps in a systematic physical examination of the newborn.

- Relate the importance of symmetry to the physical examination of the newborn infant.

- Describe common variations of the newborn considered to be within normal range.

- Discuss the significance of reflexes elicited on a neurologic assessment of the newborn.

- Describe the use of the Brazelton Neonatal Assessment Scale in the assessment of behavior.

- Discuss the development of the sensory modalities at birth.

The transition from intrauterine to extrauterine life is a very critical time for the newborn. Due to the spectacular advances in neonatology, many conditions which were previously considered hopeless have successful outcomes if early recognition of the problem occurs and is followed by timely intervention and initiation of therapy (Ziai, Clarke, and Merritt, 1984).

The nurse caring for the newborn infant assumes a very important role in the assessment process. Because the registered nurse is usually the first health care professional available to assess the neonate's adjustment during this transition, the nurse must possess both the knowledge and skills to evaluate comprehensively the newborn's physical status.

THE IMPORTANCE OF ASSESSMENT

The purpose of an objective, systematic newborn assessment is to obtain an accurate, in-depth picture of the infant in the first minutes, hours, and days of life. There are many types of assessments, including observation of physical characteristics and behavior, neurologic assessment, gestational dating, and comparisons of measurements on growth curves. All data collected influence the medical and nursing intervention the newborn receives. Each tool is designed for a specific purpose, and the use of several tools gives a comprehensive assessment of the newborn's status.

Three tools are used by nurses in data collection: interaction, measurement, and observation. The neonatal nurse uses measurement and observation. Information obtained by the nurse provides the basis for valid and reliable judgments. Powell (1981) has provided a concise summary of assessment philosophy that should assist the nurse to be comprehensive and objective:

1. Assessment is a beginning, not an end in itself.
2. One tool alone is not sufficient to evaluate the health status of an infant accurately.
3. Regular and periodic assessment is crucial in monitoring and evaluating growth and adaptation, as well as in planning anticipatory and preventive care.
4. The presence of clusters or patterns of abnormal findings alerts the health care practitioner to the possibility of a major defect.
5. Valid data from assessments are invaluable in determining a baseline of what is normal for each individual infant.
6. Parents should be included in the assessment process as active and interested participants.

CLASSIFICATION OF NEWBORN INFANTS

Determining and documenting baseline data through the use of a variety of assessment tools provides important information needed for developing an infant's individualized plan for care. According to the recommendations of the Academy of Pediatrics through its Committee on the Fetus and Newborn, all newborn infants should be classified by birth weight, gestational age, and intrauterine growth (Lubchenco, 1981). Intrauterine growth standards are determined by using birth weights of infants born at different gestational ages. However, each standard has common built-in biases, resulting from such factors as the sex, race, and socioeconomic level of the population from which the standard was compiled (Black, 1978).

Until the 1960s, birth weight was considered to be the most reliable index of an infant's maturity. Essentially, infants were divided into two groups: premature (less than 2500 g) and term (greater than 2500 g). This categorization of infants according to birth weight alone implied that all fetuses developed at the same growth rate *in utero* and that birth weight accurately reflected gestational age.

In 1961, the World Health Organization recommended that babies weighing less than 2500 g be designated as *low-birth-weight* (LBW) infants. A dividing line was also set between preterm and term birth. A preterm infant is one born before 38 weeks' gestation. Term infants are born between 38 and 42 weeks. Post-term infants are born at 42 weeks or later. Gestational weeks are calculated from the first day of the last menstrual period (Sweet, 1979; Korones and Lancaster, 1981).

Birth Weight

In the early recovery phase of the newborn, during the first hours after birth, infants are weighed, measured, and classified by birth weight and gestational age. There are a variety of intrauterine growth curves, but most newborn nurseries use the Colorado Intrauterine Growth Curve. The Colorado curve was based on data from 5635 Caucasian infants, mostly indigent, born between 1948 and 1961 at the University of Colorado Medical Center (Lubchenco et al., 1963). The growth chart is a composite of percentile curves graphing intrauterine growth by weight, length, head circumference, and weight–length ratio. For practical reasons, both sexes were combined for

548 CHANGE: THE NEONATAL PERIOD

each of the percentile charts (Lubchenco, Hansman, and Boyd, 1966).

On the Colorado Intrauterine Growth Curve, birth weights from 400 to 4000 g are plotted against gestational ages from 24 to 43 weeks or more. By definition, an infant is large for gestational age (LGA) if the birth weight is greater than the 90th percentile and small for gestational age (SGA) if the birth weight is less than the 10th percentile for all infants at that particular age (see Fig. 26–1). Babies who are categorized between the 10th and 90th percentiles are appropriate for gestational age (AGA; Korones and Lancaster, 1981).

A more simplified graph (Fig. 26–2) may be used. Infants are categorized as small, appropriate, and large for gestational age. At the bottom of the chart are preterm, term, and post-term classifications, given according to the weeks of gestation. The infant's weight and gestational age may be plotted on this chart.

Gestational Assessment

Interest in the assessment of gestational age of the newborn has increased over the past two decades. Health care personnel became aware that clinical problems differed in infants with comparable weights but different gestational ages. For example, preterm infants with normal weight for gestational age have shown respiratory difficulties, immaturity of organ systems, temperature control problems, and feeding difficulties. On the other hand, full-term infants who are small for date have shown different problems, such as hypoglycemia and polycythemia (Dubowitz and Dubowitz, 1981; see Chapter 32).

Estimation of Gestational Age

There are three basic methods for estimating gestational age: (1) calculation of the mother's menstrual dates, (2) obstetric methods, and (3) physical examination of the infant (Sullivan, Foster, and Schreiner, 1979).

Maternal History and Examination

Calculation of menstrual dates since the first day of the last menstrual period (LMP) is still the basis from which gestational age is most often calcu-

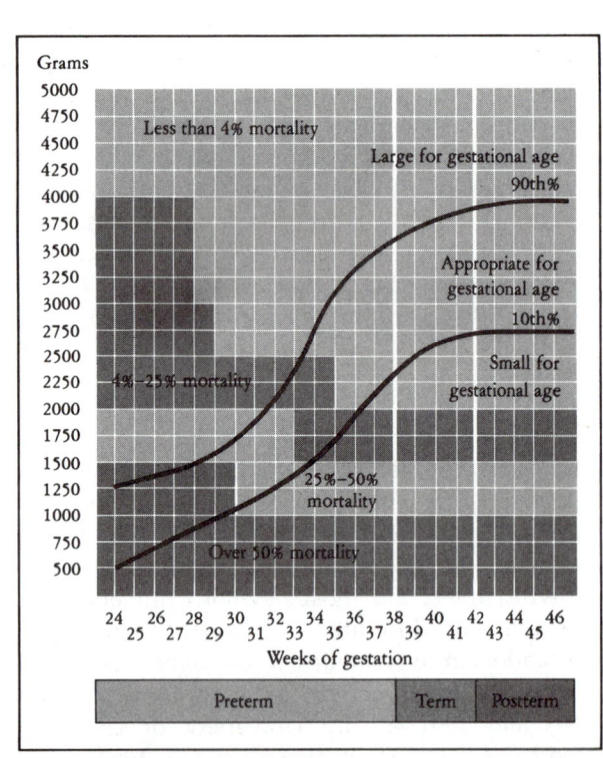

FIGURE 26–1. University of Colorado Medical Center classification of newborns by birth weight and gestational age and by neonatal mortality risk.
SOURCE: Battaglia and Lubchenco (1967).

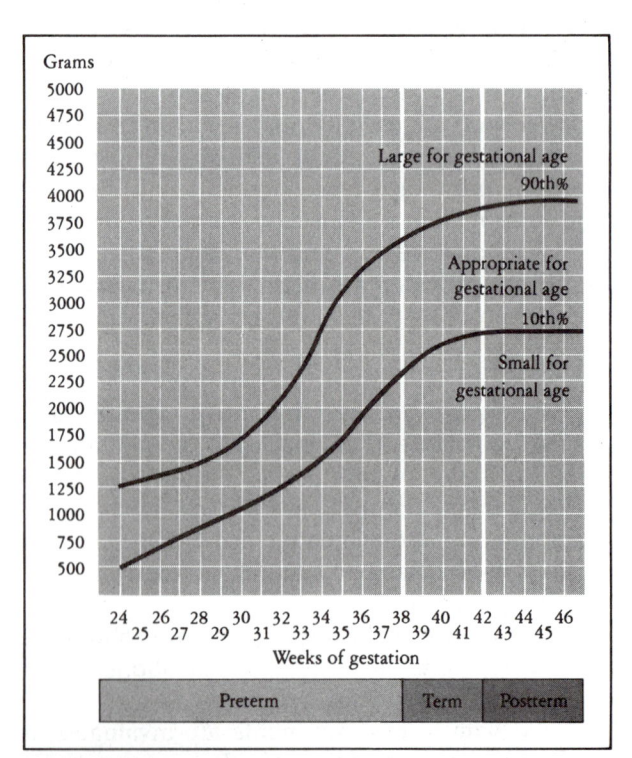

FIGURE 26–2. University of Colorado Medical Center classification of newborns by birth weight and gestational age.
SOURCE: Battaglia and Luchenco (1967).

lated. There is reason to doubt the accuracy of the dates, because accuracy is totally dependent on the mother's recall. However, it has been found that when a maternal history is obtained early in the pregnancy, the dates are valid in 75–85 percent of patients (Korones and Lancaster, 1981). Other factors that can reduce the likelihood of accuracy of the dates are (1) a short interval between pregnancies, (2) postconceptual bleeding misinterpreted as a menstrual period, (3) interruption of ovulation due to use of contraceptive drugs, and (4) absence of menstruation for several months in some nursing mothers (Black, 1978; Korones and Lancaster, 1981).

Additional data for determining fetal age can be obtained by obstetric examination. These estimates include measurement of the uterine fundus above the symphysis pubis, determination of when quickening occurred, auscultation of fetal heart tones, sonography, and amniotic fluid analyses (see Chapter 13).

Assessment of Maturity by Postnatal Examination

The physical examination of the newborn can be divided into two parts, the nonneurologic assessment, which involves a head-to-toe appraisal of the infant's physical characteristics, and the neurologic assessment, which involves a demonstration of responses that indicate the degree of neurologic integrity of the infant.

The Dubowitz scoring system, which has standardized 11 external characteristics and 10 neurologic parameters, is being used in many newborn nurseries for gestational dating of infants (see Fig. 26–3). The Dubowitz scoring system is popular because it is easy for health care personnel to use. The Dubowitz scoring system meets the following basic requirements for ease of application (Dubowitz and Dubowitz, 1981):

1. To be suitable for staff with no particular expertise in neonatal neurology, it should have a recording system that is simple and objective.
2. It should be applicable to preterm as well as full-term infants.
3. It should be reliable as soon after birth as possible so that it can be used to document the influence of drugs, hypoxia, trauma, and other environmental factors in the perinatal period and to identify and possibly prevent or reduce resulting complications.
4. The full examination and its recording should not take longer than 10–15 min to complete, so that the test can be used as a component of the routine clinical assessment of newborn infants.
5. The same examination should be suitable for repeated application for periodic examination of infants after birth.

Optimally, the nonneurologic examination should be performed within 1–2 hours after birth. Of the 11 parameters given by Dubowitz many nurses observe only the breasts, ears, genitals, sole creases, and posture. It has been shown that by observing these five main characteristics, the nurse can determine the correct age of the infant in almost all cases (Sullivan, Foster, and Schreiner, 1979).

Nurses performing the gestational age assessment should chart the results. Scores assigned to each parameter are later used to estimate the infant's gestational age. Assessment of physical characteristics and reflexes will be discussed later in this chapter.

PHYSICAL ASSESSMENT

The nurse is the member of the health care team who assumes responsibility for immediate and constant observation of the newborn. The nurse must have a thorough understanding of the physical characteristics and functions of the newborn to detect any deviation from normal. In the early recovery phase, the first 8–12 hours of the newborn's life, the nurse should review the mother's prenatal history, including her general health status during pregnancy, medications taken, and possible complications; the labor and delivery record for length of labor, intravenous fluids given, analgesia and anesthesia required, results of fetal monitoring, and complications; and the newborn's record, including the Apgar score at 1 and 5 min, results of cord blood analysis, birth weight and length, head and chest circumferences, and gestational age. The nurse then performs a detailed physical examination.

Factors That Influence Examination

When performing an examination on a newborn infant, the nurse should consider several factors that can affect the infant's responses:

1. Time in relation to feedings. The optimum time for examination is approximately 1–2 hours after a feeding.
2. Temperature of the environment. A neutral

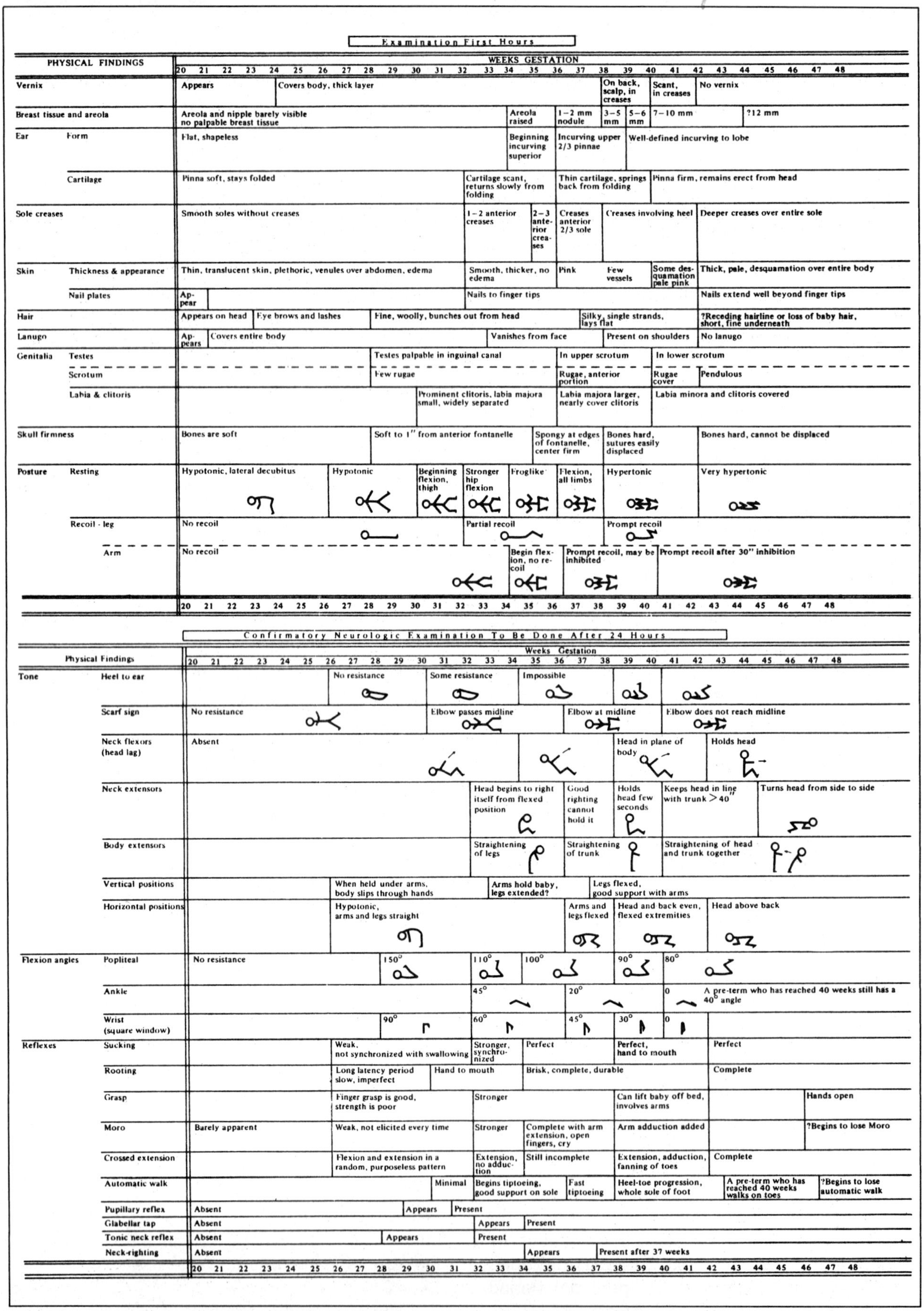

FIGURE 26-3. The Dubowitz system for clinical estimation of gestational age.

SOURCE: Dubowitz and Dubowitz (1981).

temperature is recommended, as hypothermia can result in a depressed response and hyperthermia may cause irritability.
3. State of consciousness. The infant should be in a quiet, alert state for the most effective assessment.
4. Gestational age. The infant's responses and physical appearance depend to a large degree on the maturation and age of the infant.
5. Degree of illness. When the newborn is depressed due to illness the data will not be as accurate as if the newborn is well.

Equipment

Prior to the examination the nurse should assemble the necessary equipment, including thermometer, stethoscope with neonatal diaphragm, tape measure, ophthalmoscope, and chart for recording findings. The room should be free of drafts and well lighted. A sturdy table of convenient height for the nurse is desirable, and a pad, sheet, or blanket should cover the table for the comfort of the infant. Alternatively, the infant's crib or the mother's bed may be used for the examination. An extra diaper should also be close by.

Symmetry

For the purposes of facilitating a systematic appraisal, the term *symmetry* can be used when describing equality, evenness, or balance, and *asymmetry* can be used to refer to states of inequality or difference (Powell, 1981). The nurse should observe symmetry of the newborn's movements as well as symmetry, or in some cases asymmetry, of physical characteristics.

General Appearance of the Newborn

The infant should be examined during the quiet, alert period. Before disturbing the infant, the nurse should listen to the heart rate and observe the breathing pattern. Then observations should be made relating the infant's size to the estimated gestational age; the nurse should note skin color and thickness, general nutritional status, amount of subcutaneous tissue, resting posture, and alertness. Preferably, the infant should be unclothed and in a supine position. While undressing the infant, the nurse should observe the general muscle tone and response to external stimuli. Keep in mind that the most important observations are often made without instruments and without touching the infant (Ziai, Clarke, and Merritt, 1984).

Characteristically, the normal newborn infant weighs 2500–4300 g (5.5–9.5 lb) and is approximately 34–35 cm (18–21 in) in length. The body is cylindrical in shape with the head appearing slightly larger than the chest. The average head circumference ranges from 33 to 35 cm (13 to 14 in), and the average chest circumference ranges from 30 to 33 cm (12 to 13 in). Normally, the relationship of head to chest is quite constant. If the head is slightly smaller than the chest, microcephaly is suspected, or hydrocephaly if it is significantly larger. The neck is short, giving the appearance that the head is sitting directly on the shoulders. The chest is barrel-shaped and breathing is diaphragmatic. The rib cage is narrow and cylindrical. The abdomen protrudes slightly, and the hips are narrow in relation to the chest. The arms and legs are generally flexed, and the legs appear bowed (see Fig. 26–4). The skin of the normal term infant is soft, wrinkled, velvety, and covered with varying amounts of vernix caseosa (Behrman and Vaughan, 1983). Within a few hours of birth, the skin develops an intense red color. Cyanosis of the hands and feet, or *acrocyanosis*, is frequently seen in the first hours of life. This is normal and is usually transitory.

Systematic Evaluation of the Newborn

In performing a systematic appraisal of the newborn, the nurse should proceed in an orderly manner, examining from the head downward to the toes. Skilled nurses must become thoroughly knowledgeable regarding the characteristics of the newborn. This is best done by studying the normal infant and completing hundreds of physical assessments. Once the nurse has a grasp of normal characteristics, deviations from normal are quickly recognized.

Skin

Color
The newborn assessment should begin with an evaluation of the color and appearance of the skin. The newborn is usually quite pink but flushes and pales quickly. An infant who is very ruddy and

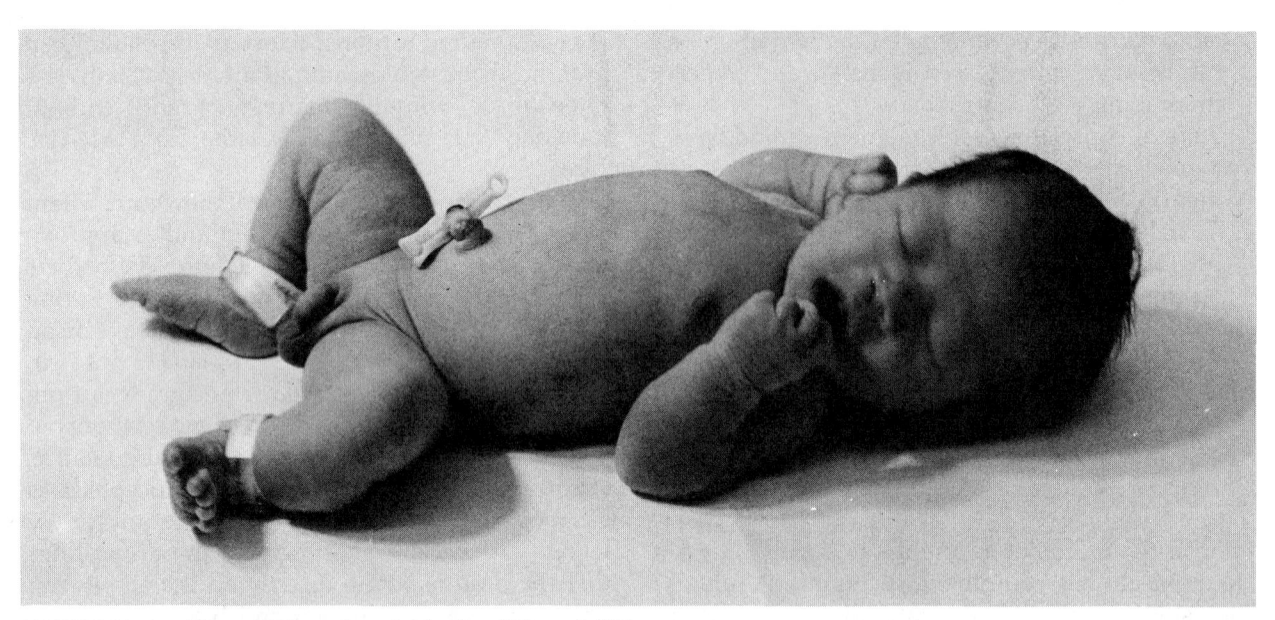

FIGURE 26-4. The normal newborn in the first 12 hours of life.

plethoric should be evaluated for polycythemia (a central hematocrit of ≥ 65%). Neonatal polycythemia occurs most commonly in infants of diabetic mothers, in those who are small for gestational age, in recipients of maternal-to-fetal transfusions or twin-to-twin transfusions, or in infants whose deliveries involved delayed clamping of the cord. The newborn who is pale may be anemic or hypotensive as a result of placental abruption, placenta previa, being a donor in a twin-to-twin transfusion, anomalous umbilical cord insertion with hemorrhage, or erythroblastosis fetalis (Gagliardi, 1983).

Acrocyanosis is a bluish coloration of the skin or mucous membrane involving the feet, hands, and circumoral area (around the lips). It is present in most infants after birth and for a short time thereafter.

A phenomenon observed in the immediate neonatal period is the Harlequin color change that peaks between 2-4 days and 3 weeks. This phenomenon is more common in the low-birth-weight infant. When the infant is placed on its side, a sharp line of demarcation bisects the baby. The upper half of the body becomes pale while the dependent half becomes intensely red. This phenomenon is attributed to a temporary imbalance in the autonomic regulatory mechanism of the cutaneous vessels (Behrman and Vaughan, 1983).

Jaundice is the most likely color change to be noted on examination. It is caused by a high indirect bilirubin and requires a level of at least 4-6 mg/100 ml before it causes visible staining of the skin. Jaundice in the first 24 hours of life is always considered abnormal. The nurse can assess for the presence of jaundice by blanching the skin over the bony prominences of the frontal bone and sternum and the cartilage of the nose. Jaundiced skin will blanch a yellowish hue.

This blanching gives the nurse a general index for decision making. The sclera of the eye is another index point; in the presence of jaundice it will appear yellow. The progression of jaundice in the newborn is from head to toe and gives us a rough estimate of the bilirubin level (e.g. to the umbilicus 8 mg/100 ml, to the knees 10 mg/100 ml, and to the feet 14 mg/100 ml). The hands and feet are the last to become jaundiced (Ziai, Clarke, and Merritt, 1984). Jaundice requires prompt evaluation of the infant's bilirubin level.

Integrity

The integrity of the skin should be evaluated. The skin is thin and almost transparent in preterm infants, becoming thicker and more nearly opaque with increasing age. Early in gestation the skin is pink and venules are prominent over the abdomen. By 40-42 weeks the skin is pale, and a few vessels are seen in the newborn (Behrman and Vaughan, 1983). Two protective coverings of the skin developed *in utero* are vernix caseosa and lanugo.

Vernix caseosa, a greasy, yellowish-white material with a pH of 7.4, is a mixture of desquamating cells and sebum. This sebaceous deposit covers the body of the fetus and serves as protection for the skin. It is seen in the creases and flexor surfaces of the newborn. The amount and distribution varies in infants. Preterm infants are generally covered with a generous amount; however, at term, vernix usually remains only in the skin creases and hair. The post-term infant may have no vernix, appearing as if freshly bathed. The post-term and the intrauterine-growth-retarded (IUGR) infant may also have dry skin, with cracking and peeling of the superficial layers.

Physiologic desquamation is present in infants of 40–42 weeks' gestational age. Shedding peaks on the eighth postpartal day. The dysmature infant, in contrast with the postmature baby, has a lean body with little subcutaneous fat, and weight is low in relation to length. In the postmature baby the skin is parchmentlike, scaly, and stained with meconium. Desquamation is a transient phenomenon (Fanaroff and Martin, 1983).

Lanugo, a fine downy hair, is found in varying amounts over the body of the newborn. The infant is covered with lanugo at 20 weeks *in utero*. The preterm infant often has generous amounts of lanugo covering scalp and brow. It may also be present over the shoulder and on the face, ear lobes, and back. Lanugo disappears from the face first, then the trunk, and finally the extremities.

Meconium Staining

Meconium staining of the infant suggests prior fetal distress. The umbilical cord, vernix, and nails are the areas where meconium staining is the most obvious. Meconium usually requires at least 6 hours of contact to stain skin (Ziai, Clarke, and Merritt, 1984).

Edema

The presence of edema should be noted. The subcutaneous tissue may be moderately edematous for several days after delivery. Edema is most noticeable about the eyelids and the dorsal aspects of the hands and feet. Generalized edema may indicate the presence of serious renal, cardiac, or other systemic disease. Localized edema of the eyelids may indicate the presence of conjunctivitis, while edema in the dorsum of the extremities may be an early finding in Turner's syndrome. Edema may be related to trauma sustained during labor and delivery, especially if it appears in relation to ecchymoses or bruising (Korones and Lancaster, 1981; see Fig. 26–5).

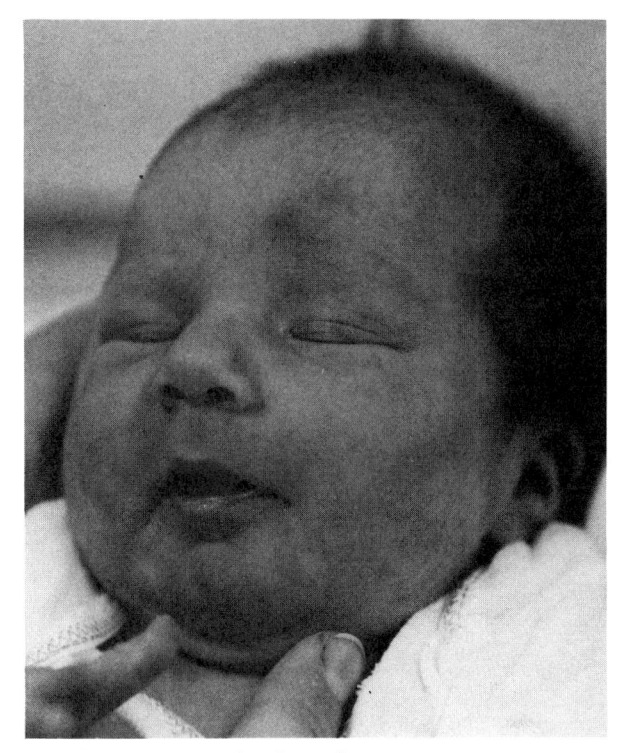

FIGURE 26–5. Facial ecchymosis due to forceps delivery.

Lesions

The skin should be observed for birthmarks, skin rashes, petechiae, excessive peeling, staining, and vesicles. The most common lesions found on the skin are erythema toxicum, milia, miliaria, Mongolian spots, capillary hemangiomas, and petechiae.

Erythema toxicum is a normal finding. This benign, self-limited eruption occurs within the first 2 days of life, but lesions may appear as late as 14 days. Erythema toxicum occurs in 30–70 percent of newborns. The lesions vary in character and number but may have any of the following characteristics: 1–3 mm in diameter, firm in consistency, pale yellow to white papules or pustules, erythematous macules up to 3 cm, or splotchy erythema (see Fig. 26–6a). The cause is unknown, although a "sensitivity" to the environment is suspected, and there are no related systemic symptoms (Behrman and Vaughan, 1983). Parents are often concerned about this rash, referred to commonly as "flea bite." The implication of this term alone brings concern. The nurse should give a clear explanation regarding this phenomenon. It should be remembered that the skin of the newborn is extremely delicate and that clothing, although new and soft, may be as rough as sandpaper to the newborn's delicate skin by comparison.

Milia are small, white papules on the chin, nose,

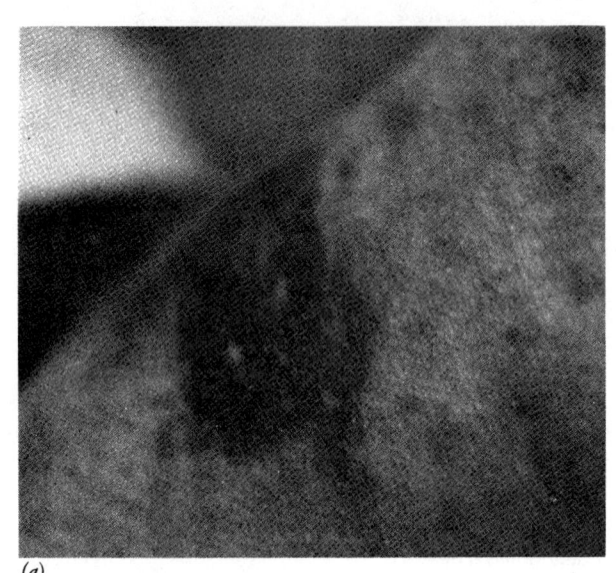

FIGURE 26-6. Skin lesions of newborns: (a) erythema toxicum, (b) milia, (c) Mongolian spots.
SOURCE: (a) and (b) courtesy of Mead Johnson Laboratories.

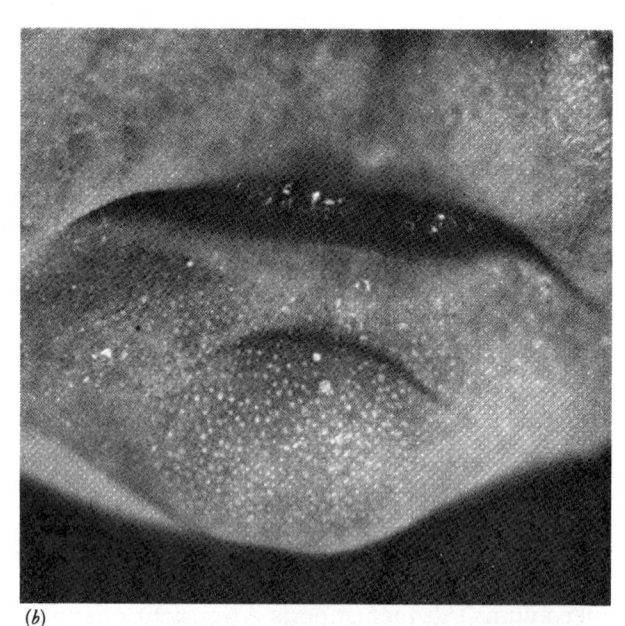

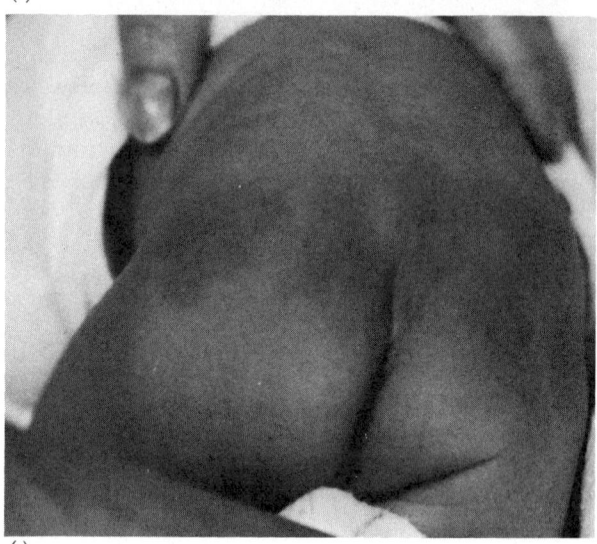

cheeks, and forehead seen in about 40 percent of infants. They represent distended sebaceous glands that disappear spontaneously within a few weeks. Milia may be few or numerous and are frequently distributed in clusters. Parents should be instructed not to squeeze these whitehead-like spots (see Fig. 26-6b).

Miliaria are lesions resulting from obstruction of the sweat glands, and are of two types: (1) *miliaria crystallia* are superficial, thin-walled vesicles without inflammation; (2) *miliaria rubra* are small, erythematous, grouped papules appearing in the folds of the skin and over the face and scalp. During the first weeks of life these lesions may be exacerbated by a warm environment. Removal to a cooler environment is usually the only treatment necessary. Miliaria is often confused with erythema toxicum (Behrman and Vaughan, 1983).

Mongolian spots are the most frequently encountered pigmented lesion seen in the newborn. Darkened areas of bluish-gray discoloration, resulting from an infiltrate of melanocytes deep in the dermis, occurs in 70 percent of black, Oriental, and American Indian infants and in 9 percent of Caucasian infants. Most of these lesions are found over the lumbosacral area and buttocks, but they may be present on the thighs, calves, and shoulders (Behrman and Vaughan, 1983; see Fig. 26-6c). The spots usually disappear during the first year of life but may remain through the preschool years.

Capillary hemangiomas, commonly referred to as

"stork bites," are found in 30–50 percent of normal newborns. These are found on the lower occiput, at the nape of the neck, on the eyelids and glabella, and above the upper lip at the cupid's bow. They are generally caused by capillary dilation, and they decrease in size and color as the child grows, usually disappearing by 2 years of age. They may become more prominent when the infant is crying.

Petechiae are pinpoint hemorrhagic areas scattered over the trunk and face as a result of pressure during descent and rotation through the birth canal. They are increased when the umbilical cord has been around the neck or when the cervix clamps down after the delivery of the head (Ziai, Clarke, and Merritt, 1984). Usually, petechiae will fade within 24–48 hours. Fresh or numerous petechiae may suggest thrombocytopenia or infection and should be reported immediately.

Head

The size, shape, symmetry, and general appearance of the head should be carefully evaluated. The head often shows pronounced effects from the labor and delivery. Overriding sutures and small or absent fontanelles are common during the first few hours of life as a result of molding during vaginal delivery (see Fig. 26–7).

Sutures and Fontanelles

Sutures and fontanelles are bands of connective tissue that separate the six major cranial bones (see Fig. 26–7). Sutures are palpable as cracks; fontanelles are broader "soft spots" (Korones and Lancaster, 1981). Fontanelles should be gently palpated, and the size and placement of both anterior and posterior fontanelles should be noted. The anterior fontanelle is 1–4 cm (1–3 fingerbreadths) in diameter. It is soft and pulsates with the infant's pulse. When the infant is quiet and in an upright position, the anterior fontanelle becomes depressed slightly. The posterior fontanelle is less than 1 cm in diameter. The lambdoid, sagittal, coronal, and metopic sutures can be clearly defined on the skull of the newborn. The anterior fontanelle is palpated at the junction of the coronal, frontal, and sagittal sutures. The posterior fontanelle is palpated at the junction of the sagittal and lambdoid sutures.

In malnourished infants the sutures might be quite wide, suggesting impaired fetal growth of the cranial bones. Intracranial pressure causes firmness and bulging of the fontanelles and may also cause enlargement of the head circumference, so the nurse needs to take daily measurements of the head circumference and record findings. The circumference is measured from occiput to frontal bones. The average head circumference is 33–35 cm (13–14 in).

An immobile, rigid suture line suggests *craniosynostosis*, the premature closure and fusion of one or more sutures. The condition occurs *in utero* but may not be evident until several weeks after birth (Bernardo, 1979).

In examination of the skull, the nurse needs to differentiate a caput succedaneum from a cephalhematoma. *Caput succedaneum* is edema of the scalp due to local pressure and trauma during labor (see Fig. 26–8a). *Cephalhematoma* is subperiosteal hemorrhage secondary to trauma of labor and delivery. The margins of the suture lines are

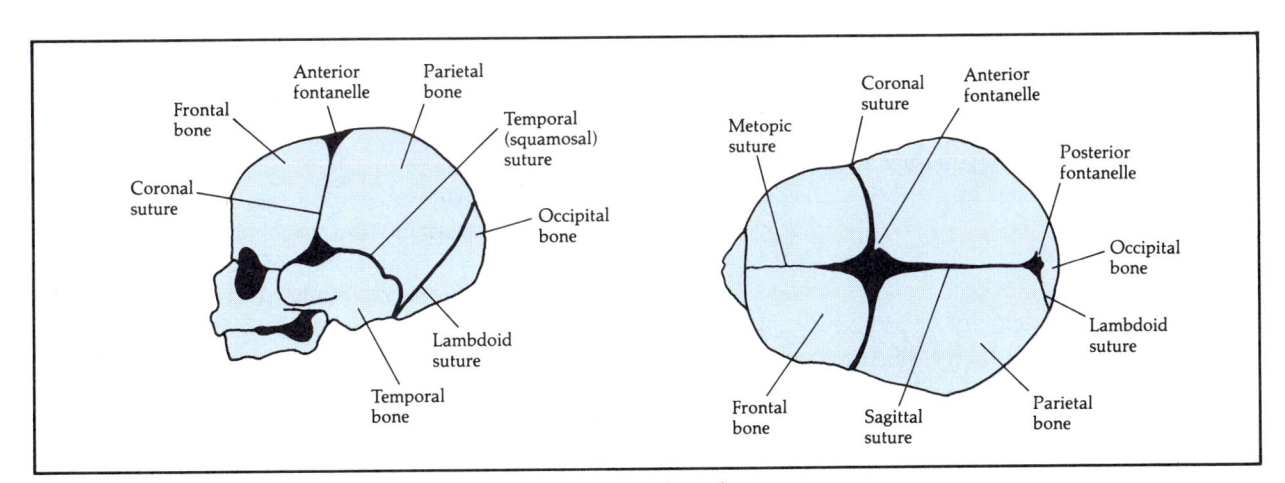

FIGURE 26–7. Neonatal cranial bones, sutures, and fontanelles from the lateral view and from above.

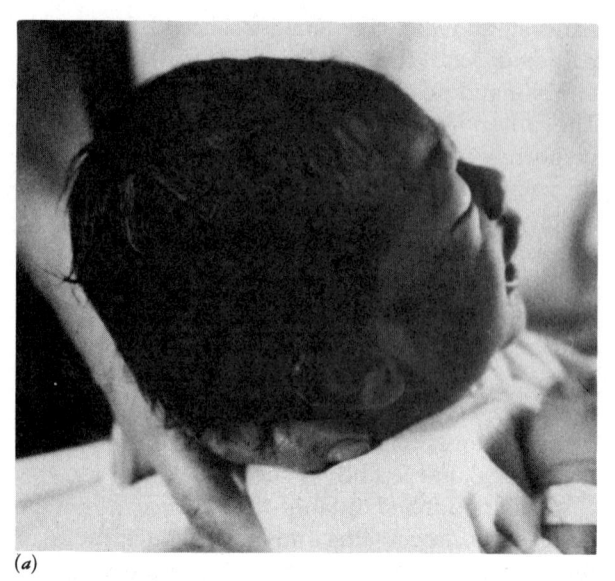

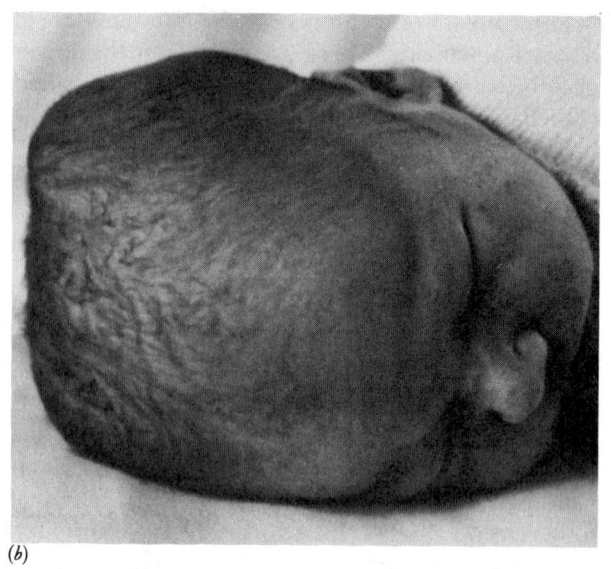

FIGURE 26–8. (a) Caput succedaneum is a diffuse, generalized swelling of the scalp, not sharply defined. (b) Cephalhematoma, subperiosteal hemorrhage, usually well defined by suture lines.
SOURCE: Courtesy Mead Johnson Laboratories.

poorly defined in caput succedaneum, as the edema is generalized. In cephalhematoma, the margins are clearly demarcated and the swelling never crosses the suture lines (see Fig. 26–8b).

Scalp

The scalp should be inspected for any laceration resulting from the site of insertion of the fetal monitoring electrode. This area needs to be cleansed and observed daily for any signs of infection. A larger, red, distinct circular area may be due to a vacuum extractor.

Hair

The more premature the infant, the finer the hair. At 33–34 weeks' gestation, the hair strands tend to be very fine, to mat together like wool, and to stick out from the head. At 40 weeks the hair lies flat in single strands. In the postmature infant a receding hairline is sometimes seen.

Facies

The face should be clearly observed for swelling, ecchymoses, or asymmetry of movement. Odd facies are often associated with specific syndromes and should alert the nurse to search for further problems. Facial paralysis is observed with asymmetry of movement, usually movement of only one side of the face when the infant cries. The unaffected side of the mouth moves normally, giving a distorted facial grimace (Koops and Battaglia, 1982). This paralysis results from pressure on the facial nerve during delivery and will disappear within a few days.

Eyes

The eyes are normally symmetrical in appearance. Puffy eyelids due to chemical conjunctivitis may result from treatment with silver nitrate eye prophylaxis. Erythrocin ointment may be used for the same purpose. The eyes of the newborn infant should never be forced open for an examination. If the room is dimly lit and the infant is in a quiet, alert state, the eyes should open spontaneously. Observation of spontaneous ocular activity is usually most reliable when the infant is being held or is nursing. Obviously, a proper eye examination cannot be carried out if the infant is screaming and crying. The presence of a red reflex should be established, and the lens checked for the presence of cataracts. The pupils should be inspected to see whether they are normally round and equal in diameter. Using an ophthalmoscope, the nurse should note pupil size and reaction to light. The pupils should react equally by constricting to the light. The red reflex should be seen bilaterally on examination by shining the ophthalmoscope light directly into the pupil. The reflection should be orange-red and fairly uniform in color. In dark-skinned infants—Indian, Mexican-American, and black—the reflex is pale. The iris appears blue. Subconjunctival hemorrhage, resulting from pressure on the fetal head during delivery, may be present. The surface of the cornea should have good luster, and the whole cornea should be absolutely transparent. Any unusual discharge should be noted.

Congenital malformations of the eyes include the rare findings of cataracts, glaucoma, and colobomas. Glaucoma presents with an enlargement of the eye due to abnormal development of the drainage mechanism of the aqueous humor (Moore, 1982). Cataracts are opacities of the lens that vary in size from pinpoint areas to total involvement of the lens. Colobomas are rare defects of the eyelids characterized by a small notch usually of the upper eyelid. In iris colobomas, one of the most common malformations of the eye, a small notch in the iris is present, giving the pupil a key-like appearance (Korones and Lancaster, 1981).

The eyes should be examined for spontaneous range of motion and movement. Common uncoordinated eye movements include *strabismus*, the inability to direct the eyes (see Fig. 26–9), and *nystagmus*, involuntary, irregular movements of the eyeball. Fixation and the ability of the infant to follow a brightly colored object or a bright light in a dimly lit room should be noted for each eye separately and both eyes together (Fanaroff and Martin, 1983).

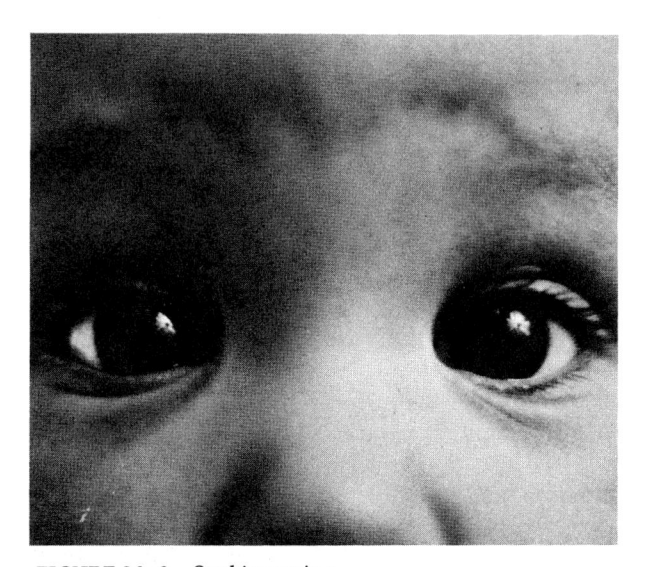

FIGURE 26–9. Strabismus is a common finding in the newborn.
SOURCE: Courtesy Mead Johnson Laboratories.

Nose

The size and shape of the nose, the presence of nasal discharge, and any obstructed breathing should be noted. Since the newborn infant is an obligatory nose breather, the nose should be checked for patency. This can be done by passing a small catheter through both nares or, when the infant's mouth is closed, pressure can be applied to one nostril and the infant's ability to breathe through the other nostril assessed. Flaring of the alae nasi occurs with increased respiratory effort (see Chapter 32). *Choanal atresia,* an obstruction of the nares by membranes or bony septa, may be present in the newborn, resulting in respiratory distress. If nasal obstruction is present, the infant may become cyanotic or apneic. If the obstruction is bilateral, this is a surgical emergency, because the infant will not breathe through his mouth on his own.

Ears

Inspection of the ear should begin with the surfaces of the *pinna,* or auricle, the projected part of the exterior ear. The position of the ears in relation to the eyes should be noted. The upper part of the ear should be level with the infant's eye. Low-set ears are often associated with other congenital abnormalities, such as urinary tract problems. The nurse should describe the pinna as to ear form and ear cartilage. The pinna should be pulled superiorly and posteriorly to allow inspection of the surfaces around the ear (Potsie and Handler, 1982).

In assessing ear form the nurse should note the incurving of the upper pinna, which begins at 33–34 weeks and is extended to the lobe by 39–40 weeks. Ear cartilage assessment involves noting the firmness of the pinna. This can be done by bending or folding the pinna forward. At 32–33 weeks the pinnas stay folded, but by 36 weeks they are firm and stand erect from the head (Lubchenco, 1981). Elasticity of the ear cartilage is important in determining gestational age (see Fig. 26–10).

The ear canal should be patent. To inspect the eardrum, the nurse should introduce the otoscope gently and carefully into the ear canal. The infant's head should be supported and the ear pulled down to visualize the eardrum. The eardrum in the newborn is grayish in color rather than pink, as it is in the adult. The sense of hearing is acute at birth, and the infant will respond to loud noises or to the gentle ringing of a bell.

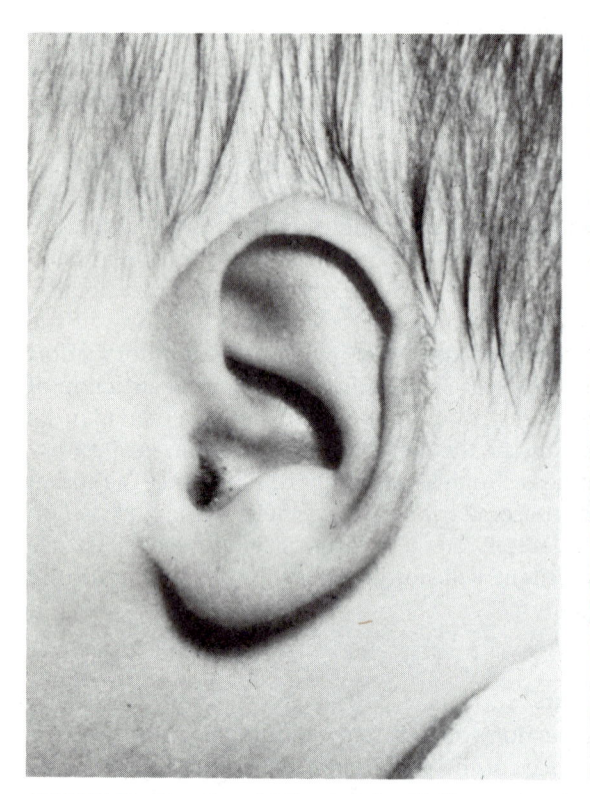

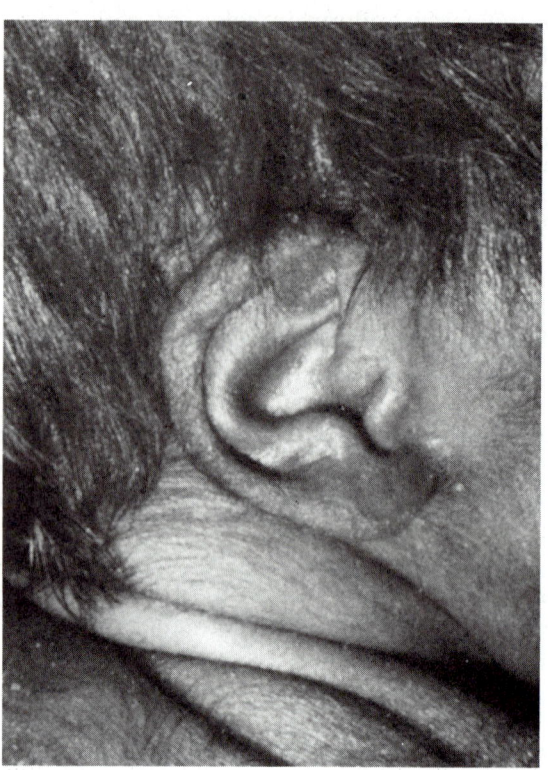

FIGURE 26–10. Ear of full-term infant (left); ear of premature infant (right).

Mouth

The mouth can most easily be inspected when the infant is crying. The lips are prominent and sensitive to touch. Sucking calluses may appear on the central portion of the upper lip within a few days after birth. The frenum of the tongue is short and tight. The size and shape of the tongue should be noted. The nurse may use a tongue depressor and light to examine the palate and mucous membranes. The soft palate, hard palate, uvula, and dental ridge should all be viewed for intactness. The nurse should feel as well as visualize the roof of the mouth for the presence of clefts. Mucous membranes are pink and moist in a well-hydrated infant. Using a pacifier or a finger, the nurse can evaluate the infant's sucking reflex. Epstein's pearls, or Bohn's nodules, are white or grayish-white pinpoint-sized cysts commonly found on the roof of the mouth at the junction of the soft and hard palates. They are asymptomatic and are shed spontaneously within a few weeks.

Natal or precocious teeth may on a very few occasions be found at birth. They are usually the lower, central incisors. This is a third set of teeth and removal is commonly done to prevent detachment and aspiration. An unusual thickening of the cheek, called the sucking fat pad, which develops soon after birth (Einhorn, 1982), exists to facilitate sucking during the first year of life. Excessive salivation should be noted, because this is an early sign of esophageal atresia.

Neck

The neck should be inspected for masses, ruptured blood vessels, limitation of movement, webbing, or shortness. The clavicles should be symmetrical, smooth, and even on palpation. A fractured clavicle, as a result of a traumatic delivery, can be felt as a crunching, or *crepitus*, at the fracture site on palpation. The arm on the affected side will have limited movement. The sternocleidomastoid muscles should be even in size and should allow for easy movement of the head from side to side (see Fig. 26–11). The neck should be observed for *torticollis*, an asymmetric deformity of the neck and head. Torticollis is characterized by lateral flexion of the head toward the involved side with rotation of the chin toward the opposite shoulder. Torticollis may be present at birth but is usually noted at 2–3 weeks.

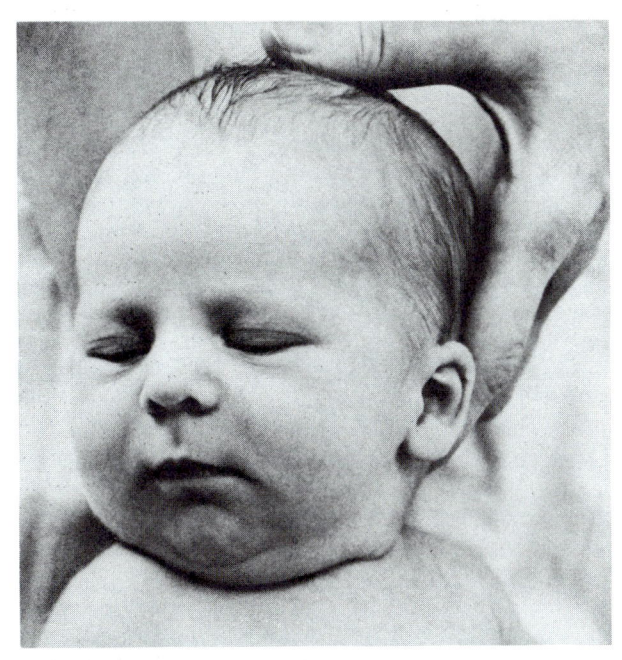

FIGURE 26-11. The neck of the newborn should allow for easy movement.
SOURCE: Courtesy Mead Johnson Laboratories.

Chest

The thorax should be inspected for shape, symmetry, position, and development of the nipples and breast tissue. The chest should be measured over the nipples on inspiration, as this is the widest area. The normal chest measures 30–33 cm (12–13 in). The nipples are present at 34 weeks' gestation, when the areola first becomes raised with visible hair follicles. At 36 weeks a 1–2 mm nodule of breast tissue is palpable, increasing to 7–10 mm by 40 weeks. When the infant is in the quiet, alert state, an assessment of heart rate and respirations should be done with a neonatal stethoscope. The respiratory rate should be counted for a full minute; 40–60 breaths/min is normal. The quality and character of respirations should be observed. The heart sounds should be evaluated for both rhythm and rate. The normal heart rate for a newborn is 120 to 160 beats/min. Any murmurs should be noted and their location, radiation, intensity, and quality should be described. Femoral pulses, normally present in all infants, should be assessed for presence, strength, and quality (Gagliardi, 1983). Radial pulses, which should be equal to each other and equal to the femoral pulses, should be assessed as well. When there is any question of unequal pulses or any evidence of cardiac shunting, the blood pressure should be taken on all four extremities. Blood pressure in the upper extremities should be slightly lower than in the lower extremities. A widening or increase in pulse pressure (the difference between systolic and diastolic pressure) may be due to a patent ductus or other left ventricular or aortic abnormality (Ziai, Clarke, and Merritt, 1984).

Abdomen

Using a light touch, the nurse should palpate the abdomen for organs and masses. The abdomen should be soft, not tight. If the abdomen is tight, bring the infant's legs up to a knee–chest position and then extend the legs to relax the abdomen.

The liver is usually palpable 1–2 cm below the right costal margin. Palpate just below the umbilicus and roll the first digit of the index finger up until the liver edge is felt. Measure with a tape measure – the edge of the liver should be 1–3 cm below the last rib. Palpate the left side for the spleen. No more than 1 cm of the spleen should be palpable. If it is, it indicates that the baby might have been exposed to an intrauterine infection.

To palpate the kidneys, support the lower back and roll the tips of the fingers gently over the kidneys. Both kidneys are usually palpable if the examination occurs immediately after birth, before the intestines fill with air. Normal kidneys will feel like a stuffed, medium-sized olive under four or five blankets (Ziai, Clarke, and Merritt, 1984) and are situated 1–2 cm above the level of the umbilicus. The bladder may be felt above the symphysis pubis as a ballottable mass in the lower abdomen.

The umbilical cord should be inspected for the presence of three vessels (see Fig. 26–12). A single umbilical artery is frequently associated with other major congenital anomalies. The cord should be dry, with no bleeding or discharge present. It begins drying within hours after birth, usually dropping off within 7–10 days.

Diastasis recti, a separation of the rectus muscle of the abdominal wall, may appear as a sausage-shaped bulge down the middle of the abdomen (see Fig. 22–27). This finding is relatively insignificant. Herniation of abdominal contents into the umbilical cord, or omphalocele, is a significant finding, and demands immediate action. Omphaloceles appear in the midline and are covered by membranes, whereas gastroschisis is a defect in the abdominal wall lateral to the midline and is not covered by umbilical cord membranes.

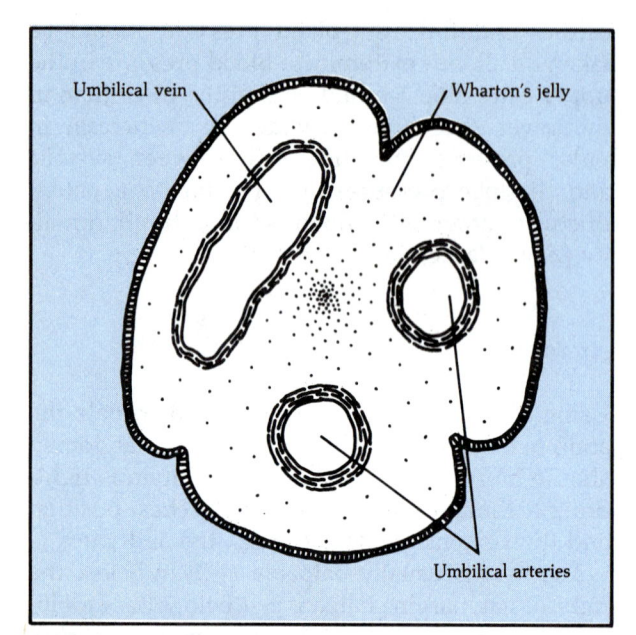

FIGURE 26-12. Cross-section of the umbilical cord. The arteries have thick walls; the lumen of the vein is larger than those of the arteries, and its wall is thin.

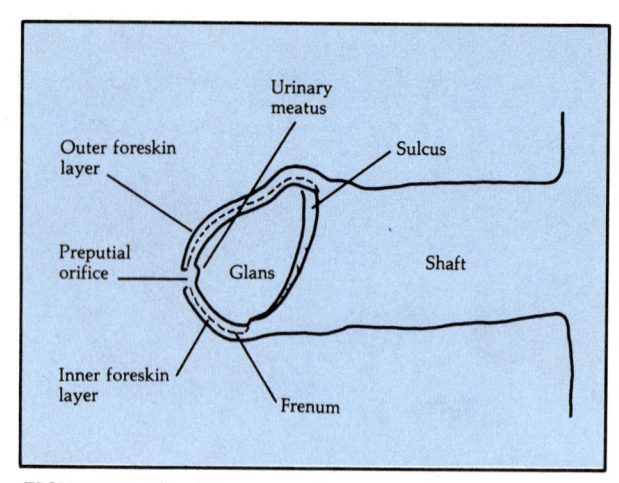

FIGURE 26-13. Diagrammatic representation of the inner and outer foreskin layers.
SOURCE: Reprinted with the permission of Edward Wallenstein.

Genitals

The genitals should be examined for gestational maturity and sexual ambiguity. At birth, the penis consists of a cylindrical shaft with a rounded end called the glans. The shaft and glans are separated by a groove called the sulcus. The entire penis – shaft and glans – is covered by a continuous layer of skin. The section of the penile skin which covers the glans is called the foreskin or prepuce. The foreskin consists of two layers – the outer foreskin and an inner lining similar to a mucous membrane (see Fig. 26-13). The penis in the normal male newborn is approximately 3–4 cm long and 1–1.3 cm wide. The prepuce usually adheres to the glans of the penis at birth. Circumcision is the surgical removal of the prepuce.

Hypospadias is characterized by placement of the urethral meatus on the ventral portion of the glans or anywhere along the ventral shaft of the penis. Hypospadias is quite common and, therefore, the location of the meatus should be checked and the male infant's stream of urine should be examined upon voiding.

The size of the scrotum varies considerably. The testicles descend into the external inguinal canal and can be palpated at the external inguinal ring at about 30 weeks. Gradually they descend toward the scrotum, and at 37 weeks they are located high in the scrotal sac. By 40 weeks the testicles are well descended. The post-term infant tends to have a pendulous scrotum that is covered with rugae (wrinkles). Rugae are first seen on the anterior scrotum at about 36 weeks and cover the entire scrotum by 40 weeks (Lubchenco, 1981). The scrotum should be inspected carefully for the presence of a hydrocele. Hydroceles are quite common at birth and must be distinguished from an inguinal hernia. Since a hydrocele is a fluid-filled sac, it can be differentiated from an inguinal hernia by dimming the room and testing to see if a light will shine through it. A hydrocele usually disappears spontaneously within a few days or weeks.

In females, the labia minora appear relatively large. The labia majora are small and widely separated at 30–32 weeks but by term have increased in size and fullness and completely cover the clitoris and labia minora (see Fig. 26-14). The clitoris is enlarged at birth. The urethra is visible below the clitoris. The vagina is a distinct orifice. There may be a tenacious white mucoid vaginal discharge that is occasionally blood-tinged. The blood-tinged discharge is thought to be due in part to a hormonal reaction transmitted from the mother.

In both sexes, rustlike stains may be seen on the diaper with the first voidings due to high concentrations of uric acid.

Assessment of the Normal Newborn 561

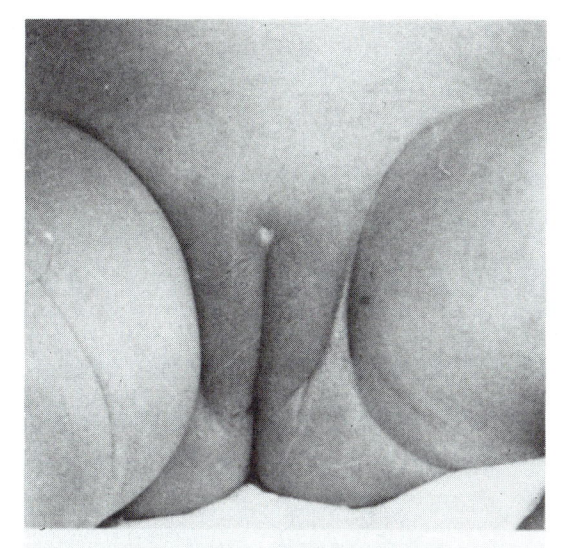

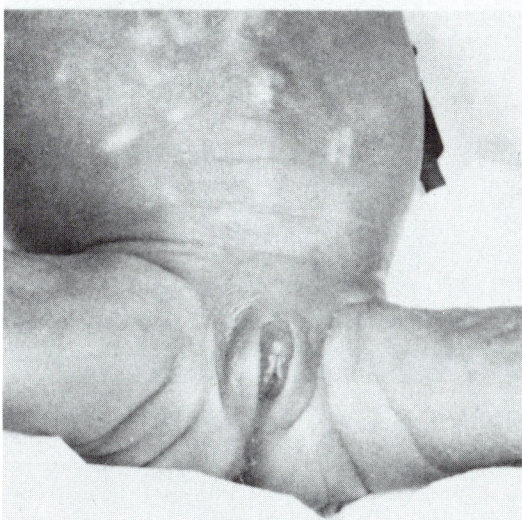

FIGURE 26–14. Female genitalia of full-term infant (top); female genitalia of premature infant (bottom).

The legs are of equal length, and the inguinal folds should be symmetrical. When the infant is in a supine position, the thighs can be flexed and the knees can be abducted through 90 degrees, until they touch the examining table. When the infant is in a prone position, the contours of the buttocks and gluteal, knee, and ankle folds are symmetrical. Trauma to the lower extremities is quite common. Approximately 5 percent of newborn infants have deformities due to positional abnormalities, intrauterine posture, or true malformations (Phibbs, 1982).

The average infant's foot is fat and wide and lacks a longitudinal arch. The relative number of creases in the feet should be observed in determining the gestational age. Wrinkling of the soles of the feet first occurs in the anterior portion and extends toward the heel as gestation progresses. There are usually one or two creases by 32 weeks. By 37–40 weeks the creases have become more numerous and cover the anterior two-thirds of the foot (see Fig. 26–15). In the postmature infant the

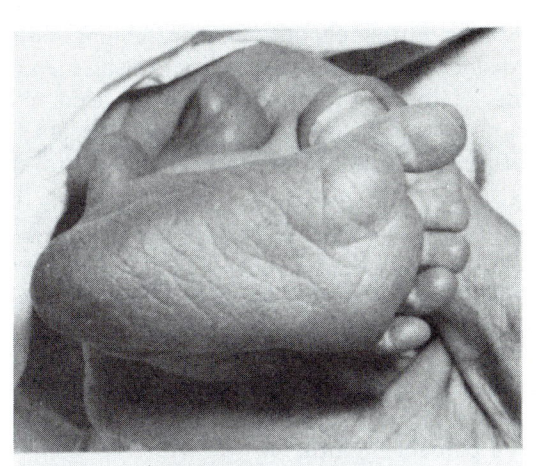

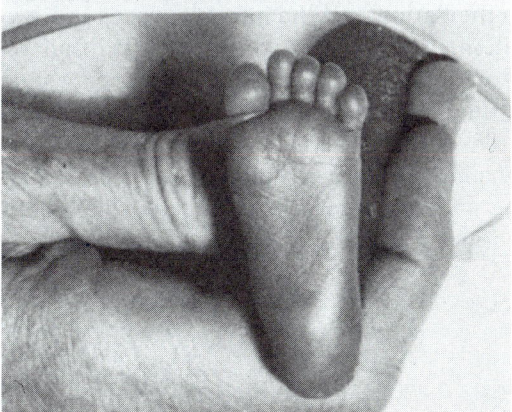

FIGURE 26–15. Foot of full-term infant (top); foot of premature infant (bottom).

Extremities

The movements of upper and lower extremities should be observed for equality and symmetry. In normal newborns the arms are of equal length. The fingers are usually kept in a flexed position in the palm of the hand. The nails appear at 20 weeks' gestation and cover the nail bed by term. Long nails extending beyond the fingertips may be observed in the post-term infant. Absent or hypoplastic nails are seen with certain syndromes. Malformations of the extremities frequently involve the hands. An excessive number of digits on the hands or feet is called polydactyly; the fusion of two digits into one is called syndactyly.

creases appear deep, and desquamation is sometimes present (Lubchenco, 1981).

Spine

The spine has two curves, dorsal and sacral. These curves are convex when observed from the posterior position. If the infant is in a sitting position, only the posterior dorsal curve will be observed. To ascertain alignment, the nurse should run a finger down the spine. At this time the back can also be checked for the presence of masses, hair tufts, dimples, or open lesions.

Buttocks

Asymmetry of the gluteal folds or inequality of the length of the legs may suggest congenital dislocation of the hips. If there is a limitation of abduction of the hips, or if only one knee can touch the table on exam, a dislocation of the hip may be suspected. The head of the femur is displaced posteriorly or is completely out of the acetabular fossa in hip dislocation. There are two diagnostic manipulations of the hip joint that must be used to be certain there is a dislocated hip–the Ortolani test and the Barlow test. The most reliable of the two tests is the Ortolani test (see Fig. 26-16). The infant should be relaxed, comfortable, and lying supine on a flat surface during the examination. The knee and hip are bent to a 90-degree angle and fully abducted. When the hip is reduced by abduction, a "click" can be heard as the femoral head enters the acetabulum. On adduction, the femoral head redislocates out of the acetabulum with a palpable "clunk."

In the Barlow test the infant is placed in a prone position. When the legs are extended and compared, the leg on the affected side appears shorter and the major gluteal folds are asymmetrical (see Fig. 26-17). Congenital dislocation of the hips is six to eight times more common in females than in males and three times greater in the left hip than in the right. Congenital hip dislocation occurs in 20–30 percent of breech deliveries (Tachdjian, 1982).

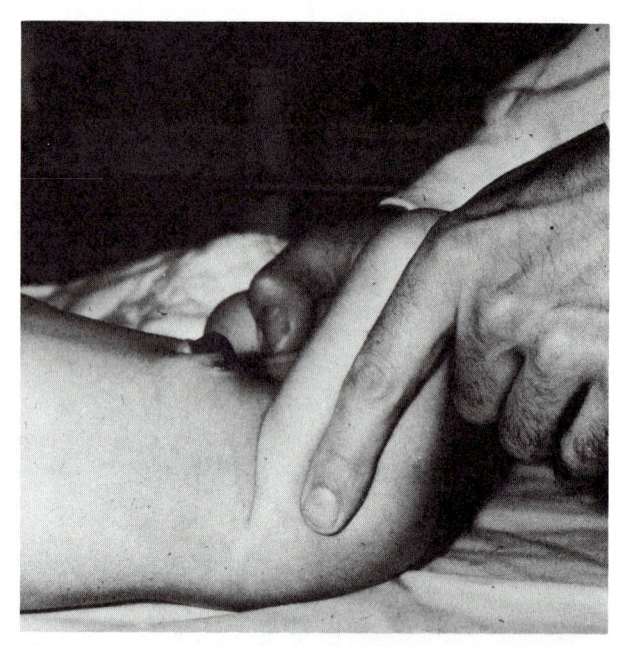

Rectum

The anus and rectum should be observed for irritation, patency, and the presence of fissures. The initial temperature reading should be taken

(a)

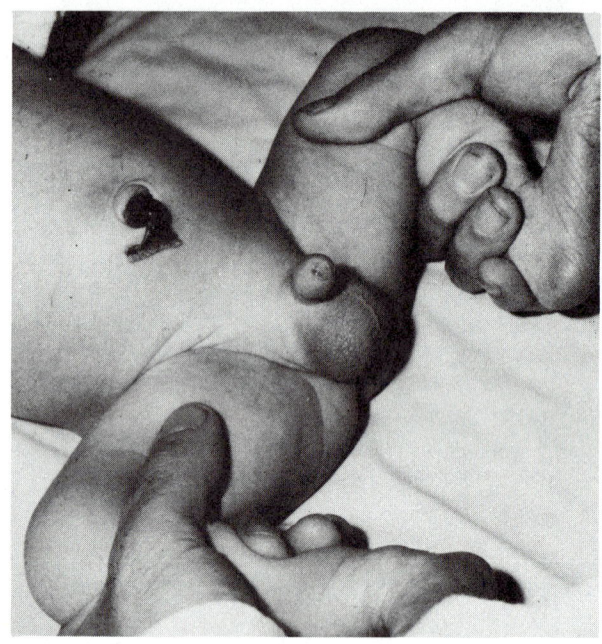

(b)

FIGURE 26–16. Method of inducing Ortolani's sign. (a) With the infant's knees bent, hips flexed to 90 degrees, the examiner's fingers are placed over the femoral head, exerting pressure downward. (b) The thighs are then fully abducted to induce the characteristic "click".
SOURCE: Courtesy Mead Johnson Laboratories.

rectally in order to rule out any anal obstruction. The passage of meconium is an almost certain indication of anal patency.

The physical assessment includes a thorough

Assessment of the Normal Newborn 563

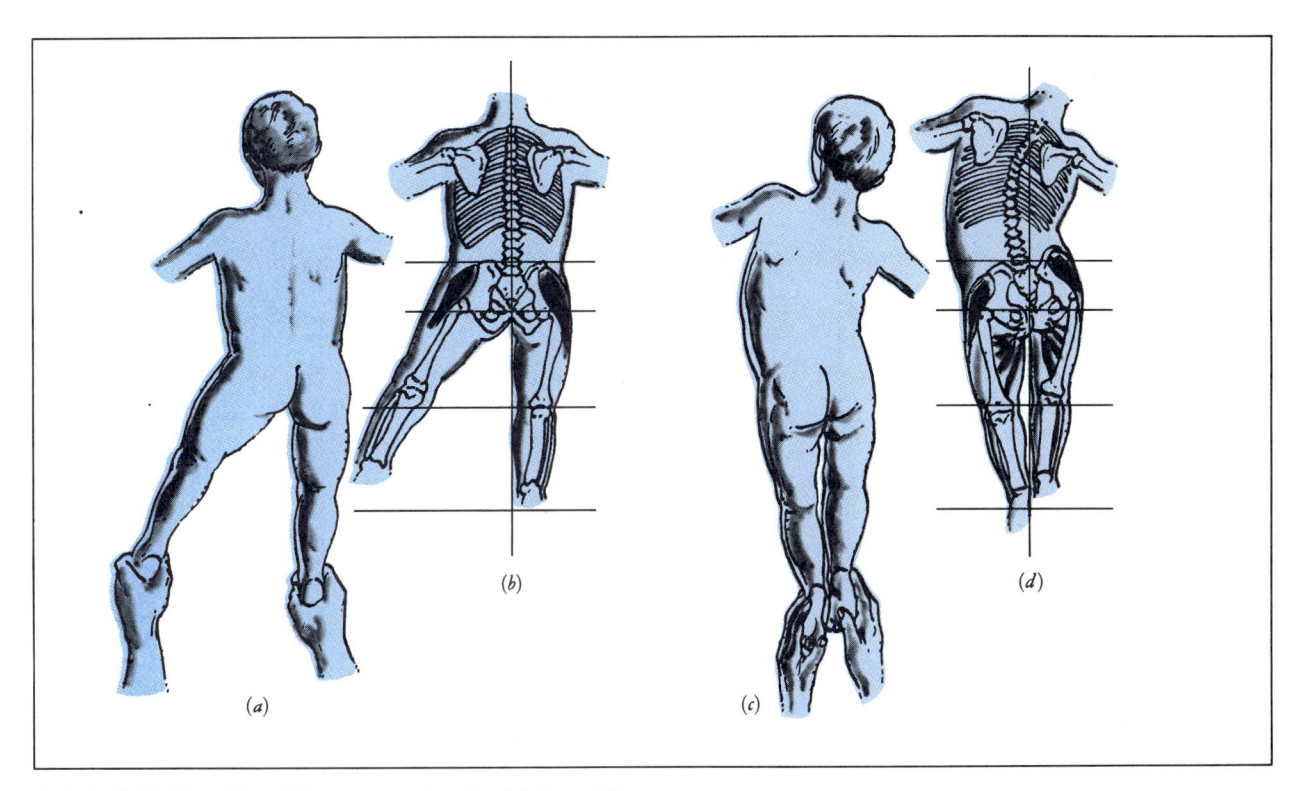

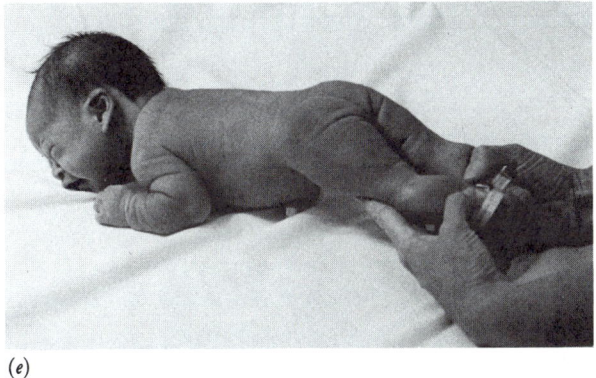

FIGURE 26-17. Congenital abduction contracture of the left hip and pelvic obliquity. (a,b) When the left hip is maintained in abduction, the pelvis is level and at a right angle to the longitudinal axis of the spine, which remains straight. (c,d) When the left leg is brought down into the weight-bearing position, parallel with the vertical axis of the trunk and the opposite extremity, the pelvis assumes an oblique position. (e) A Barlow test determines asymmetry of skin folds in congenital dislocation of the hip.
SOURCE: Rudolph and Hoffman (1982).

evaluation of the physical characteristics of the newborn infant as well as assessments of gestational age, neurologic status, and behavior, which will be covered in the following sections. A thorough basis for understanding the status of each newborn as well as early identification of problems is essential for planning effective nursing care.

NEUROLOGIC ASSESSMENT

The neurologic examination is limited to an assessment of the development of muscle tone. Posture and movements should be observed when the infant's condition has stabilized, after the first hour of life. Preferably, this examination should be done when the infant is neither very sleepy nor very hungry. This examination is often done in conjunction with the gestational age assessment. The neurologic criteria scoring (see Fig. 26-18) is done in conjunction with the external criteria scoring (see Tables 26-1a and 26-1b) as part of the Dubowitz gestational age assessment.

Posture

Posture tone and spontaneous movements should be observed for symmetry while the infant is in a quiet, restful state. The infant should be evaluated for the changes that occur with gestational age.

As gestational age increases, the limbs become more flexed. Hypotonia is present until about 30

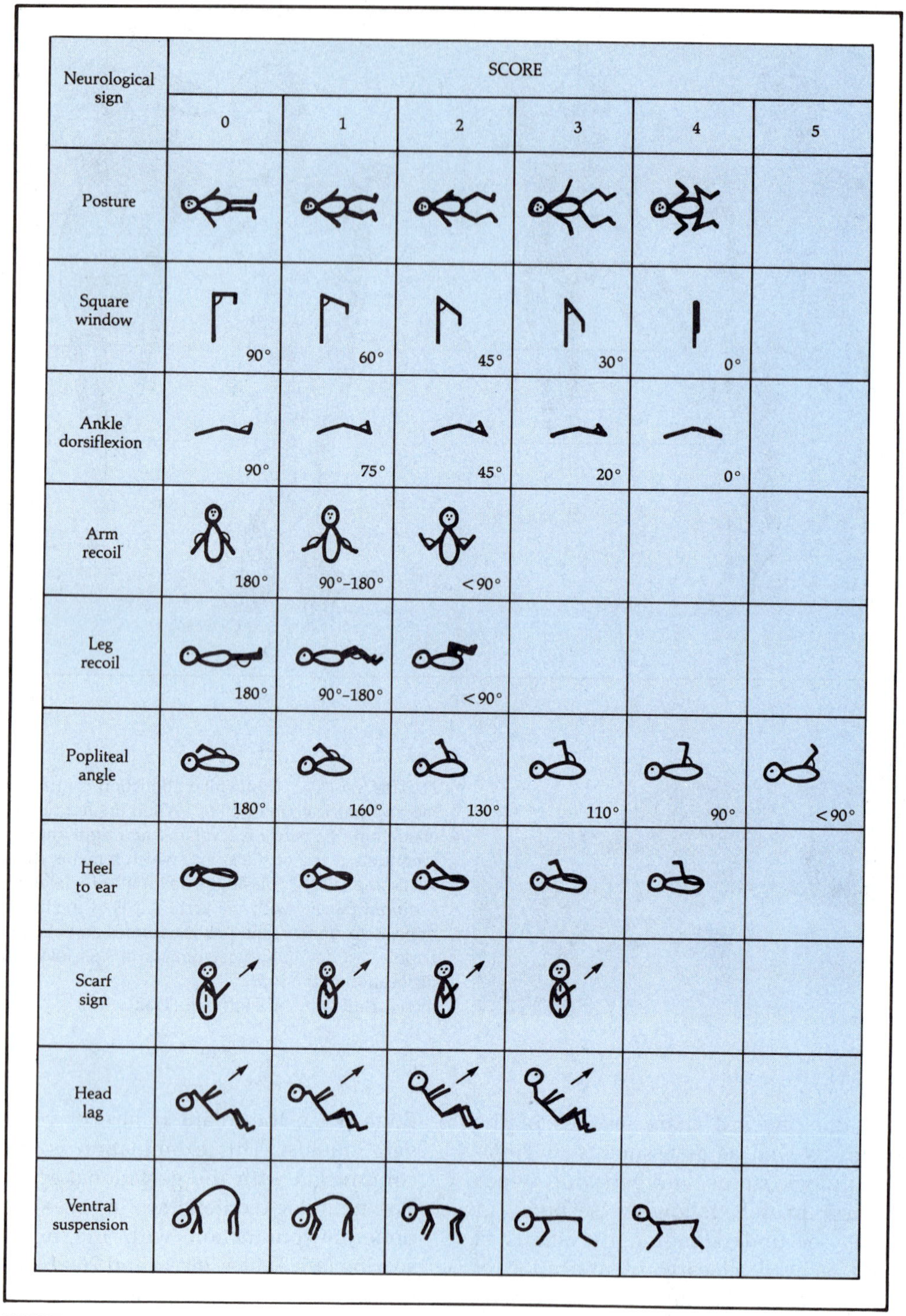

FIGURE 26–18. Scoring system of neurologic signs for assessment of gestational age.
SOURCE: Dubowitz, Dubowitz, and Goldberg (1970).

weeks' gestation, with slight flexion of the feet and knees. Flexion of the thighs and hips occurs at 34 weeks, and the characteristic frog-leg position of the legs is observed. The arms are extended. By 35 weeks the beginning of arm flexion can be seen. At 36–38 weeks the resting posture is that of complete flexion. There is about a 2-week lag between the time when resting flexion of the extremities is observed and the time when recoil after brief extension occurs. At 36–37 weeks the infant will lie in a flexion position. If the arms are extended, they will remain extended. By 40 weeks there is

SOME NOTES ON TECHNIQUES OF ASSESSMENT OF NEUROLOGIC CRITERIA
(for use in conjunction with Fig. 26–18)

Posture: Observed with infant quiet and in supine position. Score 0: Arms and legs extended; 1: Beginning of flexion of hips and knees, arms extended; 2: Stronger flexion of legs, arms extended; 3: Arms slightly flexed, legs flexed and abducted; 4: Full flexion of arms and legs.

Square window: The hand is flexed on the forearm between the thumb and index finger of the examiner. Enough pressure is applied to get as full a flexion as possible, and the angle between the hypothenar eminence and the ventral aspect of the forearm is measured and graded. (Care is taken not to rotate the infant's wrist while doing this maneuver.)

Ankle dorsiflexion: The foot is dorsiflexed onto the anterior aspect of the leg, with the examiner's thumb on the sole of the foot and other fingers behind the leg. Enough pressure is applied to get as full a flexion as possible, and the angle between the dorsum of the foot and the anterior aspect of the leg is measured (see Fig. 26–20).

Arm recoil: With the infant in the supine position the forearms are first flexed for 5 seconds, then fully extended by pulling on the hands, and then released. The sign is fully positive if the arms return briskly to full flexion (Score 2). If the arms return to incomplete flexion or the response is sluggish, it is graded as score 1. If they remain extended or are only followed by random movements, the score is 0.

Leg recoil: With the infant supine, the hips and knees are fully flexed for 5 seconds, then extended by traction on the feet, and released. A maximal response is one of full flexion of the hips and knees (Score 2). A partial flexion scores 1, and minimal or no movement scores 0.

Popliteal angle: With the infant supine and his pelvis flat on the examining couch, the thigh is held in the knee-chest position by the examiner's left index finger and thumb supporting the knee. The leg is then extended by gentle pressure from the examiner's right index finger behind the ankle and the popliteal angle is measured.

Heel to ear maneuver: With the baby supine, draw the baby's foot as near to the head as it will go without forcing it. Observe the distance between the foot and the head as well as the degree of extension at the knee. Grade according to diagram. Note that the knee is left free and may draw down alongside the abdomen.

Scarf sign: With the baby supine, take the infant's hand and try to put it around the neck and as far posteriorly as possible around the opposite shoulder. Assist this maneuver by lifting the elbow across the body. See how far the elbow will go across and grade according to illustrations. Score 0: Elbow reaches opposite axillary line; 1: Elbow between midline and opposite axillary line; 2: Elbow reaches midline; 3: Elbow will not reach midline.

Head lag: With the baby lying supine, grasp the hands (or the arms if a very small infant) and pull him slowly toward the sitting position. Observe the position of the head in relation to the trunk and grade accordingly. In a small infant the head may initially be supported by one hand. Score 0: Complete lag; 1: Partial head control; 2: Able to maintain head in line with body; 3: Brings head anterior to body.

Ventral suspension: The infant is suspended in the prone position, with examiner's hand under the infant's chest (one hand in a small infant, two in a large infant): Observe the degree of extension of the back and the amount of flexion of the arms and legs. Also note the relation of the head to the trunk. Grade according to diagrams (Fig. 5–4).

If score differs on the two sides, take the mean.

SOURCE: Dubowitz, Dubowitz, and Goldberg (1970).

TABLE 26–1a. *Scoring System for External Criteria*

External sign	Score 0	Score 1	Score 2	Score 3	Score 4
Edema	Obvious edema of hands and feet; pitting over tibia	No obvious edema of hands and feet; pitting over tibia	No edema		
Skin texture	Very thin, gelatinous	Thin and smooth	Smooth; medium thickness; rash or superficial peeling	Slight thickening; superficial cracking and peeling especially of hands and feet	Thick and parchmentlike; superficial or deep cracking
Skin color	Dark red	Uniformly pink	Pale pink; variable over body	Pale; only pink over ears, lips, palms, or soles	
Skin opacity (trunk)	Numerous veins and venules clearly seen, especially over abdomen	Veins and tributaries seen	A few large vessels clearly seen over abdomen	A few large vessels seen indistinctly over abdomen	No blood vessels seen
Lanugo (over back)	No lanugo	Abundant; long and thick over whole back	Hair thinning especially over lower back	Small amount of lanugo and bald areas	At least ½ of back devoid of lanugo
Plantar creases	No skin creases	Faint red marks over anterior half of sole	Definite red marks over > anterior ½; indentations over < anterior ⅓	Indentations over mt anterior ⅓	Definite deep indentations over > anterior ⅓
Nipple formation	Nipple barely visible; no areola	Nipple well defined; areola smooth and flat, diameter < 0.75 cm	Areola stippled, edge not raised, diameter < 0.75 cm	Areola stippled, edge raised, diameter > 0.75 cm	
Breast size	No breast tissue palpable	Breast tissue on one or both sides, < 0.5 cm diameter	Breast tissue both sides; one or both 0.5 to 1.0 cm	Breast tissue both sides; one or both > 1 cm	
Ear form	Pinna flat and shapeless, little or no incurving of edge	Incurving of part of edge of pinna	Partial incurving whole of upper pinna	Well-defined incurving whole of upper pinna	
Ear firmness	Pinna soft, easily folded, no recoil	Pinna soft, easily folded, slow recoil	Cartilage to edge of pinna, but soft in places, ready recoil	Pinna firm, cartilage to edge; instant recoil	
Genitals Male	Neither testis in scrotum	At least one testis high in scrotum	At least one testis right down		
Female (with hips ½ abducted)	Labia majora widely separated, labia minora protruding	Labia majora almost cover labia minora	Labia majora completely cover labia minora		

SOURCE: Dubowitz, Dubowitz, and Goldberg (1966).

TABLE 26–1b. Dubowitz Score/Gestational Age

Score	Weeks of Gestation
0–9	26
10–12	27
13–16	28
17–20	29
21–24	30
25–27	31
28–31	32
32–35	33
36–39	34
40–43	35
44–46	36
47–50	37
51–54	38
55–58	39
59–62	40
63–65	41
66–69	42

Scoring the Dubowitz Gestational Age Exam

The total scores for the neurologic and external criteria exams comprise a maximum of 70. Gestational age may be read by comparing the total score obtained against the weeks of gestation in Table 26–1. Utilizing these previous scoring criteria, an estimate of gestational ages is accurate within 2 weeks. With experience, this scoring can be completed in 5–8 min.

Reflexes

Many reflexes are observed in the normal newborn infant. The absence of these reflexes may indicate a depression of central or peripheral motor functions. Asymmetric responses suggest focal motor lesions, either peripheral or central. As the infant matures, the neonatal reflexes disappear in a predictable order. Abnormal persistence of these reflexes is seen in infants with general developmental lag or with central motor system lesions (Behrman and Vaughan, 1983).

Although the reflexes are interesting in themselves, assessment of them contributes very little to the detection of neurologic abnormalities in the newborn. The ages at which the newborn's reflexes normally appear and are no longer attainable are shown in Table 26–2. Their possible value as assessment tools lies in their asymmetry under certain pathologic conditions, their absence in generally unresponsive infants, and their low threshold in hyperresponsive infants (Dubowitz and Dubowitz, 1981).

1. *Moro reflex.* The most familiar reflex in the newborn infant is the Moro reflex, which is elicited by jarring the infant's bed, making a loud noise, or suddenly dropping the infant's head about 10 degrees while supporting it (see Fig. 26–21a). The infant's response is to "startle," to open the eyes wide, and then to cry. The spine is extended and the arms and legs are extended and abducted. The legs are then flexed with the arms brought forth in a clonic or jerky motion as if in an embrace.
2. *Rooting reflex.* The rooting reflex is elicited when the infant's cheek is stroked near the corner of the mouth. The infant will open its mouth and turn its head toward the response (see Fig. 26–21b).
3. *Sucking reflex.* The examiner's index finger is placed in the infant's mouth to initiate the sucking reflex. Since it is important to determine both the rhythm and strength of the

prompt recoil of the arms on extension (Black, 1978).

The normal newborn holds the head to a preferred side except when crying, at which time a midline position is assumed. The term newborn lies in a semiflexed position with the hips slightly abducted.

The arm on the side to which the head is turned is usually in a position of extension, and the opposite arm may be flexed at the elbow. The fingers are in a fist position. The trunk tends to lean to the preferred side (the side to which the head is turned). The hips are in a position of flexion and external rotation, and the knees are slightly flexed. The feet may be freely moved in all directions. Hyperextension of the head and neck and arching of the back indicate the need for further evaluation.

In a prone position the newborn infant may lift the head for a few minutes but usually lies with it rotated to the preferred side. The hips tend to be in a position of flexion and external rotation and are usually tucked or drawn up under the lower trunk, making the buttocks high. The knees are flexed and the feet turned out (see Fig. 26–19).

Muscle Tone

Muscle tone in the newborn infant is determined by the amount of resistance offered to passive movement. The nurse should assess tone in the limbs, trunk, and head (see Fig. 26–18 for scoring criteria).

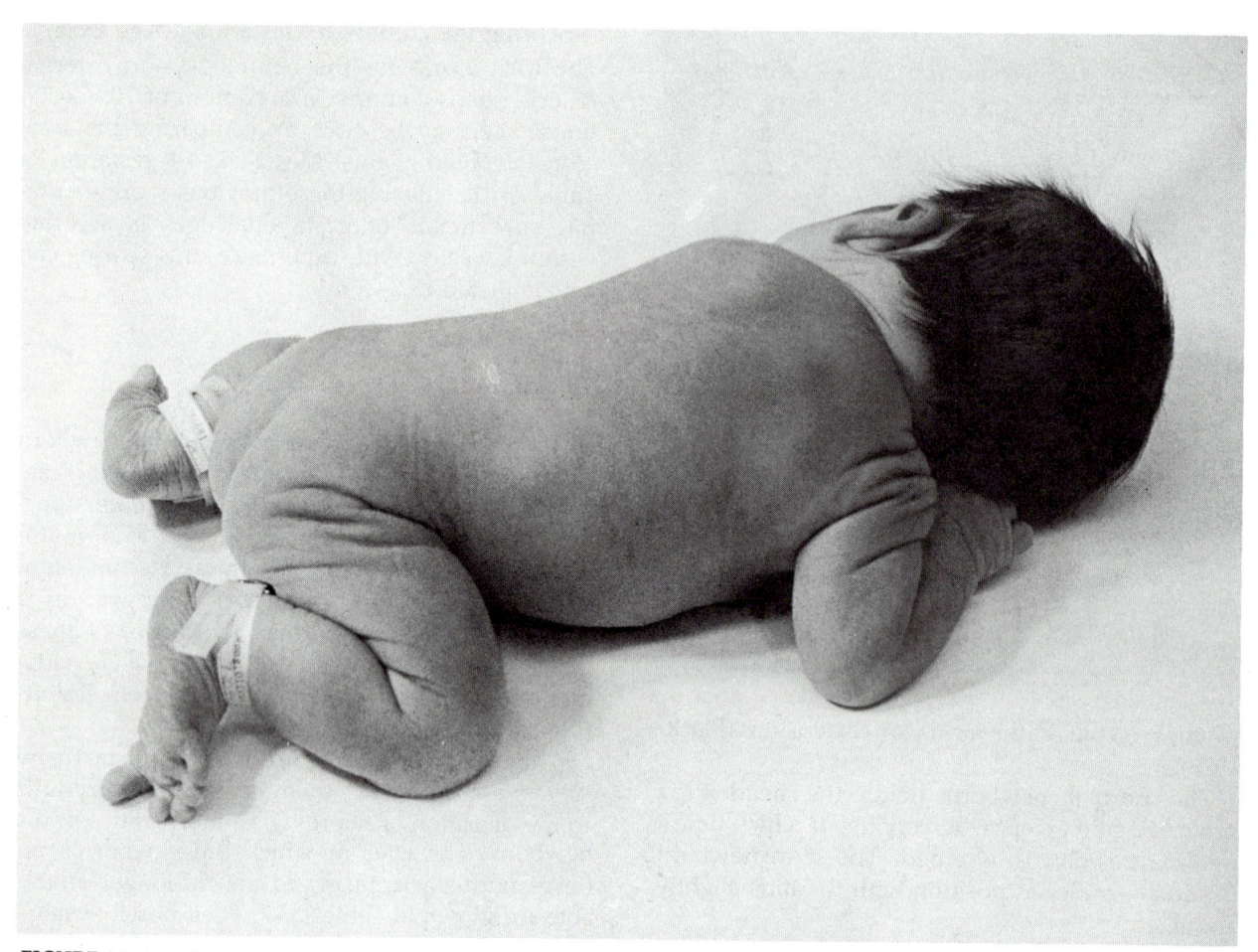

FIGURE 26-19. Newborn posture in the prone position.

TABLE 26-2. Reflexes of Neonates

Reflex	Age At Which Reflex Usually Appears	Age At Which Reflex Is Normally No Longer Obtainable
Moro	Birth	3 months
Stepping	Birth	6 weeks
Placing	Birth	6 weeks
Sucking and rooting	Birth	4 months awake 7 months asleep
Palmar grasp	Birth	6 months
Plantar grasp	Birth	10 months
Adductor spread of knee jerk	Birth	7 months
Tonic neck	2 months	6 months
Neck righting	4–6 months	24 months
Landau	3 months	24 months
Parachute reaction	9 months	Persists

SOURCE: Behrman and Vaughan (1983).

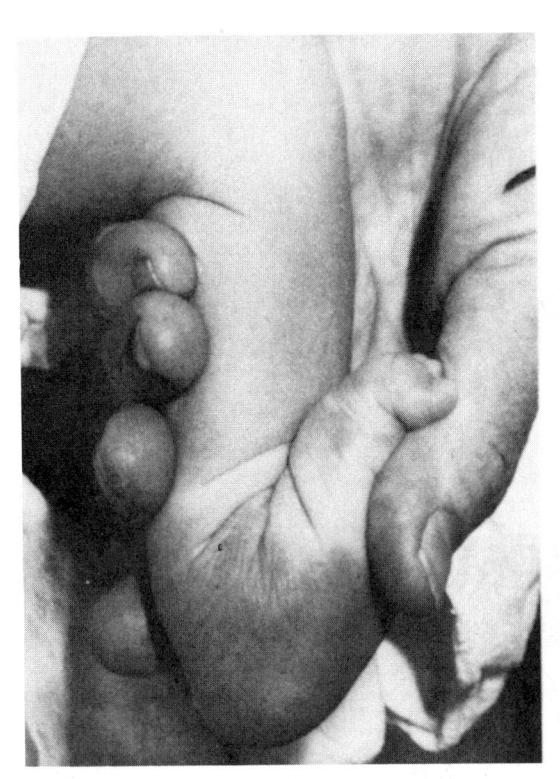

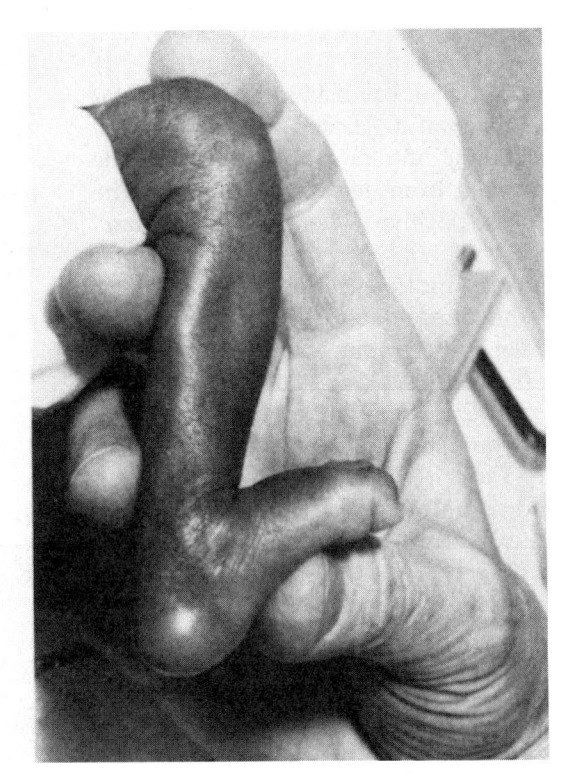

FIGURE 26-20. Dorsiflexion of foot of full-term infant (left); dorsiflexion of foot of premature infant (right).

suck, the nurse should wear either a finger cot or nonsterile glove when eliciting the sucking reflex to ensure aseptic technique. Strong, regular sucking in a sequence of five to eight movements is considered normal. The sucking will be less strong in a premature infant.

4. *Palmar grasp reflex.* To elicit this response, the examiner's index finger is placed in the infant's palm. The strength of the hold is evaluated. The full-term infant's grasp is strong enough to lift the infant off the table. The grasp should be symmetrical in strength. The premature infant will grasp the finger but will let go almost immediately (Fig. 26-21c).
5. *Plantar grasp reflex.* To elicit this reflex, the ball of the foot is pressed. The reflex is considered positive if the toes grasp the examiner's finger with prompt flexion (Fig. 26-21d).
6. *Parachute reflex.* When the infant is suspended in a prone position and is suddenly allowed to fall a short distance, the arms, hands, and fingers extend.
7. *Landau reflex.* When the infant is supported in a prone position with a hand beneath the abdomen, a normal newborn will respond by extending the head, trunk, and hips. When the examiner's hand is flexed, the infant responds by flexing the trunk and hips.
8. *Incurvation reflex.* To elicit this reflex, the examiner lifts the infant and holds it over his hand in a prone position. The amount of flexion of the head and body is noted to estimate tone. The incurvation reflex is obtained by stroking or applying intermittent pressure with the finger parallel to the spine, first on one side, then the other, watching for a movement of the pelvis toward the stimulated side.
9. *Lower-extremity reflexes.* Included in the spontaneous reflexes of the lower extremities are those of placing, stepping or walking, and dancing. *Placing* is demonstrated when the infant is held upright and the dorsum of the foot touches the underside of a surface such as a shelf. The infant will pick up the foot and place it on the top of the surface. Placing is similar to *walking*, which is observed when the infant is held in an upright position and the soles of the feet touch the surface. The infant places one foot in front of the other and "walks" slowly forward (see Fig. 26-21e). *Dancing* is observed when the infant moves

both feet alternately as if taking short, fast dance steps.
10. *Babinski reflex.* The Babinski reflex is a plantar response that can be elicited with a fingernail or the wooden end of an applicator stick. The sole is stroked from heel to toe laterally. The response is positive when the toes "fan" outward. Unilateral absence of the plantar response may indicate peripheral nerve damage on the affected leg. If the response is absent bilaterally, a spinal cord lesion may be present (Farwell, 1983, Fig. 26–21*f*).
11. *Tonic neck reflex.* The infant assumes a fencing position when supine. The head is turned to one side. The arm and leg on the side to which the head is facing are extended, and the opposite extremities are flexed. The tonic neck reflex is observed in the term newborn infant 2–4 months after birth. Like the Moro reflex, it disappears after the first few months of life if neurologic development progresses normally (Fig. 26–21*g*).

BEHAVIORAL ASSESSMENT

By the end of the gestational age assessment, the systematic head-to-toe appraisal of physical characteristics, and the neurologic examination, the nurse will have a thorough picture of the physical status of the newborn. The infant has been evaluated for both spontaneous activity and response to stimulation. The behavioral assessment adds more information to the overall evaluation of the infant's developmental status.

The newborn infant has been found to have distinct behavior patterns. In the past, the newborn was viewed as a passive recipient of care, rather than as a person with a distinct personality. The mind of the newborn was viewed as a blank tablet awaiting the imprinting of experience. However, scientific research carried out in the 1950s and 1960s has shown that newborn babies have far greater abilities than ever before imagined.

FIGURE 26–21. (*a*) The Moro reflex; (*b*) the rooting reflex; (*c*) palmar grasp reflex; (*d*) plantar grasp reflex; (*e*) walking reflex; (*f*) Babinski reflex; (*g*) tonic neck reflex.
SOURCE: Courtesy Mead Johnson Laboratories.

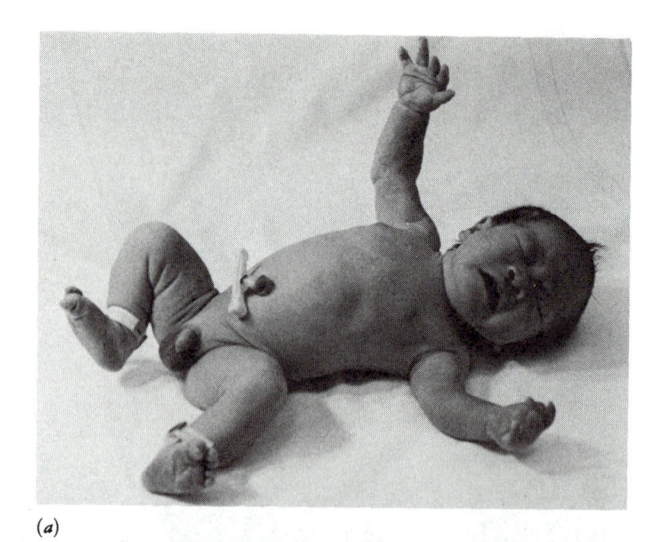

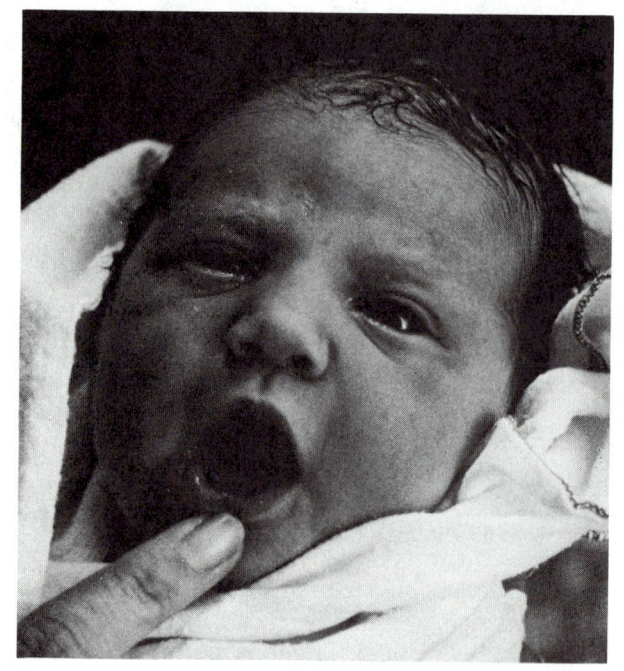

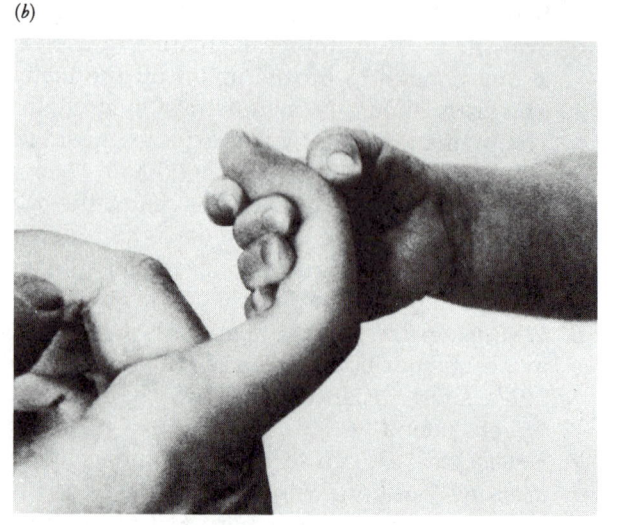

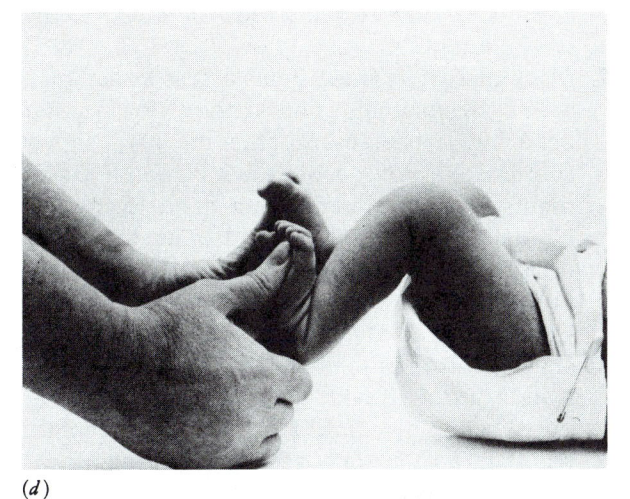

(d)

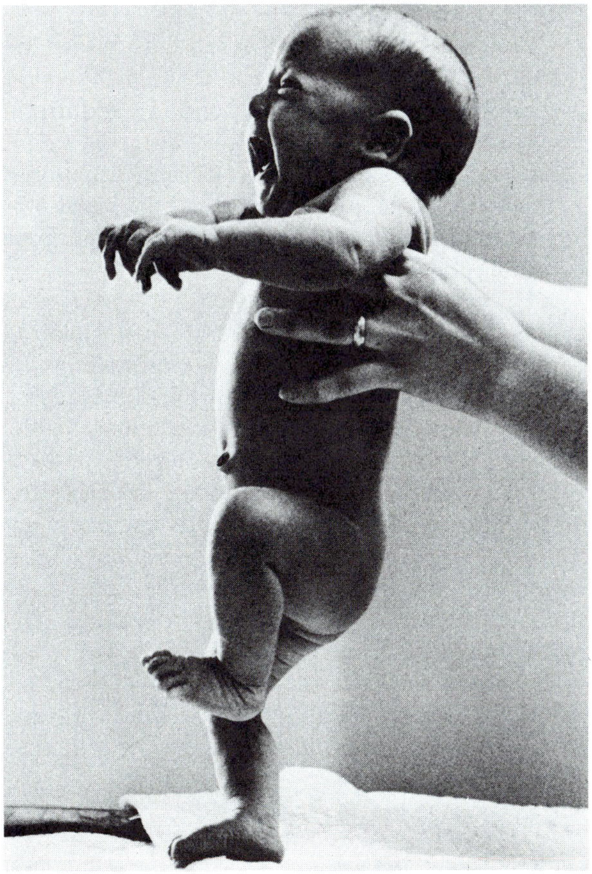

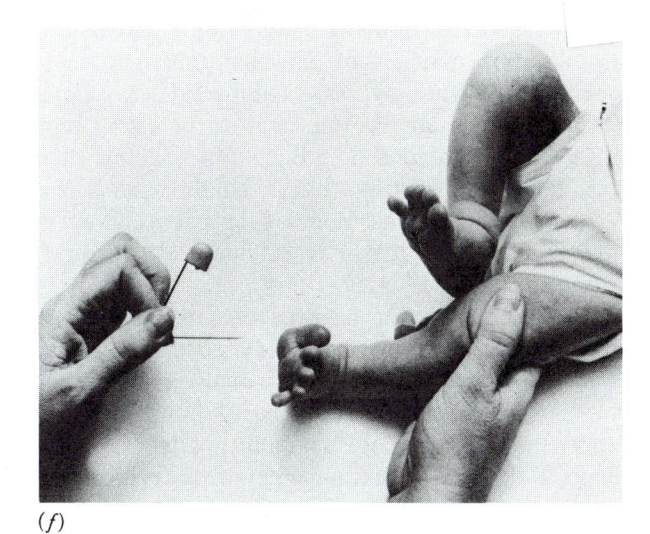

(f)

(e)

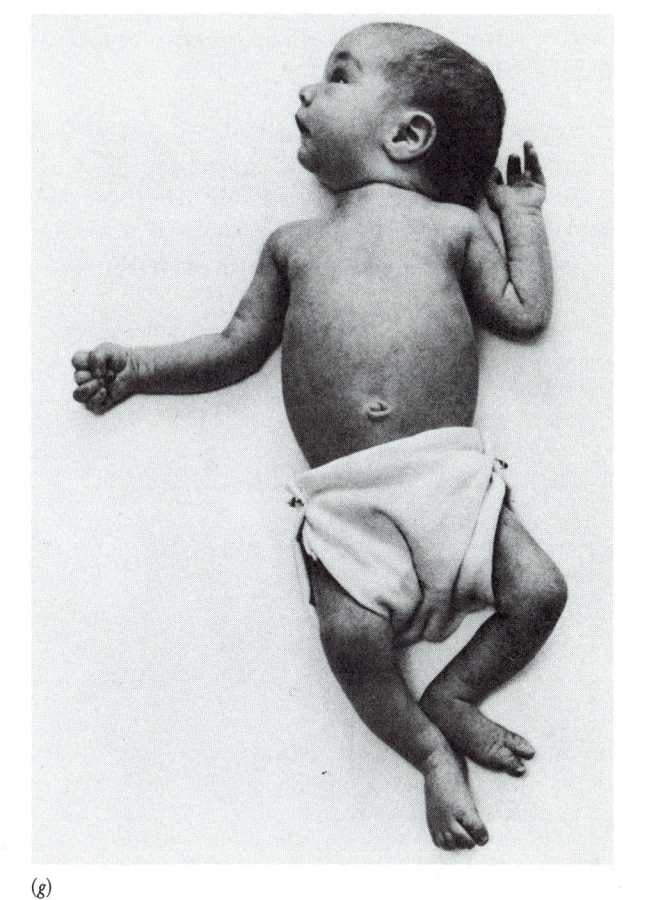

(g)

Brazelton Neonatal Behavioral Assessment Scale

The Brazelton Neonatal Behavioral Assessment Scale (BNBAS) was developed by T. Berry Brazelton and associates in the 1960s to score the newborn's interactive behavior (Brazelton, 1973). The BNBAS has been used to study normal and premature infants and to compare the behavior of infants of different cultural and ethnic populations. The scale is administered by trained testers. The examination is designed to take approximately 20 min to complete and another 10 min to score. It requires a flashlight, rattle, bell, and safety pin. The examination assesses the newborn's neurologic intactness by eliciting 20 reflex responses. However, the major part of the examination consists of 27 behavioral responses that identify the newborn's habituation, response to environmental stimuli, motor maturity, and interactive capacities. The Brazelton scale yields a profile of functioning, not a single score. The emphasis of the assessment is on process, which is evidenced as the infant integrates and organizes more complex activities.

Each of the 20 reflex measures–sucking, rooting, Moro, and so on–is scored on a scale of 0–3. These measures identify neurologic abnormalities (see Table 26–3). The 27 behavioral responses are rated on a 9-point scale (see Fig. 26–22). The 27 behavioral items can be grouped together into four behavioral dimensions: interactive capacities, motor capacities, organization of state control, and physiologic organization (Nugent, 1981):

1. *Interactive capacities.* These items assess the infant's capacity to attend to and process various visual and auditory stimuli. Alertness and orientation to stimuli are examined. Can the infant follow a stimulus with a bright-eyed, alert look? How responsive is the infant to the environment?
2. *Motor capacities.* These items assess the infant's ability to maintain tone and control motor behavior. They assess whether the infant shows coordinated motor activity with smooth movements. Can the infant bring hand to mouth? How does the infant respond to having vision occluded?
3. *Organization of state control.* These items assess the infant's ability to organize and modulate state, control irritability, and habituate. How well can the infant shut out disturbing or overwhelming stimuli? How well can the infant maintain a calm state despite increased input? How smoothly can the infant move from one state to another?
4. *Physiologic organization.* These items assess the infant's stability in response to stress. Physical symptoms associated with handling and dressing are observed. How quickly does the infant recover good skin color in stressful situations? How well is the infant able to inhibit startles or tremors in order to attend to social or inanimate stimuli?

The BNBAS has been useful in facilitating parent–infant attachment by demonstrating the behavior of the newborn infant and by teaching parents what the newborn contributes to the developing relationship (see Chapter 29).

The examiner observes the infant to assess the motor, social, interactional, and cognitive responses. For best results, the BNBAS should begin when the infant is asleep, covered, and fully clothed, preferably 2 hours after a feeding. The room should be dimly lit.

The assessment should follow an established procedure (see Table 26–4). All persons who use the scale should be trained in its proper administration.

The Infant's State

The infant's state should be observed first. *State* refers to the infant's state of consciousness. State is the single most important variable in the behavioral assessment. The infant's reactions to stimuli are interpreted within the context of whether it is in a *sleep* state or an *awake* state. State is measured on a 6-point scale. There are two sleep states and four awake states (Brazelton, 1973):

1. *Deep sleep, characterized by regular breathing.* The eyes are closed. There is no spontaneous activ-

TABLE 26–3. Elicited Responses on 20 Reflex Measures

Reflex	O[a]	L	M	H	A[b]
Plantar grasp		1	2	3	
Hand grasp		1	2	3	
Ankle clonus		1	2	3	
Babinski		1	2	3	
Standing		1	2	3	
Automatic walking		1	2	3	
Placing		1	2	3	
Incurvation		1	2	3	
Crawling		1	2	3	
Glabella		1	2	3	
Tonic deviation of head and eyes		1	2	3	
Nystagmus		1	2	3	
Tonic neck reflex		1	2	3	
Moro		1	2	3	
Rooting (intensity)		1	2	3	
Sucking (intensity)		1	2	3	
Passive movement					
Arms R		1	2	3	
L		1	2	3	
Legs R		1	2	3	
L		1	2	3	

SOURCE: Brazelton (1973).
[a] O = Response not elicited (omitted).
[b] A = Asymmetry.

Behavior Scoring Sheet

Initial State ....
Predominant State ....

Scale (Note State)	1	2	3	4	5	6	7	8	9
1. Response decrement to light (2, 3)									
2. Response decrement to rattle (2, 3)									
3. Response decrement to bell (2, 3)									
4. Response decrement to pinprick (1, 2, 3)									
5. Orientation inanimate visual (4 only)									
6. Orientation inanimate auditory (4, 5)									
7. Orientation animate visual (4 only)									
8. Orientation animate auditory (4, 5)									
9. Orientation animate visual & auditory (4 only)									
10. Alertness (4 only)									
11. General tonus (4, 5)									
12. Motor Maturity (4, 5)									
13. Pull-to-sit (3, 5)									
14. Cuddliness (4, 5)									
15. Defensive movements (4)									
16. Consolability (6 to 5, 4, 3, 2)									
17. Peak of excitement (6)									
18. Rapidity of buildup (from 1, 2 to 6)									
19. Irritability (3, 4, 5)									
20. Activity (alert states)									
21. Tremulousness (all states)									
22. Startle (3, 4, 5, 6)									
23. Lability of skin color (from 1 to 6)									
24. Lability of states (all states)									
25. Self-quieting activity (6, 5 to 4, 3, 2, 1)									
26. Hand-mouth facility (all states)									
27. Smiles (all states)									

FIGURE 26–22. Scoring of behavioral responses.
SOURCE: Brazelton (1973).

ity except startles or jerky movements at quiet, regular intervals. External stimuli produce startles with some delay. Suppression of startles is rapid, and state changes are less likely than from other states. No eye movements are visible.
2. *Light sleep, characterized by irregular respiration.* The eyes are closed. Rapid eye movements can be observed under the lids. The activity level is low, with random movements or startle equivalents often seen with a change of state. Sucking movements occur intermittently.
3. *Drowsy or semidozing.* The eyes may be open or closed with eyelids fluttering. The activity level is variable, with some mild startles. Reaction to sensory stimuli is observed, but response is

TABLE 26-4. **Steps to Follow in BNBAS**

1. Observe infant for 2 min – note state.
2. Flashlight (3–10 times) through closed lids.
3. Rattle (3–10 times).
4. Bell (3–10 times).
5. Uncover infant.
6. Light pinprick (5 times).
7. Ankle clonus.
8. Plantar grasp.
9. Babinski response.
10. Undress infant.
11. Passive movements and general tone.
12. Orientation, inanimate: visual and auditory.
13. Palmar grasp.
14. Pull to sit.
15. Standing.
16. Walking.
17. Placing.
18. Incurvation.
19. Body tone across hand.
20. Crawling-prone reflex.
21. Pick up and hold.
22. Glabella reflex.
23. Tonic deviation and reflex.
24. Orientation, animate: visual; auditory; visual and auditory.
25. Cloth on face.
26. Tonic neck response.
27. Moro response.

SOURCE: Brazelton (1973).

often delayed. State change is often observed after stimulation. Movements are usually smooth.

4. *Alert with bright look, or quiet, alert.* The infant seems to focus attention on a source of stimulation, such as an object to be sucked or a visual or auditory stimulus. Impinging stimuli may break through, but with some delay in response. Motor activity is at a minimum.
5. *Alert but agitated, or eyes open.* Considerable motor activity is observed, with thrusting movements of the extremities and even a few spontaneous startles. Reaction to external stimulation demonstrated by an increase in startles or motor activity. Discrete reactions are difficult to distinguish because of a generally high activity level.
6. *Vigorous crying.* This state is characterized by intense crying that is difficult to break through with stimulation.

Presentation of Stimuli

After an assessment of the infant's initial state, auditory and visual stimuli are presented. While the infant is still wrapped and quiet (state 1, 2, or 3), the flashlight is used as a visual stimulus, and the degree of response is noted. Next, using the rattle or, if the infant is in an alert state, the bell, the examiner notes the infant's response to auditory stimuli. The infant should then be uncovered, and any reactions to change should be recorded—for example, a change in skin color or movement from a quiet to an agitated state. While the infant is still quiet (state 1, 2, or 3), response to a light pinprick should be tested. While the infant is still dressed, clonus (ankle), foot grasp, and Babinski response should be determined.

When the infant assumes an awake-alert state, the order of administration of test items can vary. The infant can be undressed and observed, again, for state change, skin color, and response to maneuvers. In the alert state the infant can be pulled to sitting, and then standing, walking, and placing reflexes can be tested. Incurvation, body tone across the hand, and prone responses are then assessed. The response to cloth on the face, the tonic neck reflex, and the Moro reflex are tested last. Since these are disturbing to the infant, the infant's self-quieting and consolability can be assessed after these tests.

Value of the BNBAS

The BNBAS focuses on the newborn's behavior, identifying both strengths and limitations. The infant's social interaction and coping capacities are demonstrated. The scale was developed as a clinical tool for identifying neurologic and behavioral responses. The infant's habituation, orientation, and responses to stimuli are assessed. The examiner can observe motor maturity and variation in the rate and amount of change—in color, activity, and excitement, for example—during peak periods of alertness. Self-quieting abilities, consolability, and the infant's social behaviors are demonstrated (Powell, 1981).

The BNBAS is also useful in facilitating the parent–infant relationship. The examiner can demonstrate the baby's responses to the parents and thereby increase their awareness of the infant's capabilities.

Sleep/Wake Cycle

The infant's state–asleep or awake–influences every physiologic and neurosensory function. During fetal development a sleep/wake cycle is established that is still present at the time of birth. However, this cycle is disrupted almost immediately after birth. The newborn stays awake for longer periods of time, with periods of quiet alertness alternating with periods of activity. During the first 24 hours the infant experiences increased alertness. By the fifth day of life, the state cycles have stabilized (Fanaroff and Martin, 1983).

During the first week of life the term newborn spends only 8–16 percent of the day in a quiet, alert state (Fanaroff and Martin, 1983). Most of the rest of the time is spent in quiet or active sleep. The newborn spends 50 percent of the sleep cycle in active sleep. In the newborn, awakening follows active sleep, whereas the adult awakens from quiet sleep or drowsiness. Term infants awaken at approximately 4-hour intervals.

Parents need information regarding the infant's sleep/wake cycle in order to plan the newborn's care and to accommodate the other members in the household.

Table 26–5 shows the physiologic body functions that are affected by the state of the infant.

Assessment of Sensory Status

The newborn infant is more than a pink or blue bundle that cries incessantly when hungry, more than an egocentric entity demanding physical comfort. In the first days, weeks, and months of life the newborn demonstrates fascinating sensory and cognitive development.

Since the 1950s, research has shown that from birth the infant has the capacity to process external information (for example, from visual, auditory, and tactile stimuli) and the potential for interacting with the environment. The sensory system cannot be thoroughly evaluated in the newborn (Farwell, 1983), but the nurse can elicit the infant's responses to stimuli and share the information gained with parents. This serves to identify the individual needs of the infant.

Habituation

The newborn tends to respond to excessive stimulation in the environment by becoming accustomed to it; this is the process of *habituation*. When the nursery is overlighted or noisy, the infant tends to shut down its capacity to attend (Brazelton, 1981). To obtain the most accurate sensory assessment, the nurse must consider habituation and examine the infant in a semidarkened, quiet environment.

Sensory Modalities

AUDITORY. A soft rattle or bell can be used to elicit a response. A term infant is capable of responding to sound whether asleep or awake. The sleeping infant will respond to sound by eye blinking, startle response, irregular breathing, and eye opening. The response may be greater in active than in quiet sleep. The infant who is awake will

TABLE 26–5. *Physiologic Body Functions Affected by State*

Body Functions	Quiet Sleep	Active Sleep	Awake/Crying
Heart rate	Regular	Irregular	Irregular
Respirations	Regular	Irregular and faster; apnea and periodic breathing may occur	Irregular and faster
O_2 consumption	Lower	Higher	Higher (especially if crying)
Transcutaneous pO_2	Higher	Lower	
Blood pressure	Lower	Variable	Higher
Endocrine			Cortisol secretion increases with increasing arousal

SOURCE: Adapted from Fanaroff and Martin (1983).

turn its eyes and head toward the sound. Low-frequency sounds have been found to soothe the infant, whereas high-frequency sounds may cause distress, with increased heart rate and crying (Fanaroff and Martin, 1983).

VISUAL. A bright, shiny object such as a red ball can be an appropriate stimulus to test an infant's visual response. The response is best elicited if the infant is in a quiet, alert state. The infant should be held in an upright, vertical position and the object held in the midline. The newborn has the capacity to be alert to, turn the eyes and head to follow, and fixate on an object (Fanaroff and Martin, 1983).

OLFACTORY. The sense of smell is present at birth. An alcohol wipe can be used to elicit a response to smell. The newborn will respond as if offended. The nurse can observe a flaring of the nares, a blinking response, and sometimes a sneeze. Newborns will respond to the smell of milk with rooting and sucking reflexes.

GUSTATORY. Infants respond differently to sweet versus plain liquids. To assess an infant's preference for liquids, give first feedings of sterile water. Most infants will take a few initial sucks and then show little interest. Follow sterile water with glucose water and note the infant's sucking. Most infants will show a preference for sweet liquids.

TACTILE. Touch is the most developed sense at birth. The premature infant at 28 weeks' gestation can differentiate touch from pain. Touch results in alerting or slight motor activity, while pain results in withdrawal or crying. At 32 weeks rooting is elicited by perioral stimulation, and at 35–36 weeks the infant will rapidly turn its head away from a pinprick over the side of the face (Avery, 1981).

When an infant is quiet, a rapid, intrusive tactile stimulation will elicit an alert state. When the infant is upset, a slow, modulated tactile stimulation tends to soothe the infant. A patting motion of three times per minute has been found to be soothing, whereas five to six times per minute is found to be an alerting stimulus (Brazelton, 1981). A crying newborn will respond to touch and will almost always stop crying when held.

To assess the infant's tactile response to painful stimuli, the nurse can apply a light pinprick (5–10 times) to both hands and feet in succession. Normal response is the withdrawal of the pricked extremity and a facial grimace or cry (Volpe, 1981; Farewell, 1983). The infant's response to pain can be tested by observation of withdrawal and the emotional reaction to the pinprick. This maneuver tests the intactness of peripheral pain fibers and of pain pathways up to the level of the thalamus (Behrman and Vaughan, 1983).

Of all the sensory modalities in the newborn, touch can be evaluated the most accurately.

Examination at Discharge

At the time of discharge the nurse should examine the newborn in the presence of the parents. This examination should be thorough, yet concise. Having both parents present gives the nurse an opportunity to identify their concerns and engage them in problem solving. It also allows the parents to get to know their infant and to begin to understand the common variations of normalcy. This is a very good time to share observational data from others on the health care team regarding the individuality of their infant and to offer anticipatory guidance related to its care (see Chapter 29).

SUMMARY

Because the registered nurse is usually the first health care professional to assess the neonate's adjustment to extrauterine life, the nurse must possess both the knowledge and skills to evaluate comprehensively the newborn's physical status. The purpose of an objective, systematic assessment of the newborn is to obtain an accurate, in-depth picture of the infant in the first few minutes, hours, and days of life. Determining and documenting baseline data through the use of a variety of assessment tools provides important information needed for developing an infant's individualized plan of care.

According to the recommendations of the Academy of Pediatrics through its Committee on the Fetus and the Newborn, all newborn infants should be classified by birth weight, gestational age, and intrauterine growth (Lubchenco, 1981). By the end of the gestational age assessment, the systematic head-to-toe appraisal of physical characteristics, and the neurologic examination, the nurse will have a thorough picture of the physical status of the newborn.

REFERENCES

American Academy of Pediatrics. 1971. *Standards and recommendations for hospital care of newborn infants.* 5th ed. Evanston, Ill.: American Academy of Pediatrics.

American Academy of Pediatrics. 1986. *Care of the uncircumcised penis.* Elb Grove Village, Ill.: American Academy of Pediatrics.

American Academy of Pediatrics, Committee on Fetus and Newborn, 1975. Report of the ad hoc task force on circumcision. *Pediatrics.* 56:610–611.

American Academy of Pediatrics and American College of Obstetricians and Gynecologists. 1983. *Guidelines for perinatal care.* March of Dimes Publication.

Avery, G. B. 1981. *Neonatology: Pathophysiology and management of the newborn.* 2nd ed. Philadelphia: J. B. Lippincott.

Battaglia, F. C., and Lubchenco, L. O. 1967. A practical classification of newborn infants by weight and gestational age. *J. Pediatrics.* 71(2):159–163.

Behrman, R. E., and Vaughan, V. C., eds. 1983. *Nelson textbook of pediatrics.* 12th ed. Philadelphia: W. B. Saunders.

Bernardo, M. L. 1979. Craniosynostosis: The child's care from detection through correction. *MCN.* 4(4): 234–237.

Black, M. 1978. Assessment of weight and gestational age. *Nurs. Clin. N. Amer.* 13:13–22.

Brazelton, T. B. 1973. *Neonatal behavioral assessment scale.* Philadelphia: J. B. Lippincott.

Brazelton, T. B. 1981. Behavioral competence of the newborn infant. In *Neonatology: Pathophysiology and management of the newborn,* 2nd ed., ed. G. B. Avery. Philadelphia: J. B. Lippincott.

Candy, M. M. 1979. Birth of a comprehensive family-centered maternity program. *J. Obstet. Gynecol. Neonatal Nurs.* 8(2):80–84.

Clark, A. L.; Affonso, D. D.; and Harris, T. R. 1979. *Childbearing: A nursing perspective.* 2nd ed. Philadelphia: F. A. Davis.

Crelin, E. S. 1969. *Anatomy of the newborn: An atlas.* Philadelphia: Lea and Febiger.

Dubowitz, L., and Dubowitz, V. 1977. *Gestational age of the newborn.* Menlo Park, Calif.: Addison-Wesley.

Dubowitz, L., and Dubowitz, V. 1981. *The neurological assessment of the preterm and full-term newborn infant.* Philadelphia: J. B. Lippincott.

Dubowitz, L.; Dubowitz, V.; and Goldberg, C. 1970. Clinical assessment of gestational age in the newborn infant. *J. Pediatrics.* 77(1):1–10.

Einhorn, A. H., ed. 1982. The newborn infant. In *Pediatrics,* 17th ed., eds. A. M. Rudolph and J. E. Hoffman. Norfolk, Conn.: Appleton-Century-Crofts.

Erickson, M. P. 1978. Trends in assessing the newborn and his parents. *MCN.* 3(2):99–103.

Eyres, P. J. 1972. The role of the nurse in family-centered nursing care. *Nurs. Care N. Amer.* 7(1):27–39.

Fanaroff, A., and Martin, R. J. 1983. *Behrman's neonatal–perinatal medicine: Diseases of the fetus and infant.* 3rd ed. St. Louis: C. V. Mosby.

Farwell, J. 1983. Maturational and neurobehavioral assessment of the newborn. In *Principles and practice of perinatal medicine: Maternal–fetal and newborn care,* eds. J. B. Warshaw and J. C. Hobbins. Menlo Park, Calif.: Addison-Wesley.

Fitzpatrick, E.; Reeder, S. R.; and Mastroianni, L. 1971. *Maternity nursing.* 12th ed. Philadelphia: J. B. Lippincott.

Gagliardi, J. V. 1983. Initial assessment of the newborn. In *Principles and practice of perinatal medicine: Maternal–fetal and newborn care,* eds. J. B. Warshaw and J. C. Hobbins. Menlo Park, Calif.: Addison-Wesley.

Hennel, M. 1968. Family-centered maternity nursing in practice. *Nurs. Clin. N. Amer.* 3(2):289–298.

Herrmann, J., and Light, I. J. 1971. Infection control in the newborn nursery. *Nurs. Clin. N. Amer.* 6(1):55–65.

Hilliard, M. E. 1968. The changing role of the maternity nurse. *Nurs. Clin. N. Amer.* 3(2):277–288.

Jensen, M. D.; Benson, R. C.; and Bobak, I. M. 1977. *Maternity care: The nurse and the family.* St. Louis: C. V. Mosby.

Klaus, M. H., and Kennell, J. H. 1982. *Parent–infant bonding.* 2nd ed. St. Louis: C. V. Mosby.

Koops, B. L., and Battaglia, F. C. 1982. The newborn infant. In *Current pediatric diagnosis and treatment,* 7th ed., eds. C. H. Kempe, H. K. Silver, and D. O'Brien. Los Altos, Calif.: Lange Medical Publications.

Korones, S. B. 1976. *High-risk newborn infants.* St. Louis: C. V. Mosby.

Korones, S. B., and Lancaster, J. 1981. *High-risk newborn infants: The basis for intensive nursing care.* 3rd ed. St. Louis: C. V. Mosby.

Lubchenco, L. O. 1981. Assessment of weight and gestational age. In *Neonatology: Pathophysiology and management of the newborn,* 2nd ed., ed. G. B. Avery. Philadelphia: J. B. Lippincott.

Lubchenco, L. O.; Hansman, C.; Dressler, M.; and Boyd, E. 1963. Intrauterine growth as estimated from liveborn birth-weight data at 24 to 42 weeks of gestation. *Pediatrics.* 32:793–800.

Lubchenco, L. O.; Hansman, C.; and Boyd, E. 1966. Intrauterine growth in length and head circumference as estimated from live births at gestational ages from 26 to 42 weeks. *Pediatrics.* 37:403–408.

Luciano, K. B. 1972. Components of planned family-centered care. *Nurs. Clin. N. Amer.* 7(1):41–52.

Moore, K. 1982. *The developing human: Clinically orientated embryology.* 3rd ed. Philadelphia: W. B. Saunders.

Nugent, J. K. 1981. The Brazelton neonatal behavioral assessment scale: Implications for intervention. *Pediatric Nurs.* 7(3):18–21.

Parker, S., and Brazelton, T. B. 1981. Newborn behavioral assessment: Research, prediction, and clinical use. *Children Today.* 2–4.

Paukert, S. E. 1979. One hospital's experience with

implementing family-centered maternity care. *J. Obstet. Gynecol. Neonatal Nurs.* 8(6):351–358.

Phibbs, R. H., ed. 1982. The newborn infant. In *Pediatrics*, 17th ed., eds. A. M. Rudolph and J. E. Hoffman. Norfolk, Conn.: Appleton-Century-Crofts.

Potsie, W. P., and Handler, S. D., eds. 1982. Pediatric otorhinolaryngology. In *Pediatrics*. 17th ed., eds. A. M. Rudolph and J. E. Hoffman. Norfolk, Conn.: Appleton-Century-Crofts.

Powell, M. L. 1981. *Assessment and management of developmental changes and problems in children*, 2nd ed. St. Louis: C. V. Mosby.

Reed, B.; Sutorius, J.; and Coen, R. 1971. Management of the infant during labor, delivery, and in the immediate neonatal period. *Nurs. Clin. N. Amer.* 6(1):3–14.

Reeder, S. J.; Mastroianni, L.; and Martin, L. L. 1983. *Maternity nursing*. 15th ed. Philadelphia: J. B. Lippincott.

Rich, O. J. 1969. Hospital routines as rites of passage in developing maternal identity. *Nurs. Clin. N. Amer.* 4(1):101–109.

Rudolph, A. M., and Hoffman, J. E., eds. 1982. *Pediatrics*. 17th ed. Norfolk, Conn.: Appleton-Century-Crofts.

Scharping, E. M. 1983. Physiological measurements of the neonate. *MCN.* 8(1):70–73.

Sullivan, R.; Foster, J.; and Schreiner, R. L. 1979. Determining the newborn's gestational age. *MCN.* 4(1):38–45.

Sweet, A. Y. 1979. Classification of the low-birth-weight infant. In *Care of the high-risk neonate*, 2nd ed., eds. M. H. Klaus and A. A. Fanaroff. Philadelphia: W. B. Saunders.

Tachdjian, M. O., ed. 1982. Orthopedic problems in childhood. In *Pediatrics,* 17th ed., eds. A. M. Rudolph and J. E. Hoffman. Norfolk, Conn.: Appleton-Century-Crofts.

Torrance, J. T. 1968. Temperature readings of premature infants. *Nurs. Research.* 17:312.

Van Leeuwen, G. 1973. The nurse in prevention and intervention in the neonatal period. *Nurs. Clin. N. Amer.* 8(3):509–520.

Volpe, J. J. 1981. *Neurology of the newborn*. Philadelphia: W. B. Saunders.

Weinstein, R. A.; Boyer, K. M.; and Linn, E. S. 1983. Isolation guidelines for obstetric patients and newborn infants. *Am. J. Obstet. Gynecol.* 146(4):353–360.

Wheeler, W. 1972. Recollections of 40 years of hospitalization of children. *Pediatric Research.* 6:840–842.

Wolff, P. H. 1959. Observations on newborn infants. *Psychosomatic Med.* 21:110.

Ziai, M.; Clarke, T.; and Merritt, T. 1984. *Assessment of the newborn: A guide for practitioners*. Boston: Little, Brown.

27
Care of the Normal Newborn

BEHAVIORAL OBJECTIVES

Upon completion of this chapter, the reader should be able to:

- List the two most important priorities in infant care and identify at least two nursery plans that address each one.

- Describe the purpose and function of the observational nursery, the central nursery, and rooming-in.

- Define family-centered care and give an example of how the nurse can promote this philosophy when providing routine care to the normal newborn

ROUTINE CARE OF THE NORMAL NEWBORN

Most infants delivered in a hospital environment are admitted into the regular, or well-baby, newborn nursery. These infants remain in the nursery for the duration of their mother's hospitalization, usually 1–4 days, depending on the mode of delivery (vaginal or cesarean). If the delivery occurs in an alternative birth center, discharge may occur as early as 4–6 hours after birth. After immediate care is delivered to the newborn (see Chapter 19) and once a thorough physical assessment has been completed, if the infant is identified as a healthy full-term newborn, routine care is provided until the time of discharge. *Routine care* is defined as that care provided to all newborns in the course of a few hours, an 8-hour shift, or a few days by the nursing staff that is caring for that particular infant. This care includes observation of the infant's appearance, activity, and color; care of the skin; care of the circumcision; assessment of temperature, feeding and bowel and bladder function; weighing; and transportation to the mother for breastfeeding and bottle-feeding, as well as maintaining supplies and records. These routines should be considered standing orders (American Academy of Pediatrics, 1971).

Because infants are unable to communicate verbally, it is of paramount importance that nurses be aware of any changes in the infant's activity or behavioral patterns (see Chapter 29). The method of care delivery depends on the concept of care being implemented at a particular hospital. These concepts of care—the central nursery, rooming-in, and family-centered care—will be discussed in detail later in this chapter.

Regardless of the type of care the newborn receives, the two most important care issues are safety and prevention of infection. Both of these issues are addressed through (1) the physical designs of nurseries, (2) the equipment used in nurseries, (3) the policies and procedures adopted by the hospitals that provide newborn care, and (4) the training and expertise of the nursing staff.

The course of neonatal care is determined primarily by the infant's ability to adapt to extrauterine life. Ideally, the physical design of the facility for care of the newborn allows uninterrupted clinical observation throughout the newborn's hospitalization. In an effort to provide guidance for hospital care of newborn infants, the American Academy of Pediatrics (1971) has developed standards and recommendations for nursery areas in all hospitals.

Safety of the Newborn

The location of the newborn service should be close to the maternity service, to reflect the concept of continuity of care and to allow the mother immediate access to her infant should the infant need to be evacuated in an emergency. The lighting in the nursery should be bright enough, with shadow-free illumination, to allow for detection of cyanosis and jaundice. The color of the nursery walls and the type of paint used should also be considered, since they can contribute to color distortion. White or pink-white colors of nonglossy or flat paint should be used (American Academy of Pediatrics, 1971). The environmental conditions of temperature and ventilation should be comfortable for working personnel, but temperature instabilities in newborns should be considered, and temperature and ventilation should be maintained at a level that will prevent excessive heat loss or gain for each infant. To allow for this flexibility, it is ideal for the ventilation and heat units in the nursery to be separate from the main hospital systems. Windows in the nurseries may also contribute to changes in environmental conditions, so window coverings and placement of the infants in relation to the windows must be considered and monitored at all times. An emergency system (for example, a call light or call button) should be available so any person can call for help in an emergency without leaving the infant alone.

Resuscitation equipment should be immediately available. This can be accomplished by having oxygen and air outlets and suction available from a central source or a portable source (for example, a crash cart). All nursery personnel must be trained and competent in infant resuscitation. Infants should never be left unattended by the nursery staff or by their parents during the initial hospital stay after birth.

Any electrical equipment utilized or stored in the nursery should be checked on a regular basis for adequacy of grounding. This equipment should be placed in an area that makes it easily accessible to be applied to the infant, but where it does not pose any danger to the infant. The use of extension cords and adaptors is discouraged, and most hospitals require that all equipment be tested and approved by their engineering or biomedical departments prior to being used on patients. Other nursery equipment, such as bassinets and scales, should be sturdy and secure so it is not potentially hazardous to the newborn.

Many nurseries have two doors to allow for safe and rapid evacuation of infants in an emergency. All nursery personnel should be trained in emergency procedures for fire, bomb threats, earthquakes, or other disasters. Practice drills should be conducted randomly to ensure patient safety. Since it would be difficult either to remove all infants from their bassinets or to push all bassinets out at the same time, infant evacuation aprons have been developed (see Fig. 27–1). These aprons allow for one person to be able to safely carry out from four to six infants at a time. The ideal situation would be for each mother to be able to be evacuated with her infant. Most hospitals have specific policies regarding safety of the newborn.

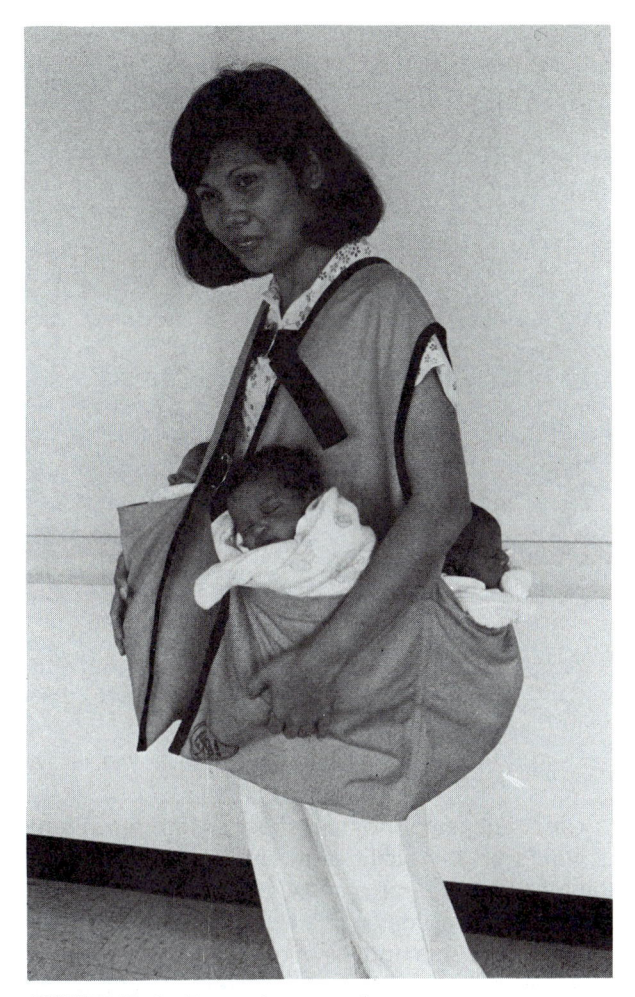

FIGURE 27-1. Evacuation apron for infants.

Any person coming in contact with the nursery should be familiar with these policies.

All newborns should have two identical identification bands on their wrist and ankle indicating the mother's name, admission number, infant's sex, and date and time of birth. These should be applied in the delivery room. Each time the infant is taken to the mother the infant's band should be matched against the mother's band to verify the correct identity of the infant.

Prevention of Infection

In the late 1930s and early 1940s, epidemic diarrhea was commonplace in the newborn nurseries of many obstetric hospitals all over the country. A few years later the staphylococcus epidemic became a threat to newborn infants (Wheeler, 1972). In today's modern nurseries, the prevention of infection is of utmost importance in caring for the newborn. Everyone who is in contact with infants must assume the responsibility of keeping the newborn free of contamination. This includes parents as well as personnel (Herrmann and Light, 1971; Reeder, Mastroianni, and Martin, 1983).

The practical problems of caring for large numbers of infants make maintenance of a germ-free environment unrealistic. In addition, once infants are discharged to go home, they face the microbial challenges of the outside world. Nursery procedures are, at best, attempts to prevent exposure of the newborn to those organisms that are most likely to cause disease (Herrmann and Light, 1971)—organisms from other newborns.

Most of the common infectious agents responsible for colonization and for disease in the nursery are transmitted from infant to infant by the hands of nursery personnel (American Academy of Pediatrics, 1971). Haire and Haire (1971) indicated that the central nursery, not contact with the parents, is one of the chief sources of staphylococcal contamination. Thorough handwashing with antiseptic detergents or soaps is essential in the prevention of infection. A 2-min scrub to the elbows should be done with a soft brush prior to entering the nursery. Additionally, hands should be washed carefully just before and just after caring for each infant (see Fig. 27-2). Care should be taken that clean hands do not touch contaminated equipment. If cover gowns are used over street clothes, gowns should be changed after the nurse finishes caring for one baby and before he or she begins to care for the next. A gown should never be used for a period longer than 8 hours. Most nurseries require that nonnursery personnel (including parents) use cover gowns over their street clothes when they enter the nursery. A cover gown may provide the visitor/staff with a false sense of security; organisms are transmitted chiefly by airborne droplets or skin contact, neither of which are controlled by the cover gown (Renaud, 1983). Good handwashing is the only protection for the infant. Most nursery personnel usually change their street clothes into clean scrub clothes while they work in the nursery, but this is done primarily for the protection of the nurse's clothes or to keep consistency among the nursery staff. As with the use of cover gowns, scrub clothes are not an effective primary infection control measure. All personnel working in the nursery with infants should be free of any infection.

The physical design of the nursery can also contribute to the prevention of infection. Sinks should be readily accessible, to facilitate and encourage frequent handwashing. Soap and towel

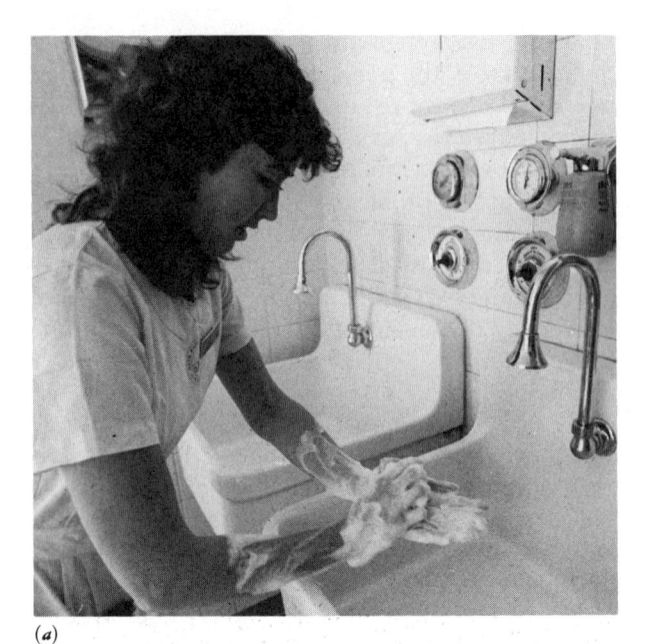

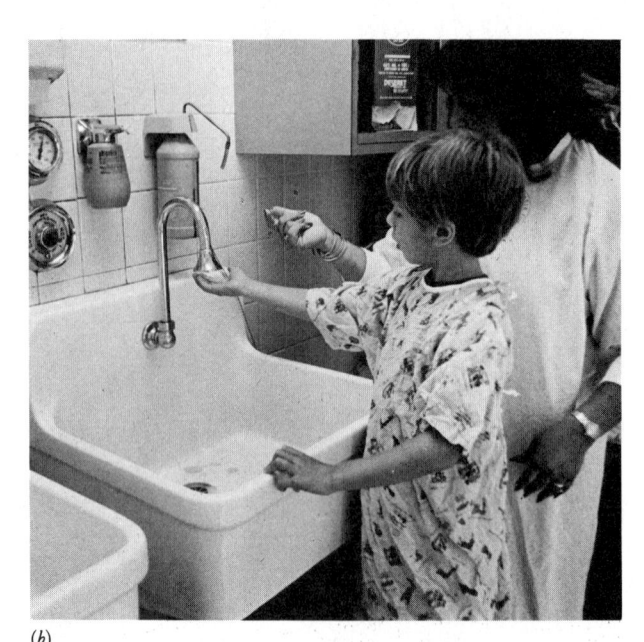

FIGURE 27–2. (a) Care of the newborn includes thorough handwashing. (b) Siblings must be aware that proper hygiene is essential prior to handling the newborn.

dispensers should be kept well stocked. The American Academy of Pediatrics (1971) recommends that one sink be available for each six infants inside each nursery area. Equipment should be designed for ease of cleaning. Trash and dirty diaper receptacles should be kept near the sink and should have covers. Only 8–12 bassinets should be in each nursery, and a minimum of 20 square feet of floor space per infant is recommended (American Academy of Pediatrics, 1971).

The number of persons entering the nursery area can also affect the likelihood of infection. Concern about protecting infants from contagious diseases led to what appear to have been bizarre policies of isolation and separation. In the early 1940s, visiting hours were no longer than 30–60 min per week, and maternity hospitals gathered full-term infants in large nurseries in a fortresslike arrangement (Klaus and Kennell, 1982). Today some nurseries still limit visitation to parents only, but most hospitals allow 24-hour visiting. Special arrangements are often made for siblings to visit in the mother's room, and often grandparents are also included. It is recommended that siblings be screened for colds, running noses, and other signs of contagion prior to their being allowed to visit in the maternity area. Siblings should also wear cover gowns and wash their hands prior to being with the new baby.

The management of a suspect or infected infant depends on the facilities available, the species of the infecting organism and the source of infection. Table 27–1 provides some isolation guidelines for obstetric patients and newborns.

Some nurseries utilize a system of cohorting babies in a particular nursery in an attempt to minimize the risk of infection. Under this system, all newborns are admitted into the same nursery until the nursery is at maximum capacity (usually 8–12 babies). Then the nursery closes to new admissions until all infants have been discharged from that particular room and the room (floor, walls, and windows) has been thoroughly cleaned and disinfected. Other nurseries do not necessarily have specific systems for thorough cleaning and disinfection, and often low-census times (when few infants are in the nursery) are used to accomplish these tasks. Regardless of the specific policies of a particular hospital, every person who comes in contact with any infant should be aware of the potential risks of infection and should exercise good aseptic technique and sound judgment in handling the infant.

Infants born outside the hospital environment are usually not admitted into the regular well-baby nursery. They are often admitted directly into, and cared for in, an observation nursery, where they can be monitored closely for any evidence of infection.

Text continued on page 590.

TABLE 27–1. Isolation Guidelines for Obstetric Patients and Newborn Infants

Infection	Maternal Isolation (Duration)[a]	Newborn Isolation (Duration)[a]	Mother–Infant Contact	Breast-Feeding	Comments
Amnionitis	None[b]	None	Permitted	Permitted	See "Endometritis" if fever continues postpartally.
Antibiotic-resistant bacteria					
Mother	WSP (DH)		Permitted	Permitted	Includes methicillin-resistant *Staphylococcus aureus* and aminoglycoside-resistant enteric bacilli and *Pseudomonas aeruginosa* cultured from surface sites or infected lesions.
Newborn infant		II	Permitted	Permitted	
Campylobacter diarrhea. See Diarrhea					
Chickenpox					
Mother	SI (C)	I	After VZIG	After VZIG	Varicella zoster immune globulin (VZIG) for infant if onset of maternal disease is less than 5 days before delivery or within 48 hours after delivery. Continue maternal SI until rash crusted. Exclude susceptible personnel.
Newborn infant	None	I	In isolation room	Permitted	Continue SI until rash crusted. Exclude susceptible personnel.
Chlamydia					
Mother					
Carriage	None	None	Permitted	Permitted	
Newborn infant					
Conjuntivitis or pneumonia	None	None	Permitted	Permitted	
Congenital infection, unknown etiology	None	SI (DH)	In isolation room	Permitted	Exclude pregnant personnel from contact with infant. If etiology established, see relevant category. If syphilis and rubella excluded, isolation may be discontinued.
Cytomegalovirus					
Mother	None	None	Permitted	Permitted	Breastfeeding is prohibited if mother has an acute cytomegalovirus syndrome. Exclude pregnant personnel from contact with infected mother or infant.
Newborn infant	None	None	Permitted	Permitted	

[a] WSP = Wound and skin precautions (gown and glove); SI = strict isolation (gown, glove, and mask); EnP = enteric precautions (gown and glove); BP = blood precautions (glove); RI = respiratory isolation (mask). Specific operational details can be found in *Isolation Techniques for Use in Hospitals*. DI = Duration of illness (for draining lesions, until drainage stops). DH = Duration of hospitalization. DIP = Duration of expected incubation period (after perinatal exposure to infected mother). C = Duration given under "Comments." U = Until 24 hours of appropriate therapy. I = Type I nursery isolation (isolation room and gown: glove and contact precautions); II = type II nursery isolation (newborn nursery of ICN placement OK with gown and glove and contact precautions).
[b] Drainage or infected lesions should be contained by clean, dry dressings or perineal pads. Personnel should wear gloves or use "no touch" technique when handling soiled dressings or pads.
[c] Fresh cover gown (and careful handwashing) for mother before contact with neonate.

Continued

TABLE 27-1. Continued

Infection	Maternal Isolation (Duration)[a]	Newborn Isolation (Duration)[a]	Mother–Infant Contact	Breast-Feeding	Comments
Diarrhea					
Mother					
Infectious etiology suspected or confirmed	EnP (C)	II	With EnP[c]	After mother asymptomatic[c]	Continue maternal EnP while cultures positive or symptoms persist.
Antibiotic associated	EnP (C)	None	With EnP[c]	After mother asymptomatic[c]	Continue EnP while *Clostridium difficile* toxin assay positive or symptoms persist.
Newborn infant					
Infectious etiology suspected or confirmed	None	II	In nursery with EnP	After full-strength enteral feeding tolerated	Continue EnP while cultures positive or symptoms persist. If cases cluster, cohort affected infants.
"Dirty" delivery	None	None	Permitted	Permitted	Includes infants exposed to nonmaternal flora during delivery. On admission, such infants should be bathed. If infection is suspected or found in mother or infant see appropriate category.
Endometritis	None[b]	None	Permitted	Permitted	See instructions for sitz or tub cleaning. See Streptococcal disease, group A or Staphylococcal disease if these pathogens cultured or suspected.
Enterovirus					
Mother	None	II	Permitted[c]		
Newborn infant	None	II	In nursery with EnP		
Escherichia coli diarrhea. See Diarrhea					
Gonococcal infection					
Mother					
Untreated or less than 24 hours of treatment	None	None	After 24 hours of appropriate treatment	After 24 hours of appropriate treatment	Treat infant prophylactically with 50,000 U of aqueous crystalline penicillin G intramuscularly or intravenously (20,000 U if low birth weight).

[a] WSP = Wound and skin precautions (gown and glove); SI = strict isolation (gown, glove, and mask); EnP = enteric precautions (gown and glove); BP = blood precautions (glove); RI = respiratory isolation (mask). Specific operational details can be found in *Isolation Techniques for Use in Hospitals.* DI = Duration of illness (for draining lesions, until drainage stops). DH = Duration of hospitalization. DIP = Duration of expected incubation period (after perinatal exposure to infected mother). C = Duration given under "Comments." U = Until 24 hours of appropriate therapy. I = Type I nursery isolation (isolation room and gown: glove and contact precautions); II = type II nursery isolation (newborn nursery of ICN placement OK with gown and glove and contact precautions).

[b] Drainage or infected lesions should be contained by clean, dry dressings or perineal pads. Personnel should wear gloves or use "no touch" technique when handling soiled dressings or pads.

[c] Fresh cover gown (and careful handwashing) for mother before contact with neonate.

TABLE 27-1. Continued

Infection	Maternal Isolation (Duration)[a]	Newborn Isolation (Duration)[a]	Mother–Infant Contact	Breast-Feeding	Comments
Newborn infant Conjunctivitis or scalp abscess	None	II	Permitted	Permitted	Culture and treat parents before infant is discharged from hospital.
Hepatitis Mother Type A	EnP (C)	None	After prophylaxis of infant[c]	After prophylaxis of infant[c]	Give infant immune globulin (IG), 0.5 ml/kg of body weight intramuscularly. Continue EnP until maternal aminotransferase levels normal.
Type B, acute	BP (C)	None	After first dose of prophylaxis[c]	After first dose of prophylaxis[c]	Give infant hepatitis B immune globulin (HBIG), 0.5 ml intramuscularly (repeat 3 and 6 months later). Continue BP until mother HBsAg negative and HbsAb positive.
Type B, chronic antigen carrier (HBsAg positive)	BP (DH)	None	After first dose of prophylaxis[c]	After first dose of prophylaxis[c]	Give infant HBIG as above. Discontinue breastfeeding by 6 months of age.
Unknown type or non-A, non-b	EnP, BP (C)	None	With EnP[c]	No	Consider giving infant IG (or HBIG), 0.5 ml intramuscularly. Continue EnP and BP until maternal aminotransferase levels normal.
Herpes simplex Mother Genital, delivery by cesarean section	None[b]	None	Permitted[c]	Permitted[c]	See instruction for sitz or tub cleaning. If rupture of membranes occurred less than 6 hours before cesarean section, isolate infant as for vaginal delivery.
Genital, vaginal delivery	None[b]	II	In nursery in WSP[c]	Permitted[c]	See instruction for sitz or tub cleaning.

[a]WSP = Wound and skin precautions (gown and glove); SI = strict isolation (gown, glove, and mask); EnP = enteric precautions (gown and glove); BP = blood precautions (glove); RI = respiratory isolation (mask). Specific operational details can be found in *Isolation Techniques for Use in Hospitals*. DI = Duration of illness (for draining lesions, until drainage stops). DH = Duration of hospitalization. DIP = Duration of expected incubation period (after perinatal exposure to infected mother). C = Duration given under "Comments." U = Until 24 hours of appropriate therapy. I = Type I nursery isolation (isolation room and gown: glove and contact precautions); II = type II nursery isolation (newborn nursery of ICN placement OK with gown and glove and contact precautions).

[b]Drainage or infected lesions should be contained by clean, dry dressings or perineal pads. Personnel should wear gloves or use "no touch" technique when handling soiled dressings or pads.

[c]Fresh cover gown (and careful handwashing) for mother before contact with neonate.

Continued

TABLE 27-1. Continued

Infection	Maternal Isolation (Duration)[a]	Newborn Isolation (Duration)[a]	Mother–Infant Contact	Breast-Feeding	Comments
Oral or cutaneous	None[b]	None	Permitted[c]	Permitted[c]	Mother should wear mask and not kiss neonate if herpes labialis present, glove if herpetic whitlow present, and cover any other cutaneous herpetic lesions with a clean dry dressing. Breastfeeding is prohibited if herpetic breast lesions are present.
Newborn infant	None	I	In nursery in SI	No	
Herpes zoster					
Mother	WSP (C)	None	Permitted if lesions covered[b]	Permitted if lesions not on breast[b]	Continue WSP until rash is crusted. Exclude susceptible personnel. Disseminated disease requires SI—see comment under Chickenpox regarding VZIG.
Influenza					
Mother	RI (DI)	None	After temperature less than 38.5°C for 48 hours	After temperature less than 38.5°C for 48 hours	Consider febrile respiratory illnesses to be influenza during community outbreaks (Nov.–March only).
Newborn infant	None	II	In nursery with WSP	Permitted	
Listeria					
Mother	None	None	Permitted	Permitted	
Newborn infant	None	None	Permitted	Permitted	
Necrotizing enterocolitis					
Newborn infant	None	None	Permitted	After full-strength enteral feeding tolerated	If cases cluster, institute cohorting for affected infants (see policy for diarrhea).
Respiratory infection					
Mother	None	None	Permitted; mother should wear mask and wash hands	Permitted; mother should wear mask and wash hands	See Streptococcal disease, group A, Pharyngitis, Enterovirus, Influenza, or Tuberculosis if these pathogens cultured or suspected.

[a] WSP = Wound and skin precautions (gown and glove); SI = strict isolation (gown, glove, and mask); EnP = enteric precautions (gown and glove); BP = blood precautions (glove); RI = respiratory isolation (mask). Specific operational details can be found in *Isolation Techniques for Use in Hospitals*. DI = Duration of illness (for draining lesions, until drainage stops). DH = Duration of hospitalization. DIP = Duration of expected incubation period (after perinatal exposure to infected mother). C = Duration given under "Comments." U = Until 24 hours of appropriate therapy. I = Type I nursery isolation (isolation room and gown: glove and contact precautions); II = type II nursery isolation (newborn nursery of ICN placement OK with gown and glove and contact precautions).
[b] Drainage or infected lesions should be contained by clean, dry dressings or perineal pads. Personnel should wear gloves or use "no touch" technique when handling soiled dressings or pads.
[c] Fresh cover gown (and careful handwashing) for mother before contact with neonate.

TABLE 27–1. Continued

Infection	Maternal Isolation (Duration)[a]	Newborn Isolation (Duration)[a]	Mother–Infant Contact	Breast-Feeding	Comments
Respiratory syncytial virus					
Newborn infant	None	II	In nursery with WSP	Permitted	
Rotavirus diarrhea. See Diarrhea					
Rubella					
Mother	RI (C)	None	After rash clears	After rash clears	Continue RI until rash clears. Exclude susceptible personnel.
Newborn infant (congenital)	None	I	In nursery in SI	Permitted	Congenitally infected infants may shed virus for up to 2 years. Exclude susceptible personnel.
Salmonellosis. See Diarrhea					
Shigellosis. See Diarrhea					
Staphylococcal disease					
Mother					
Mastitis	None[b]	None	Permitted[c]	Permitted[c]	
Wound infection, draining lesion, or toxic shock syndrome	WSP (DI)	None	After 48 hours of appropriate therapy[c]	After 48 hours of appropriate therapy[c]	Mother-infant contact permitted only if draining lesions adequately contained by dressing.
Newborn infant					
Pneumonia	None	I	In nursery in isolation	Permitted	
Skin lesions	None	I	In nursery in isolation	Permitted	If cases cluster, cohort infected infants and contact Infection Control and Chief of Pediatrics.
Streptococcal disease, group A					
Mother					
Endometritis or wound infection	WSP (DI)	II	After 48 hours of appropriate therapy[c]	After 48 hours of appropriate therapy[c]	

[a] WSP = Wound and skin precautions (gown and glove); SI = strict isolation (gown, glove, and mask); EnP = enteric precautions (gown and glove); BP = blood precautions (glove); RI = respiratory isolation (mask). Specific operational details can be found in *Isolation Techniques for Use in Hospitals*. DI = Duration of illness (for draining lesions, until drainage stops). DH = Duration of hospitalization. DIP = Duration of expected incubation period (after perinatal exposure to infected mother). C = Duration given under "Comments." U = Until 24 hours of appropriate therapy. I = Type I nursery isolation (isolation room and gown: glove and contact precautions); II = type II nursery isolation (newborn nursery of ICN placement OK with gown and glove and contact precautions).

[b] Drainage or infected lesions should be contained by clean, dry dressings or perineal pads. Personnel should wear gloves or use "no touch" technique when handling soiled dressings or pads.

[c] Fresh cover gown (and careful handwashing) for mother before contact with neonate.

Continued

TABLE 27–1. Continued

Infection	Maternal Isolation (Duration)[a]	Newborn Isolation (Duration)[a]	Mother–Infant Contact	Breast-Feeding	Comments
Pharyngitis	RI	None	After 24 hours of appropriate therapy[c]	After 24 hours of appropriate therapy[c]	
Newborn infant Omphalitis	None	II	In nursery	After 48 hours of appropriate therapy	
Wound infections Mother	WSP (DI)	None	After temperature less than 38.5°C for 24 hours[c]	After temperature less than 38.5°C for 24 hours[c]	See Streptoccal disease, group A, Staphylococcal disease, or Gonococcal infection if these pathogens suspected or cultured. Minimal infections, such as stitch abscesses, do not require isolation
Newborn infant	None	II	In nursery with WSP	In nursery with WSP	See Streptococcal disease, group A, Staphylococcal disease, or Gonococcal infection if these pathogens suspected or cultured. Serous drainage of umbilical stump, circumcision site, or scalp monitor site should be cultured but does not require isolation unless there is apparent clinical infection.
Streptococcal disease, group B Mother Colonization	None	None	Permitted	Permitted	
Endometritis. See Endometritis Newborn infant Colonization	None	None	Permitted	Permitted	
Sepsis or meningitis	None	None	Permitted	Permitted	If cases cluster, cohort infected and colonized infants. Contact Infection Control and Chairman of Pediatric Committee.

[a]WSP = Wound and skin precautions (gown and glove); SI = strict isolation (gown, glove, and mask); EnP = enteric precautions (gown and glove); BP = blood precautions (glove); RI = respiratory isolation (mask). Specific operational details can be found in *Isolation Techniques for Use in Hospitals*. DI = Duration of illness (for draining lesions, until drainage stops). DH = Duration of hospitalization. DIP = Duration of expected incubation period (after perinatal exposure to infected mother). C = Duration given under "Comments." U = Until 24 hours of appropriate therapy. I = Type I nursery isolation (isolation room and gown: glove and contact precautions); II = type II nursery isolation (newborn nursery of ICN placement OK with gown and glove and contact precautions).

[c]Fresh cover gown (and careful handwashing) for mother before contact with neonate.

TABLE 27–1. Continued

Infection	Maternal Isolation (Duration)[a]	Newborn Isolation (Duration)[a]	Mother–Infant Contact	Breast-Feeding	Comments
Syphilis					
Mother					
Mucocutaneous	WSP, BP (U)	BP (U)	After 24 hours of appropriate therapy	After 24 hours of appropriate therapy	
Newborn infant					
Mucocutaneous	BP (U)	II, BP (U)	After 24 hours of appropriate therapy	After 24 hours of appropriate therapy	
Seropositive, no lesions	BP (U)	BP (U)	Permitted	Permitted	
Toxic shock syndrome. See Staphylococcal disease					
Toxoplasmosis					
Mother	None	None	Permitted	Permitted	
Newborn infant	None	None	Permitted	Permitted	
Tuberculosis					
Mother					
Positive skin test, asymptomatic	None	None	Permitted	Permitted	Obtain chest x-ray film for mother if positive skin test represents recent conversion (less than 2 years) or is of unknown duration.
Pulmonary, on effective treatment more than 2 weeks	None	None	Permitted	Permitted	
Pulmonary, inadequate treatment (or noncompliance)	RI (C)	None	After mother on appropriate treatment for at least 2 weeks	After mother on appropriate treatment for at least 2 weeks	Consider isoniazid or bacille Calmette Guérin (BCG) prophylaxis for infant. Continue isolation until mother on effective treatment for at least 2 weeks.
Urinary tract infection					
Mother	None	None	Permitted	Permitted	

Varicella. See Chickenpox

SOURCE: Weinstein, Boyer, and Linn (1983).

[a] WSP = Wound and skin precautions (gown and glove); SI = strict isolation (gown, glove, and mask); EnP = enteric precautions (gown and glove); BP = blood precautions (glove); RI = respiratory isolation (mask). Specific operational details can be found in *Isolation Techniques for Use in Hospitals.* DI = Duration of illness (for draining lesions, until drainage stops). DH = Duration of hospitalization. DIP = Duration of expected incubation period (after perinatal exposure to infected mother). C = Duration given under "Comments." U = Until 24 hours of appropriate therapy. I = Type I nursery isolation (isolation room and gown: glove and contact precautions); II = type II nursery isolation (newborn nursery of ICN placement OK with gown and glove and contact precautions).

CONCEPTS FOR CARE FOR THE NEWBORN

Admission/Transitional/Observation Nursery

Some of the protections offered new babies are provided by special nursery areas designed for temporary placement and monitoring of newborns immediately after delivery. Depending on the hospital, these particular nurseries are often called the *admit* or *admission nursery*, the *transitional nursery*, or the *observation nursery*. These nurseries allow for the close monitoring of infants during the crucial first hours when they are making the transition into extrauterine life (see Chapter 25). Infants are initially admitted into this type of nursery for a period of 4–24 hours, until the presence or absence of problems is determined. It is in this nursery that immediate care is delivered to the newborn (see Chapter 19). Some hospitals utilize the transitional nursery to observe infants who are suspected of having an infectious condition or to admit infants born outside the hospital environment.

The routine care provided in this nursery includes frequent (every 15 min to 1 hour) monitoring of infant activity, color, and vital signs (most important, temperature), a physical and gestational age assessment, eye prophylaxis, and vitamin K administration. The first feeding and first bath are usually also done during the time the infant is in this nursery. This allows for close evaluation of the infant's response to any treatments and provides the nurse with the opportunity to assess the infant's suck, swallow, and gag reflexes.

Immediately after delivery, the infant is placed nude in a radiant warmer that provides overhead heat and allows for close observation. If these warming tables are not available, infants may instead be placed in bassinets with some type of controlled overhead heat source (see Fig. 27–3).

It usually is not until about 3–6 hours after birth that the infant's temperature is stable enough for the first bath to occur. The bath, to cleanse the infant of maternal blood, stool, and so on, is often given under the available additional heat source. After the bath, the infant should be dressed and the temperature should be monitored for the duration of the infant's stay in that particular nursery.

Once the infant is bathed and dressed, the first feeding is usually initiated. If the infant is to breastfeed, he or she may have already done so in the delivery room, in which case the baby usually is taken to the mother for more breastfeeding on a demand basis (see Chapter 21). If the infant is to bottle-feed, it is recommended that sips of sterile water be given first in case the infant should have difficulty swallowing and aspirate.

After careful monitoring during the transitional period, the infant should be transferred to the regular newborn nursery. When a hospital has limited space, both transitional and well-baby routine care may be delivered in the same nursery area. This is certainly acceptable, provided it is clearly understood that more frequent, careful monitoring will occur in the initial hours after birth.

If there is any question of infection and the infant is admitted into an observation nursery, the infant may be kept until the presence or absence of infection is determined. Once a definite diagnosis of infection is made, the infant should be placed in an *isolation nursery*, a separate room or designated area that separates the infected infant from the others (Reeder, Mastroianni, and Martin, 1983) if this is deemed necessary per the infection control guidelines in Table 27–1.

Central Nursery

The concept of the central nursery was first developed in the early and mid-1900's in response to the rampant epidemics that were seen among hospitalized infants. This type of nursery was designed for the care of a variable number of healthy newborns (Reeder, Mastroianni, and Martin, 1983; see Fig. 27–4). The care in this area is usually provided by a few people, and there is usually no need for bulky equipment. There must be at least 2–3 feet in all directions between bassinets, and one nursing staff member is required for each 6–8 infants, limiting the number of infants for each individual room to 6–8, 12–16, or 18–24 (American Academy of Pediatrics and American College of Obstetricians and Gynecologists, 1983). The infant care in this area may be delivered in one room or in more rooms, depending on the size of the hospital and on its specific needs.

With the central nursery concept, an infant may remain in the nursery entirely and only be brought out to the mother's room at feeding times, or the infant may be with the mother in a modified rooming-in situation and may be returned to the

(a) *(b)*

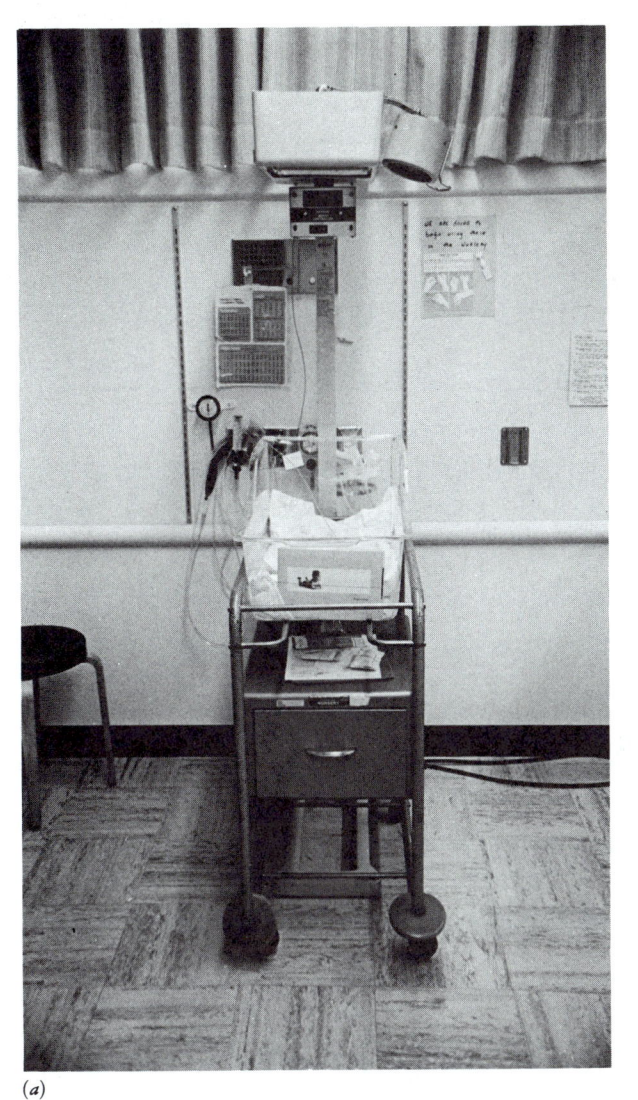

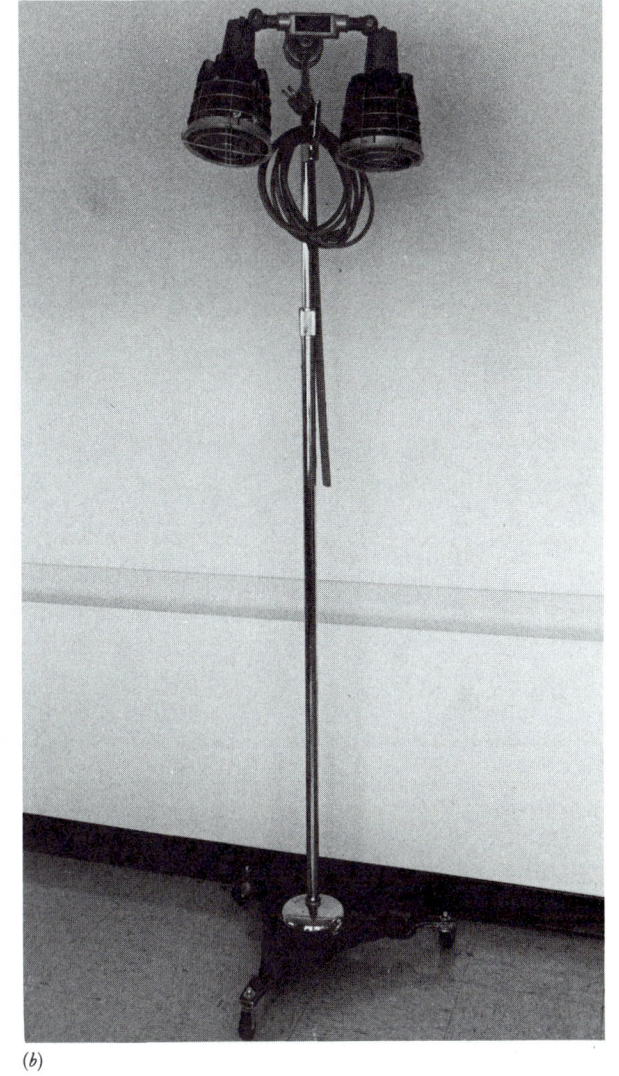

FIGURE 27–3. *(a)* Overhead heat element that fits over a bassinet. *(b)* Emerson light.

central nursery only at night or at the mother's request.

Each infant's individual bassinet should have space for storage of routinely used supplies such as blankets, shirts, diapers, formula, soap, tape measure, comb or brush, towelettes, wipes, thermometer with lubricant, etc. There should be no exchange of supplies between infants' bassinets by mothers or nursing personnel (McKay and Phillips, 1984).

Rooming-In

Rooming-in began in the late 1940s. Its purpose was to offset rigid infant-care patterns that had been established earlier through the use of the central nursery (Hilliard, 1968). *Rooming-in* is the plan of having the new infant share the mother's hospital room so that mother and infant may be cared for together (Reeder, Mastroianni, and Martin, 1983; see Fig. 27–5). Special features of rooming-in are (American Academy of Pediatrics, 1971):

1. It provides the mother and infant with a natural mother–infant experience while under the care of maternity personnel.
2. It fosters infant feeding on a permissive plan.
3. It facilitates instruction of mothers and fathers in infant care.
4. It reduces the incidence of cross-infection among infants.

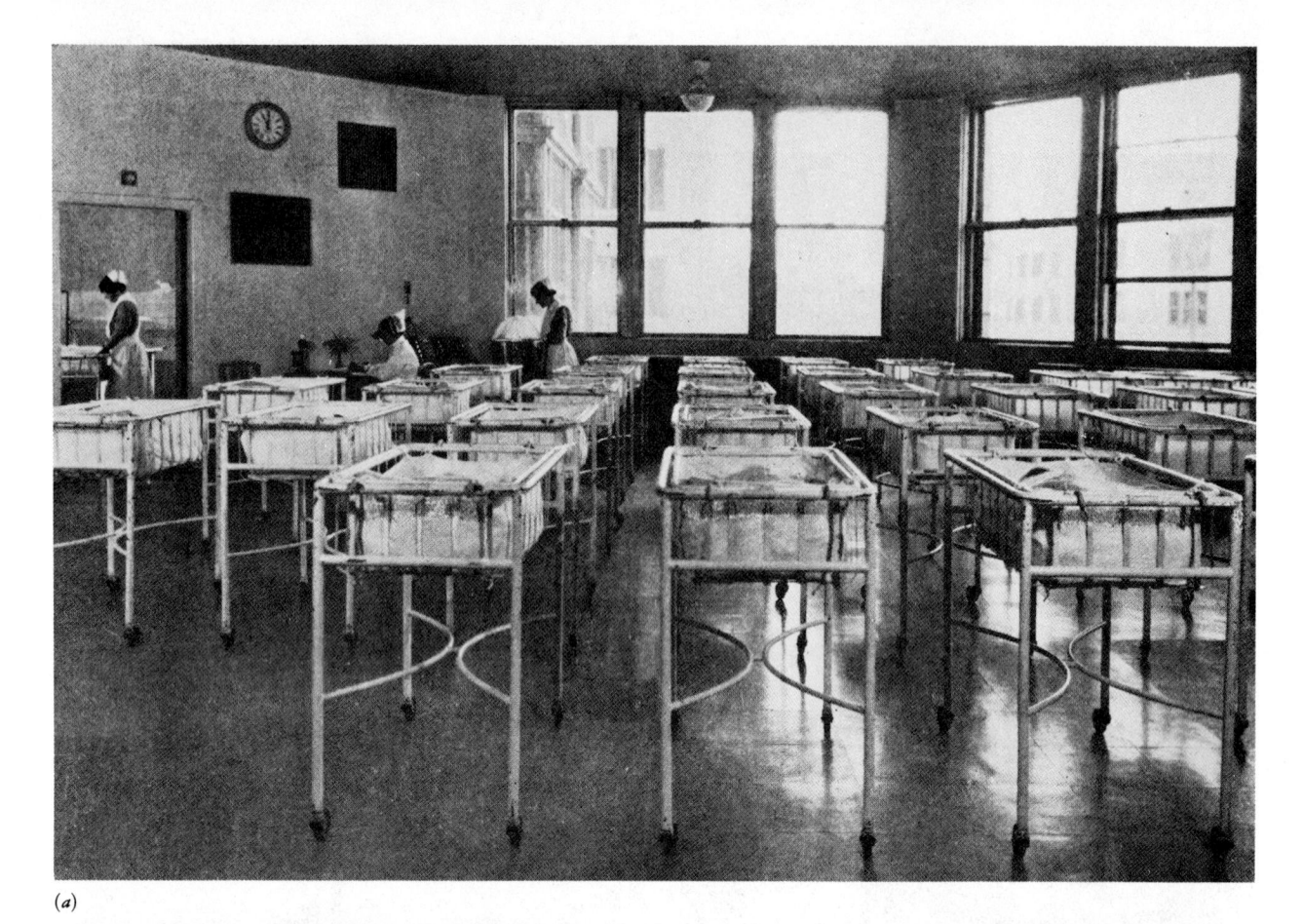

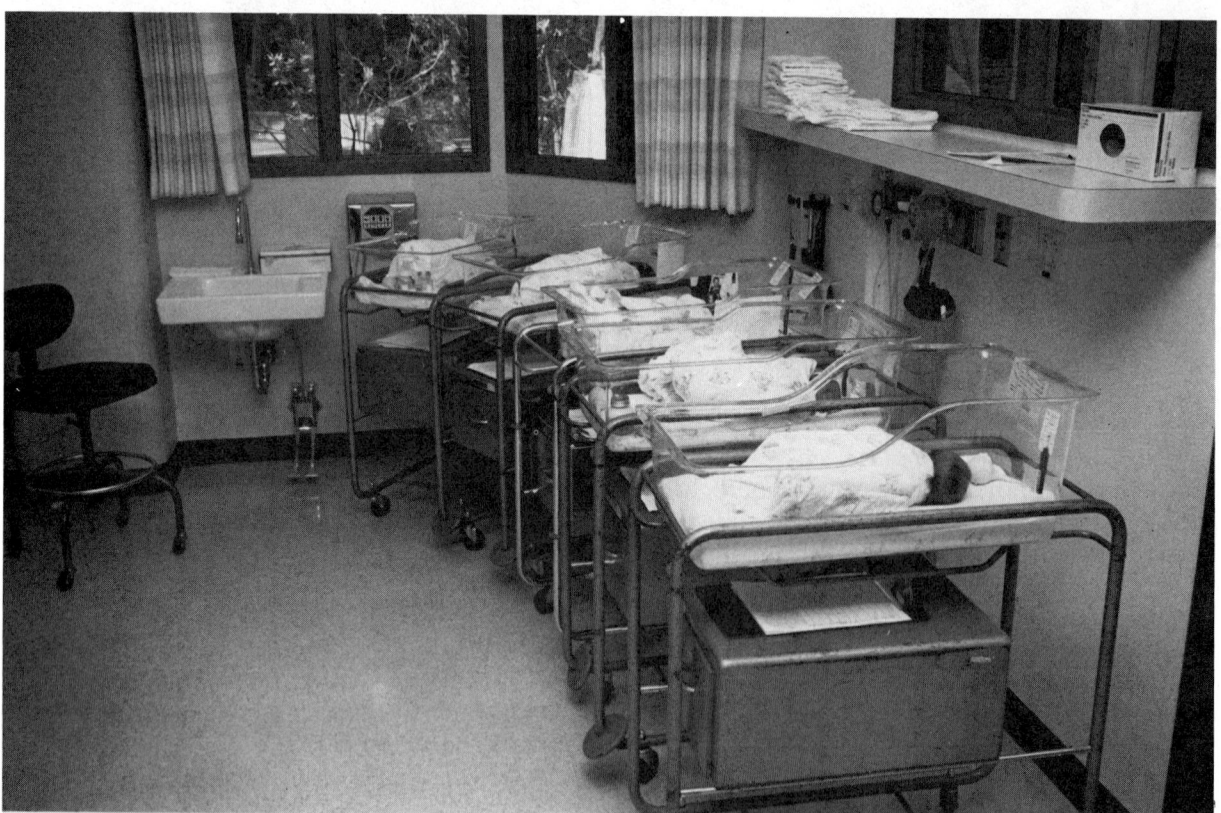

FIGURE 27–4. (a) Central nursery, 1940s. (b) Central nursery, 1980s. Note fewer babies, because babies are rooming-in with their mothers.
SOURCE: (a) Maternity Hospital, Western Reserve University Hospitals, Cleveland, Ohio.

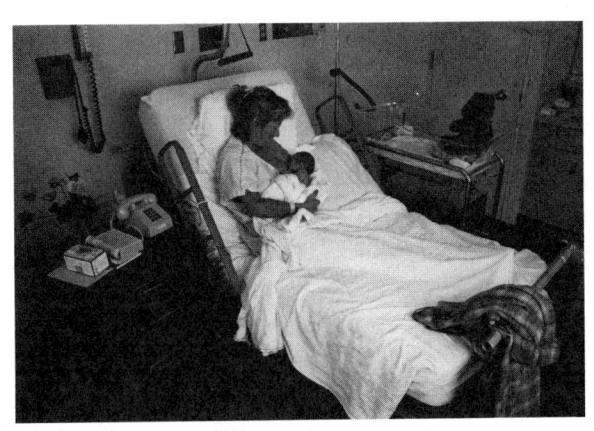

FIGURE 27-5. Mother with bassinet at her bedside in a rooming-in situation.

Rooming-in can occur under different types of plans. It may be continuous, 24 hours a day, with the infant constantly at the mother's beside, or it can be modified and intermittent, with the infant returning to the central nursery during specified times during the day and evening and at night to allow the mother uninterrupted sleep. It has been suggested that the infant should remain with the mother for a minimum of 5 hours a day so that the mother can learn about the infant's needs and activities (Klaus and Kennell, 1982). If rooming-in is continuous, some hospitals limit the visitors to the father, and possibly, the grandparents and siblings. All visitors should be instructed in proper handwashing technique (American Academy of Pediatrics, 1971).

To ensure safety of the infant in a rooming-in situation, it is important that certain criteria be met before rooming-in is authorized. Klaus and Kennell (1982) recommend the following criteria:

1. Apgar score at 5 min greater than 7.
2. Weight over 5 lb but under 9.5 lb.
3. Heart rate between 110 and 170 beats/min.
4. Respiratory rate 37-70 breaths/min.
5. Color normal.
6. Infant able to breathe without difficulty.

Complete rooming-in with minimal separation of mother and baby during the waking hours promises the best results for future parenting (Mahan, 1981). In a randomized study with a carefully matched control group, it was concluded that rooming-in mothers felt more confident and competent in baby care than other mothers and thought they would need less help in caring for their infants at home (Greenberg, Rosenberg and Lind, 1973).

In mother-baby care, sometimes called dyad or couplet care, the postpartum mother and her infant are cared for together by the same nurse. Such an arrangement can improve continuity of care, communication and teaching while avoiding overlap of responsibilities and duplication of services. One nurse usually cares for three to four "pairs." Dyad care may be provided on a 24-hour or 16-hour basis depending on the needs of the mother at a particular hospital. In the 16-hour model, the newborn nursery functions as it does under the rooming-in plan. Nursery care on a 24-hour basis will still be needed for infants being adopted and those receiving phototherapy.

If the infant meets the above criteria and the decision is to room-in, all further examinations and assessments are done in the mother's room by the nurses and pediatricians. Klaus and Kennell (1982) further recommend that the following criteria for infants be utilized to allow for early discharge of rooming-in patients if they do desire:

1. Infant at least 6 hours old.
2. Birth weight over 5 lb but under 9.5 lb.
3. Vital signs normal.
4. Physical examiniation by pediatrician normal.
5. Hematocrit between 45 and 65%.
6. Dextrostix over 45 mg/dl.
7. If mother Rh negative, cord blood shows no signs of incompatibility.
8. No complications requiring additional observation.
9. At least one feeding observed by the nurse.
10. Mother able to demonstrate she can handle and care for the infant.
11. Birth certificate complete.

Five factors contributing to the trend toward early postpartum discharge are:

1. Demonstrated patient safety measured by low complication and rehospitalization rates.
2. Patient satisfaction and family well-being.
3. Changes in attitudes toward birth and newborn care. Attitudes have shifted from an illness to a wellness orientation.
4. Controlling costs and providing low-cost care.
5. Availability of community home health care agencies (Patterson, 1987).

Family-centered maternity/newborn care can be defined as the delivery of safe, quality health care while recognizing, focusing on, and adapting to both the physical and psychosocial needs of the client–patient, the family, and the newly born. The emphasis is on the provision of maternity/newborn health care which fosters family unity while maintaining physical safety (McKay and Phillips, 1984).

Regardless of where the infant is cared for, family-centered care, based on the concept of keeping the family together as a unit as much as possible, should be encouraged (Hennel, 1968). Planned family-centered care suggests a multidimensional concept of nursing care that embraces the family in its entirety during all phases of the experience of birth and postpartal hospitalization. It suggests that the nursing care provided to a family be goal-directed toward the family's well-being. The various components of family-centered care are reflected in the philosophies of the obstetric and neonatal (pediatric) departments and nursing service. This type of philosophy emphasizes the worth of the individual infant as a member of a family, and it means that significant family members are included in establishing objectives to meet the health care needs of the infant (Luciano, 1972) (Fig. 27–6).

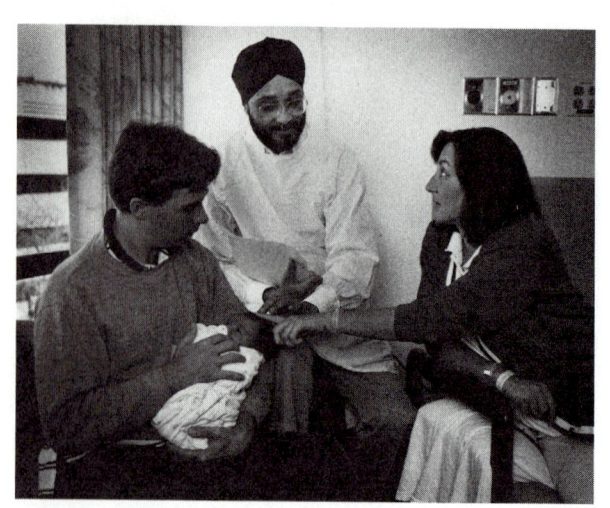

FIGURE 27–6. Pediatrician involving parents in identifying health care needs of infant.

General Infant Care Routines

Infant care has changed in recent years. For comparison, it is of particular interest to note the recommended daily routine of a newborn in 1943 (Zabriskie and Eastman, 1943):

6:00 a.m.	First feeding.
9:00 a.m.	Cod-liver oil in orange juice (when awake). Bath usually precedes next feeding.
10:00 a.m.	Second feeding, followed by nap.
2:00 p.m.	Third feeding, followed by nap. Exercise and play with infant after nap.
6:00 p.m.	Fourth feeding, then to bed.
10:00 p.m.	Fifth feeding.
2:00 a.m.	Sixth feeding (if the baby is awake).

It seems that in 1943 infants were primarily fed and occasionally held and stimulated. Today's daily infant-care routines involve the need for more nursing skills and assessment.

Observation of Skin Color, Appearance, and Activity

These characteristics should be noted on an ongoing basis, every time the infant is fed or when vital signs are taken. Skin color is particularly important in assessing for pallor, cyanosis, and jaundice. Jaundice is a common occurrence in neonates. The serum bilirubin level must exceed 4–6 mg/100 ml before it is visible as pigment in the skin. In full-term infants, a peak bilirubin level is reached on the third or fourth day after birth. This is known as *physiologic jaundice*. If jaundice is present in the first 24 hours of life, it is *pathologic jaundice*, and further evaluation and intervention are required. A serum bilirubin level of more than 12–14 mg/100 ml may require the use of phototherapy to help break down bilirubin in the skin and tissue (Korones, 1976; see Fig. 27–7). Phototherapy is applied by exposing the nude infant's skin to light. The average fall in pigment concentration is 3–4 mg/100 ml after 8–12 hours of therapy (Korones, 1976). Most jaundiced term infants, otherwise healthy, will remain under phototherapy for 2–3 days. The infant's eyes should be shielded during the treatment (see Chapter 32). The infant needs to be carefully observed for hyperthermia, loose stools, and increased loss of water through the skin. Daily fluid intake should be increased while the infant is under phototherapy (Korones, 1976). Other outward signs indicating possible illness, such as dyspnea, cyanosis, vomiting, hemorrhage, pallor, and twitching, must be reported and investigated promptly.

Care of the Skin

The condition of the skin should be carefully noted every time the infant is dressed or changed. A

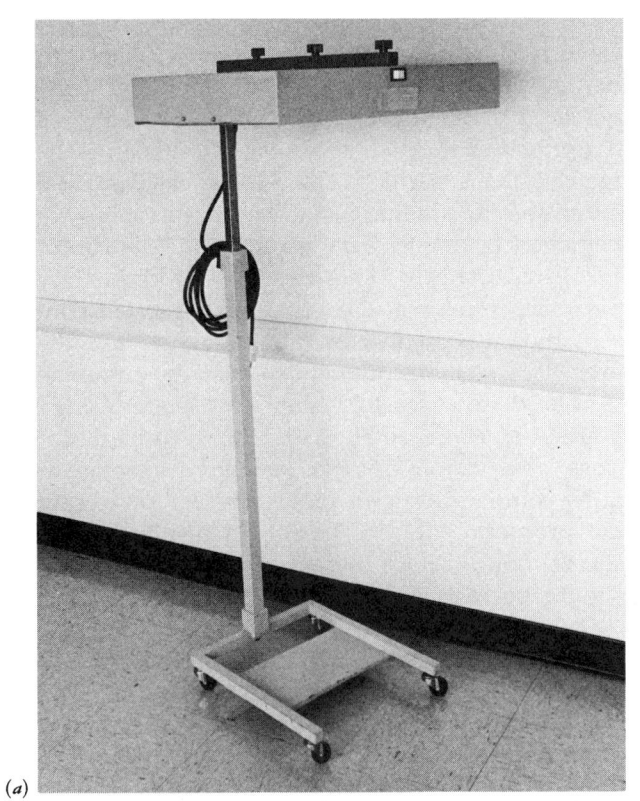

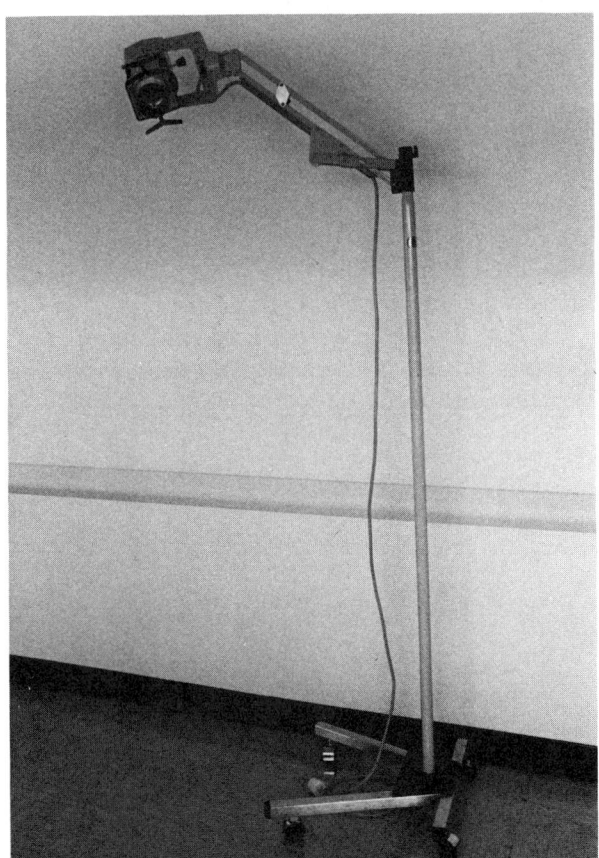

FIGURE 27-7. Photo therapy lamps.
(a) Olympic fluorescent light.
(b) Cavitron light.

sponge bath is usually given every other day or as needed, should the infant spit up or stool excessively. Chapter 24 describes the bathing procedure in detail. There should be as little rubbing as possible to prevent irritation of the skin, and care should be taken to prevent chilling the infant during the bath.

Temperature

An infant's temperature should be monitored every 4–8 hours. Consideration should be given to the taking of the axillary temperature of normal newborn infants. The thermometer should be held in place high in the axilla by pressing the infant's arm gently but tightly against it and the side of the body for 3 min (Torrance, 1968).

Weighing

All infants should be weighed daily, at the same time each day. Care should be taken to ensure accuracy of the scale and to avoid chilling the infant during weighing, since the infant should be weighed nude.

Transportation

The infant should be transported in its own bassinet, for both safety and hygiene reasons. Each time the infant is transported to the mother's room, the mother's arm band should be checked against the infant's for proper identification. If the mother comes to the nursery door for her infant, her identification should also be checked prior to allowing her to take the infant back to her room. Many hospitals will not allow the mother to carry the infant back to her room but do allow her to wheel the bassinet.

Feeding

The routine for feeding and how frequently it is done depend on whether the infant is being breastfed or bottle-fed. Most nurseries maintain a 4-hour feeding schedule for bottle-fed infants unless otherwise ordered. This means that in a central nursery situation the infant is brought out to the mother every 4 hours. To make it easy for the nursing staff to take numerous babies out to their mothers, all infants are usually on a single feeding schedule adopted for that particular nursery. If the infant is breastfed, feeding is done on a demand schedule, and if the infant is not already rooming-in with the mother, the nurse wheels the infant in the bassinet to the mother every time the infant appears to be hungry. Whether the infant's feeding is followed by supplemental formula or water depends on the physician's order. However, it has been documented that healthy, exclusively breastfed infants do not need supplementation. Water or other fluids are all that are necessary to maintain adequate hydration, even in a hot climate (Brown et al., 1986).

Nurse's Record

The nurse's notes should include observations about the infant's weight, temperature, respiratory rate, pulse, dyspnea, cyanosis, jaundice (including "present" or "absent" in each note), pallor, plethora, edema, lethargy, twitching, condition of skin, condition of umbilical cord, feeding (type, volume offered, amount taken, how taken, volume retained), vomiting, stools (time of passage and character of each), urine (number of times and character of stream), abdominal distention, bowel sounds, condition of sutures and fontanells, condition of circumcision (if applicable), treatments and medication, and other noteworthy manifestations (cry absent or excessive, type of salivation, "not behaving normally," "doing poorly," "stable, doing well").

Other important documentation related to assessment of parent–infant attachment should also be included. Some nurseries have separate sheets for this type of charting. The nurse's recorded observations should begin upon the infant's arrival at the nursery and continue as frequently as is warranted, but at least once each shift. The observations should be identified by date and time of day. Each note should be signed by the nurse caring for that particular infant and each signature should also have a title after it (for example, M. Smith, R.N.) for identification purposes.

Aside from the physical care of the infant, the education of the parents regarding infant care is of paramount importance and is definitely part of the daily routine (see Chapter 24). The nurse is responsible for providing this parent teaching. The parents should be involved in as much care of the infant as possible, to help them prepare for taking over full responsibility of the infant when they get home (Reeder, Mastroianni, and Martin, 1983). Documentation of what was taught, what the parents understand, and what needs to be reinforced should be done at least once during every shift.

Circumcision

Circumcision is an elective procedure that is carried out to remove by surgery that section of the penile skin called the foreskin. The procedure is performed by the pediatrician or obstetrician at the request of the parents. There is no valid medical indication for circumcision (American Academy of Pediatrics, Committee on the Fetus and Newborn, 1975), but many parents elect this procedure for personal or religious reasons. An informed consent should be signed by one parent prior to the procedure. It is recommended that the circumcision be done at least 12 hours (but preferably 24 hours) before the infant's discharge, to allow for close observation of any bleeding problems or other complications. To prevent aspiration during the procedure, the infant should not be fed for several hours before the circumcision. The infant should be restrained in a supine position on a circumcision board (see Fig. 27–8); Reeder, Mastroianni, and Martin, 1983). The infant should not be left unattended at any time.

Hospitals have different policies and procedures regarding preparing the penis prior to the procedure. The physician uses sterile gloves, instruments, and drapes during the procedure. The Gomco clamp and Plastibell are two methods of circumcision (Reeder, Mastroianni, and Martin, 1983). The nurse should observe the circumcision carefully at each diaper change, and care should be taken to prevent the penis from sticking to the diaper. Some nurseries advocate the use of sterile Vaseline gauze or a petroleum jelly dressing for this purpose. The nurse should closely monitor the infant's voiding after the procedure.

Care of the uncircumcised penis is quite easy. External washing and rinsing on a daily basis is all that is required. No attempt should be made to

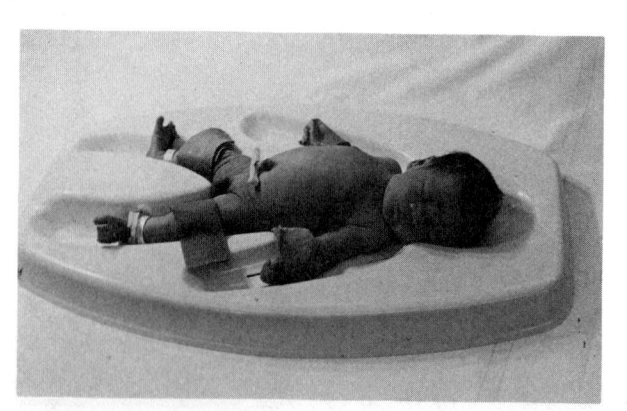

FIGURE 27–8. Infant on circumcision board.

retract the foreskin forceably. This may harm the penis, causing pain, bleeding, and possibly adhesions. Separation of the foreskin from the glans may take years (see Chapter 26; American Academy of Pediatrics, 1986).

SUMMARY

The physical care given to the newborn is directed toward protecting and nurturing the infant. These actions are interrelated in promoting infant well-being (Clark, Affonso, and Harris, 1979). Through established daily routines of care, the newborn can be carefully monitored for early signs and symptoms of potential problems. The nurse plays a key role in maintaining these routines. The multidisciplinary care provided should be carried out through a many-faceted approach that is directed toward family-centered care. This concept of care allows for the family's involvement in the care of their infant in preparation for establishing routines once the infant is at home.

REFERENCES

American Academy of Pediatrics. 1971. *Standards and recommendations for hospital care of newborn infants*. 5th ed. Evanston, Ill.: American Academy of Pediatrics.

American Academy of Pediatrics. 1986. *Newborns: Care of the uncircumcised penis*. Elb Grove, Ill.: American Academy of Pediatrics.

American Academy of Pediatrics, Committee on the Fetus and Newborn. 1975. Report of the ad hoc task force on circumcision. Evanston, Ill. *Pediatrics*. 56:610–611.

American Academy of Pediatrics and American College of Obstetricians and Gynecologists. 1983. *Guidelines for perinatal care*. Evanston, Ill. March of Dimes Publication.

Avery, G. B. 1981. *Neonatology: Pathophysiology and management of the newborn*. 2nd ed. Philadelphia: J. B. Lippincott.

Battaglia, F. C., and Lubchenco, L. O. 1967. A practical classification of newborn infants by weight and gestational age. *J. Pediatrics*. 71(2):159–163.

Behrman, R. E., and Vaughan, V. C., eds. 1983. *Nelson textbook of pediatrics*. 12th ed. Philadelphia: W. B. Saunders.

Bernardo, M. L. 1979. Craniosynostosis: The child's care from detection through correction. *MCN*. 4(4): 234–237.

Black, M. 1978. Assessment of weight and gestational age. *Nurs. Clin. N. Amer.* 13:13–22.

Brazelton, T. B. 1973. *Neonatal behavioral assessment scale*. Philadelphia: J. B. Lippincott.

Brazelton, T. B. 1981. Behavioral competence of the newborn infant. *Neonatology: Pathophysiology and management of the newborn*, 2nd ed., ed. G. B. Avery. Philadelphia: J. B. Lippincott.

Brown, K. H.; de Kanashio, H. C.; del Aguila, R., et al. 1986. Milk consumption and hydration status of exclusively breast-fed infants in a warm climate. *J. Pediatrics*. 108:677–680.

Candy, M. M. 1979. Birth of a comprehensive family-centered maternity program. *J. Obstet. Gynecol. Neonatal Nurs.* 8(2):80–84.

Clark, A. L.; Affonso, D. D.; and Harris, T. R. 1979. *Childbearing: A nursing perspective*. 2nd ed. Philadelphia: F. A. Davis.

Dubowitz, L., and Dubowitz, V. 1977. *Gestational age of the newborn*. Menlo Park, Calif.: Addison-Wesley.

Dubowitz, L., and Dubowitz, V. 1981. *The neurological assessment of the preterm and full-term newborn infant*. Philadelphia: J. B. Lippincott.

Dubowitz, L.; Dubowitz, V.; and Goldberg, C. 1970. Clinical assessment of gestational age in the newborn infant. *J. Pediatrics*. 77(1):1–10.

Einhorn, A. H., ed. 1982. The newborn infant. In *Pediatrics*, 17th ed., eds. A. M. Rudolph and J. E. Hoffman. Norfolk, Conn.: Appleton-Century-Crofts.

Erickson, M. P. 1978. Trends in assessing the newborn and his parents. *MCN*. 3(2):99–103.

Eyres, P. J. 1972. The role of the nurse in family-centered nursing care. *Nurs. Care N. Amer.* 7(1):27–39.

Fanaroff, A., and Martin, R. J. 1983. *Behrman's neonatal–perinatal medicine: Diseases of the fetus and infant*. 3rd ed. St. Louis: C. V. Mosby.

Farwell, J. 1983. Maturational and neurobehavioral assessment of the newborn. In *Principles and practice of perinatal medicine: Maternal–fetal and newborn care*, eds. J. B. Warshaw and J. C. Hobbins. Menlo Park, Calif.: Addison-Wesley.

Fitzpatrick, E.; Reeder, S. R.; and Mastroianni, L. 1971. *Maternity nursing*. 12th ed. Philadelphia: J. B. Lippincott.

Gagliardi, J. V. 1983. Initial assessment of the newborn. In *Principles and practice of perinatal medicine: Maternal–fetal and newborn care*, eds. J. B. Warshaw and J. C. Hobbins. Menlo Park, Calif.: Addison-Wesley.

Greenberg, M.; Rosenberg, J.; and Lind, M. 1973. First mothers rooming-in with their newborns: Its impact upon the mother. *Am. J. Orthopsychiatry*. 43(5): 783–788.

Haire, D., and Haire, J. 1971. *Implementing family centered care with a central nursery*. Bellevue, Wa.: International Childbirth Education Association.

Hennel, M. 1968. Family-centered maternity nursing in practice. *Nurs. Clin. N. Amer.* 3(2):289–298.

Herrmann, J., and Light, I. J. 1971. Infection control in

the newborn nursery. *Nurs. Clin. N. Amer.* 6(1):55–65.

Hilliard, M. E. 1968. The changing role of the maternity nurse. *Nurs. Clin. N. Amer.* 3(2):277–288.

Jensen, M. D.; Benson, R. C.; and Bobak, I. M. 1977. *Maternity care: The nurse and the family.* St. Louis: C. V. Mosby.

Klaus, M. H., and Kennell, J. H. 1982. *Parent–infant bonding.* 2nd ed. St. Louis: C. V. Mosby.

Koops, B. L., and Battaglia, F. C. 1982. The newborn infant. In *Current pediatric diagnosis and treatment,* 7th ed., eds. C. H. Kempe, H. K. Silver, and D. O'Brien. Los Altos, Calif.: Lange Medical Publication.

Korones, S. B. 1976. *High-risk newborn infants.* St. Louis: C. V. Mosby.

Korones, S. B., and Lancaster, J. 1981. *High-risk newborn infants: The basis for intensive nursing care.* 3rd ed. St. Louis: C. V. Mosby.

Lubchenco, L. O. 1981. Assessment of weight and gestational age. In *Neonatology: Pathophysiology and management of the newborn,* 2nd ed., ed. G. B. Avery. Philadelphia: J. B. Lippincott.

Lubchenco, L. O.; Hansman, C.; Dressler, M.; and Boyd, E. 1963. Intrauterine growth as estimated from liveborn birth-weight data at 24 to 42 weeks of gestation. *Pediatrics.* 32:793–800.

Lubchenco, L. O.; Hansman, C.; and Boyd, E. 1966. Intrauterine growth in length and head circumference as estimated from live births at gestational ages from 26 to 42 weeks. *Pediatrics.* 37:403–408.

Luciano, K. B. 1972. Components of planned family-centered care. *Nurs. Clin. N. Amer.* 7(1):41–52.

Mahan, C. 1981. Ways to strengthen the mother–infant bond. *Contemp. Ob./Gyn.* 17:177–187.

McKay, S., and Phillips, C. 1984. *Family-centered maternity care: Implementation strategies.* Rockville: Aspen Publications.

Nugent, J. K. 1981. The Brazelton neonatal behavioral assessment scale: Implications for intervention. *Pediatric Nurs.* 7(3):18–21.

Parker, S., and Brazelton, T. B. 1981. Newborn behavioral assessment: Research, prediction, and clinical use. *Children Today.* 2–4.

Patterson, P. K. 1987. A comparison of postpartum early and traditional discharge groups. *QRB.* 365–371.

Paukert, S. E. 1979. One hospital's experience with implementing family-centered maternity care. *J. Obstet. Gynecol. Neonatal Nurs.* 8(6):351–358.

Phibbs, R. H., ed. 1982. The newborn infant. In *Pediatrics,* 17th ed., eds. A. M. Rudolph and J. E. Hoffman. Norfolk, Conn.: Appleton-Century-Crofts.

Potsie, W. P., and Handler, S. D., eds. 1982. Pediatric otorhinolaryngology. In *Pediatrics.* 17th ed., eds. A. M. Rudolph and J. E. Hoffman. Norfolk, Conn.: Appleton-Century-Crofts.

Powell, M. L. 1981. *Assessment and management of developmental changes and problems in children.* 2nd ed. St. Louis: C. V. Mosby.

Reed, B.; Sutorius, J.; and Coen, R. 1971. Management of the infant during labor, delivery, and in the immediate neonatal period. *Nurs. Clin. N. Amer.* 6(1):3–14.

Reeder, S. J.; Mastroianni, L.; and Martin, L. L. 1983. *Maternity nursing.* 15th ed. Philadelphia: J. B. Lippincott.

Renaud, M. 1983. Effects of discontinuing cover gowns on a postpartal ward upon cord colonization of the newborn. *J. Obstet. Gynecol. Neonatal Nurs.* Nov./Dec.:399–401.

Rich, O. J. 1969. Hospital routines as rites of passage in developing maternal identity. *Nurs. Clin. N. Amer.* 4(1):101–109.

Rudolph, A. M., and Hoffman, J. E., eds. 1982. *Pediatrics.* 17th ed. Norfolk, Conn.: Appleton-Century-Crofts.

Scharping, E. M. 1983. Physiological measurements of the neonate. *MCN.* 8(1):70–73.

Sullivan, R.; Foster, J.; and Schreiner, R. L. 1979. Determining the newborn's gestational age. *MCN.* 4(1):38–45.

Sweet, A. Y. 1979. Classification of the low-birth-weight infant. In *Care of the high-risk neonate,* 2nd ed., eds. M. H. Klaus and A. A. Fanaroff. Philadelphia: W. B. Saunders.

Tachdjian, M. O., ed. 1982. Orthopedic problems in childhood. In *Pediatrics,* 17th ed., eds. A. M. Rudolph and J. E. Hoffman. Norfolk, Conn.: Appleton-Century-Crofts.

Torrance, J. T. 1968. Temperature readings of premature infants. *Nurs. Research.* 17:312.

Van Leeuwen, G. 1973. The nurse in prevention and intervention in the neonatal period. *Nurs. Clin. N. Amer.* 8(3):509–520.

Vezeau, T., and Hallsten, D. 1987. Making the transition to mother–baby care. *MCN.* 12:193–198.

Volpe, J. J. 1981. *Neurology of the newborn.* Philadelphia: W. B. Saunders.

Weinstein, R. A.; Boyer, K. M.; and Linn, E. S. 1983. Isolation guidelines for obstetric patients and newborn infants. *Am. J. Obstet. Gynecol.* 146(4):353–360.

Wheeler, W. 1972. Recollections of 40 years of hospitalization of children. *Pediatric Research.* 6:840–842.

Wolff, P. H. 1959. Observations on newborn infants. *Psychosomatic Med.* 21:110.

28

Infant Nutrition

BEHAVIORAL OBJECTIVES

Upon completion of this chapter, the reader should be able to:

- Discuss the growth and developmental needs of infants during the first year of life.

- Discuss the importance of anthropometric measures, clinical observations, laboratory data, and dietary analysis in assessing an infant's nutritional status.

- List caloric requirements necessary for an infant to achieve maximal weight gain.

- Define the principle nutrient standards available in infant formulas.

- Differentiate nutritional components of special formulas and human milk for the preterm and full-term infant.

- Identify feeding difficulties encountered with very small infants requiring alternate methods of feeding.

- Compare the protein, fat, and carbohydrate contents of the three major types of standard commercial formulas.

- Identify the two most common metabolic disorders that require special formulas during the infant's first year of life.

At the beginning of the human life cycle, each infant bears the imprint of the physical resources provided by the mother and the heritage of generations before her. It is upon these resources and this unique heritage that the child's individual life experiences will develop. In exquisite form and function, the newborn infant displays the tremendous growth that has already taken place during fetal life.

The guiding and development of growth in the child's first year of life are of vital import for the whole of life to follow. Nutritional support provides the fundamental base for the initiation and development of this human growth process. Physiologic growth of the infant depends upon special chemical substances – *nutrients* – in the child's diet and on the biochemical processes of metabolism that ensure that the right elements will be in the right place at the right time for the formation and maintenance of all body tissues. However, nutrition is far more than a physical process alone. Many social and psychologic influences and relationships, along with the infant's culture and environment, affect food and feeding practices and nurture individual growth potential. Thus, nutrition and food and feeding practices during the highly significant first year of life (referred to as the infant year) cannot exist apart from this broader, overall growth and development. The *whole* process produces the *whole* person.

INFANT GROWTH AND DEVELOPMENT NEEDS

Human growth and development is a specific, highly individualized process. Although we can discuss general nutritional needs during the infant year, wide individual variations exist within so-called "normal" ranges. The wise practitioner will never lose sight of the individual infant's unique needs and growth potentials.

Physical Growth

The first year of life is one of rapid growth. During this early period, the infant shows remarkable changes in form and function.

Birth weight is a function of the mother's prepregnancy weight status and her weight gain during pregnancy. After birth, a period of "catch-up" or "lag-down" growth may occur as the infant tends toward a genetically predetermined channel of growth. This process may take from a few months to a year or more. Weight loss is normal following birth and is usually regained by the tenth day. Growth then proceeds at a rapid but decelerating rate. In general, by 4–5 months of age the infant will have doubled his/her birth weight and at 1 year of age will have tripled it. Thus a baby weighing 3.2 kg (7 lb) at birth will weigh approximately 6.4 kg (14 lb) at 4–5 months and about 9.5 kg (21 lb) at 1 year (Pipes, 1985).

Infants generally increase in length by 50 percent in the first year, from an average of 50 cm (20 in) at birth to approximately 75 cm (30 in). Body composition changes along with body size; water as a percentage of body weight decreases during the first year, from 70 percent to about 60 percent. Lean body mass gradually increases in the first year, and fat accumulates rapidly for the first 9 months, at which point it accounts for approximately 25 percent of body weight (Pipes, 1985).

The most critical period for brain growth begins prenatally and continues up to the age of around 18 months. Increases in brain mass are indicated by the rapid increase in head circumference, which will achieve two-thirds of its postnatal growth by age 2 years. Malnourished children are known to have smaller head circumferences than their well-nourished counterparts (Pipes, 1985).

Assessment of Growth

In general clinical practice, a child's growth pattern is regularly compared with percentile growth curves derived from the measurement of large numbers of children. Older growth charts have not proved satisfactory for current use because the data were derived from only two small nonrepresentative groups of children in Boston and Iowa (Stuart and Meredith, 1948). Currently used growth charts, developed by the National Center for Health Statistics (NCHS), reflect a broader database for measuring growth patterns in American children today (Hamill et al., 1979). These improved charts are based on more valid data from large numbers of a nationally representative sample of children. These charts are provided in two age intervals: birth to 36 months, and 2–18 years, with separate curves for girls and boys.

Several measurements of height and weight taken at different ages are used to assess whether the infant's growth is progressing as expected. It is important to realize, however, that growth tends to occur in spurts and may not follow the smooth curve that is pictured in growth charts. Effective use of these charts requires that measurements be taken by the same procedures by which the reference data were obtained (Pipes, 1985).

1. *Length.* The recumbent length of an infant is best measured by use of a measuring board. One adult holds the crown of the infant's head gently against an immovable headboard while the measurer extends the infant fully and moves a footboard toward the heels of the infant. Measurements are read to the nearest ⅛ inch and repeated until two readings agree to within ¼ inch (US Department of Health and Human Services, 1981).
2. *Weight.* Infants should be weighed nude using calibrated beam balance scales. Weight on pediatric scales should be read to the nearest ½ ounce; it is necessary to repeat the adjustment of the fractional weight until two readings agree within ½ ounce (US Department of Health and Human Services, 1981).
3. *Head circumference.* Measurement of the head circumference is accomplished by passing a cloth, metal, or paper tape over the most prominent part of the occiput and just above the supraorbital ridges. NCHS head circumference grids are most commonly used for children less than 3 years of age (Pipes, 1985).
4. *Other measurements.* Occasionally measurements of the abdomen, chest, and leg (calf) circumference may be used to provide additional information regarding growth progress. *Midarm circumference* can be used to monitor muscle mass accretion; it is taken at the midpoint between the shoulder joint and the elbow. Obesity may be distinguished from overweight through measurements of *skinfold thickness;* the most common site is the *triceps skinfold* (Cooper and Heird, 1982). At the same midarm point used for the circumference measurement, the nurse places a thumb and forefinger around a fold of the skin and gently pulls it away from the underlying triceps muscle. At this point the nurse applies a standard caliper, such as the Lange caliper, with the axis of the caliper perpendicular to that of the arm. For greater accuracy this measure should be taken several times, with a mean of these measurements used for monitoring purposes.

Mental and Psychosocial Growth

The infant's growing abilities to communicate and to respond to parental care are measures of mental growth. It was formerly thought that mental growth and learning were fairly minimal during the first year of life. However, there is mounting evidence that a great deal of development occurs in mental growth and learning ability during the infant year (see Chapter 29). Fundamental nutritional intake provides the basic elements for brain growth, while food and feeding practices serve as tools and stimuli for the learning process.

The infant's emotional growth can be measured in his/her growing capacity for love and affection and his/her ability to handle frustration and anxiety. This gradual development begins early in the infant year and is largely focused on the satisfaction of physical needs, especially adequate food intake to meet hunger needs, given in a warm, supportive environment.

The foundation of a child's social and cultural growth is also laid during the infant year. This social development is measured in terms of ability to relate to others and to participate in the group culture and living pattern. Many social and cultural behaviors, learned first through early relationships with parents and family, focus on food habits and feeding patterns, which in turn influence other areas of behavior. Early play behaviors in the infant year, as well as food patterns and feeding practices, are highly purposeful developmental activities. As the child's contacts broaden, relationships develop with persons outside the family and others in the community.

NUTRITIONAL REQUIREMENTS

Normal growth and development of the healthy infant requires sufficient energy for rapid growth, high-quality protein for developing tissues, sufficient fluid to serve tissue needs, and adequate minerals and vitamins to supply specific structural and metabolic processes.

Energy Needs

Total energy needs in relation to body size are relatively great during the infant year. However, infants can vary greatly in energy needs, depending on growth progress and general physical condition. The daily kilocalorie requirement is spent to meet basal metabolic needs, additional physical activity, and tissue growth, as well as to compensate for fecal loss of nutrients. Most of the required kilocalories are involved in the accelerated metabolic activities of food digestion, absorption, and metabolism. Term infants are estimated to need about 115 kcal/kg per day for the first 6 months and about 105 kcal/kg per day from 6 months to 1 year of age; preterm infants may require considerably more to achieve a desirable rate of growth (Kennaugh and Hay, 1987). Kilocalories are provided in the form of carbohydrates, proteins, and fats.

Carbohydrates

Carbohydrates are the primary energy source, sparing proteins for essential tissue growth. Lactose is the major carbohydrate in the newborn's diet: a disaccharide composed of glucose and galactose, it provides about 40 percent of the calories in human milk or "humanized" formula. Glucose is readily absorbed into the bloodstream; galactose is cleared from the circulation by the liver, where it contributes to glycogen storage, and thus it is a source of glucose between feedings. The central nervous system of the neonate is dependent upon glucose as an energy source, and lack of an appropriate energy supply can quickly prove damaging to brain tissues (Kennaugh and Hay, 1987).

Protein

Protein supplies the basic growth element of the body. The essential amino acids necessary for body tissue synthesis and maintenance must come from proteins of high biologic value. Such proteins are found in the infant's initial food – milk – as well as in the mixed diet during the latter half of the first year. Protein also supplies needed amino acid elements for such body fluids and secretions as enzymes, hormones, lymph, and plasma. For these body tissue proteins to be synthesized, essential amino acids must be supplied in proper amounts, proportion, and timing. The regular infant feedings provide for these needs.

The infant's overall growth is the final determinant of protein requirements. During the first 6 months of life, an infant requires 2.2 g/kg per day. During the second 6 months, as the rate of growth gradually decreases somewhat, the daily requirement drops to 2.0 g/kg. By and large, the healthy, active, growing infant will consume the necessary amount of kilocalories and protein in the intial milk and in the added variety of solid foods provided in a mixed diet during the second half of the year. However, in population groups where these needed foods are not as readily available in the quantities and forms needed, malnutrition problems may occur.

Fats

Fats are an important source of energy, fat-soluble vitamins, hormones, and essential fatty acids in the diet of the newborn. The essential fatty acids, as phospholipids, are important components of cell membranes in the infant's rapidly growing tissues (Kennaugh and Hay, 1987). *Linoleic acid* is the major essential fatty acid and provides 8–10 percent of the fat calories in human milk. Linoleic acid deficiency produces a characteristic eczema. Fat supplies approximately 50 percent of the calories in human milk.

Water

Water is second only to oxygen as an essential requirement for life. The infant's need for water is especially great in comparison to that of an adult. For example, in the infant, water composes 70–75 percent of the total body weight, whereas in the adult water makes up only about 60–65 percent of total body weight. Moreover, in the infant a relatively large amount of the total body water is *outside* the cells and thus more vulnerable to loss.

The infant's water requirement is directly related to caloric intake and the specific gravity of the urine. In general, an infant consumes an amount of water equivalent to 10–15 percent of body weight daily. In comparison, daily adult consumption is about 2–4 percent of body weight. The approximate daily infant need for water is 150 ml/kg (2.25 oz/lb). Breastfed infants generally obtain sufficient water from breast milk and do not require supplementation.

The kidneys of the neonate are functionally immature, and infants are susceptible to water imbalance. Water intoxication leading to hyponatremia, irritability, and coma has been reported in infants who were fed water after each feeding, or water as a milk substitute (Pipes, 1985).

Minerals

All of the major minerals and most of the known trace minerals are essential in overall metabolism.

Several specific minerals are needed in special cases, as will be seen in the discussion of small, underdeveloped infants. However, two of these basic minerals – calcium and iron – are of particular importance in the general nutritional needs for healthy growing infants.

Calcium

Calcium is the most abundant mineral in the body, almost all of it being contained in the skeletal mass, or bone compartment. Calcium, with phosphorus, in the form of hydroxyapatite, is essential for the rapid bone mineralization that takes place during the infant year. In the newborn infant only the central sections of the large bones are mineralized; thus, an x-ray taken at this time would present the appearance of a collection of disconnected, separate bones. Calcium is also essential for muscle contraction, blood coagulation, nerve irritability, tooth development, and heart muscle action. The infant's first food – milk – satisfies this major need for calcium, as do additional sources in the mixed diet during the second half of the year.

Iron

Iron is an essential trace element, necessary for the synthesis of hemoglobin. As such, it is a major component of the body's system for supplying cell oxygen requirements. In the cells, iron is also a component of oxidative enzymes necessary for cell metabolism. During fetal growth, a 6 months' supply of iron is stored in the fetal liver. Because the first infant food, milk, is low in iron, the infant needs solid food additions at about 6 months of age to supply this mineral. Iron-fortified cereals introduced at this time and, at a later date, egg yolks and meat, will satisfy this need. Although the amount of iron in human milk is low, its bioavailability is high in comparison to that of the iron in cow's milk or commercial formulas. For breastfeeding infants, about 40–50 percent of the available iron is absorbed, in contrast to the iron of commercial formulas, of which less than 10 percent is absorbed (Sunshine, 1983).

Vitamins

Because of their essential roles as coenzymes in cell metabolism and as structural factors, vitamins are necessary for normal growth and maintenance of body tissues. Here we shall briefly discuss several of the vitamins particularly needed for growth.

Vitamin A (Retinol)

Vitamin A is a necessary component of visual purple, a pigment that regulates the eye's adaptation to light and dark. This pigment begins to develop prior to birth. After the infant is born, vitamin A continues the development of this essential pigment, enabling the infant to distinguish degrees of light as visual adaptation develops. Vitamin A is also necessary for bone mineralization and tooth development; it is an essential agent in the development of specialized cells in the gums that help in the tooth mineralization and development process. Vitamin A also plays a role in the formation and maturation of other epithelial tissues, such as the skin, eyes, and mucosal linings of the digestive, respiratory, urinary, and reproductive tracts.

B-Complex Vitamins

B-complex vitamins serve as coenzyme factors in various processes involved in energy and protein metabolism. Three vitamins associated with these processes are thiamin, niacin, and riboflavin.

1. *Thiamin* is specifically involved in carbohydrate metabolism and also in caloric intake. That is, the need for thiamin increases as the caloric need increases. Thus, during the rapid growth period of infancy, when energy demands are relatively large, thiamin is particularly needed as an important coenzyme factor in the growth of tissue, to provide for increased anabolic activity and meet increased energy demands.
2. *Niacin* also serves as a coenzyme factor in important metabolic activities related to both protein and energy metabolism. It is required for cellular oxidation of numerous substrate fuels and tissue growth materials.
3. *Riboflavin* also functions as a coenzyme factor in metabolism, in various reactions involving amino acids and fatty acids as well as carbohydrate metabolites.

Several other B vitamins are essential to the proper formation of red blood cells and hence are especially important during the infant growth year. *Vitamin B$_{12}$* (cobalamin) is a cofactor in the synthesis of heme, the nonprotein part of hemoglobin. *Folic acid* (folacin) also functions along with vitamin B$_{12}$ in the development of hemoglobin. During the prenatal period, there is an increased need for folic acid in the maternal diet to meet fetal growth demands, and these needs continue during the period of infant growth. A deficiency of folic acid is associated with megaloblastic anemia, especially in infancy.

A deficiency of *vitamin B₆* (pyridoxine) is associated with nerve and muscle irritability and hypochromic anemia. Convulsive disorders in infants have been attributed to the inadvertent use of pyridoxine-deficient formulas.

Vitamin C (Ascorbic Acid)

Vitamin C plays several important roles during the rapid infant growth period:

1. *Tissue strength.* Vitamin C provides an essential material for the formation of intercellular cement substance in all tissues. It is thus especially needed during rapid tissue growth periods.
2. *Iron absorption.* Vitamin C aids in the absorption of essential iron by providing additional acid medium to change ferric iron, the form in foods, to ferrous iron, the form necessary for absorption.
3. *General metabolism.* Vitamin C is an active participant in a number of other general metabolic activities, such as bone mineralization and enzyme systems. For example, it is closely involved as a coenzyme in the cell metabolism of the two amino acids phenylalanine and tyrosine, both of which are essential for growth.

Vitamin D (Cholecalciferol)

Vitamin D is necessary for the absorption and utilization of calcium and phosphorus needed for bone development and other body functions.

Vitamin K (Menadione)

Vitamin K is a necessary agent in the liver's formation of prothrombin, an essential substance in the blood-clotting mechanism. A lack of vitamin K is not usually a continuing dietary problem because it is synthesized by intestinal microorganisms. However, because the newborn lacks these microorganisms, vitamin K is routinely given at birth to avoid any immediate hemorrhagic tendencies.

Vitamin E (Ergesterol)

Vitamin E has important growth-associated functions in its major role as an antioxidative agent. It protects the polyunsaturated fatty acids that make up cell walls and other vital tissue membranes from oxidative deterioration. It is especially required in the diets of premature infants, who may be receiving increased amounts of polyunsaturated fatty acids in special formulas. The increased intake of polyunsaturated fats requires an increased intake of vitamin E for protection from breakdown. Hemolytic anemia from vitamin E deficiency has been observed in premature infants. Vitamin E supplements are used to avoid this problem.

Hypervitaminosis

Care must be taken to avoid excess intake of two of the fat-soluble vitamins, A and D. An excess of these vitamins may occur when they are given to an infant in large quantities for prolonged periods of time because of parents' misunderstanding of directions from the practitioner or because of ignorance or carelessness. Parents must be counseled to use only the amount directed and no more, as supplements of these vitamins are now provided in concentrated products to be taken only in drops.

Vitamin excesses have clear toxic symptoms. Symptoms of vitamin A toxicity include loss of appetite, drying and cracking of the skin, slow growth, swelling and pain of long bones, bone fragility, and enlargement of the liver and spleen. Vitamin D toxicity symptoms include weight loss, nausea, diarrhea, polyuria, nocturia, and eventual calcification of soft tissues such as those of the renal tubules, bronchi, blood vessels, heart, and stomach.

Recommended Dietary Allowances

A summary of the nutritional needs for infant growth, as recommended by the National Research Council, is presented in Table 28–1. The protein allowances are based on basal energy requirements, with appropriate increments for growth. Some allowance is added to cover individual variability within a large population. These overall allowances also include safety margins to cover variations in groups of healthy normal infants. Remember, therefore, that these are *population guidelines*, not necessarily specific individual requirements, for needed amounts of nutrients that the infant can obtain from milk as an initial food and from a mixed diet during the last 6 months of the infant year. As we shall see, in cases

TABLE 28-1. Recommended Daily Dietary Allowances for Growth of Infants

Nutrients	Birth–0.5 Years	0.5–1 Year
Weight		
lb	13	20
kg	6	9
Height		
in	24	28
cm	60	71
Energy (kcal)	kg × 115	kg × 105
Protein (g)	kg × 2.2	kg × 2.0
Fat-soluble vitamins		
Vitamin A		
(µg RE)	420	400
(IU)	1400	2000
Vitamin D (µg)[a]	10	10
Vitamin E (mg TE)	3	4
Water-soluble vitamins		
Vitamin C (mg)	35	35
Folacin (µg)	30	45
Niacin (mg)	6	8
Riboflavin (mg)	0.4	0.6
Thiamin (mg)	0.3	0.5
Vitamin B_6 (mg)	0.3	0.6
Vitamin B_{12} (µg)	0.5	1.5
Minerals		
Calcium (mg)	360	540
Phosphorus (mg)	240	360
Iodine (µg)	40	50
Iron (mg)	10	15
Magnesium (mg)	50	70
Zinc (mg)	3	5

SOURCE: Williams (1985).
[a] As cholecalciferol; 10 µg cholecalciferol = 400 IU vitamin D.

of special need, supplementation of specific nutrients may be required.

Assessment of Nutritional Status

The goal of nutritional assessment is to determine whether the infant's nutritional needs are being met or if the child is at risk of developing nutrition-related problems later on. The nurse can utilize information from several sources in order to achieve this goal.

Anthropometric Measures

The infant's weight and recumbent length, crown to heel, are measured at birth and at frequent intervals as a basis of monitoring individual growth patterns. Other measurements, such as head circumference, are also commonly used to determine growth trends and nutritional adequacy.

Clinical Observations

Besides body measurements of physical growth, various clinical signs may be observed as measures of nutritional status. These signs include general vitality; condition of various tissues, such as gums and teeth, skin, hair, and eyes; and development of muscles and general nervous control. A number of these clinical observations and signs of nutritional status are summarized in Table 28–2.

Laboratory Data

Other measures of nutritional status are reflected in various laboratory tests, including blood and urine studies to determine levels of vitamins, hemoglobin, and similar substances. In addition, x-rays of the bones in the hands and wrists may be used to indicate degree of ossification and overall bone development.

Dietary Analysis

Analysis of the infant's food intake and general eating pattern provides an additional measure of nutritional adequacy. A standardized nutrition history form is useful for recording specific information regarding quantity and quality of food ingested as well as preparation and storage practices, financial resources, and other aspects of daily living that will have an effect upon the infant's food intake (Murray and Glassman, 1982). An example of a nutrition screening form for use in infancy is shown in Figure 28–1. In some clinical settings, comprehensive nutritional analyses are quickly performed by using a computer and various nutrition data bases.

Infant Feeding

The first year of life is one of rapid change in physical characteristics and neuromotor development. To appreciate the enormity of this change, one need only consider that infants who at birth

TABLE 28-2. *Clinical Signs of Nutritional Status*

Parameter	Good	Poor
General appearance	Alert, responsive	Listless, apathetic, cachexic
Hair	Shiny, lustrous; healthy scalp	Stringy, dull, brittle, dry, depigmented
Neck (glands)	No enlargement	Thyroid enlarged
Skin (face and neck)	Smooth, slightly moist, good color; reddish-pink mucous membranes	Greasy, discolored, scaly
Eyes	Bright, clear; no fatigue circles beneath	Dryness, signs of infection, increased vascularity, glassiness, thickened conjunctiva
Lips	Good color, moist	Dry, scaly, swollen; angular lesions (stomatitis)
Tongue	Good pink color, surface papillae present, no lesions	Papillary atrophy, smooth appearance; swollen, red, beefy (glossitis)
Gums	Good pink color; no swelling or bleeding, firm	Marginal redness or swelling, receding, spongy
Teeth	Straight, no crowding; clean, no discoloration; well-shaped jaw	Unfilled caries, absent teeth, worn surfaces, mottled, malpositioned
Skin (general)	Smooth, slightly moist, good color	Rough, dry, scaly, pale, pigmented, irritated; petechiae, bruises
Abdomen	Flat	Swollen
Legs, feet	No tenderness, weakness, or swelling; good color	Edema, calf tender, tingling, weakness
Skeleton	No malformations	Bowlegs, knock-knees, chest deformity at diaphragm, beaded ribs, prominent scapulas
Weight	Normal for height, age, body build	Overweight or underweight
Posture	Erect, arms and legs straight, abdomen in, chest out	Sagging shoulders, sunken chest, humped back
Muscles	Well developed, firm	Flaccid, poor tone; undeveloped; tender
Nervous control	Good attention span for age; does not cry easily; not irritable or restless	Inattentive, irritable
Gastrointestinal function	Good appetite and digestion; normal, regular elimination	Anorexia, indigestion, constipation, or diarrhea
General vitality	Good endurance, energetic; sleeps well at night; vigorous	Easily fatigued, no energy, looks tired, apathetic

SOURCE: Williams (1985).

FIGURE 28-1. Infant nutrition screening form. ▶

INFANT NUTRITION SCREENING FORM

Name: _____ Chron. Age − Months Premature = Corrected Age Date: _____

☐ ☐ ☐   Evaluator: _____

FOODS

Circle infant's corrected age in months	1 2 3 4 5 6 7 8 9 10 11 12	Assessment Acceptable	Not Acceptable	Intervention	Identified Problem ( )
Breastmilk: F/D ____ Min/F ____		Supplement Vitamins & Iron Brand: ____		Supplement Vitamins & Iron	☐
Formula: F/D ____ oz/F ____ Total ____		Plain, Iron Iron Supplement Brand: ____		Formula w/iron or plain w/iron drops	☐
Water		Plain	Sugar, honey, Karo	Plain	☐
Infant Cereal		Spoon	In bottle adult cereal	Spoon, infant	☐
Fruits and Vegetables		Spoon	Strained food in bottle	Spoon	☐
Meat, Poultry/Alt.		Spoon	Strained food in bottle	Spoon	☐
Breads/Starches		Finger Foods, toast, crackers, Cornbran, Cheerios	Sugar coated cereals, cake, cookies	Dry toast, crackers, Cornbran, Cheerios	☐
Juices		Infant or Adult dil. w/ Vit. C	Kool-aid, Tang, soda, iced tea	Infant or Adult diluted w/ Vit. C	☐
Egg Yolk		Cooked yolk	Egg whites whole eggs	Cooked yolk	☐
Dessert/Snacks		Pudding Plain Yogurt	Candy, chips, sweets	Plain yogurt, fruit	☐
Milk		Whole milk	Nonfat milk	Formula to 1 year	☐
Fluoride Supplement?		Yes	No	If no, refer to Physician	☐

☐ Food Groups can be introduced   ☐ Food groups should not yet be introduced

Brand of formula _____ RTF Conc. Powder How mixed? _____ Correctly? Yes No ☐

SKILLS

Age/Weight	Formula/Food	Assessment	Intervention	Identified Problem ( )
8 lbs.	20-23 oz. formula	Completes bottle in 20-30'? Yes No Holds baby while feeding? Yes No	>30 → evaluate suck-swallow Encourage/demo holding	☐
12 lbs.	28-32 oz. formula	Completes bottle in 20-30'? Yes No Holds baby while feeding? Yes No	>30 → evaluate suck-swallow Encourage/demo holding	☐
4 to 6 mo.	30-32 oz. + strained foods	Hold head upright? Yes No Food stays in mouth? Yes No	Start Solids	☐
7 to 9 mo.	28-30 oz. + Junior foods	Picks up small objects? Yes No Holds own bottle? Yes No	Start finger feeding Evaluate cup introduction	☐
10 to 12 mo.	22-28 oz. + Junior + table foods	Drinks from cup? Yes No Eats lumpy food? Yes No	Encourage self-feeding, introduce table foods & textures	☐

Problems with diarrhea or constipation? Yes No _____ ☐

Bottle taken to bed? Yes No _____ ☐

GROWTH

Measurements	Assessment Lt., Wt., or Wt./Lt.			Intervention
NCHS Growth Chart Lt. ____ ____% Wt./Lt. ____% Wt. ____ ____%	Falling off curve? ☐ Yes ☐ No	>95% ☐ Yes ☐ No	Excessive gain ☐ Yes ☐ No	Refer None needed

Refer to Nutitionist if: Foods—3 or more identified problems   Skills—discretion of evaluator   Growth—referral needed, per above

Other— _____

Comments: _____

Referred to: _____

Pat Morris, R.D., M.P.H., Memorial Hospital Medical Center of Long Beach © 1983.

are only prepared to suck liquids from a nipple are by 1 year of age attempting to feed themselves table food using culturally appropriate utensils (Pipes, 1985).

Physiological Considerations

The growth rate during infancy, especially during the first 4–6 months, is rapid. As a result, the young infant's energy needs are high, requiring an RDA of 115 kcal/kg per day. To meet rapid growth needs during these first 6 months of life, the recommended protein allowance is 2.2 g/kg per day.

In comparison with the limited capacities of preterm and SGA babies, full-term infants have the ability to digest and absorb proteins, moderate amounts of fat, and simple carbohydrates. Full-term infants have some difficulty with starch digestion, since amylase, the starch-splitting enzyme, is not yet produced. However, as starch is later introduced, this enzyme functions well.

The renal system of the full-term infant functions well, but the need for water relative to size is greater than that of older children or adults. This additional water is needed to manage adequate renal excretion. Because the first teeth do not erupt until about the fourth month, the initial food, i.e. milk, is liquid. Solid food additions are not recommended until 6 months of age, since breast milk or prepared formula provide all the growth requirements to that point and the enzyme systems are not fully developed to handle other foods until then.

Another physiologic characteristic of the newborn infant is the *rooting reflex*, which helps to ensure adequate food intake. Also, the somewhat recessed lower jaw is a natural adaptation for feeding at the breast.

PSYCHOSOCIAL NEEDS

Throughout the human life cycle, food and the feeding process serve not only to meet essential nutritional requirements for growth and physical maintenance of the body but also to strengthen psychosocial development. This is particularly true during the initial stage of the infant growth year when fundamental patterns are laid down.

Over the past 30 years, Erik Erikson's theory of human personality development has greatly influenced our view of the life cycle (Erikson, 1963; Hall, 1983). This leading American psychoanalyst has identified eight stages of human growth, each of which is characterized by a basic psychosocial problem. Success in handling the developmental problem at each stage has a positive ego value, while failure has a negative ego value. Erikson has identified the basic developmental task at the beginning of life (Stage 1) as the struggle of *trust versus distrust*. Thus, it is especially important that trust be established in the infant year, as it lays the foundation for continuing personality growth.

Feeding is the infant's primary means of establishing human relationships, especially with the mother or other feeding adult. If the infant's needs for food and love are recognized and satisfied during the early days with the mother and other family members, trust will develop. Evidence of this trust can be seen in the infant's increasing ability to wait for feedings until they are prepared.

Successful feeding depends upon the caretaker being sensitive and responsive to the infant's preferences regarding timing, amount, tempo, and eating ability in feedings. Mothers who breast- or bottle-feed effectively exhibit certain behaviors: they feed the infant upon demand; they hold their infants close to them, yet still allow a range of movement; they allow their infants to set the pace of the feeding; they talk and smile to their infants, yet avoid engaging in behaviors that will disrupt the feeding; and they allow their infants to decide when the feeding is finished. In these positive feeding relationships, infants learn to be aware of their feelings, discover that they are capable of conveying their needs, and develop trust that their needs will be met. Infants who are consistently frustrated in feeding or who are force-fed will learn to associate hunger with anxiety (Satter, 1986).

Support of Successful Feeding

Studies have indicated that between 40 and 60 percent of all mothers have decided upon their mode of infant feeding prior to becoming pregnant, and by far the majority of mothers have made their decision before delivery. Nurses and midwives are perceived as being more helpful in providing information regarding feeding than are physicians (Simopoulos and Graves, 1984). The nurse can help set the mother up for success in feeding by providing her with the information she needs in order to decide upon her method of infant feeding and then providing her, after delivery, with whatever support she needs in order to implement her decision.

The clinician may inadvertently put stress on the feeding relationship in the process of inquiring about feeding habits or offering nutrition advice. Intervention should focus on enhancing the parent's awareness of the infant's feeding cues and ability to respond appropriately to them. Table 28–3 outlines strategies useful in managing feeding issues.

Breastfeeding

Human breast milk provides the ideal food for young infants. It carries many advantages for overall infant nutrition (Sunshine, 1983):

1. Breast milk contains numerous immune factors, including *Lactobacillus bifidus*, a growth factor that interferes with the development of potentially pathogenic organisms, and other immunoglobulins, antiviral substances, and complements.
2. Breast milk confers numerous nutritional benefits, including an ideal ratio of nutrients in proportion to the growing infant's requirements.
3. Breast milk provides allergy protection, since allergy to human milk is essentially unknown, and breastfeeding during the first 6 months delays the introduction of other possible allergens in solid food additions until they are more readily tolerated by the infant.
4. Breastfeeding promotes mother–infant bonding, which is an extremely important aspect of the mother–infant relationship.

Today, as in times past, the process of breastfeeding can be successfully initiated and maintained by the great majority of women who try (see Chapter 21).

Nutritional support for the lactation process is provided by the continuation of the optimum diet the mother followed during her pregnancy with an additional increase of 500 cal. More calories are required to meet the energy demands of lactation and to increase the energy value of the breast milk. Also, since milk is a fluid, increased attention to fluid intake is necessary (see Chapter 12).

A diet of breast milk alone is usually sufficient to meet all the nutrient needs for the infant's first 6 months of life (Fig. 28–2). However, a few nutrient supplements may be indicated in some cases (American Academy of Pediatrics, 1980):

1. *Vitamin K.* For the neonate, parenteral administration of vitamin K is needed because the content of vitamin K in human milk is low and because infants consume relatively small amounts of human milk during the first few days of life.
2. *Vitamin D.* The amount of vitamin D activity in human milk is greater than previously recognized. However, infrequent cases of rickets have occurred in breastfed infants, particularly when they have had limited exposure to sunlight. To avoid this possible problem, supplementation with 400 IU vitamin D (10 μg cholecalciferol) per day is advised.
3. *Iron.* There is controversy about iron supplementation for the breastfed infant. Usually, there is sufficient fetal iron storage to meet needs during the first 4–6 months of life. However, in some cases, 7 mg of iron daily is recommended during the first 6 months.

TABLE 28–3. Strategies for Support of a Positive Feeding Relationship

1. Education of the parents regarding the natural sequence of growth and the process of food regulation
2. Encouraging parents to recognize and respect their infant's messages regarding hunger, satiety, and food preference
3. Teaching parents appropriate food selection for the nutritional needs and developmental readiness of the child
4. Anticipation of feeding difficulties in the case of infants who are sick or have congenital anomalies
5. Being mindful of family dynamics when it is necessary to institute a modified diet for an infant
6. Distinguishing feeding problems that are simply the result of lack of information from those which are secondary to a disturbed family environment. The latter require a family referral to a mental health worker for psychosocial evaluation

SOURCE: Satter (1986).

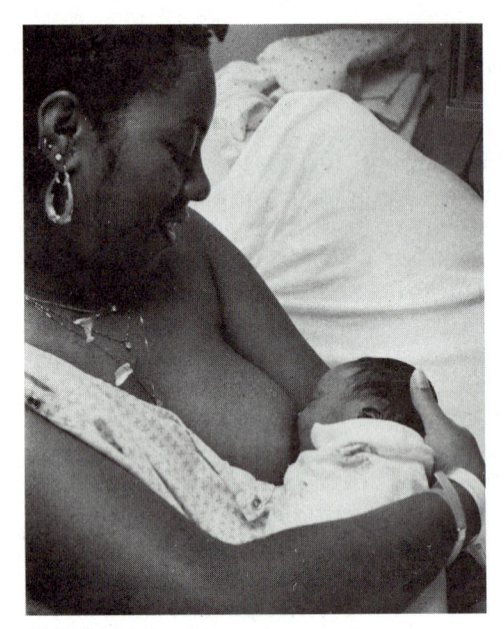

FIGURE 28–2. Human breast milk fills all nutrient needs.

4. *Fluoride.* Controversy also exists about fluoride supplementation. Recently, however, the American Academy of Pediatrics (1979) has published a revised dosage schedule for fluoride supplementation. Because the fluoride content of human milk is low, a supplement of 0.25 mg/day, administered with an appropriate dropper, is recommended beginning at about 2 weeks of age for the breastfed infant.

Formula Feeding

Since ancient times, women have sometimes been obliged, for whatever reason, to find an alternative to breastfeeding. Throughout most of history, the best alternative was another lactating woman, the wet nurse. Contracts detailing the duties and fees of wet nurses from ancient Mesopotamia, Egypt, and Greece are still in existence, and even well into the nineteenth century these women enjoyed a professional status. Those parents who could not afford a wet nurse often looked to the milk of other animals. Although cow's milk has been employed most universally in feeding infants, in some places and times the milk of goats, asses, horses, camels, pigs, reindeer, sheep, dogs, elephants, and llamas was more readily available (Radbill, 1981). Infant mortality was high when using these substitute milks, until it was recognized that human milk has a low protein concentration, and the other milks were subsequently diluted. In order to support adequate growth, an increase in caloric density was indicated, and sugars or cereals were added to the diluted milks. Infant mortality remained high among artificially fed infants until the twentieth century ushered in some advances that made formula feeding safer and more convenient. Electric refrigeration allowed formulas to be kept relatively free of bacteria. Techniques were developed to improve the digestibility of cow's milk protein through modification by heat or lactic acid. Good rubber nipples made bottle feeding much easier. Vitamin, and later, mineral supplementation of formulas became common. In the last 40 years, as the special characteristics of human milk have increasingly come to light, manufacturers have altered the composition of formula to resemble human milk more closely and have provided a wide array of formulations for infants with special needs (Barness, 1987).

Surveys indicate that the incidence and duration of breastfeeding are increasing in the United States (Martinez and Nalezienski, 1979). Prevailing medical opinion, as voiced by both the American Academy of Pediatrics and the American Medical Association, favors breastfeeding of infants whenever possible (American Academy of Pediatrics, 1976). None the less, there are instances, as with galactosemia, where neither cow's milk nor human milk can be used. Also, there may be other cases in which breastfeeding is inappropriate or undesired by the mother. Furthermore, the practice of giving sample formula packs to mothers leaving the maternity ward after delivery has contributed to the early change from breastfeeding to formula feeding (Bergevin, Dougherty, and Kramer, 1983). For whatever reason, if the mother does not choose breastfeeding or stops early, bottle feeding of an appropriate formula is an acceptable alternative. Of these mothers, by far the majority – about 90 percent – use a commercial formula, with the few remaining ones using a home-prepared evaporated milk formula.

Standard Infant Formulas

Recognizing the suitability of human milk for infants, companies producing commercial formulas have focused on developing products that simulate human milk and provide comparable nutritional benefits (Anderson, Chinn, and Fisher, 1982). The basic protein component is usually derived from cow's milk, soy protein, protein

TABLE 28-4. A Comparison of Types of Formulas Manufactured for Full-Term Infants

Type of Formula (Use)	Protein Content	Fat Content	Carbohydrate Content
Milk-based (routine)			
Source	Nonfat cow's milk	Vegetable oils	Lactose
g/100 kcal	2.2–2.3	5.4–5.5	10.5–10.8
% kcal	9	48–50	41–43
Whey-adjusted (routine)			
Source	Nonfat cow's milk plus demineralized whey	Vegetable and oleo oils	Lactose
g/100 kcal	2.2	5.4	10.8
% kcal	9	48	43
Soy isolate (cow's milk sensitivity)			
Source	Soy isolate	Vegetable oils	Corn syrup solids and/or sucrose
g/100 kcal	2.7–3.2	5.1–5.6	9.9–10.2
% kcal	12–13	45–51	39–40
Casein hydrolysate (protein sensitivity, galactosemia)			
Source	Casein hydrolysate	Corn oil or corn oil plus medium-chain triglycerides	Tapioca starch and glucose, sucrose, or corn syrup solids
g/100 kcal	2.8–3.3	3.9–4.0	13.1–13.6
% kcal	11–13	35	52–54
Meat-based (cow's milk sensitivity, galactosemia)			
Source	Beef hearts	Sesame oil and beef heart fat	Tapioca starch and sucrose
g/100 kcal	4.0	4.8	9
% kcal	16	47	37

SOURCE: Williams (1985).

hydrolysate, or meat base. The three major types of standard commercial formulas for full-term infants – milk-based, whey-adjusted, and soy-isolate – are described in Table 28–4. Note that some of the milk-based formulas are whey-adjusted to more nearly approximate the protein ratio in human milk.

The standards for nutrient levels required in infant formulas have been set by the Infant Formula Act of 1980. This regulation was based on recommendations from the American Academy of Pediatrics (1976). Table 28–5 compares these standards with the RDAs recommended by the National Research Council for infants from birth to 6 months.

Currently, most infant formulas for home use are either ready-to-feed liquids or concentrated preparations to be diluted with water. About 40 percent of the formulas are of the ready-to-feed-package form, over 50 percent are concentrated liquids, and less than 10 percent are powdered forms to be mixed with water.

Two physical characteristics of commercial infant formulas are of concern to practitioners (Anderson, Chinn, and Fisher, 1982):

1. OSMOLALITY. This measure of the osmotic pressure exerted by a solution is a function of its density of solute particles. Minerals and carbohydrates are the main determinants of osmolality in milk- and soy-based formulas. Solutions of high osmolality draw water into the small intestine,

TABLE 28–5. *Nutrient Standards for Formulas Manufactured for Healthy, Full-Term Infants*

Nutrient	RDA (1980) 0–6 Months	Nutrient Requirements of the Infant Formula Act of 1980 Minimum	Maximum
Energy (kcal)	570–870	670	
Protein (g)	13.2	12.1	30.2
Essential fatty acids (linoleate; % kcal)	3.0	2.7	
Fat-soluble vitamins			
A (IU)	1400 (420 µg)	1675 (503 µg)	5025 (1508 µg)
D (IU)	400 (10 µm)	268	670
E (IU)	4.5	4.7	
K (µg)	12.0[a]	27.0	
Water-soluble vitamins			
C (mg)	35.0	54.0	
B_1 (thiamin) (µg)	300.0	268.0	
B_2 (riboflavin) (µg)	400.0	402.0	
B_6 (pyridoxine) (µg)	300.0	235.0	
B_{12} (µg)	0.5	1.0	
Niacin (mg)	6.0	1.68	
Folacin (µg)	30.0	27.0	
Pantothenic acid (mg)	2.0[a]	2.0	
Biotin (µg)	35.0	10.0	
Choline (mg)		47.0	
Inositol (mg)		27.0	
Minerals			
Calcium (mg)	360.0	350.0	
Phosphorus (mg)	240.0	168.0	
Magnesium (mg)	50.0	40.0	
Iron (mg)	10.0	1.0[b]	
Iodine (µg)	40.0	34.0	
Zinc (mg)	3.0	3.4	
Copper (µg)	500–700[a]	402.0	
Manganese (µg)	500–700[a]	34.0	
Sodium (mg)	115–350[a]	134.0	402.0
Potassium (mg)	350–925[a]	536.0	1340.0
Chloride (mg)	275–700[a]	369	1005.0
Fluoride (µg)	100–500[a]		
Chromium (µg)	10–40[a]		
Selenium (µg)	10–40[a]		
Molybdenum (µg)	30–60[a]		

SOURCE: Williams (1985).
[a] Based on estimated safe and adequate daily dietary intakes. Some figures are given in ranges because of a lack of information on which to base allowances.
[b] Based on iron content of nonfortified infant formula (0.15 mg/100 kcal). The Committee on Nutrition recommends that infants receive 1.0 mg/100 kcal formula.

thus causing diarrhea and possible dehydration and electrolyte imbalance. The Committee on Nutrition of the American Academy of Pediatrics (1976) has set a standard for osmolality of formulas for use by healthy infants at a level no more than 400 mOsm/l. The osmolality of human milk has been measured at 285–300 mOsm/kg water, and osmolalities of a number of ready-to-feed and reconstituted liquid concentrate formulas fall within an approximate range of 225–320 mOsm/kg water, which is well below the maximal concentration indicated by the Committee on Nutrition. In comparison, however, specialized high-caloric dietary products used under direct medical supervision for special conditions may well exceed the osmolality of 400 mOsm/l recommended by the American Academy of Pediatrics. The use of such concentrated formulas would thus need to be carefully monitored.

2. STABILITY. Infant formulas are mixtures of proteins, carbohydrates, emulsified fats, minerals, and vitamins. Thickening or stabilizing agents are often used to prevent separation of these components and to add stability for longer shelf life. In the United States, the use of such stabilizing agents in formulas is governed by FDA standards. However, European formulas do not contain such agents because they are thought not to be recommended for infants younger than 4 months of age. In any case, it is important that any infant formula be used only within the dates specified on the product.

Evaporated Milk Formulas

In a few cases, usually because of economic constraints, the mother may use a home-prepared evaporated milk formula. Such formulas are made using approximately 1.5 parts evaporated milk, 2 parts water, and 3 percent carbohydrate, supplemented with vitamin C and iron because cow's milk is low in both of these nutrients. Honey and Karo syrup should not be used for infants under 1 year of age because of the danger of infant botulism.

Cow's Milk

Regular unmodified cow's milk is not suitable for infants during the early months of life for two reasons:

1. The solute load of regular milk is too heavy for the infant renal system to handle.
2. Cow's milk that has been pasteurized but not more expensively heat treated provokes gastrointestinal blood loss.

Studies have also shown that use of unmodified cow's milk in young infants induces trace mineral deficiencies of both copper and zinc (Report: Perils of Cow's Milk, 1983). Unmodified cow's milk is tolerated, however, by the infant 6 months of age or older.

The US Department of Agriculture authorizes the use of regular whole fluid milk as well as evaporated milk and commercial infant formulas beginning at 6 months of age for infants in the Special Supplemental Food Program for Women, Infants, and Children (WIC). Since regular milk is low in vitamin C and iron, the mixed diet begun at this age should include a variety of food sources for these nutrients, such as fruit juices and iron-fortified cereals.

During the first year of life, infants should definitely *not* use milks of reduced fat content such as skim or 2 percent milk because (1) skim milk contains *insufficient energy* to supply maintenance or growth caloric requirements, causing the use of body fat to make up the deficit; and (2) the fat portion of milk is necessary as a source of the essential fatty acid linoleic acid, which is necessary for the growth and development of body tissues.

Feeding Techniques

Just as in breastfeeding, the infant being fed a formula should be cradled in the arm for the close human touch and warmth the infant requires (Fig. 28–3). The bottle should be inclined to keep the nipple filled with milk, thereby minimizing the swallowing of air. When the infant is satisfied, no extra milk should be forced, regardless of the amount remaining in the bottle. Any remaining formula should be thrown away and not refrigerated for re-use. A healthy infant fed on demand will take the amount of formula needed. During and after each feeding, the infant should be held erect against the feeder's shoulder to expel any swallowed air.

Solid Food Additions

For the first 6 months of life, the optimal single food for the infant is human milk, with appropri-

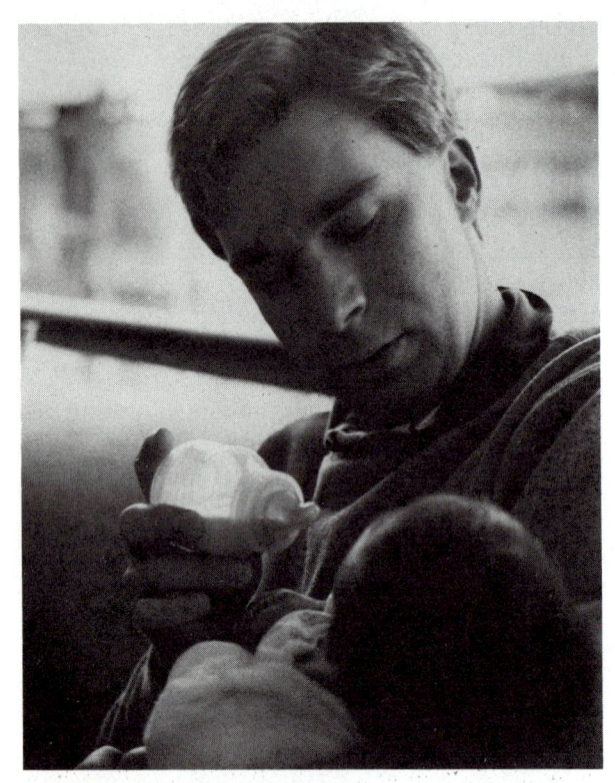

FIGURE 28-3. The bottle-fed infant receives nutritional support and close paternal contact during the feeding.

ate alternative formula feeding when necessary. There is no nutritional need for introducing other foods to infants before 6 months of age. After that time, solid foods can be gradually added. By the time infants are 6 months old they can handle solid foods through mastication and swallowing and can communicate desire and interest in food, thus participating in feeding, which is a learning and socialization process as well as a source of nutritional support. If solid foods are withheld until this time, there is less tendency to overfeed an infant. As solid food is gradually added, the amount of milk the infant consumes will gradually decrease accordingly.

There is no one specific sequence of food additions that must be followed. The responses and needs of the individual infant serve as a basis for choices, with food becoming a source of enjoyment and bonding of warm family relationships. Usually, single foods are introduced first, one at a time, in small amounts, so that any possible adverse reaction to an offending food can easily be identified.

Traditionally, the initial transition food is iron-fortified infant cereal with the addition of a little breast milk or formula, then fruits, vegetables, egg yolks, and meat. Consistency of the food should reflect the infant's eating abilities. In the beginning, the mother gives small amounts, usually before the milk feeding when the infant's appetite is greatest. Over time, she introduces a wide variety of foods and helps the infant develop an enjoyment of a large number of them.

A variety of commercial baby foods are available, prepared today without the formerly used ingredients of sugar, salt, and monosodium glutamate. However, some mothers choose to prepare their own baby food, which can easily be done by cooking and straining vegetables and fruits, freezing a batch at a time in ice cube trays, then storing the cubes in plastic bags in the freezer. In this way, a single cube can be reheated conveniently for use at a feeding.

In general, two basic guidelines are useful in adding solid foods to the infant's diet:

1. The infant needs the required nutrients, not any one food per se.
2. Learning development uses food as one of its main tools.

Food not only provides physical sustenance but also meets other personal and cultural needs. Good food habits begin at birth and continue as the child grows older. By the time infants are about 8–9 months old, they should have achieved a fairly good ability to eat so-called family foods — chopped cooked foods, simply seasoned – without need for special infant preparation.

SMALL, UNDERDEVELOPED INFANTS

Tiny, underdeveloped babies born too soon and too small present special problems in nutritional care. Both the preterm infant and the small-for-gestational-age (SGA) infant require careful and vigorous nutritional support to survive (see Chapter 32).

Physical Characteristics

Each year, approximately 16 million babies are born abnormally small because they have suffered growth retardation in the womb. In the United States, this intrauterine growth retardation occurs in about 5 percent of all pregnancies and increases the risk of death for fetuses in late pregnancy and newborns approximately five-fold (Miller, 1983a). Another 4 percent of all live newborns are premature and are also at risk in the period following birth.

Preterm infants vary in weight and development but are usually considered *preterm* if they are born at fewer than 270 days of gestation or weigh less than 2500 g (5.5 lb). The *small-for-gestational-age* (SGA) infant may be one who has reached full term but is retarded in growth and has a low birth weight. The SGA infant can be defined as one whose size is less than its genetic potential. These small babies usually have a low birth weight of 2500 g (5.5 lb) or less (see Chapter 32). The overall percentage of premature babies in the newborn population varies little around the world, but the incidence of SGA babies has increased to six times higher in underdeveloped or developing countries than in more economically developed areas of the world.

Although the cause of intrauterine growth retardation is unknown, investigators speculate that nutrition is involved in two ways: either there has been a limitation of essential nutrients in the maternal diet, or there has been a restricted transfer of nutrients from the mother to the fetus through the blood flow from the mother (Miller, 1983b). One possible explanation is that during pregnancy the mother's blood vessels are incompletely transformed into arteries capable of supplying blood to the uterus and the placenta.

Preterm and SGA infants have different body compositions than those of full-term infants. Both types of underdeveloped babies have similarities in appearance, but SGA infants have a distinctive marasmic malnourished look and often appear older than their weights would indicate. They have a much smaller energy reserve than a normal newborn and thus are less well equipped to withstand stress before and during birth.

Both types of underdeveloped infants present "catch-up" problems in growth and nutrition. The preterm infant arrives when some organs, especially the brain, are still at critical developmental stages of cell division. In general, all of these tiny infants are fragile and face survival hazards. Their body composition differs in several ways from that of full-term infants:

1. They have much more water in their body weight and less protein and minerals.
2. They have very little subcutaneous fat to use for fuel and maintenance of body temperature.
3. Their bones are poorly calcified.
4. Their digestive and absorptive abilities, as well as renal function, are limited.
5. Their neuromuscular systems are incompletely developed, making normal sucking mechanisms weak.
6. Their livers are immature and thus lack developed enzyme systems or adequate iron stores.

Food and Feeding

Throughout the neonatal period and for many weeks afterward, optimum nutrition is crucial for the infant's survival and sound growth and development. If these "tiniest babies" are to survive, they require special feeding. Consideration has to be given to the type of milk and to the methods of feeding used.

The length of gestation and adequacy of intrauterine growth may alter the infant's nutrient needs and selection of the most effective feeding method. Premature infants generally require 120 kcal/kg per day to achieve satisfactory weight gain; some infants, due to intrauterine growth retardation or respiratory illness, may have even higher energy needs. A range of protein intake, from 3.5 to 4 g/kg per day is recommended to allow for tissue growth without the complication of protein overload. Whey-predominant milk is recommended because preterm infants lack the enzymes to oxidize certain amino acids found in higher quantities in casein (Anderson, 1987).

Type of Milk

Neonatologists disagree about whether to feed breast milk or formula to preterm or SGA infants. Breast milk has certain advantages. It is empirically safe, since potentially toxic metabolic disturbances are unlikely, and it has the advantage of being biologically compatible if produced by the infant's own mother. In addition, use of breast milk contributes greatly to the mother's involvement in the care of her infant at a critical time in the establishment of important mother–infant bonding. Current studies indicate that milk from mothers of full-term infants is inappropriate for preterm infants (Gross, 1983). However, studies have shown that milk produced by mothers of preterm infants may be better suited to the needs of the tiny infant, since in comparison to full-term milk it has a higher protein and mineral content, and its fat is more digestible (Brooke, 1983). Preterm infants, however, show improved growth when fed with special preterm formulas or with fortified preterm milk. Two supplements are presently available to add to human milk: Human Milk Fortifier (Mead Johnson) and Natural Care (Ross Laboratories) (Kennaugh and Hay, 1987; see Fig. 28–4).

Mothers who wish to breastfeed require education and emotional support from the health care team. Although she may not be able to provide for all of her infant's nutritional needs as she might like, the mother should be reassured that she is doing a wonderful job of providing for her infant (Anderson, 1987).

For a variety of reasons a large number of preterm infants receive special formulas at some stage of their development. Several newer commercial formulas in wide use have demonstrated that they are nutritionally adequate and safe. They are nutrient-dense to allow for small volumes of intake in the face of increased need. Their protein is predominantly whey protein. Some of the carbohydrate is supplied in the form of glucose polymers to decrease the osmolality and reduce the lactose load. Medium-chain triglycerides (MCT) are added to facilitate the absorption of calories, protein, and calcium (Anderson, 1987). When these formulas are used appropriately for individual need, they support growth at intrauterine rates (Brady et al., 1982). The special formulas include Enfamil Premature Formula with Whey, Similac Special Care, and "Premie" SMA. Soy formulas are not recommended because their protein composition does not meet the growth needs of the preterm infant, and because phytates contained in the formula bind calcium and phosphorus, making these vital minerals unavailable to the infant (Anderson, 1987).

Methods of Feeding

Initial feeding difficulties are encountered with very small infants, and decisions concerning the method of feeding will vary according to the condition of the individual infant.

Parenteral feeding is frequently the main source of nutrition for the first few days of the preterm infant's life. The major goal is to provide enough fluids, electrolytes, and glucose for maintenance. The focus then shifts to growth, and protein, fat, vitamins, and minerals will be added to the intravenous solution. Parenteral feedings are slowly decreased and enteral feedings increase (Anderson, 1987).

Premature infants have been fed by tube for several weeks after birth. Considerable controversy exists regarding the best placement and timing of tube feedings. Feedings may be supplied via the nasogastric, orogastric, nasoduodenal, or nasojejunal routes. Many clinicians prefer orogastric feedings because most preterm newborns are nose-breathers. Transpyloric feedings are associated with higher complication rates than gastric feedings, but they may be indicated if the infant has a delayed gastric emptying time, has severe reflux, or is receiving continuous positive airway pressure (CPAP). Debate also occurs over gavage (intermittent gastric bolus) or continuous gastric feeding. Clearly, more research is needed in this area (Pereira and Barbarosa, 1986).

Total parenteral nutrition (TPN) with central line placement is usually reserved for infants who will be unable to receive enteral feedings for a long period of time. Though not without complications, total parental nutrition may be the feeding method of choice in the case of infants with gastrointestinal abnormalities, infants who require bowel rest due to short bowel syndrome or necrotizing enterocolitis (NEC), and infants with severe respiratory disease who cannot tolerate enteral feeding. Nutrient requirements are altered somewhat with parenteral nutrition, and the infant must be monitored closely for imbalances (Anderson, 1987).

For some infants, bottle feeding, using either an appropriate special preterm formula or the mother's preterm breast milk, may work quite well.

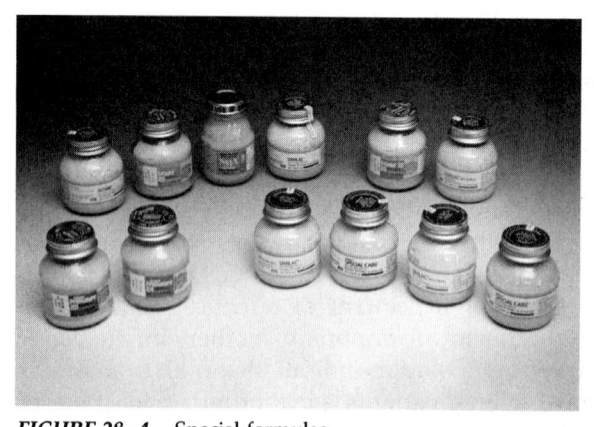

FIGURE 28–4. Special formulas available for infants.

Workers have found that SGA infants can sustain regular weight gain through bottle feedings if they are generally healthy and weighed between 1800 and 2500 g at birth. Also, these premature infants apparently can thrive on a modified demand feeding schedule.

Studies have found that mothers of low-birth-weight infants may tend to be more active during feedings, and that in response the infants eat less, possibly because the activities are tiring for the infants. The perception that their infants are "at risk" may lead these mothers to increase their attempts to promote food intake, through jiggling the nipple or the infant and forcing the nipple into the infant's mouth (Satter, 1986). Mothers of tiny infants may need special guidance in learning to trust their infants' feeding cues.

As the premature infant grows older, parents will need reminding that their "4-month-old" infant who was born 2 months premature is physiologically a 2-month-old, presenting the tongue-thrust reflex that is a sign of lack of preparedness for spoon feedings. Thus, recommendations for continued infant feeding must be made on the basis of the individual infant's physiologic, or "corrected," age rather than on the chronologic age (Ernst et al., 1983).

In summary, general trends in current use in feeding premature infants include:

1. More bottle feeding and breastfeeding to avoid potential hazards of tube feeding, following brief initial use of intravenous feeding.
2. On-demand oral feeding to prevent overfeeding or underfeeding and to reduce health care costs in hospital nurseries.
3. At-home feeding practices based on "corrected" chronologic age rather than "birth" age, delaying the start of solid foods until at least "corrected" age 4 months, cow's milk until "corrected" age 6 months or more, and low-fat milk (if used at all) until at least "corrected" age 2 years (Gibson and DeWolfe, 1981; Ernst et al., 1983).

Nutrient Supplements

Because of the increased demands of a more rapid growth rate and less complete intestinal absorption, preterm infants require proportionately greater amounts of key nutrients. Thus, the American Academy of Pediatrics (1980) recommends that during the first few weeks of life, before the infant is able to consume about 300 kcal/day or reach a body weight of 2.5 kg, it receive a multivitamin supplement providing the equivalent of the Recommended Dietary Allowances (RDA) for full-term infants. This supplement should include vitamin E in an easily absorbed form, since preterm formulas usually include more polyunsaturated fatty acids and iron, both of which require additional vitamin E for antioxidation protection. Also, because folic acid deficiency has been reported in some preterm infants, this vitamin should be included in the supplement. (Folic acid is not included in liquid multivitamin mixes because of its lack of stability, and will need to be added in the hospital pharmacy preparation.) Iron supplementation is best delayed until after the first few weeks of life because extra iron may predispose to anemia when there is insufficient absorption of vitamin E. Neonatal iron stores are usually sufficient during this period of time.

After several weeks, when the infant is consuming more than 300 kcal/day or when the body weight exceeds 2.5 kg, the multivitamin supplement is no longer needed; nevertheless, it is a convenient method for providing a few specific nutrients, such as vitamin D, iron, and folic acid, that may still be required.

INFANT NUTRITIONAL THERAPY NEEDS

Quality patient care focuses on two main factors: (1) determining the particular needs of the individual patient, and (2) planning wise care to meet those needs. This is especially true when infants are ill. These small patients cannot communicate with us through language, so we need to make special observations and relate to them and their parents in a supportive manner that facilitates teamwork. Ill children require not only physical care but much emotional support as well as sound nutritional support for healing and continued growth maintenance. Food and its nutrients are essential to physical and emotional recovery from illness. The biochemical base of health and recovery functions at the tissue level through the mediums of many chemical nutrients and their metabolic interactions. Whether delivery is through regular oral feeding or an intravenous or tube route, these nutrients essential to life and growth must be obtained. This nutrient delivery requires careful planning and attention to special needs.

Planning Nutritional Care

Using the nutritional assessment methods described earlier in this chapter, the nurse and nutritionist must gather information about the infant's nutritional status and food patterns. Close observations of food and fluid intake are necessary; these observations should be carefully recorded for analysis by the health care team. The ill infant's physical growth and psychosocial development require careful monitoring.

An initial exploration of the needs of the infant must also center upon any necessary diet modifications required by the illness. What is the illness? Is it long- or short-term? Is it a simple disorder or is it serious or even terminal? Does it require any modification in food texture, nutrient content, or mode of feeding? Does it hinder eating ability in any way? Have all of these needs been discussed with the health care team?

Throughout the assessment and care of an ill infant, close family involvement is necessary. Home care of the infant provides helpful background for planning nutritional care during a period of hospitalization for illness or for investigation of physical needs. If the infant requires any special diet modifications, they must be discussed with the parents, and ways of meeting these adjustments must be explored in relation to family eating patterns in order to meet continuing needs after hospitalization. Parents also need an opportunity to express their anxieties about the infant. Practitioners can provide support and guidance while educating parents about normal growth and development needs of their infant as well as those imposed by the illness.

Special Infant Needs

Low Birth Weight

As indicated earlier, over the past decade tremendous progress has been made in the care of low-birth-weight infants. Improved nutritional management and feeding techniques, together with other aspects of care such as attention to respiratory and environmental needs, have produced an increase in survival rate from 10 percent or less in 1970 to about 90 percent in 1980 (Brady et al., 1983; Paige, 1983). Some of these small babies may do well on breast milk, if it is the mother's own premature milk especially adapted for the infant's stage of development. However, many infants require and thrive on one of the special newly developed commercial formulas (see Table 28–3). Tube feeding or parenteral nutritional support may be used. Some low-birth-weight infants are started on regular-strength formulas (67 kcal/dl), building up to earlier use of a higher-energy special premature infant formula (80 kcal/dl).

Failure to Thrive

Sometimes pediatricians use a brief period of hospitalization to investigate and classify infants who fail to thrive normally. The general term *failure to thrive* has been used to describe any infant or older child who does not measure up to usual growth and development standards. Fomon (1974) defines children at risk as those having:

> a rate of gain in length and/or weight less than the value corresponding to two standard deviations below the mean during an interval of at least 56 days for infants less than 5 months of age and during an interval of at least 3 months for older infants.

During the period of hospitalized investigation, the nurse and the nutritionist play important roles, providing necessary nutrition assessment to help identify underlying causes of feeding problems.

A number of factors may be involved in failure to thrive:

1. *Neuromotor problems.* There may be problems associated with poor sucking ability, retention of primitive reflexes that should have diminished at an earlier age, or abnormal postural tone during feeding. In some cases, the problems with eating, chewing, and swallowing may be so severe as to compromise the infant's nutrient intake.
2. *Dietary practices.* Some infants may have had inappropriate formula feeding because of improper dilutions in mixing or other practices that result in an inadequate caloric intake. For example, cases of iatrogenic kwashiorkor were observed in California from the use of nondairy creamers, rather than milk, for infant formula preparations (Report: Iatrogenic kwashiorkor in California, 1981).
3. *Clinical disease.* The presence of a central nervous system disorder, endocrine disease, congenital defect, or partial intestinal obstruction may contribute to limited food intake.
4. *Nutrient losses or unusual needs.* Some infants receive a diet insufficient for growth promotion because of inadequate nutrient absorp-

tion and therefore excessive fecal loss. In other cases a hypermetabolic state resulting from underlying disease may create an increased caloric need that is not being met.
5. *Psychosocial problems.* Early feeding problems during infancy may be the result of psychosocial factors within the family. This may be especially true during the later part of infancy when a mixed diet is begun and food rejection by the infant occurs during the learning stage. Milk intake may be erratic and reduced, and the infant may be uninterested in many of the new foods offered. In most cases, these behaviors are normal and transient, but in some disturbed parent–child relationships they may become exaggerated.

The full rehabilitation of infants who fail to thrive requires not only careful and optimal nutritional support but sensitive correction of social and environmental factors surrounding the problem. Often failure to thrive results from a complex of factors with no easy solution. Thus, careful history taking and supportive nutritional guidance throughout, together with warm, sensitive care, are necessary to influence normal growth patterns.

Gastrointestinal Problems

Simple functional vomiting – regurgitation or "spitting up" – is common in young infants. It is usually due to gastric distention from overfeeding or air swallowing during feeding, or from extended crying. The infant may not have had effective burping or may have been left in a supine rather than a prone position after feeding. Also, feedings that are too hot may induce vomiting. Milk at room temperature is ideal, and even cold feedings usually cause no difficulty.

Sometimes simple physiologic constipation may occur in ill or hospitalized infants, usually resulting from the stress of separation from the usual home and family environment or from changes in feeding patterns. Such constipation is usually corrected by reducing the milk intake somewhat, increasing the carbohydrate intake, increasing the intake of fruits and vegetables in older infants, and increasing the water intake. Other functional problems may include so-called "infantile colic." This continuous crying is not uncommon in newborns and seldom lasts beyond the third month of life. It is more common in first-born infants and seldom occurs in subsequent siblings. Parents may require counseling and attention from the supportive health care team (see Chapter 21).

Diarrhea in infants, especially if prolonged and associated with infection, can become a critical medical emergency. Fluid and electrolyte reserves may be rapidly depleted because of the infant's relatively high body water content and large area of intestinal mucosa in proportion to body surface area. Pediatricians have usually relied on intravenous feedings of fluid and electrolytes and have withheld oral feedings. However, recent studies have revealed that oral rehydration therapy with earlier solid feedings achieves successful results with no intravenous therapy in infants 3 months of age and older (Santosham et al., 1982). According to these studies, glucose-electrolyte oral solutions can completely replace intravenous fluids in the majority of generally well-nourished children. This regimen has proved successful as a means of treating acute infant diarrhea in both sophisticated and sanitized medical centers of the Western world and rural areas in other countries. In fact, Panamanian children used in this study for comparison received not only oral rehydration therapy but also critical kilocalories within a few hours in the form of rice, bananas, and apple sauce (Santosham et al., 1982; Carpenter, 1982).

Zinc depletion has also been observed in infants with chronic diarrhea, manifested by an acrodermatitis-like skin rash and low serum alkaline phosphatase levels (Rothbaum, Maur, and Farrell, 1982). This deficiency is corrected with an increased zinc supplementation of 200–300 µg/kg per day. A primary concern with infant diarrhea, as well as with other general gastrointestinal problems, is preventing malnutrition and ensuring appropriate growth progress.

Conditions Requiring Special Formulas

A number of conditions screened at birth or manifested in early infancy require special formulas because of intolerance to cow's milk or human milk. These conditions include genetic disease and allergy.

Genetic Disease

In cases of inborn errors of metabolism, the infant is unable to metabolize specific nutrients and hence these nutrients must be excluded or adjusted in the feeding plan. Two such conditions serve as examples here: phenylketonuria and galactosemia.

PHENYLKETONURIA (PKU). This condition results from a defective gene controlling the synthesis of the liver enzyme phenylalanine hydroxylase, which oxidizes *phenylalanine*, an essential amino acid, to *tyrosine*, another amino acid. When the controlling enzyme is missing, the reaction cannot proceed normally, phenylalanine accumulates in the blood, and its alternative metabolites, the phenyl acids, are excreted in the urine. One of these acids, *phenylpyruvic acid*, is a phenylketone – hence the name *phenylketonuria*.

Mandatory screening of all newborns detects PKU infants at birth so that a low-phenylalanine diet may be initiated immediately to avoid the profound effects of mental retardation that can occur in uncontrolled PKU as the infant grows older. Dietary management is built on two basic components:

1. *Breast milk or a special milk substitute formula.* Breast milk has relatively low levels of phenylalanine; total or partial breastfeeding can be encouraged as long as the infant's phenyalanine levels are closely monitored (Berger, 1981). Special milk-substitute formulas are available for the PKU infant. In the United States, the formula is usually made from Lofenalac, a special casein hydrolysate product balanced with carbohydrates, fats, vitamins, and minerals. One measure of Lofenalac powder in 60 ml (2 oz) of water makes a formula of 20 kcal/30 ml (1 oz) that is well accepted by the infant. A small calculated measure of milk, usually evaporated milk, is added to the Lofenalac formula to adjust the phenylalanine content according to individual need (Acosta and Wenz, 1978). Another product, Milupa, a European formula now marketed in the United States, is made up of a mixture of amino acids excluding phenylalanine. It is useful with older infants, allowing a greater variety of other foods to supply the limited phenylalanine allowance in the diet.
2. *An expanded low-phenylalanine diet.* During the second half of the infant year, solid foods are added to the diet as calculated according to their phenylalanine content. These food additions are selected from a list of low-phenylalanine food exchange groups or equivalents (Schuett, 1981). Sensitive family counseling and instruction are required for good control.

Studies have indicated that the dietary control of PKU during the first year of life is directly related to three factors: (1) the parents' understanding of the diet; (2) the appropriateness of the dietary prescriptioin to the needs of the individual infant; and (3) the frequency of infection (Acosta, Wenz, and Williamson, 1978). On the metabolic clinical care team, the physician, nutritionist, and nurse carry primary responsibilities, with supportive care from social services and various behavioral therapists as needed. In many places, wise and experienced parents have formed parents' groups and work with the medical care team to provide initial and continuing care so that the PKU infant grows and develops normally.

GALACTOSEMIA. This genetic disease is also caused by a missing enzyme, in this case affecting carbohydrate metabolism. The missing enzyme, *galactose-1-phosphate uridyl transferase* (G-1-PUT), is one of the three enzymes controlling steps in the conversion of galactose to glucose; thus, regular milk cannot be used and all forms of milk and lactose must be removed from the diet. In this galactose-free diet a milk-substitute formula, usually with a soy base, is used. Such formulas are complete protein hydrolysate products free of galactose. They include Nutramigen, Isomil, Neomullsoy, Prosobee, Soyalac, and meat-based formulas. Breastfeeding, of course, cannot be used. In the latter half of the infant year solid foods added to the infant's diet must be selected from those containing no lactose.

Food Allergy

The term *food allergy* should be used only for food intolerance or hypersensitivity caused by a normal immunologic reaction to specific constituents of food or their digestive products. Thus, food allergy is distinct from food intolerances caused by non-immunologic mechanisms, such as cow's milk intolerance due to lactase deficiency.

The care of an allergic infant is often frustrating and formidable because a wide variety of environmental, emotional, and physical factors influence the infant's reaction, and an appropriate dietary regimen is sometimes difficult to find. Sensitivity to protein substances is a common basis of food allergy, so the early foods of infants are frequent offenders.

Cow's milk has long been a common cause of allergic disease in young infants. It usually brings on gastrointestinal difficulties such as vomiting and diarrhea in sensitive infants. Soybean formulas have frequently been used as substitutes for cow's-milk formulas. However, the Committee on Nutrition of the American Academy of Pediatrics (1981) has recommended against routine use of soy formulas in the management of cow's milk allergy. Since cow's milk allergy can cause small bowel damage which may lead to an increased uptake and immunologic response to otherwise non-allergenic proteins, a protein hydrolysate formula is recommended. If symptoms subside on the milk-free formula, a trial on milk may follow to determine whether it does indeed cause the symptoms to reappear. Only then is the diagnosis of milk allergy well established. Other symptoms, such as skin problems or respiratory difficulties, may also result from milk allergy.

In the second half of the infant year when solid food additions are made, certain foods are delayed because they have been shown to be frequent allergens in sensitive infants. These foods include wheat, egg white, and citrus fruits. As the food choices in the infant's diet are expanded one by one, a given food can be identified as an offending substance and eliminated from use for the time being. As the infant grows older, the allergic reaction to the given food may wane, and the food may be gradually reinstated in the diet.

The education of the parents and family of an allergic infant should include a knowledge and understanding of the allergic state and the many factors that influence it. Guidance should be provided in the substitution of special food products and the use of special recipes that can be provided for the infant's mother.

SUMMARY

The first year of an infant's life is a time of rapid growth. Physiologic growth is dependent on the nutrients in the food the child eats. However, growth and development involve far more than the physical process. It encompasses social and psychologic influences and relationships, the whole of the environment and culture that nurtures the individual growth potential. Nutritional resources to meet physical growth are conditioned by the food habits and feeding practices that are psychosocially and culturally derived. The nurse plays a vital role in early nutritional assessment and in implementing growth and development needs that will enable the infant to arrive at his or her maximum potential in the adult years.

REFERENCES

Acosta, P. B., and Wenz, E. 1978. *Diet management of PKU for infants and preschool children.* DHEW Pub. No. HSA 78-5209. Washington, D.C.: U.S. Government Printing Office.

Acosta, P. B.; Wenz, E.; and Williamson, M. 1978. Methods of dietary inception in infants with PKU. *J. Am. Diet. Assoc.* 72(2):164.

American Academy of Pediatrics, Committee on Nutrition. 1976. Commentary on breastfeeding and infant formulas, including proposed standards for formulas. *Pediatrics.* 57:278.

American Academy of Pediatrics, Committee on Nutrition. 1979. Fluoride supplementation: Revised dosage schedule. *Pediatrics.* 63:150.

American Academy of Pediatrics, Committee on Nutrition. 1980. Vitamin and mineral supplement needs of normal children in the United States. *Pediatrics.* 66(6):1015.

American Academy of Pediatrics, Committee on Nutrition. 1983. Soy-protein formulas: Recommendations for use in infant feeding. *Pediatrics.* 72(3):359–363.

Anderson, D. M. 1987. Nutrition care for the premature infant. *Top. Clin. Nutr.* 2(1):1–9.

Anderson, S. A.; Chinn, H. I.; and Fisher, K. D. 1982. History and current status of infant formulas. *Am. J. Clin. Nutr.* 35(2):381.

Barness, L. A. 1987. History of infant feeding practices. *Am. J. Clin. Nutr.* 46:168–70.

Berger, L. R. 1981. When should one discourage breastfeeding. *Pediatrics.* 67(2):300–302.

Bergevin, V.; Dougherty, C.; and Kramer, M. S. 1983. Do infant formula samples shorten the duration of breastfeeding? *Lancet.* 1(8334):1148.

Brady, M. S.; Rickard, K. A.; Ernst, J. A.; Schreiner, R. L.; and Lemons, J. A. 1982. Formulas and human milk for premature infants: A review and update. *J. Am. Diet. Assoc.* 81(5):547.

Brooke, O. G. 1983. Nutrition in the preterm infant. *Lancet.* 1(8323):514.

Carpenter, C. C. J. 1982. Oral rehydration: Is it as good as parenteral therapy? *New Engl. J. Med.* 306:1103.

Cooper, A., and Heird, W. C. 1982. Nutritional assessment of the pediatric patient including the low-birth-weight infant. *Am. J. Clin. Nutr.* 35(5):1132.

Erikson, E. 1963. *Childhood and society.* New York: W. W. Norton.

Ernest, A. E.; McCabe, E. R. B.; Neifert, M. R.; and O'Flynn, M. E. 1980. *Guide to breastfeeding the infant with PKU.* DHHS Pub. No HSA 79-5110. Washington, D.C.: U.S. Government Printing Office.

Ernst, J. A., et al. 1983. Feeding practices of the very low-birth-weight infant within the first year. *J. Am. Diet. Assoc.* 82(2):158.

Fomon, S. J. 1974. *Infant nutrition.* Philadelphia: W. B. Saunders.

Gibson, R. S., and DeWolfe, M. S. 1981. The food

consumption patterns and nutrient intakes of some Canadian low-birth-weight infants during the first twelve months of infancy. *Can. J. Pub. Health.* 72(4):273.

Gross, S. J. 1983. Growth and biochemical response of preterm infants fed human milk or modified infant formula. *New Engl. J. Med.* 308(5):237.

Hall, E. 1983. A conversation with Erik Erikson. *Psych. Today.* 17(6):22.

Hamill, P. V., et al. 1979. Physical growth: National Center for Health Statistics percentiles. *Am. J. Clin. Nutr.* 32:607.

Kennaugh, J. M., and Hay, W. W. 1987. Nutrition of the fetus and newborn. *West. J. Med.* 147(4):435–448.

Lambert-Lagace, L. 1983. *Feeding your child.* New York: Beaufort Books.

Martinez, G. A., and Nalezienski, J. P. 1979. The recent trend in breastfeeding. *Pediatrics.* 64:686.

Miller, J. A. 1983a. The littlest babies. *Science News.* 124(16):250.

Miller, J. A. 1983b. Small-baby biology. *Science News.* 124(17):266.

Murray, C. A., and Glassman, M. S. 1982. Nutrient requirements during growth and recovery from failure to thrive. In *Failure to thrive in infancy and early childhood: A multidisciplinary team approach,* ed. P. J. Accardo. Baltimore: University Park Press.

Paige, D. M., ed. 1983. *Manual of clinical nutrition.* Pleasantville, N. J.: Nutrition Publications.

Pereira, G. R., and Barbosa, N. M. M. 1986. Controversies in neonatal nutrition. *Pediatr. Clin. North Am.* 33(1):65–89.

Pipes, P. L. 1985. *Nutrition in infancy and childhood.* 3rd ed. St. Louis: C. V. Mosby.

Radbill, S. X. 1981. Infant feeding through the ages. *Clin. Pediatr.* 20(10):613–621.

Report: Iatrogenic kwashiorkor in California. 1981. *Nutr. Rev.* 39(11):397.

Report: Perils of cow's milk. 1983. *Nutrition and the MD.* 9(5):3.

Rothbaum, R. J.; Maur, R. P.; and Farrell, M. K. 1982. Serum alkaline phosphatase and zinc undernutrition in infants with chronic diarrhea. *Am. J. Clin. Nutr.* 35:595.

Roy, S., III. 1983. Perspectives on adverse effects of milks and infant formulas used in infant feeding. *J. Am. Diet. Assoc.* 82(4):373.

Santosham, M., et al. 1982. Oral rehydration therapy of infantile diarrhea: A controlled study of well-nourished children hospitalized in the United States and Panama. *New Engl. J. Med.* 306:1070.

Satter, E. M. 1986. The feeding relationship. *J. Am. Diet. Assoc.* 86(3):352–356.

Schuett, V. E. 1981. *Low protein food list.* Madison: University of Wisconsin.

Simopoulos, A. P., and Grave, G. D. 1984. Factors associated with the choice and duration of infant feeding practice. *Pediatrics.* 74(Suppl.):603–614.

Smith A. E., and Klotz, R. 1982. Use of a nutritional products formulary as a patient care and cost-containment tool in a pediatric hospital. *Nutr. Support Services.* 2(10):6.

Stuart, H. C., and Meredith, H. V. 1948. Use of body measurements in the school health program. *Am. J. Pub. Health.* 36:1365.

Sunshine, P. 1983. Advantages of breastfeeding in infant nutrition. *Nutrition and the MD.* 9(5):1.

Suskind, R. M., ed. 1981. *Textbook of pediatric nutrition.* New York: Raven Press.

US Department of Health and Human Services. 1981. *A guide to pediatric weighing and measuring.* DHSS Publication No. 740-010/4557. Washington, D.C.: US Government Printing Office.

Ziegler, E. E.; Biga, R. L.; and Fomon, S. J. 1981. Nutritional requirements of the premature infant. In *Textbook of pediatric nutrition,* ed. R. M. Suskind. New York: Raven Press.

29

Infant Attachment and Stimulation

BEHAVIORAL OBJECTIVES

Upon completion of this chapter, the reader should be able to:

- Define infant attachment and its role in the parent–infant relationship.

- Discuss past hospital practices that interfered with infant attachment and identify present hospital practices that help to promote this attachment.

- Describe the pattern of behavior that occurs when a mother first becomes "acquainted" with her infant.

- List those factors that have been found to influence parent–infant attachment.

- Discuss differences between parent–infant attachment of a term infant and of a premature infant.

- Discuss sensorimotor intelligence of the newborn, including assimilation and accommodation.

- Discuss the sensory status of the newborn and its effect on the process of developing social interaction.

- Name the key factors to be included in an infant stimulation program.

■ Discuss the nurse's role in educating parents about their infant's ability to interact.

It has long been known that babies require touching, cuddling, and loving attention if they are to thrive. This close contact may be as important to the parents' well-being as to the infant's. There are certain processes parents and their newborn go through during the first few hours and days of life that may be the key to how well the parents will respond to their infant later in their lives and how well the infant will in turn respond to the parents (Clark and Affonso, 1976). The importance of interaction between parents and their infant during the first few weeks is significant (Rubin, 1963; Klaus et al., 1970, 1972; Salk, 1970; Klaus and Kennell, 1982). Delay in initiation of the parent–infant relationship, especially beyond the first 24 hours, can create an environment in which a maladaptive parent–infant relationship can develop. Such an environment can affect both the infant's and parents' future growth and development, and so can ultimately affect society. The goal should be to prevent maladaptation and send confident, content parents home with their thriving infant. In order to attain this goal, it is important for the nurse to understand parent–infant attachment. *Attachment* is a bond that develops between the parents and their infant. A *bond* can be defined as a unique and special type of relationship between two people that is specific and endures over time. The parents' bond to their infant may be the strongest of all human ties. It is the power of this attachment that enables the parents to make the unusual sacrifices necessary in caring for their infant day after day, night after night: changing diapers, attending to crying, protecting from danger, and giving feedings in the middle of the night regardless of how tired they are (Klaus and Kennell, 1982).

Maternal attachment is evaluated in terms of such attachment behaviors as fondling, gazing, kissing, holding close, and looking *en face* (Fig. 29–1). However, these behaviors correspond to behaviors that might be called "affectionate" in contemporary Western society and do not necessarily have equal importance in other cultures (Goldberg, 1972). Variations in attitudes and behaviors that may result from cultural influences need to be carefully understood (see Chapter 6).

Childbirth is an emotional and immeasurably complex event, and the experience means a great deal to the individuals involved, both at the time of birth and later (Macfarlane, 1977). Influences on

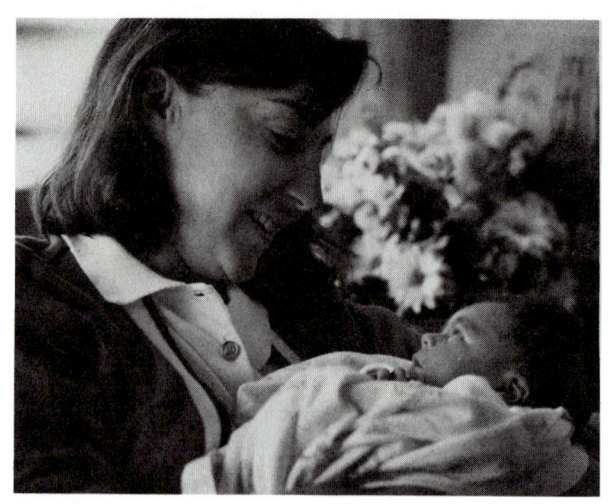

FIGURE 29–1. En face is a behavior that bonds mother and infant.

the outcome of a pregnancy and delivery begin at the time the mother herself is conceived. The genes the mother inherits from her parents, her own development inside the uterus with all its complex changes, the hazards of her own delivery, her social and biologic experiences during infancy, childhood, and adolescence – all form a basis for her mental and physical health as an adult (Macfarlane, 1977). Many other factors as well, such as where she lives, the people she grows up with, and her social and economic status, affect the mother's experience of giving birth and bringing up her own children (Macfarlane, 1977). There are no rights and wrongs in childbearing, just differences. Until these differences are fully understood, all behavior should be considered meaningful and should not be ridiculed or ignored (Clark, Affonso, and Harris, 1979). Knowledge about maternal behavior in animals and how it relates to human maternal behavior also contributes to our understanding of parent–infant attachment.

MATERNAL BEHAVIOR IN ANIMALS

Several different kinds of animals have been studied to facilitate a more focused approach to the problem of experimenting with different factors involved in parent–infant relationships and the effects of each of them. This research is done not to explain human behavior but rather to view human beings within the context of species-specific behavior (Klaus and Kennell, 1982). The requirements of caring for the young seem to have led to the existence of similar maternal behaviors in humans and other animals.

The evolutionary importance of certain reproductive changes in mammals (internal fertilization, the development of the amniotic egg, and the development of the placenta) has been described by Kaufman (1970). He states that, of equal significance, mammals also evolved a behavior program of reproductive economy, i.e. a higher order of parental care of the young after birth, without which the human species could not have evolved as it has. Care of the very young was already evolved in fish, reptiles, and especially birds, but what made possible the tremendous advance in mammals was the system of feeding the infant, through special glands, a substance (milk) that contains everything needed for growth and development. It is the improved feeding arrangement that keeps the young physically close to the mother and safer from harm.

Of particular importance is that the close physical relationship and the shared personal experience of mammary feeding constitute a degree of contact and intimacy that creates a new kind of bond, one with durable characteristics. Rheingold (1963) and Rosenblatt (1975) both noted the development of this new kind of *affectional bond* in mammals. Rheingold (1963) found that the first stage of attachment is primarily a stage of close mother–infant contact. In his studies with rats, Rosenblatt (1975) found that prepartum maternal behavior is hormonally determined. After parturition, however, it appears to be regulated chiefly by stimuli from the pups. Maternal behavior in the rat consists of four principal components: nursing or crouching over the young, retrieving pups to the nest, body and genital licking of pups, and nest building. The size of the litter, age of pups, amount of externally induced stress, and other factors can affect the mother–infant interaction. A period of special vulnerability to disruption of the mother–infant relationship shortly after parturition corresponds to the period of transition from hormonal to nonhormonal regulation of maternal behavior.

In lower primates the infant clings to its mother, but in higher primates, such as the gorilla and human being, the infant is unable to cling, so the mother must carry the baby. In these more advanced species the mother plays a more important role in maintaining contact with the infant, and the infant's survival is dependent on the mother's attachment (Trause, Klaus, and Kennell, 1982).

Detailed observations of various animal species have shown that there are species-specific patterns of parturitive behavior (see Table 29–1).

HUMAN MATERNAL ATTACHMENT BEHAVIOR

Development of the Attachment Process

The process of maternal–infant attachment is an involved one that begins with pregnancy but is formulated prior to the actual pregnancy. Pregnancy is a developmental task of a woman's life through which the woman can attain motherhood. Pregnancy is well recognized as a time of normal psychologic turmoil, and much of the turmoil is centered around the mother–infant relationship (Bibring, Dwyer, and Huntington, 1961; Brazelton, 1963). Pregnancy involves four psychologic tasks:

1. Accepting the fact of pregnancy;
2. Believing the existence of the baby;
3. Visualizing the baby; and,
4. Preparing oneself to mother the child (Shields, 1974).

These tasks are usually not completed until months or even years after delivery. However, the role change is stabilized once a woman identifies herself as someone's mother (see Chapter 11). This identification process may be affected by factors present prior to the actual pregnancy. According to Klaus and Kennell (1982), certain determinants – the mother's care by her own mother, endowment or genetics of the mother, practices of culture, relations with family and husband, experiences with previous pregnancies, and the planning and events during pregnancy – are ingrained and unchangeable. The events occurring after birth, which involve the psychologic tasks of the mother of visualizing her baby and preparing herself to mother the child, are also important in the formation of a mother's attachment to her infant; however, these can be altered by such factors as behavior and attitudes of doctors, nurses, and hospital personnel; whether or not there is separation from the infant during the first days of life; practices of the hospital; the nature and temperament of the infant; and whether the baby is healthy, sick, or malformed (Klaus and Kennell, 1982).

Klaus and Kennell further believe that a mother can elicit certain behaviors from her infant. These behaviors include eye-to-eye contact; cry; initiation in secretion of oxytocin, and an increase in prolactin levels if breastfeeding; odor; and entrainment. By *entrainment* is meant that when in a quiet, alert state, the infant moves in rhythm with the moth-

TABLE 29–1. *Species-specific Mothering Behaviors*

Animal	Preparation for Birth	Birth Site	Birth	Protection of Young	Nursing	Stimulation of Young	Other Observations
Domestic cat	Genital licking	Warm, dark place	Licks self, young, and floor of birth site; eats placenta	Retrieves vocalizing young	Initiates by presenting; begins 30 min to 12 hours postpartum	Licking	
Laboratory rat	Builds nest; anogenital licking	Birth nest	Eats placenta	Nests; retrieves; attacks intruders	Drapes herself over litter	Licking	At first somewhat afraid of young
Goat	Separates from herd	Secluded	Self-licking; licks newborn all over	Butts away all intruders; moves toward vocalizing kids	Adjusts position; accepts only own young	Licking	Attempts to steal other young before birth
Sheep	Separates from herd	Domestic: indoor shelter Big horn: inaccessible mountain area	Licks anal areas; licks newborn all over	Moves toward bleating lamb	Adjusts position; accepts only own young	Licking	
Primates North Indian langur				Keeps to herself for first hours		Licking, grooming, manipulating, stroking	Allows other females to hold on first day
Rhesus monkey	Explores genitals; removes mucus manually	Floor of cage or metal bar	Squats; pulls fetus forward; eats placenta; licks young	Holds young close, cradles, avoids others for a long time; retrieves and restrains		Grooming	
Chimpanzee	Moves away from herd		Carries placenta by umbilical cord	Stays away from group for several days; 5 months before allows others to touch			

SOURCE: Trause, Klaus, and Kennell (1982).

er's speech. The infant in turn elicits such behaviors from the mother as eye-to-eye contact, high-pitched voice, entrainment, time giver, odor, heat, and T and B lymphocytes, macrophages, and bacterial flora (if breastfeeding), which are important in providing the baby with protection against enteric pathogens.

There is evidence of an early sensitive period in the mother (Salk, 1970; Klaus et al., 1972; Kennell, Trause, and Klaus, 1975; de Chateau, 1977; Lozoff et al., 1977; Klaus and Kennell, 1982) and of an early responsive state of consciousness in the human infant (Desmond, Rudolph, and Phitaksphraiwan, 1966; Brazelton, 1973). This responsive state in the newborn has been identified as a quiet, alert state. Both the early sensitive period in the mother and the quiet, alert state in the infant have been found to occur shortly after birth, before 12 hours in the mother and within 1 hour in the infant. Since both the infant and the mother are responsive to each other in the first hour after birth, it seems that this first hour is the optimal time for an affectional bond to develop. If the father is also present at this time, the role he plays in parent–infant bonding is significant.

Parent–Infant Attachment Behaviors

Every baby is born with a sensitivity to love and touch, and every baby's primary sense organ is its skin. The mothering activity of touch is viewed as an act of feeling something with the body, the important word being *feeling*. Although touch is not in itself an emotion, it induces neural, glandular, muscular, and mental changes that in combination we call emotion (Montagu, 1971). Thus, touch is not experienced physically as sensation but more *affectively* as emotion. Touch is a vital part of the nurturing process. For the mother, maternal touch has many meanings: it is communicative and informative, and it is a form of loving, perhaps the only way a mother can show her newborn infant her love. It can also be an avenue of control over physical and emotional closeness to and distance from the infant. Mothering activities involving close contact include stroking, caressing, patting, and rhythmic motions of the mother's body. Being stroked, caressed, cuddled, and cooed to, the infant develops a feeling of being loved and thus learns to love others (Montagu, 1971) (Fig. 29–2). Maternal touch of the newborn may occur more often than any other maternal behavior, and in its direct relationship to maternal "knowing" of

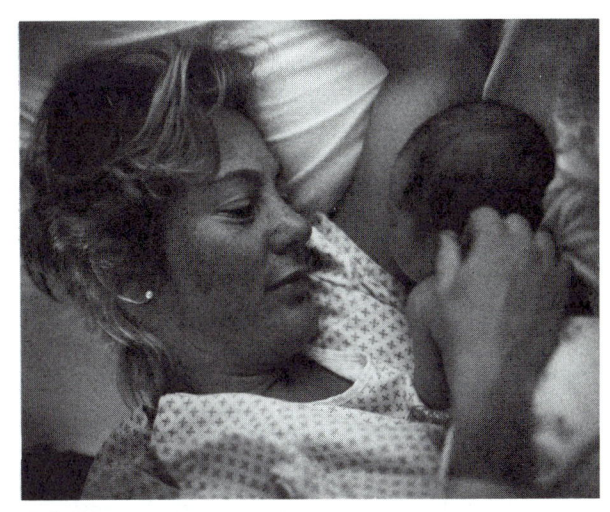

FIGURE 29–2. Being stroked, caressed, cuddled and cooed to brings a sense of being loved to the infant.

the infant, it may reflect progressive attainment of some of the complex developmental tasks of mothering (Dunbar, 1976).

Besides touch, eye-to-eye contact also appears to be important. The role of eye-to-eye contact in maternal–infant attachment has been identified by Robson (1967) as an important variable in nonverbal transactions between a mother and her newborn infant. The eye, in comparison with other parts of the body, has a remarkable array of interesting qualities: (1) it is a shiny globe; (2) it is mobile, while at the same time being fixed in space; and (3) its pupil has the capacity to vary in diameter. These qualities make the mother's eyes a rich stimulus, appealing to the infant and vice versa. The basic and primary activity in the infant's exploration of his environment is his visual contact (Rheingold, 1961). It has been observed that a newborn infant's eyes can fix on and follow a visual object for several minutes within a short period of 1–3 hours immediately after birth (Brazelton, 1973).

Attachment between parents and their infant is the beginning step of a "claiming" process that occurs immediately after birth, in which the parents claim the infant as being theirs. The methods by which the parents claim their infant can be altered by many factors. However, even though not all parents will have the same orderly and predictable pattern of behavior when first examining their newborn, certain rules and expectations of parents have been established. These patterns of behavior were first identified by Rubin (1961) and later further explored by Klaus and his associates (1970) and Macfarlane (1977). The findings of these various studies had a tremendous impact on hospital practices, recommending changes to make the birth process and postpartum experience more humane, less medically managed, and more family involved (Paukert, 1982).

In an effort to identify specific behaviors of a human mother with her infant immediately after delivery, Klaus et al. (1970) conducted a study in which they observed 9 mothers of premature infants on their first three visits to the nursery and 12 mothers of full-term normal infants during the first contact after delivery. All women were well at the time of labor and all were delivered vaginally, with the exception of one of the mothers in the premature group who was delivered by cesarean section. Social and economic status of both groups covered a wide range, and at the time of study all mothers planned to keep their infants. At delivery, all infants were well and free of anomalies. Behavior of the mother and infant was recorded by a time-lapse camera that took a picture every second. The mothers in both groups were aware that they were being photographed. Every fifth frame for the first 10 minutes of each 15-minutes film was analyzed in detail, and the mother's remarks to her infant were on audiotape. The full-term infants and their mothers were filmed by a camera placed 8–10 feet from the foot of the bed, beginning 30 minutes to 13 hours after delivery, with the mean time being 5.3 hours after delivery. The bed was flattened, the infant was nude (with heat being provided by an overhead warmer panel), and the infant's head was placed about 6–8 inches from its mother at the level of her shoulder. All mothers were on their sides, with their "uninteracting" arm to their side (Klaus, personal communication). Within each frame of film, the following activities were looked for and analyzed: movement of the infant; position of the mother's fingertips and palms on the trunk; extremities or head of the infant; and maternal smiling, physical support, and encompassment of the infant. The amount of time spent by the mother in an *en face* position, defined by Robson (1967) as when the mother's face is rotated so that her eyes and those of the infant's meet fully in the same vertical plane of rotation, was also measured.

The findings of the study revealed that each mother went through an "orderly and predictable" pattern of behavior when she first examined her newborn infant. First, the mother touched the hands and feet of the naked baby with her fingertips. Then, within 4–5 minutes, she began to caress and massage the baby's trunk and body with the palms of her hands, showing increasing excitement as she did this. Finally, the mother and the infant established eye-to-eye contact. The examination of the infant by the mother continued for a few minutes and then diminished as the mother dozed off with her naked baby at her side. During the 10 minutes of filming there was a marked increase noted in the time that the mother positioned herself and her baby so that they could look into each other's eyes (if the baby's eyes were open): from 0 to 3 minutes there was a 10 percent total observation time noted in *en face* position, from 3 to 6 minutes, 17 percent, and from 6 to 9 minutes, 23 percent (Klaus et al., 1970).

At the same time that the mother positioned herself and her baby so that they could look into each other's eyes, she showed intense interest in waking her infant in an attempt to get him to open his eyes. This interest was verbalized by almost 75 percent of the other mothers. Some of the verbalizations made by the mothers were: "Open your eyes; oh, come on now, open your eyes," and "If you open your eyes, I'll know you're alive." The behaviors of fingertip touching, palm touching, and eye-to-eye contact were usually accomplished by the mothers of the full-term infants within the first 10 minutes of the initial contact. Rubin (1961) had previously described these specific behaviors, but noted that touching the infant with the palm and close contact developed only after several days; these observations varied from those of Klaus and his associates (1970).

As follow-up work to the study by Klaus et al., Macfarlane (1977) observed 12 mothers and their infants in the delivery rooms of a large maternity hospital immediately after birth, starting from the time the baby's head was delivered, through the infant's being given to the mother and sometimes to the father, to the time the infant was taken away to be washed and weighed. Macfarlane's observations differed in many ways from those of Rubin and of Klaus and his associates. All of the babies in Macfarlane's study were well wrapped, and the only exposed parts were the head and sometimes the hands and feet. He noted that when holding their babies, the mothers spent nearly 75 percent of the time looking at them, and one-third of that time smiling or laughing. Nine of the twelve mothers talked directly to their babies, and on average all mothers spent about 80 percent of the time with both hands supporting or holding the baby, though the variation was large—0–100 percent. Many of the mothers did start by touching the babies with their fingertips, but few progressed to stroking with the palms of the hands and few manipulated the hands and feet. Macfarlane felt that this progression was hampered in most cases because the baby was wrapped up.

Macfarlane found that the time between the delivery and the time the baby was given to the mother to hold was from 1 minute 25 seconds to 9 minutes, with an average for the group of about 3.5 minutes. The delay was attributed to clearing the mouth of the infant and observing the infant to make sure breathing was adequate. The babies were with their mothers for an average of 6.5 minutes, but it varied between 1 and 15.5 minutes.

Like Klaus and his associates, Macfarlane noted the mother's intense interest in the baby's eyes. This was verbalized by the mothers asking their infants to open their eyes while in the *en face* position. Although the *en face* position was identified by Rubin (1961), and also observed by Robson (1967) and Klaus et al. (1970), Goldberg (1972) found in her studies in Zambia that eye-to-eye contact rarely occurs between mother and infant and is not reliably associated with other social interaction. This might raise the question of whether Zambian mothers, who are in constant skin-to-skin contact with their infants (they carry their infants on their backs continuously), are less attached to them than the mothers in the United States because of the absence of the eye-to-eye contact behavior. This possible misinterpretation of the process of maternal-infant attachment comes about because people in the United States seem to rely on face-to-face exchanges with infants more than people in other societies, many of which emphasize reciprocal bodily interactions. As evidenced by the various studies of Rubin (1961), Klaus et al. (1970), Goldberg (1972), and Macfarlane (1977), there are societal differences among the maternal-infant attachment behaviors that occur after delivery. The processes that determine the different characteristics of mother-infant relationships in humans must be defined before maternal behaviors truly representative of the species can be identified.

Infant Attachment and the Premature Infant

The pattern of behavior established by mothers of premature infants differs from what has been observed in mothers of full-term infants. With the full-term infant the mother is found to have a rapid progression from fingertip to palm and encompassing contact within a period of 10 minutes during their first contact. Mothers of premature infants who were studied over their first three contacts (over a period of from 1 to 17 days), exhibited an attenuated sequence of the behavior observed in the mothers of full-term infants during the first contact. The progression from fingertip to palm contact did not occur during the first three contacts. Instead, fingertip contact continued to increase in the second and third contacts. The behavior of the mother of a premature infant is arrested at a stage that is normally quickly passed in the mother of a full-term infant (Klaus et al., 1970).

Although research on parent-infant attachment has focused mainly on the parents of full-term infants, there has been some observation of the ways in which the parent of a premature infant manages to meet the needs of this immature, sleepy, unpredictable, and fragile infant (Klaus and Kennell, 1982).

From the early 1900s through the late 1940s, D. Martin Couney and his staff of skilled nurses cared for premature infants in incubators in exhibit halls (Silverman, 1979). These infants were touched only during feedings and bathing. The infants were fed breast milk from wet nurses through feeding bottles (if they were able to suck), through drops into their mouth, or with a nasal spoon. The parents of these infants were not allowed to care for or even touch their infants; they only visited them and looked through the same viewing windows used by the public. The care of the infant never cost the parents any money, and Dr. Couney was puzzled (and hurt) by what he felt was an inappreciative attitude on the part of parents. Some parents visited their infants infrequently, and when it came time to send the infants home, many parents were reluctant to assume their parental responsibilities (Silverman, 1979).

Even after the first premature nursery opened in New York City at Cornell's New York Hospital in the late 1940s, it was not until 1960 that parents were allowed in the nursery to touch and be with their infants (Silverman, 1979).

The first recorded observations of parental reactions to the birth of a premature infant were made by Prugh in 1953, before parents were allowed to enter the premature nursery. Prugh stressed that it was essential for the mother to see her premature infant as soon as possible to minimize her fears and to assist her in beginning to experience the maternal feelings that she expected but was denied because of not having close contact with her infant. The reactions of mothers of premature infants were viewed as acute reactions to trauma rather than in the context of an ongoing pathologic process.

Four psychologic tasks that the mother of a premature infant must master to establish a healthy mother–infant relationship have been identified (Kaplan and Mason, 1960):

1. At the time of birth the mother must prepare for the possible loss of the infant whose life is in jeopardy. This is known as *anticipatory grief*.
2. The mother must face and acknowledge her maternal failure to give birth to a normal, full-term infant.
3. The mother must resume the process, which has been interrupted, of relating to the infant.
4. The mother must come to understand how a premature infant will differ from a full-term infant in terms of special needs and growth patterns.

A major impetus to the study of parent–infant bonding, particularly with premature infants, occurred when staffs of intensive care nurseries observed that small prematures who were sent home intact and thriving would sometimes return to the emergency rooms failing to thrive or battered by their parents. This was felt to occur, in part, as a result of the separation between the parents and infant at the time of birth (Klaus and Kennell, 1982). As health professionals interested in preventing psychologic disorders in children, nurses should be alert to any signs of stress or failure in the interactional process between an infant and the parents.

THE IMPORTANCE OF INFANT STIMULATION

An infant is born equipped with a number of behavioral systems that are ready to be activated and that can have a significant impact in early life. Each system is already biased to be activated by stimuli falling within one or more broad ranges and is strengthened or weakened by stimuli of other sorts (Bowlby, 1969). Auditory stimuli that arise from the human voice, visual stimuli that arise from the human face, and kinesthetic stimuli that arise from touch are some examples of infant stimulation. All of the stimuli arise from parental behavior. Parental behavior is believed to be learned. Those behaviors that cannot be practiced cannot be learned, and since the infant is wholly dependent on the parents to meet all physical and emotional needs, the strength and durability of the attachment is vital, and parenting behaviors must be practiced.

In the 1960s and 1970s ways were devised to measure what the newborn could see and hear. Electrodes were used to measure the infant's heart rate; sucking strength was recorded by means of pacifiers connected to electronic equipment; and computers interpreted data. Within one decade the obviously incompetent neonate became the "amazing newborn" (Pines, 1982). In the 1980s research has tended to focus on the newborn's ability to process information, with studies conducted on the infant's cognition and ability to understand and remember.

Sensorimotor Intelligence

According to Jean Piaget's theory, cognitive development consists of four stages (see Table 29–2). The first stage is the period of sensorimotor intelligence; it lasts from birth to 2 years of age. An infant first learns about the world through sensory impressions and motor activities. The first stage in the sensorimotor period is the reflex stage. During this stage, usually the first month of life, the infant learns to differentiate between certain stimuli and accommodate to them. According to Piaget, human beings adapt to their world through the interrelated processes of assimilation and accommodation. *Assimilation* is the process through which new information is absorbed from the environment. *Accommodation* is the process through which an individual adjusts to the new information assimilated. Assimilation and accommodation allow infants to integrate new learning with old and thus adapt to their ever-expanding environment (Freiberg, 1983). More complex levels of organization in learning take place as the infant matures and as the brain and nervous system grow and develop.

The concepts of equilibrium and disequilibrium have been introduced by Piaget to help explain cognitive development. *Equilibrium* is a state of relative balance between assimilation and accommodation of environmental stimuli. *Disequilibrium* exists when the balance is upset by new information requiring additional mental effort. As learning takes place, the mind fluctuates between equilibrium and disequilibrium. Stimulus–response learning closely parallels Piaget's theory of equilibrium–disequilibrium. For example, when new

TABLE 29-2. *Piaget's Four Stages of Cognitive Development*

Period	Description	Substages
Sensorimotor period	In which the apparatus of the senses and of the musculature become increasingly operative	Reflexes Primary circular reactions Secondary circular reactions Coordination of secondary schemas Tertiary circular reactions Invention of new means through mental combinations
Preoperational period	In which the child has the emerging ability to think mentally	Preconceptual phase Intuitive phase
Concrete operations period	In which the child learns to reason about what he or she sees and does in the here-and-now world	
Formal operations period	In which people have the ability to see logical relationships among diverse properties and to reason in the abstract	

SOURCE: Freiberg (1983).

information (a stimulus) upsets the equilibrium, new learning accommodation (a response) is required in order to restore the balance (Freiberg, 1983).

Infants are capable of stimulus–response learning. For example, they can anticipate being picked up by associating auditory stimulation with this behavior (Thoman, Korner, and Beason-Williams, 1977). After only a few days of experiencing being placed in a feeding position, newborns have exhibited anticipatory sucking movements, demonstrating classical conditioning (Brazelton, 1981). Research among Navaho and Caucasian newborns has shown a difference in the effects of environment on behavior. When Navaho infants were wrapped and tied onto a cradle board (a practice seen sporadically on reservations), most of them calmly accepted it. Some even showed unrest when they were off and demanded to be put back on. Caucasian infants, on the other hand, resisted loudly (Freedman, 1979).

The more awareness parents have of the competencies of their newborn infant, the more responsive they are to the infant. They need to know that the newborn can discriminate various stimuli and has the ability to be selective. The infant can respond to his or her own mother's odor. The infant prefers bright-colored objects and is selectively attentive to the contour and characteristics of the human face. The baby is selectively responsive to sounds that are rhythmical, soft, high-pitched, and human (Affonso, 1976; Thoman, Korner, and Beason-Williams, 1977).

Knowledge of the abilities of the newborn to follow a voice, habituate to repeated stimuli, and exhibit reflex behavior increases a parent's involvement in the infant's care. This has been found to be particularly true of fathers (Metzl, 1980; Myers, 1982; Perry, 1983).

Reciprocity

The newborn is an active participant in the parent–infant interaction. The infant's responses influence the parent's responses. *Reciprocity* between parent and infant is an adaptive process consisting of mutually satisfying behaviors (Anderson, 1981). This process is cyclic in nature (see Fig. 29–3).

The infant has the ability to give cues that indicate existing needs. The parent interprets the cues, engages in problem solving, and offers appropriate stimulation to the infant. The infant absorbs the stimuli and reacts to them. If satisfied, the infant responds by becoming relaxed and appearing content. The infant's positive response indicates to the parents that they have satisfactorily and successfully stimulated the infant. They are motivated to respond again when the infant

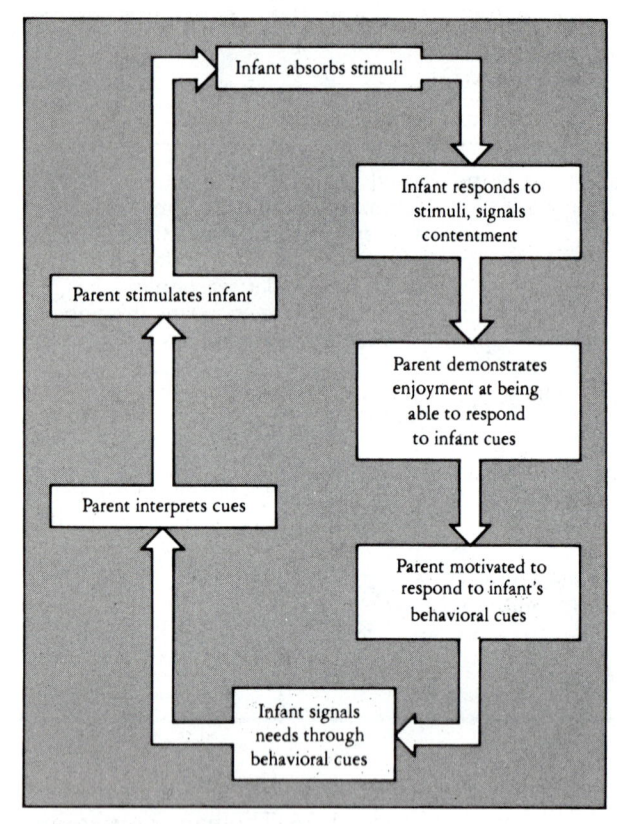

FIGURE 29–3. Response to stimulation: reciprocal responses of parent and infant.

gives a behavioral cue indicating a need. This parent–infant interchange is the key to the development of a dynamic reciprocal relationship.

MATERNAL ACTIONS AND THEIR EFFECTS ON INFANTS

Tactile Stimulation

Infants respond to touch. The most sensitive areas are the face (especially around the mouth), the palms, the soles, the genital area, and along the spinal column (Reeder, Mastroianni, and Martin, 1983). Babies respond to slow, modulated tactile stimulation, such as gentle rubbing and stroking, and are observed to relax and reduce their activity level in response to this stimulation. The tactile sense is initially probably the most important. Even the smallest of infants that are placed in isolettes have been found to scoot around until they come in contact with the side or the end of the crib before relaxing and going to sleep. Providing an infant with tactile stimulation such as stroking provides muscular and sensory stimulation, relaxation, and passive movement (Blackburn, 1983). Infants enjoy being held and talked to simultaneously. Holding and talking to babies are frequently observed forms of maternal behavior. Research has demonstrated that babies who were repeatedly picked up and held to the shoulder while being exposed to mother-talk were more alert, kept their eyes open more, and cried less (Thoman, Korner, and Beason-Williams, 1977).

Auditory Stimulation

The infant's response to sound begins during the third trimester. There are reliable differences in infant readiness to respond to auditory stimuli. Infants who respond readily to auditory stimuli also tend to engage in visual activity (Blackburn, 1983). Newborns have been observed to prefer a maternal voice more often than a nonmaternal voice. By recording the sucking activity of newborns in the quiet, alert state, observers have demonstrated that infants at 3 days of age can distinguish their mother's voice from those of others. Given the voice of another female, the newborn will try to mimic its own mother's voice (DeCasper and Fifer, 1980). Infants prefer voices with inflection over monotones. They can discriminate tone frequencies and pitch. Loud sounds tend to arouse the infant, whereas soft tones tend to relax the infant and produce sleep.

Entrainment, the rhythm or tune of body movement present during adult communication, has been observed in the newborn. As early as the first days of life the newborn moves in precise and sustained rhythm in synchrony with the articulated structure of adult speech. Audio tapes containing American English, isolated vowel sounds, tapping sounds, and Chinese language excerpts were played for infants from 12 hours to 2 days of age. Films of these infants document that they responded to the spoken words and moved in response to them. For example, when the word "come" was spoken, the infant's head was observed to move, the left elbow extended slightly, the shoulders rotated in synchronous rhythm alternately, the hips rotated, and the great toe extended. These findings reveal that the organization of the newborn's motor behavior is entrained by and synchronized with the organized speech behavior of the adults in his or her environment. If the infant moves in precise rhythm with the speech structure of the culture, then he or she participates developmentally through complex, sociobiologic entrainment processes in linguistics (Condon and Sander, 1974).

The infant moves in rhythm to the mother's voice and is affected by her, and the infant's movements may reward the mother and stimulate her to continue (Klaus and Kennell, 1982). Studies of newborns in various ethnic groups show striking differences in temperament and behavior in the first few days of life. In the past it was thought that mothers who tended to vocalize less to their infant (for example, Japanese mothers) might possibly condition their babies toward quietude. However, babies have been found to have striking differences in temperament and behavior as early as the first few days of life. Research has shown that mothers and babies probably condition each other. The naturally quiet Japanese babies affect the mother's behavior as much as the mothers affect their babies (Freedman, 1979).

Stimulation of Preterm Infant

The preterm infant misses the final weeks of intrauterine stimulation. Stimulation for these infants should begin as soon after birth as possible. With the use of ultrasonography it is possible to obtain data on fetal activity and behavior so that stimulation programs for the preterm infant can be developed based on fetal environment (Field, 1980).

The preterm infant has an immature central nervous system and is not as responsive as the term newborn. However, the value of stimulating the preterm infant has been demonstrated and reported in the literature (Scarr-Salapatek and Williams, 1973; Powell, 1974; Rose et al., 1980). High-risk infants seldom have periods of visual alertness. Health care providers can assist such an infant who is in a drowsy or active-awake state to an alert state by unwrapping (at least the upper arms) the infant; placing the infant in an upright position; talking to the infant; varying the pitch or tempo of the voice; showing their face to the infant; eliciting the rooting, sucking, grasping reflexes; and shading the infant's eyes or positioning the infant away from bright lights (Blackburn, 1983).

A group of preterm infants who were given tactile stimulation over only a brief period of time each day were observed to take more formula, show an increase in weight gain, and stool more frequently than infants not receiving stimulation (Rausch, 1981).

Developmental intervention is a new method to improve the care of preterm infants. Cole and Frappier (1985) piloted an individualized developmental intervention approach. They used the Assessment of Preterm Infant Behavior (APIB) scale to determine the infant's current behavioral functioning. The program that they implemented was to be a model for use with hospitalized, high-risk premature infants. The goals were to strengthen the focus on developmental aspects of care and to increase linkages and information-sharing among service providers.

The APIB scale was based on the Brazelton Neonatal Behavioral Assessment Scale (see Chapter 26) and was useful in documenting the individuality of the preterm newborn. By observing the infant's behavioral reactions to stimuli, individual needs were met.

Nurses, by demonstrating the APIB scale to parents, were able to assist them in reading their infant's cues more accurately and, thus, interacting more appropriately with their neonate. Parents were found to have a renewed sense of confidence with the improved quality of the interaction and thereby were in more control of the caregiving of their infant.

Tactile and kinesthetic stimulation combined with visual and auditory stimulation in preterm infants produce developmental gains. During feeding times a group of infants weighing 1200–1800 g were given a prescribed enrichment program in addition to their standard care. The program included visual stimulation with brightly colored mobiles and 5 minutes of soothing and rubbing by the nurse. During feeding time the nurses rocked the infants while talking and singing to them. The infants in the treatment group had significantly higher developmental scores than those infants receiving only standard care (Leib, Benfield, and Guidubaldi, 1980). According to Gorski, however, the immature infant can only afford to take in a small amount of stimuli at one time and only in one modality (touch, visual, or auditory), and is only able to gradually take in two or more stimuli presented simultaneously (rocking and singing, or looking, singing, and rocking) without becoming overloaded (Blackburn, 1983).

A new, computerized system is now available in intensive care nurseries to monitor and measure infant moods and levels of distress of preterm infants. These infants are unable to reveal their responses (eye contact, sucking, smiling, and crying) as readily as term infants. Therefore, the preterm infant is less able to signal clearly to caregivers to satisfy their needs. By analyzing continuous data regarding preterm infants' physiologic responses to tactile stimulation, the interrelationships between caregiver and preterm infant can be examined (Gorski et al., 1983a, b). Harrison (1985), in her review of the literature of 24 studies of the effects of supplemental stimulation on premature infants over the past 20 years, found that extra tactile, auditory, gustatory, and visual stimulation, either alone or in combination, might have beneficial effects. These effects include increased weight gain, earlier hospital discharge, enhanced auditory and visual responsiveness, advanced social and neurological development, and decreased irritability and wakefulness.

INFANT CHARACTERISTICS AFFECTING RELATIONSHIPS

Appearance

The general appearance of the infant is important to parents. Any deviation from normal – even a deviation as simple as the shape of the infant's head or uncoordinated eye movement – can cause concern. When the infant is premature or at risk, these concerns become exaggerated. Parents need information regarding the infant's physical characteristics, gestational age, and developmental level to allay their concerns.

The infant's behavior is also of concern to parents. During pregnancy the infant has been fantasized to look and act a certain way. When actual appearance and behavior deviate from preconceived images, parents need time to adjust to the reality of the actual infant. They may have expected a quiet, cuddly infant, and when theirs is hyperactive and resistant to attempts at soothing, they need specific information regarding the normalcy of these responses.

Visual Responses

A newborn can pursue slowly moving objects within a few hours after birth and can follow an object by turning his/her head at 2–3 days of life. Newborns have been found to prefer human faces to visual images. Normal infants were studied at 9 minutes of life and were found to turn their eyes and head significantly to follow facelike stimuli (Fig. 29–4; Goren, Sarty, and Wu, 1976). Infants have been observed to focus best when held vertically in a midline position.

Newborns have preferences for complex (checkerboard, bullseye) patterns versus simple patterns,

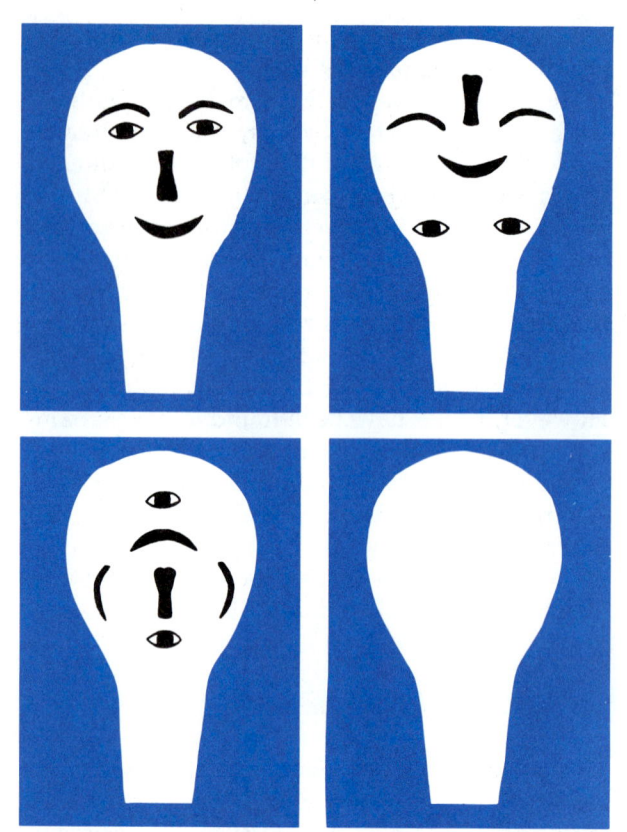

FIGURE 29–4. The stimuli: face *(top left)*, moderately scrambled face *(top right)*, scrambled face *(bottom left)*, and blank *(bottom right)*.

moving versus stable objects, black and white contrast versus monochromes, for bright colors, and for contour changes (Blackburn, 1983). By 6 weeks of age infants have been observed to differentiate objects by form and motion, and they can discern black and white patterns of dots, checks, and stripes, from simple to complex (Greenberg and O'Donnell, 1972; see Fig. 29–5).

Olfactory Abilities

At 5 days of life newborn infants can distinguish their own mother's breast pads from those of other lactating mothers (Macfarlane, 1975; Schaal et al., 1980). Thus, a mother can be reassured that her infant does recognize her as the primary caregiver.

Gustatory Responses

Infants' differential response to taste has been studied by feeding them with monitored nipples and recording sucking responses. Infants fed a saline solution were found to resist. When cow's

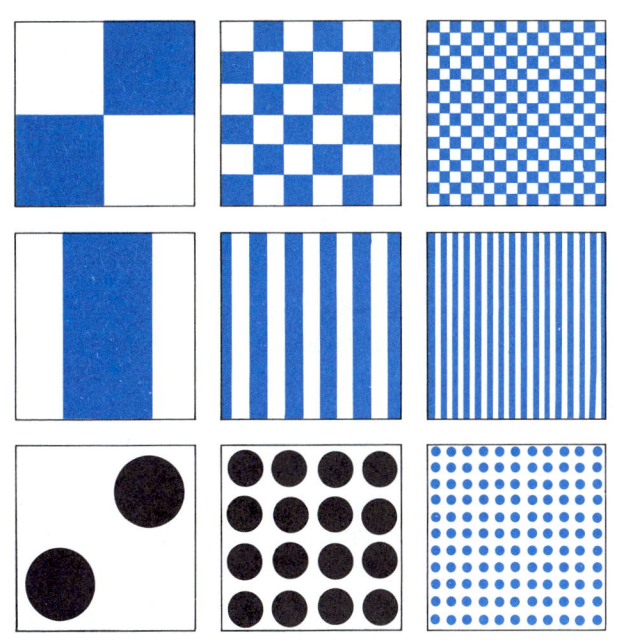

FIGURE 29-5. Stimuli discerned by 6-week-old infants.
SOURCE: Greenberg and O'Donnell (1972).

milk formula was given, infants sucked in a continuous fashion but registered a recognition when formula changed to breast milk. Infants had larger sucking bursts when given sweet fluids rather than saline fluids (Brazelton, 1981). The fact that infants prefer milk, either formula or breast, is a positive factor in the reciprocal response between mother and infant.

Physiologic State and Responsiveness

Communication of the nurse's observations of the state of the newborn can help parents. For example, if the infant is observed to be overresponsive, easily upset, and intensely active, this information should be shared with parents. They should expect that the baby might cry for unpredictable reasons and may not be easily consoled. The nurse should suggest soothing measures for parents to perform, such as swaddling the infant and using a pacifier, cradle, or rocking chair. This information will tend to reduce feelings of anxiety and guilt that arise in the parents when they are unable to soothe their baby. When an infant is hard to arouse, unresponsive, inactive, and reacts with dullness to visual and auditory stimuli, parents need to know. Parents tend to leave the dull, seemingly uninterested baby alone. Unless parents are alerted to their baby's state, these unresponsive babies may set a tone for decreased parent–infant interaction. The nurse needs to help parents understand that the dull baby needs *more* stimulation. Many times, as the physiologic status of the baby improves (SGA, mild placental insufficiency) with rehydration and nutrients, its responsiveness and ability to interact with the environment will increase. Parents then view the infant's increasing responsiveness as an indication of their success, and the parent–infant interaction is reinforced (Brazelton, 1981).

Smiling

Mothers look for response from their newborns and seek approval for their attempts to meet the infant's needs. Mothers enjoy seeing the infant smile (Fig. 29-6). Smiling in the newborn can be either spontaneous or elicited. The preterm infant lacks many of the reflexes that elicit early attachment. After 32 weeks' gestation the preterm infant will open its eyes, grimace, smile, and yawn – all reflex responses. Spontaneous smiling is seen in the term newborn during periods of active sleep or drowsiness in the first days and weeks of life. After 3–4 weeks smiling can be elicited by auditory

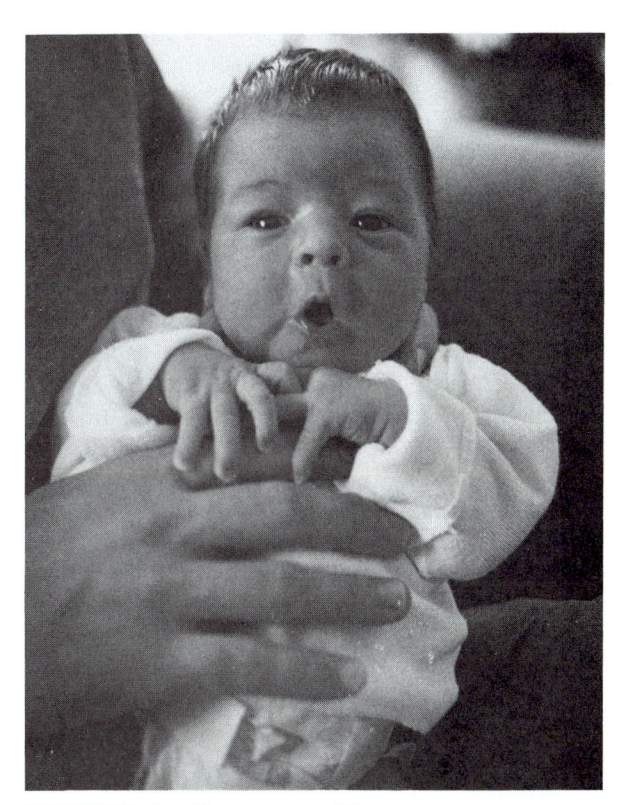

FIGURE 29-6. The response of the newborn is important in mother-infant attachment.

or tactile stimulation. The true sociable response, in which the infant responds with an alert smile, bright eyes, and grin, occurs about 8–12 weeks after birth (Fanaroff and Martin, 1983).

Nurses should be aware that mothers need the confirmation from the baby that spontaneous smiling affords. The mother interprets the smile as affirmation that she is giving the baby enjoyment. To inform the mother that this smile is "only a reflex response" does not support or encourage the mother.

Crying

The newborn responds to external stimuli (tactile, auditory, and visual) in the first days of life by crying. After 34 weeks' gestation, 80 percent of newborn infants will cry when the Moro reflex is elicited (Fanaroff and Martin, 1983). Babies cry when uncomfortable and when disturbed. Parents may interpret crying as an indication of rejection if the baby cries during diaper change or when being held. Since the parent–infant relationship is reciprocal, parental anxiety can be sensed by the infant, altering not only the parent's response to the infant but also the infant's response to the parent (Newton, 1983). Nurses can provide support for parents by helping them understand the purpose of the baby's cry, ways to interpret the various types of cry, and techniques to soothe their infant.

THE NURSE'S ROLE

Education of Parents

The Brazelton Neonatal Behavioral Assessment Scale (BNBAS) has been useful in documenting objective data about infant behavior (see Chapter 26). The use of the BNBAS has been shown to establish communication between tester and parent. When the nurse is tester, he or she can discuss information regarding the infant's uniqueness with the parents. Mothers who have assessed their male newborn infants with the BNBAS have been found to spend more time looking at their babies, talking to them, and playing with them, rather than just holding them (Liptak et al., 1983).

Mothers need to be taught about their newborn's sensory capacities. When mothers understand and observe that the infant is capable of visually following a moving object, able to orient to sound, and alert to surroundings, they express amazement and can be drawn into further stimulation activities. Mothers who are taught to administer the BNBAS tend to have better interactions with their infants than those mothers not receiving the intervention. They are:

1. More sensitive to the unique abilities of their infant;
2. More interested in observing the developmental process; and,
3. More active in providing stimulation to facilitate development (Widmayer and Field, 1981).

When a mother perceives her newborn as not being cuddly or as being overreactive, she needs to know that the infant responds the same way with other caregivers. Parents can profit from knowing what responses their infant has to external stimuli as well as how they can stimulate certain responses in their newborn (Powell, 1981).

Parents need information about how to stimulate their newborn. Nurses should assist parents in making decisions that are informed regarding sensory stimulation of their infant. These decisions should be based on available evidence and with full consideration of the individualistic needs of the infant (Koniak-Griffin and Ludington-Hoe, 1988). Babies request new stimulation by utilizing vocal or physical messages. This request can occur with a long, searching gaze with direct eye-to-eye contact, or by smiling and by cooing. A baby may also move physically by turning the head or by stretching the fingers or toes toward a person or object that appears enticing. When the parent establishes patterns of interaction for approaching the infant, for beginning each waking cycle, and for concluding each cycle, it will provide a source of continuity and routine so that the infant can begin to anticipate certain steps in the parent's method of nurturance (Fig. 29–7). For instance, the parent may decide to be physically and emotionally reassuring to the newborn who has awakened by holding the baby up against the left side of the body while talking quietly and rubbing the baby's head or back in a slow, gentle rhythm. This method allows the baby a period of transition between sleep and the fully awake state. The parent may wish to spend the first few moments with this method and then proceed to changing the diaper and providing more stimuli – talking more excitedly, touching the baby's fingers, toes, and chest, etc.

Another possible approach to use in the transition period between sleep and wakefulness is the body massage of the infant. The parent may wish to use oil or lotion. The baby can be gently

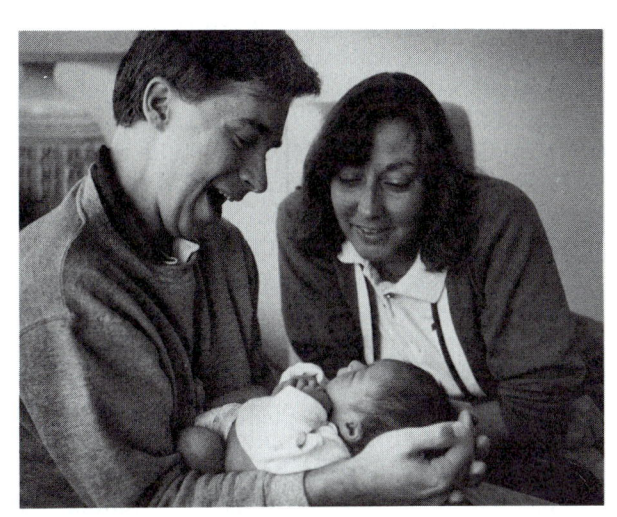

FIGURE 29-7. Parents establish patterns of interaction with the newborn.

abilities and inabilities. Too often, parents may perceive that because the infant cannot sit up in a straight manner or immediately grab for or grasp an object that there is little the infant is capable of accomplishing. The nurse is able to point out the infant's capabilities and demonstrate stimulation techniques to assist in the baby's motor development. The parents can be encouraged to use these stimulation techniques and to begin to notice the initial accomplishments of their infant. The nurse can demonstrate methods of exercising the infant with leg and arm flexion and with auditory or visual stimuli to encourage the baby to turn and reach toward an object.

Implementation of a Stimulation Program

Parents need to know specific ways to stimulate the infant to become more socially responsive. Goals for implementing an individualized stimulation program for parents are (1) to increase the involvement of fathers (Fig. 29-4), (2) to encourage parental visitation, and (3) to decrease parental anxiety. Premature infants can also be part of a stimulation program (Fig. 29-9). Parents are provided with practical help and emotional support.

A stimulation program should include:

1. The same caregiver each shift/each day to provide continuity of care for the infant.
2. Help for the infant in establishing the same wake/sleep cycle by covering the baby's eyes at night and dimming the room light.
3. Making the baby attractive with knitted caps, colorful ribbons, decorated name cards.

awakened in a head-to-toe fashion while receiving gradually increased auditory or visual stimuli. At the conclusion of an awake state, the parent may wish to utilize a rhythmic movement such as rocking or lightly patting the baby's bottom while the baby is in the prone position, to aid the baby into sleep. A massage at the conclusion of the awake cycle could also relax the baby for sleep. Other methods of stimuli – soft music or rotating mobiles, for example – can be successfully paired to bring about sleep (Fig. 29-8).

The parents can choose or develop a variety of techniques to care for their infant. It is important that the parents start developing a system of care in which they feel comfortable and to which the baby responds in a positive manner.

Other capabilities of the infant involve motor

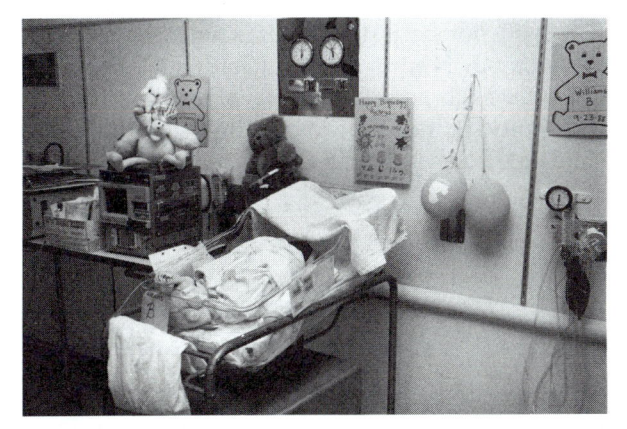

FIGURE 29-8. Stimuli around the baby's crib will personalize his/her environment.

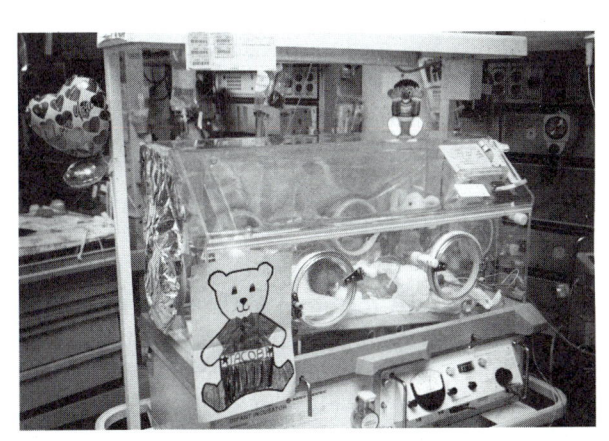

FIGURE 29-9. Premature infants can be a part of a stimulation program.

4. Colorful mobiles placed in the baby's line of vision. These should be hung from the crib's side since limited strength of the neck muscles make midline vision difficult (Coyner, 1978).
5. A pacifier for the gavage-fed infant so that sucking will be associated with feeding.
6. Touching and handling. Give parents a schedule to follow (for example, stroke arm and leg 5 seconds each; cuddle baby for 3–4 minutes; rock baby for 5–10 minutes).
7. Talking to baby while holding the baby in a vertical position at a 12- to 15-inch midline plane (for example, repeat baby's name three to four times in a soft voice or repeat the phrase "pretty baby" three to four times; sing two to three verses of "Rock-a-Bye Baby").

Chaze and Ludington-Hoe (1984) developed an infant stimulation care plan for use in the NICU. Their care plan reflects a possible method of infant stimulation for use in the nursery regime. The stimuli presented are visual, tactile, auditory, vestibular, olfactory, and gustatory. A variety of stimulation approaches are suggested in the care plan and the nurse has the opportunity to choose the one that best meets each infant's state or condition.

The nurse can assist parents in appreciating the uniqueness of their own infant. As a role model, the nurse interacts with infant and parents. The nurse can address the baby by the name chosen by the parents, thus reinforcing the idea that this is a separate, unique individual. Parents will begin to call the baby by name much more rapidly when they hear the nurse doing so.

Infants respond differently to stress. For instance, some infants are very vocal and some are not. Methods used to calm an aroused infant will need to be specific for each individual infant. Among methods that can be used to calm an infant are swaddling, music, rhythmic motion, visual stimulation, and sucking. Again, the message by the nurse must be one that helps the parents to feel that they can gain an understanding of their particular infant by a gradual learning process.

SUMMARY

It is important to foster an affiliation and attachment between parents and their infant. Early parent and infant contact is very important in the establishment of a healthy long-term relationship. As indicated by Klaus and Kennell (1982), there is a sensitive period for both mother and infant in the first minutes and hours of life, during which it is necessary that close contact be made to allow for optimal growth and development. Babies who are not touched lose, and the loss can never be recovered. Giving a baby twice what he need later does not make up for what he needs earlier. The baby also plays a vital role in the interaction process, since infants have the capability of interacting with their parents.

Nurses are in an important position to help parents interact with their infants. Nurses are immediately available after birth, when it is crucial for the claiming process for attachment to occur. Nurses can encourage parents to see and touch their infants, and they can help parents to become aware that their newborn has a potential for interaction. Parents need to appreciate that the best source of stimulation they can offer their infants is themselves.

In dealing with mothers and their newborn infants, nurses should be aware of the need for maternal–infant claiming and interaction, and of the need of the infant for physical contact. The infant requires body contact as well as a positive maternal–infant attachment to ensure healthy neurophysiologic and psychologic growth and development. Nurses also need to be aware of the fact that mothers differ in their initial contact and claiming behaviors, and that an attempt should be made to identify the particular pattern of behavior of a mother prior to intervening. Nurses should value the significance of feedback in the interaction process and appreciate the fact that parents need feedback regarding their efforts to interact with their infants.

Nurses need to facilitate healthy mother–infant interaction. An atmosphere conducive to promoting parent–infant and maternal–infant attachment seems to be one where there is freedom of the parents to interact with their infant – where they will not be judged, but where they will be understood. Nurses are the health providers that can offer such an atmosphere, since they provide continuity of health care during childbirth and child-rearing experiences.

REFERENCES

Affonso, D. 1976. The newborn's potential for interaction. *J. Obstet. Gynecol. Neonatal Nurs.* 5(6):9–14.

Anderson, C. J. 1981. Enhancing reciprocity between mother and neonate. *Nurs. Research.* 30(2):89–93.

Bibring, G. L.; Dwyer, T. F.; and Huntington, D. S. 1961. A study of psychological processes of pregnancy and of the earliest mother–child relationship. *Psychoanalytic Study Child.* 16:9–24.

Blackburn, S. 1983. Fostering behavioral development of high-risk infants. *J. Obstet. Gynecol. Neonatal Nurs.* 12(3) Suppl. 76s–86s.

Bowlby, J. 1969. *Attachment and loss: Attachment,* Vol. 1. New York: Basic Books.

Brazelton, T. B. 1973. *Neonatal behavioral assessment scale.* Philadelphia: J. B. Lippincott.

Brazelton, T. B. 1976. The parent–infant attachment. *Clin. Obstet. Gynecol.* 19(2):373–389.

Brazelton, T. B. 1981. Behavioral competence of the newborn infant. In *Neonatology: Pathophysiology and management of the newborn,* 2nd ed., ed. G. B. Avery. Philadelphia: J. B. Lippincott.

Brown, J., and Hepler, R. 1976. Stimulation – a corollary to physical care. *Am. J. Nurs.* 76(4):578–581.

Buckner, E. B. 1983. Use of Brazelton Neonatal Behavior Assessment in planning care for parents and new borns. *J. Obstet. Gynecol. Neonatal Nurs.* 12(1):26–29.

Chaze, B. A., and Ludington-Hoe, S. 1984. Sensory stimulation in the NICU. *Am. J. Nurs.* 84(1):68–71.

Clark, A., and Affonso, D. 1976. Infant behavior and maternal attachment: Two sides of the coin. *MCN.* 2(March/April):95–99.

Clark, A.; Affonso, D.; and Harris, T. R. 1979. *Childbearing: A nursing perspective.* 2nd ed. Philadelphia: F. A. Davis.

Cole, J. G., and Frappier, P. A. 1985. Infant stimulation reassessed. A new approach to providing care for the preterm infant. *J. Obstet. Gynecol. Neonatal Nurs.* 14(6):471–477.

Condon, W. S., and Sander, L. W. 1974. Neonate movement is synchronized with adult speech: Interactional participation and language acquisition. *Science.* 183(11):99–101.

Coyner, A. B. 1978. Meeting developmental needs of neonates. *Perinatal Health Promotion.* 1:79–90.

DeCasper, A. J., and Fifer, W. P. 1980. Of human bonding: Newborns prefer their mothers' voices. *Science.* 208(6):1174–1176.

deChateau, P. 1977. The importance of the neonatal period for the development of synchrony in the mother–infant dyad: A review. *Birth Fam. J.* 4(1):10–22.

Desmond, M. M.; Rudolph, A. J.; and Phitaksphraiwan, P. 1966. The transitional care nursery: A mechanism of a preventive medicine. *Pediatric Clin. N. Amer.* 13:651.

Dunbar, J. 1976. First encounters of mothers with their infants. *MCN.* 5(1):1–4.

Fanaroff, A., and Martin, R. J. 1983. *Behrman's neonatal–perinatal medicine: Diseases of the fetus and infant.* 3rd ed. St. Louis: C. V. Mosby.

Field, T. 1980. Supplemental stimulation of preterm neonates. *Early Human Devel.* 4(3):301–314.

Freedman, D. G. 1979. Ethnic differences in babies. *Human Nature.* 2:36–43.

Freiberg, K. L. 1983. *Human development: A life-span approach.* 2nd ed. Monterey, Calif.: Wadsworth Health Science Division.

Gay, J. 1981. A conceptual framework of bonding. *J. Obstet. Gynecol. Neonatal Nurs.* 10(6):440–444.

Gibes, R. M. 1981. Clinical use of the Brazelton Neonatal Behavioral Assessment Scale in nursing practice. *Pediatric Nurs.* 7(3):23–26.

Goldberg, S. 1972. Infant care and growth in urban Zambia. *Human Devel.* 15:75–89.

Goren, C. G.; Sarty, M.; and Wu, P. Y. K. 1976. Visual following and pattern discrimination of facelike stimuli by newborn infants. *Pediatrics.* 56:544–549.

Gorski, P. A.; Hole, W. T.; Leonard, C. H.; and Martin, J. A. 1983a. Direct computer recording of premature infant and nursery care: Distress following two interventions. *Pediatrics.* 72(2):198–202.

Gorski, P., 1983b. Caregiver-infant interaction and the immature nervous system: A touchy subject. Presented at Johnson & Johnson Round Table #10 on Touch. Key Largo, Fla., October 2–6.

Greenberg, D. J., and O'Donnell, W. J. 1972. Infancy and the optimal level of stimulation. *Child Devel.* 43:639–645.

Harrison, L. 1985. Effects of early supplemental stimulation programs for premature infants: Review of the literature. *Matern. Child Nurs. J. Summer.* 14(2):69–90.

Kaplan, D. N., and Mason, E. A. 1960. Maternal reactions to premature birth viewed as an acute emotional disorder. *Am. J. Orthopsych.* 30:539–552.

Kaufman, C. 1970. In *Parenthood: Its psychology and psychopathology,* eds. E. Anthony and T. Benedek. Boston: Little, Brown.

Kennell, J. H.; Trause, M. A.; and Klaus, M. H. 1975. Evidence for a sensitive period in the human mother. In *Parent–infant interaction.* CIBA Foundation Symposium 33. Amsterdam: Elsevier.

Klaus, M. H., and Kennell, J. H. 1982. *Parent–infant bonding.* 2nd ed. St. Louis: C. V. Mosby.

Klaus, M. H.; Kennell, J. H.; Plumb, N.; and Zuehlke, S. 1970. Human maternal behavior at the first contact with her young. *Pediatrics.* 46(2):187–192.

Klaus, M. H.; Jerauld, R.; Kreger, N. C.; McAlpine, W.; Steffa, M.; and Kennell, J. H. 1972. Maternal attachment: Importance of the first postpartum days. *New Engl. J. Med.* 286:460–463.

Koniak-Griffin, D., and Ludington-Hoe, S. 1988. Developmental and temperament outcomes of sensory stimulation in healthy infants. *Nurs. Res.* 37(2):70–76.

Leib, S. A.; Benfield, G.; and Guidubaldi, J. 1980. Effects of early intervention and stimulation on the preterm infant. *Pediatrics.* 66(1):83–90.

Liptak, G. S.; Keller, B. B.; Feldmann, A. W.; and Chamberlin, R. W. 1983. Enhancing infant development and parent–practitioner interaction with the Brazelton Neonatal Assessment Scale. *Pediatrics.* 72(1):71–78.

Lozoff, B.; Brittenham, G. M.; Trause, M. A.; Kennell, J.

H.; and Klaus, M. H. 1977. The mother–newborn relationship: Limits of adaptability. *J. Pediatrics.* 91(1):1–12.

Macfarlane, A. 1977. *The psychology of childbirth.* Cambridge, Mass.: Harvard University Press.

Macfarlane, J. A. 1975. Development of social preferences in the human neonate. In *Parent–infant interaction.* CIBA Foundation Symposium 33. Amsterdam: Elsevier.

Metzl, M. N. 1980. Teaching parents strategy for enhancing infant development. *Child Devel.* 51(2): 538–586.

Miranda, S. 1970. Visual abilities and pattern preferences of premature infants and full-term neonates. *J. Exper. Child Psych.* 10:189–205.

Montagu, A. 1971. *Touching: The human significance of the skin.* New York and London: Columbia University Press.

Myers, B. J. 1982. Early intervention using Brazelton training with middle-class mothers and fathers of newborns. *Child Devel.* 53(2):462–471.

Nelson, D.; Heitman, R.; and Jennings, C. 1986. Effects of tactile stimulation on premature infant weight gain. *J. Obstet. Gyncol. Neonatal. Nurs.* 15(3): 262–267.

Newton, L. D. 1983. Helping parents cope with infant crying. *J. Obstet. Gynecol. Neonatal Nurs.* 12(3): 199–203.

Paukert, S. 1982. Maternal–infant attachment in a traditional hospital setting. *J. Obstet. Gynecol. Neonatal Nurs.* 11(1):23–26.

Perry, S. E. 1983. Parents' perceptions of their newborn following structured interactions. *Nurs. Research.* 32(4):208–212.

Pines, M. 1979. A head start in the nursery. *Psychol. Today.* 13:56–68.

Pines, M. 1982. Baby, you're incredible. *Psychol. Today.* 16:48–53.

Powell, L. F. 1974. The effect of extra stimulation and maternal involvement on the development of low-birth-weight infants and on maternal behavior. *Child Devel.* 45(1):106–113.

Powell, M. L. 1981. *Assessment and management of developmental changes and problems in children.* 2nd ed. St. Louis: C. V. Mosby.

Prugh, D. 1953. Emotional problems of the premature infant's parents. *Nurs. Outlook.* 1:461–464.

Rausch, P. D. 1981. Effects of tactile and kinesthetic stimulation on premature infants. *J. Obstet. Gynecol. Neonatal Nurs.* 10(1):34–37.

Reeder, S. J.; Mastroianni, L.; and Martin L. L. 1983. *Maternity nursing.* 15th ed. Philadelphia: J. B. Lippincott.

Rheingold, H. L. 1961. The effect of environmental stimulation upon social and exploratory behavior in the human infant. In *Determinants of infant behavior,* vol. 1, ed. B. M. Fosse. New York: John Wiley & Sons.

Rheingold, H. L. 1963. *Maternal behavior in mammals.* New York: John Wiley & Sons.

Robson, K. S. 1967. The role of eye-to-eye contact in maternal–infant attachment. *J. Child Psychol. Psychiatry.* 8:13–25.

Rose, S. A.; Schmidt, K.; Riese, M. L.; and Bridger, W. H. 1980. Effects of prematurity and early intervention on responsibility to tactile stimuli: A comparison of preterm and full-term infants. *Child Devel.* 51(2):416–425.

Rosenblatt, J. S. 1975. Prepartum and postpartum regulation of maternal behavior in the rat. In *Parent–infant interaction.* CIBA Foundation Symposium 33. Amsterdam: Elsevier.

Rubin, R. 1961. Basic maternal behavior. *Nurs. Outlook.* 9(11):683–686.

Rubin, R. 1963. Maternal touch. *Nurs. Outlook.* 11(Nov.):828–831.

Salk, L. 1970. The critical nature of the postpartum period in the human for the establishment of the mother–infant bond: A controlled study. *Dis. Nerv. System.* 31(11):110–116.

Scarr-Salapatek, S., and Williams, M. L. 1973. The effects of early stimulation on low-birth-weight infants. *Child Devel.* 44(1):94–101.

Schaal, B. 1980. Les stimulations olfactives dans les relations entre l'enfant et la mere. *Reprod. Nutr. Devel.* 20:843–858.

Shields, D. 1974. Psychology of childbirth. *Canad. Nurse.* 70:24–26.

Silverman, W. A. 1979. Incubator-baby side shows. *Pediatrics.* 64(2):127–141.

Thoman, E. B.; Korner, A. F.; and Beason-Williams, L. 1977. Modification of responsiveness to maternal vocalization in the neonate. *Child Devel.* 48:563–569.

Trause, M. A.; Klaus, M. H.; and Kennell, J. H. 1982. Maternal behavior in mammals. In *Parent–infant bonding.* 2nd ed., eds. M. H. Klaus and J. H. Kennell. St. Louis: C. V. Mosby.

Widmayer, S. M., and Field, T. M. 1981. Effects of Brazelton demonstrations for mothers on the development of preterm infants. *Pediatrics.* 67(5): 711–714.

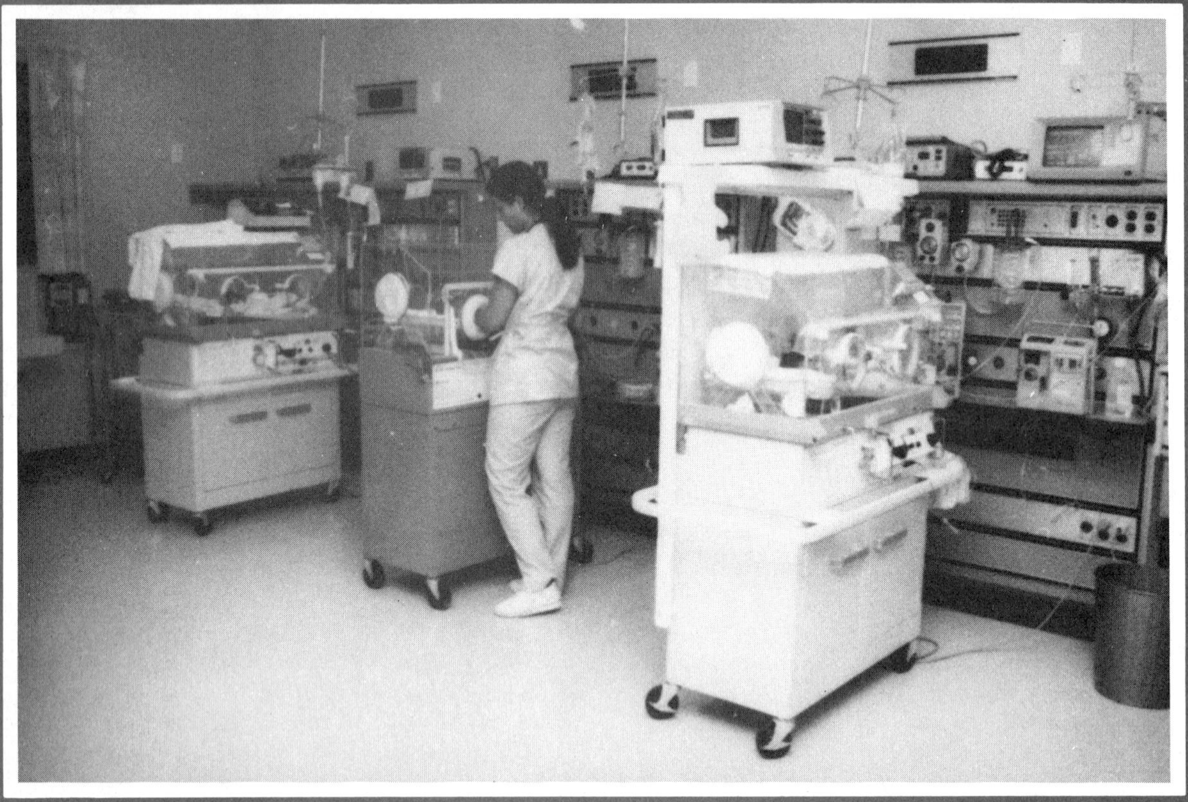

UNIT SIX

HIGH RISK MOTHER, INFANT AND FAMILY

30

Problems During Pregnancy

BEHAVIORAL OBJECTIVES

Upon completion of this chapter, the reader should be able to:

- Distinguish between the types of hypertensive disorders of pregnancy.

- Discuss the nursing care of the patient with premature labor.

- Discuss the effects of diabetes mellitus on the mother and fetus.

- Identify common infections in pregnancy and discuss their effects on both the mother and fetus.

- Compare and contrast abruptio placentae and placenta previa and discuss the nursing care of each.

- List factors that predispose women to the development of postpartum complications.

- Explain the pathophysiology associated with each of the postpartum complications considered.

- Formulate a nursing care plan for a patient exhibiting problems during postpartum, to include: potential problems and assessment, expected outcomes, nursing interventions, and rationale.

Complications during pregnancy may pose a threat to the woman or her infant. Ideally, no woman should die as a result of a complication of childbirth. In 1982 the reported maternal mortality in the United States was 8.9 per 100,000 live births. The leading causes of maternal death were hemorrhage, hypertension that is either induced or aggravated by pregnancy, and infection. All of these conditions are treatable; thus, with prompt detection and proper prenatal care for all pregnant women, maternal mortality can be reduced.

Both maternal and perinatal mortality rates have dropped greatly in the last century. Perinatal mortality consists of stillbirths and deaths occurring in the first 28 days of life. The reported perinatal mortality rate for 1980 was 12.6. With improvements in prenatal care and with intensive neonatal care available for all babies, these rates can be reduced even further.

HYPERTENSIVE STATES IN PREGNANCY

Hypertension occurs in 6–8 percent of all pregnancies. In the past, the term *toxemia* was used as a broad label for any of several hypertensive states that occur in pregnancy. The main characteristics of toxemia are hypertension, generalized edema, and proteinuria. It was hypothesized that these cardinal symptoms developed in response to a toxic substance produced during pregnancy that promoted vasospasm of the blood vessels. However, no such substance has been isolated, and the underlying etiology for hypertension in pregnancy remains unknown.

In 1972 the Committee on Terminology of the American College of Obstetricians and Gynecologists proposed a classification system to replace the broad term *toxemia*. According to this new system, hypertension in pregnancy is defined as a diastolic blood pressure of at least 90 mm Hg or a systolic blood pressure of at least 140 mm Hg. The term may also be applied to a rise in the systolic pressure over the prepregnant level. These elevated findings must be present on at least two separate occasions a minimum of 6 hours apart.

In some women hypertension occurs only during pregnancy. If hypertension develops during the latter half of pregnancy or during the first 24 hours after delivery with no other symptoms, it is labeled *gestational hypertension*. This type of hypertension disappears within 10 days of delivery. Some women have symptoms of hypertension that persist beyond the postpartum period. These women usually had persistent hypertension prior to the pregnancy. If a woman displays hypertension before the 20th week of pregnancy or persistent hypertension beyond the 42nd day of the postpartum period, it is termed chronic hypertensive disease.

Edema and proteinuria often occur alone or in association with hypertension. The term *gestational edema* is used to describe the occurrence of a generalized and excessive accumulation of fluid in the tissue that is greater than +1 pitting edema after 12 hours of bedrest or the occurrence of a weight gain of 5 lb or more in 1 week. *Proteinuria* is defined as more than 0.3 g protein/liter in a 24-hour specimen or greater than 1.0 g/liter in at least two random urine specimens collected at least 6 hours apart. If the proteinuria occurs only during pregnancy and in the absence of hypertension, edema, or known renal-vascular disease, it is termed *gestational proteinuria*.

The development of either proteinuria, edema, or both with the presence of hypertension due to pregnancy is termed *preeclampsia* or *pregnancy-induced hypertension* (PIH). This condition typically occurs after the 20th week of gestation but may develop earlier in the presence of trophoblastic disease. If these symptoms develop in a patient with chronic hypertensive, vascular, or renal disease, the condition is classified as *superimposed preeclampsia*. The patient with this problem displays hypertension prior to the pregnancy, and the blood pressure increases with pregnancy so that a 30 mm Hg rise in the systolic pressure or a 15 mm Hg rise in the diastolic pressure is seen.

Preeclampsia can progress to the point that convulsions occur. If a convulsion occurs that is not attributable to a cerebral disorder such as epilepsy or cerebral hemorrhage, the classification changes to *eclampsia*. Often the eclampsia is superimposed on a patient with known chronic hypertensive, vascular, or renal disease.

Risks to Mother and Infant

Hypertension during pregnancy can pose a serious threat to both mother and fetus. Eclampsia is one of the three leading causes of maternal mortality. These maternal deaths result from intracranial hemorrhage, aspiration pneumonias, and congestive heart failure. Women with eclampsia are also more prone to premature separation of the placenta, which may cause death due to hypovolemic shock.

The risk to the infant is also increased with

hypertensive states during pregnancy. Infants of hypertensive mothers are usually small for gestational age and are often born early because of placental insufficiency. They are also prone to develop hypoxia and acidosis during maternal convulsions. Therefore, these infants should be monitored closely in the newborn period for complications (see Chapter 32).

Medical Intervention

The goal behind the medical interventions used in preeclampsia and eclampsia is to minimize adverse effects on the mother and fetus. This goal is accomplished by interventions that stabilize the blood pressure within an acceptable range and restore adequate perfusion to all organs.

Recognition of Signs and Symptoms

Early recognition of the signs and symptoms of preeclampsia is an essential component in the management of pregnant women.

Vasospasm is the underlying cause of the signs and symptoms that are displayed in the hypertensive condition of pregnancy. Although it has been established that vasospasm is present in preeclampsia, the precipitating cause for this change in vascular tone has not been proven. Currently, the roles of nutritional, endocrine, and genetic mechanisms are being investigated as possible etiologic factors in the vasospasm.

Whatever the causes of the vasospasm seen in preeclampsia/eclampsia, the resulting physiologic changes have been established. Hypertension is an early sign of preeclampsia. It results from an increase in peripheral vascular resistance that is promoted by the vasospasm. Other symptoms associated with hypertension include blurred vision and headaches. Thus, all pregnant women should be questioned regarding eye symptoms and headaches. In addition, all patients should have their blood pressure taken on each prenatal visit.

Besides hypertension, another cardinal symptom of preeclampsia/eclampsia is proteinuria. If vasospasm and the resulting hypertension continue, the amount of blood supplied to the kidneys is reduced. This lowering of renal perfusion causes degenerative changes in the glomerulus. The result of these degenerative changes is increased permeability of the glomerular membrane, causing protein to be spilled into the urine. This proteinuria promotes loss of serum proteins, thus lowering the colloid osmotic pressure. As a result of the altered pressure, fluid is drawn from the capillaries into the tissues. The resulting edema is manifested by swelling in the feet, hands, and face. In addition to observing these areas for edema, the nurse should monitor the patient's weight on each prenatal visit and assess reflexes.

Perfusion to the placenta is also reduced in preeclampsia. Therefore, the fetus may experience a reduction in oxygen and nutritional supplies, resulting in intrauterine growth retardation (see Chapter 32). Changes in the placenta itself may occur. Often the placenta is smaller and shows premature aging. There is also an increased incidence of premature separation of the placenta in women with preeclampsia/eclampsia. Therefore, the physician may order serum or urinary estriol levels in the last trimester to determine the functional status of the placenta. Oxytocin challenge tests may also be ordered to determine the ability of the fetus to withstand the stress of labor, which will further compromise the uteroplacental blood supply (see Chapter 13).

Treatment

Once a diagnosis of hypertension during pregnancy has been made, the woman should be carefully monitored. Hospitalization is usually prescribed so that feedback regarding the effectiveness of the prescribed therapy can be obtained. Strict bedrest is used in the treatment of preeclampsia. Such bedrest, particularly if the woman reclines on her left side, will increase renal and uterine blood flow. This increase in renal perfusion will promote diuresis, thus promoting a lowering of the blood pressure.

Medications used in the treatment of preeclampsia/eclampsia include sedatives, antihypertensives, and anticonvulsants (see Table 30–1). Diuretics, which have been overused in the past, are usually avoided, as research indicates these agents can reduce renal and uteroplacental perfusion.

Magnesium sulfate is the drug of choice in the treatment of preeclampsia. This drug depresses the conduction of impulses at the myoneural junction and decreases the hyperreflexia commonly seen in preeclampsia. Magnesium sulfate also has some vasodilating effects, which tend to lower the blood pressure and increase the blood flow to the kidneys and uterus. Also, the drug has a depressing effect on the central nervous system, so it serves as an anticonvulsant.

Magnesium sulfate may be administered intra-

CASE PRESENTATION:

PREECLAMPSIA

Mrs. R. is 18 years old (gravida 1, para 0), and is in her 32nd week of gestation. She has been receiving regular prenatal care with a normal course of pregnancy thus far. Her present weight gain for the pregnancy is 18 lb. Her blood pressure has ranged between 110/70 and 120/80 on each of her previous visits. Her urine has been negative for protein and glucose. All other laboratory values have remained within normal limits.

When Mrs. R. appears for her routine prenatal visit, she complains of headaches and of swelling in the hands and face for the past 3–4 days. Assessment reveals the following data:

1. Blood pressure 120/100.
2. Urine positive for protein (2+), negative for glucose.
3. Pitting edema in the extremities 3+.
4. Weight gain of 4 lb in the last week.
5. Negative funduscopic exam.
6. Reflexes without clonus 3+.

After the examination the physician admits Mrs. R. to the hospital for close observation and bedrest.

NURSING CARE PLAN OF MRS. R.:

PREECLAMPSIA

Nursing Diagnosis	Expected Outcome	Nursing Interventions	Rational
1. Alteration in blood pressure due to preeclampsia	1. The patient will follow prescription – bed modification for daily activities; the blood pressure will return to normal prepregnant range	1a. Monitor BP every 2 hours b. Assess for headache, blurred vision, or epigastric pain every 4 hours c. Maintain seizure precautions: padded tongue blade, padded side rails, suction available at bed side, dim lighting d. Maintain complete bedrest e. Administer prescribed sedatives and anticonvulsant	1. To decrease BP to within normal range and to assess mother for worsening condition should BP continue elevated
2. Alteration in renal function due to preeclampsia (2+ protein in urine)	2. The patient will modify diet to comply with plan; the urine will become negative for protein	2a. Assess the urine for protein every 4 hours b. Turn to left side every 4 hours for 15 min c. Encourage a high-protein diet d. Encourage 240 ml water every 2 hours while awake e. Maintain intake and output record	2. To evaluate renal status
3. Alteration in fluid volume due to preeclampsia (1+ pitting edema)	3. The patient will modify diet to eliminate excessive sodium; the extremities will have no pitting edema; a weight loss of at least 2 lb will occur in 24 hours	3a. Assess the extremities for edema every 4 hours b. Weigh daily c. Maintain bedrest d. Avoid excess of sodium	3. To evaluate for the presence of edema and any complications
4. Alteration in reflex activity due to preeclampsia (hyperreflexia)	4. The patient will comply with the prescribed modification in daily activities; the reflexes will return to a normal state; no seizure activity will occur	4a. Assess knee, biceps, and ankle reflexes every 4 hours b. Promote bedrest in quiet, dimly lit room c. Limit visitors d. Administer prescribed anticonvulsant medication e. Maintain seizure precautions	4. To assess for worsening of condition and early intervention
5. Potential for fetal compromise due to impaired perfusion	5. The patient will recognize and report any change in fetal activity	5a. Auscultate FHTs every hour b. Observe for onset of labor c. Question patient regarding fetal movement	5. To assess for fetal well-being with early intervention

TABLE 30-1. Medications Used in the Treatment of Preeclampsia/Eclampsia

Drug	Classification	Nursing Implications
Amobarbital (sodium amytal)	Sedative and anticonvulsant	1. Check respirations prior to administration; should be greater than 12. 2. Keep side rails in place.
Valium (diazepam)	Tranquilizer	1. Check respirations prior to administration; should be greater than 12. 2. Observe fetus for effects of the drug.
Apresoline (hydralazine)	Antihypertensive	1. Monitor blood pressure and pulse every 30 min. 2. Be alert for irregularities in the pulse.

Magnesium sulfate	Antihypertensive and anticonvulsant	1. Prior to administration, check:
		  a. Respirations (should be greater than 12).
		  b. Urinary output (should be greater than 20 ml/hour).
		  c. Reflexes.
		2. Administer with z-tract technique if given i.m.
		3. Have antidote (calcium gluconate) available at bedside.
		4. Keep side rails in place.

Phenobarbital	Sedative and anticonvulsant	1. Check respirations prior to administration; should be greater than 12. 2. Observe fetus for bleeding, as drug may reduce the vitamin K-dependent coagulation factors. 3. Keep side rails in place.

muscularly or through an intravenous infusion pump. Whenever the drug is administered intramuscularly, a 3-inch, 20-gauge needle should be used. Because this drug can be extremely irritating to the tissues, the z-tract technique should be used.

When administering magnesium sulfate the nurse should make certain observations to prevent buildup of toxic levels in the patient. As the drug builds up, the patellar reflex will begin to diminish or will become completely absent. Respiration may also be affected as central nervous system depression increases. These symptoms are more likely to occur in the patient with oliguria (decreased urinary output), since the drug is excreted in the urine. Therefore, if the urinary output is below 20 ml/hour, the respiratory rate is 12 or less, or the patellar reflex is absent, the nurse should notify the physician, as the medication may need to be held.

In addition to making pertinent observations of patients receiving magnesium sulfate, nurses should also take other precautions. Calcium gluconate, which is the antidote for magnesium sulfate, should be readily available to administer if symptoms of toxic levels of magnesium sulfate appear. Often a small tray that contains syringes, alcohol sponges, magnesium sulfate, and calcium gluconate is kept at the bedside of preeclamptic patients. These patients should also have a padded tongue blade at the bedside for immediate use if a convulsion should occur. Other common seizure precautions, such as padded side rails and a quiet, dimly lighted room, are advised.

PREMATURE LABOR

Premature labor is defined as the onset of labor after the 28th week but before the 37th week of pregnancy. Progressive dilatation and regular uterine contractions (contractions that occur at least once every 10 min and last for 30 sec) are characteristic signs that distinguish preterm labor from false labor. The incidence of preterm delivery in the United States is 5–8 percent of all deliveries (Cohen and Friedman, 1983).

CASE PRESENTATION:

PREMATURE LABOR

S.B. is 20 years old (gravida 2, para 1) and is in the 30th week of gestation. She has been seeing her obstetrician regularly since she first learned of her pregnancy. Her blood pressure has remained within normal limits and her urine has been negative for protein and glucose. However, 1 week ago she arrived at the clinic with a temperature of 101.2°F, chills, and complaints of urinary frequency. A urinalysis revealed bacteria TNTC (too numerous to count). She was treated with Macrodantin and encouraged to drink at least 2000 ml of fluid per day.

A few days later she arrived at the clinic with complaints of backache and low abdominal pain. She also stated she was having some mild uterine contractions. Her urinalysis revealed bacteria. A pelvic exam done at this time revealed a 2-cm dilatation of the cervix. The membranes were intact. Uterine contractions were occurring at a frequency of every 5–8 min and lasted approximately 20–30 sec. The physician ordered hospitalization with bedrest and prescribed a ritodrine infusion.

NURSING CARE PLAN OF S.B.:

PREMATURE LABOR

Nursing Diagnosis	Expected Outcome	Nursing Interventions	Rationale
1. Discomfort due to presence of pain in lower abdomen	1. The patient will verbalize a lessening of pain after implementation of plan of care; she will have relaxed facial features and body posture; vital signs will remain within normal limits	1a. Assess for presence of pain every hour b. Palpate for bladder distention every 4 hours c. Encourage position changes d. Backrub as needed	1. To provide patient comfort and to alleviate any pain that is present
2. Onset of premature labor	2. The patient will follow the prescribed modifications in daily activities; uterine contractions will decrease in frequency and duration until completely absent	2a. Monitor uterine contractions with external monitor b. Administer prescribed medications for halting labor c. Check BP, pulse, and respirations every 15 min d. Report immediately any irregularities in the pulse e. Check IV rate and infusion site every 15 min	2. To assess for presence of premature labor and to provide early intervention

Risks to Mother and Infant

Premature labor holds no more risk for the mother than labor at term. However, preterm labor can pose a serious threat to the infant. Preterm labor is a contributing factor to infant mortality, with the principal causes of death among premature infants being anoxia, birth injuries, hyaline membrane disease, bronchopneumonia, and septicemia. These complications are primarily the result of prevalent immaturity of the various organ systems. Generally, the lower the birth weight and gestational age, the poorer the prognosis for the infant.

Medical Intervention

One of the first priorities for the physician is to determine whether it is in the mother's and baby's best interests to halt the labor process. In situations where there is serious maternal disease, such as preeclampsia, hemorrhage, or renal disease, attempting to stop labor may be contraindicated. Interventions aimed at stopping labor would also be contraindicated in situations in which the fetus is compromised and would have a better prognosis if delivered, such as abruptio placentae and erythroblastosis fetalis. Ruptured membranes, which increase the possibility of uterine and fetal infection, are another contraindication to stop premature labor.

If a decision is made to attempt to stop labor, the physician may prescribe one of several medications. Drugs currently in use include ritodrine, terbutaline, and isoxsuprine. Ethanol, which was used in the past, is not used as frequently today because of its depressant effect on the fetus.

Ritodrine and terbutaline are β-mimetic drugs. These drugs stimulate beta-adrenergic receptors which are located in the uterus. These drugs also stimulate beta-adrenergic receptors located in other smooth muscle organs which accounts for the side-effects associated with these drugs.

Ritodrine hydrochloride is administered intravenously using a recommended protocol of 0.1 mg (100 μg/min). This initial dose is increased by 0.05 mg (50 μg/min) every 10 min until the uterine contractions stop or the maximum dose of 0.35 mg (350 μg/min) is reached. This infusion level is then maintained at that level for 12 hours. The patient is next started on the drug orally in an initial dose of 10 mg which is administered 30 min before stopping the intravenous infusion. The oral regimen is 10 mg every 2 hours for 24 hours. The dosage is then adjusted to 10–20 mg every 4–6 hours, depending on the patient's response. The maximum daily oral dose should not exceed 120 mg.

Terbutaline sulfate (Brethine) has not been approved by the FDA and has no standard protocol for its use. Like Ritodrine, it is initially given intravenously and increased gradually to a maximum dose. Once the intravenous route is discontinued, the drug is given orally.

The side-effects of the β-mimetic drugs related to the cardiovascular system include tachycardia, hypotension, chest tightness or actual chest pain and, in rare cases, pulmonary edema. Hypokalemia may also be produced which can lead to cardiac arrhythmias. The nurse should monitor the patient carefully for signs and symptoms of toxic levels. The pulse and blood pressure should be monitored as frequently as every 10 min when these drugs are being given intravenously. Measures to minimize hypotension should be instituted. These include absolute bedrest, preferably on the left side, Trendelenburg position, and TED stockings. If hypotension or tachycardia should occur that is uncorrected by a side-lying position and adequate fluid hydration, a beta-blocker agent such as propranolol (Inderal) may be prescribed to counteract the effect of the β-mimetic drugs.

Magnesium sulfate is another drug often prescribed to halt premature labor. This drug appears to act as an antagonist of calcium, thereby inhibiting myometrial contractability. Gabbe, Niebyl, and Simpson (1986) recommend a 4-g loading dose given over 20 min, followed by an infusion of 2 g/hour, dropping to 1 g/hour after contractions cease. Whenever magnesium is administered, the nurse should monitor for signs of toxicity. These include diminished respirations (less than 12 per min) and diminished or absent reflexes. Because the drug is excreted in the urine, the nurse should ascertain that the urinary output is adequate when administering this drug.

The physician may order bedrest in addition to pharmacologic agents in an attempt to stop premature labor. Bedrest alone will halt premature labor in 50 percent of cases. Whenever bedrest is prescribed, the nurse should encourage the woman to lie on her side with her head flat or only slightly raised on a small pillow. This position will enhance blood flow to the uterus.

DIABETES MELLITUS

Diabetes mellitus, a disorder of carbohydrate metabolism that results from a deficiency of insulin, is a

TABLE 30–2. Diabetes Classification System for Pregnancy

Class	Characteristics	Insulin-dependent?
A	Presence of abnormal glucose tolerance with normal fasting blood glucose levels. The glucose tolerance test returns to normal after termination of the pregnancy.	No
B	The onset of diabetes mellitus prior to pregnancy and after 20 years of age. The disease has been present less than 10 years.	Yes
C	The onset of diabetes mellitus occurred between the ages of 10 and 19 and has had a duration of 10–19 years.	Yes
D	The onset of diabetes mellitus occurred prior to 10 years of age and has been present for more than 20 years. Peripheral vascular disease, retinal changes, and hypertension are present.	Yes
E	All of the characteristics of class D, plus calcification of the pelvic vessels.	Yes
F	All the characteristics of Class E, plus neuropathy.	Yes

SOURCE: White (1965).

challenging high-risk obstetric condition. Typically, diabetes is classed as Type I, or insulin-dependent, and Type II, or noninsulin-dependent. White (1965) developed a classification system for pregnant women with diabetes. This system is summarized in Table 30–2.

Risks to Mother and Infant

The presence of diabetes mellitus poses a threat to both maternal and fetal well-being. Although maternal mortality for the pregnant diabetic has decreased in recent years, pregnant diabetic women have a higher mortality rate than the general obstetric population. This increased maternal mortality rate may be related to the increased incidence of preeclampsia/eclampsia, infection, and hemorrhage that occurs in pregnant diabetics.

The offspring of diabetic mothers are also in a high-risk category. The fetal mortality rate is 10 times that of fetuses of nondiabetic mothers. After birth, there is also a higher risk: infants of diabetic mothers have two to five times the mortality rate of infants of nondiabetic mothers. Complications seen in infants of diabetic mothers include hypoglycemia, hypocalcemia, hyperbilirubinemia, and respiratory distress syndrome. These infants also have a higher incidence of congenital anomalies, with 6–8 percent exhibiting congenital abnormalities. Macrosomia is seen in infants born to mothers in classes A through C, and intrauterine growth retardation is seen in infants whose mothers are in classes D through F.

Medical Intervention

The prime objective in the medical management of pregnant diabetics is to maintain the blood glucose within an acceptable range. Ideally, the range should be 120–150 mg/100 ml after fasting and 150–180 mg/100 ml on a 2-hour postprandial test.

Stabilization of the blood glucose level is often difficult in pregnancy because of the profound changes in metabolism that take place. During the first half of pregnancy, there is a tendency to fasting *hypoglycemia*. The increased demands to provide glucose to the developing fetus lead to a lowering of the maternal blood glucose level. The National Diabetes Data Group (1979) define fasting hyperglycemia during pregnancy as a woman with a plasma level of 105 mg/dl or higher. In a nonpregnant woman, hyperglycemia is defined as a level of 140 mg/dl or higher. This tendency to hypoglycemia may be even more pronounced if the patient is diabetic. Another factor that contributes to hypoglycemia in early pregnancy is nausea and vomiting, particularly when insulin is being used. In the presence of nausea the patient may reduce her intake of carbohydrates. If this reduc-

CASE PRESENTATION:

DIABETES MELLITUS

Ms. S. is 21 years old (gravida 1, para 0), and is in her 26th week of pregnancy. Ms. S., who has had diabetes mellitus Type I since age 12, fits into Class B of White's classification system.

Ms. S.'s blood sugar has been stabilized thus far with adjustments in her insulin dosage. Her urine has remained between 0 and 2+ for glucose, and negative for acetone.

When Ms. S. arrived at the clinic, she complained of nausea, vomiting, and polyuria. Her vital signs were a temperature of 101.4°F, pulse 90, and respiration 24. Fetal heart tones were 132 and regular. Her skin was warm and dry and exhibited poor turgor. The nurse also noted Kussmaul type respirations and an acetone odor to Ms. S.'s breath. Lab work revealed a hematocrit of 36 percent, glucose 400 mg/100 ml (fasting specimen), and urine 4+ glucose and 3+ ketones. Blood gases were pH 7.28, with pCO_2 28 mm Hg. The physician ordered immediate hospitalization for stabilization of her diabetes mellitus.

NURSING CARE PLAN OF MS. S.

DIABETES MELLITUS

Nursing Diagnosis	Expected Outcome	Nursing Interventions	Rationale
1. Fluid volume deficit	1. The patient will drink at least 200 ml/hour when awake; complications of fluid volume deficits will be prevented	1a. Assess temperature and skin turgor every 4 hours b. Encourage fluids (200 ml/every hour while awake) c. Keep track of intake and output d. Administer PRN medication as needed for nausea	1. To assess for and maintain an adequate fluid in take and good skin turgor
2. Alterations in homeostasis due to ketoacidosis	2. The patient's blood glucose level will return within normal limits; condition of ketoacidosis will be corrected; Kussmaul respirations will cease; blood gases will return to normal; urine will be free of glucose and acetone	2a. Monitor respirations for rate and pattern every 15 min until stabilized b. Check each voided specimen for glucose and ketones c. Monitor I.V. site and rate every hour d. Administer insulin as ordered	2. To maintain homeostasis and prevent ketoacidosis
3. Alteration in nutrition due to diabetes mellitus	3. The patient will follow prescribed diet; blood glucose will return to normal levels	3a. Review the effect of diabetes on carbohydrate and fat metabolism b. Discuss the effect of pregnancy on diabetes c. Consult a dietician to work with patient on prescribed ADA diet	3. To maintain normal glucose level through diet and adequate nutrition
4. Potential for recurrence of ketoacidosis or insulin shock	4. The patient will state the signs and symptoms of ketoacidosis and insulin shock; the patient will comply with treatment plan regarding insulin administration and urine testing	4a. Review signs and symptoms of ketoacidosis and insulin shock b. Observe patient administer insulin and check her urine prior to hospital discharge	4. To educate patient about signs and symptoms of ketoacidosis and early intervention
5. Potential fetal distress	5. The patient will be monitored on a more frequent basis; a viable infant will be delivered	5a. Assess FHTs every 30 min until ketoacidosis stabilized b. Reinforce importance of prenatal visits c. Teach patient to report any significant increase or decrease in fetal activity	5. To prevent fetal distress and insure the delivery of a healthy infant

tion of carbohydrates is prolonged, a state of ketoacidosis may develop.

Dietary management is essential in minimizing hypoglycemia and ketoacidosis. The physician will prescribe caloric intake based on the individual's prepregnant weight and daily activities. Usually, a caloric intake between 25 and 50 cal/kg per day is ordered. This caloric intake is distributed throughout the day and evening so that a smooth blood sugar curve can be maintained.

In addition to restriction of caloric intake, the intake of carbohydrates, fats, and proteins is also regulated. Although the prescribed content of the diet may vary, usually about 1.5 g/kg per day of protein and 3 g/kg per day of carbohydrates is prescribed. The remaining calories are allocated to fat intake.

During pregnancy there is also a tendency toward *hyperglycemia*, particularly in the latter half of gestation. Several hormonal factors contribute to this diabetogenic effect. Growth hormone and cortisol, two hormones whose secretion is increased in pregnancy, are capable of elevating the blood glucose level. Other hyperglycemic factors are the placental hormones—estrogen, progesterone, and human placental lactogen.

Pregnancy also affects insulin, the pancreatic hormone responsible for the lowering of the blood glucose level. In pregnancy the effectiveness of this hormone is decreased, leading to a diminished ability of the tissues to use insulin. This state, termed *insulin resistance*, increases with the progression of pregnancy.

When hyperglycemia occurs in pregnancy, the signs and symptoms seen in untreated diabetes will be present: polyuria (excessive urine production), glycosuria (glucose in the urine), and polydipsia (excessive thirst). If the hyperglycemia continues, the patient may develop ketoacidosis as her body begins to use fats and proteins in an attempt to supply the cells with glucose.

The diabetic pregnant patient must be carefully supervised so that complications can be detected early. Visits are scheduled at least every 2 weeks for the first 32 weeks, and then weekly. During these visits, special attention is given to the levels of glucose in the blood and urine. The insulin dosage is adjusted as needed, based on the laboratory findings. NPH and Lente Iletin are the insulins used most frequently in pregnancy. However, the physician's choice of insulin is based on the individual patient. Table 30-3 summarizes the various types of insulins and their peak times of action.

In addition to monitoring the patient for signs of hypoglycemia and hyperglycemia, the nurse should observe her for other complications that occur more frequently in pregnant diabetics, including urinary tract infections, hydramnios (excess of amniotic fluid), and preeclampsia/eclampsia.

Early delivery may be planned for the diabetic woman, particularly if she is in class B through F. Women in these classes are often delivered early because of the increased incidence of fetal death in the last weeks of pregnancy. A cesarean section may be required, since women in classes A through C often have large babies.

INFECTIONS

Urinary tract infections are a common type of infection in pregnancy. In fact, approximately 10 percent of pregnant women develop a urinary tract infection. These infections are also common in the immediate postpartal period. In some women, asymptomatic bacteria (a colony count of 100/ml or more) are found. Other women display the common symptoms of urinary tract infection: urinary frequency, dysuria, and fever.

Several factors predispose pregnant women to urinary tract infections. Progesterone, one of the principal hormones of pregnancy, causes dilation of the ureters, which increases the possibility for bacteria to ascend to the kidney and produce pyelonephritis. Also, as the uterus increases in size, the ureters may be displaced, which may impede the flow of urine from the kidney to the bladder. A third contributing factor is the lowered renal threshold for glucose during pregnancy. This physiologic change may produce glycosuria, which encourages the growth of bacteria.

Vaginal infections are another common type of infection during pregnancy. Monilial, or yeast, infections are caused by *Candida albicans*, an organism commonly found in the intestinal tract. Trichomonas infections are produced by the protozoan *Trichomonas vaginalis*. This organism may be transmitted sexually, and treatment of the partner is required to prevent reinfection of the pregnant woman.

Other sexually transmitted diseases found in pregnant women include gonorrhea and syphilis. Gonorrhea, an infection caused by the bacterium *Neisseria gonorrhoeae*, may be asymptomatic in women. All pregnant women should be screened for gonorrhea on their initial prenatal visit. Physicians may draw a blood sample to determine the presence of gonorrheal antibodies or they may

TABLE 30–3. Some Insulin Products (U-100)

Product	Origin	Purified[a]	Onset Of Action (Hours)[b]	Duration of Action (Hours)[b]
Rapid-acting				
Regular				
Actrapid – Novo	Pork	Yes	0.5	8
Iletin II – Lilly	Pork	Yes	0.5–1	5–7
Velosulin – Nordisk	Pork	Yes	0.5	8
Mixtard – Nordisk (30% reg, 70% NPH)	Pork	Yes	0.5	24
Iletin II – Lilly	Beef	Yes	0.5–1	5–7
Iletin I – Lilly	Beef, pork	No	0.5–1	5–7
Insulin – Squibb	Beef, pork	No	0.5–1	6
Zinc suspension				
Semitard (semilente) – Novo	Pork	Yes	1.5	16
Iletin I (semilente) – Lilly	Beef, pork	No	1–3	12–16
Insulin (semilente) – Squibb	Beef	No	0.5–1	12–16
Intermediate-acting				
Globin				
Insulin – Squibb	Beef, pork	No	2	24
NPH				
Insulatard – Nordisk	Pork	Yes	1.5	24
Insulin – Squibb	Beef, pork	No	1–1.5	24
Zinc suspension				
Monotard (lente) – Novo	Pork	Yes	1.5	22
Lentard (lente) – Novo	Beef, pork	Yes	2.5	24
Iletin II (lente) – Lilly	Pork	Yes	1–3	24–28
Iletin II (lente) – Lilly	Beef	Yes	1–3	24–28
Iletin I (lente) – Lilly	Beef, pork	No	1–3	24–28
Insulin (lente) – Squibb	Beef	No	1–3	24–28
Long-acting				
Zinc suspension				
Ultratard (ultralente) – Novo	Beef	Yes	4	36
Iletin II (PZI) – Lilly	Pork	Yes	4–6	36+
Iletin II (PZI) – Lilly	Beef	Yes	4–6	36+
Iletin I (ultralente) – Lilly	Beef, pork	No	4–6	36+
Insulin (ultralente) – Squibb	Beef	No	4–8	36+
Insulin (PZI) – Squibb	Beef, pork	No	4–8	36+

SOURCE: *Medical Letter on Drugs and Therapeutics* (1981).
[a]Less than 10 ppm proinsulin.
[b]Onset and duration can vary widely with different doses and different patients.

take a cervical smear. The physician will also screen the pregnant woman for syphilis on her first prenatal visit. Syphilis, which is caused by the spirochete *Treponema pallidum,* can be diagnosed with the Venereal Disease Research Laboratories (VDRL) test or the reactive plasma reagin (RPR) test.

Other sexually transmitted diseases are not as easy to detect through routine screening procedures. These include genital herpes and condylomata acuminata. Genital herpes is caused by the herpes simplex virus Type II. This disease, which is reported by Perley and Bills (1983) to affect between 5 million and 20 million adults in the United States, is incurable. It is diagnosed by tissue cultures or with a Papanicolaou (Pap) test or cytologic test. Serum antibody titers may also be used. However, only the tissue culture will differentiate herpes Type I from Type II. Condylomata acuminata are warts that occur in the vulvar area. They are believed to be transmitted by a virus that has yet to be identified. These warts, which resemble skin warts, grow rapidly during pregnancy and may spread to the vagina and cervix.

Toxoplasmosis is one of four diseases of the TORCH complex: toxoplasmosis, rubella, cytomegalovirus, and herpes. These diseases are grouped together under this acronym because they can cause severe damage to a developing embryo or fetus. This disease, caused by the protozoan *Toxoplasma gondii,* can be contracted from eating poorly cooked meat or through contact with feces of an infected animal, usually a cat.

Rubella (German measles), another disease of the TORCH complex, is caused by the rubella virus. Women can be screened with a serologic test to determine whether they have immunity to the disease. In women who are susceptible to the disease, another test after exposure to the virus will show an increased titer if infection has occurred.

Cytomegalic inclusion disease is a sexually transmitted disease that may be caused by one of at least six strains of the cytomegalovirus. Cytomegalic inclusion disease is confirmed by the presence of the cytomegalovirus in the urine or the presence of cytomegalovirus antibodies in the blood.

Risks to Mother and Fetus

The risks to the mother and fetus depend on the specific infectious process and the time in gestation that the infection occurs (see Table 30–4).

Medical Intervention

Medical intervention is aimed at treatment of the infectious process while minimizing the potential hazards to the mother and fetus. The type of intervention depends on the etiologic agent involved.

Urinary tract infections are treated with antibiotics following a urine culture to determine the specific causative organism. Most bacteria that cause urinary tract infections in pregnancy will respond to the short-acting sulfonamides and somewhat less often to ampicillin. Macrodantin is recommended in a treatment regimen of 100 mg/day for 10 days and sulfisoxazole (Gantrisin) 1 g four times a day (Pritchard, MacDonald, and Gant, 1980). The sulfonamides may cause hyperbilirubinemia in the newborn when used late in pregnancy, since they interfere with the protein binding of bilirubin. Tetracyclines, which are used in the treatment of urinary tract infections in nonpregnant women, are contraindicated in pregnancy, as they may cause discoloration of the fetal teeth.

In addition to being given appropriate antibiotic therapy, women with urinary tract infections should be encouraged to drink at least 3000 ml of fluid per day unless some other contraindication is present. They should also be assessed for signs of premature labor, which occurs more frequently in women with urinary tract infections.

Monilial infections may be treated with either gentian violet or nystatin (Mycostatin). Gentian violet, which will stain the skin and clothes a deep purple, is applied with a swab or vaginal applicator. Nystatin may be prescribed in the form of vaginal tablets or suppositories. During treatment of vaginal infections, the patient should abstain from intercourse. She should be taught proper genital hygiene (to wipe from front to back) and told to wash her hands following elimination and the application of the prescribed medications, since the infection can be spread by contaminated hands.

Trichomonas infection is often treated with metronidazole (Flagyl). This drug can cross the placenta and is therefore avoided during the first trimester, when the possibility of teratogenicity is present. Other drugs that may be used as a vaginal suppository include furazolidone (Tricofuron) and Vagisec. The partner or partners should also be treated, to prevent reinfection with the *Trichomonas* organism.

Penicillin is the drug of choice for the treatment of both gonorrhea and syphilis. For the treatment

TABLE 30-4. *Effects of Infections During Pregnancy*

Infection	Maternal Effects	Fetal Effects
Condylomata acuminata	Vulvar warts; may require cesarean section	None noted
Cytomegalovirus disease	Asymptomatic or mimics mononucleosis	Increase in perinatal mortality; fetal malformations
Gonorrhea	Asymptomatic or vaginal discharge; scarring of the fallopian tubes, which can affect ability to conceive	Fetal death, mental retardation, ophthalmia neonatorum
Herpes simplex Type II	Vulvovaginitis	Increased perinatal mortality; fetal malformations
Influenza	Can produce critical illness if pneumonia develops	Fetal death and congenital anomalies

Hepatitis
  Infectious (Type A)
  Serum (Type B)
	Abortion or premature labor	Fetal death, fetal deformities, congenital hepatitis

Monilial vaginitis	Thick, irritating vaginal discharge	Thrush
Poliomyelitis	More susceptible during pregnancy	Increased perinatal mortality
Rubella (German measles)	Fever and typical rash, abortion	Increased perinatal mortality and congenital defects
Rubeola (3-day measles)	Fever and typical rash, abortion	Increased perinatal mortality; congenital or neonatal infection will produce rash
Syphilis	May be asymptomatic or produce primary and secondary lesions	Fetal death, congenital syphilis
Toxoplasmosis	Asymptomatic	Increased perinatal mortality, congenital anomalies, congenital toxoplasmosis
Urinary tract infections	Asymptomatic or fever, chills, dysuria, urinary frequency, and pain; abortion and premature labor	No effects unless sulfonamides are used in late pregnancy; they may cause jaundice
Varicella	Typical lesions; may precipitate shingles	Fetal death, growth retardation, and fetal malformations

CASE PRESENTATION:

INFECTION

Mrs. K. is 25 years old (gravida 3, para 2) and is in the 24th week of gestation. Both of her previous pregnancies were full term with no prenatal complications. Her current pregnancy had been uneventful until recently.

Now Mrs. K. is complaining of urinary frequency and pain. Her temperature is 100.4°F. She says she has had these symptoms for a couple of days. A urinalysis reveals 4+ bacteruria. The physician prescribes Gantrisin 1 g four times a day on an outpatient basis and instructs her to return in 1 week.

NURSING CARE PLAN OF MRS. K.:

URINARY TRACT INFECTION

Nursing Diagnosis	Expected Outcome	Nursing Interventions	Rationale
1. Alteration in urine due to infection	1. The patient will become negative for bacteria in the urine after complying with plan of care	1a. Obtain urine for ordered urinalysis b. Assess urinalysis reports for progress c. Assess urine culture reports d. Encourage fluids (200 ml/every hour while awake) e. Teach proper perineal wiping technique (front to back) f. Encourage patient to wear cotton panties g. Administer prescribed antibiotic	1. To assess for presence of urinary tract infection and implement nursing inter ventions to minimize further complications
2. Alteration in urinary elimination due to infection	2. The patient will have no increased urinary frequency after complying with plan of care	2a. Assess for urinary frequency every 4 hours	2. To continually assess for presence of urinary tract infection
3. Discomfort due to pain related to urinary tract infection	3. The patient will verbalize a lessening of pain after complying with plan of care	3a. Assess for pain every 4 hours b. Administer prescribed analgesic	3. To provide comfort measures to patient experiencing pain from urinary tract infection
4. Alteration in regulatory mechanism of temperature due to infection	4. The patient will become afebrile	4a. Assess temperature every 4 hours b. Maintain cool room c. Administer prescribed antibiotics	4. To maintain patient afebrile

of uncomplicated gonorrhea, the Center for Disease Control (1979) recommends aqueous procaine penicillin G in a dose of 4.8 million units divided into two injections, given intramuscularly. They also recommend that 1 g probenecid (Benemid) be given orally just prior to the injections. If the patient is allergic to penicillin, then erythromycin, cefazolin, or streptomycin may be used.

In the treatment of syphilis during the incubation period, the Center for Disease Control (1979) recommends the same therapy as for gonorrhea. If the syphilis is past incubation but has been present less than a year, penicillin G benzathine in a dosage of 2.4 million units total, half in each buttock, or aqueous penicillin G 600,000 units per day for 8 days is recommended. With syphilis that has been present longer than a year, higher total dosages may be required and are administered over a period of time. Treatment of the partner or partners should be done to prevent reinfection of the pregnant woman.

There is no specific therapy for genital herpes or for condylomata acuminata. Treatment is aimed at relieving vulvar pain and itching. With both of these infections a cesarean section may be required.

With diseases of the TORCH complex that are contracted early in pregnancy, therapeutic abortion should be considered. There is no specific drug therapy to counteract the effects of rubella, cytomegalovirus, or herpes. With toxoplasmosis the physician may prescribe a combination of pyrimethamine and a sulfonamide or the antibiotic spiramycin in an attempt to reduce the frequency of congenital infection.

POSTPARTAL INFECTION

Puerperal infection has been defined by the Joint Commission on Maternal Welfare as the incidence of a persistent temperature greater than 100.4°F (38°C) orally, with the elevation occurring on any 2 of the first 10 postpartum days, exclusive of the first 24 hours (Eschenbach and Wager, 1980; McKenzie, 1983).

Postpartum infection is largely confined to the genital tract, although the source may be extragenital, and it is most likely to be wound related (see Fig. 30–1). Fever in the postpartum period is found to be a reliable indicator of an offending organism (Eschenbach and Wager, 1980).

A number of factors clearly predispose to the development of postpartum infection; some are antepartal or general risk factors, while others are of intrapartal etiology. These factors are summarized in Table 30–5. Contributing antepartal factors are primarily indirect but may affect the ability of the host to respond to infectious organisms. Three main intrapartal factors have been identified: (1) introduction of pathogenic bacteria into the upper genital tract, (2) trauma with delivery that devitalizes tissue, and (3) hemorrhage. The uterus is considered sterile prior to rupture of the membranes. Despite the use of sterile equipment, use of antiseptic solutions, and attention to principles of asepsis, it is unlikely that any vaginal examination or procedure is truly aseptic. It is therefore essential to consider risk versus benefit when determining the frequency of exams, especially in women with ruptured membranes. Patient education about the process of infection is also very important (see Fig. 30–2).

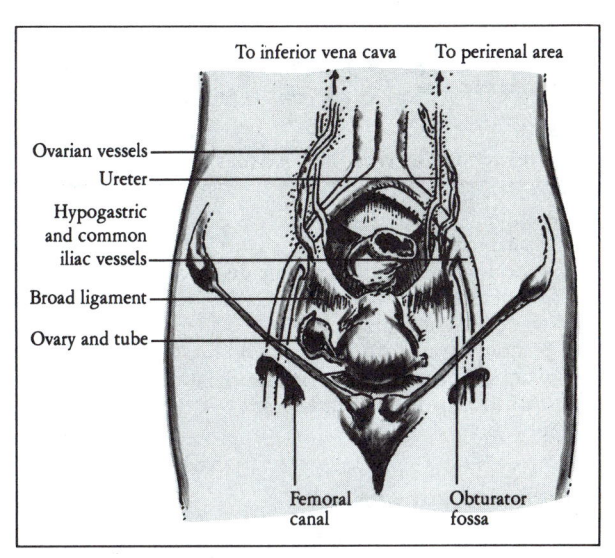

FIGURE 30–1. Modes and sites of spread of uterine infection.
SOURCE: Charles and Klein (1973).

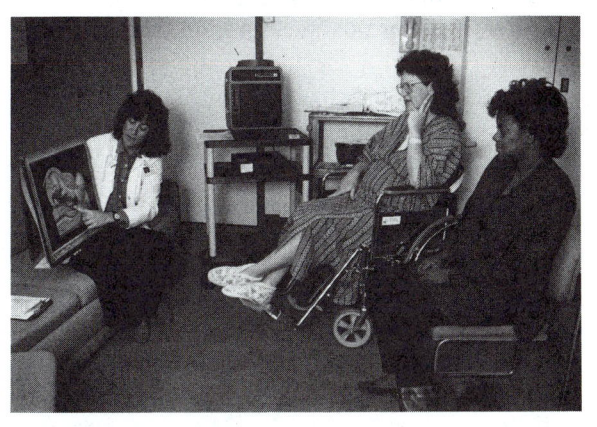

FIGURE 30–2. Nurse providing education regarding risks of infection.

TABLE 30–5. Predisposing Risk Factors to Puerperal Infection

Antepartum/General Risk Factors

Anemia
Poor nutritional status
General debilitation – chronic disease
Lack of prenatal care
Low socioeconomic status
Obesity
Sexual intercourse with or immediately preceding rupture of the membranes
Diabetes

Intrapartum/Delivery

Prolonged rupture of the membranes with repeated vaginal examinations (more than 24 hours)
Chorioamnionitis
Intrauterine fetal monitoring
Intrauterine manipulation or operative delivery
Trauma during labor and delivery
Manual removal of the placenta
Retained placental fragments
Hematomas
Droplet infection in hospital personnel
Breaks in aseptic technique and handwashing
Improper perineal care

SOURCES: Adapted from Eschenbach and Wager (1980); MacKenzie (1978).

Hemorrhage and trauma to tissue increase infection risk by providing additional access portals and by necessitating further manipulation of tissue for repair, thereby potentially introducing contaminants via an ascending route. Hematoma formation, possible with genital tract trauma, can also provide excellent growth media to support opportunistic or nosocomial (hospital-acquired) organisms (Eschenbach and Wager, 1980).

Usual forms of postpartum infection include:

1. Endometritis (involving the endometrium, decidua, and adjacent myometrium).
2. Pelvic thrombophlebitis (involving the exposed placental site and increasing risk for septic embolism).
3. Peritonitis (from lymphatic transfer via the uterine wall or operative delivery).
4. Pelvic cellulitis (involving the pelvic connective tissue via lymphatic transfer from cervical lacerations or secondary to pelvic thrombophlebitis).

Etiology/Diagnosis

Common pathogens responsible for infection are those that inhabit the lower genital tract and bowel, as well as nosocomial organisms. Portals of entry are most often moist, dark, and susceptible to bacterial invasion: the placental site, the perineal body, episiotomy or lacerations, the urinary tract, the vagina, the breasts, and the lymphatic system along uterine veins. Table 30–6 lists bacteria that are commonly found, along with recommended antibiotic therapy based on sensitivities. Cultures are necessary to diagnose the offending organism, plan management, and select appropriate antibiotic therapy (McKenzie, 1983).

Incidence

Puerperal infection occurs in 6 percent of all deliveries (Eschenbach and Wager, 1980; McKenzie, 1983).

Pathophysiology/Clinical Aspects

Following delivery, infectious access to the body may occur through numerous sites. Once placental detachment occurs, the site becomes an excellent culture medium for bacteria as well as a portal of entry for pathogenic organisms. The infectious/inflammatory process may remain localized in particular wound sites or may become systemic via blood and lymphatics to the varying types of puerperal infection.

Patients with postpartum infection will show an elevated temperature approximately 48 hours postpartum and exhibit tenderness to uterine palpation. Lochia will give off an offensive odor caused by the invasion of anaerobic bacteria. Elevation of the white blood cell count is common. Absence of many of these symptoms does not necessarily indicate absence of postpartal infection, nor does it suggest that the infectious process is less severe (Pritchard, MacDonald, and Gant, 1985).

Genital Infections

Pelvic cellulitis commonly causes sustained fever in the postpartum period and manifests in tenderness of one or both sides of the abdomen on vaginal exam.

Septic thrombophlebitis is characterized by repeated chills, severe temperature swings, and a

TABLE 30-6. Pathogens Identified in Puerperal Infection: Recommended Antibiotics and Sensitivities

Common Pathogenic Bacteria	Penicillin G	Chloramphenicol	Clindamycin	Tetracycline	Cephalothin	Gentamicin	Kanamycin	Erythromycin	Ampicillin
Anaerobic									
Peptostreptococcus	S	S	S	S-R	S	R	R	S-R	S
Peptococcus	S	S	S	S-R	S	R	R	S-R	S
Bacteroides fragilis	R	S	S	S-R	R	R	R	S-R	R
Clostridium perfringens	S	S	S	S-R	S	R	R	S-R	S
Clostridium (other)	S	S	S-R	S	S	R	R	S	S
Aerobic									
E. coli	R	S	R	S-R	S	S	S	R	S-R
Klebsiella	R	S	R	S	S	S	S	R	R
Enterobacter	R	S-R	R	S-R	R	S	S-R	R	R
Proteus mirabilis	R	S	R	R	S-R	S	S	R	S-R
Pseudomonas	R	R	R	R	R	S	R	R	R
Hemolytic Streptococcus									
Group A and B	S	S	S	S	S	R	R	S	S
Group D	S-R	S-R	R	S-R	S-R	R	R	S-R	S-R
Staphylococcus aureus	R	S	S	S	S	S	S	S	R
Neisseria gonorrhoeae	S	S	R	S	S	R	R	S	S

SOURCE: Adapted from Pritchard, MacDonald, and Gant (1985).
S = The great majority of strains sensitive to the antibiotic.
R = The great majority of strains resistant to the antibiotic.
S-R = Different strains variably sensitive.

tendency for distant spread (especially to the pulmonary veins). Hypotension may be seen with cases of septic bacterial shock. Cases of this type of infectious process may be prolonged.

Symptoms of postpartal *peritonitis* are similar to those of surgical peritonitis except that the abdomen may be less rigid. Pain will be present and may be severe. Ileus causes bowel distention and eventually nausea and vomiting, which may be projectile; severe diarrhea and fluid or electrolyte disturbances may follow (Pritchard, MacDonald, and Gant, 1985).

Extragenital Infections

Extragenital postpartum infections that must be considered when a patient becomes febrile are pyelonephritis, mastitis, upper respiratory infection, and abdominal wound abscesses.

Pyelonephritis is diagnosed with urine culture (collected via catheter) showing bacteriuria and pyuria (pus cells in urine); it may cause costovertebral angle or flank tenderness.

Mastitis presents with sustained temperature elevation, and the mother usually complains of flu-like symptoms. Examination of the breasts usually reveals a tender, reddened, raised area. Introduction of infection is generally via sore, cracked nipples. Emptying of the breasts should be encouraged to prevent stasis of milk and to increase comfort. Breastfeeding can continue unless an abscess is present. Wound abscess may be evident on inspection and most likely will require incision and drainage. The most common offender in mastitis is *Staphylococcus*, which responds well to penicillinase-resistant antibiotics (cephalosporins) and does not interfere with breastfeeding.

Therapy

Antibiotic therapy is recommended for all puerperal infections and is based on culture and sensitivity reports. Prior to the availability of laboratory results but following specimen collection, the physician may begin therapy utilizing a broad-spectrum antibiotic to decrease morbidity and increase patient comfort (Eschenbach and Wager, 1980; McKenzie, 1983).

Other therapeutic measures include ensuring adequate fluid and nutritional intake and rest to improve host response; supportive care measures and analgesics to increase comfort and mobility; isolation and aseptic technique as appropriate; and continued observation of body systems to prevent or recognize progression of infection (McKenzie, 1983).

Puerperal infection can present in the immediate postpartum period or within the first 2–3 days after delivery. Nursing knowledge and assessment of the various signs and symptoms is of paramount importance if complications are to be prevented. Early diagnosis and treatment can result in a favorable prognosis, with the majority of the time in the postpartal period being spent by the mother in adjusting to her new infant.

HEMORRHAGIC DISORDERS

The leading causes of bleeding in the first half of pregnancy are abortion, ectopic pregnancy, and hydatidiform mole. In the latter half of pregnancy they are abruptio placentae and placenta previa.

Abortion refers to the termination of a pregnancy prior to the age of viability of the fetus. Abortions are classified as either *spontaneous* (those occurring naturally) or *induced* (those that result from artificial intervention).

Ectopic pregnancy is the implantation of the blastocyst at any site outside the uterus. Sites include the ovary, abdomen, and fallopian tube. Tubal implantation is the most common type and occurs in 90 percent of the cases of ectopic pregnancy.

Hydatidiform mole, a degenerative disorder of the trophoblast, occurs in approximately one out of every 1500 pregnancies in the United States (Pritchard, MacDonald, and Gant, 1985). In this disorder the trophoblastic villi degenerate and the cells fill with clear fluid to form clusters of vesicles that resemble a cluster of grapes. Although there is no fetus present, the vesicles grow at a rapid rate, causing the uterus to enlarge.

Abruptio placentae is the premature separation of a normally implanted placenta. This disorder occurs in 0.5 percent of deliveries and is seen most frequently in women with hypertension during pregnancy (Pritchard, MacDonald, and Gant, 1985). Marginal placental separation is the most

---

CASE PRESENTATION:

PUERPERAL INFECTION

F.D. is 36 years old (gravida 3, para 1), with premature rupture of membranes at 38 weeks' gestation. She was delivered by primary cesarean section at 2 hours postrupture, because of a history of genital herpes and a positive culture 1 week prior to delivery. Delivery and immediate recovery were uneventful. Patient and infant were isolated as per hospital protocol for active herpes simplex. Following the operative delivery, the patient was started on Piperacil, 2 g IV every 6 hours, prophylactically. On the second postpartum day, Ms. D. reached a temperature of 102–103°F (orally). On exam, her lungs were found to be clear, the abdomen soft, the uterus nontender, and the wound site intact. Lochia was appropriate and without foul odor; calves were negative for Homans' sign. The white blood count was 8000–9000, with no bands. Gentamicin was added to her regimen following uterine, blood, and urine cultures.

On the third postoperative day, her temperature remained at 102°F. The white blood count was then 12,000 with three bands, and the lochia had assumed a foul odor. A tentative diagnosis of endometritis was made. On the fourth postoperative day the patient had a mildly tender uterus, a temperature of 100.4°F (with afebrile periods), and continued foul lochia. Preliminary cultures were without definitive findings. By the fifth day, Ms. D. was afebrile with resolving uterine tenderness and decreasing lochial odor. She reported an absence of malaise and myalgia and was discharged with her infant on day 6.

NURSING CARE PLAN OF MS. D.:

PUERPERAL INFECTION

Nursing Diagnosis	Expected Outcome	Nursing Interventions	Rationale
1. Potential subinvolution/impaired healing due to endotoxin effect on uterine tissue	1. Patient will show appropriate reduction in uterine size, with no excessive bleeding; wound healing will proceed normally	1a. Palpate fundus and note its size, consistency, tenderness, response to massage; assess amount, type, and odor of lochia b. Observe wound/incision c. Notify physician appropriately; follow lab tests to monitor presence of infection; administer antibiotics as ordered – note response d. Isolate as appropriate – adhere to aseptic technique	1a. To monitor involution process b. To assess would healing and rule out infection c. To initiate early diagnosis and provide necessary treatment d. To protect other mothers and infants from infection
2. Fever/malaise/myalgia related to presence of pathogen and physiologic response	2. Temperature will be within normal limits; patient will report reduced or absent discomfort	2a. Assess heart rate, temperature, BP every 2–4 hours b. Question patient as to signs and symptoms of infection (i.e. generalized malaise, muscle ache); notify physician and document c. Plan care and visitations d. Administer antipyretics as ordered e. Assist in repositioning and offer K-pad to areas of discomfort	2a. To monitor patient's vital signs for presence of infection b. To assess and rule out possibility of infection c. To maximize rest periods d. To decrease temperature e. To aid patient with comfort measures
3. Potential fluid, electrolyte, and nitrogen imbalance due to decreased fluid and nutrients and increased insensible loss due to fever	3. Fluids will be in balance; electrolytes will be within normal limits; nitrogen will be in balance; intake will be appropriate	3a. Monitor intake and output: Measure urine every shift Push fluids with nutritional electrolyte value as appropriate Give small, frequent feedings Increase protein, carbohydrate content b. Obtain/arrange for lab screening as ordered	3a. To maintain fluid and electrolyte balance and to avoid dehydration b. To monitor for fluid and electrolyte imbalances
4. Potential progression of infection to more serious sequelae (e.g. peritonitis)	4. Symptoms will be resolved; there will be no serious complications or symptoms	4a. Monitor for sustained fever despite pharmacologic therapy; continued subinvolution; deep flank pain; signs of ileus; signs and symptoms of septic shock b. Notify physician promptly	4a. To monitor for any complications of infection b. To initiate early diagnosis and treatment

common cause of spotting at 7 months' gestation or later.

Placenta previa is a placenta that is implanted in an abnormal site within the uterus. The placenta typically implants in the upper portion of the uterus, well away from the cervix. With placenta previa, however, it implants near or over the cervix. This can produce bleeding at the time the cervix begins to dilate. The four types of placenta previa are defined by Pritchard, MacDonald, and Gant as follows:

1. *Total placenta previa:* the cervical internal os is completely covered by the placenta.
2. *Partial placenta previa:* the internal os is partially covered by the placenta.
3. *Marginal placenta previa:* the edge of the placenta is at the margin of the internal os.
4. *Low-lying placenta:* the region of the internal os is encroached upon by the placenta, so that the placental edge may be palpated by the examining finger introduced through the cervix.

Risks to Mother and Infant

Hemorrhage is still the leading cause of maternal mortality, although the availability of blood and blood products has greatly reduced the number of such maternal deaths. Hemorrhage is also responsible for a large number of fetal deaths. When hemorrhage occurs in early pregnancy, the pregnancy often terminates spontaneously or requires medical intervention that terminates it, as with ectopic pregnancy. Low implantation of the placenta decreases its vascularity and may cause some intrauterine growth retardation in the infant.

Medical Intervention

The primary objective with any patient who is bleeding is to stop the bleeding and counteract the effects of hypovolemic shock. When the patient is pregnant, two lives may be affected by the loss of blood. Therefore, the nurse and physician must assess both the fetus and the mother and consider both in the determination of the plan of care.

In ectopic pregnancies there is often no sign until the patient begins to bleed. Most often, the bleeding occurs when the fallopian tube is no longer able to accommodate the growing embryo and ruptures. In most cases the patient will have missed only one menstrual period and may not be aware that she is pregnant. The bleeding is often dark and may vary in amount, depending on whether there is a gradual loss of blood from a small rupture or an acute loss from a large rupture. In addition to the bleeding, which may produce the characteristic signs of shock, the patient will complain of unilateral pain over the affected tube. Upon examination the physician may feel an adnexal mass. Once a preliminary diagnosis of tubal pregnancy is made, a laparotomy is done. Blood transfusions may be required prior to the surgery to stabilize the patient. In most cases a salpingectomy, or removal of the affected fallopian tube, is required. In rare cases the products of conception can be evacuated from the tube and the tube left in place.

CASE PRESENTATION:

PLACENTA PREVIA

D.B. is 30 years old (gravida 5, para 4), in her 35th week of pregnancy. D.B. has a good obstetric history. All previous pregnancies have gone to term and resulted in viable infants. In this pregnancy D.B. has had no significant problems. Her blood pressure has remained within an acceptable range. The urine has remained free of glucose and acetone. All other laboratory results have been within normal limits.

D.B. presents at the emergency room with complaints of a sudden gush of bright red blood. A small amount of bright red vaginal bleeding is present. When questioned, D.B. says she has had no pain. The abdomen is soft with no distention noted. The vital signs are blood pressure of 120/84, temperature of 98.8°F, pulse of 90, and respirations of 22. The fetal heart tones are 132 and regular. The physician plans to admit D.B. for bedrest and observation. The tentative diagnosis is placenta previa.

NURSING CARE PLAN OF D.B.:

PLACENTA PREVIA

Nursing Diagnosis	Expected Outcome	Nursing Interventions	Rationale
1. Potential for fluid volume deficit due to hypovolemic shock	1. The patient will exhibit no further vaginal bleeding; the patient will have no signs of fluid volume deficit	1a. Assess for vaginal bleeding every 15 min, then every 30 min b. Monitor BP, pulse, and respiration every 15 min, then every 30 min if stable c. Assess for other signs of shock every 15 min, then every 30 min d. Record intake and output e. Do *not* perform vaginal exam f. Obtain hematocrit, hemoglobin, and Rh as ordered g. Type and cross-match 2 units of blood as ordered h. Start an intravenous solution as prescribed (use 16-gauge needle in case blood must be transfused) i. Maintain complete bed rest with the head elevated 20–30 degrees j. Assess consistency of abdomen every 30 min	1. To prevent hypovolemic shock and continually assess for vaginal bleeding
2. Potential for fetal distress due to inadequate placental perfusion secondary to fluid volume deficit	2. FHTs will remain stabilized between 120 and 140; no increased or decreased fetal activity will occur; a viable infant will be delivered	2a. Assess FHTs every 30 min if no more bleeding occurs b. Monitor with external monitor if vaginal bleeding or labor should occur c. If signs of fetal distress occur, turn mother to left side, start O$_2$ and notify M.D. immediately	2. To assess for fetal distress and implement early intervention to ensure delivery of a healthy infant
3. Potential for surgical intervention	3. The patient will display an understanding of the possible need for surgery	3a. Allow nothing by mouth (NPO) b. Prepare for double setup exam (vaginal and abdominal delivery) c. Prepare for possibility of cesarean section	3. To have patient prepared for possibility of emergency cesarean section

For ectopic pregnancies that occur in the ovary, an oophrectomy (removal of the ovary) is required. In abdominal ectopic pregnancies the placenta is implanted on some abdominal organ, such as the liver or intestine. During surgery the cord is cut flush with the placenta, which is left in place. The placenta will then dissolve and be absorbed. This is done because an attempt to remove the placenta may cause massive hemorrhage.

In hydatidiform mole pregnancies the primary objective is to evacuate the uterus. If caught early enough, a dilatation and curettage may be performed. However, if the mole is too large for this method and the uterus is to be preserved, a hysterotomy may be performed. In older women who desire no further pregnancies, a hysterectomy is the treatment of choice, since choriocarcinoma, a malignant condition of the trophoblast, often follows molar pregnancies. After the initial treatment, women who have not had a hysterectomy are followed closely for a year to detect the presence of increased levels of human chorionic gonadotropin (HCG), which is indicative of choriocarcinoma. Because a pregnancy will also produce elevated levels of HCG, the patient should be instructed not to become pregnant for a year following termination of the molar pregnancy.

In late pregnancy, bleeding is evaluated to determine the etiology, which will influence the treatment prescribed. Table 30–7 compares the signs and symptoms of abruptio placentae and placenta previa. With both of these bleeding disorders, prompt intervention may be required to save the fetus if distress should occur.

In placenta previa the extent of the previa determines whether the patient will be allowed to deliver vaginally or will require a cesarean section. With total placenta previa, a cesarean section will always be required if the fetus is viable. With the other types of placental previa the amount of placenta involved and the condition of the fetus will determine whether a cesarean section is needed. If the bleeding from a placenta previa occurs before term, the patient may be hospitalized for bedrest and closely monitored for signs of fetal distress, which may occur as the cervix begins to dilate. Any woman with placenta previa should have blood available in case the need for surgery should arise.

In abruptio placentae the degree of placental separation and the condition of the fetus influence the medical management. In cases in which the placental separation is not severe, bedrest and close observation may be prescribed. However, with pronounced amounts of placental involvement the fetus is in jeopardy and an immediate cesarean section may be necessary.

Two potential problems that are of great concern to the physician and nurse managing a pregnancy complicated by abruptio placentae are *couvelaire uterus* and *disseminated intravascular coagulation defect* (DIC). A couvelaire uterus is a uterus that has become ecchymotic and has lost its ability to contract because of the filling of the myometrial wall with blood. In abruptio placentae, in which there has been concealed hemorrhage, the blood is often forced into the uterine wall. With couvelaire uterus a hysterectomy may be required if the uterus will not contract and bleeding continues after delivery.

Disseminated intravascular coagulation is a pathologic form of clotting. In this disorder, which

TABLE 30–7.	Comparison of Abruptio Placentae and Placenta Previa	
Characteristic	*Abruptio Placentae*	*Placenta Previa*
Pathology	Sudden separation of a normally implanted placenta	Abnormal implantation of the placenta
Vaginal bleeding	May not be present if concealed behind placenta; if present, it will appear dark	Abrupt in onset and will be bright red in color
Pain	Typically manifests as a sharp, stabbing pain in abdomen	None
Uterus	Myometrium may fill with blood, producing a hard, boardlike abdomen	Soft unless uterine contractions are present

may be precipitated by abruptio placentae, preeclampsia/eclampsia, hydatidiform mole, or a dead fetus *in utero,* there is uncontrolled hemorrhage. Treatment is to replace the lost blood with fresh blood if possible. Frozen plasma is required to supply necessary clotting factors and to replace volume. In addition, cryoprecipitate may be ordered to supply fibrinogen and factor VIII.

POSTPARTAL HEMORRHAGE

Postpartal hemorrhagic disorders are among the leading causes of maternal mortality and protracted recovery in the postpartal period. If left untreated, hemorrhage from sites within the genital tract leads to cardiovascular collapse and may trigger a cluster of serious sequelae, including defects in the coagulation system. In this section we will discuss phenomena commonly responsible for postpartal hemorrhage, and recommended management.

Etiology/Diagnosis

During normal pregnancy, a number of hematologic adaptations occur, thus safeguarding hemostasis at the time of delivery and during the immediate postpartum period. The blood volume is generally expanded approximately 1500 ml (or 40–50 percent), depending on the size and prepregnancy blood volume of the woman. In addition, the concentration of plasma coagulation factors is increased, notably fibrinogen and factors VII, VIII, IX, and X (Pritchard, 1973; Lange and Dynesius, 1973; Laros and Alger, 1979).

Estimated blood loss during and following normal vaginal delivery is approximately 600 ml, compared to approximately 1000 ml for cesarean section. Many factors may singly or in combination significantly increase this loss. They include uterine atony, adherent placental fragments, failure of involution of the placental site (subinvolution), trauma to the genital tract with incisions or lacerations, coagulopathy, and uterine inversion. Predisposing factors are summarized in Table 30–8.

If excessive bleeding is suspected, it is imperative to locate the source and treat appropriately. If the source is traumatic, steps must be taken to repair the tissue or, if this fails, to ligate the involved vessels. With atony, oxytocin or Methergine (ergot derivatives) may be given. Whenever oxytocin is administered intravenously, it should not be injected as a bolus directly into the vein or IV line because this may cause acute hypotension and cardiac arrest (Knuppel and Drukker, 1986). Prostaglandins have also been used to improve muscle tone. These drugs can be administered intravenously, intramuscularly, or as a vaginal suppository, depending on the drug used. Retained or adherent placental fragments dictate exploration, removal, and uterine massage; pharmacologic therapy may also be indicated. In all cases, volume replacement must be concomitant (Pritchard, 1973; Watson, 1980).

TABLE 30–8. Factors Predisposing to Postpartal Hemorrhage

Prepregnancy

Fibroid uterus

Grand multiparity

Previous postpartal hemorrhage from uterine atony

Coagulation defects:
  Acquired
  Congenital

Antepartum/Intrapartum

Hypotonic myometrium
  General anesthesia (especially with halogenated compounds)
  Poorly perfused myometrium (hypotension due to hemorrhage or conduction anesthesia)
  Overdistended uterus (large fetus, multiple fetuses, polyhydramnios)
  Prolonged labor
  Rapid labor
  Labor with vigorous oxytocin stimulation
  Chorioamnionitis

Retention of placental tissue
  Abnormally adherent placenta
  Accessory lobes

Trauma to the genital tract
  Large episiotomy
  Lacerations of cervix, vagina, perineum
  Uterine rupture
  Operative abdominal delivery
  Operative vaginal delivery
  Forceps manipulations
  Delivery through an incompletely dilated cervix
  Vaginal delivery after cesarean section

Uterine inversion (due to atony, removal of adherent placenta, excessive cord traction)

SOURCE: Pritchard, MacDonald, and Gant (1985).

Incidence

Estimated blood loss exceeding 500–600 ml during and following a vaginal delivery and 1000 ml during and following a cesarean section occurs in 3–5 percent of all deliveries (McKenzie, 1983).

Pathophysiology/Clinical Aspects

Normally, a decrease in the volume of the uterus occurs with fetal delivery, and the implantation site reduces in area, facilitating shearing of the placenta from the decidual lining (Pritchard, 1973); thus, the process of involution begins. Immediately following delivery of the placenta, contractions of the myometrium compress and constrict the exposed, severed vessels of the implantation site to minimize blood loss. When placental delivery is incomplete, effective myometrial contraction and, therefore, constriction of vessels at the implantation site is impeded. Under these circumstances, continued and severe blood loss may occur. Even when the placenta has been examined for intactness, retained placental fragments may be recovered from the uterus, especially with the presence of succenturiate or accessory lobes (Woodling et al., 1976).

Women with predisposing factors must be closely observed. In anticipation of possible hemorrhage, an intravenous route appropriate for fluid and blood product administration, as well as blood product availability, may be established. The size and location of the fundus and the volume of lochia must be monitored, since a uterus may be palpably firm and yet be insidiously filling with or sequestering blood and clots. Also of significance in postpartum hemorrhage is failure of the pulse and blood pressure to reflect more than moderate alterations until large amounts of blood volume have been lost (Pritchard, MacDonald, and Gant, 1985).

In the absence of apparent atony and with a firm fundus at or below the umbilicus, excessive blood loss from other sources must be considered and investigated. Trauma to the genital tract may be induced by operative or instrumental delivery or may occur with spontaneous delivery of the fetus. It is not uncommon for lacerations of the upper vaginal tract to go unnoticed until heavy bleeding ensues. Inspection of the genital tract and appropriate repair should proceed quickly, along with adequate fluid replacement. Differential diagnosis to rule out other, though rare, causes of postpartum hemorrhage, such as uterine rupture, abnormal implantation of the placenta, coagulopathy, and uterine inversion (occult or complete), must be undertaken (Watson, 1980).

The seriousness of the deleterious effects of hemorrhage to the woman depend greatly on the maternal blood volume, the extent of pregnancy-induced volume expansion, and the presence or absence of anemia at the time of delivery.

Management of postpartal hemorrhage to prevent severe hypovolemia and shock consists of meticulous attention to volume replacement to prevent circulatory collapse (see Table 30–9 for symptoms of shock). A large-bore intravenous access route is essential to deliver crystalloid solutions and blood products. It is not uncommon to place additional intravenous lines and a central venous pressure catheter to facilitate volume administration and gauge fluid replacement needs more accurately. An indwelling urinary catheter is inserted to determine urinary output. Renal blood flow is especially sensitive to changes in blood volume and may be reflected in quantity and specific gravity of urine. Urine flow, when carefully measured, has proved to be extremely valuable in monitoring perfusion of the kidney and other vital organs affected by volume depletion (Pritchard, 1973; Watson, 1980).

Treatment of severe postpartal hemorrhage with hypovolemic shock is aimed at refilling the vascular compartment as quickly as possible. Lactated Ringer's solution (crystalloid) and blood products are delivered via several peripheral IV lines to keep urinary output at least 30 ml/hour (ideally 60 ml/hour) and hematocrit at 30 percent or slightly greater. A central venous pressure (CVP) or Swan Ganz pulmonary artery catheter should be in place to evaluate fluid needs and to guard against pulmonary edema resulting from overzealous volume expansion (Pritchard, 1973; Watson, 1980).

Further management of severe hemorrhage with shock in the postpartum period may include exploration of the abdomen to rule out rupture of the uterus; ligation of the uterine or internal iliac arteries; intramyometrial prostaglandin $F_2\alpha$ or intramuscular prostaglandin $F_2\alpha$ ester; hysterectomy; or use of a gravity suit to facilitate stabilization and return to normal hemostasis (Watson, 1980).

Rarely, with severe hemorrhage, the coagulation mechanism is activated, precipitating disseminated intravascular coagulation (DIC), or consumptive coagulopathy. This syndrome may markedly increase blood loss due to lack of available clotting factors; it must be treated promptly with replacement of blood (to keep hematocrit greater than 32 percent), platelets (to keep count greater than 75,000), and cryoprecipitate (to restore fibrinogen levels to greater than 100 mg/100 ml). Obstetric conditions increasing the risk of DIC are (Watson, 1980):

1. Pregnancy-induced hypertension
2. Abruptio placentae

CASE PRESENTATION:

POSTPARTAL HEMORRHAGE

A.M. is 28 years old (gravida 3, para 2). She arrived in the labor and delivery suite at 8 cm dilated, +1 station, with intact membranes, having begun labor 1 hour prior to admission. She was taken to the delivery room, where an amniotomy was performed, with rapid progression to complete dilation. While awaiting placental delivery, the physician inspected the cervix and vaginal vault and found them to be intact. There were no signs of placental separation (gushing blood, lengthening of the cord, rise of fundus into abdominal cavity).

Thirty minutes after delivery the physician gently explored the uterus, but attempts to facilitate completion of separation and expulsion were not met with success. The fundus was soft and only temporarily responsive to massage. Brisk blood flow prevented further exploration or visualization. The anesthesiologist was notified. A 16-gauge catheter was placed, with blood drawn for cross match, and lactated Ringer's solution was infused. Blood pressure and heart rate remained close to intrapartal values (100–110/60–70; 90–110). Although she was responsive to questioning and pain, Mrs. M.'s response time was decreasing.

By 50 min postdelivery, the estimated blood loss approached 2000 ml. Type-specific uncrossed, matched blood was ordered by the anesthesiologist, who performed a rapid-sequence induction (general anesthesia) to allow the obstetrician an opportunity to explore without impediment. The placenta was found to be firmly adherent with some areas of detachment (placenta accreta) and was manually removed with the aid of curretage. A Foley catheter was placed, returning 100 ml dark amber urine, which was emptied. Two units of whole blood were administered rapidly. A central venous pressure (CVP) catheter was placed. Total fluid intake to this point consisted of 4 liters of lactated Ringer's solution and 2 units of whole blood, for a total of 5000 ml. Initial CVP was 12 cm H_2O and the intravenous fluid rate was decreased.

The patient was extubated and transferred to the recovery room 90 min postdelivery, with oxygen running. Vital signs were blood pressure 84/56; heart rate 130; respiratory rate 14 and regular; CVP 13.5 cm H_2O; and a small quantity of urine in the urometer. Intravenous fluids were running at TKO (to keep open) rate and the patient was responsive to command. Fundus was firm ↑ 1 U. Initial laboratory values showed hematocrit at 24 percent and platelets at 130,000.

Over the next hour, the CVP gradually rose to 15.6 cm H_2O, and the chest presented with bilateral rales and decreased breath sounds in the bases; respiratory rate increased to 24, blood pressure to 90/62, and heart rate to 140. Fundal height and lochia remained appropriate. Urinary output was 25 ml. Intravenous fluids were continued at TKO. Lasix 20 mg IV was administered, and a unit of packed red blood cells was superimposed at a slow rate.

Over the next 6 hours, the vital signs returned to intrapartum values, urinary response to Lasix was remarkable, and the chest improved. By 10 hours postdelivery the patient was awake and alert, with stable fundus, stable vital signs, appropriate urine output, and a clear chest. She was transferred to a postpartum room. Repeat hematocrit was 30 percent at 12 hours postdelivery, with a platelet count of 200,000. An additional unit of packed cells was administered. Mrs. M. continued to improve over the next 48 hours and was discharged with her infant on the fourth postpartum day with a hematocrit of 36 percent and platelet count of 250,000.

NURSING CARE PLAN OF MRS. M.:

HEMORRHAGE

Nursing Diagnosis	Expected Outcome	Nursing Interventions	Rationale
1. Excessive blood loss	1. Blood loss will be corrected	1. Facilitate voiding; give frequent uterus massage and instruct patient in same	1. To minimize blood loss, prevent hemorrhage
2. Uterine atony	2. Uterine tone will be restored	2. Note whether uterus boggy, and massage fundus	2. To monitor for uterine atony
3. Retained placenta accreta, accessory lobes	3. Placenta will be expelled	3. Note whether clots expressed, and check for tissue	3. To monitor for possible retained placental fragments
4. Laceration of cervix or vagina; occult/overt uterine inversion	4. Tissue will be repaired; uterine position/tone will be restored	4. Note whether uterus firm without increase in flow on uterine massage	4. To monitor blood loss
5. Presence of hemorrhage	5. Condition will be treated	5. Note whether vaginal flow is bright red, dark, or absent with increasing uterine size	5. To assess presence of hemorrhage
6. Potential hypovolemic shock due to severe loss of circulating volume	6. Circulatory volume will be restored; excessive bleeding will cease	6a. Make sure adequate IV is in place (large bore) fluid load with crystalloid solution (D.LR, LR); clot for type and crossmatch b. Monitor blood pressure and quality of respirations, pulse rate and quality c. Measure output – catheterize as ordered d. Assess skin for pallor, cyanosis, coldness, clamminess e. Observe for changes in level of consciousness f. Count pads and weigh contents (1 lb of weight = 1 pt of fluid) g. Trendelenburg position; O$_2$/mask at 7 liters/min	6a. To maintain open IV line should immediate fluids or blood be needed b. To monitor for presence of shock f. To assess amount of blood loss g. To minimize blood loss

NURSING CARE PLAN OF MRS. M.: Continued

HEMORRHAGE

Nursing Diagnosis	Expected Outcome	Nursing Interventions	Rationale
		h. Administer IV oxytocin, blood, and Methergine as ordered i. Keep patient NPO until bleeding subsides j. Provide constant attendance; explain all procedures to reduce anxiety k. Obtain appropriate labs as ordered.	h. To help contract uterus i. To keep patient from aspirating if surgery needed j. To provide support k. To monitor any changes
7. Potential coagulopathy due to reduction in clotting factors	7. Clotting factors (platelets, fibrinogen, fibrin split products) will be within normal limits	7a. Note lab values—keep physician informed b. Observe for bleeding from venipuncture sites, hematuria, ecchymosis, excessive lochial flow c. Prevent injury	7a. To assess any change b. To monitor for potential coagulopathy c. To prevent further problems with bleeding
8. Potential pulmonary edema with fluid overload	8. Pulmonary edema will be absent with chest clear; CVP will be within normal limits; there will be no shortness of breath or tachypnea	8a. Observe closely for increased respiration rate, shortness of breath, moist breath sounds, increasing CVP, decreasing urinary output b. Administer diuretics as appropriate and document response	8a. To monitor for possible pulmonary edema b. To aid in elimination of excessive fluids that could contribute to pulmonary edema

3. Retained placental tissue
4. Sepsis
5. Massive transfusion of stored blood
6. Acquired coagulopathies (Von Willebrand's disease; thrombocytopenia purpura; idiopathic thrombocytopenia purpura)
7. Amniotic fluid embolism

Nursing care of the postpartum patient mandates close observation of hemodynamic status. Early recognition of excessive blood loss, identification of the source of hemorrhage, and prompt intervention to reduce blood loss and reestablish circulating volume are essential to appropriate nursing management.

PULMONARY EMBOLISM: THROMBOEMBOLIC DISEASE

Venous thromboembolic disease is a common complication of the postpartum period. Thromboses with a significant potential for creating pulmonary emboli may originate in the deep veins of the leg, thigh, or pelvis. Thrombophlebitis that involves the more superficial vessels is less likely to generate pulmonary emboli. Nevertheless, the greatest danger from postpartum venous thromboses is, in fact, pulmonary embolism. Embolism of the pulmonary artery obstructs circulation to the lungs, reduces cardiac output, and may cause

TABLE 30-9. Symptoms of Shock

Parameter	Mild	Moderate	Severe	Irreversible
Respirations	Rapid, deep	Rapid, becoming shallow	Rapid, shallow, may be irregular	Irregular or barely perceptible
Pulse	Rapid, tone normal	Rapid, tone may be normal but is becoming weaker	Very rapid, easily collapsible, may be irregular	Irregular apical pulse
Blood pressure	Normal or hypertensive	69–90 mm Hg systolic	Below 60 mm Hg systolic	None palpable
Skin	Cool and pale	Cool, pale, moist, some cyanosis	Cold, clammy; cyanosis of lips and fingernails	Cold, clammy, cyanotic
Urine output	No change	Decreasing to 10–20 ml/hour	Oliguric (less than 10 ml) to anuric	Anuric
Level of consciousness	Alert, oriented; diffuse anxiety	Oriented; mental cloudiness or increasing restlessness	Lethargy; reacts to noxious stimuli; comatose	Does not respond to noxious stimuli
Central venous pressure	May be normal	3 cm H_2O		0–3 cm H_2O

SOURCE: Wagner (1973).

profound cardiorespiratory collapse (Laros and Alger, 1979).

Incidence/Diagnosis

The reported incidence of pulmonary embolism during the postpartum period is 0.6 percent. It is a leading cause of nonobstetric postpartum death, with puerperal patients outnumbering antepartal patients three to one. The incidence of pulmonary embolism depends heavily on whether deep vein thrombosis (DVT) is adequately treated. Without treatment, 24 percent of patients with DVT will develop pulmonary emboli (Laros and Alger, 1979). Untreated pulmonary embolism can result in a mortality rate of 50 percent (Knuppel and Drukker, 1986). Diagnosis is difficult; careful examination and screening for risk factors are essential.

The risk of thromboembolic disease and subsequent pulmonary embolism is increased by cesarean section (ninefold over vaginal delivery), forceps delivery, advanced maternal age, increased parity, and estrogen suppression of lactation. Other reported risk factors include a history of prior thromboembolism; trauma or infection; obesity; congestive heart failure; dehydration; shock; and anemia (especially sickle cell).

Deep vein thrombosis is seen most frequently on the second postpartum day and demands prompt anticoagulant therapy to prevent pulmonary embolism (Laros and Alger, 1979). When pulmonary embolism develops, tachypnea becomes the most significant sign (see Table 30–10 for common signs and symptoms of pulmonary embolism.) Pulmonary embolism may or may not result in infarction. Small emboli may become lodged peripherally and precipitate infarction accompanied by pleural signs that include cough, hemoptysis, pleuritic chest pain with splinting, and a friction rub. However, the majority of emboli do not produce infarction, so these symptoms may be absent, with only tachycardia or atelectic rales and apprehension presenting. Multiple small emboli may mimic a major embolus.

Pathophysiology/Clinical Aspects

Pregnancy produces significant alterations in the coagulation mechanism, with all factors increased except XI and XIII. A hypercoagulable state is achieved, preparing the woman for placental sep-

TABLE 30–10. Signs and Symptoms of Pulmonary Embolism

Observations	Percentage of Patients Indicating Findings with Pulmonary Embolus
Tachypnea	81
Dyspnea	81
Pleuritic pain	72
Apprehension	59
Cough	54
Tachycardia	43
Hemoptysis	34
Temperature over 37°C	34

SOURCE: Adapted from Laros and Alger (1979).

TABLE 30–11. Coagulation Factors and Pregnancy

Factor/Activity	Effects of Pregnancy
Platelets	Slow decrease during pregnancy; further decrease after delivery; marked increase 3rd–5th postpartum day; no change in adhesiveness
Fibrinogen	Marked increase during antepartum period; no change during labor, but prompt decrease after placental delivery; incease to predelivery level by day 3–5 with slow decrease thereafter
Prothrombin	No change
V	Immediate increase after placental delivery; slow decrease to normal by day 7
VII, IX, X	Progressive increase during pregnancy; gradual decrease in puerperium
VIII	Progressive increase during pregnancy; decrease after delivery with secondary increase, then gradual decrease
XI, XIII	Decrease during pregnancy; gradual increase to normal in puerperium
Fibrin split products	Increase in labor and immediately postpartum
Fibrinolysis	Decrease after first trimester with prompt increase to normal after delivery

SOURCE: Laros and Alger (1979).

aration at delivery. The noted diminution of platelets, fibrinogen, and factor VIII is thought to represent localized intravascular coagulation at the implantation site, with the increased fibrin split products suggesting local fibrinolysis (see Table 30–11 for a summary of alterations in coagulation factors).

A triad of factors are postulated in the activation of intravascular clot formation: (1) injury to the vessel wall, (2) stasis, and (3) changes in local clotting factors. Various arguments can be made to support the potential presence of this pathogenic state in pregnancy (Laros and Alger, 1979):

1. Vein distensibility is present from the first trimester (alterations in vessel integrity).
2. The rate of venous return from the lower extremities is reduced by 50 percent, creating stasis of varying degrees (this occurs in the third trimester and is due to uterine mechanical obstruction). A tendency toward increasing stasis manifests with the restriction in activity level enforced with complications of pregnancy.
3. The hypercoagulable state and increased fibrinolysis during pregnancy complete the triad.

Once significant pulmonary embolism has occurred, and depending on the presence or degree of obstruction, several mechanical factors produce the main sequelae (Courtney, 1974):

1. Abrupt decrease in blood flow to the left side of the heart, with decreased left ventricular outflow, precipitates peripheral vascular collapse.
2. Sudden onset of pulmonary hypertension with acute cor pulmonale and right heart failure contributes to pulmonary edema.
3. Disturbance of the ventilation/perfusion ratio creates hypoxemia, manifesting in cyanosis (decreasing arterial oxygen saturation and hyperpnea), restlessness, convulsions, and coma.

Findings

In addition to physical examination and consideration of risk factors, specific laboratory evaluation

CASE PRESENTATION:

PULMONARY EMBOLISM

G.F., a 32-year-old (gravida 3, para 2), was admitted to the labor and delivery suite at 8 cm cervical dilation with a bulging bag of waters. Her contractions were every 10–15 min, 20–30 sec in duration, and less than adequate quality. Mrs. F. was 5'0" and appeared, by abdominal exam, to have an exceptionally large infant. The physician was notified of her arrival and was provided with a status report. Upon his arrival, an amniotomy was performed, revealing meconium-stained amniotic fluid. The internal fetal monitor was applied and oxytocin augmentation infusion was initiated at 2 mu/min. The patient progressed slowly to complete dilation and was transferred to the delivery room.

Delivery of the head was uneventful; however, this was followed by impaction of the shoulders. Fundal pressure and traction facilitated delivery of the shoulders 5 min after delivery of the head. The infant weighed 10 pounds, 8 ounces. Immediate positive pressure O_2 resuscitation of the neonate met with good response. Shortly after spontaneous delivery of the placenta, the patient had a grand mal seizure followed by respiratory then cardiac arrest. Immediate cardiopulmonary resuscitation efforts were instituted, including ventilation and drug therapy, without response. A cardiologist was called and a transvenous pacemaker was placed. Electrical-mechanical dissociation was evident. Forty minutes following initiation of CPR the patient was pronounced dead. On postmortem, amniotic fluid debris, including meconium, was isolated in the pulmonary arteries.

NURSING CARE PLAN:

PULMONARY EMBOLISM

Nursing Diagnosis	Expected Outcome	Nursing Interventions	Rationale
1. Respiratory distress due to a reduction in pulmonary perfusion with impaired gaseous exchange	1. Respiratory rate will be within normal limits; respiratory disorders will be absent; arterial blood gases will be within normal limits	1a. Evaluate respiratory status b. Assess vital signs every shift c. Observe for cyanosis of mucous membranes d. Note hemoptysis, evidence of pulmonary edema (CVP) e. Administer O_2 as ordered f. Administer analgesics as ordered g. encourage bedrest	1a. To monitor for respiratory distress b. To monitor any hypotension c. To assess respiratory distress d. To assess any evidence of pulmonary embolus e. To increase oxygen saturation and reduce respiratory effort f. To decrease anxiety g. To decrease metabolic demands, allow clot organization

NURSING CARE PLAN: Continued

PULMONARY EMBOLISM

Nursing Diagnosis	Expected Outcome	Nursing Interventions	Rationale
2. Potential adverse effect due to heparin therapy	2. Unusual bleeding will be absent and lochial flow appropriate; incision site or perineum will lack evidence of hematoma formation or excessive ecchymosis	2a. Observe puncture sites; note intactness/condition of abdominal incision or perineum; follow response to therapy in thrombin clotting time, activated clotting time, prothrombin time, partial thromboplastin time b. Notify physician of signs of excessive bleeding – abnormal values out of anticipated therapeutic range c. Provide for safe environment d. Instruct patient in purpose of heparin therapy and potential side effects; emphasize importance of taking care to prevent injury; observe for excessive lochial flow	2a. To assess for effects of heparin b. To initiate early treatment if lab values not within therapeutic range c. To ensure patient safety d. To decrease patient anxiety and to ensure patient safety
3. Anxiety/apprehension due to impaired respiratory status and discomfort	3. Patient/family will be able to ventilate fears, concerns, informational needs; will verbalize understanding of rationale for plan of care	3. Explain all procedures; reassure patient; make sure O_2 and necessary supportive equipment/meds are immediately available; administer morphine sulfate	3. To decrease anxiety and apprehension
4. Potential cardiorespiratory (CR) collapse due to obstructed flow of oxygenated blood	4. There will be no C-R collapse; no symptoms indicative of worsening in patient's condition	4. Observe for worsening of respiratory difficulty, increased cyanosis, profound drop in BP, increased heart rate, seizure activity, change in level of consciousness; institute emergency therapy (CPR) if indicated, and summon help	4. To monitor and continuously assess for any evidence of cardiorespiratory collapse

may facilitate confirmation of a pulmonary embolus. These laboratory findings are listed in Table 30-12.

Management

Supportive Therapy

Oxygen therapy is especially important, with the aim to increase or maintain the pO_2 greater than 70 mm Hg. Postpartum oxygen administration may be required if pulmonary edema accompanies embolism. Narcotics such as Demerol or morphine are used to alleviate pain and apprehension. Bedrest is indicated for 5-7 days and allows time for initial organization of the clot. Straining at defecation should be avoided, and stool softeners as well as an increase in dietary fiber should be prescribed. Isuprel is recommended for hypotension (2-4 mg in 500 ml D_5W drip by titration).

Fluid administration is monitored by means of a CVP line. Aminophylline may be used to reduce bronchospasm while facilitating diuresis and is of benefit in relieving pulmonary edema. Digoxin is given for cardiac failure but is rarely helpful. Antibiotics are reserved for septic emboli (Laros and Alger, 1979).

Pharmacologic Therapy

Heparin, the drug of choice for acute pulmonary embolism, acts to interfere with fibrin formation. Because of its large molecular size, it is not excreted in the breast milk. It can be reversed rapidly by protamine sulfate 1 mg per 100 units of administered heparin (if using a continuous infusion, twice the amount necessary to neutralize the hourly dose is adequate). No greater than 50 mg of protamine sulfate should be given over a 10-min period, since protamine itself may cause bleeding.

For a pulmonary embolus, a loading dose of 10,000-15,000 units is given intravenously and initially facilitates relief of vasospasm as well as inhibiting the larger amounts of clotting factors. The maintenance dose is delivered by a controlled infusion device only. A number of laboratory tests facilitate the adjustment of maintenance dosing: TCT (thrombin clotting time - to achieve 2-3 times control); ACT (activated clotting time - to achieve 1.5-2.5 times control); and PTT (partial thromboplastin time). These tests are performed several times a day. Once a stable dosage is achieved, testing may be reduced to once daily or every other day (Laros and Alger, 1979).

The major risk of anticoagulant therapy is bleeding; the patient must be counseled on avoiding injury and monitored closely while on intravenous heparin. Hemocrit and hemoglobin measurements may reveal concealed hemorrhage (Pritchard, MacDonald, and Gant, 1985).

CAUTIONS. Heparin should not be mixed in glucose solutions as it loses its activity in the presence of glucose; however, it is safe in various salt

TABLE 30-12. Laboratory Findings

Laboratory Study	Findings with Pulmonary Embolus
Arterial pO_2	80 mm Hg on room air
EKG	Abnormal in 90% of cases - tachycardia with massive embolism; nonspecific T wave inversion; R+ axis deviation
Chest x-ray	Infiltration; elevation of diaphragm; areas of increased radiolucency; pleural effusion
Lung scan	Hypoperfusion
Angiography	Radiographic evidence of embolism/obstruction
Other:	
White blood count (WBC)	Always elevated
Serum LDH	Always elevated
Bilirubin	Always elevated
Erythrocyte sedimentation rate	Always elevated
Fibrin split products	Always present

SOURCE: Laros and Alger (1979).

solutions. To protect against accidental overdose, no greater than a 6-hour dose should be utilized at any one time. In patients with renal disease, heparin clearance and excretion are reduced and lower doses are used (less than standard 15–20 U/kg/per hour).

Continuous intravenous heparin is administered for an acute pulmonary embolus or until symptoms have resolved and there is no evidence of recurrence. The patient is then placed on subcutaneous heparin or oral Coumadin for 3–6 months if long-term management is required.

Subcutaneous heparin is given every 12 hours, with the patient instructed in self-administration into the anterior abdominal wall. The patient must also be cautioned about the use of aspirin and preparations containing aspirin (Laros and Alger, 1979). Local hematoma is avoided by applying ice to the site and rotating sites each day. Intramuscular use of heparin is contraindicated because of an increased incidence of hematoma formation.

Alternative Therapies

FIBRINOLYTIC AGENTS. Two agents, streptokinase and urokinase, are available. They act to increase plasmin formation and, therefore, clot lysis. Both drugs produce rapid resolution of pulmonary emboli. Unfortunately, both are contraindicated during pregnancy and the first 10 postpartum days. If used with patients who have undergone anticoagulation, great caution must be exercised, since this combination significantly increases the risk of overanticoagulation and bleeding.

ANTIPLATELET AGENTS. Antiplatelet agents play a role in resolving arterial emboli but are of little benefit in the treatment or prophylaxis of DVT. Dextran is the most commonly used drug and must be given intravenously; however, it is less effective than subcutaneous heparin.

SURGICAL INTERVENTION. Pulmonary embolectomy is considered only in patients with angiographic evidence of massive embolism of the main pulmonary artery and failure to maintain adequate cardiac output despite therapeutic measures. This therapy requires thoracotomy and cardiopulmonary bypass but may be lifesaving (Laros and Alger, 1979).

Amniotic Fluid Embolus

Another source of pulmonary embolism – one with catastrophic consequences – is amniotic fluid embolus (AFE). AFE occurs in 1 out of 10,000–30,000 deliveries and accounts for 4–6 percent of all maternal deaths (Courtney, 1974; Pritchard, MacDonald, and Gant, 1985). Entry of amniotic fluid and debris into the maternal circulation is fatal in 80 percent of all cases (Pritchard, 1973). Amniotic fluid has been shown to possess potent procoagulant properties (Phillips and Davidson, 1972). Infusion of amniotic fluid causes overwhelming mechanical blockage of the pulmonary vessels and is thought to also induce an anaphylactoid reaction because of particulate matter (vernix, lanugo, meconium) (Courtney, 1974).

AFE is frequently associated with tumultuous labors of women delivering at term or post-term, intrauterine fetal death, multiparity, advancing age of the mother, and delivery of large infants. Diagnosis is commonly made postmortem; however, if the patient survives, a definitive diagnosis is made by placing a catheter into the right heart and pulmonary vasculature to sample blood for amniotic fluid debris (Courtney, 1974).

AFE presents with chills, shivering, severe dyspnea, respiratory distress (with perhaps arrest), circulatory collapse, cyanosis, and, not uncommonly, convulsions and coma (Pritchard, 1973; Courtney, 1974; Resnik et al., 1976). Embolism may come immediately after delivery or may be delayed because of trapping of the amniotic fluid in the uterine veins after delivery and gradual release into the circulation with the reduction in uterine tone (Courtney, 1974).

The response to pulmonary embolism with amniotic fluid is acute and overwhelming. Resuscitative therapy is required, with occasional pulmonary embolectomy undertaken if supportive services are available. Mortality and morbidity associated with this condition are high. Those patients who do survive tend to develop acute DIC with hemorrhage and uterine hypotonia that is resistant to treatment (Pritchard, 1973; Courtney, 1974; Resnik et al., 1976).

Pulmonary embolism poses a serious threat to the well-being and life of the patient during the postpartum period. The nurse must be cognizant of the factors that predispose the postpartum individual to deep vein thrombosis and subsequent pulmonary embolism. In addition, the nurse must continually evaluate the patient for evidence of suggestive thromboembolic phenomena.

SUMMARY

The major problems of the prenatal and postpartal period have been identified and defined. Undetected, these conditions can lead to poor maternal and neonatal outcomes. Some problems occur as a result of preexisting medical conditions, others develop in the course of the pregnancy or puerperineum. Early prenatal care plays a significant role in detecting any problems that develop. The nurse also plays a significant role in assessing the patient and preparing her and her family for possible complications with the infant. Early detection and prompt treatment are essential for ensuring a decrease in both infant and maternal morbidity and mortality.

REFERENCES

Anderson, W. R., and Davis, J. 1968. Placental site involution. *Am. J. Obstet. Gynecol.* 102:23–33.

Attwood, H. D. 1972. Amniotic fluid embolism. *Pathology Annuals.* 7:145–172.

Benedetti, T. J., and Carlson, R. W. 1979. Studies of lalloid osmotic pressure in pregnancy-induced hypertension. *Am. J. Obstet. Gynecol.* 135:308–311.

Byrne, J. J. 1973. Thromboembolism in pregnancy. In *Obstetrical and perinatal infections,* eds. D. Charles and M. Finland. Philadelphia: Lea & Febiger.

Carson, S. L., and Balognese, R. J. 1977. Postpartum uterine atony treated with prostaglandins. *Am. J. Obstet. Gynecol.* 129:918–919.

Cavanaugh, D.; Woods, R. E.; and O'Conner, T. C. F. 1978. *Obstetric Emergencies.* 2nd ed. Hagerstown, Md.: Harper & Row.

Center for Disease Control. 1979. Recommended Schedules. Publication 97–796. Atlanta, Georgia.

Charles, D., and Kelin, T. A. 1973. Postpartum infection. In *Obstetrical and perinatal infections,* eds. D. Charles and M. Finland. Philadelphia: Lea & Febiger.

Chesley, L. C. 1978. *Hypertensive Disorders in Pregnancy.* New York: Appleton-Century-Crofts.

Cohen, W. R., and Friedman, E. 1983. *Management of Labor.* Baltimore: University Press.

Colman, R. M., and Gibson, J. 1953. Pyrexia in the puerperium. *Lancet.* 649–652.

Condie, R. G. 1976. A serial study of coagulation factors XII, XI, and X in plasma in normal pregnancy and in pregnancy complicated by preeclampsia. *Brit. J. Obstet. Gynecol.* 83:636–639.

Courtney, L. D. 1974. Amniotic fluid embolism. *Obstet. Gynecol. Survey* 29:169–177.

Cryer, P. S., and Kissane, J. M., eds. 1980. Unexplained fever in the postpartum period. *Am. J. Med.* 69:443–450.

DePalma, R. T., et al. 1980. Identification and management of women at high risk for pelvic infection following cesarean section. *Obstet. Gynecol.* 55 (supplement): 1855–1915.

Dixon, R. E. 1973. Disseminated intravascular coagulation: A paradox of thrombosis and hemorrhage. Significance in obstetrics and gynecology. A review. *Obstet. Gynecol. Survey.* 28:385–393.

Eschenbach, D., and Wager, G. 1980. Puerperal infections. *Clin. Obstet. Gynecol.* 23:1003–1037.

Ferris, T. F. 1975. Toxemia and hypertension. In *Medical complications during pregnancy,* eds. G. Burrows and T. Ferris. Philadelphia: W. B. Saunders.

Filker, R., and Money, G. R. G. 1979. The significance of temperature during the first 24 hours postpartum. *Obstet. Gynecol.* 53:358–361.

Fliegner, J. R. 1971. Postpartum broad ligament haematomas. *J. Obstet. Gynecol. Brit. Commonwealth.* 78:184–189.

Fliegner, J. R. 1978. Third stage management: How important is it? *Med. J. Australia.* 190–193.

Fox, H. 1972. Placenta accreta, 1945–1969. *Obstet. Gynecol. Survey.* 27:475–490.

Gabbe, S. G.; Niebyl, J. R.,; and Simpson, J. L. 1986. *Obstetrics Normal and Problem Pregnancies.* New York: Churchill Livingstone.

Gibbs, R. S. 1976. Treatment of refractory postpartum fever. *Clin. Obstet. Gynecol.* 19:83–85.

Gibbs, R. S.; Jones, P. M.; and Wilder, C. J. 1978. Antibiotic therapy of endometritis following cesarean section: Treatment success and failures. *Obstet. Gynecol.* 52:31–37.

Gibbs, R. S.; O'Dell, T. N.; MacGregor, R. R.; Schwarz, R. H.; and Marton, H. 1976. Treatment of refractory postpartum fever. *Clin. Obstet. Gynecol.* 19:83–95.

Goplerud, C. P., and White, C. A. 1965. Postpartum infection: A comparative study for the period 1926 through 1961. *Obstet. Gynecol.* 25:227–231.

Goplerud, C. P.; Ohm, M. J.; and Galask, R. P. 1976. Aerobic and anaerobic flora of the cervix during pregnancy and the puerperium. *Am. J. Obstet.* 126:858–865.

Green, S. L., and Sarubbi, F. A. 1977. Risk factors associated with past cesarean section febrile morbidity. *Obstet. Gynecol.* 49:686–690.

Harwick, H. J.; Purcell, R. H.; Iuppa, J. B.; and Fekety, F. R. 1971. Mycoplasma hominis and postpartum febrile complications. *Obstet. Gynecol.* 37:765–768.

Hendricks, C. H., and Brerner, W. E. 1970. Cardiovascular effects of oxytocic drugs used postpartum. *Am. J. Obstet. Gynecol.* 108:751–760.

Hughes, E. C., ed. 1972. *Obstetric-Gynecologic Terminology.* Prepared by the Committee in Terminology of the American College of Obstetricians and Gynecologists. Philadelphia: F. A. Davis.

Hume, M. 1975. Vascular disease. In *Medical complications of pregnancy,* eds. G. Burrow and T. F. Ferris. Philadelphia: W. B. Saunders.

Iffy, L.; Kaminetzky, H. A.; Maidman, J. E.; Lindsey, J.; Arrata, W.S.M. 1979. Control of perinatal infection by traditional preventive measures. *Obstet. Gynecol.* 54:403–411.

Jenkins, D. M., and Soltan, M. L. 1980. Plasma prolactin and puerperal blood pressure. *Brit. J. Obstet. Gynecol.* 87:597–599.

Jones, M. B. Hypotensive disorders of pregnancy. *J. Obstet. Gynecol. Neonatal Nurs.* 8(2):92–96.

Kitzmiller, J. L.; Lang, J. E.; Yelenosky, P. F.; and Lucas, W. E. 1974. Hematologic assays in preeclampsia. *Am. J. Obstet. Gynecol.* 118:362–367.

Klotz, T. A. 1982. Diagnostic Advances, Therapeutic Guidelines. *Contemp OB/Gyn* 19:18.

Knuppel, R. A.; and Drukker, J. E. 1986. *High Risk Pregnancy. A Team Approach.* Philadelphia: W. B. Saunders.

Lange, R. D. and Dynesius, R. 1973. Blood volume changes during normal pregnancy. *Clin. Haematology.* 2:433–451.

Laros, R. K., and Alger, L. S. 1979. Thromboembolism and pregnancy. *Clin. Obstet. Gyncol.* 22:871–888.

Ledger, W. J., and Kriewall, T. J. 1973. The fever index: A quantitative indirect measure of hospital-acquired infections in obstetrics and gynecology. *Am. J. Obstet. Gynecol.* 115:514–520.

Ledger, W. J.; Norman, M.; Gee, C.; and Lewis, W. 1975. Bacteremia on an obstetrical-gynecologic service. *Am. J. Obstet. Gynecol.* 121:205–212.

Ledger, W. J.; Reite, A.; and Headington, J. T. 1971. A system for infectious disease surveillance on an obstetric service. *Obstet. Gynecol.* 37:769–778.

Levinoson, G., and Schneider, S. 1979. *Anesthesia for obstetrics.* Baltimore: Williams & Wilkins.

MacKenzie, M. R. 1973. Disorders of immunohaematology in pregnancy. *Clin. Haematology.* 2:515–523.

McCormack, W. M.; Lee, Y.; Lin, J.; and Ranken, J. S. 1973. Genital mucoplasmas in postpartum fever. *J. Infect. Dis.* 127:193–196.

McKenzie, C. A. M. 1983. Postpartal crises. In *High risk perinatal nursing*, eds. K. W. Vestal and C. A. M. McKenzie. Philadelphia: W. B. Saunders.

Mead, P. B. 1974. Practical application of antibiotics in prevention and treatment of pelvic infections. *J. Reprod. Med.* 13:135–141.

Mead, P. B., and Gump, D. W. 1976. Antibiotic therapy in obstetrics and gynecology. *Clin. Obstet. Gynecol.* 19:109–129.

Milwidsky, A.; Beller, U.; Palti, Z.; and Mayer, M. 1982. Protease and protease inhibitory activity in pregnant and postpartum involuting uterus. *Am. J. Obstet. Gynecol.* 143:906–911.

Morgan, M. 1979. Amniotic fluid embolism. *Anaesthesia.* 34:20–32.

National Diabetes Data Group. 1979. Classification of diabetes mellitus and other categories of glucose intolerance. *Diabetes* 28:1039.

Nocheles, T. 1973. Obstetric complication associated with haemoglobinopathies. *Clin. Haematology.* 2:497–513.

O'Reilly, R. A. 1973. Problems of hemorrhage and thrombosis in pregnancy. *Clin. Haematology.* 2:543–562.

Peck, T. M., and Arias, F. 1979. Hematologic changes associated with pregnancy. *Clin. Obstet. Gynecol.* 22:785–798.

Perley, N. Z., and Bills, B. J. 1983. Herpes genitalis in the childbearing cycle. *MCN.* 8:123.

Phelan, J. P., and Yurth, D. A. 1982. Severe preeclampsia, I: Peripartum hemodynamic observations. *Am. J. Obstet. Gynecol.* 144:17–22.

Phillips, L. L., and Davidson, E. C. 1972. Procoagulant properties of amniotic fluid. *Am. J. Obstet. Gynecol.* 113:911–919.

Pipkin, F. B., and Symonds, E. M. 1978. Sequential changes in the human renin-angiotensin system following delivery. *Brit. J. Obstet. Gynecol.* 85:821–827.

Pirani, B. B., and MacGillivray, J. I. 1975. The effect of plasma retransfusion on the blood pressure in the puerperium. *Am. J. Obstet. Gynecol.* 121:221–226.

Pritchard, J. A. 1973. Haematological problems associated with delivery, placental abruption, retained dead fetus and amniotic fluid embolism. *Clin. Haematology.* 2:563–586.

Pritchard, J. A. 1975. Standardized treatment of 154 consecutive cases of eclampsia. *Am. J. Obstet. Gynecol.* 123:543–552.

Pritchard, J. A. 1983. Hypertension: Pregnancy-induced or preexisting. In *Common Problems in Obstetrics.* Symposium presented by the American College of Obstetricians and Gynecologists, Nevada.

Pritchard, J. A., MacDonald, P. C., and Gant, N. F. Ed. 1985. *Williams Obstetrics.* 17th ed. New York: Appleton-Century-Crofts.

Rafferty, T., and Berkowitz, R. L. 1980. Hemodynamics in patients with severe toxemia during labor and delivery. *Am. J. Obstet. Gynecol.* 138:263–270.

Read, J. A.; Cotton, D. Z.; and Miller, F. C. 1980. Placenta accreta: Changing clinical aspects and outcome. *Obstet. Gynecol.* 56:31–34.

Resnik, R.; Swartz, W. H.; Plumer, M. H.; Benirschke, K.; and Stratthaus, M. E. 1976. Amniotic fluid embolism with survival. *Obstet. Gynecol.* 47:295–298.

Roberts, J. M., and Perloff, D. L. 1977. Hypertension and the obstetrician-gynecologist. *Am. J. Obstet. Gynecol.* 127:316–325.

Sabath, L. D. 1973. Use of antibiotics in obstetrics. In *Obstetrical and perinatal infections*, eds. D. Charles and M. Finland. Philadelphia: Lea & Febiger.

Schulman, H., and Zatuchni, G. 1964. Pelvic thrombophlebitis in the puerperal and postoperative gynecologic patient. *Am. J. Obstet. Gynecol.* 90:1293–1296.

Sharman, A. 1953. Postpartum regeneration of the human endometrium. *J. Anatomy.* 87:1–10.

Sonstegard, L. 1979. Pregnancy-induced hypertension: Prenatal nursing concerns. *MCN.* 4 (March/April):90–97.

Speroff, L. 1973. Toxemia of pregnancy. *Am. J. Cardiology.* 32:582–591.

Steer, C. M., and Petrie, R. H. 1979. A comparison of magnesium sulfate and alcohol for the prevention of premature labor. *Am. J. Obstet. Gynecol.* 54:220.

Stubblefield, P. G. 1978. Pulmonary edema occurring after therapy with dexamethasone and terbutaline for premature labor: A case report. *Am. J. Obstet. Gynecol.* 132:341.

Sweet, R. L., and Ledger, W. J. 1973. Puerperal infections morbidity: A two-year review. *Am. J. Obstet. Gynecol.* 117:1093–1100.

Tichy, A. M., and Chong, D. 1979. Placental function and its role in toxemia. *MCN.* 4:84–97.

Ueland, K. 1982. Personal communication.

Wagner, M. M. 1973. In Royce, J., Shock: Emergency nursing implications. *Nurs. Clin. N. Amer.* 8:380.

Wallace, R. J.; Alpert, S.; Browne, K.; Lin, J. L.; and McCormack, W. M. 1978. Isolation of mycoplasma hominis from blood cultures in patients with postpartum fever. *Obstet. Gynecol.* 51:181–185.

Watson, P. 1980. Postpartum hemorrhage and shock. *Clin. Obstet. Gynecol.* 23:985–1001.

Watson, P.; Besch, N.; and Bowes, W. A., Jr. 1980. Management of acute and subacute puerperal inversion of the uterus. *Obstet. Gynecol.* 55:12–16.

Weiss, R. R., et al. 1976. Erythrocyte 2,3-diphosphoglycerate in normal and hypertensive gravid women and their newborn infants. *Am. J. Obstet. Gynecol.* 124:692–696.

Wheeler, L., and Jones, M. B. 1981. Pregnancy-induced hypertension. *J. Obstet. Gynecol. Neonatal Nurs.* 10:212–232.

White, P. 1965. Pregnancy and diabetes: Medical aspects. *Med. N. Am.* 49:1016.

Woodling, B. A., Kroener, J. M., Puffer, H. W., Furukawa, S. B., Anderson, G., Ochoa, R. G., and Warner, N. E. 1976. Gross examination of the placenta. *Clin. Obstet. Gynecol.* 19(1):21–44.

Zuspan, F. P. 1978. Problems encountered in the treatment of pregnancy-induced hypertension. *Am. J. Obstet. Gynecol.* 131:591–597.

31

Problems During the Intrapartal Period

BEHAVIORAL OBJECTIVES

Upon completion of this chapter, the reader should be able to:

- Define cesarean section, induction, dystocia, and fetal distress.

- Identify prenatal and intrapartal risk factors that may contribute to complications during labor and delivery.

- Describe abnormal labor patterns and discuss nursing interventions for them.

- Identify the major indications for a cesarean section and describe preparations and procedure for a cesarean section.

- Describe the various methods of induction and differentiate between induction and augmentation of labor.

- Discuss the nursing responsibilities during oxytocin administration.

- Describe nursing interventions to relieve fetal distress.

- List factors that contribute to intrapartal hemorrhage.

- Identify signs and symptoms of hemorrhage and describe nursing care of a parturient who is hemorrhaging.

- Describe the effects of labor complications on the mother and family and discuss providing emotional support when complications occur.

Interference with the normal process of labor can be required at any point. Because labor complications can have profound effects on both mother and neonate, numerous screening tools have been developed to predict perinatal mortality and morbidity. It is estimated that 70–80 percent of all observed perinatal mortality and morbidity can be identified with the appropriate application of antepartal and intrapartal risk screening (Aubry and Pennington, 1973; Hobel et al., 1973).

During labor, high-risk characteristics are not equally hazardous for mother or fetus, and thus astute maternal–fetal assessment skills are required by the nurse (Johnson, 1986; Warshaw and Hobbins, 1983; Ouimette, 1986). Risk characteristics rarely affect only the other or fetus. Generally, the risk characteristic is maternal in nature and has a physical affect on the fetus as well as the entire family (Hall, 1986). The nurse must be knowledgeable about possible risk factors and prepared to provide care when complications arise unexpectedly.

The actual rate of intrapartal complications varies among hospitals, practitioners, and prevailing medical philosophies and practice. Most mothers (82–85 percent) with a medically uncomplicated pregnancy are also able to deliver without complications (Mehl et al., 1977; L'Esperance, 1979; Adams, 1983). The labor complication rate in low-risk mothers has been found to range from 4.6 percent at a hospital staffed with family practice physicians to 31.0 percent at a perinatal center. There appears to be a positive correlation between the rate of labor complication and the rate of operative interventions (drug induction of labor, forceps delivery, and cesarean section). At these particular hospitals staffed with family practice physicians, the 3-year average rate was 5.5 percent for cesarean section, 12.7 percent for forceps deliveries, and 11.3 percent for drug-induced labor. From 1977 to 1979 the induction rate decreased from 13.1 to 8.4 percent (Adams, 1983). Approximately 6–13 percent of all births are achieved by labor induction (Lange et al., 1982; Lumley, 1982).

Labor complications often require rapid clinical judgments. The nurse must take action on the basis of sound theoretical grounds and thoroughly assess maternal–fetal well-being. Assessment includes observation, interviewing, and physical examination, and provides the basis for specific nursing diagnosis and intervention. Following any nursing intervention for a labor complication or variation a thorough evaluation is necessary. The evaluative process must be ongoing and result in the systematic comparison of maternal–fetal status with intervention outcomes. In addition, fetal status can be determined by a variety of biophysical and biochemical means that the nurse must be able to understand and interpret (see Chapter 13).

Effective communication is necessary for the accurate recording and reporting of labor variations or interferences. Such communication facilitates decision making and implementation of nursing care and medical management. To reduce maternal apprehension or stress, the nurse should provide adequate explanation and reassurance. Childbirth educators and physicians can emphasize prenatally that labor variations or interferences occasionally occur and are generally easily managed without neonatal problems. Additionally, the parents should participate in decision making (except in extreme emergencies). The family or father should be informed of maternal and infant status as soon as possible, to allay possible anxiety or fear. The same physical comfort measures required in the nursing support of normal labor are necessary (see Chapter 17). In addition, the nurse must be aware that the labor may be more prolonged and/or painful, and thus the mother may be more apprehensive, requiring constant care and attention. The nurse must recognize the unique needs of the childbearing family when stressful labor complications arise and assist the family in the decision-making process to promote a meaningful and positive birth regardless of delivery method.

This chapter examines the interventions of cesarean section and labor induction and describes such labor complications as dystocia, fetal distress, and hemorrhagic disorders.

CESAREAN SECTION

A *cesarean section* is a surgical procedure in which the fetus is delivered through abdominal and uterine incision. The term *primary* cesarean section refers to a woman's first cesarean, regardless of previous births. A *repeat* cesarean section refers to subsequent cesarean sections. An *elective* cesarean section is one that has been planned prior to the onset of labor or prior to rupture of the membranes.

The term *cesarean* comes from *cadare*, meaning

"to cut." It is also thought to come from a law in early Roman times making postmortem cesarean sections mandatory to try to save the fetus if the pregnant woman died. It was not the method of birth of Julius Caesar, as is commonly believed. In the past, cesarean section carried high risks to the mother. Infection and hemorrhage were the primary reasons for maternal death. But with the advent of antibiotics, transfusions, and improved anesthesia, maternal mortality rates dropped significantly.

Among the terms that have been used for cesarean section are cesarean birth, cesarean delivery, and cesarean childbirth. The rationale for using these alternative terms has been to deemphasize the surgical aspect of the delivery. In fact, a cesarean section is not even referred to as abdominal surgery. As a result, some people may erroneously conceptualize "section" as implying something different from other major abdominal surgical procedures.

The cesarean section rate in the United States has increased dramatically in the last 15 years. In 1970 the cesarean rate was reported at 5.5 percent. At present, the rate varies from approximately 9 percent at community hospitals to 25 percent at larger high-risk centers (Quilligan and Keegan, 1981; Jones, 1983). The cesarean birth rate in 1980 was estimated to be 15.5 percent based on a survey of 64 U.S. hospitals (Bottoms, Rosen, and Sokal, 1980). Presently, the cesarean section has become the most frequent inpatient operative procedure in the United States with 18 percent of all live-births in 1981 and 21 percent in 1983 delivered by this method (Rutkow, 1986) (see Fig. 31–1).

The economic implications are tremendous as the cesarean section rate has continued to rise in the U.S. as well as Canada (Young, 1986). The approximate cost of a cesarean birth was $4000 in 1984. In 1989 the cost rose to $9000.

A variety of consumer advocacy groups have come into being to provide peer support and reproductive information for women requiring cesarean section, and they have influenced birth practices in many hospitals. This has also been thought to affect a decline in the number of cesarean births in the late 1980s. Among the altered birth practices that have been instituted are allowing the father in the operating room, providing mirrors for the mother to view the cesarean procedure, and creating cesarean childbirth classes. Additionally, cesarean section prevention groups have been organized to call attention to the increasing rate of cesarean births and to critically examine obstetrical intervention. The unquestioning acceptance of cesarean section as the indicated delivery has been addressed by such organizations. There has been an effort to increase the focus of cesarean birth in prenatal education to provide the childbearing family with pertinent information for the decision-making process in operative procedures for birthing (Young and Ahrens, 1986).

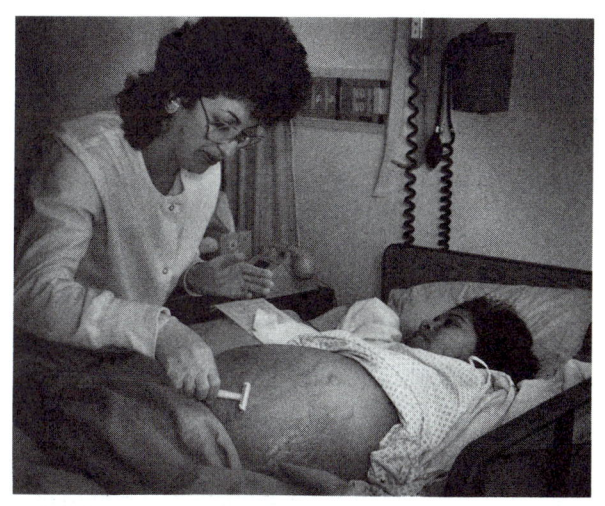

FIGURE 31–1. Nurse preparing abdomen of mother in preparation for cesarean.

Indications

A number of obstetric and nonobstetric factors are involved in the decision to perform a cesarean section.

Obstetric Factors

DYSTOCIA. Dystocia is a major indication for cesarean section. *Dystocia* is defined as abnormal labor or failure of labor progression because of mechanical abnormalities. The most common type of dystocia contributing to a cesarean section is *cephalopelvic disproportion* (CPD), also referred to as fetopelvic disproportion. Simply stated, the maternal pelvis is unable to accommodate the fetal head. Dystocia is the largest single cause (34 percent) of the increase in the rate of cesarean sections (Bottoms, Rosen, and Sokal, 1980). Functional dystocia in nulliparous women resulting in a cesarean section has been correlated with decreased cervical dilatation at admission, large birth weights, and maximum doses of oxytocin and prolonged administration of oxytocin (Seitchil, 1986).

Many physicians have cited "failure to progress" as another major reason for a cesarean section. This is a collective term usually referring to cephalopelvic disproportion, contracted or small pelvis, and uterine inertia. The use of such phrases may be attributed to the decreased use of pelvimetry and utilization of standard labor progression curves as advocated by Friedman and Sachtleben (1976).

ABNORMAL PRESENTATION. Changes in the management of abnormal fetal presentation have also contributed to the increase in the cesarean section rate. Breech presentation delivered by cesarean section has increased from 15 percent in 1970 to 67.2 percent in 1980 (Taffel and Placek, 1983). An abnormal presentation will often necessitate a cesarean section because the techniques of external and internal inversion are not performed by many physicians. Transverse and brow-face presentations have commonly been the reason for cesarean section. However, it is changes in management of breech presentations that have had the greatest effect on cesarean birth rates. In fact, an 18.8 percent increase in the rate of cesarean sections has been attributed to breech presentation (Bottoms, Rosen, and Sokal, 1980). This change in practice has resulted from the lower morbidity rate for infants delivered by cesarean section versus breech vaginal delivery. Generally, a cesarean is performed for a breech presentation when the woman is primiparous, the fetus is preterm, or the fetal head is hyperextended. Some practitioners have dealt with breech presentations by attempting external version near term, with betamimetics to relax the uterus. Confirmation of breech presentation at 36 weeks' gestation may be the appropriate time to discuss external version, since virtually all malpositioned fetuses will remain malpositioned at that point (Hughey, 1985). The external version method has been suggested as a means to transform the high-risk breech population into a low-risk cephalic group (Young and Ahrens, 1986). This approach needs further investigation to determine its safety and efficacy.

REPEAT CESAREANS. Repeat cesarean sections have also been a major reason for the increased cesarean rate. The general practice of performing a repeat cesarean section unless the patient is in advanced, active labor has been challenged in the United States. It had been believed that the risk of uterine rupture is too great to allow a previous cesarean section patient to labor and deliver vaginally. However, the rate of uterine rupture is greater with the classical incision (to be described later), varying from 0 to 9 percent, than with the lower uterine segment incision, for which the rate is 0.5 percent (Quilligan and Keegan, 1981). Thus, a vaginal delivery may be attempted when a classical incision has not been previously performed and there is no current reason for a cesarean, such as cephalopelvic disproportion. In a study involving 226 patients with a previous low transverse cesarean section, 38.5 percent were able to deliver vaginally (Saldana, Schulman, and Reuss, 1979). It has been estimated that the repeat cesarean section rate could be as low as 10 percent with appropriate vaginal births.

Guidelines for attempting a vaginal birth after a cesarean should include: (1) absence of the original indication for the previous cesarean; (2) absence of current obstetric or medical complications; (3) a low segment uterine incision for the previous cesarean; and (4) patient desire (Saldana, Schulman, and Reuss, 1979; Pauerstein, 1981).

ACOG (The American Association of Obstetricians/Gynecologists) established guidelines for repeat cesareans which suggest a vaginal delivery may be attempted in certain situations (Young and Ahrens, 1986). It is strongly recommended that the laboring patient be carefully monitored for signs of uterine rupture or fetal distress. The capability of performing an immediate repeat cesarean is necessary during the trial of labor. Labor following a previous cesarean section is unique due to negative feelings (e.g. fear, guilt, grief, etc.) from the previous birth experience and special restrictions due to defensive medical practice (Young and Ahrens, 1986).

The number of repeat cesareans will decrease as vaginal births after cesareans become more prevalent. Childbearing patterns are changing, resulting in women delaying childbearing and electing to have only one child, which will also decrease the repeat cesarean rate (Placek and Taffel, 1980).

The timing of elective repeat cesarean sections is important – it is imperative that such cesareans be performed only when the fetus is capable of extrauterine life. Many practitioners are now waiting until the patient has begun labor or has ruptured membranes before performing a repeat cesarean section. Some practitioners have advocated that amniocentesis be performed to ensure fetal lung maturation prior to the cesarean (Porreco, 1980). Because amniocentesis is not without risk, other practitioners advocate at least a minimum of clinical estimation of gestation and ultrasonography prior to an elective cesarean section (Chervenak and Shamsi, 1982).

FETAL DISTRESS. Fetal distress has been implicated as the major cause of the increased rate of cesarean sections. With the advent of electronic fetal monitoring in the 1970s, fetal distress or fetal intolerance to labor has been easier to establish. The increased use of electronic fetal monitoring has paralleled the increase in cesarean sections, prompting many to believe that monitoring has caused the increased numbers of cesareans. This is a plausible but untested belief. Past studies often compared monitored high-risk groups with unmonitored low-risk groups. Thus, an accurate determination of the extent to which the increase in cesarean section rates has been due to electronic monitoring detecting fetal distress has not been determined, as the groups studied were dissimilar initially.

The reality is that primary cesareans performed solely for fetal distress accounted for only 5 percent of the increase in the cesarean section rate (Hughey et al., 1977). Frequently, fetal distress coincides with dystocia and breech presentation.

Many practitioners advocate continuing routine electronic fetal monitoring as an effort to decrease perinatal morbidity until further research can determine whether risks of monitoring outweigh the benefits. Additionally, many practitioners now correlate fetal distress noted by monitoring with fetal blood scalp sampling in an effort to perform a cesarean section only when necessary (see Chapter 16).

OTHER FACTORS. Other obstetric factors that are indications for a cesarean section include placenta previa, abruptio placentae, prolapse of the umbilical cord, and moderate to severe erythroblastosis fetalis. Some maternal infections, such as genital herpes, may also warrant a cesarean section.

Certain maternal medical diseases may necessitate a cesarean section. Maternal diabetes, for example, has been a common indication for a cesarean. However, with improved prenatal diabetic management, diabetic mothers are less likely to have overly large infants and are thus able to have a vaginal delivery. Other maternal medical diseases that may lead to a cesarean include pregnancy-induced hypertension, cardiovascular abnormalities, and hepatic abnormalities.

Nonobstetric Factors

Nonobstetric reasons for the increased cesarean section rate can be classified as sociodemographic factors. That is, a physician may be more apt to perform a cesarean because of such factors as maternal age, the malpractice climate, the type of hospital where his or her practice is based, and various economic factors (Marieskind, 1982).

There is a positive relationship between maternal age and the cesarean section rate: the rate increases until age 40 (see Fig. 31–2). These data may indicate an increase in obstetric or medical complications for the older woman.

The present malpractice climate has been cited by many practitioners as a major influence for the increase in cesarean section rates (Marieskind, 1982). Many physicians perform a cesarean to ensure a healthy infant and to prevent a possible parental lawsuit (Guillemin, 1981).

Cesarean birth rates differ with the type of hospital. In 1978, larger urban hospitals had a significantly higher rate of cesareans (17 percent) than smaller hospitals (10.1 percent). Overall, private hospitals had a slightly higher rate of cesareans (16.4 percent) than nonprofit, voluntary hospitals (15.8 percent) (Placek and Taffel, 1980). The difference in rates for the various types of hospitals may be a result of variations in the type

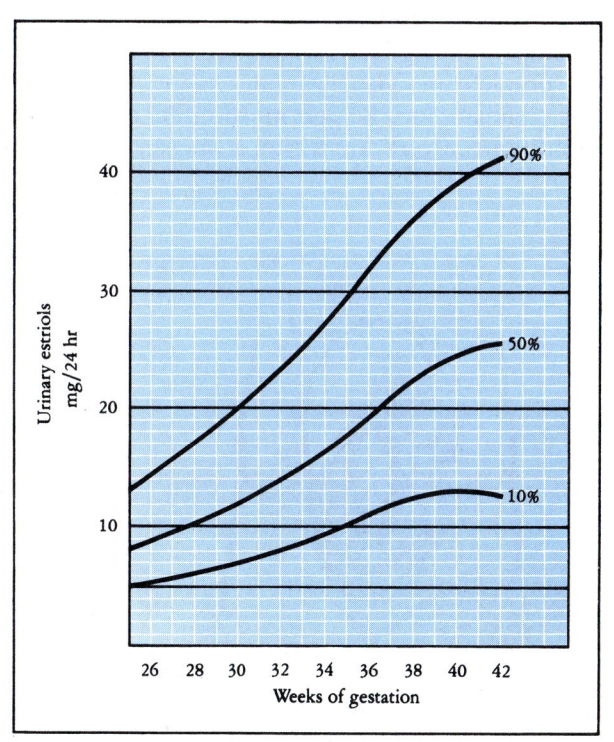

FIGURE 31–2. Graph showing the positive relationship between maternal age and cesarean section rate.
SOURCE: Placek and Taffel (1980).

of specialized practitioners at each site, the philosophies or training of those practitioners, or economic factors.

Several economic factors have been implicated in the increased cesarean section rate. Although a cesarean is a more involved procedure than a vaginal delivery, it may take less time than the management of labor, and most practitioners receive a higher fee for a cesarean than for a vaginal delivery. Additionally, the cesarean section patient has a longer hospital stay (usually 5 days), thus decreasing the number of empty hospital beds. Interestingly, some women request a cesarean section despite the physician's recommendation for a continued trial of labor/vaginal delivery (Johnson et al., 1986).

Description of Procedure

Abdominal Incision

A cesarean section can involve either a vertical or a transverse abdominal incision. The vertical incision, frequently used in the past, has the advantage of rapid entry and good visualization of abdominal contents. However, many women are now opting for a transverse or Pfannenstiel incision for cosmetic reasons. The incision is crescent shaped at the pubic hair line and is barely visible postoperatively. This incision requires more time to complete and visualization is slightly limited. If the cesarean must be performed under emergency conditions, a vertical incision is chosen.

Uterine Incision

There are several types of uterine incisions. The classical incision, a vertical incision in the body of the uterus (see Fig. 31-3), is rarely used today because of the higher incidence of postoperative morbidity, increased operative bleeding, an increased possibility of peritonitis, and an increased incidence of uterine rupture in subsequent pregnancies. Vertical incision is indicated in cases of emergency delivery, transverse lie, some previous classical scars, some uterine malformations, placenta previa, and difficult exposure of the lower uterine segment.

Lower-segment uterine incisions are the most frequently performed (see Fig. 31-4). They include transverse (the procedure of choice by most practitioners) and vertical incisions. The transverse incision has the advantage of less bleeding, reduced likelihood of placental incision, and reduced peritonitis. In a vertex presentation the fetus is directly under the incision and thus is easily delivered. A vertical incision into the lower uterine segment is indicated with a large fetus, malpresentation, some fetal anomalies, and occasionally placenta previa. There are disadvantages to both incisions, including bleeding, extension of incision into cervix or bladder, and difficulty if adhesions are present.

Extraperitoneal Cesarean Section

With the extraperitoneal approach, the peritoneum is dissected from the bladder, which allows

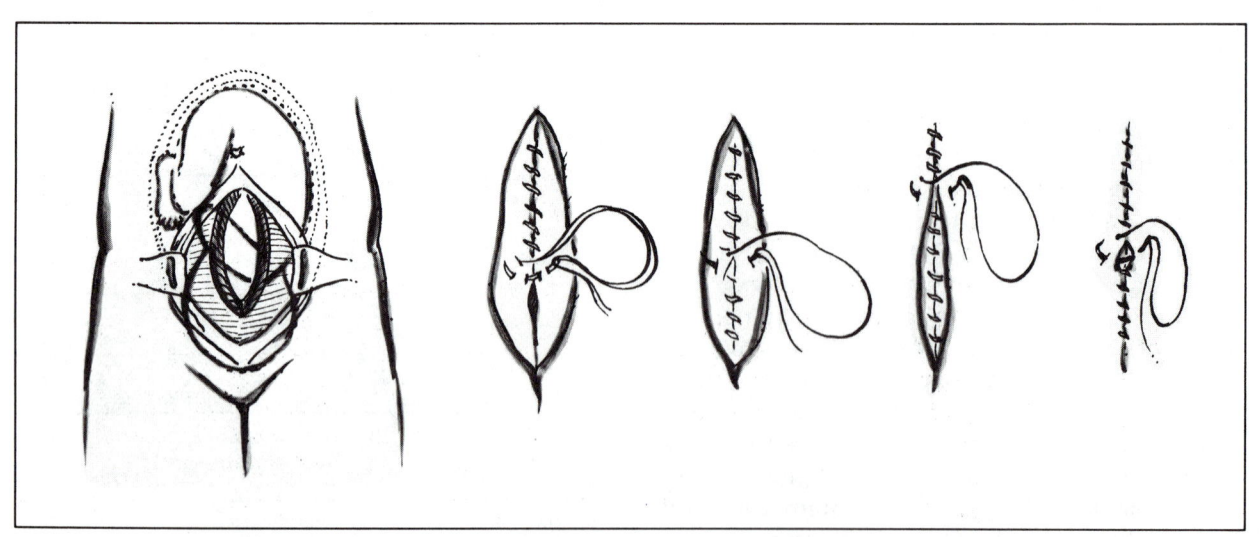

FIGURE 31-3. Classic cesarean section.
SOURCE: Sandberg (1978).

longer than 12 hours (even more so when labor is present); (3) uterine infection is present; and, (4) the patient has had multiple cervical examinations. The procedure is contraindicated with placenta previa, fetal distress, a large fetus, and the need for coincident exploration or surgery. The extraperitoneal approach has increased in popularity among some practitioners because of the decreased risk of peritonitis and of such postoperative complications as abdominal gas, abdominal distention, and paralytic ileus.

Cesarean Hysterectomy

A cesarean hysterectomy is the surgical removal of the uterus following an abdominal delivery. It is the indicated procedure in some cases of uterine rupture, uterine tumors, uncontrollable uterine bleeding, infection, and placenta accreta (abnormal adherence of the placenta to the uterine wall). The cesarean hysterectomy has a high complication rate that is due primarily to infection and hemorrhage (the result of increased pelvic vascularity).

Possible Complications

Infection

The most common postoperative complication of a cesarean is infection, primarily endometritis. Urinary tract infections are also common, probably resulting from the use of a catheter for 24–72 hours postoperatively. Women undergoing an emergency cesarean or having prior ruptured membranes are more at risk for infection than women having a planned cesarean section. The postcesarean infection rate at most hospitals is 20 percent for patients with labor prior to cesarean and 85 percent for patients with labor and ruptured membranes over 6 hours prior to cesarean (Rudd et al., 1982).

There has been some controversy over the risk factors involved in postoperative infection. Among the factors that have been implicated are maternal age, weight, socioeconomic status, and anemia; the use of general anesthesia; rupture of membranes; and internal fetal monitoring. An infection rate of 25 percent for emergency cesareans versus 9 percent for planned cesareans was found in a Swedish hospital (Hagglund et al., 1983). It has been suggested that cesareans tend to be performed more frequently on those patients at risk

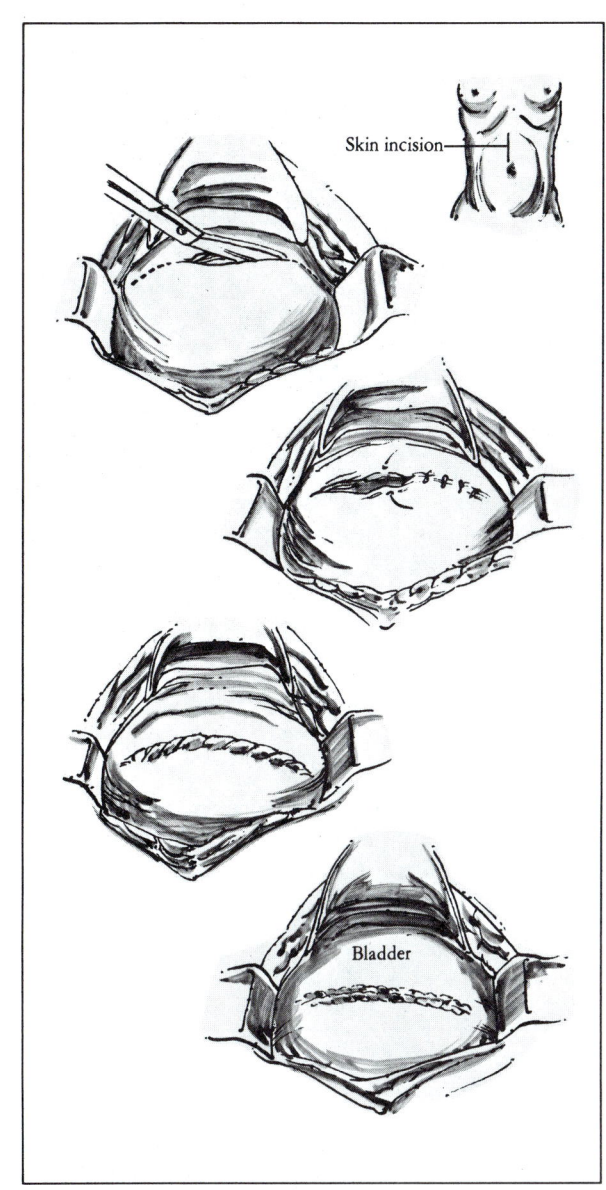

FIGURE 31–4. Transverse uterine incision with vertical skin incision.
SOURCE: Sandberg (1978).

for access to the uterus without entry into the peritoneal tissue. This approach was fairly common in the preantibiotic era because uterine and amniotic contaminants never entered the peritoneal space. Another approach is the *peritoneal exclusion*, in which the peritoneal cavity is entered but repaired prior to the uterine incision.

The extraperitoneal cesarean requires skill but can be performed rapidly if the practitioner is experienced. The extraperitoneal approach should be considered when: (1) labor has been established for 12 hours; (2) membranes have been ruptured

CASE PRESENTATION:

CESAREAN BIRTH

Mrs. M. is a 30-year-old woman (gravida 2, para 1) presenting at the maternity unit. She is admitted for a planned repeat cesarean section for the following morning. She is at 40 weeks' gestation, verified by two sonograms earlier in the pregnancy and by size (fundal height is 39 cm), as she is unsure of the date of her last menstrual period. She was delivered by emergency cesarean section 2 years ago after the discovery of a prolapsed umbilical cord. At that time she had a classical uterine incision under general anesthetic, delivered a healthy 7 pound, 1 ounce male, and had an uneventful postpartum course.

Mrs. M. and her husband attended cesarean childbirth classes, and Mr. M. plans to attend the cesarean birth. In conjunction with their physician, they have chosen an epidural as their anesthesia. The pregnancy has progressed without complications and Mrs. M. appears calm on admission.

NURSING CARE PLAN OF MRS. M.:

PLANNED CESAREAN SECTION

Nursing Diagnosis	Expected Outcome	Nursing Interventions	Rationale
Preoperative 1. Potential for preoperative apprehension from lack of knowledge about cesarean procedure and postoperative course	1. Mother will verbalize understanding of surgical procedures and postoperative course; she will be familiar with hospital routines and unit; her apprehension will be reduced	1a. Orient mother to room and hospital routines b. Assess and record vital signs, including fetal heart rate c. Measure and record fundal height d. Obtain urine and blood specimens (usually urinalysis, CBC, blood type, and RH factor) e. Provide preoperative teaching, including surgical preparation, surgery, anesthesia, postoperative course f. Obtain and witness consents according to hospital policy	1a. To reduce apprehension b. To establish baseline for future comparisons c. To provide estimate of gestational age d. To establish baseline body function and status for future comparisons e. To reduce apprehension f. To ensure patient understanding
2. Potential for alterations in self-concept	2. Mother will be aware of bodily changes with pregnancy and cesarean; she will have a positive self-concept and birth experience	2a. Encourage verbalization of questions and concerns b. Involve family members in care and discussions c. Discuss realistically the reasons for cesarean as	2a. To reduce fear and isolation, to allow patient to validate, change, or reduce anxiety and thoughts b. To provide opportunity to assess family interac-

NURSING CARE PLAN OF MRS. M.: Continued.

PLANNED CESAREAN SECTION

Nursing Diagnosis	Expected Outcome	Nursing Interventions	Rationale
		an alternate means of childbirth	tion and expand their knowledge base c. To promote positive self-concept and reduce social stigma sometimes associated with a cesarean
3. Potential for complications, perioperative and postoperative	3. Preoperative preparation will be completed; mother and fetus will tolerate surgery and not develop complications	3a. Shave operative area as per hospital policy b. Insert retention catheter – to gravity drainage c. Administer preoperative medication as ordered (e.g. antacid, analgesic) d. Initiate intravenous therapy as ordered e. Position mother on left side f. Remove dentures, contact lenses, rings, nail polish	3a. To improve visualization of operative site and decrease potential of infection, as hair harbors bacteria b. To improve visualization and prevent accidental perforation c. To reduce chance of aspiration pneumonia; to reduce anxiety d. To maintain fluid and electrolyte balance e. To prevent supine hypotension f. To prevent intubation difficulties, corneal abrasions, secure valuables, and allow for visualization of nail bed perfusion
Postoperative 1. Potential for undetected complications with involution or hemostasis	1. The uterus will remain firm, be in midline position and at the umbilicus; involution will proceed normally and be complete at 6 weeks; lochia rubra will be present for 2 days, serosa from 3rd to 10th day; alba will cease by 6th week	1a. Check fundal consistency and position; record b. Massage uterus if soft after pain medication c. Check vaginal flow, color, amount; record d. Check abdominal dressing for any bleeding; record e. Obtain vital signs as per policy	1a. To find uterine contractility, which promotes hemostasis b. To promote uterine contractility (but can cause discomfort at operative site) c. To detect excessive bleeding or passage of tissue d. To detect incisional bleeding e. To detect present or potential problems (e.g. hemorrhage, infection)
2. Potential for fluid volume deficit or excess	2. The fluid and electrolyte balance will be maintained	2a. Check IV solution, rate, and site b. Offer oral fluids as ordered	2a. To ensure proper solution and rate; to detect infiltration or phlebitis b. To promote gastro-

Continued

NURSING CARE PLAN OF MRS. M.: Continued.

PLANNED CESAREAN SECTION

Nursing Diagnosis	Expected Outcome	Nursing Interventions	Rationale
		c. Observe status of mucous membranes d. Give blood and blood products as ordered e. Observe urinary output; should be minimum of 30–60 ml/hour f. Record intake and output as ordered	intestinal activity and hydration c. To determine hydration level d. To replace volume loss or to promote coagulation properties e. To determine fluid status f. To provide baseline data; to allow for detection of abnormalities
3. Potential for alteration in pulmonary status related to anesthetic and immobility	3. Respiratory rate will remain at 16–24/min Breath sounds will be clear and equal bilaterally	3a. Have patient turn, cough, or "huff" and deep breathe every 2 hours when awake b. Ambulate as per order or policy c. Splint incision with pillow when patient is coughing or deep breathing	3a. To provide adequate ventilation and promote movement of pulmonary secretions, to prevent atelectasis and pneumonia b. To promote adequate ventilation in all lobes c. To decrease discomfort and strain on incisional area
4. Potential for alteration in vascular status related to immobility and increased clotting rate	4. Blood pressure will remain within normal range; transient bradycardia (60–70 beats/min) up to 6–8 days; hematocrit a minimum of 32%; hemoglobin minimum of 10 g/dl; no phlebitis postpartally	4a. Obtain vital signs as per policy b. Obtain hematocrit and hemoglobin as ordered and monitor values c. Check extremities for Homan's sign, warmth, edema, erythema, or tenderness d. Apply TEDS (support stockings) as ordered; encourage limb exercise while in bed; ambulate per order	4a. To detect abnormalities and provide baseline data b. To detect blood loss or anemia c. To detect possible thrombophlebitis d. To prevent venous stasis
5. Potential alteration in elimination related to pregnancy and surgery	5. Urinary output should be >30 ml/hour; urinalysis within normal limits; catheter removed by 2–3 days without cystitis; flatus passed by 2nd or 3rd day; normal bowel pattern within 5–6 days	5a. Insert indwelling catheter to gravity drainage; monitor patency b. Provide aseptic catheter care c. Monitor passage of flatus and stool; monitor for bowel sounds and abdominal distention d. Encourage abdominal tightening exercises (Chapter 22); ambulate as ordered	5a. To prevent urine stasis or reflux b. To prevent infection, as urine is excellent medium for bacterial growth c. To detect possible paralytic ileus or bowel obstruction d. To stimulate and enhance bowel function

NURSING CARE PLAN OF MRS. M.: Continued.

PLANNED CESAREAN SECTION

Nursing Diagnosis	Expected Outcome	Nursing Interventions	Rationale
6. Potential for alteration in comfort related to postoperative pain	6. Mother will experience little discomfort; she will be well rested	6a. Administer pain medication as required b. Offer pain medication as required; encourage mother to take pain medication before pain is severe c. Position patient and provide for a quiet environment d. Monitor pain medication and its use if mother is lactating	6a. To reduce pain threshold and promote relaxation b. Patient may not realize the need for prompt pain relief postoperatively or may be reluctant to ask; pain relief and relaxation are better achieved when pain is moderate c. Distraction and improper body alignment cause discomfort and interfere with relaxation d. Many drugs are secreted in breast milk
7. Potential for alteration in coping mechanisms and parenting	7. Parental bonding and infant caretaking patterns will be established; parents will be knowledgeable of abnormal infant responses and normal growth and development	7a. Provide for early parent–infant contact b. Encourage continued infant contact and caretaking c. Instruct parents on caretaking, abnormal infant responses, and normal growth and development d. Monitor parent–infant interaction e. Observe patient–family interaction and assess support system and coping mechanisms f. Promote maternal comfort and rest g. Encourage verbalization of feelings and provide opportunity for questions h. Demonstrate infant care and provide positive reinforcement	7a. To allay parental concern of infant's welfare and to promote bonding b. To allow for parental responsibility and to promote bonding c. To provide parents with basis to make comparisons and detect potential problems d. To detect abnormal parenting behaviors e. To detect potential problems in family structure, behavior, or coping strategies f. To facilitate bonding and healing process for increased parental responsibilities g. To clear confusion and misconceptions h. To provide role model

for infection, rather than the intervention being the actual cause of the infection.

The use of perioperative antibiotics, either intravenously or by irrigation into the operative site, has been questioned by both obstetricians and pediatricians. Some practitioners prefer to administer the antibiotic after the cord is clamped, while others prefer administration before, to allow the potentially affected fetus to benefit from the antibiotics. However, the antibiotic may be metabolized differently in the fetus than in an adult and can be potentially harmful. It is therefore suggested that perioperative antibiotics be administered after clamping of the cord, since the maternal benefits will occur regardless of when the cord is clamped and any potential harmful effects to the neonate can be avoided (Cunningham et al., 1983).

To prevent endometritis, the use of antibiotic irrigation of the operative site has also been advocated. The exact pharmacokinetics of this technique are under investigation. It is known that the antibiotic is absorbed systemically; however, the exact mechanism and levels are unknown. The irrigation is believed to prevent bacterial growth at the traumatized tissue sites, which have little vascularization. The procedure is not without risk, since allergic drug reactions or the emergence of drug-resistant organisms may result (Duff et al., 1982).

Gastrointestinal Disturbances

Gas accumulation is a frequent postoperative complaint of cesarean patients. It is usually relieved by ambulation, lying on the left side, and drinking fluids through a straw. It is important for the nurse to thoroughly assess gastrointestinal function postoperatively by ascultating for bowel sounds in all four quadrants and determining flatus and stool expulsion. Paralytic ileus will occasionally develop, especially if the bowel was handled extensively during the operation or if infection is present. Signs of ileus are the absence of bowel sounds and abdominal distention. The problem is generally treated with nasogastric suction and the cessation of oral intake. Actual bowel obstruction rarely occurs; when it does, an immediate surgical consultation is necessary.

Pulmonary Disturbances

Atelectasis (lung collapse) is a frequent complication and can be the cause of a fever within the first 24 hours postoperatively. Coughing and deep breathing should be encouraged as soon as the patient is able to cooperate. Many practitioners institute intermittent positive-pressure breathing four times a day to prevent atelectasis. Frequent position changes and early ambulation assist in maintaining adequate pulmonary expansion and hygiene.

Pulmonary embolism is a postoperative complication that can be life threatening. The clinical course and treatment are dependent on the clot size (see Chapter 30).

Psychosocial Considerations

A cesarean section can evoke many feelings for both mother and father. The mother may initially feel a sense of relief that the birth is imminent but then may experience fear, anger, guilt, or confusion. The father may feel helpless, disappointed, angry, and confused. Generally, the parents have anticipated sharing and participating in the birth experience and they have not psychologically prepared themselves for a cesarean.

Research suggests that cesarean-delivered women may experience anger, depression, and a loss of self-esteem, and that they perceive a social stigma attached to cesarean delivery (Marut and Mercer, 1979; Fawcett, 1981; Bradley, Russ, and Warynca, 1983; Cranley, Hedahl, and Pegg, 1983). The woman who undergoes a planned cesarean may have less fear regarding the infant's or her own safety and may view the experience more positively if she has a supportive person attending the delivery and if she receives regional anesthesia versus a general anesthetic.

Earlier mother–infant contact has been encouraged for cesarean mothers. In the past, contact did not occur until many hours after the birth, whereas vaginally delivered mothers had immediate contact or contact within 1–2 hours. More positive maternal perceptions of infants have been reported during the first few days postpartum for cesarean mothers having earlier infant contact than for mothers with delayed contact (McClellan and Cabianca, 1980).

Further research is still needed to understand fully the needs of the cesarean patient and of the father. Nevertheless, there are many obvious nursing implications based on current findings. These include: (1) involving the parents in the birth experience; (2) educating and supporting the parents both prior to the cesarean and postpartally; (3) allowing the parents to express their concerns and feelings; and, (4) offering information on cesarean section support groups.

It is important that all factors regarding the need for a cesarean be considered. Once the need is established, minimizing the potential maternal complications becomes a priority. Recently, potential sequelae in subsequent pregnancies following a cesarean section have received attention, indicating that the mean length of gestation is shorter, and problems arise during the pregnancy, labor, and delivery as a result of the operation (Hemminki, 1987). There are also risks to the infant, primarily respiratory distress. This risk occurs because the infant does not receive the squeezing effect on the chest during the delivery that it would during a vaginal delivery. This squeezing or mechanical pressure normally allows the infant to expel the amniotic fluid present in the lungs. If this fluid is not expelled, the infant may develop respiratory distress.

INDUCTION OF LABOR

Artificial induction of labor is initiated by pharmacologic or mechanical means. The pharmacologic or medical method involves the administration of *uterotonic agents* (oxytocin or prostaglandin). The mechanical or surgical method involves *amniotomy* (rupture of the amniotic membranes) or "stripping" the amniotic membranes from the lower uterine segment. *Augmentation* of labor is the enhancement of already established labor by pharmacologic or mechanical means. Labor augmentation may also be referred to as *assisted* labor. Generally, labor patterns are augmented by the use of oxytocin infusion or an amniotomy.

An *elective induction* is an induction of labor for social or convenience factors as opposed to obstetric indications. Elective induction of labor has decreased in the past 20 years because of such potential hazards as prematurity, uterine rupture, and fetal distress (Niswander and Patterson, 1963; Lumley, 1982). Elective inductions are no longer advocated unless the woman lives a long distance from the hospital or has a history of rapid labors. The practice of amniotomy is also being questioned, and careful analysis is needed to determine whether its benefits outweigh its possible harmful effects (Simkin, 1982).

The only uterotonic agent currently approved in the United States for labor induction or augmentation by intravenous infusion is oxytocin. However, the use of prostaglandin in other countries is common.

Indications

The artificial initiation of labor may be indicated for several obstetric reasons. The most frequent reasons include prolonged rupture of membranes, postmaturity (over 42 weeks' gestation), maternal diabetes or hypertension, a positive oxytocin challenge test (OCT), and fetal demise. An amniotomy may be performed for induction or for inspection of the fluid, for placement of a fetal scalp electrode, for scalp sampling, and for insertion of an intrauterine pressure catheter.

Oxytocin is contraindicated with an overdistended uterus, cephalopelvic disproportion, fetal distress, and previous uterine surgery. Contraindications for an amniotomy include unengaged vertex presentation, presentation other than vertex, and a nondilated cervix.

Prior to labor induction, a cervical assessment should be done (Lange et al., 1982). This assessment is referred to as the determination of cervical "ripeness". The degree of cervical ripeness is directly related to the initiation of spontaneous labor and the success of labor induction. Artificial induction may fail even with the use of oxytocin and amniotomy if the cervix is firm, posterior, uneffaced, or closed. Various scoring systems have been designed to determine the degree of cervical inducibility. Generally, the numerical scoring system consists of five categories: (1) cervical dilation; (2) cervical effacement; (3) cervical position; (4) cervical consistency; and, (5) fetal station (Bishop, 1964; Calder, Embrey, and Hillier, 1974; Wingerup, 1979).

Description of Procedure

Oxytocin

The administration of oxytocin for induction should only be intravenous. Oxytocin is a potentially dangerous drug; it is capable of causing uterine hyperstimulation, fetal distress, placental abruption, or water intoxication. Endogenous oxytocin is released by the pituitary gland, but its role in spontaneous labor is not clearly understood. Intramuscular or buccal oxytocin is not advocated since absorption rates are unpredictable.

Exogenous oxytocin is delivered with an infusion pump to ensure a constant and controllable rate. Most hospitals advocate the use of a protocol such as that listed in Table 31–1. Generally, a "piggy-back" setup is used, with a 5% dextrose in water solution in the main intravenous line and the oxytocin in a 5% dextrose in electrolyte solution in a secondary line. With this setup the oxytocin solution can be discontinued immediately while keeping the main infusion line intact.

The nurse should obtain frequent maternal blood pressure and pulse rates (every 15–30 min) during the oxytocin infusion. In large amounts, oxytocin can cause smooth muscle relaxation in blood vessels, resulting in tachycardia and hypertension. For future comparisons, a baseline assessment (30 min) of fetal heart tones, uterine status, and maternal vital signs is recommended prior to the oxytocin infusion. Electronic fetal monitoring is strongly encouraged to detect fetal distress or uterine hypersensitivity. Initially, oxytocin is infused in a low dose (0.5–2.0 milliunits/min) and slowly increased if untoward effects are unobserved.

Amniotomy

An amniotomy is performed after the fetal station, fetal presentation, and cervical status are determined. During a sterile vaginal examination, then the practitioner guides an amnihook or similar instrument into place and perforates the membranes. The nurse observes and records the fluid characteristics (color, odor, consistency, and amount), notes the time of procedure, and assesses fetal heart tones following the procedure. The patient will expel amniotic fluid after each contraction, necessitating clean peri-pads or linens for comfort.

Prostaglandin

The role of prostaglandins in spontaneous labor is not clearly understood. Prostaglandin, administered in a variety of forms, has resulted in successful labor induction and in cervical softening. Prostaglandin E_2 has been administered orally, intravenously, intravaginally, intracervically, and extraamniotically with general success rates of 85 percent (Ueland and Conrad, 1983).

Outside of the United States prostaglandin has been used routinely to induce labor. It has been given through a variety of routes, with the oral route most common and easiest to use.

In the United States prostaglandin has generally been used for elective abortions. Recently, there has been research in which prostaglandin has been used as a cervical priming agent prior to labor induction. An intravaginal suppository and oral preparations of prostaglandin are effective methods of cervical priming (Steiner and Creasy, 1983).

Locally administered prostaglandin intracervical suppositories or gels that avoid the extraamniotic space are believed to have a cervical ripening effect independent of uterine contractility (Laube, Zlatnik, and Pitkin, 1986). Systemic maternal side-effects include fever, nausea, vomiting, and diar-

---

CASE PRESENTATION:

INDUCTION

Mrs. K. is a 23-year-old woman (gravida 1, para 0) with prolonged ruptured membranes. The membranes have been ruptured 6 hours without any labor prior to hospitalization. The fluid was a large amount, clear, nitrazine positive, and without odor. Mrs. K.'s vital signs are a temperature of 98°F, pulse 76, respirations 20, and blood pressure 118/78, and the fetal heart rate is 158 beats/min. Mrs. K. is at 39 weeks' gestation based on her LMP, and the fundal height is 39.5 cm. A speculum and pelvic examination upon admission reveals the cervix to be 1 cm dilated and 100 percent effaced, and the head at minus 1 station.

Mrs. K. and her husband have attended childbirth classes at the hospital. They planned on a birthroom delivery under local anesthesia. A baseline electronic fetal monitoring tracing is obtained upon admission and reveals normal fetal activity and heart rate. No contractions are palpated or found with an external tocodynamometer. Mrs. K. is encouraged to ambulate and to have clear liquids as tolerated. A pelvic examination 14 hours after the rupture of membranes reveals no cervical change. The physician orders an oxytocin induction as per hospital protocol. The maternal vital signs and fetal heart rate remain stable.

NURSING CARE PLAN OF MRS. K.:

OXYTOCIN INDUCTION

Nursing Diagnosis	Expected Outcome	Nursing Interventions	Rationale
1. Potential for inadequate or absence of spontaneous labor	1. A normal labor pattern will be established resulting in a vaginal delivery; mother and infant will have no adverse effects from the induced labor	1a. Apply fetal monitor and palpate uterus for possible contractions b. Obtain and record vital signs c. Explain procedure and reason to patient; describe the contractions d. Initiate mainline (primary) IV e. Position patient in left lateral f. Prepare oxytocin solution as per protocol or order; place oxytocin solution on infusion pump; secure oxytocin infusion tubing and needle to port closest to vein site g. Maintain primary IV at slow rate	1a. To provide baseline data; patient may not perceive contractions b. To provide baseline data and detect any abnormalities c. To reduce apprehension and promote relaxation d. To maintain fluid and electrolyte balance and establish a primary intravenous route for continued therapy when oxytocin is discontinued e. To promote venous return f. Oxytocin is a potent uterogenic agent with potential side-effects and must be administered in small controlled doses; if complications arise, it can be discontinued immediately g. To ensure patency and prevent fluid overload
2. Potential for hypotension, tachycardia, uterine hypersensitivity, and fetal distress related to oxytocin administration	2. Vital signs and fetal heart rate will remain within normal limits; contractions will occur every 3–4 min lasting 60 sec	2a. Initiate oxytocin infusion as per order or protocol b. Increase oxytocin as per order or protocol until contractions occur every 3 min; then maintain at that level c. Discontinue immediately if contractions are longer than 60 sec or occur more frequently than every 3 min, or if fetal distress is encountered	2a. To control administration and dosage b. Optimal cervical dilatation is achieved when contractions occur every 3–4 min and are 50–60 mm Hg pressure; adequate uterine relaxation between contractions allows for uteroplacental perfusion c. To avoid compromised uteroplacental perfusion or fetal intolerance to labor, potentially resulting in fetal hypoxia, uterine rupture, or placental abruption
3. Potential for fluid volume excess	3. Patient's fluid and electrolyte balance will remain stable; patient will not have signs of water intoxication (headache, vomiting)	3a. Monitor IV intake – not to exceed 150 ml/hour b. Limit oral intake c. Administer oxytocin in a normal saline or electrolyte solution d. Monitor urine output e. Observe for signs of water intoxication	3. To prevent water intoxication: oxytocin has an antidiuretic effect in large amounts

> **TABLE 31–1. Protocol for Oxytocin Administration**
>
> *Equipment*
>
> *Primary intravenous line*
> 1. 20 gauge catheter
> 2. I.V. solution administration set
> 3. Dextrose 5% in electrolyte solution
>
> *Secondary (oxytocin) intravenous line*
> 1. Infusion pump
> 2. Lactated Ringer's solution (500 ml with 10 units of Pitocin added)
> 3. Mini dripper burette
>
> *Procedure*
>
> 1. Obtain maternal vital signs, obtain fetal heart rate, and assess labor status.
> 2. Apply electronic fetal monitor 20 min prior to oxytocin infusion.
> 3. Initiate primary IV and place oxytocin solution needle at the closest part of the venous catheter site.
> 4. Initiate oxytocin infusion as ordered. Suggested dose progression:
>
> | | | |
> |---|---|---|
> | 2:00 P.M. | 1.0 mu = | 3 mgtts/min |
> | 2:10 P.M. | 2.0 mu = | 6 mgtts/min |
> | 2:20 P.M. | 4.0 mu = | 12 mgtts/min |
> | 2:40 P.M. | 8.0 mu = | 24 mgtts/min |
> | 2:50 P.M. | 9.0 mu = | 27 mgtts/min |
> | 3:00 P.M. | 10.0 mu = | 30 mgtts/min |
> | 3:10 P.M. | 11.0 mu = | 33 mgtts/min |
>
>   increasing by 1.0 mu up to 20.0 mu/min every 10 min.
> 5. If hypersensitivity or fetal distress are encountered, discontinue oxytocin infusion and notify practitioner.
> 6. Record all findings on chart.

rhea. Additionally, uterine hyperstimulation, refractory to conservative management, is possible and, therefore, caution is warranted for fetal risk due to potential placental insufficiency (Laube, Zlatnik, and Pitkin, 1986; Trofatter et al., 1985). The use of prostaglandin for labor induction or cervical priming may become an alternative to oxytocin in the United States after further research has been completed.

Laminaria Tents

The use of *Laminaria digitata*, a dried and sterilized Japanese seaweed, to prime the cervix for induction has been controversial. Laminaria has been primarily used for cervical priming in second trimester abortions. It is placed intracervically and removed the next day, prior to the procedure. It has also been used in the same hospitals as a cervical priming agent prior to labor induction. Various research studies have shown anything from no demonstrable infections or other side-effects (Gower, Toraya, and Miller, 1982) to a 60 percent maternal infection rate and a 20 percent neonatal infection rate (Kazzi, Bottoms, and Rosen, 1982). Further research is necessary to fully understand the risks and benefits of using laminaria for preinduction cervical priming.

Possible Complications

Oxytocin

A major maternal complication with the administration of oxytocin is uterine hypersensitivity. This could result in uterine rupture, placental abruption, cervical laceration, or postpartal hemorrhage. Maternal apprehension may be another complication, resulting from lack of knowledge about the procedure and a concern for fetal well-being if the induction fails. Some mothers have reported that induced labor is more painful than previous labors, and it has been found that women with induced labors receive more analgesia and anesthesia than women with spontaneous labor (Oakley, 1983). The differences between spontaneous and induced labor need more systematic investigation to understand both the physiologic and psychologic components of each. The possible fetal complication is fetal distress resulting from inadequate uteroplacental circulation during uterine hypersensitivity.

Amniotomy

An amniotomy may produce maternal or fetal complications. Infection is the most common complication. The longer the membranes are ruptured, the greater the incidence of infection. A minimum of sterile vaginal examinations is suggested to help prevent ascending infection.

If the vertex is not engaged or the presentation is not vertex, the risk of umbilical cord prolapse exists. Compression of the cord by two bony surfaces could cause immediate fetal compromise. It has also been suggested that amniotomy produces a higher incidence of fetal head trauma, such as molding and caput succedaneum (Caldeyro-Barcia, Schwarcz, and Belizan, 1974). This idea has generally been supported by Baumgarten (1976) and Martell, Belizan, and Nieto (1976). Use of amniotomy as a means to shorten labor is a controversial issue. Labor following an amniotomy does not differ from spontaneous labor if the cervix is "ripe" (Friedman, 1978).

Prostaglandin

Like any uterotonic agent, prostaglandin is a potent uterine stimulant and should be used with caution. Constant surveillance for uterine hypersensitivity and fetal distress is strongly advised. Additionally, when given intravenously, prostaglandin has specific side-effects, such as gastrointestinal disturbances (nausea and diarrhea) and local phlebitis. Gastrointestinal disturbances can frequently be prevented by prophylactic drug therapy.

In short, the practice of labor induction is not without risk. It should only be initiated when indicated. The responsibility of the nurse caring for the mother being induced is significant. The nurse must consider the risks, possible complications, and maternal emotional responses, as examined in the Nursing Care Plan for Mrs. K.

DYSTOCIA

As noted earlier, *dystocia* is defined as abnormal labor or failure of labor progression because of mechanical abnormalities. Dystocia can result from uterine, fetal, or pelvic factors.

Causes of Dystocia

Uterine dystocia, also referred to as uterine dysfunction, involves inefficient contractions that prohibit normal labor progression. Uterine dystocia can be classified as primary (developing from the onset of labor) or secondary (developing after established normal labor). The ineffectual contractions can present as hypertonic, hypotonic (most common), or dystonic.

Hypertonic contractions, sometimes referred to as "colicky" labor, are of excessive intensity. These contractions are reported to be extremely painful and are ineffectual. Hypertonic contractions are associated with the onset of labor and are the least common type of uterine dystocia. *Hypotonic* contractions are weak, infrequent, irregular, and ineffectual. These contractions generally occur after the onset of established labor. Some practitioners feel that such contractions are a protective mechanism for maternal or fetal well-being resulting from labor intolerance. Hypotonic contractions can also be the result of excessive or untimely analgesic or of false labor. *Dystonic* contractions are asymmetrical and ineffectual. They result from certain uterine segments that contract independently or may remain in a contracted state.

Annular uterine strictures can also result in uterine dystocia. In normal labor, the lower uterine segment is passively retracted by fundal contractions. Occasionally, the junction of the lower uterine segment and fundus is obstructed by a pathologic retraction ring, or Bandl's ring. This ring develops with prolonged labor and can indicate imminent rupture. At this point, a cesarean is necessary.

Fetal factors that can produce dystocia include abnormal presentation or position, certain anomalies, and cephalopelvic disproportion. An abnormal presentation is any presentation other than a vertex and an abnormal position is any position other than occiput anterior. With abnormal presentations or positions engagement may not be accomplished or labor progression may be slow. Among fetal anomalies that can produce dystocia are hydrocephaly, abdominal mass, and myelomeningocele. Cephalopelvic disproportion (the inability of the maternal pelvis to accommodate the fetus) will result in dystocia and must be resolved by a cesarean section.

Pelvic factors that can produce dystocia include pelvic contraction and maternal pelvic masses. The interior of the pelvis may have a decreased diameter, producing an inlet, midpelvic, or outlet contraction. Among reasons for pelvic contraction are fractures, malignancy, and congenital rickets (vitamin D deficiency). Maternal pelvic masses can result from cervical stenosis, malignancies, or congenital abnormalities.

A full bladder or rectum may also impede labor progress and can easily be rectified. The patient should be encouraged to void at least every 2 hours during labor. An enema may be necessary, and some practitioners order enemas routinely.

Risks to Infant

Dystocia, regardless of cause, is potentially dangerous to the fetus and can result in neonatal morbidity. The most common risk is fetal distress (to be discussed in the next section) or intolerance of the prolonged labor. Prolonged fetal distress can result in low Apgar scores, central nervous system impairment, and developmental delay. Dystocia with prolonged rupture of membranes also increases the risk of neonatal sepsis. Head trauma (molding, caput succedaneum, cephalhematoma) may result from prolonged head compression. Large neonates may have the risk of brachial plexus damage, Erb's palsy, spinal cord or vertebral damage, and fractures when a vaginal delivery is attempted. Infants with shoulder dystocia are at risk for a fractured clavicle.

Once the cause of dystocia is determined, the appropriate action can be taken. The intervention is specific to the cause of dystocia and should be initiated as soon as possible to prevent any neonatal morbidity.

Medical Intervention

Uterine Dystocia

The uterus at the peak of an efficient and well-coordinated contraction is firm and not easily indented upon palpation. The uterus with an inefficient or weak contraction can easily be indented and is softer upon palpation. Uterine pressure is measured in either Montevideo units (M units) or mm Hg. Contractions for cervical dilatation must be a minimum of 15 mm Hg, and for normal labor progression pressures should be 50–60 mm Hg or 140–180 M units occurring every 3 min.

Hypertonic contractions without normal cervical dilatation are determined by palpation or by an intrauterine pressure catheter. Generally, the intervention for hypertonic labor consists of sedation and pain relief. A sedative or narcotic of short-acting duration may be administered. The fluid and electrolyte balance is often maintained by intravenous infusion. After rest has been achieved, a normal labor pattern is usually established. Because the patient may experience considerable anxiety during the hypertonic labor, she will need support and guidance to alleviate her anxiety or fear so she can achieve the needed rest.

Hypotonic labor may be either primary (at the onset of labor) or secondary (developing after a normal labor pattern). For intervention purposes, hypotonic labor is also classified by relationship to the phase of labor. Comparing the labor progression to established labor curves determines the specific phase and length of the dystocia (Hendricks, Brenner, and Kraus, 1970; Friedman, 1978). Using labor curves, or *partography*, can aid in determining the cause of dystocia, which mandates the intervention necessary.

Hypotonic contractions in the latent phase of labor (longer than 20 hours in the nullipara or longer than 14 hours in the multipara) are frequently treated with induced rest. This is accomplished by administering a short-acting sedative or narcotic. Usually after rest has been provided, a normal labor pattern is established.

Hypotonic contractions during the active phase result in cervical dilatation of less than 1–2 cm for nulliparas and 1.5 cm for multiparas. The hypotonic labor may be treated conservatively at first (sedation, supportive intravenous fluids, ambulation, and reassurance). If these measures do not initiate normal labor pattern, oxytocin is necessary. Oxytocin administration is the usual intervention for inefficient contraction in the active phase. Oxytocin should only be administered after fetal malposition or cephalopelvic disproportion has been excluded as the cause of the dystocia.

Dystocia in the transition or deceleration phase can result in either labor prolongation or an arrest (Friedman, 1978). An arrest of labor is when progress has ceased. During transition dystocia is commonly the result of sedation or conduction anesthesia. If this has been the case, a normal labor pattern will usually continue when the effects of the sedative have subsided. Oxytocin administration can be initiated once cephalopelvic disproportion or fetal malposition is excluded.

Occasionally, second-stage dystocia is encountered for reasons other than fetal malposition or cephalopelvic disproportion. These reasons include weak abdominal muscles, maternal fatigue, anesthesia effects blocking maternal pushing efforts, and maternal fear or discomfort. As a result, the mother may not or will not push effectively during second stage. The nurse must guide or coach the patient to push effectively and allay her fears. Forceps may be applied if the mother is unable to push effectively because of fatigue or anesthesia effects.

Dystonic contractions may be treated with either sedation or oxytocin. A rest period may be all that is necessary for a normal labor pattern to ensure, or oxytocin administration may help to coordinate the uterine contractions. The fluid and electrolyte balance should be maintained with intravenous fluids. A cesarean section may be indicated if all types of uterine dysfunction do not respond to medical intervention.

Fetal Factors

The type of medical intervention for cases of dystocia caused by fetal factors is specific to each cause. Abnormal presentations such as breech, shoulder, brow, or face are generally indications for a cesarean section because of the associated risks of neonatal morbidity during version or vaginal delivery (see Fig. 31–5). As noted earlier, the management of a breech presentation has changed over the past several years, with many practitioners now performing a cesarean section to

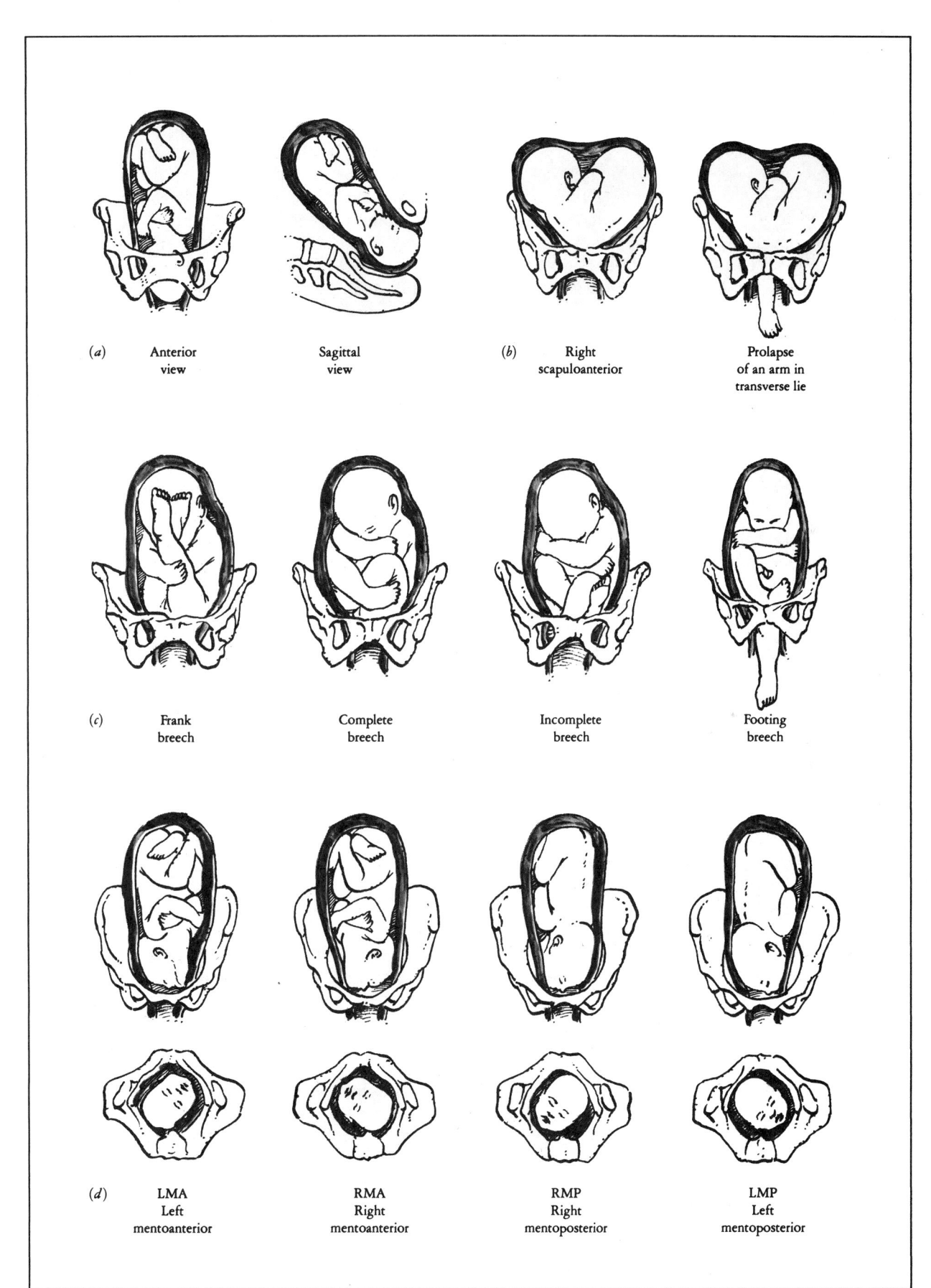

FIGURE 31–5. Abnormal presentations requiring cesarean section. (a) Brow presentation; (b) transverse presentation; (c) breech presentations; (d) face presentations.

decrease the risk of neonatal morbidity associated with a vaginal delivery.

Virtually all shoulder or persistent brow presentations are delivered by cesarean section because of the associated high rate of perinatal morbidity with vaginal delivery (Rovinsky, 1981). A brow presentation may convert to an occiput or face presentation (because of the instability of the position) and result in an easier vaginal delivery.

Face presentations result from a deflexion of the head as the result of a contracted pelvis. They are more common in multiparas and occur at the rate of approximately 0.2 percent. A vaginal delivery may be accomplished if the pelvis is adequate and if normal labor ensues. The practitioner may attempt manual flexion of the fetal head or delivery by forceps. A cesarean section is indicated if the pelvis is not adequate. The face generally has edema and ecchymoses as a result of prolonged pressure on the presenting part. The nurse should reassure the parents that this is a temporary condition.

Fetal malrotations that most commonly cause dystocia are occiput posterior and occiput transverse. These positions are associated with a pelvis that is not gynecoid and occur in approximately 25 percent of cases (Rovinsky, 1981). Usually, the fetal head rotates spontaneously as it reaches the pelvic floor; however, in 6 percent of cases the head remains posterior. Of those cases that are persistent occiput posterior, a vaginal delivery may sometimes be possible (usually with multiparas), although there is the risk of perineal lacerations or fetal head trauma.

The intervention for a persistent occiput posterior or transverse position is generally manual or forceps rotation and delivery. The *Scanzoni maneuver* is the application of one set of forceps to rotate the head and another to deliver the head (Rovinsky, 1981). A cesarean section may be necessary if the head remains in a malposition after a "trial of forceps." The mother generally experiences back pressure or back labor and will need back rub, a side-lying or modified knee–chest position, and reassurance to increase her comfort.

Forceps application is an operative procedure

CASE PRESENTATION:

DYSTOCIA

P.L. is a 29-year-old female (gravida 1, para 0) with labor for 7 hours prior to hospitalization. She has had back labor from the onset. She is at 38 weeks' gestation by dates, the fundal height is 39 cm, and the fetus is in vertex presentation. The initial pelvic examination reveals the cervix to be 4 cm dilated and 100 percent effaced and the fetal head at minus 1 station. The membranes rupture spontaneously 1 hour after admission. The fluid is a large clear amount, nitrazine positive, fern positive, and without odor. A pelvic exam is done to rule out cord prolapse and to determine cervical progress. There is no cord prolapse, the fetal head is at 0 station, and the cervix is 5 cm dilated. The fetal head is in occiput posterior position.

The first stage of labor progresses within a normal time limit. P.L. continues to experience back labor, which is relieved somewhat by changing position, back massage, pressure on the sacral area, and breathing techniques. P.L.'s labor coach is assisting with comfort techniques.

After 12 hours of labor P.L. is 10 cm dilated and is encouraged to bear down with her contractions. She pushes for 1 hour without advancing or rotating the infant's head. The nurse encourages her to push in a side-lying position to facilitate rotation of the fetal head. P.L. continues pushing for another 2½ hours. The fetal head descends to plus 1 station but is still in a persistent occiput posterior position. The physician attempts to rotate the fetal head manually without success. The physician suggests a forceps delivery, as P.L. is fatigued and no longer able to push effectively. P.L. and her labor coach agree to a forceps delivery under spinal anesthesia. The labor coach is allowed in the delivery room after the anesthesia has been administered. The physician rotates and delivers the fetal head by a Scanzoni maneuver. A viable female, 7 pounds, 4 ounces with Apgars of 7 and 9, is delivered. The infant has a moderate degree of molding, and the parents are told that this is a temporary condition.

NURSING CARE PLAN OF P.L.:

DYSTOCIA

Nursing Diagnosis	Expected Outcome	Nursing Interventions	Rationale
1. Potential for prolonged or abnormal labor related to uterine, pelvic, or fetal factors	1. A normal labor pattern will ensue and delivery will be achieved either spontaneously or operatively; the mother and infant will survive the birth with no adverse effects	1a. Monitor contractions for intensity, frequency, and duration b. Monitor cervical progress and compare with standard labor curves c. Monitor fetal heart rate in relation to contractions d. Monitor fetal presentation, position, descent, caput, and molding e. Monitor mother's degree of fatigue, hydration status, and vital signs	1a. To determine whether the dystocia is due to uterine factors; uterine rupture is possible if dystocia is prolonged b. To determine the presence and degree of dystocia and to detect if dystocia is due to cervical stenosis or cervical abnormalities c. To determine fetal tolerance to labor d. To determine whether dystocia is caused by fetal or pelvic factors e. Maternal effort and energy is required in second stage labor for fetal descent; uterine rupture can be sudden and cause rapid changes in vital signs
2. Potential for apprehension or fear related to labor variation	2. Mother and family will understand reasons for dystocia and interventions	2a. Explain reasons for dystocia and specific interventions to parents b. Offer information as to progress and fetal status c. Allow parents to participate in decision making when possible d. Explain procedures and operative management e. Offer comfort and support measures (back rub, change of position) f. Allow verbalization of feelings and offer reassurance	2a-d. Knowledge will allay apprehension and promote relaxation; adequate knowledge will allow for accurate decision making and facilitate compliance with labor management e. To promote relaxation and decrease discomfort f. To promote positive self-concept, as labor variation may be unexpected; to clear misunderstanding

requiring skill on the part of the practitioner to prevent fetal or maternal damage. There are several different types of forceps, but they all have a fetal or cephalic curve and a maternal or pelvic curve to facilitate the delivery with minimal or no trauma (see Fig. 31–6). The forceps blades are applied singularly, locked together, and traction is used for the delivery. The most common forceps

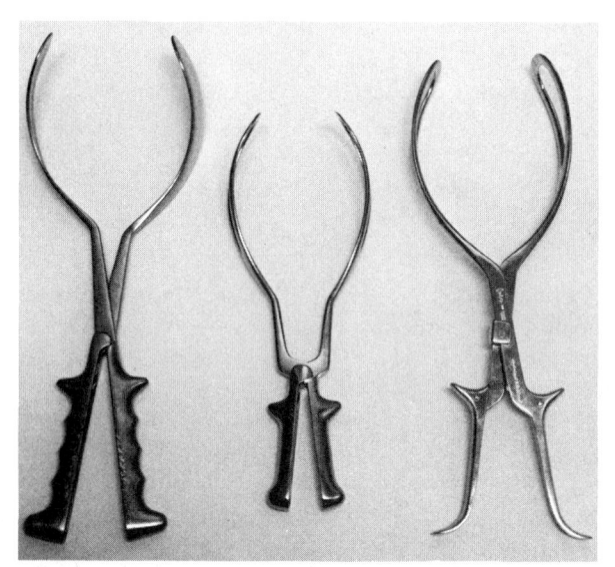

FIGURE 31-6. Types of forceps: *(left)* Tucker-McLean forceps; *(middle)* Simpson forceps; *(right)* Kielland forceps.

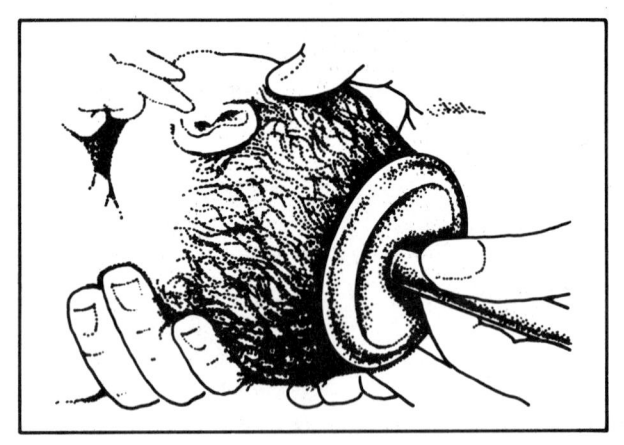

FIGURE 31-7. Ideal positioning of vacuum cup.
SOURCE: Courtesy of Appleton-Century-Crofts.

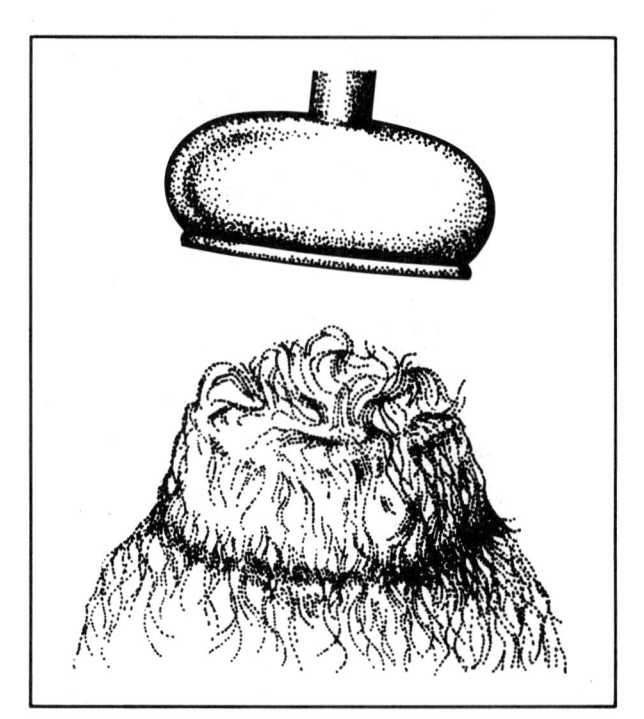

FIGURE 31-8. Chignon immediately after birth.
SOURCE: Courtesy of J. L. Waeltz.

delivery is a low, or outlet, application. This is when the fetal head is at the perineal floor. Midforceps application is used when the fetal head is engaged and when the largest diameter is past the pelvic inlet. The application of high forceps (head not engaged) is not advocated because of the high rate of perinatal morbidity.

Vacuum extraction can be used as an alternative to forceps application in some cases. Vacuum extraction involves a metal or plastic cup being applied to fetal head; suction is then initiated by a pump that withdraws air between the head and the cup (Figs. 31-7, 31-8). Traction can also be applied after the vacuum has been slowly increased to ensure a firm attachment to the head. The lithotomy position facilitates traction in backward and downward plane during vacuum extraction (Galvan and Broekuizen, 1987). Vacuum extraction has been popular in countries other than the United States, although U.S. practitioners have been showing an increased interest in this procedure (Greis, Bienarz, and Scommegna, 1981). With vacuum extraction, risks to the fetus include cephalhematomas, scalp lacerations, edema, and intracranial hemorrhage (Fig. 31-9). The nurse should observe the neonate for jaundice, cerebral irritation, and potential infection of the application site post-vacuum extraction (Galvan and Broekiuzen, 1987). The use of vacuum extraction needs further research to determine whether it is an effective and safe alternative to forceps.

Shoulder dystocia occurs with the delivery of the head and neck of a large fetus with the shoulders at the pelvic brim or outlet. Medical intervention involves manually bringing the posterior arm down and across the chest without force and easing the anterior shoulder through the pelvis and out. Sometimes the practitioner can ease the shoulders out by a side-to-side rocking motion. To prevent fetal compromise, a deliberate clavicular fracture may be necessary if other efforts fail.

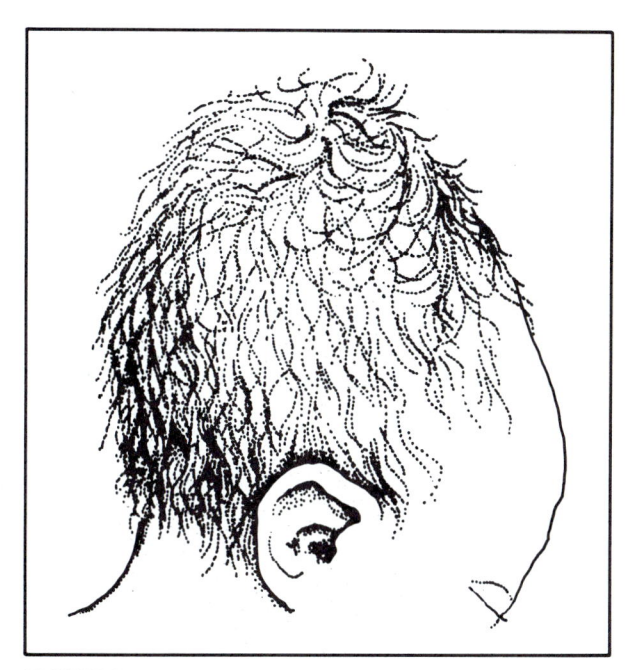

FIGURE 31–9. Regression of chignon.
SOURCE: Courtesy of J. L. Waeltz.

Pelvic Dystocia

Pelvic anomalies or obstruction by soft tissue masses virtually necessitate a cesarean section to prevent fetal or maternal morbidity. Soft tissue masses can be detected by ultrasonography and occasionally through palpation.

Because dystocia, whatever the cause, has various fetal and maternal risks associated with it, immediate intervention is necessary. The mother will need support and guidance as well as comfort measures when dystocia is encountered. Furthermore, electronic fetal monitoring may be required to ensure constant fetal surveillance, since fetal well-being is paramount.

FETAL DISTRESS

Fetal distress is a state characterized by sustained abnormal heart rate patterns resulting from hypoxia. The fetus may be stressed or show signs of intolerance to labor (transient periodic changes) prior to actually being in distress. Fetal distress may result from a variety of factors that produce hypoxia. Maternal factors include hypertension, hypotension, respiratory dysfunction, cardiac abnormalities, and general anesthesia. Fetal factors causing hypoxia include cord compression, prematurity, anemia, and cord abnormalities. Placental factors that can cause fetal distress include inadequate blood flow in the intervillous space, resulting from inadequate uterine relaxation between contractions, and placental insufficiency from aging or calcifications.

The diagnosis of fetal distress is frequently made on the basis of abnormal fetal heart rate patterns obtained during electronic fetal monitoring.

It is critically important to distinguish maternal and fetal heart rate tracings since interventions are frequently performed based on electronic monitor tracings. To differentiate maternal–fetal impulses, if suspicion warrants, pressure applied to the fetal head transvaginally will cause an increase in heart rate (Herbert, Stuart, and Butler, 1987).

Early decelerations are thought to be a result of head compression; they coincide with the contraction and are uniformly shaped. Late decelerations are believed to result from uteroplacental insufficiency and are ominous if prolonged. These decelerations are uniformly shaped, but they occur after the acme or peak of the contraction. Variable decelerations are suspected to be the result of cord compression; they occur irrespective of uterine activity and are variable in shape. Decreased beat-to-beat variability (less than 5 beats/min) can also aid in determining fetal distress. The presence of meconium-stained fluid indicates a period of stress for the fetus, but it must be taken into account with heart rate patterns.

Fetal blood scalp sampling has become more prevalent in combination with electronic fetal monitoring to assess for fetal distress. After cervical dilation of 3–4 cm a small blood sample is obtained from the fetal scalp using a sterile endoscopic cone. The sample is obtained using a microscalpel, and a layer of silicon gel allows the blood to form beads, enhancing collection in heparinized tubes. The blood is analyzed for pH level, pO_2, pCO_2, and bicarbonate ion excess. The pH is the easiest result to analyze and is the usual determinant of fetal distress. With hypoxia, acid levels increase and lower the body pH. Scalp blood pH values below 7.20 are associated with ominous heart rate patterns or fetal distress. The normal range of pH of fetal blood is between 7.25 and 7.35, with transient decreases associated with contraction (Kublis, Hon, and Khayin, 1969). There is always a small possibility that pH values will be falsely positive or negative; thus, careful evaluation of maternal status and direct fetal electrocardiogram patterns are indicated. Serial pH levels are suggested but may be impractical.

Experience with the procedure of continuous fetal tissue pH monitoring in the United States has proved promising. A continuous pH monitoring electrode is attached to the fetal scalp with a probe placed just slightly below the skin surface to provide pH values of the fetal blood. This procedure has the potential of providing precise changes in pH over a period of time that will allow a more definitive diagnosis of fetal distress. At this point the procedure is experimental, but most of the problems encountered have been technical.

Currently, continuous fetal scalp transcutaneous carbon dioxide measurement is being investigated as a more accurate method of fetal well-being and can provide data for carbon dioxide levels from placental to lung breathing if the electrode remains attached from labor to delivery (Lofgren, 1987). Fetal blood gas status is more accurately judged by transcutaneous carbon dioxide measurement or fetal blood scalp sampling than Apgar scoring or fetal heart rate tracing (Lofgren, 1987; Ingemarsson and Arulkumaran, 1986; Low et al., 1986). Further research is needed to determine the benefit versus risk potential of continuous fetal pH monitoring.

Risk to Infant

Prolonged fetal hypoxia and resulting acidosis may lead to low Apgar scores, neonatal apnea and bradycardia, central nervous system damage, or fetal demise. The longer the period of hypoxia, the greater the fetal risk of CNS damage or death. Research has associated low Apgar scores and the need for vigorous resuscitation with developmental delays and CNS damage. An estimated 20–40 percent rate of cerebral palsy has been noted because of intrapartal hypoxia. Additionally, intrapartal hypoxia has an "all or nothing" effect (that is, either complete recovery or death) on the neonate.

It is recommended that further research be done on electronic fetal monitoring and that it be done on a selective basis rather than routinely (Haverkamp and Orleans, 1982). Thus, high-risk mothers should be monitored continuously, whereas low-risk mothers should have an initial monitoring period, followed by close observation and repeated intervals of fetal heart rate assessment.

Abnormal fetal acid-base balance in low-risk groups have been found to be common, transient, and of an innocuous respiratory type without fetal distress (Ingemarsson, 1986). Fetal acid-base assessment demonstrating significant metabolic acidosis is the most accurate indicator of fetal hypoxia, with baseline fetal heart rate tachycardia and appearance of decelerations rather than disappearance of accelerations as the earlier sign of fetal compromise (Low et al., 1986).

CASE PRESENTATION:

FETAL DISTRESS

M.J. is a 31-year-old woman (gravida 3, para 2) at 41 weeks' gestation. She had an uneventful prenatal course. She did not attend childbirth education classes for this pregnancy. Her sister is her labor coach. She has been separated from her husband for 6 months.

M.J. has been in labor for 2 hours, with spontaneous rupture of membranes occurring 1 hour prior to the onset of labor. Upon admission to the birthing center, initial examination reveals a vertex presentation, 4 cm dilatation, 100 percent effacement, and the fetal head at plus 1 station. Her contractions are every 3–4 min, lasting 60 sec, and of moderate intensity. Her vital signs are blood pressure 108/64, pulse 86, respirations 24, and temperature 98.4°F, and the fetal heart rate is 146 beats/min.

When the electronic fetal monitor is applied for a baseline tracing, several variable decelerations are noted. An internal scalp electrode is applied, with cervical dilatation at 9 cm. She is positioned in a left lateral recumbent position. The variable decelerations continue and become more severe. She is placed in a right lateral recumbent position and an intravenous infusion of dextrose 5% is initiated. Oxygen is administered at 7 liters/min via a face mask. The variable decelerations decrease in severity and in frequency. She expresses an urge to push and is found to be fully dilated and at plus 2 station. She has six more contractions and spontaneously delivers a viable male with cord wrapped tightly two times around the neck (nuchal cord).

NURSING CARE PLAN OF M.J.:

FETAL DISTRESS

Nursing Diagnosis	Expected Outcome	Nursing Interventions	Rationale
1. Fetal distress related to head compression, cord compression, or uteroplacental insufficiency	1. The mother will have a basic understanding of potential causes of fetal distress and treatment; FHR will remain in normal range (120–160 beats/min) with good variability (5 beats/min); fetal asphyxia will be prevented	1a. Monitor fetal heart for baseline, beat-to-beat variability, and periodic changes b. Monitor fetal heart with uterine contractions c. Monitor and palpate contractions as to intensity, frequency, and duration d. Interpret tracings and notify physician as needed	1a. To allow for detection of any abnormality and provide baseline data b. Contractions interrupt uteroplacental perfusion and fetus must rely on placental fetal reserve for oxygenation c. Hypertonic contractions compromise uteroplacental perfusion, thus can cause fetal hypoxia d. To prevent fetal hypoxia
2. Potential for fetal asphyxia related to altered uterine-placental or cord blood flow	2. The neonate will not have adverse sequelae	2a. Discontinue oxytocin administration if being infused b. Change position to left lateral for early and late decelerations; attempt different positions (left, right, knee–chest) for variable decelerations c. Stay with patient; have someone notify physician d. Initiate an i.v. or increase rate e. Administer oxygen at 7–8 liters/min f. Check monitor for malfunctioning and apply to internal scalp electrode g. Prepare for fetal scalp blood sampling and explain procedure to parents if performed h. Prepare for operative intervention as indicated i. Provide rapid explanations and reassurance to parents j. Assess maternal vital signs	2a. Oxytocin may cause uterine hypersensitivity and compromise uteroplacental perfusion b. To promote venous return; may relieve cord compression c. To provide prompt intervention, constant patient support d. To increase fluid volume to ensure adequate uterine perfusion e. Small increases in maternal O_2 aid in elevating fetal O_2 due to disassociation curve and fetal hemoglobin concentration f. Variability can be accurately determined only with a scalp electrode; monitors can malfunction at any point g. Fetal scalp blood sampling correlates fetal distress with fetal pH levels h. Prolonged fetal distress can result in asphyxia i. To allay fears, improve compliance j. To detect maternal disorders (e.g. uterine rupture)

Medical Interventions

When fetal distress is suspected, immediate intervention must be initiated to prevent neonatal morbidity or fetal demise. Many hospitals have protocols or standing orders for the nurse to follow if fetal distress is encountered. Frequently, it is the nurse who is present when fetal distress is originally detected. The nurse must stay with the patient and summon assistance from the physician or midwife (see the accompanying Nursing Care Plan for fetal distress).

Oxytocin Discontinuation

The discontinuation of oxytocin is essential whenever fetal distress is suspected. The fetal intolerance of labor may be transient; thus oxytocin may be resumed after a complete evaluation. The necessity of close observation and monitoring during oxytocin infusion has already been emphasized.

Increased Uterine Blood Perfusion

Specific interventions are essential if the uterine blood flow is compromised as a result of maternal hypertension, hypotension, or volume deficit (shock). Maternal hypertension related to preeclampsia should be treated with appropriate medication to decrease the blood pressure slowly. Maternal hypotension caused by pressure on the inferior vena cava from the gravid uterus can be treated by placing the patient in a left lateral recumbent position. This is commonly referred to as *supine hypotension syndrome* and can easily be prevented. Intravenous fluid or blood products may be administered for volume expansion in cases of severe preeclampsia or hemorrhage with resulting shock.

Oxygen Administration

Fetal hypoxia can be somewhat relieved by the administration of 100% oxygen to the mother via face mask or nasal cannula. Generally, the oxygen is delivered at 7–8 liters/min. This does not increase maternal oxygen concentrations significantly, but it can effectively raise fetal blood oxygen concentration. This is because fetal oxygen values are in the range where the oxygen disassociation curve is steep; that is, small increases in fetal pO_2 increase the hemoglobin saturation (Iffy and Kaminetzky, 1981). Therefore, with a higher fetal hemoglobin concentration, a higher level of fetal blood oxygen can be achieved with small increases of fetal pO_2.

Umbilical Cord Compression

Partial or complete cord prolapse must be ruled out when fetal distress is suspected. If a cord prolapse is found by vaginal examination, the woman can be placed in a modified knee–chest or modified Trendelenberg position. A sterile hand in the vagina and cervix must place constant pressure on the presenting fetal part for disengagement. An emergency cesarean section is indicated in cases of cord prolapse.

When there is no cord prolapse but cord compression is suspected based on variable deceleration heart rate patterns, changing the maternal position may be helpful. This would include maternal left or right lateral recumbent, supine, or Trendelenberg positions.

Operative Procedures

When conservative interventions fail to resolve the fetal distress, operative procedures are indicated. Forceps or vacuum extraction to achieve a rapid vaginal delivery is indicated if the fetal head is low in the pelvis. An emergency cesarean section is the procedure of choice when forceps or vacuum extraction cannot rapidly or reasonably deliver the distressed fetus.

To summarize, the nurse has the initial responsibility for intervention when fetal distress is encountered. The nurse must be cognizant of the risk factors that can lead to fetal distress and must carefully monitor the patient for any signs of distress. The nurse should be knowledgeable about fetal heart rate patterns and should seek assistance when needed. The capability of performing a cesarean section is essential; thus, adequate personnel and equipment must be available. Additionally, the nurse must give rapid and brief explanations as well as reassurance to the patient during episodes of fetal distress.

HEMORRHAGIC DISORDERS

Hemorrhagic disorders during the intrapartal period comprise abnormal bleeding from the onset of labor to the fourth stage (1 hour after delivery). Shock can result if the hemorrhage is severe, thereby reducing blood volume. With a blood volume deficit, there is decreased venous return to the heart and cardiac output is diminished. Compensation is immediate, as a result of reflex activation of adrenergic receptors releasing catecholamines. This release causes tachycardia and vasoconstriction.

The signs and symptoms are dependent upon the severity of the bleeding. Mild hemorrhage is defined as approximately 15–25 percent blood loss, resulting in a minimal decrease in blood pressure and slight tachycardia. Moderate hemorrhage, 25–35 percent blood loss, results in marked tachycardia (100–120 beats/min) and the systolic blood pressure at 90–100 mm Hg. Severe hemorrhage, up to 50 percent blood loss, results in severe tachycardia (over 120 beats/min) and the systolic blood pressure at 60 mm Hg (Danforth, 1977). The patient experiencing moderate to severe blood loss may manifest such symptoms as restlessness, stupor, diaphoresis, pallor, and decreased renal function.

Intrapartal hemorrhage can result from a variety of maternal or placental factors. Predisposing maternal factors include hypertension (regardless of cause), dystocia, uterine overdistention, diabetes, previous history of bleeding, cervical and vaginal lacerations, and uterine rupture. Placental factors include placenta previa, abruptio placentae, placenta accreta, and retained fragments.

The etiology of abruptio placentae is unknown. It is associated with trauma, hypertension, a short umbilical cord, precipitous labor, and uterine anomalies. Bleeding with abruptio can be concealed by the fetal head, the placenta, or membranes, or it may be apparent externally. The woman usually experiences sudden and severe abdominal pain and the uterus is rigid upon palpation. The average total blood loss fetal death is 2.5 liters and the incidence for a pregnancies (Hayashi, 1986).

Placenta accreta results when the placental villi become firmly attached or invade the myometrium. The degree of hemorrhage and the successful manual removal of the placenta depends upon the penetration of the placenta into the uterine wall. *Placenta accreta vera* is contact of the villi but not penetration of the myometrium. *Placenta increta* is the invasion of the endometrium by the villi. *Placenta percreta* is invasion of the villi through the myometrium to adjacent structures. The etiology of placenta accreta is unknown. It is associated with placenta previa and previous uterine surgery. Placenta accreta may involve only

---

CASE PRESENTATION:

HEMORRHAGE

J.B. is a 35-year-old woman (gravida 4, para 3) who has been admitted with sudden abdominal pain. She is at 39 weeks' gestation with an unremarkable prenatal course. She was admitted directly into the labor unit via ambulance and appears to be in severe pain. She is restless and complains of excruciating pain in the lower abdomen. She had no contractions prior to the episode of sudden pain. Her vital signs are blood pressure 96/50, pulse 102, respirations 30, and temperature 97.2°F, and the fetal heart rate is 80 beats/min. Upon examination, the uterus is palpated as a separate mass from the fetus. Preparations for an emergency laparotomy/possible hysterectomy are made. An intravenous line of dextrose 5% in water and oxygen at 7 liters/min have been initiated. Blood is obtained for type, Rh, crossmatch, cell blood count, and clotting studies.

She is taken to the operating room while her husband signs a consent for surgery. A nurse remains with the husband to provide an explanation and inform him of maternal and infant progress. The neonatal and anesthesia team are present as the mother enters the operating room. A Foley catheter is inserted as the general anesthetic is administered. The laparotomy reveals the fetus to be completely out of the uterus and unresponsive. The female infant is resuscitated and taken to the neonatal intensive care unit in stable condition. The father is able to visit the baby 30 min after the birth. A hysterectomy is performed, with central venous pressure monitoring during the procedure. J.B. receives 2 units of whole blood while in the operating room. She is admitted into the recovery room in stable condition.

NURSING CARE PLAN OF J.B.:

HEMORRHAGE

Nursing Diagnosis	Expected Outcome	Nursing Interventions	Rationale
1. Potential for risk factors associated with obstetric hemorrhage (uterine rupture, placental abruption, etc.)	1. The mother will not have excessive or uncontrolled bleeding; maternal vital signs and fetal heart rate will remain within normal limits	1a. Thoroughly assess for presence of risk factors b. Observe for restlessness, anxiety, or sudden pain c. Obtain vital signs every hour unless abnormal d. Monitor fetal heart rate and uterine activity e. Prepare equipment for emergency cesarean if indicated f. Notify practitioner of any problems	1a. To obtain objective assessment and force attention on risk factors b. To look for signs of uterine rupture, abruptio placentae, or blood loss c. To establish baseline data and to detect abnormalities d. To establish baseline data and to detect abnormalities e. Prompt action may prevent maternal or fetal morbidity or demise f. Adequate information facilitates accurate decision making
2. Potential for fluid volume deficit related to blood loss	2. Mother and infant will survive the birth without adverse effects; urine output will be at least 50 ml/hour; CVP will be 5–10 cm H_2O	2a. Observe and report any unusual bleeding; monitor vital signs and fetal heart rate; assist physician in correcting cause of bleeding b. Insert retention catheter; monitor output and specific gravity c. Observe for skin color and changes d. Monitor level of consciousness e. Monitor CVP f. Administer blood and blood products as ordered g. Administer oxygen as ordered h. Prepare patient for emergency cesarean if indicated i. Provide rapid explanation to mother	2a. Uncontrolled or excessive bleeding can result in hypopvolemia; if the hypovolemia is severe, blood will be shunted to organs that require the most oxygen, thus resulting in tissue damage b. Blood flow is decreased to the kidney with hypovolemia, and tissue damage results in the inability to concentrate urine c. Skin reflects perfusion and oxygenation levels; diaphoresis results from sympathetic stimulation of sweat glands d. Decreased cerebral blood flow decreases level of consciousness e. To evaluate venous return and heart function to pump blood f. To expand volume and restore clotting factors g. To provide fetus with increased oxygen levels and correct maternal hypoxia if present h. Prompt action can help to prevent maternal and fetal compromise; hemorrhage or fetal distress may be managed by operative intervention i. To reduce fear and facilitate cooperation with management

segments of the placenta and result in retained placental fragments.

Certain maternal or placenta factors that cause intrapartal hemorrhage can lead to *disseminated intravascular coagulation* (DIC). DIC is an abnormal, diffuse form of clotting in which the clotting factors are rapidly consumed, resulting in widespread internal and external bleeding. Either primary fibrinolysis or intravascular clotting occurs, causing a reduction of circulating fibrinogen levels to 100 mg/100 ml or less. The predisposing hemorrhage factors of DIC include abruptio placentae, uterine rupture, pregnancy-induced hypertension, and shock. DIC is suspected with profuse bleeding from the uterus, episiotomy, lacerations, puncture sites, or mucous membranes. The diagnosis of DIC is confirmed by assessing fibrinogen levels and administering a clot observation test.

Risks to Mother and Infant

The maternal risk of hemorrhage depends on the severity of the hemorrhage. Mild hemorrhage may reduce hemoglobin and hematocrit levels slightly. Moderate or severe hemorrhage will produce shock and, if uncorrected, can cause maternal cellular damage and ultimately death.

Maternal hemorrhage resulting in decreased uteroplacental perfusion can lead to fetal hypoxia. The degree of fetal hypoxia is directly related to the degree of maternal hemorrhage. Uncorrected moderate or severe maternal hemorrhage can ultimately result in fetal distress or fetal death.

Medical Intervention

The treatment of maternal hemorrhage involves correcting the cause and providing blood replacement as indicated. The treatment of hemorrhage resulting from maternal factors is specific to each factor. Hemorrhage can often be prevented if the predisposing factors, such as maternal hypertension, dystocia, and diabetes, are managed appropriately. Uterine overdistention and a previous history of bleeding or coagulation defects will necessitate close observation in labor. Cervical or vaginal lacerations will need prompt repair. Uterine rupture is a serious complication requiring an emergency cesarean section.

The intervention for maternal hemorrhage caused by placental factors is again specific to the cause. Placenta previa and abruptio placentae necessitate a cesarean section. Placenta accreta generally necessitates a hysterectomy, regardless of whether delivery is vaginal or abdominal. Retained placental fragments require manual removal under an anesthetic.

Supportive interventions should be initiated concurrent with determining and treating the primary causes of moderate to severe maternal hemorrhage. An intravenous line in a large vein with a large-bore plastic cannula should be established. Maternal blood should be drawn for type, crossmatch, and Rh factor. Oxygen should be administered at 7–8 liters/min via a face mask or cannula. The mother should be in a left lateral position to prevent supine hypotension. Central venous pressure (CVP) monitoring may be initiated to maintain the normal range of 6–12 cm H_2O.

Blood replacement therapy may be initiated to maintain the hematocrit at 30 percent and urinary output at 30–60 ml/hour. It is also necessary to note the patient's religious convictions prior to blood replacement therapy.

Medical interventions for DIC include treatment of the primary cause, administration of whole blood and components, and occasionally intravenous heparin. The heparin is thought to arrest intravascular coagulation and fibrinolysis. The various blood components may include platelets, cryoprecipitate, or fresh frozen plasma. Currently, blood transfusion practices emphasizes the administration of packed red blood cells to improve oxygen delivery and volume replacement in cases of hemorrhage rather than fresh frozen plasma (Hayashi, 1986). Additionally, as with other hemorrhagic disorders, general supportive mechanisms (such as intravenous and oxygen therapy) should be instituted promptly.

SUMMARY

The intrapartal period is usually uncomplicated and often requires little or no medical intervention. However, it is not a period without risks for the mother or fetus. A gamut of complications of varying severity can occur and can be potentially hazardous to the mother or fetus. It is a time that requires astute nursing assessment and prompt intervention to prevent maternal–fetal compromise.

Frequently, the mother and family anticipate an uncomplicated birth. Feelings of helplessness, frustration, and failure are common. Thus, the nurse must provide emotional support to promote a meaningful childbirth experience and a positive beginning for the new family.

REFERENCES

Adams, J. 1983. The use of obstetrical procedures in the care of low-risk women. *Women and Health.* 8(1):25–28.

Aubry, R., and Pennington, J. 1973. Identification and evaluation of high-risk pregnancy: The perinatal concept. *Clin. Obstet. Gynecol.* 16(1):3–27.

Baumgarten, K. 1976. Advantages and disadvantages of low amniotomy. *J. Perinatal Med.* 4(3):11.

Bishop, E. 1964. Pelvic scoring for elective induction. *Obstet. Gynecol.* 24:266–268.

Bottoms, S.; Rosen, M.; and Sokal, R. 1980. The increase in the cesarean birth rate. *New Engl. J. Med.* 302(10):559–563.

Bradley, C.; Ross, S.; and Warynca, J. 1983. A prospective study of mothers' attitudes and feelings following cesarean and vaginal births. *Birth.* 10(2):79–83.

Calder, A.; Embrey, M.; and Hillier, K. 1974. Extraamniotic prostaglandin E for induction of labour at term. *J. Obstet. Gynaecol. Brit. Commonwealth.* 81:39.

Caldeyro-Barcia, R.; Schwarcz, R.; and Belizan, J. 1974. Adverse perinatal effects of early amniotomy during labor. In *Modern perinatal medicine,* ed. L. Gluck. Chicago: Year Book Medical Publishers.

Chervenak, R., and Shamsi, H. 1982. Is amniocentesis necessary before elective repeat cesarean section? *Obstet. Gynecol.* 60(3):305–308.

Cranley, M.; Hedahl, K.; and Pegg, S. 1983. Women's perceptions of vaginal and cesarean deliveries. *Nurs. Research.* 32(1):10–15.

Cunningham, F.; Leveno, K.; DePalma, R.; Roark, M.; and Rosenfeld, C. 1983. Perioperative antimicrobials for cesarean delivery: Before or after cord clamping? *Obstet. Gynecol.* 62(2):151–154.

Danforth, D. 1977. *Obstetrics and Gynecology.* 3rd ed. Baltimore: Harper & Row.

Duff, P.; Gibbs, R.; Jorgensen, J.; and Alexander, G. 1982. The pharmacokinetics of prophylactic antibiotics administered by intraoperative irrigation at the time of cesarean section. *Obstet. Gynecol.* 60(4):409–412.

Fawcett, J. 1981. Needs of cesarean birth parents. *J. Obstet. Gynecol. Neonatal Nurs.* 10(5):372–376.

Friedman, E. 1978. *Labor: Clinical evaluation and management.* 2nd ed. New York: Appleton-Century-Crofts.

Friedman, E., and Sachtleben, M. 1976. Station of the fetal presenting part. *Obstet. Gynecol.* 47(2):129–136.

Galvan, B. and Broekhuizen, F. 1987. Obstetric vacuum extraction. *J. Obstet. Gynecol. Neonatal Nurs.* July/August: 242–248.

Gower, R.; Toraya, J.; and Miller, J. 1982. Laminaria for preinduction cervical ripening. *Obstet. Gynecol.* 60(5):617–619.

Greis, J.; Bienarz, J.; and Scommegna, A. 1981. Comparison of maternal and fetal effects of vacuum extraction with forceps or cesarean deliveries. *Obstet. Gynecol.* 57(5):571–577.

Guillemin, J. 1981. Cesarean section. *Babies by Cesarean: Who Chooses, Who Controls.* 11(3):15–18.

Hagglund, L.; Christensen, K.; Christensen, P.; and Kamme, C. 1983. Risk factors in cesarean section infection. *Obstet. Gynecol.* 62(2):145–150.

Haverkamp, A., and Orleans, M. 1982. An assessment of electronic fetal monitoring. *Women & Health.* 7(3/4):115–134.

Hayashi, R. 1986. Hemorrhagic shock in obstetrics. *Clin. Perinat.* 13(4):744–762.

Hemminski, E. 1987. Pregnancy and birth after cesarean section. *Birth.* 14(1):12–17.

Hendricks, C.; Brenner, W.; and Kraus, G. 1970. Normal cervical dilatation pattern in late pregnancy and labor. *Am. J. Obstet. Gynecol.* 106(7):1065–1082.

Herbert, W.; Stuart, N.; and Butler, L. 1987. Electronic fetal heart rate monitoring with intrauterine fetal demise. *J. Obstet. Gynecol. Neonatal Nurs.* July/August:249–252.

Hobel, C.; Hyvarinen, M.; Okada, D.; and Oh, W. 1973. Prenatal and intrapartum high-risk screening. *Am. J. Obstet. Gynecol.* 117(1):1–9.

Hughey, M. 1985. Fetal position during pregnancy. *Am. J. Obstet. Gynecol.* 153:885–886.

Hughey, M.; LaPata, R.; McElin, T.; and Lussky, R. 1977. The effect of fetal monitoring on the incidence of cesarean section. *Obstet. Gynecol.* 49(5):513–518.

Iffy, L., and Kaminetsky, H. A., eds. 1981. *Principles and practice of obstetrics and perinatology.* New York: John Wiley & Son.

Ingemarsson, I., and Arukumaran, S. 1986. Fetal acid–base balance in low-risk patients in labor. *Am. J. Obstet. Gynecol.* 155:66–69.

Johnson, S. 1986. *Nursing assessment and strategies for the family at risk.* Philadelphia: J. B. Lippincott.

Johnson, S.; Elkins, T.; Strong, C.; and Phelan, J. 1986. Obstetric decision making: Responses to patients who request cesarean delivery. *Obstet. Gynecol.* 67:847–850.

Jones, H. 1983. Cesarean section in modern-day obstetrics. *North Carolina Med. J.* 44(3):100–102.

Kazzi, G.; Bottoms, S.; and Rosen, M. 1982. Efficacy and safety of laminaria digitata for preinduction ripening of the cervix. *Obstet. Gynecol.* 60(4):440–443.

Kublis, F.; Hon, E.; and Khayin, A. 1969. Observations on heart rate and pH in the human fetus during labor. *Am. J. Obstet. Gynecol.* 104:1190–1206.

Lange, A.; Secher, N.; Westergaard, J.; and Skovgard, I. 1982. Prelabor evaluation of inducibility. *Obstet. Gynecol.* 60(2):137–147.

Laub, D.; Zlatnik, F.; and Pitkin, R. 1986. Preinduction cervical ripening with prostaglandin E_2 intracervical gel. *Obstet. Gynecol.* 68:54–57.

L'Esperance, C. 1979. Homebirth – a manifestation of aggression? *J. Obstet. Gynecol. Neonatal Nurs.* 4(8):227–230.

Lofgren, O. 1987. Continuous transcutaneous carbon dioxide measurement from the fetal scalp during labor and during the first minutes of extrauterine life. *J. Perinat. Med.* 15:37–44.

Low, J.; McGrath, M.; Marshall, S.; Fisher, F.; and Karchmar, J. 1986. The relationship between antepartum fetal heart rate, intrapartum fetal heart rate, and fetal acid–base status. *Am. J. Obstet. Gynecol.* 154:796.

Lumley, J. 1982. Antepartum fetal heart rate tests and induction of labour. *Women & Health.* 7(3/4):9–29.

Marieskind, H. 1982. Cesarean section. *Women & Health.* 7(3/4):179–198.

Martell, M.; Belizan, J.; and Nieto, F. 1976. Blood acid-base balance birth in neonates from labors with early and late ruptures of membranes. *J. Pediatrics.* 89:963–967.

Marut, J., and Mercer, R. 1979. Comparison of primiparas' perceptions of vaginal and cesarean births. *Nurs. Research.* 28(5):260–266.

McClellan, M., and Cabianca, W. 1980. Effects of early mother–infant contact following cesarean birth. *Obstet. Gynecol.* 56(1):52–55.

Mehl, L.; Peterson, G.; Whitt, M.; and Hawes, W. 1977. Outcomes of elective home births: A series of 1,146 cases. *J. Reprod. Med.* 19(5):281–290.

Niswander, K., and Patterson, R. 1963. Hazards of elective induction of labor. *Obstet. Gynecol.* 2:228–233.

Norwood, C. 1984. *How to avoid a cesarean section.* New York: Simon and Schuster.

Oakley, A. 1983. Social consequences of obstetric technology: The importance of measuring "soft" outcomes. *Birth.* 10(2):99–108.

Ouimette, J. 1986. *Perinatal nursing.* Boston: Jones and Bartlett.

Pauerstein, C. 1981. Labor after cesarean section. *J. Reprod. Med.* 26(8):409–412.

Perkins, R. 1980. Role of extraperitoneal cesarean section. *Clin. Obstet. Gynecol.* 23(2):583–596.

Placek, P., and Taffel, S. 1980. Trends in cesarean section rates for the United States, 1970–1978. *Public Health Reports.* 95(6):540–548.

Porreco, R. 1980. Timing of repeat cesarean section. *Clin. Obstet. Gynecol.* 23(2):499–506.

Quilligan, E., and Keegan, K. 1981. Cesarean section. *Perinatal Press.* 5(8):111–116.

Rovinsky, J. 1981. Abnormalities of position, lie, presentation, and rotation. In *Principles and practice of obstetrics and perinatology,* eds. L. Iffy and H. A. Kaminetsky. New York: John Wiley & Sons.

Rudd, E.; Cobey, E.; Long, W.; Dillon, M.; and Matthews, M. 1982. Prevention of endomyometritis using antibiotic irrigation cesarean section. *Obstet. Gynecol.* 60(4):413–416.

Rutkow, I. 1986. Obstetric and gynecologic operations in the US. 1979 to 1984. *Obstet. Gynecol.* 67:755–759.

Saldana, L.; Schulman, H.; and Reuss, L. 1979. Management of pregnancy after cesarean section. *Am. J. Obstet. Gynecol.* 135(5):555–561.

Seitchik, J.; Holden, A.; and Castilo, M. 1986. Amniotomy and oxytocin treatment of functional dystocia and route of delivery. *Am. J. Obstet. Gynecol.* 155:585–592.

Simkin, P. 1982. Amniotomy. *Women & Health.* 7(3/4):103–112.

Steiner, A., and Creasy, R. 1983. Methods of cervical priming. *Clin. Obstet. Gynecol.* 26(1):37–46.

Taffel, S., and Placek, P. 1983. Complications in cesarean and noncesarean deliveries: US, 1980. *Am. J. Pub. Health.* 73(8):856–860.

Trofatter, K.; Bowers, D.; Gall, S.; and Killam, A. 1985. Preinduction cervical ripening with prostaglandin E_2 gel. *Am. J. Obstet. Gynecol.* 153:268–271.

Ueland, K., and Conrad, J. 1983. Characteristics of oral prostaglandin E_2-induced labor. *Clin. Obstet. Gynecol.* 26(1):87–94.

Warshaw, J., and Hobbins, J. 1983. *Principles and practice of perinatal medicine.* Menlo Park, Calif.: Addison-Wesley.

Wingerup, L.; Andersson, K. E.; and Ulmsten, U. 1979. Ripening of the cervix and induction of labor in patients at term by single intracervical application by prostaglandin E_2 in viscous gel. *Acta Obstet. Gynecol. Scand.* 84(Suppl.):11–14.

Young, D., and Ahrens, J. 1986. Health education and cesarean childbirth. In *Health education for women,* ed. V. Littlefield. New York: Appleton-Century-Crofts.

32
The High-risk Newborn

BEHAVIORAL OBJECTIVES

Upon completion of this chapter, the reader should be able to:

- Define, using gestational weeks or growth parameters: (a) the premature infant, (b) the small-for-gestational age infant, and (c) the postmature infant.

- List two of the physical characteristics observed in infants from each of the three classifications.

- List one physiologic "handicap" for the premature infant from each of the following areas: (a) temperature regulation, (b) liver function, (c) renal function, (d) metabolism, (e) immune system, (f) respiratory system, (g) digestive system, (h) central nervous system, and (i) skin.

- Describe the impact that chronic intrauterine malnutrition and chronic intrauterine hypoxia can have on the fetus and newborn.

- Define *asphyxia* and outline its impact on the newborn.

Pregnancy and birth have different meanings to different people, depending on their culture, economic status, psychologic background, age, prior life experiences, and other factors. Nevertheless, it can generally be agreed that for all pregnancies the desired outcome is the same: a healthy, robust baby with all the potential to become a productive member of the parents' society.

Unfortunately, problems can occur prior to, during, and after the birth that can alter this desired outcome for the parents, for society, and most important, for the baby. These problems can result from a wide variety of factors, including social, economic, and cultural influences as well as genetic, metabolic, physiologic, and environmental ones.

Examples of unexpected outcomes at birth include (1) premature infants (birth prior to 37 weeks' gestation); (2) postmature infants (birth after 42 weeks' gestation); (3) small-for-gestational-age infants; and (4) infants with congenital anomalies or birth defects (see Chapter 13).

Statisticians sometimes use the classification of *low-birth-weight* (LBW) infants for high-risk infants who weigh less than 2500 g (5 lb, 8 oz). The infants in this classification can be premature, postmature, or small for gestation. The incidence of low-birth-weight infants has remained essentially unchanged in recent years. Approximately 8 percent of all births, or 250,000 infants per year, are LBW infants. Of this group, 40,000–45,000 infants die in the first month of life. This number is equal to the number of term fetuses that die *in utero* yearly (Behrman, 1983). Another 60,000 of the LBW infants are thought to be at higher risk for serious lifetime disabilities, but identification of these infants is difficult and sometimes impossible during the neonatal period.

Improvement in the medical and nursing care for infants who are at risk during the first few days or months of life has become a sophisticated and ever-changing addition to the health care system. In the past several decades, the field of neonatology and the formation of neonatal intensive care units has provided hope and improved outcome for many infants.

The impact of the problems that can occur during the neonatal period and the impact of the neonatal intensive care unit are keenly felt by the families of high-risk infants. Not achieving their goal of a healthy newborn can be a serious blow both to parents and to other family members. They may be in a state of crisis, concerned for their fragile newborn and, sometimes, guilty over misconceptions about their role in this unexpected happening. However, most parents retain all the hope they can that, although difficulty has marked their infant's beginning, perhaps he or she will survive to become an important member of their family in years to come.

THE PREMATURE INFANT

Prematurity is defined as birth at or prior to 37 weeks' gestation. This definition replaced the previous one based solely on birth weight. Until the late 1960s all infants born with weights less than 2500 g were considered premature. However, the work of Lubchenco and Dubowitz, which utilized both physical and neurological assessment to determine maturity, dramatically illustrated that weight alone does not always reflect maturity (Lubchenco et al., 1963; Dubowitz, Dubowitz, and Goldberg, 1970). Although premature infants are usually smaller than term infants, some infants weighing more than 2500 g may also exhibit immature neurologic and physical characteristics. These immature characteristics place them at an increased risk when compared with infants of similar weight born at term. Thus, weight alone is not a sufficient criterion for determination of prematurity.

Premature births accounted for 8.9 percent of the birth rate in 1978, according to the National Center for Health Statistics. The mortality rate for premature infants has declined from 16 to 10 per 1000 births. However, prematurity is still associated with 70 percent of all neonatal deaths and infants with permanent neurologic damage.

Physical Characteristics

Physical characteristics of prematurity are more pronounced in the very premature infant of 28 weeks' gestation than in the slightly premature infant of 36 weeks' gestation. The most apparent differences are observed in body hair (lanugo), ear development, genitals, breast tissue, sole creases, vernix, nail length, fat distribution, and skin.

The premature infant is covered with lanugo, while the full-term infant usually has lanugo covering only the shoulders and upper back. The premature infant's ear has incomplete pinna formation and less cartilage and may stay folded, unlike the ready recoil upon folding noted in the more mature infant. The premature male has undescended testicles with a few rugae (folds and creases) on the scrotum. In the very immature male, the testes are still in the inguinal canal. The premature female has pronounced prominence of the clitoris and labia minora when compared to the term female, in which the labia majora covers these structures. Breast tissue is absent in the premature; definition of the areola develops with advancing gestational age. Well-defined, complete creasing of the soles of the feet does not occur until 40 weeks' gestation; the 28-week infant has a completely smooth sole. Vernix accumulation peaks at about 36 weeks and is found only in the creases of a term infant. Nails do not extend to the finger or toe tips in the premature, but subtleties in nail length are not helpful in determining gestational age. The premature infant has less body fat and appears lean when compared to the term infant. Lack of fat, coupled with a difference in skin thickness, gives the premature infant a ruddy red appearance, with clearly visible veins and capillaries. Because premature skin is thin and translucent, visual evaluation of oxygenation is difficult, as the premature may appear pink even when actual central oxygenation is low.

Reflexes and muscle tone provide additional contrasts between premature and term infants. The premature has less flexion; flexion progresses from heel to head with advancing gestational age. The premature infant has a predominance of muscles of extension, whereas flexors dominate in the more mature infant. There is less resistance in the premature infant when an extremity is taken through a range of motion, as the elbow is when demonstrating the Scarf sign (see Chapter 26). Such reflexes as sucking, swallowing, grasping, and the Moro reflex are slow, incomplete, or absent in the premature infant while readily elicited in the healthy term infant.

Observation of respiratory pattern and auscultation of bowel sounds provide additional differences. Compared to the term infant, respiratory rate is slightly higher in the healthy premature and the pattern of breathing is more irregular, with frequent short respiratory pauses. Bowel sounds are softer and less frequent in the premature because of decreased bowel musculature and peristalsis.

Physiologic Characteristics

With these physical and neurologic differences in mind, the nurse can assess maturity of the infant and better anticipate and screen for the physiologic "handicaps" that are associated with prematurity. Although the mechanisms, frequency, and treatment of these physiologic handicaps are not completely understood, we shall examine them in the following areas: temperature regulation, liver function, metabolism, renal function, immune system, respiratory system, cardiovascular system, digestive system, central nervous system, and skin.

Temperature Regulation

The premature infant has two handicaps related to thermoregulation: (1) a large body surface area compared to body mass, which increases radiant and conductive heat losses, and (2) reduced brown fat stores, usually deposited in the last weeks of gestation. Thus, the premature is deprived of both insulation and a potential energy source for rapid heat production. In addition, immature vasomotor control does not allow the premature to vasoconstrict peripheral blood flow and conserve body heat for maintenance of core temperature. For this reason, acrocyanosis (blueness of hands and feet) is not observed in the premature. Premature infants are also at risk for overheating, since sweat glands produce little or no sweat for cooling. These handicaps in temperature regulation mandate that nurses incorporate thermoregulation as a priority in all aspects of caring for the premature infant.

Common problems associated with cold stress include increased oxygen consumption (see Fig. 32–1), increased glucose consumption with associated hypoglycemia, poor weight gain, acidosis,

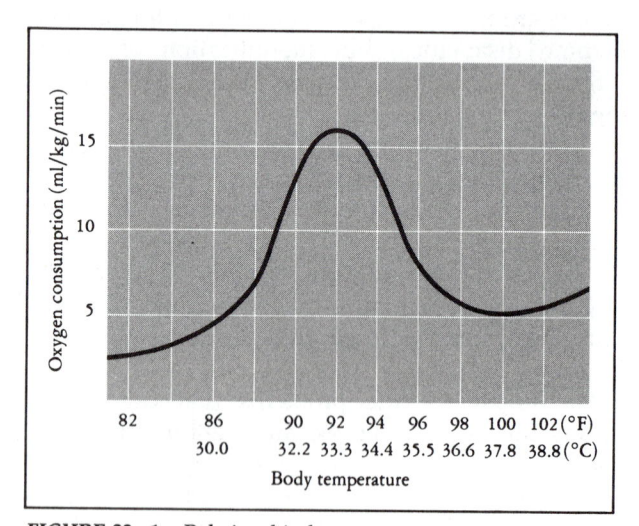

FIGURE 32–1. Relationship between body temperature and oxygen consumption.
SOURCE: The National Foundation/March of Dimes (1976). March of Dimes. Clinical Education Aids. The National Foundation–March of Dimes, White Plains, N.Y. 1976.

and decreased surfactant production. Problems associated with overheating include increased insensible water loss through the skin, increased oxygen consumption, apnea, and burns.

Although perhaps simple in concept, providing and maintaining a "neutral thermal environment" remains one of the biggest challenges in providing care for the premature infant. The neutral thermal environment charts (see Tables 32–1 and 32–2) provide a guide, as does a knowledge of temperature norms.

The nurse should completely understand the use and maintenance of heating devices available in the clinical setting. Providing thermoregulation for premature infants involves the use of external heat sources, including radiant warming tables, incubators (or Isolettes – see Fig. 32–2), and heat lamps with bassinets for larger prematures.

When using an incubator, the nurse selects an environmental temperature based on the infant's weight and age. The incubator is preheated to the desired temperature, as are the bed linens and weighing scale. On arrival in the nursery, the infant is weighed on the warmed scale and placed in the warmed incubator. Very small prematures are usually attached to a "servocontrol" mechanism that allows for feedback between the infant's skin temperature and the heating device; as the skin temperature falls below a preset level, the warming element heats up. An appropriate skin temperature that has been shown to provide a neutral thermal environment is 36.5°C. The tem-

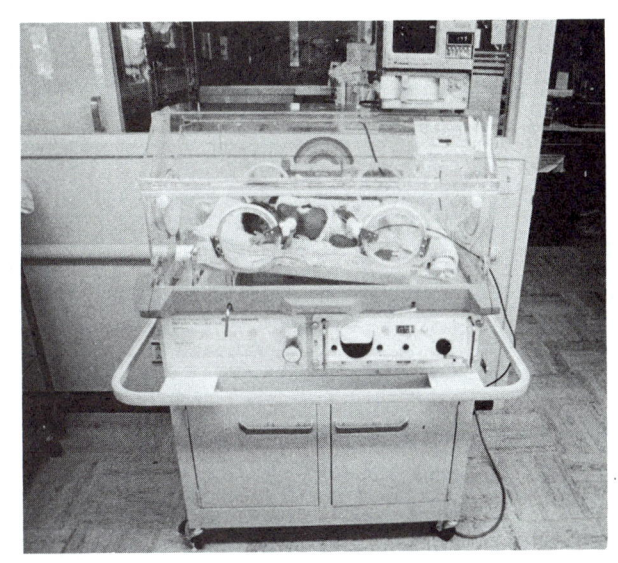

FIGURE 32–2. Thermoregulation maintained via an isolette.

TABLE 32–1. *Incubator Air Temperatures, First 24 Hours*

Birth Weight		Temperatures			
		°C Median ± Range		°F Median ± Range	
g	lb	Median	Range	Median	Range
	1	35.5	0.5	96.0	0.9
500		35.5	0.5	96.0	0.9
	2	35.0	0.5	95.0	0.9
1000		34.9	0.5	94.9	0.9
	3	34.2	0.5	93.6	0.9
1500		34.0	0.5	93.2	0.9
	4	33.7	0.5	92.7	0.9
2000		33.5	0.5	92.3	0.9
	5	33.3	0.7	92.0	1.3
2500		33.2	0.8	91.8	1.4
	6	33.1	0.9	91.6	1.6
3000		33.0	1.0	91.4	1.8
	7	32.9	1.1	91.2	1.9
3500		32.8	1.2	91.0	2.1
	8	32.8	1.3	91.0	2.3
4000		32.6	1.4	90.7	2.5
	9	32.5	1.4	90.5	2.5

SOURCE: American Academy of Pediatrics (1977).

TABLE 32–2. Incubator Air Temperatures, According to Age and Birth Weight

Age	Weight Under 1500 g °C Median ± Range	Weight Under 1500 g °F Median ± Range	Weight 1501–2500 g °C Median ± Range	Weight 1501–2500 g °F Median ± Range	Over 36 Weeks' Gestation and Weight Over 2500 g °C Median ± Range	Over 36 Weeks' Gestation and Weight Over 2500 g °F Median ± Range
1 day	34.3 0.4	93.8 0.7	33.4 0.6	92.1 1.1	33.0 1.0	91.4 1.8
2 days	33.7 0.5	92.7 0.9	32.7 0.9	90.9 1.6	32.4 1.3	90.4 2.3
3 days	33.5 0.5	92.3 0.9	32.4 0.9	90.4 1.6	31.9 1.3	89.4 2.3
4 days	33.5 0.5	92.3 0.9	32.3 0.9	90.2 1.6	31.5 1.3	88.6 2.3
5 days	33.5 0.5	92.3 0.9	32.2 0.9	90.0 1.6	31.2 1.3	88.1 2.3
6 days	33.5 0.5	92.3 0.9	32.1 0.9	89.8 1.6	30.9 1.3	87.6 2.3
7 days	33.5 0.5	92.3 0.9	32.1 0.9	89.8 1.6	30.8 1.4	87.4 2.5
8 days	33.5 0.5	92.3 0.9	32.1 0.9	89.8 1.6	30.6 1.4	87.0 2.5
9 days	33.5 0.5	92.3 0.9	32.1 0.9	89.8 1.6	30.4 1.4	86.7 2.5
10 days	33.5 0.5	92.3 0.9	32.1 0.9	89.8 1.6	30.2 1.5	86.4 2.7
11 days	33.5 0.5	92.3 0.9	32.1 0.9	89.8 1.6	29.9 1.5	85.8 2.7
12 days	33.5 0.5	92.3 0.9	32.1 0.9	89.8 1.6	29.5 1.6	85.1 2.8
13 days	33.5 0.5	92.3 0.9	32.1 0.9	89.8 1.6	29.2 1.6	84.6 2.8
14 days	33.4 0.6	92.1 1.1	32.1 0.9	89.8 1.6		
15 days	33.3 0.7	92.0 1.3	32.0 0.9	89.6 1.6		
4 weeks	32.9 0.8	91.2 1.4	31.7 1.1	89.0 1.9		
5 weeks	32.1 0.7	89.3 1.3	31.1 1.1	87.9 1.9		
6 weeks	31.8 0.6	89.2 1.1	30.6 1.1	87.1 1.9		
7 weeks	31.1 0.6	87.9 1.1	30.1 1.1	86.2 1.9		

SOURCE: American Academy of Pediatrics (1977).

perature probes that are used for "servocontrol" should be set at this temperature. Axillary temperatures are taken every 30 min until stabilized in the range of 97.4–98.8°F (36.4–37°C). Rectal temperatures may be used, but there is usually no difference noted between axillary and rectal, and the frequent taking of rectal temperatures can damage delicate rectal mucosa. Axillary temperatures, taken for 3 min, have been shown to be an effective way to monitor temperature in neonates. Even after initial stabilization, all care and treatment activities must include the prevention of heat losses and careful temperature monitoring for the remainder of the hospitalization.

Liver Immaturity

The premature infant's liver has lower enzyme levels and in general performs all its functions less efficiently than the liver of a term infant or adult. The most common problems associated with this decreased liver function are hyperbilirubinemia, decreased production of clotting factors and albumin, and poor drug clearance. (Poor drug clearance will be discussed in the section on renal immaturity.)

Hyperbilirubinemia in the neonatal period refers to elevated levels of unconjugated bilirubin, a waste product of red cell destruction. Laboratory data refer to this as "indirect bilirubin" as compared to "direct bilirubin", which refers to levels of bilirubin that have been conjugated by the liver. This distinction is important, since conjugated bilirubin does not cause kernicterus, the brain-damaging condition caused by excessively high levels of unconjugated bilirubin.

The problem of hyperbilirubinemia in the premature is compounded by lower levels of liver enzymes needed for conjugation. An additional problem is poor bowel motility, which impedes excretion of bilirubin in the stool once it has been conjugated. Prematures therefore attain higher mean peak bilirubin levels than term infants, and their hyperbilirubinemia and resultant jaundice last longer. Their lower serum albumin levels also place them at greater risk of having free bilirubin, which can pass the blood–brain barrier.

Treatment includes use of phototherapy lights (see Fig. 32–3) and, if serum bilirubin levels become extremely high, an exchange transfusion. During this procedure the baby's total blood volume (approximately 100 ml/kg body weight) is exchanged with donor blood. This exchange transfusion is done in very small increments, usually 5–10 ml amounts, to avoid dramatically altering blood pressure and perfusion during the procedure.

Decreased production of clotting factors requires that gentle handling of premature infants be coupled with close observation for bruising. If any birth asphyxia has occurred, the liver may be further compromised by liver ischemia, which will greatly increase the risks of all these problems.

Metabolic Immaturity

Hypoglycemia and hypocalcemia are the two most common metabolic problems associated with prematurity. They result from decreased stores of glycogen and calcium, ordinarily laid down in the fetus during the last trimester. Routine screening for low glucose levels, using the Dextrostix© or ChemStrip© determination method, is common practice and is essential in the care of premature infants until feedings have been well established. In extremely premature infants, this screening is of continued importance if intake of either oral or intravenous nutrients is interrupted for even a short time, since glycogen stores are not readily available for rapid conversion to glucose.

Serum glucose, or blood glucose levels, should remain between 50 and 100 mg/100 ml (or Dextrostix between 45 and 130) for optimal physiologic balance. Hypoglycemia, or blood glucose levels less than 25 mg/100 ml, in the premature can lead to seizures and brain damage if left untreated. Therefore, this aspect of care is critically important for all prematures.

Because of decreased calcium stores in the premature infant, it is also essential to obtain serum calcium levels. Normal serum calcium levels should be above 7 mg/100 ml. A range of 8–10 mg/100 ml is preferred. Hypocalcemia can result in jitteriness and tremulousness, apnea, and seizures. Until feedings can provide adequate dietary calcium, intravenous supplementation must be given. It is also important to recognize that serum levels may be maintained by bones' giving up calcium to maintain homeostasis. Thus, a finding of normal serum levels does not alter the need to provide calcium supplementation for optimal care in the premature infant.

Renal Immaturity

The premature infant's kidneys do not clear wastes efficiently, have a reduced glomerular filtration rate, and are less efficient at reabsorption of glucose, amino acids, and bicarbonate. Problems associated with inefficient waste clearance are metabolic acidosis, elevated phosphorus levels, and poor drug clearance. A reduced glomerular filtration rate can lead to edema and fluid overload. Inefficient reabsorption of glucose can lead to glycosuria and poor weight gain. Loss of bicarbonate in the urine further aggravates metabolic acidosis.

Intervention includes meticulous fluid calculations and the routine use of infusion pumps for all intravenous therapy. Intake and output determinations are essential. Weighing a dry diaper before placing it on the infant, then weighing it after the

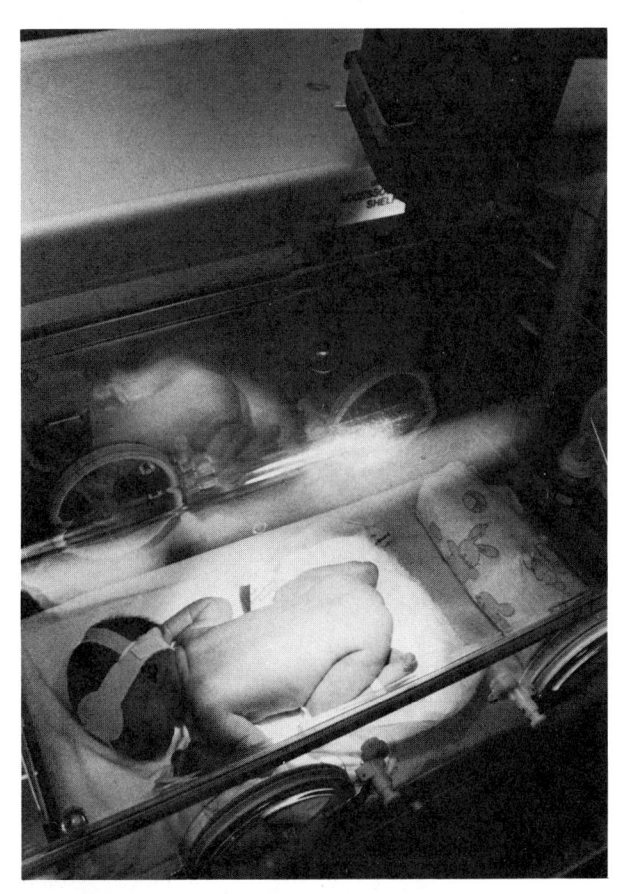

FIGURE 32–3. Premature infant under phototherapy.

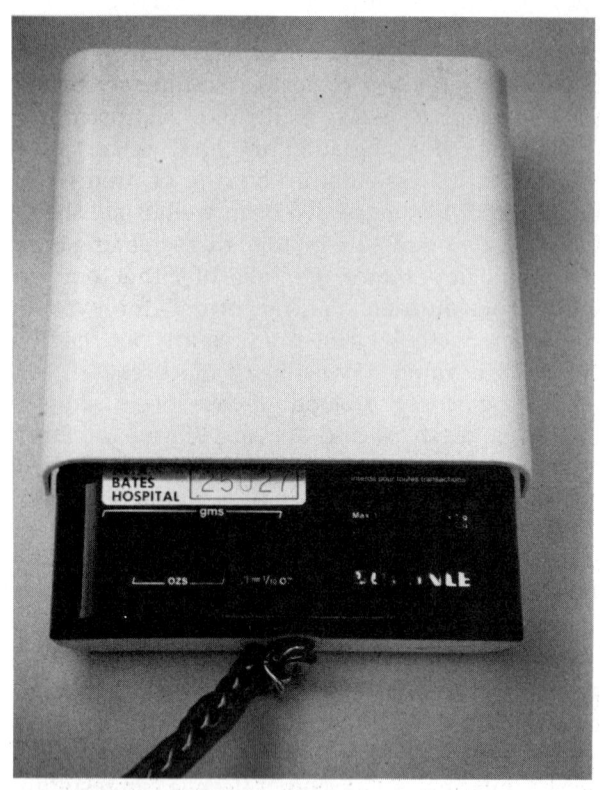

FIGURE 32-4. Scale to weigh diaper.

infant has urinated and subtracting the difference (1 g = 1 ml) is accepted in most nurseries as a reliable way to determine urinary output (see Fig. 32-4). Daily or twice daily weighing provides additional information for renal function evaluation. Blood determination of pH or bicarbonate levels may be needed, particularly in infants who remain on intravenous therapy, have associated respiratory problems, or show poor weight gain on adequate caloric intake. It is also of benefit to spot-check urine for glucose (using Testape or Clinitest) and to obtain specific gravities using the refractometer method (which needs only a drop of urine) (see Fig. 32-5).

Because of poor clearance of drugs by both kidney and liver in the premature, drug doses must be accurately calculated based on body weight, and serum drug levels must be obtained to determine each infant's individual response to the drug. Premature infants are at great risk to develop drug toxicity due to renal immaturity even when "safe" doses and administration techniques are used.

Treatment for problems associated with renal immaturity includes fluid restriction, reduced drug doses based on drug level determinations, bicarbonate supplementation to correct deficits, and reduced protein intake. There are additional risks if the infant has suffered any degree of perinatal asphyxia, because of the likelihood that renal ischemia has occurred and further compromised renal function. In these cases, anuria or oliguria (urine less than 1 ml/kg per hour) can lead to fluid overload and compromised cardiac and respiratory function.

Immune System Immaturity

Immune function is poor in all infants, but the premature's risk for infection is thought to be 10-16 times greater than the term infant's. This greater risk is due in part to low IgG levels. This immunoglobulin is received transplacentally from the mother, with the most significant rise in levels of IgG occurring in the last trimester. In addition, the white blood cells of a premature are not as competent in identification and phagocytosis of bacteria. The major problem associated with this decreased immune activity is the increased likelihood of bacterial, viral, and fungal infections.

All prematures should be considered at great risk for infection. Strict handwashing, individual isolation techniques, and meticulous cleaning of equipment (especially humidified oxygen delivery devices) are essential when caring for the premature. Nurseries should develop infection control policies that specify which infants require isolation from others and that outline conditions preventing personnel from safely working with the premature infants (see guidelines in Chapter 27).

Evaluation of each premature who enters the nursery involves taking a birth history, reviewing

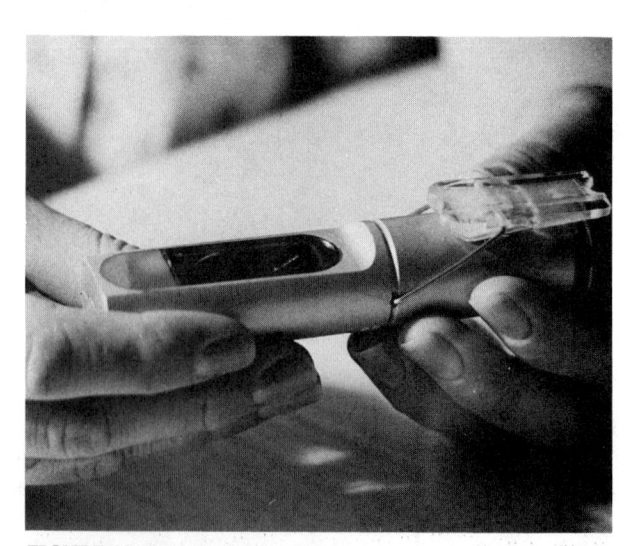

FIGURE 32-5. A refractometer.

the maternal condition prior to and during delivery, and obtaining physical assessment and laboratory data prior to deciding which medical intervention is most appropriate. Because prematures are unable to localize infection due to poor white cell function, known colonization from an infected mother is treated aggressively. Treatment with broad-spectrum antibiotics, such as ampicillin and gentamicin, is started for infants in whom infection is suspected after completion of the septic work-up. This work-up includes blood, spinal fluid, and urine cultures, a complete blood count, and a chest x-ray. Because pneumonia cannot be easily distinguished from hyaline membrane disease, infants with abnormal chest x-rays are usually treated with antibiotics until cultures prove negative or until a specific organism with known sensitivities is isolated. Since most infections in premature infants are systemic, delay in antibiotic administration until culture reports are available is unwise. Such a delay can result in septic shock and death of an infected infant.

Respiratory Immaturity

Immaturity of the respiratory system is one of the major threats to survival for premature infants. *Respiratory distress syndrome* (RDS) and *hyaline membrane disease* (HMD) are terms used interchangeably to define the leading cause of death in premature infants. Levels of *surfactant*, a phospholipid that stabilizes alveolar expansion, remain low until about 36 weeks' gestation. Surfactant production can also be adversely affected if birth asphyxia occurs, which accounts for some severe cases of HMD in more mature infants. Other factors, such as weak respiratory muscles, less rigid rib cages, weak cough and gag reflexes, and immaturity of the respiratory center in the brain, can lead to hypoventilation with subsequent hypoxemia, carbon dioxide retention, and apnea.

Respirations are characterized by a period of rapid breathing followed by a short respiratory pause, with a higher average rate than in term infants. The correct term for this breathing pattern is *periodic breathing;* it does not have the same clinical significance as the Cheyne-Stokes respirations observed in adults. This periodic breathing pattern is physiologic and changes to a more regular pattern as the infant matures.

Interventions include positioning the infant to improve airway clearance, maintaining airway patency, head-up positioning to reduce risk of diaphragm compression and aspiration of gastric contents, and frequent assessment of respiratory rate, effort, grunting, flaring, retractions, and breath sounds. Although the color of the skin and mucous membranes should be noted, color is not a reliable indicator of adequate arterial oxygen saturation. Blood gas determinations are used to evaluate oxygenation, carbon dioxide retention, and acidosis. Arterial blood samples are needed to determine accurate pO_2 levels. Warmed heelstick samples (warming promotes arterialization of the capillaries) may be used to assess CO_2 and pH levels.

Infants with evidence of respiratory failure require vigorous and skilled interventions. It is important to be prepared to provide immediate care to the infant (see Fig. 32–6). These include insertion of an umbilical artery catheter for frequent arterial blood gas determinations; transcutaneous monitoring of oxygen or carbon dioxide levels (a probe heats up the skin surface and arterializes vessels while pO_2 levels are determined through the skin by sensors); and initiation of some degree of ventilatory assistance. This assistance can consist of increasing environmental oxygen via a plexiglas hood enclosing the infant's head, providing continuous positive airway pressure (CPAP) via nasal prongs, mask, or endotracheal tube; or delivering intermittent mandatory ventilation (IMV) via endotracheal tube and an infant ventilator (see Fig. 32–7). For more in-depth information about care of infants with respiratory failure, see the suggested readings list at the end of the chapter.

Apnea, defined as respiratory pauses longer than 15 sec or any respiratory pause with associated bradycardia, is another respiratory problem frequently encountered in the care of premature infants. Treatment of apnea usually begins with tactile stimulation at the time of the episode, accompanied by careful recording of the length of the apnea episode, any associated bradycardia and color change, and the infant's response to intervention. If episodes become frequent, with more pronounced bradycardia and color changes, intervention becomes more aggressive. Pathologic causes for the apnea, such as seizures, infection, anemia, and hypoglycemia, must first be ruled out. If pathology has been ruled out, treatment is focused on the symptoms. Recommendations include treatment with central nervous system stimulants, such as drugs in the xanthine group (for example, theophylline or caffeine), to increase minute volume of ventilation. Also recommended is vestibular stimulation, such as that provided by oscillating mattresses.

If apnea becomes too severe, compromising the

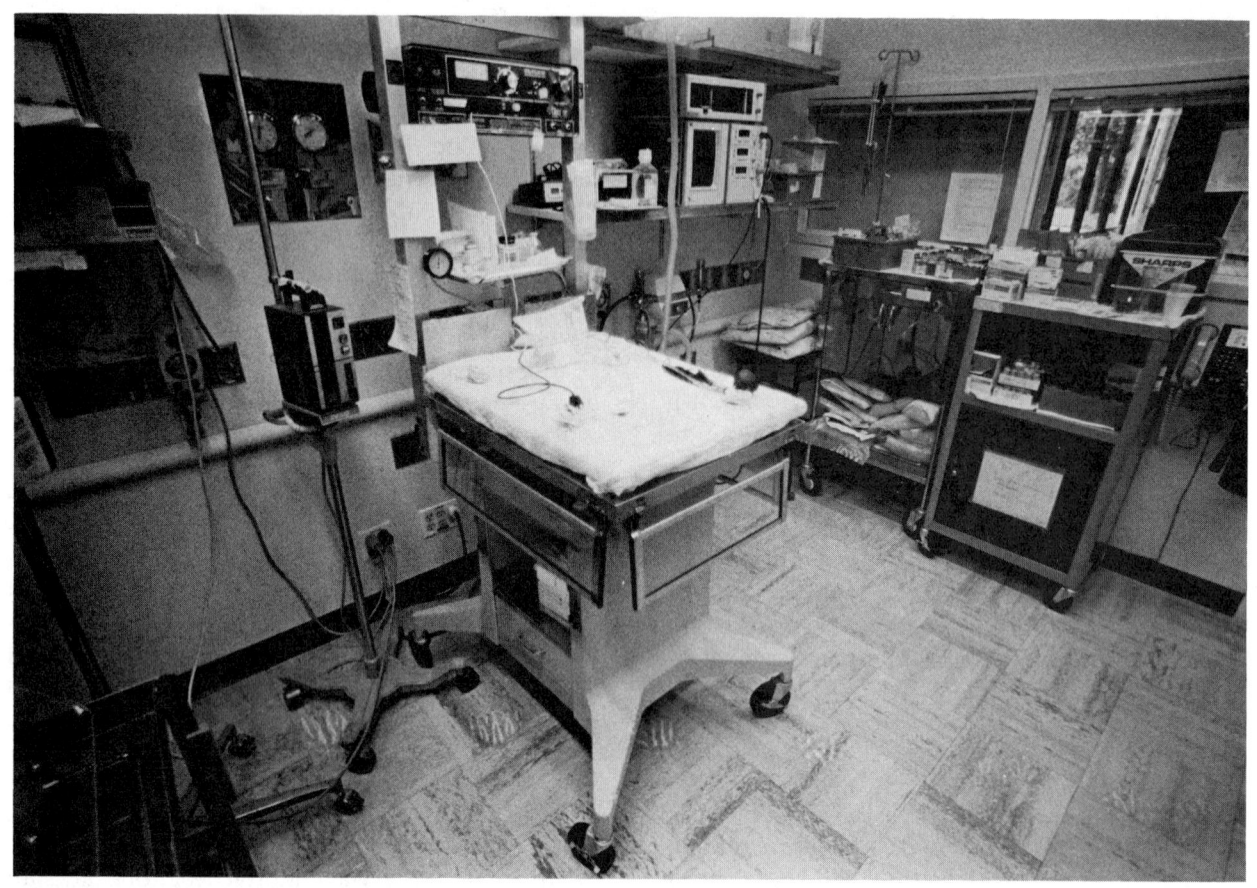

FIGURE 32–6. High-risk setup for intensive care nursery.

infant with frequent hypoxic episodes, intubation and mechanical ventilation with an infant respirator may be required. Because apnea is frequently encountered in premature infants, nurseries caring for prematures must be equipped with cardiorespiratory monitors to detect this life-threatening complication.

Cardiovascular Immaturity

The premature has a tendency toward persistence of fetal circulation, with delayed closure of the patent ductus arteriosus (PDA), relative higher pulmonary artery pressure, and increased capillary fragility. Problems associated with these characteristics include pulmonary edema and heart

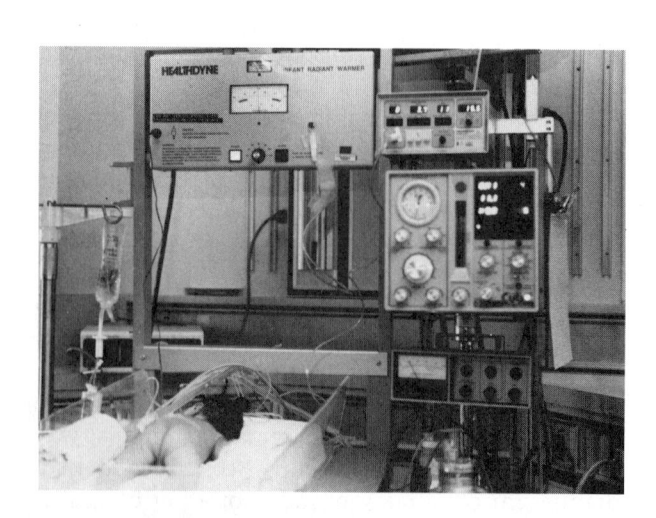

(a)

FIGURE 32–7. (a) Baby in head oxygen.

(b) Infant on ventilator.

failure due to increased pulmonary blood flow through the PDA, and a predisposition toward bruising and hemorrhage.

Intervention includes frequent assessment of cardiovascular status. This assessment should include recording heart rate and blood pressure, listening for heart murmurs, and evaluating quality of pulses and blood perfusion. Problems associated with a PDA usually manifest in the first 1–2 weeks of life and are characterized by a continuous systolic heart murmur, widened pulse pressure (difference between systolic and diastolic pressures), and bounding pulse. There may also be decreased urine output, rapid weight gain due to fluid retention, increased respiratory rate and effort and, often, increased oxygen needs. Treatment includes a cardiology evaluation, with EKG, echocardiogram, and chest x-ray to assess for pulmonary edema. Conservative medical management includes fluid restriction, diuretic therapy, and rarely, digitalization. If conservative medical management fails, indomethacin may be given, which helps to close the PDA by means of its prostaglandin-inhibiting properties. If indomethacin fails to close the PDA, surgical ligation may be required.

The problems associated with capillary fragility are, in part, addressed through gentle handling and avoidance of blood pressure swings. However, bruising can occur through even the best of deliveries. The bruised infant may require early initiation of phototherapy, since extravascular blood increases the bilirubin load to the liver. Preventing blood pressure swings includes slow administration of volume-expansion agents such as blood products, albumin, and fluids. If frank bleeding occurs, blood is replaced by slow transfusion. Massive blood loss may require faster replacement to prevent shock and tissue ischemia.

Two problems that are related to vascular fragility and immaturity but that affect other organ systems are intraventricular hemorrhage and retinopathy. Since better diagnostic techniques such as cranial ultrasonography and CAT scans have become available, *intraventricular hemorrhage* (IVH) and hemorrhage involving other cerebral structures have recently been identified as high-incidence phenomena, occurring in 40–50 percent of all infants weighing less than 1500 g (Brann and Schwartz, 1983). Effects on neurodevelopmental outcome range from no harm to hydrocephalus with serious motor or cognitive sequelae. Contributing factors to the development of IVH include asphyxia, swings in blood pressure, and capillary fragility. Prevention is aimed at reducing perinatal asphyxia, careful monitoring of blood pressure to avoid rapid shifts in either direction, and avoiding a head-down position. Early diagnosis is helpful in determining the extent of injury and in the early detection of hydrocephaly.

Retinopathy of prematurity (ROP), formerly known as retrolental fibroplasia (RLF), has recently been noted in increasing numbers in small, immature infants. When identified in the 1950s, RLF was thought to be caused by administration of oxygen in too high levels. In the 1960s, high arterial oxygen levels were thought to be the cause. Careful monitoring of arterial blood gases would supposedly eradicate this condition. However, in very immature infants, vascular instability and fragility are now thought to be the overriding factors in the pathogenesis of this condition – hence the change in name to retinopathy of prematurity. Careful monitoring of arterial oxygen levels is still indicated, and keeping paO$_2$ in the lower ranges of normal is accepted practice in an attempt to prevent or diminish the effects of this condition. In addition, the use of vitamin E to reduce severity of the retinopathy is being researched (Hittner et al., 1981). Some nurseries are currently using high doses of vitamin E on small infants to try to diminish the effects.

Digestive Immaturity

Digestive function is slow and generally inefficient in the premature infant. Sucking and swallowing reflexes remain weak and poorly coordinated until about the 34th week of gestation. After this time, feedings by mouth should be approached with caution, and close observation is needed to prevent aspiration. Once the infant is stronger, he or she may be allowed to breastfeed (see Fig. 32–8). Gastric emptying time is slow compared to that of term infants, and bowel motility is decreased and uncoordinated, leading to abdominal distention and failure to pass stool. Digestive enzyme levels are low and can lead to malabsorption of oral nutrients and to slow weight gain. Because bacterial colonization in the bowel is delayed, vitamin K production is inefficient and requires supplementation.

In the very immature infant, poor bowel motility may make the digestion of oral nutrients impossible. Changes in diet are unsuccessful because the intestinal tract is simply unable to propel the nutrients. Other feeding intolerances are due to the infant's inability to digest and absorb nutrients properly and efficiently. The use of supplemental intravenous therapy and special feeding tech-

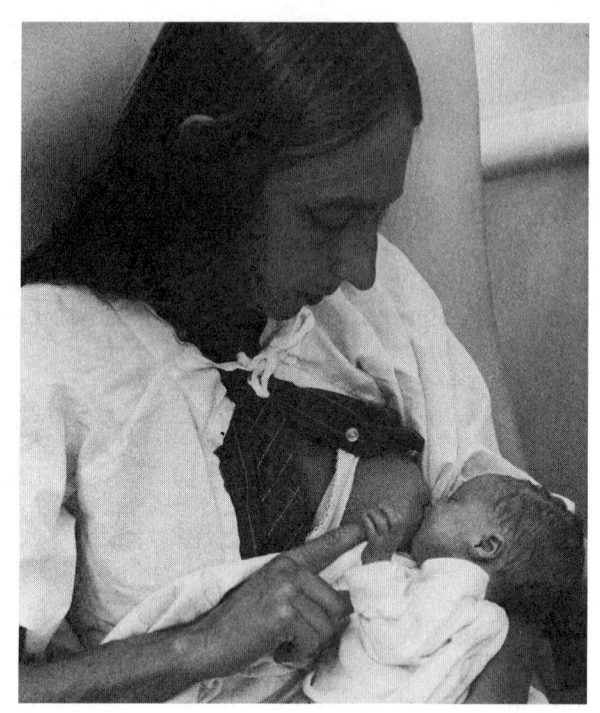

FIGURE 32-8. Mother breastfeeding her premature infant.

niques such as gavage feedings and continuous infusion feedings may be necessary (see Fig. 32–9). If the infant cannot suck adequately, intermittent gavage feedings may be preferred. The procedure for inserting the gavage tube is safe and easily taught (Babson et al., 1975):

1. Place the infant on its side or back. The infant's hands may need to be restrained to keep it from pulling the tube out during the feeding.
2. Insert a soft French 8 or 5 catheter through the mouth, for a distance equal to that from the bridge of the nose to the xiphoid process.
3. Closely observe the infant for any choking or gasping that may indicate possible tracheal entry. It is not unusual for the infant to gag as the tube is being passed.
4. Attach a syringe to the feeding tube and slowly push 1–2 ml of air into the tube at the same time you listen over the stomach with a stethoscope. If the tube is correctly placed into the stomach, you will hear a swish of air.
5. Once you are sure you are in the infant's stomach, aspirate gently. If there is feeding residual of 1–2 ml, the amount of the feed-

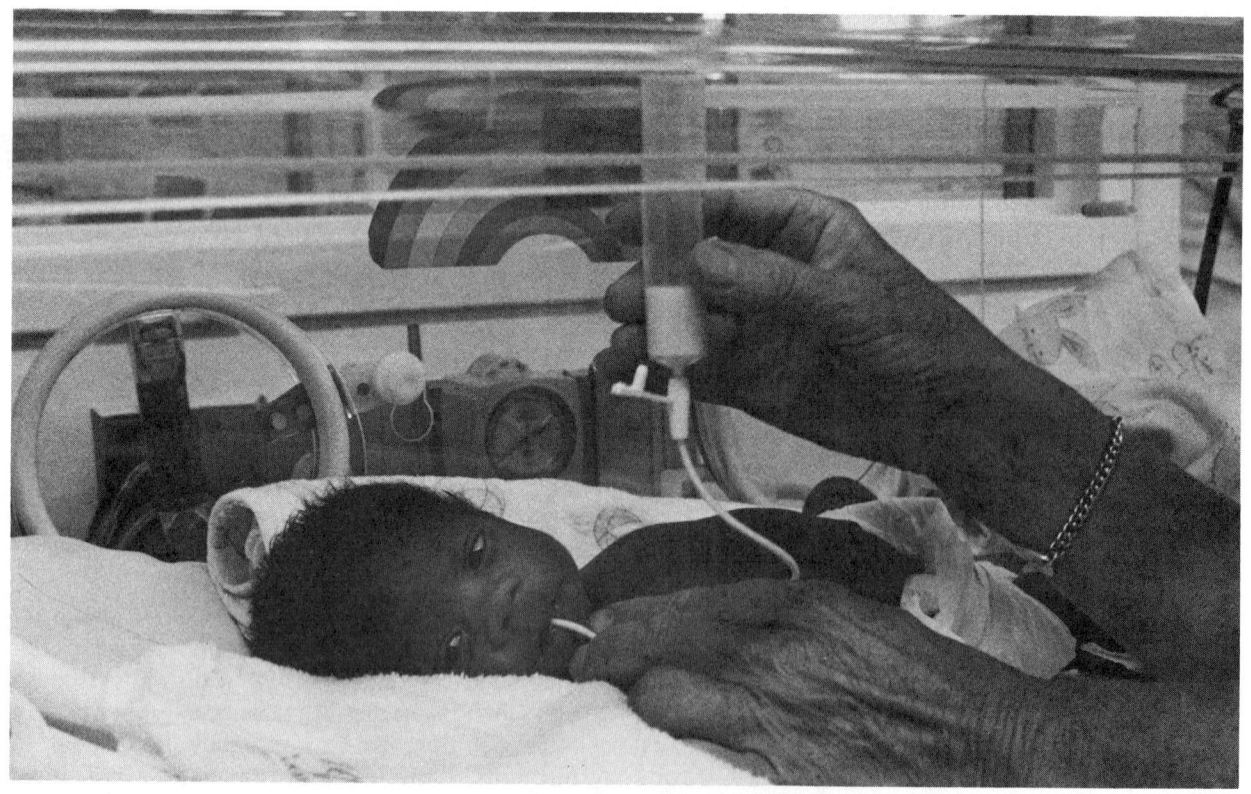

FIGURE 32-9. With a gavage feeding, the formula or breast milk flows in by gravity.

ing may be decreased by the amount of the residual. Unless the residual is very mucousy, it should not be discarded. Rather, it should be refed to the infant with the new feeding. Any residual of more than 2 ml should be reported to the physician prior to the next feeding.
6. Remove the barrel of the syringe (detach tube from syringe while doing this). Pour the feeding through the barrel of the syringe and allow the milk to run slowly, with no pressure and minimal elevation of the syringe.
7. Once the feeding is complete, or if the feeding needs to be interrupted, pinch to close the tube and withdraw it quickly.

Total parenteral nutrition, with intravenous preparations of amino acids, glucose, fat, vitamins, and minerals, has been successful in recent years in providing optimal nutritional status until the gastrointestinal tract matures enough to receive adequate nutrients. The role of nutrition in the recovery from illness, in general well-being, and in eventual outcome must not be underestimated when caring for the premature infant.

Premature infants are at risk for developing *necrotizing enterocolitis* (NEC). This disease is thought to occur as a result of damage to the bowel wall from ischemia. When the infant is fed, undigested nutrients allow for bacterial overgrowth, hydrogen gas is produced, and gas and bacteria invade the wall of the bowel. This invasion eventually leads to perforation through the bowel wall and necrosis of intestinal tissue. All prematures are considered at risk for developing NEC. Nursing surveillance includes measuring stomach residuals and stool frequency to determine bowel motility; observation for abdominal distention, with frequent abdominal girth measurements; and testing stools for blood.

Unfortunately, even with the cautious use of oral feedings and vigorous surveillance, NEC strikes suddenly and accounts for high mortality and morbidity among prematures. Abnormal abdominal x-rays, distention, vomiting, bloody diarrhea, and stomach residuals are vigorously treated with discontinuation of oral feeding, nasogastric decompression, broad-spectrum antibiotic coverage, and frequent abdominal x-rays to follow disease progression. Surgery is required in severe cases: The necrotic bowel is resected and viable bowel is externalized as a temporary ostomy until the disease subsides.

Central Nervous System Immaturity

The central nervous system of the premature has profound effects on all organ systems, yet its role is probably one of the least understood and researched. However, current work being done by neurologists and developmental specialists is centered on improving our knowledge of, and therefore our ability to protect, the young brain.

The most readily observed sign of the premature infant's immature central nervous system is an inability to interact with the environment in the same way that a term infant does. The premature infant spends more time in active sleep, spends minimal time in a quiet, alert state, and is unable to signal needs in a way that is easily interpreted by caretakers and parents (High and Gorski, 1983). Jerky, uncoordinated movements are often misinterpreted as seizures by parents and staff alike. The ability to recover from nursing interventions and social interactions is poor and can result in physiologic decompensations such as paleness, tachypnea, even apnea, and bradycardia.

It is essential for nurses to become familiar with the normal behavior of the premature, not only to comfort and guide parents but to distinguish normal behavior from abnormal. Reflexes, for example, are weak and slow, but their complete disappearance may signify problems. Tone and reflexes, including response to pain, should be regularly evaluated and documented. To promote parent-infant interaction, parents are encouraged to visit the infant regularly to learn premature infant behavior and cues (see Fig. 32–10). Research is still needed in this area. At this time, specific handling for optimal protection of the central nervous system without neglecting the sensory experiences necessary for development is not clear.

Skin Immaturity

The skin of a premature infant is thin and permeable. The bond between dermal and epidermal layers is fragile. The protective "acid mantle" covering the epidermis takes longer to recover after it has been altered by soaps and other topical agents. Problems include poor reliability of skin color to determine oxygenation, skin loss due to removal of adhesives, bacterial invasion of skin after removal of the acid mantle, and exaggerated absorption of topically applied agents.

Intervention requires that knowledge of these

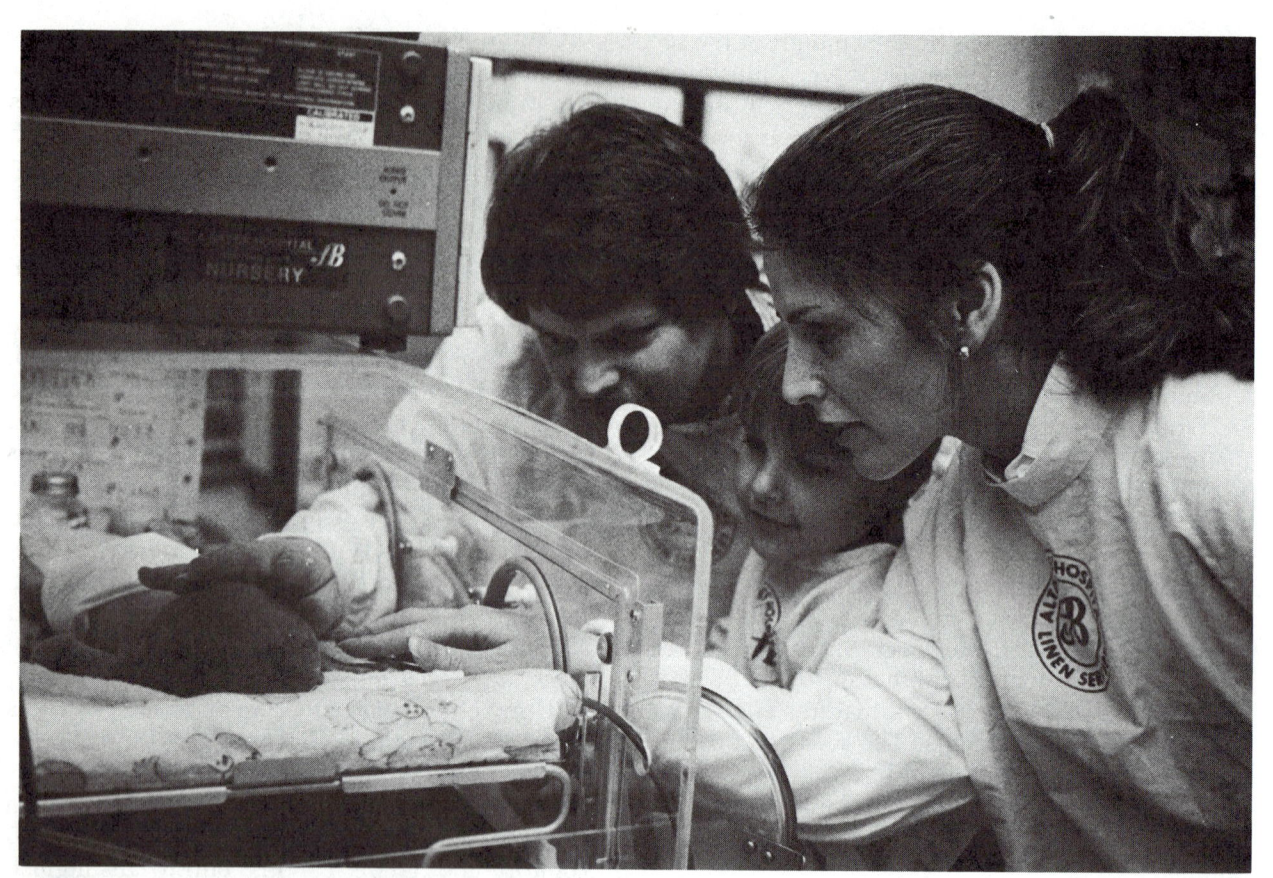

FIGURE 32–10. Parents and sibling visiting a premature infant.

handicaps be incorporated into nursing practice. Use of adhesives should be minimized. When absolutely necessary, adhesives should be chosen that are hypoallergenic and that can be removed with the least trauma (Kuller, Lund, and Tobin, 1983; Lund et al., 1986). Use of topical agents should be minimized. If essential, as in Betadine prepping for procedures, the agent should be removed immediatley after the procedure. To maintain the acid mantle and its barrier function for infection, bathing frequency should be reduced to one to two times weekly, and a neutral pH soap should be used.

To summarize, these physiologic "handicaps" exist in varying degrees in all premature infants but are most pronounced in the very premature infant of 30 weeks' gestation or less. It is imperative that every premature infant be observed and assessed for complications arising from these physiologic handicaps to prevent catastrophic complications that can ultimately lead to long-term handicaps.

THE SMALL-FOR-GESTATIONAL-AGE INFANT

This section focuses on the population of infants who, although small, are actually older than their weight would suggest. Many different terms have been used to describe these infants: "pseudomature", small for dates, dysmature, victims of chronic fetal distress, victims of intrauterine growth retardation (IUGR), and small for gestational age (SGA). Perhaps the concept of the "runted" infant, pictured as smaller and weaker but with the same degree of maturity as larger litter mates, best describes the infant who is SGA. Throughout the rest of this section the designations SGA and IUGR will be used.

The standard definition of an SGA infant is any infant whose birth weight falls at or below the tenth percentile on the intrauterine growth curve (see Chapter 26). Premature, term, or postmature

CASE PRESENTATION:

THE PREMATURE INFANT

Baby boy H. is a 1500 g (3 lb, 5 oz) infant born by spontaneous vaginal delivery to a 21-year-old primigravida after 6 hours of labor. Membranes spontaneously ruptured 12 hours prior to delivery, and attempts to stop premature labor were unsuccessful. Dates and gestational exam confirmed the infant to be 33 weeks' gestation and appropriate for gestational age. Apgar scores were 6 and 8; mask oxygen was administered for poor color in the delivery room. Upon arrival in the nursery, Baby Boy H. was placed in a hood with 30% oxygen on a radiant warming table. Admission assessment included a temperature of 97.4°F, heart rate of 168, respiratory rate of 66, and blood pressure of 48/32. His color was pale pink in 30% oxygen, his breath sounds were equal with poor air entry by auscultation, and substernal and intercostal restrictions were noted. Dextrostix was 45, pulses were equal, and extensive bruising was noted on the right arm and scalp.

Because of respiratory effort, rate, and color, along with the added finding of a borderline Dextrostix, an umbilical artery catheter was placed to allow for blood gas sampling and administration of fluids and glucose. The infant was thoroughly dried and the environmental heat was increased. He was placed in a head-up position, and a nasogastric tube was passed to aspirate stomach contents. He was placed on a cardiorespiratory monitor, and the umbilical artery catheter was connected to a transducer for continuous blood pressure monitoring. A 10% dextrose solution was administered by infusion pump, and preweighed diapers were used to begin urine output measurement.

Blood gases revealed mild hypoxemia and carbon dioxide retention, and the hood oxygen was increased to 40%. Environmental oxygen was measured continuously by an oxygen analyzer, and levels were recorded every hour and with each change. A chest x-ray revealed underaeration consistent with mild hyaline membrane disease. The infant was placed on "special care status" with hourly vital signs.

During the first 24 hours, respiratory rate and effort continued to be abnormal. Oxygen needs were determined by blood gas analysis every 4 hours in addition to continuous transcutaneous oxygen monitoring. Acceptable pO_2 parameters were ordered by the physician, and hood oxygen levels were adjusted according to the infant's pO_2 readings on the transcutaneous monitor. Fluids were limited to 60 ml/kg per day; weights were obtained daily. Blood specimens for electrolytes, calcium, and glucose were obtained, in addition to blood and urine cultures to rule out infection. Since the chest x-ray was abnormal, ampicillin and gentamicin were begun. Gentamicin levels were obtained before and after the third dose to determine drug levels and renal clearance.

On the second day, jaundice was observed on the infant's face and upper chest, and a serum bilirubin level was obtained and phototherapy initiated. Feedings were delayed because of an absence of bowel sounds and continued tachypnea and respiratory effort. Intravenous fluids were adjusted based on weight, output, and serum electrolyte determinations.

On day 3, hood oxygen levels were decreased to 25%, as pO_2 levels consistently were above 70 in higher oxygen amounts. Retractions and the respiratory rate decreased, so gavage feedings of water, then breast milk, were initiated. To decrease risk of aspiration, stomach residuals were checked before each feeding and the infant was positioned on his side after feedings. Initial volumes were small (5 ml), so intravenous fluids were continued to provide adequate hydration and caloric intake. Jaundice had progressed to the level of the knees, and the indirect bilirubin level was 9.0, so phototherapy was continued.

On the fourth day the infant's chest x-ray showed clear lung fields, and supplemental oxygen was no longer needed to maintain the pO_2 in the 60–70 range. The umbilical artery catheter was removed, and feeding volumes were adjusted to meet fluid needs. Jaundice had progressed to full body length and phototherapy was continued. The indirect bilirubin had reached 11.2.

During the entire 4 days, vital signs had been monitored every 1–2 hours; Dextrostix were obtained every 4 hours, with an increase to every 2 hours after intravenous fluids were discontinued; oxygen analyzer levels were recorded hourly; and physical assessment was done each shift by the infant's nurse. The mother was encouraged to visit, touch, and hold her infant. Visitation was not limited, so the father was able to bring a friend to visit upon request. Explanations and realistic optimism about the infant's condition and treatment had been provided to the parents and repeated often.

By day 7, bilirubin levels began to fall and feedings providing 150 ml/kg per day and 100 cal/kg per day were given. Weight loss had stopped, and the infant began to gain 10–20 g each day.

This infant's clinical course represents the middle of the spectrum of premature birth and the associated physiologic problems encountered. The infant remained in the special care nursery for 31 days. At discharge he weighed 2060 g (4 lb, 8½ oz) and was taking all feedings at the breast. Close monitoring of physical and laboratory parameters prevented serious complications associated with the risks present at this infant's birth.

NURSING CARE PLAN OF BABY BOY H.:

THE PREMATURE INFANT

Nursing Diagnosis	Expected Outcome	Nursing Interventions	Rationale
1. Potential cold stress	1. Infant's temperature will remain within acceptable range for his weight; infant will not suffer cold stress	1a. Place infant in incubator or on radiant warming table; monitor axillary temperature every 1–2 hours, then every 4 hours b. Use servocontrol mechanism for very small or unstable infants. Set probe at 36.5°C c. Keep away from windows; use heat shield or double-wall incubator (for under 1200 g infants) d. Use knit caps e. Warm linen and scales f. Work through portholes or put sides of radiant warming table up; place table away from doors g. Use neutral thermal environment chart to determine appropriate setting for incubator h. Use incubator until infant reaches weight of 1800–2000 g i. When infant is placed in bassinet, check temperatures more frequently; weight gain should also be monitored since cold stress can decrease weight gain	1a. To be able to closely monitor infant and prevent hypothermia, since infant is unable to maintain own temperature b. To determine if infant temperature is in normal range. To maintain thermal neutrality c. To decrese radiant heat loss d. To prevent heat loss from head (large surface area with premature infant) e. To reduce conductive heat loss f. To prevent drafts g. To prevent cold stress by reducing convective heat loss h. To allow infant to gain as much weight as possible so that he may maintain his own temperature in an open crib i. To ensure temperature stability and assess for cold stress
2. Potential for developing hyperbilirubinemia	2. Problems with jaundice will be resolved without further complications	2a. Assess skin for presence of jaundice every 4–8 hours b. Begin phototherapy if ordered by physician c. Ensure adequate hydration	2a. To notify physician so serum bilirubin levels are monitored b. To treat jaundice c. Use of phototherapy may contribute to dehydration

NURSING CARE PLAN OF BABY BOY H.: *Continued*

THE PREMATURE INFANT

Nursing Diagnosis	Expected Outcome	Nursing Interventions	Rationale
		d. Cover eyes with patches e. Remove all clothes, including diapers	d. To protect eyes from any damage from use of lights e. To let infant's total body be exposed to phototherapy treatment
3. Potential for hypoglycemia and hypocalcemia	3. Infant's Dextrostix will remain within normal limits; infant's serum calcium level will remain within normal limits	3a. Initiate Dextrostix protocol every hour until stable; every 2 hours 4 times; every 4 hours 4 times; every 8 hours unless complications arise b. Assess for decreased tone, seizures, hypoventilation, apnea, and bradycardia c. Administer glucose infusions accurately d. Administer i.v. calcium if not on adequate feedings; heart rate monitoring indicated during calcium infusions	3a. To observe for signs and symptoms of hypoglycemia b. To observe for signs and symptoms of hypocalcemia
4. Alteration in urinary eliminations; potential for fluid volume deficit or excess	4. Infant will be able to tolerate and clear the numerous drugs utilized; infant's urinary output will be within normal limits	4a. Obtain serum drug levels, especially gentamicin, phenobarbital b. Include infusion pump on all i.v.s; weigh wet diapers c. Make sure all fluid rates and drug doses are calculated precisely according to weight and delivered precisely	4a. To assess infant's renal ability for drug clearance b. To maintain accurate intake and output c. To provide adequate fluids and prevent fluid overload
5. Potential for infection	5a. Infant will remain free of signs and symptoms of infection while in the hospital	5a. Assess infant for signs and symptoms of infection: hypothermia, hyperthermia, lethargy, irritability, poor feeding, apnea, bradycardia, open wounds	5a. To identify onset of infection b. To prevent cross-contamination by personnel between infants c. To prevent contamination

Continued

NURSING CARE PLAN OF BABY BOY H.: Continued

THE PREMATURE INFANT

Nursing Diagnosis	Expected Outcome	Nursing Interventions	Rationale
		b. Use strict handwashing technique: 3 min scrub upon entry to the nursery and scrub between infants c. Use individual isolation technique for each infant d. Prevent skin breakdown e. Do not allow nursery personnel with upper respiratory infections or herpes lesions to work in nursery	d. Breaks in skin are good source of infection e. Infant has small amount of IgG and is therefore susceptible to infection
6. Ineffective breathing patterns; impaired gas exchange	6. Infant will remain free of any respiratory distress; infant's blood gases will remain within normal limits	6a. Use cardiorespiratory monitor; check breath sounds, respiratory rate, skin color, mucous membrane color, and any evidence of respiratory distress b. Make sure suction equipment is available at all times; make oxygen bag and mask available at all times; ensure availability of ventilatory assistance (especially hood oxygen)	6a. To assess and observe for any signs of respiratory distress b. To suction and resuscitate infant should he develop respiratory distress and need some ventilatory assistance
7. Potential for cardiac output alterations; potential for injury	7. Infant will remain free of cardiovascular complications due to immaturity	7a. Handle gently; avoid use of tight tourniquet; avoid head-down position; give volume expanders and blood products slowly to avoid rapid blood pressure swings b. Assess for heart murmur; full, bounding pulses; active precordium; wider pulse pressure; increased oxygen needs; rapid weight gain	7a. To prevent trauma due to capillary fragility b. To observe for signs and symptoms of patent ductus arteriosus (PDA) c. To assess perfusion

NURSING CARE PLAN OF BABY BOY H.: Continued

THE PREMATURE INFANT

Nursing Diagnosis	Expected Outcome	Nursing Interventions	Rationale
		c. Monitor blood pressure every 1 hour until stable	
8. Alteration in nutrition: less than body requirements	8. Infant will experience some problems with feedings due to digestive immaturity but will not develop any complications; infant will gain weight appropriately	8a. Delay nipple feedings until 34 weeks' corrected age and respiratory status stable b. Offer pacifier when NPO, and during gavage feeds c. Observe for coordination of suck and swallow, color changes; offer frequent rest periods if needed d. Hold infant during gavage feedings if possible e. Assess tolerance of feedings: check for abdominal distention, gastric residuals, emesis	8a. To prevent infant from tiring easily from weak suck reflex b. To have infant associate sucking with fullness; to meet sucking needs c. To prevent infant from tiring easily d. To promote bonding and to have ready access to infant if problems develop during gavage feeding e. To prevent infant from developing necrotizing enterocolitis (NEC)
9. Sleep pattern disturbances; potential for parenting alterations	9. Infant will have some degree of CNS immaturity but will not develop any complications; infant will respond appropriately to environmental and parental stimulation	9a. Teach parents about normal premature behavior and development and discuss how their infant is unique within this scheme b. Do not disturb during sleep unless absolutely necessary c. Offer sensory stimuli one at a time to prevent CNS overload (i.e. just voice or visual, not both at the same time) until infant becomes more mature and physiologically stable d. Assess for paleness, tachypnea, splayed fingers	9a. To prepare parents for some differences they may notice in infant's behavior b. To minimize fatigue in infant and to be alerted to signs of overstimulation

Continued

NURSING CARE PLAN OF BABY BOY H.: Continued

THE PREMATURE INFANT

Nursing Diagnosis	Expected Outcome	Nursing Interventions	Rationale
10. Potential for skin integrity impairment	10. Infant's skin will remain intact	10a. Decrease amount of tape and other adhesive to minimum; consider the use of pectin barriers under adhesives; bathe with a neutral pH soap only twice a week; water bath or no bath at other times; apply topical agents sparingly and remove immediately; avoid perfumed soaps, creams, and lotion; use non-perfumed emollient on cracked skin areas only	10a. To maintain skin integrity and acid mantle

infants can all be small for their determined gestational age. Small-for-gestational-age infants account for 1.5–2 percent of all births, and intrauterine growth retardation accounts for a large percentage of intrauterine deaths (stillbirths) as well. Overall mortality for SGA infants is 3.4 percent, with deaths from asphyxia 10 times higher than for appropriate-for-gestational-age (AGA) infants. There is also an increased rate of congenital anomalies among SGA infants (Avery, 1981).

Etiology

Causes of IUGR fall into two main categories: inadequacy of the provision of nutrients and transfer of oxygen, and fetal factors.

Inadequate supply of nutrients and oxygen can be due to maternal, environmental, or placental factors. Maternal factors include:

1. Severe undernutrition during pregnancy.
2. Conditions that decrease uterine blood flow, such as preeclampsia, toxemia, chronic hypertension, or the later diabetic stages (D, E, F, R).
3. Small maternal stature.
4. Maternal smoking greater than 20 cigarettes per day.
5. Lower socioeconomic class.
6. Adolescence of mother.
7. Grand multiparity.
8. Use of narcotics.
9. Sickle cell anemia.

Environmental factors include:

1. Living at high altitudes (infants born at 5000 feet have an average weight of 200 g less than those born at sea level).
2. Teratogenic factors such as alcohol, Dilantin, irradiation, and so on.

Placental factors include:

1. Infarcts in the placenta.
2. Premature placental separation.
3. Placental aging in a post-term (greater than 42 weeks') gestation.
4. Single umbilical artery.
5. Hemangiomas.

The fetal factors contributing to intrauterine growth retardation include intrauterine infections such as cytomegalovirus, toxoplasmosis, rubella, and hepatitis; genetic aberrations such as achondroplastic dwarfism and Russell-Silver dwarfism; chromosomal abnormalities or variations such as osteogenesis imperfecta and Cornelia de Lange syndrome; and multiple-gestation pregnancy. Twins will develop appropriately until about 30 weeks' gestation, or until the total fetal weight reaches 3 kg. After this time, the weight of one or both fetuses will drop off its original growth curve, indicating IUGR secondary to crowding in the uterine cavity. With twins, the placental transfusion syndrome, an inequality in placental circulation, may also contribute to IUGR of one or both twins.

Depending on the stage of gestation in which the growth retardation occurs, some organs may be spared during the growth reduction period. For example, the brain, heart, and pancreas may seem to be larger than the infant needs, but the liver, spleen, adrenal glands, and thymus will be decreased in size. If intrauterine growth retardation occurs early in gestation, as with some viral infections or teratogenic agents, all organs will be significantly smaller because of a decrease in cell size as well as cell number.

When the weight, length, and head circumference of an SGA infant are all below the 10th percentile, this indicates a reduction in cell number as well as cell size. Early gestational events of a long-term or chronic nature are thought to be responsible for this type of growth retardation. Congenital anomalies are also most likely to occur in the first trimester.

SGA infants may vary within their own ranks. In some SGA infants, only weight is less than the 10th percentile – head circumference and length are appropriate for the infant's determined gestation. This type of SGA infant has appropriate organ size and cell numbers but an inadequate increase in cell size. This type of IUGR occurs in the later part of gestation, when fetal growth is normally the greatest. If IUGR occurs during the post-term (greater than 42 weeks') gestation, the skull is usually a normal size but there are signs of fat depletion and muscle loss.

Physical Characteristics

The physical characteristics of SGA infants may vary depending on the causes and the stage of occurrence of IUGR, but most SGA infants look something like a thin, emaciated "little old man", with dry, cracked, and peeling skin that may look loose because of the absence of fat and musculature. Meconium staining in the amniotic fluid may leave greenish stains on the fingernails and the base of the umbilical cord. The cord itself may be thin or shriveled and should be examined to determine the number of vessels. (All infants should have two umbilical arteries, but SGA infants may have only one.)

These infants have decreased muscle mass and may appear to have a concave, or scaphoid, abdomen. Hair is sparse and skull sutures and fontanelles are wide and large, indicating growth of brain tissue in spite of decreased bone growth. Muscle tone may be tight, with flexion noted in arms and legs. Such findings may be unexpected in infants who are this small. SGA infants may appear hyperalert and active and may suck hungrily.

Physiologic Characteristics

Because SGA infants may also be premature or postmature, they are subject to the problems associated with these gestational categories. Since the problems of prematurity and postmaturity are discussed in detail elsewhere in this chapter, this section focuses on the specific alterations and neonatal problems that occur as a result of the factors contributing to intrauterine growth retardation.

Chronic Intrauterine Malnutrition

Chronic intrauterine malnutrition is responsible for (1) decreased glycogen stores, (2) decreased muscle mass, (3) decreased fat stores, and (4) a generalized reduction in the total body stores of other nutrients, such as minerals and trace minerals.

The most common problems associated with this chronic malnutrition are hypoglycemia and hypothermia. Hypoglycemia, as covered in the section on prematurity, should be determined immediately following delivery, using the Dextrostix screening method. Intravenous glucose should be initiated immediately for the preterm or severely asphyxiated SGA infant. Early oral feedings may be used for term SGA infants if their general condition permits. Dextrostix monitoring should continue for at least 48–72 hours, and longer if instability is noted. Hypothermia, a problem resulting from decreased fat stores and muscle mass, can be treated with the use of radiant warming tables, incubators, or careful drying and wrapping for slightly larger infants.

Chronic Intrauterine Hypoxia

Chronic intrauterine hypoxia is responsible for metabolic and blood constituent alterations that can seriously affect the fetus, and therefore the newborn, in several ways. The most serious problem associated with chronic or acute hypoxia is neonatal asphyxia, which affects all organ systems. As detailed in the discussion on postmaturity, asphyxia can result in cerebral edema, seizures, myocardial dysfunction, a return to fetal circulation due to severe pulmonary hypertension, and renal tubular necrosis; there may be an impact on other organ systems as well. Evaluation for meconium staining and potential meconium aspiration syndrome, which can accompany asphyxia in the fetus, is also important.

A problem associated with chronic intrauterine hypoxia commonly seen in SGA infants is polycythemia. *Polycythemia* is defined as a central hematocrit of 65 percent or greater. "Central" refers to a sample obtained by venipuncture or arterial puncture, since heelstick samples may run 5–10 percent higher than central specimens. Although polycythemia may be seen in AGA infants as a result of delayed cord clamping or cord milking, the SGA infant is at higher risk. This is because increased red cell mass is a common compensatory mechanism in response to chronic hypoxia and placental insufficiency. Excess numbers of red blood cells lead to an elevation in blood viscosity throughout the body. As the hyperviscous cells move through the body, sludging of cells in capillaries can occur in vital organs, which can impede normal circulation. Thus, polycythemia can result in respiratory distress and cyanosis, renal vein thrombosis, congestive heart failure, and seizures. Hyperbilirubinemia resulting from red cell destruction greater than the liver can handle is also seen, as are hypoglycemia, hypocalcemia, and poor feeding behavior.

To treat polycythemia, red cell mass is reduced to a hematocrit of less than 60 percent. This is accomplished by performing a partial exchange transfusion. During this procedure, a calculated amount of the infant's blood volume is removed in small increments (5–10 ml) and is replaced with equal amounts of fresh-frozen plasma or a saline/albumin solution. Thus, the red cell mass is reduced and replaced with plasma, thereby lowering the hematocrit while maintaining blood pressure and fluid volume. Treatment of nonsymptomatic infants remains controversial.

Increased Incidence of Congenital Anomalies

Another problem of SGA infants is an increased incidence of congenital anomalies. Some anomalies are associated with maternal intrauterine viral and bacterial infections during pregnancy, such as those seen in the TORCH syndrome (TO = toxoplasmosis, R = rubella, C = cytomegalovirus, H = herpes). The spectrum of clinical alterations or findings associated with congenital infections is broad and includes microcephaly, cataracts, enlarged liver and spleen, increased white blood cells, decreased platelet count resulting in petechiae or bluish discoloration, elevated direct bilirubin, and encephalitis. Some infants may present in later infancy with mental retardation, spastic diplegia, deafness, blindness, and other sensorineural deficits. Diagnosis of congenital virus is made on the basis of elevated titers, indicating an early or late exposure to the suspected virus. Treatment is supportive and is based on the symptoms exhibited by the infant.

Congenital anomalies seen in SGA infants can also be due to a chromosomal defect in the infant. Infants with trisomy 13, 15, 18, or 21 are commonly noted to have some degree of intrauterine growth retardation. The trisomy infants may have malformed or low-set ears; microcephaly; cleft lip or palate; a heart murmur with associated congenital heart defect; or hand, finger, and foot abnormalities. Diagnosis is made by obtaining a blood-sample chromosome culture that yields the abnormal trisomy pattern. Outcome for infants with trisomy 13, 15, or 18 is grim. These infants usually do not survive beyond 1 year of age, and many die in the neonatal period. Trisomy 21, or Down's syndrome, results in moderate mental retardation, but survival is good if associated anomalies, such as heart lesions or intestinal blockages, are treated. Other chromosomal conditions resulting in an infant with growth retardation include the dwarfing syndromes, osteogenesis imperfecta, and Cornelia de Lange syndrome. There are many others as well, and diagnosis is usually made by a geneticist on the basis of physical characteristics.

Congenital anomalies not associated with teratogens, viruses, or chromosome problems may also be seen. These include defects of the gastrointestinal tract, such as omphalocele, tracheoesophageal fistula, and others; congenital heart disease (seen in 6 percent of infants with IUGR); and

CASE PRESENTATION:

THE SGA INFANT

Baby girl W., born at 37 weeks' gestation, weighed only 1250 g (2 lb, 12 oz). Because of poor uterine growth, serial sonograms were obtained on this gravida 2, para 0, mother; sonograms indicated decreased head growth. A nonstress test at 36 weeks was normal, but by 37 weeks it became suspicious, with decreased fetal movement noted. Delivery by cesarean section was chosen to reduce the risk of intrauterine asphyxia during labor. Apgar scores were 7 and 9. The baby was small and emaciated, with cracked and peeling skin. Petechiae were noted on the abdomen, and the skin had a ruddy, red appearance. Only one umbilical artery was noted. The Dubowitz exam for gestational maturity confirmed the gestational age at 37-38 weeks; weight and length were well below the 10th percentile, and the head circumference was just above the 10th percentile. The infant had a shrill cry and a hyperalert appearance, with flexed extremities.

Initial Dextrostix obtained at 15 min was 25. An intravenous infusion was started in the scalp and a bolus of 10 ml of 10% dextrose/water was delivered. Intravenous fluid of 10% dextrose/water at 5 ml/hour (100 ml/kg per day) was started, since there was no evidence of respiratory distress. The Dextrostix 30 min later was 45-90 but within the next 30 min had dropped to the 25-45 range. Another bolus of 5 ml 10% dextrose was given and i.v. changed to 12.5% dextrose/water, and the rate was increased to 6 ml/hour. During this time the infant was dried thoroughly and placed on a radiant warming table with the skin probe set at 98°F. Initial temperature was 97°F, heart rate was 170, respiratory rate was 48, and blood pressure was 65/48 using a Dinamap electronic blood pressure cuff.

Initial hematocrit obtained by heelstick was 75 percent. The baby continued to be very irritable, with some grunting and nasal flaring noted. An umbilical arterial catheter was placed and a blood gas sample was obtained. The results showed a pO_2 of 52, pCO_2 of 40, pH of 7.28, base excess of −10, and a central hematocrit of 70 percent. A partial exchange transfusion was done; 25 ml of blood was exchanged for 25 ml of fresh-frozen plasma in 5-ml increments. The infant tolerated the procedure well and the hematocrit at the end of the procedure was 53 percent. Physical exam revealed a heart murmur, and pulses were palpable but not full or bounding. No other congenital anomalies were noted. A future cardiology work-up with echocardiography was planned. A complete blood count was obtained and showed a slightly low white blood cell count and a platelet count of 70,000 (normal is 150,000-200,000). Blood and urine cultures, as well as TORCH titers, were sent despite a negative maternal history for infection during pregnancy. Ampicillin and gentamicin were begun.

On day 3 a cardiology work-up and echocardiogram indicated a small atrial septal defect. No intervention or treatment was needed, since there was no evidence of congestive heart failure. The blood culture report was negative and platelet count was 140,000, so antibiotics were discontinued. Feedings, initiated on day 2, were going well, so intravenous fluids were discontinued. Dextrostix was stable at 45-90. The infant displayed a lack of suck-swallow coordination, so gavage feedings were used.

By day 6 slow weight gain was noted, approximately 10 g/day, so feedings were increased to 170 ml/kg per day to deliver nearly 120 cal/kg per day. Nipple feedings were initiated every other feeding with success. This tiny but mature infant seemed to enjoy nippling.

On day 8 weight gain was still slow, so the infant formula was changed to a 24 cal/oz concentration for better caloric intake. TORCH titers were negative for congenital viral syndrome, so etiology of the intrauterine growth retardation remained unknown. The infant was irritable, jittery, and difficult to soothe. She appeared to frown when approached socially, then averted her eyes quickly from her caretaker's face. She responded well to swaddling and decreased sensory stimulation. Her parents were involved in the infant's care, and her behavior patterns were described to them to prevent them from interpreting her behavior as rejection.

This infant was hospitalized for nearly 6 weeks, primarily to gain enough weight to maintain her temperature and show continued growth. Her behavior gradually became more sociable, with less severe response to sensory stimuli. Consistent care by her primary nurse and parents improved the amount of social interaction the infant was able to handle. Follow-up was arranged (1) in the neonatal follow-up clinic for neurobehavioral assessment, (2) in the cardiology clinic for evaluation of the atrial septal defect, and (3) with the family's pediatrician for growth assessment and well-baby care.

NURSING CARE PLAN OF BABY GIRL W.:

AN SGA INFANT

Nursing Diagnosis	Expected Outcome	Nursing Interventions	Rationale
1. Potential for cold stress	1. Infant will maintain stable temperature	1a. If infant less than 1800–2000 g, place in incubator or on warming table; check temperature every 1–2 hours until stable b. Place knit cap on infant's head c. Determine neutral thermal environment optimal for infant	1. To prevent unnecessary heat loss and to maintain infant's temperature
2. Potential for hypoglycemia	2. Infant will maintain blood glucose levels within normal ranges	2a. Initiate Dextrostix screening protocol; report all levels less than 45; if less than 25, immediate intervention required b. If IV fluids required, use continuous infusion pump c. Observe for decreased tone, seizures, hypoventilation, apnea, and bradycardia	2. To prevent hypoglycemia and associated problems due to decreased glycogen stores; to observe for signs and symptoms of hypolycemia
3. Alteration in tissue perfusion; alteration in cardiac output	3. Infant will have normal tissue perfusion, cardiac output, and gas exchange; infant's hematocrit will be decreased to within normal range without complications from polycythemia	3. Initiate partial exchange transfusion if Hct is greater than 65 percent and infant is symptomatic; tachypnea, cyanosis, seizures	3. To prevent potential complications from polycythemia
4. Alterations in nutrition (less than body requirements)	4. Infant will gain and maintain weight once adequate fluid	4a. Maintain infant in neutral thermal environment	4a. To decrease caloric expenditure b. To ensure that in-

NURSING CARE PLAN OF BABY GIRL W.: Continued

AN SGA INFANT

Nursing Diagnosis	Expected Outcome	Nursing Interventions	Rationale
	and caloric intake is established	b. After adequate caloric intake calculated, see that total amount is received by infant; decrease caloric expenditure by decreasing environmental stress and sensory overload (caloric needs may exceed the usual 120 cal/kg per day; use of 24 cal/oz formula may be indicated)	fant receives adequate calories to allow for weight gain and growth
5. Potential congenital anomalies	5. In the presence of any congenital anomalies, infant will be treated as soon as possible and further complications will be prevented	5a. Assess for presence of any obvious or hidden anomalies b. Meet with parents if congenital anomalies are present c. Consider TORCH titers and genetic work-up	5a. To detect any problems as soon as possible and implement early intervention b. To provide early emotional support to parents and encourage appropriate grieving c. To determine cause of anomalies
6. Potential for sleep pattern disturbances; potential for activity intolerance	6. Infant's irritability will decrease, and response to sensory stimulation will be within normal limits	6a. If infant fatigued, hyperalert, excessively crying, or arching, decrease stimulation by offering only one sensory experience at a time b. Try swaddling c. Provide consistent caretakers who are familiar with infant's cues	6a. To minimize irritability b. To decrease sensory stimuli and promote feeling of security c. To provide infant with familiar faces and consistent care
7. Parenting alterations potential	7. Parents will be knowledgeable about infant's behavior	7a. Provide education about SGA behavior patterns	7a. To prevent parents from interpreting behavior as rejection; to provide early emotional support to parents and prepare them for caring for their infant at home

central nervous system defects, such as anencephaly. These problems are also associated with growth retardation in the fetus.

Treatment begins with a thorough evaluation for congenital anomalies in all infants, particularly those who are small for gestational age. This assessment should include an accurate maternal history for viral infections or teratogenic agents, polyhydramnios (indicative of gastrointestinal blockage or swallowing disorder in the fetus), and oligohydramnios (indicative of genitourinary abnormality). Evaluation of the head and scalp is done to assess fontanelle and suture size, head circumference measurement, wide-set eyes, low-set or deformed ears, cleft lip or palate, and small or absent chin. A nasogastric tube is passed to determine patency of the nares and esophagus. The abdomen is palpated to determine the size of the liver and spleen, as well as the presence or absence of kidneys. Distention can indicate gastrointestinal blockage. The umbilical cord is evaluated to determine whether three vessels are present. Chest and heart are auscultated to determine whether heart murmurs are audible, and pulses are palpated for fullness and equality. The extremities are evaluated for any abnormal findings.

Identification of infants who are small for gestational age is important in the immediate neonatal period to prevent morbidity associated with some of the common physiologic problems they may experience. The outcome for these infants is as variable as the many causes of intrauterine growth retardation, but developmental follow-up is important for any infant experiencing moderate to severe growth retardation. In addition, SGA infants may pose a problem for parents because of their irritable, demanding, and unsociable behavior patterns. Counseling parents about these characteristics and providing information about the environmental impact on irritability can help parents cope during the first few months of handling the SGA infant at home. Parents should also be told that the irritable, demanding behavior usually decreases during the first year of life in most SGA infants.

THE POSTMATURE INFANT

Postmature infants are defined as those born after the 42nd week of gestation. Although only 4–6 percent of all pregnancies are post-term, these infants account for approximately 15 percent of perinatal mortality; therefore, they require identification, close observation, and monitoring during the neonatal period (Affonso and Harris, 1980).

Maternal factors associated with post-term pregnancy include previous history of post-term delivery, primigravida, or maternal age of less than 25 years. If the post-term pregnancy is associated with prolonged labor or toxemia, the chance of poor outcome is increased. If the obstetric history includes recent maternal weight loss, oligohydramnios, meconium staining of amniotic fluid, or abnormal fetal heart pattern, the risk of poor outcome increases significantly.

Physical Characteristics

Among the physical characteristics associated with postmaturity is reduced subcutaneous tissue, with pale loose skin. Prolonged exposure to amniotic fluid results in wrinkled, macerated skin at birth, which later becomes cracked and peels off in sheets (see Fig. 32–11). Advanced maturity also leads to increased alertness, long curved nails, absence of vernix, and mature genitals.

Meconium staining is another common finding. Staining that is yellow and evenly dispersed throughout the amniotic fluid usually indicates that hypoxia occurred hours prior to delivery. Green, particulate meconium staining is seen when hypoxia and passage of meconium have occurred just prior to delivery.

Physiologic Characteristics

Physiologic characteristics of the postmature infant are primarily associated with placental insufficiency due to placental aging and with birth asphyxia. These characteristics will be discussed in two major categories: (1) problems associated with insufficient nutrient supply, resulting in neonatal hypoglycemia and hypothermia; and (2) problems associated with insufficient oxygen supply during labor and delivery, resulting in birth asphyxia.

Insufficient Nutrient Supply
During prolonged gestation, nutrient supply may be inadequate. To survive *in utero*, the fetus utilizes body stores of glycogen and fat to meet energy needs. Once these stores are depleted, the fetus may begin consuming its own muscle mass. Uncomplicated birth at this time most commonly leads to problems with hypoglycemia and hypothermia due to lack of sufficient glycogen, fat, and

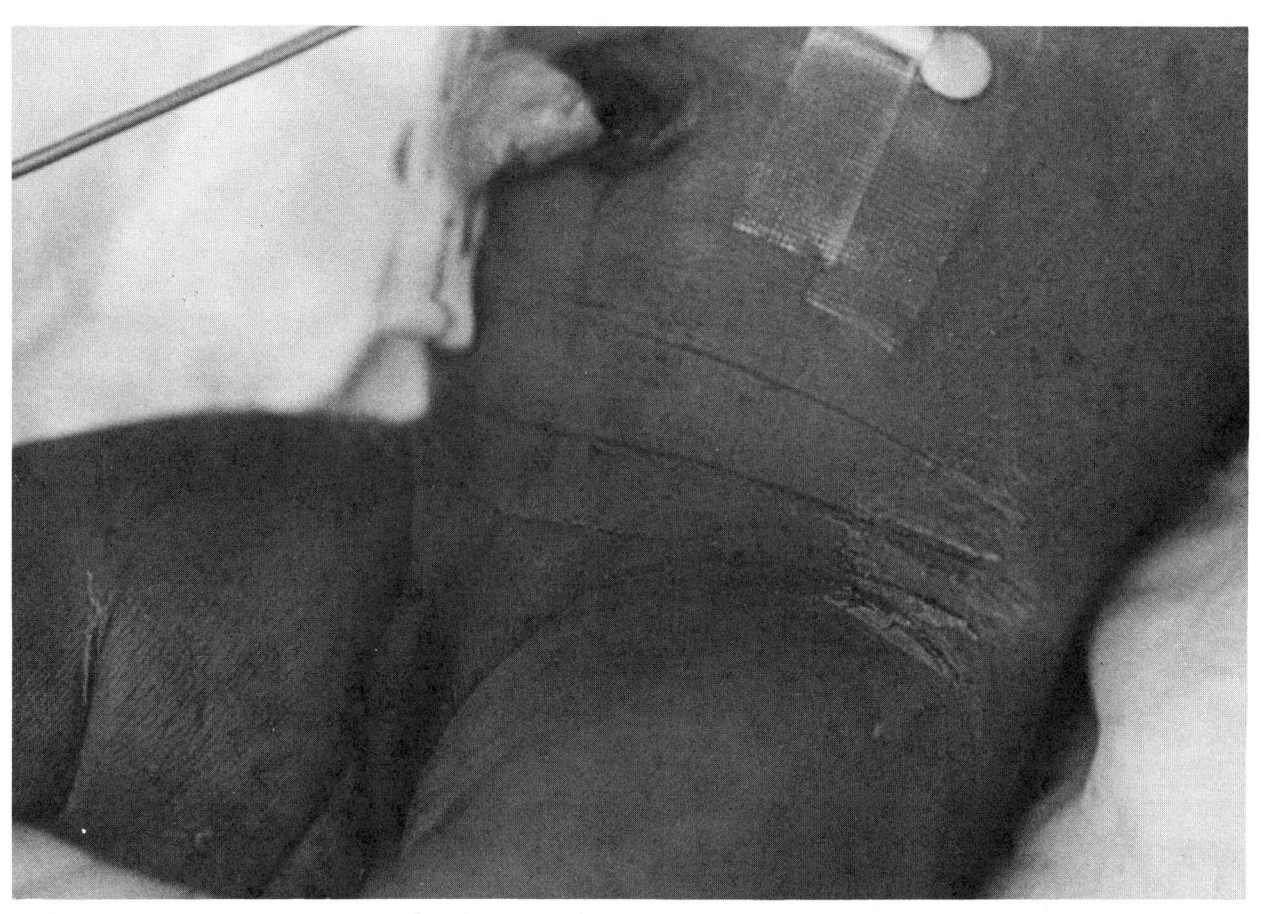

FIGURE 32-11. The dry, cracking skin of a postmature infant.

muscle mass. Intervention includes thermal support after delivery and surveillance with glucose screening, such as Dextrostix. If blood sugar is low, feedings are started early. In extreme cases, intravenous glucose may be administered. Cold stress should be avoided, as it will lead to additional demands for glucose.

Insufficient Oxygen Supply

If nutrient supply deficiency and hypoxia have been severe *in utero*, the infant will not be able to withstand the stresses of labor and delivery. Intrauterine hypoxia causes relaxation of the anal sphincter and passage of meconium. Close to 50 percent of postmature infants exhibit some degree of meconium staining at birth. With severe hypoxia the infant's respiratory center is stimulated and meconium is aspirated into the trachea prior to or during delivery. *Meconium aspiration syndrome* involves respiratory distress and failure, air trapping with potential for pneumothorax, and persistence of fetal circulation due to pulmonary hypertension. Cerebral edema, seizures, anuria, and multiple organ system ischemia are also seen, depending on the degree and severity of asphyxia.

Prevention of asphyxia involves close monitoring of the post-term fetus *in utero*. Stress and nonstress testing provide information about fetal well-being. Even if stress testing results are normal, it is imperative that labor be monitored closely. Abnormal fetal heart patterns, particularly late decelerations or loss of beat-to-beat variability, usually indicate a compromised fetus and the need for intervention. If intervention at this point is not successful, birth asphyxia or fetal death will occur.

The postmature, asphyxiated infant requires close observation and aggressive intervention. Delivery room intervention includes tracheal visualization and suctioning. For moderate asphyxia, defined as Apgar scores of 4–6, oxygen is administered by bag and mask ventilation after suctioning. In severe asphyxia, defined as Apgar scores of 1–3, ventilation is ideally given via endotracheal tube coupled with correction of acidosis with bicarbonate or ventilation, intravenous glucose administration, and cardiac compressions. Several of the suggested reading listed at the end of the

CASE PRESENTATION:

THE POSTMATURE INFANT

Baby girl T. was born to an 18-year-old primigravida by spontaneous vaginal delivery. Her mother was 42½ weeks pregnant by dates, and delivery was complicated by late decelerations in the fetal heart rate. Apgar scores were 4 and 5, and because thick neconium staining was observed, the infant's trachea was suctioned three times and oxygen was given by mask to improve color. Baby girl T. was taken to the nursery, placed on a radiant warmer, attached to a cardiorespiratory monitor, and given hood oxygen of 30%. Blood gases and Dextrostix were obtained by warmed heelstick specimen. Dextrostix result was 25, and the blood gas indicated a pH of 7.05 with a combined respiratory and metabolic acidosis. Oxygen levels in the blood could not be evaluated by this technique, but because of continued cyanosis the infant was placed in a 100% oxygen hood.

The physician in attendance consulted by phone with the regional intensive care nursery. He was advised to place an umbilical artery catheter, infuse a bolus of 10% dextrose, and obtain an arterial blood sample to assess oxygen needs. An x-ray was obtained to determine position of the arterial catheter and determine the extent of lung disease. The arterial blood sample revealed hypoxemia, and the infant was immediately intubated and hand ventilated until the transport team from the intensive care nursery arrived.

On team arrival, it was noted that generalized seizures, systemic hypotension with a blood pressure of 40/22, and continued hypoxemia were present. Repeat chest x-ray revealed collapse of the right lung due to a tension pneumothorax. A chest tube was placed and the infant was loaded with phenobarbital to begin seizure control. A repeat Dextrostix and calcium level were obtained to rule out metabolic cause for the seizures. A vasopressor, dopamine, was started by constant infusion to increase systemic blood pressure, and intravenous fluids were increased to 15% dextrose due to continued low Dextrostix. Fluid rates were adjusted to restrict intake, because of the risk of cerebral edema secondary to asphyxia.

The infant was transported to the intensive care nursery in critical condition. On arrival at the nursery, the infant was again placed on a radiant warmer. Ventilation was continued by means of an infant ventilator. Monitoring included continuous cardiorespiratory readout; continuous readout of systolic, diastolic, mean, and pulse pressures; and continuous readout of transcutaneous O_2 and CO_2. Nursing care included complete thermal support, Dextrostix analysis every hour, and head-to-toe assessment with emphasis on reflexes, tone, breath sounds, heart sounds, pulse quality, and perfusion. Strict control of intake and output was instituted, and fluids remained restricted. Laboratory screening included surveillance for infection, with blood and urine cultures, complete blood count, BUN and creatinine levels, and baseline electrolyte and calcium levels. An electroencephalogram (EEG) showed continued seizure activity, and cerebral edema was suspected on the basis of fullness of fontanelle and splitting of sutures.

The infant remained on full ventilatory support with few spontaneous respirations. Suctioning of the endotracheal tube continued to produce green-tinged mucus. A chest x-ray on admission showed diffuse patchy densities consistent with severe meconium aspiration. The pneumothorax was successfully evacuated. The chest tube remained in place connected to suction.

During the next 3 days the infant's tone slowly improved. Oxygen needs steadily decreased and spontaneous respirations increased, allowing respiratory support to be weaned from 80 breaths/min down to 20 breaths/min. Urine output remained poor – less than 1 ml/kg per hour – and fluid restriction continued. The infant had developed generalized edema and the phenobarbital level was above the toxic range because of poor drug clearance. Phenobarbital was held on day 3, and continued drug levels were obtained to determine when to reinstitute the drug. Seizures could not be recognized clinically but were still seen on repeat EEG.

All nutrients were delivered intravenously because of the risk of introducing oral nutrients into a gastrointestinal tract that had most likely had ischemic insult secondary to hypoxia at birth. The infant's skin began to dry and crack, and bathing was avoided because of the additional drying effects of soap. Antibiotics were stopped on day 4 when all culture reports were negative and the repeat complete blood count was normal. Dextrostix screening was reduced to every 4 hours, but complete thermal support continued by means of the servocontrol radiant warmer.

On day 5 the endotracheal tube was removed and the infant was placed in hood oxygen. Blood gas determination and transcutaneous monitoring of O_2 and CO_2 were continued, to assess oxygen needs. Neurologic evaluation revealed response to pain, return of all reflexes, normal EEG, and visual alertness when awake. The chest tube and arterial catheter were removed on day 7, and feeding of water was given by gavage because of continued tachypnea. Intravenous supplementation of fluids and calories continued because of the limited oral intake. The chest x-ray remained abnormal, which was clinically evident by oxygen needs, tachypnea, and mild dyspnea. Phenobarbital was continued at low maintenance doses at the recommendation of the neurologist.

During days 8, 9, and 10 there was gradual improvement of respiratory status, with adequate oxygenation in room air and decreased dyspnea and tachypnea. Feedings were increased and cautiously attempted by bottle and then breast. Intravenous supplementation was no longer needed by day 10. Dextrostix determination was discontinued after normal values were obtained before the first two feedings off intravenous supplement. The infant was weaned to an open crib, and temperature was maintained by using a knitted cap and warmed blankets.

By day 14 the infant had begun to gain weight daily, and all treatments had been stopped except phenobarbital. Parent teaching was completed. The infant was discharged with instructions for follow-up care that included a 1-week appointment with her pediatrician, a 1-month evaluation with a neurologist, and developmental evaluation. The parents had been taught how to observe breathing rate and pattern, to recognize normal color, and to administer phenobarbital safely, as well as normal infant care, including safety precautions. Because of continued dry skin, bathing with soap only twice weekly was recommended, and parents were advised to continue to dress the infant in warm clothes because of decreased body stores for insulation and heat production.

This infant represents the more critical end of the postmature spectrum, but not the most catastrophic. She responded well to aggressive medical management, and her rapid recovery probably indicated a short-term asphyxia. Her early symptoms indicated multiple organ ischemia from hypoxic insult prior to and during delivery.

NURSING CARE PLAN OF BABY GIRL T.:

A POSTMATURE INFANT

Nursing Diagnosis	Expected Outcome	Nursing Interventions	Rationale
1. Potential for hypoglycemia	1. Infant will not develop hypoglycemia; blood glucose will remain within normal ranges	1a. Initiate Dextrostix protocol every hour until stable, then every 2–4 hours until feedings are well established b. Assess infant for poor tone, jitteriness, and seizures c. Administer glucose as ordered i.v. or p.o. for abnormal levels of glucose	1. To observe for signs and symptoms of hypoglycemia
2. Potential for hypothermia	2. Infant will maintain temperature within normal ranges	2a. Provide complete thermal support until needs are evaluated; check temperature every hour until stable b. If infant is sick, continue thermal support to reduce metabolic demands c. Use knit caps, warm linens and scales; avoid drafts; dry infant immediately if wet; keep crib away from windows d. Wean thermal support gradually, using infant's temperature, warmth of extremities, and weight gain as guidelines	2. To maintain neutral thermal environment for infant to maximize growth potential, as infant is unable to regulate own temperature; to minimize heat loss
3. Ineffective breathing patterns; impaired gas exchange	3. Infant will not develop respiratory distress and associated complications	3. Use cardiorespiratory monitor; make sure that suction and emergency oxygen equipment are available at bedside and that ventilatory assistance (oxygen hood, bag/mask setup) is available at all times	3. To assess respiratory status and ensure appropriate resuscitation if infant develops respiratory problems

Continued

NURSING CARE PLAN OF BABY GIRL T.: *Continued*

A POSTMATURE INFANT

Nursing Diagnosis	Expected Outcome	Nursing Interventions	Rationale
4. Potential for impairment of skin integrity	4. Infant's skin will be maintained intact	4a. Observe skin for dryness, cracking, peeling, staining, or breakdown b. Reduce use of soap and drying agents such as Betadine; consider HEB cream for actual breakdown c. Instruct parents in bathing and skin care prior to discharge	4a. To identify indications of skin breakdown b. To maintain infant's skin integrity c. To prevent skin breakdown
5. Potential for birth injury	5. Injury to infant will be prevented; infant will be assessed and treated for any birth injury	5a. Report abnormal findings and assist with definitive testing for birth injury b. Continue reflex/tone assessment to determine improvement/deterioration c. Observe for strength of grasp, abnormal contours of bony structures, hematomas d. Be familiar with and initiate clinical management of injury	5. To prevent injury to infant; to identify problems and implement early interventions
6. Potential for decreased cardiac output	6. Infant will remain free of cardiovascular complications	6a. Control intake and output, using weighed diapers b. Delay oral feedings if bowel sounds not present c. Handle gently to avoid bruising or hemorrhage d. Measure head circumference daily and assess fontanelles and sutures e. Measure blood pressure; assess tissue perfusion; observe for signs of organ ischemia (i.e. lowered urinary output and bowel sounds, prolonged bleeding times, seizures)	6. To assess cardiovascular status and prevent associated complications

chapter give a detailed guide to delivery room resuscitation and care of the infant.

Postasphyxia care includes fluid restriction to reduce effects of cerebral edema and renal ischemia, cardiorespiratory monitoring, frequent Dextrostix determination, arterial blood gases, complete thermal support, delay of oral feeding (because of asphyxiated compromise to the intestinal tract), and chest x-rays to determine presence of meconium or pulmonary air leak. Ongoing treatment is individualized based on clinical, x-ray, and laboratory findings.

The spectrum of illness in postmature asphyxiated infants is broad, but because of the high morbidity and mortality rate, these infants should all be carefully monitored until successful adaptation to extrauterine life has been ensured.

SUMMARY

The goal of every parent is to have a healthy infant. However, there are interferences during pregnancy that may result in the birth of a premature infant, a growth retarded infant, or a postmature asphyxiated infant. Early identification of these infants allows for early intervention to prevent some expected complications. The nurse working in the nursery plays an important role in caring for these infants to allow them maximum potential for future growth and development.

SUGGESTED READINGS

Fanaroff, A., and Martin, R., eds. 1983. *Behrman's neonatal–perinatal medicine: Diseases of the fetus and infant*. 3rd ed. St. Louis: C. V. Mosby.

Gregory, G. 1979. *Neonatal pulmonary care*. Menlo Park, Calif.: Addison-Wesley.

Harrison, H. 1983. *The premature baby book*. New York: St. Martin's Press.

Klaus, M., and Fanaroff, A. 1979. *Care of the high-risk neonate*. 2nd ed. Philadelphia: W. B. Saunders.

Korones, S. 1981. *High-risk newborn infants*. 2nd ed. St. Louis: C. V. Mosby.

Oehler, J. 1981. *Family-centered neonatal nursing care*. Philadelphia: J. B. Lippincott.

REFERENCES

Affonso, D., and Harris, T. 1980. Postterm pregnancy: Implications for mother and infant, challenge for the nurse. *J. Obstet. Gynecol. Neonatal Nurs.* 9(3):139–145.

Avery, G. 1981. *Neonatology: Pathophysiology and management of the newborn*. 2nd ed. Philadelphia: J. B. Lippincott.

Babson, S.; Benson, R.; Pernoll, M.; and Benda, G. 1975. *Management of high-risk pregnancy and intensive care of the neonate*. St. Louis: C. V. Mosby.

Barden, T. P. 1983. Obstetric management of prematurity, part 2. In *Behrman's neonatal–perinatal medicine: Diseases of the fetus and infant*, 3rd ed., eds. A. Fanaroff and R. Martin. St. Louis: C. V. Mosby.

Berhman, R. 1983. The field of neonatal-perinatal medicine. In *Behrman's neonatal–perinatal medicine: Diseases of the fetus and infant*, 3rd ed., eds. A. Fanaroff and R. Martin. St. Louis: C. V. Mosby.

Brann, A., and Schwartz, J. 1983. Central nervous system disturbances. In *Behrman's neonatal–perinatal medicine: Diseases of the fetus and infant*, 3rd ed., eds. A. Fanaroff and R. Martin. St. Louis: C. V. Mosby.

Dubowitz, L. M. S.; Dubowitz, V.; and Goldberg, C. 1970. Clinical assessment of gestational age in the newborn infant. *J. Pediatrics.* 77(1):1–10.

Haddock, B.; Vincent, P.; and Merrow, D. 1986. Axillary and rectal temperatures of full-term infants: Are they different? *Neonatal Network.* 5(1):33–39.

High, P. C., and Gorski, P. A. 1983. Womb for improvement: Recording environmental influences on infant development in the intensive care nursery. In *Environmental neonataology*, eds. A. W. Gottfried and J. F. Gaiter. Baltimore: University Park Press.

Hittner, H. M., et al. 1981. Retrolental fibroplasia: Efficacy of vitamin E in a double-bind chemical study of preterm infants. *New Engl. J. Med.* 305(23):1365–1371.

Kuller, J.; Lund, C.; and Tobin, K. 1983. Improved skin care for premature infants. *MCN.* 8(3):200–203.

Lubchenco, L. O.; Hansman, C.; Dressler, M.; and Bay, A. E. 1963. Intrauterine growth as estimated from liveborn birthweight data at 24 to 42 weeks of gestation. *Pediatrics.* 32:793–800.

Lund, C.; Kuller, J.; Tobin, C.; Lefrak, L.; and Franck, L. 1986. Evaluation of a pectin-based barrier under tape to protect neonatal skin. *J. Obstet. Gynecol. Neonatal Nurs.* 15(1):39–44.

Malin, S., and Baumgart, S. 1987. Optimal thermal management for low birth weight infants nursed under high-powered radiant warmers. *Pediatrics.* 79(1):47–54.

March of Dimes. Clinical Education Aids. The National Foundation—March of Dimes. White Plains, NY 1976.

Stephens, S., and Sexton, P. 1987. Neonatal axillary temperatures: Increases in readings over time. *Neonatal Network.* 5(6):25–29.

33

Resuscitation of the High-risk Newborn

BEHAVIORAL OBJECTIVES

Upon completion of this chapter, the reader should be able to:

- List at least four physiologic characteristics of the newborn that make resuscitation different from adults.

- Describe three prepartum, intrapartum, and postpartum conditions or situations that would alert caregivers to the potential for newborn problems.

- List the equipment necessary for newborn resuscitation.

- Demonstrate how to assess a newborn rapidly to determine the need for rescue or resuscitation.

- Describe four situations in the first 48 hours of life that require rescue interventions.

- Recite the ABCs of newborn resuscitation and explain each step.

- Demonstrate bag and mask ventilation, tactile stimulation, and cardiac compressions on a resuscibaby.

- Describe the correct positioning for a newborn being intubated.

- List the preferred venipuncture sites in the newborn.

- List three drugs used in newborn resuscitation, their doses, dilutions, and routes of administration.

At no other time in the newborn period is the nurse's need for rapid assessment, thoughtful planning, appropriate intervention, and thorough evaluation more critical. Nurses in the newborn area are expected to be skilled observers, alert to an impending disastrous situation. Once a problem situation is identified, the nurse must have the knowledge base to plan appropriate care, the ability to assign and delegate tasks, and the skill to treat and protect the tiny patient. Newborn infant nurses will complete the nursing process by evaluating the situation for future interventions. Evaluation of this emergency can reveal problem areas that need refinement.

The literal definition of resuscitation is the reestablishment of heart and lung function after cardiac arrest or sudden death. In adults, there are few instances where resuscitative interventions are required before full cardiac arrest has been experienced. Newborn infants are quite different. They are often found blue, apneic, and flaccid, with a heart rate over 40. We commonly call the interventions on these infants resuscitation, yet there has not been a cardiac arrest. The more correct terminology would be rescue, where the focus is preventing cardiac arrest by facilitating ventilatory and cardiac support.

This chapter describes a systematic approach to newborn resuscitation. The words rescue and resuscitation will be used interchangeably. Identification of prepartum, intrapartum, and postpartum conditions which predispose the newborn to complications will be covered. This will aid the nurse in anticipation of high-risk situations. Resuscitative techniques, including bag and mask ventilation, endotracheal intubation, cardiac compressions, venous access, and drug therapy are also included.

In-depth pathophysiology of perinatal depression and asphyxia are not covered in this chapter. Citations in the reference section are recommended for any nurse who will need more information and spend a great deal of time in the newborn area.

PHYSIOLOGIC DIFFERENCES OF THE NEWBORN

The newborn is not a miniature adult. There are characteristics of the newborn that require special consideration. These unique characteristics make rescue interventions quite different from adult resuscitations.

1. Newborns generally are born with healthy hearts. Unless there is a congenital cardiac anomaly, the cardiac muscle itself is quite healthy and resilient. This is why most newborn arrests are respiratory and not cardiac.
2. Newborns have a larger surface area to body size ratio than adults. This allows more area for heat and insensible water loss. During an emergency situation, it is easy to forget this principle and expose the baby to undue cold stress and fluid loss. Preventing heat loss will be a major consideration during infant resuscitation because cold stress increases oxygen consumption and leads to acidosis (Behrman, 1983).
3. Newborns and small infants have a large head size to body size ratio. The head, unlike other areas of the body, has no insulating fat layer. Most newborns have little or no hair to prevent heat loss through the scalp. Stocking caps (see Fig. 19–6) and head coverings can be used to help insulate the head and prevent heat loss.
4. Even in full-term newborns, most organ systems are not fully developed. It is important to keep this generalization in mind when providing therapy to the newborn to prevent possible complications, e.g. immaturity of the hepatic and renal system complicates drug therapy by prolonging excretion and metabolism of certain drugs. Immaturity of the immune system prevents the newborn from mounting a full-blown immune response to infection and, therefore, sepsis can be overwhelming before being detected.
5. Newborn infants are preferential nose breathers. The primary airway of a newborn is nasopharyngeal rather than oral. Occlusion of the nares can lead to apnea.
6. Newborns are small, helpless, and at our mercy. It is easy to become too aggressive and even rough with the newborn, inflicting unintentional injuries.

IDENTIFYING INFANTS AT RISK

Anticipating and preparing for an emergency situation helps the participants feel calm and in control. Advanced preparation saves critical seconds and thereby increases the chance for a successful outcome. During pregnancy, delivery, and shortly after birth there are many markers that alert us to the possibility that a newborn may require rescue or resuscitative intervention. By learning these markers and how to recognize them, nurses can anticipate problem situations and be prepared when they occur.

Prepartum (Maternal)

During pregnancy certain conditions predispose the maternal/fetal unit to physiologic and metabolic stressors which may interfere with a smooth transition to extrauterine life. These conditions include:

- maternal age greater than 35 years or younger than 15 years;
- maternal diabetes;
- maternal hemorrhage or anemia;
- maternal drug or substance use;
- lack of prenatal care;
- poly- or oligohydramnios;
- maternal cardiovascular disease;
- prolonged rupture of membranes;
- uterine abnormalities;
- Rh or type incompatibility;
- multiple gestation;
- maternal hypertension;
- previous pregnancy complication;
- previous fetal loss or neonatal death (Avery, 1987).

Most institutions have policies and guidelines which require the presence of pediatric personnel at the delivery of such a high-risk mother. Whether it is mandatory or not, the nurse must be prepared for the possibility of an adverse outcome.

Intrapartum

During labor and delivery certain factors can alert the health care team that the newborn is experiencing difficulty and may require rescue or resuscitative intervention at delivery. These conditions include:

- abnormal fetal presentations;
- intrauterine growth retardation;
- maternal infection;
- prolonged or difficult labor;
- prolonged rupture of membranes;
- prolapse of the umbilical cord;
- maternal sedation;
- cesarean section;
- fetal heart rate abnormalities;
- intrapartum bleeding (Avery, 1987).

As with the prepartum conditions, the health care team should recognize that when these conditions are present, the newborn may have difficulty adapting to extrauterine life. Awareness helps the nurse to prepare for the high-risk delivery.

Postpartum

Shortly after birth the newborn may exhibit signs that indicate an underlying problem. The transitional nursery concept is based on the understanding that major physiologic transitions to extrauterine life are nearly completed by 4-6 hours of age and that most newborn problems can be identified by then (Britton and Britton, 1984). In most institutions newborns are kept under close scrutiny during this time period and released to rooming-in or regular nursery after a successful transitional period. During this observational period the nurse may note several conditions in the newborn which alert her to developing problems. These conditions place the newborn in a high-risk category and would once again allow the nurse to make preparations in anticipation of needed rescue or resuscitative intervention. These conditions include:

- meconium staining;
- seizure activity;
- failure to maintain a normal body temperature;
- cardiac arrhythmias;
- prematurity;
- postmaturity;
- respiratory difficulty/apnea;
- anomalies of the upper airway;
- failure to tolerate feedings;
- extreme color changes;
- neurological depression (Avery, 1987).

PREPARATION FOR RESUSCITATIVE INTERVENTIONS

Preparation for resuscitation begins long before high-risk patient identification. Each institution should conduct periodic equipment checks and annual recertification of personnel. Institutions should have policies that delineate how and when these checks and recertifications are performed.

Personnel recertification can be accomplished by staging a mock code with the equipment that will actually be used in an emergency situation. Nursing staff must be proficient at bag and mask ventilation and familiar with the supplies, drugs, and equipment necessary for newborn life support.

Equipment such as radiant warmers, laryngoscopes, and newborn resuscitation bags must be checked on a daily basis to ensure proper function. These checks should be documented in a permanent hospital record.

When a high-risk situation is identified or anticipated, the nurse should assemble the equipment necessary for emergency intervention, turn on heat lamps or the radiant warmer, heat towels and blankets, notify the necessary personnel, review drug dosages and routes of administration, and go through the resuscitation equipment stocking list (see Table 33-1) to be sure that everything is available, within easy reach, and ready to go. Remember, preparation and organization help participants in an emergency situation to feel calm and in control.

CRITERIA FOR RESUSCITATION

Deciding when intervention is necessary and when it is not is complex in the newborn because of their unique characteristics. Nursing assessment and skills must be rapid and accurate if interventions are to be successful. There are two categories of newborns who require intervention: newborns in the delivery room at birth, and newborns in the nursery after birth. The Apgar scoring system and its use in newborn resuscitation is covered in Chapter 19. Table 33-2 presents resuscitative interventions for each Apgar score and can be used as a quick reference.

Newborns with Apgar scores of 8 and 9 are in good condition and require only removal of oral secretions, drying, and warming. Newborns with Apgar scores of 5, 6, and 7 are mildly depressed and require minimal interventions which include drying, suctioning, stimulation, and blow by oxygen. Newborns with Apgar scores of 3 and 4 have moderate depression and require more aggressive therapy which includes bag and mask ventilation. Newborns with very low scores of 0-2 have severe perinatal depression and require full-blown resuscitative efforts, including endotracheal intubation and cardiac drugs.

The assignment of Apgar scores is best done by the person attending to the newborn. Whether this person be a nurse anesthetist, an anesthesiologist,

---

TABLE 33-1. Neonatal Resuscitation Equipment Stocking List

Light source
Heat source
Dry, warm, soft blankets
Treatment bed/table with removable sides
Clock with second hand or timer
Wall suction
Oxygen: compressed (0-15 liters flow)
Air: compressed (0-15 liters flow)

Stethoscope
0.5 liter anesthesia bag with flow adjustment valve and manometer
0.5 liter self-inflating resuscitation bag with 100% O_2 adaptor
1 premature size face mask
1 newborn size face mask
Size 0 oral airway
Size 1 oral airway
Laryngoscope with Miller 0 and 1 curved and straight blades
Suction catheters (2 each of 5 fr, 8 fr, and 10 fr)
Sterile H_2O for suction
Sterile NS ampules for suction lubrication
Bulb syringe
Cord clamp and sterile scissors

Extra batteries and bulbs for laryngoscope
Non-cuffed endotracheal tubes (2 each of 2.5, 3.0, 3.5, 4.0) with vocal cord marker
2 stylets
Liquid skin barrier
Adhesive tape 1" and 0.5"
Alcohol swabs
Betadine swabs
1-cc, 3-cc, 10-cc, and 20-cc syringes
25-g and 18-g needles
16-g intracath (over-the-needle intravascular catheter)
3-way stopcock

Epinephrine
Normal saline i.v. solution
Ringer's lactate
5% albumin
Sodium bicarbonate
Naloxone hydrochloride

TABLE 33-2. Resuscitation by Apgar Score

Appearance or color	Completely pink or acrocyanosis Score 1–2	Cyanosis Score 0–1	Cyanosis or pale Score 0–1	Pale Score 0
Pulse or heart rate	100–160 Score 2	Over 100 Score 2	100–40 Score 1	0–40 or absent Score 0–1
Grimace or reflex response	Minimal grimace cough or sneeze Score 1–2	Minimal grimace or no response Score 0–1	No response Score 0	No response Score 0
Muscle tone or activity	Well flexed, resists extension of extremity Score 2	Some flexion or some spontaneous activity Score 1–2	Some flexion or limp Score 0–1	Minimal tone or limp Score 0–1
Respirations or respiratory effort	Strong cry, rhythmic breathing Score 2	Weak cry or periodic breathing Score 1	Gasping or absent Score 0–1	Gasping or absent Score 0–1
Apgar score Management	8–9 1. Keep dry and warm 2. Clear airway if needed	5–7 1. Keep dry and warm 2. Clear airway 3. Tactile stimulation 4. Blow by oxygen with 100% FIO_2	3–4 1. Keep dry and warm 2. Clear airway 3. Begin assisted bag and mask ventilation with 100% FIO_2	0–2 1. Keep dry and warm 2. Clear airway 3. Endotracheal intubation 4. Assisted ventilation with 100% FIO_2 5. Epinephrine if 0 HR – increase ventilation after 15 sec

a delivery room nurse, or a doctor is irrelevant. The important thing is that the person who is caring for and observing the newborn makes the assignment.

The 1-min Apgar indicates the newborn's status *in utero* immediately prior to delivery. The 5-min score reflects the newborn's adaptation to extrauterine life and response to resuscitation efforts. The major transitions to extrauterine life which must occur include the establishment of rhythmic breathing patterns, opening the pulmonary circulation, clearing fetal lung fluid, and closing of the fetal shunts (foramen ovale and ductus arteriosus). These physiologic changes generally take place within the first few minutes of life. Factors which aid these transitions include cold and tactile stimulation, changes in the blood gases after the umbilical cord is clamped, vaginal squeeze that occurs at birth, lung expansion, blood flow, and pressure changes in the heart and lungs. If asphyxia is present at the time of birth, hypoxia and hypercarbia can depress the central nervous system and decrease respiratory efforts. This leads to acidosis which keeps the pulmonary vascular resistance high. High resistance in the blood vessels of the lungs can decrease the blood flow. If breathing is delayed and the blood flow in the lungs is reduced, there may be a delay in closure of the foramen ovale and ductus arteriosus, as well as the ductus venosus. If these fetal shunts remain patent, right to left shunting will occur with mixing of venous and arterial blood. This chain of events must be broken as quickly as possible if the newborn is to be prevented from sustaining long-term injuries from birth asphyxia or perinatal depression (Behrman, 1983). *Resuscitative interventions are never delayed until the 1-min Apgar score is assigned in a newborn who obviously requires intervention right from the moment of birth.*

Situations that occur in the newborn nursery which may lead to rescue or resuscitative interventions include apneic episodes, choking or aspiration, seizures, and cardiac arrest.

In the well-baby nursery, and postpartum unit for rooming-in patients, there should be a well-stocked resuscitation cart accessible to all patients. Personnel in these areas should maintain certification in newborn resuscitation. The emergency equipment should be checked on a daily basis and documented just as the equipment in the delivery room is checked and maintained.

RESUSCITATION TECHNIQUES

The basic steps in resuscitation are the same regardless of whether the resuscitation occurs in the delivery room or in the nursery. If rescue interventions are to be successful, all members of the health care team must be skilled at CPR, have an organized approach, and be careful, experienced observers.

The basic objectives for newborn resuscitation include:

1. Expanding the lungs to provide adequate ventilation. The chest should move with each breath given and good breath sounds should be heard bilaterally with a respiratory rate of at least 40 per min.
2. Assuring adequate cardiac output with the heart rate above 120 per min. There should be a palpable radial pulse and adequate peripheral perfusion with brisk capillary filling.
3. Correcting or preventing acidosis by adequately ventilating the newborn so that the PCO_2 is below 50 mm Hg.
4. Avoiding hyperthermia or hypothermia. Cold stress causes acidosis which decreases circulation and increases oxygen consumption. Hyperthermia can lead to apnea and increased oxygen consumption. The newborn should be maintained in a neutral thermal environment during resuscitation (Klaus and Fanaroff, 1986).

All resuscitative interventions, whether in the delivery room or in the nursery, should be done using the same approach. To make it easy to remember when time is short and clear thinking is imperative, this approach is called the ABCs of neonatal resuscitation. Each letter stands for a particular action or observation. For the purpose of literary clarity and to facilitate learning, the steps are outlined in a sequential fashion. Rescue interventions and assessments are usually instituted simultaneously. Remember too, that if the patient's condition fails to improve, the intervention may be ineffective because the operator or the equipment is faulty. Continual reassessment of previous steps must be ongoing throughout the process.

ABCs OF NEONATAL RESUSCITATION

A. Assessment/Airway/Agitation

Assessment is always the first step in rescue or resuscitation. The newborn should be observed briefly for color, tone, and activity. Then vital signs, including heart rate, respiratory rate and effort, and capillary refill should be taken rapidly. (Capillary refill is assessed by blanching the blood from an area of the skin with the index finger for approximately 3 sec. At the end of 3 sec, remove the finger and watch for blood to flush back into the area. Capillary refill should be less than 2 sec.) Next, check the airway for patency. Clear the nasopharyngeal and oral airway of secretions. Assess the airway for proper alignment (see Fig. 33–1); hyperflexion and hyperextension of the neck can compromise the airway. Agitate or stimulate the newborn by rubbing the back briskly to induce crying and thereby respiratory effort. When these interventions fail to bring on spontaneous, rhythmic respirations and good color, move on to step B.

B. Breathing

Ventilate the newborn. Apply a resuscitation bag and mask. To assure adequate ventilation, use

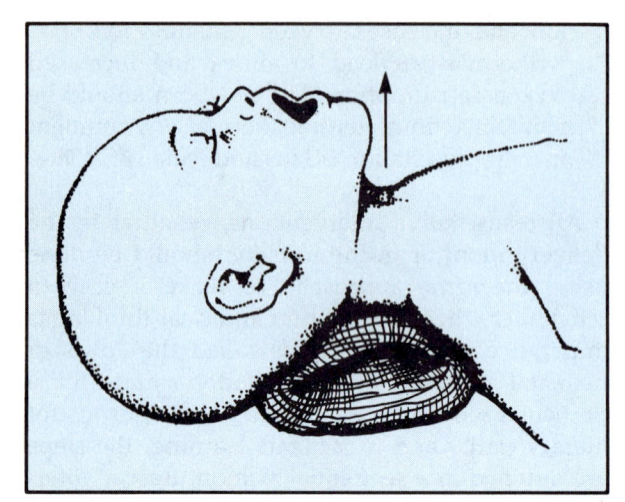

FIGURE 33–1. Appropriate sniff position for intubation. Note that the neck is not hyperextended; the roll provides stabilizing support. This demonstrates proper alignment.
SOURCE: Fletcher and MacDonald (1983).

enough pressure to raise the chest slightly (see Fig. 33–2). Unless otherwise indicated, begin with 100% oxygen. Give approximately 60 breaths/min (bpm) for 1 min to blow off CO_2 that has accumulated and then continue at 40 BPM. If efforts are successful, the newborn's color should improve within the first minute. When the newborn begins to breathe on his own, stop bagging and continue mask continuous positive airway pressure (CPAP) until the newborn's color and tone are good and his/her capillary refill is adequate. When the mask is removed from the newborn's face, watch closely for color change in room air. If bag and mask ventilation with 100% oxygen and a clear airway fail to provide adequate ventilation, i.e. raising the chest and improving the skin color, then endotracheal intubation must be performed to assure patency of the airway. Endotracheal intubation should be performed by a skilled professional with the proper size endotracheal tube (see Fig. 33–3) for the newborn being resuscitated. Intubation is performed according to Fig. 33–5. If bag and tube ventilation fail to improve the newborn's status and the heart rate remains low, move on to the next step.

C. Cardiac/Circulation

If the newborn's heart rate falls below 60, or if the heart rate is below 80 and not improving, cardiac compressions should be instituted (American Medical Association, 1986). Cardiac compressions are performed according to Fig. 33–4. An assistant should check the newborn's peripheral pulse (femoral, carotid, brachial, or radial) and capillary refill to assess the effectiveness of compressions. The

Guidelines for Endotracheal Tube Size

Tube Size, mm (Inside Diameter)	Infant Weight, g	Suction Catheter Size
2.5	<1,000	5 F
3.0	1,000-2,000	6 F
3.5	2,000-3,000	8 F
4.0	>3,000	8 F

SOURCE: AMA Standards for CPR and ECC, 1986.

FIGURE 33–3. Guidelines for endotracheal tube size.
SOURCE: American Medical Association (1986).

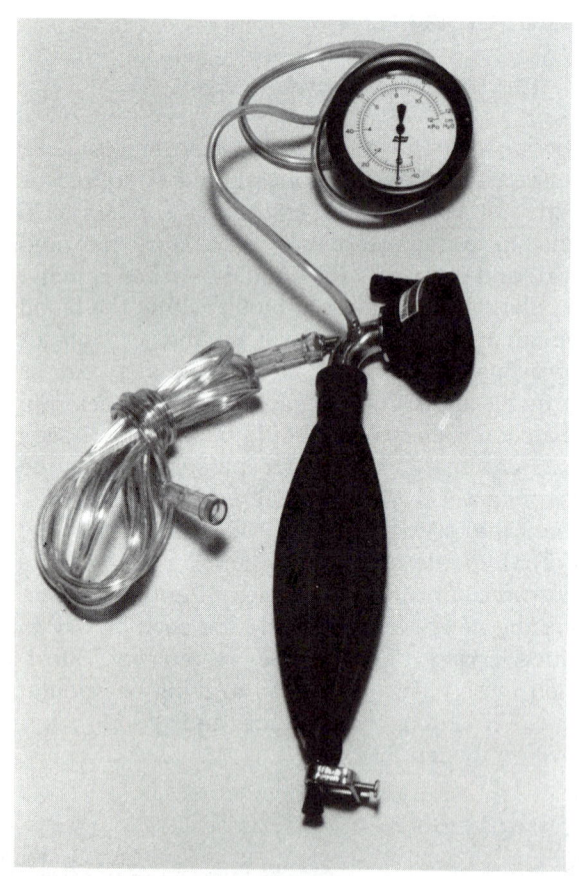

FIGURE 33–2. Resuscitation bag and mask setup with manometer.

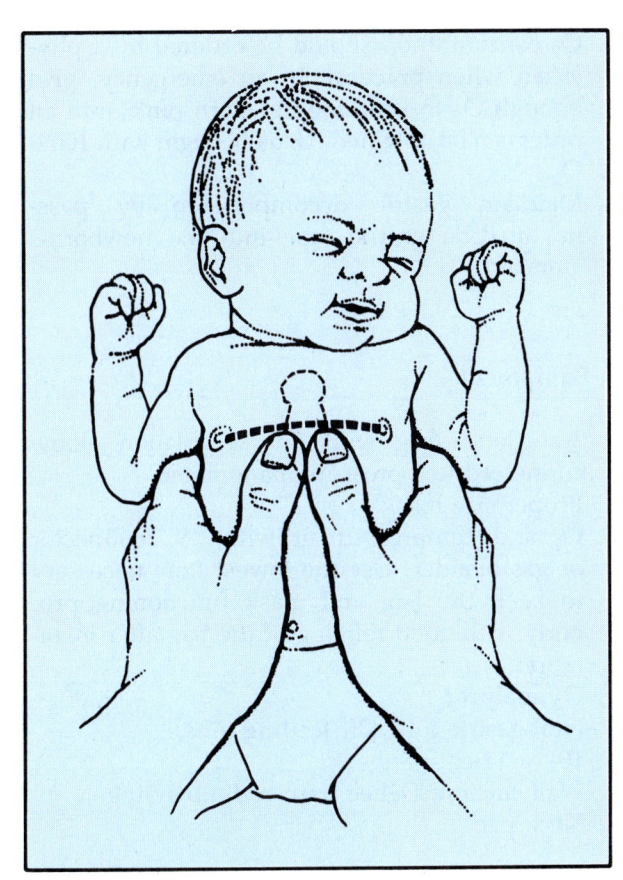

FIGURE 33-4. Hand position for cardiac compressions in a newborn.
SOURCE: American Medical Association (1986).

goal of cardiac compression is to circulate the newborn's blood. Newborns with poor or no circulation look pale rather than cyanotic. Cyanosis infers that the newborn's blood is being circulated but not oxygenated. Cardiac compressions are performed at approximately 120 per min or 2 per sec. Cardiac compressions will always be accompanied by ventilation. Coordination of ventilation and compressions in the tiny newborn should be attempted but may be difficult because of the high rates. Compression should be interrupted periodically to assess the newborn's spontaneous heart rate. Compression should be discontinued when the newborn's own heart rate is above 80.

The majority of newborn resuscitations will end at this point. Drug therapy in newborn resuscitation is rarely necessary, but if the previous interventions fail to revive the infant, move to step D.

D. Drugs

Epinephrine is the first pharmacologic agent to be considered in infant resuscitation. When this medication is prescribed, the route may be IV or via the endotracheal tube. Studies have shown that the use of endotracheal epinephrine during resuscitation is an accepted mode of therapy (Lindemann, 1982). Newborn strength epinephrine (1:10,000) should be drawn up in a 1-cc syringe. The dose is .1–.3 ml/kg per dose. Epinephrine is an endogenous catecholamine which enhances the oxygen delivery to the cardiac muscle, improves contractility of the heart, and stimulates spontaneous contractions, thereby increasing the heart rate (American Medical Association, 1986). If the newborn does not have an IV, one should be started. Venous access can be achieved as demonstrated in Fig. 33–11.

At this point in the resuscitation, it is important to recall the newborn's history. The history will help the rescue team decide what the next drug should be. Two other drugs that could be used at this point are volume expanders (if hypovolemia is suspected) and naloxone hydrochloride (if depression is thought to be a result of maternal narcotics). It should be kept in mind that naloxone can induce withdrawal in the newborn whose mother abuses narcotics and should be used with caution in these situations. Naloxone can be given intravenously, via the endotracheal tube, or if perfusion is adequate, IM or sub-Q. Volume expanders must be given intravenously (American Medical Association, 1986).

Sodium bicarbonate therapy may be useful in prolonged resuscitations. It is given for correction of documented metabolic acidosis. It should be kept in mind that if adequate ventilation is not provided, bicarbonate will not correct the newborn's pH (American Medical Association, 1986). In rare cases of newborn cardiac failure, drugs such as isoproterenol, calcium, and atropine may be requested by the resuscitating physician. Drug cards can be prepared and kept on the resuscitation cart.

E. Environment

Throughout the resuscitative process, it is important to remember the helplessness of the patient. The environment should be controlled for humidity and temperature, to assure that the newborn does not undergo unnecessary metabolic stress secondary to hypothermia or hyperthermia. The principles of heat loss and methods of maintaining a neutral thermal environment are outlined in Chapter 19 and should be reviewed at this time.

Two other environmental hazards secondary to resuscitation are sharp objects (needles, lancets, etc.) that may have been inadvertently left in the newborn's bed, and bruises or abrasions that result from undue roughness during rescue interventions. As always, the nurse must provide a safe environment for the patient and should be alert to the development of these problems and prevent them.

Newborn resuscitation is a process which contains many steps. However, all steps will not be necessary in all cases. When the newborn exhibits normal color, tone, heart rate, and respiratory effort, interventions should be stopped and the newborn kept under close scrutiny. The resuscitation outline (Fig. 33–5) depicts a cascade of resuscitative events. This outline may be used with simulated case presentations as an exercise for reviewing and practicing resuscitation.

Once newborn stabilization has been achieved, the caregivers should begin the evaluation process by recording the events in the patient's chart. A careful review can reveal where education and preparation is needed to prevent delays or problems with future resuscitations.

The health care team can now assess the newborn to determine what underlying problems exist that may have precipitated the failure.

PROCEDURES NEEDED IN NEONATAL RESUSCITATION

Bag and Mask Ventilation

Purpose

To initiate or maintain adequate ventilation by opening alveoli and keeping them open.

Guidelines

1. Ventilation may be initiated by a physician, nurse, or adequately trained person with documentation under the direction of a licensed professional.
2. Continuous positive airway pressure (CPAP) should be set at 4–6 cm H_2O pressure unless otherwise indicated by a physician.
3. O_2 concentration should be ordered by a physician when practical. In an emergency, give enough O_2 to keep the newborn pink until an order can be obtained. Usually begin with 100% O_2.
4. Maintain gastric decompression by passing an oral gastric tube into the newborn's stomach.

Equipment

1. Anesthesia bag with flow regulation elbow connected to a pressure manometer.
2. Proper size mask.
3. O_2 and compressed air with "Y" connector or gas blender. Use the lowest flow necessary to keep the bag and mask functioning properly with good refilling of the bag after inspiration.
4. O_2 analyzer.
5. Oral gastric tube (8fr feeding tube).
6. 10- or 12-cc syringe.
7. Wall suction, DeLee trap, or Bulb syringe.
8. Neck pad.

Procedure

1. Adjust the gas flow to obtain the desired O_2 concentration. Check for correct functioning of the equipment. Set the CPAP to the desired pressure by holding a hand over the mask and adjusting the flow regulation valve.
2. Position the newborn on a neck pad in the sniffing position, chin up and neck extended (see Fig. 33–1).
3. Pass the oral gastric tube into the newborn's stomach and decompress with the syringe.
4. Suction any secretions from the mouth and nose.
5. Place the mask over the nose and mouth snugly. Adjust the flow regulation valve to obtain a CPAP of 4 cm of H_2O pressure.
6. Place manometer in clear view.
7. Squeeze the bag to give only as much pressure as is necessary to adequately raise the newborn's chest (usually less than 35 cm H_2O pressure). Allow equal time for inspiration and expiration unless otherwise indicated.
8. Continue bagging and/or CPAP according to physician's order, or until the newborn is breathing rhythmically on his/her own.

Resuscitation Outline

1. **Quick assessment**

2. **Suction upper airway with bulb, DeLee or wall suction.**

3. **Dry or stimulate and keep warm by maintaining neutral thermal range.**

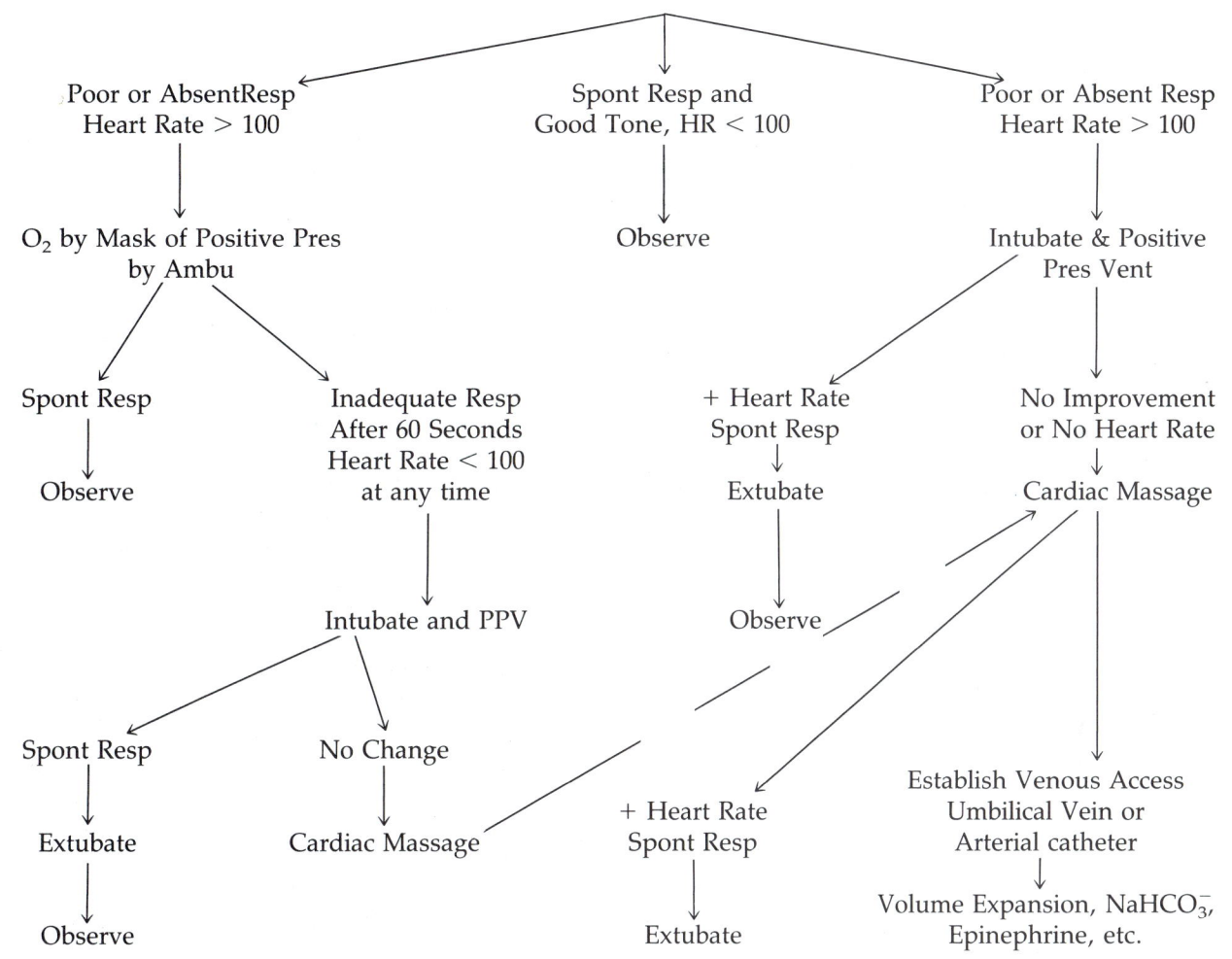

```
            Poor or Absent Resp          Spont Resp and           Poor or Absent Resp
              Heart Rate > 100          Good Tone, HR < 100         Heart Rate > 100
                    │                         │                            │
                    ▼                         ▼                            ▼
          O₂ by Mask of Positive Pres       Observe             Intubate & Positive
                 by Ambu                                             Pres Vent
                  │                                                     │
          ┌───────┴────────┐                                   ┌────────┴─────────┐
          ▼                ▼                                   ▼                  ▼
      Spont Resp    Inadequate Resp                        + Heart Rate      No Improvement
          │         After 60 Seconds                       Spont Resp        or No Heart Rate
          ▼         Heart Rate < 100                            │                  │
       Observe         at any time                          Extubate         Cardiac Massage
                           │
                           ▼
                   Intubate and PPV                          Observe
                    │           │
              ┌─────┴──┐        ▼
              ▼        ▼     Cardiac Massage
          Spont Resp  No Change
              │        │                        + Heart Rate      Establish Venous Access
              ▼        ▼                        Spont Resp        Umbilical Vein or
          Extubate  Cardiac Massage                  │            Arterial catheter
              │                                      ▼                  │
              ▼                                  Extubate                ▼
           Observe                                             Volume Expansion, NaHCO₃⁻,
                                                                    Epinephrine, etc.
```

FIGURE 33–5. Resuscitation outline.
SOURCE: Adapted from Schreiner, R. L., Neonatology for the Pediatrician Medical Education Resources Program, Indiana University School of Medicine, 1978, p. 187.

Endotracheal Intubation

Purpose
To establish or maintain a direct airway; to deliver prescribed amounts of O_2 at prescribed pressures, via anesthesia bag or ventilator; and to perform pulmonary toilet, or to obtain tracheal culture.

Guidelines

1. A physician, nurse practitioner, nurse anesthetist, or registered nurse with special training and documentation should perform the procedure.

2. The newborn should be on a cardiorespiratory

monitor before the procedure begins, or an assistant can continuously monitor the heart rate by stethescope. If bradycardia develops, stop and ventilate with bag and mask until the heart rate recovers. If available, a pulse oximeter may be used to assess the newborn's O_2 saturation during the procedure. Endotracheal tube placement should be confirmed by a radiograph as soon as possible after the procedure is completed.

Equipment

1. Anesthesia bag, appropriate size mask, and manometer.
2. Oxygen and air source with adjustable flow.
3. Sterile laryngoscope with Miller 0 and 1 blades.
4. Endotracheal tubes, sizes 2.5, 3.0, 3.5, and 4.0.
5. Sterile wire stylette.
6. Sterile saline.
7. Sterile suction catheters, 5fr and 8fr.
8. Sterile water, 4-oz bottles for rinsing suction tubing.
9. Wall suction set on low (80 cm H_2O).
10. Ventilator and respiratory therapist (if required).
11. Liquid skin barrier.
12. 0.5" adhesive tape.
13. Scissors.
14. Heat source.
15. Light source.
16. Diaper pad for head support.
17. Stethoscope.
18. Sterile gloves.
19. Surgical mask.

Procedure

1. Check the laryngoscope to assure proper function. The light should be continuous and bright.
2. Determine the proper tube insertion depth from the "lip to tip" measurement chart. Record this length in the patient's record (see Fig. 33–6).
3. An assistant should hold the newborn on a flat surface with the head and shoulders slightly elevated in the "sniffing" position (see Fig. 33–1).
4. An anesthesia bag with 100% O_2 should be within easy reach, preset, and flowing.

GROSS ESTIMATE OF ET TUBE INSERTION DEPTH

ET Tube Length "Lip to Tip" Chart

Weight	Length (cm)
1000 g	7
2000 g	8
3000 g	9

FIGURE 33–6. Estimate of the distance from the newborn's lip to the tip of the endotracheal tube.
SOURCE: Tochen (1979).

5. Wall suction should be turned on with a suction catheter attached. The bottle of sterile water should be open and ready to be used for rinsing the catheter.
6. Suction the mouth and oral pharynx to remove all secretions. This will improve visualization.
7. The laryngoscope is held in the left hand with the thumb and first two fingers. Open the newborn's mouth with the index finger of the right hand and insert the blade between the gums. Raise and move the tongue to the right so that the epiglottis is in clear view. Lift up the epiglottis with the laryngoscope to expose the vocal cords (see Fig. 33–7).
8. Gentle pressure over the external larynx with the little finger of the left hand will aid visualization of the glottis.
9. Introduce the endotracheal tube with the right hand from the right side of the mouth. Do not put the tube down the visualization tunnel of the laryngoscope blade. Visualize the vocal cords and advance the endotracheal tube through the cords to the black vocal cord line on the ET tube.
10. After the endotracheal tube is inserted and held gently but firmly in place, the laryngoscope is carefully withdrawn.
11. The assistant should check for equal breath sounds with a stethoscope and for adequate ventilation of the lungs while bagging.
12. Hold the endotracheal tube firmly against the gum to prevent extubation while stabilization is achieved with tape.

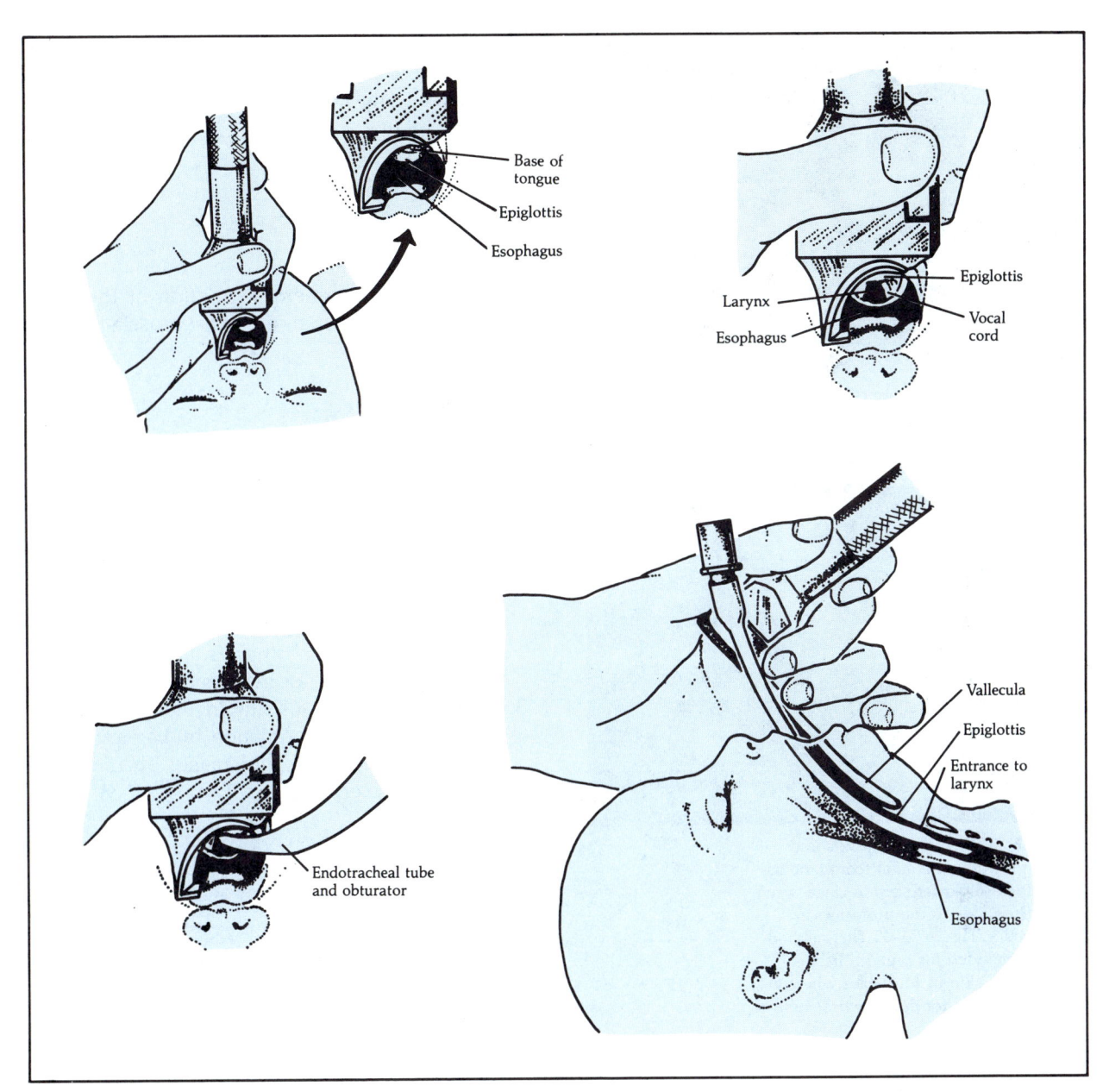

FIGURE 33–7. Endotracheal intubation.
SOURCE: Klaus and Fanaroff (1979).

13. Tape the tube securely using one of the following techniques:
    a. Paint the upper lip and cheeks with tincture of benzoin or a liquid skin barrier and allow to dry until "sticky" to touch (see Fig. 33–8). With 0.5" adhesive tape, tape the endotracheal tube to the upper lip (see Fig. 33–9). Beginning at the tube, wrap the tape clockwise twice around the tube, and then anchor the tape on the maxilla and cheek (see Fig. 33–10). Use a second piece of tape and repeat the process counterclockwise, ending on the opposite cheek.
14. Continue to bag the newborn at the prescribed settings until mechanical ventilation is available or ventilation is no longer needed.
15. Recheck the lung fields for equal, bilateral breath sounds with a stethoscope.
16. Assist with x-ray (AP and lateral) to assure proper tube position.

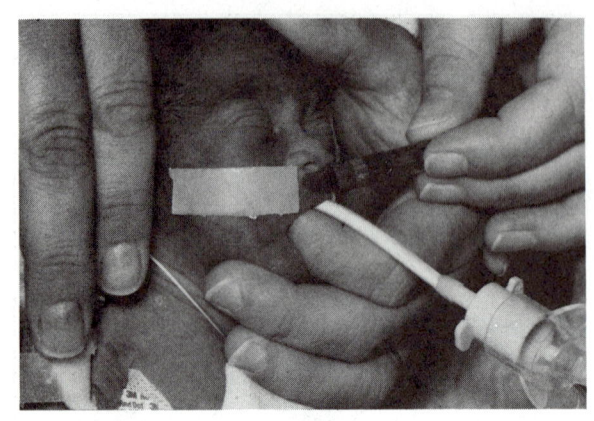

FIGURE 33-8. Tincture of benzoin applied to upper lip and cheeks.

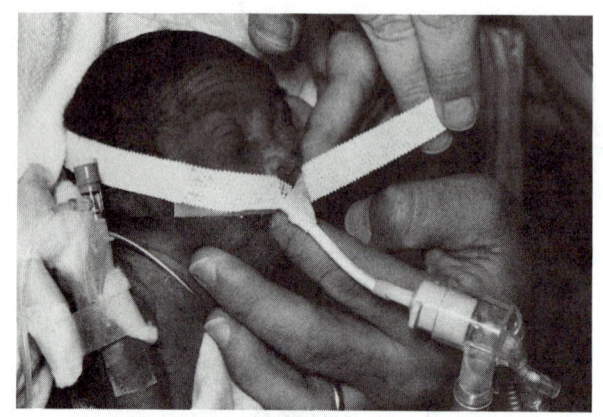

FIGURE 33-9. Apply maxilla and cheek protectors made of foam tape or a pectin-base barrier strip to clean, dry skin. Then tape to the protectors as described in Figure 33-7. This method is recommended for preterm babies with fragile skin or for babies where a prolonged need for endotracheal tube is thought likely.

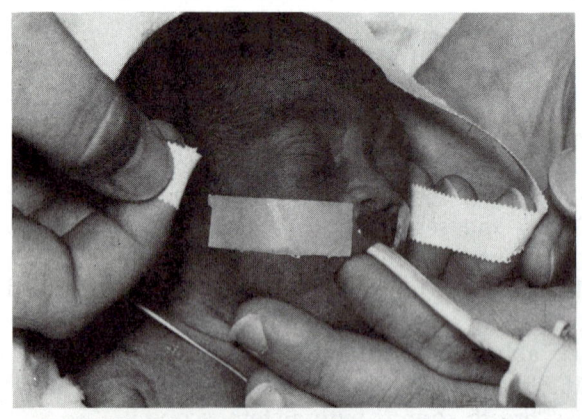

FIGURE 33-10. Wrap tape around endotracheal tube and then anchor on maxilla and cheek.

17. Record the procedure in the nurse's notes. Include the tube size and gum line marker as well as any complications noted during the placement.

Cardiac Compressions

Purpose

To establish or augment circulation of the blood through the body when the heart muscle fails as a pump.

Guidelines

1. Any individual with training can initiate or assist with closed chest cardiac compressions.
2. Initiate compressions if the newborn's heart rate is 60 bpm or less, and if the heart rate is 80 or less and not recovering. If the newborn has brief episodes of bradycardia and recovers to over 100 bpm by other interventions, then compressions are not indicated.
3. Cardiac compressions should always be done in conjunction with ventilation by bag and endotracheal tube or bag and mask. The newborn should be receiving 100% O_2.

Equipment

1. Heat source.
2. Firm surface padded with a dry blanket or towel.
3. Cardiorespiratory monitor.
4. Stethoscope.

Procedure

1. Assess or validate the newborn's heart rate by auscultation over the apex of the heart with the stethoscope.
2. Place both thumbs over the newborn's sternum, either side-by-side or one on top of the other. The palms and fingers should encircle the rib cage supporting the back as shown in Figure 33-4.
3. The thumbs should be in line with or just below the nipples to avoid compression of the xiphoid end of the sternum. If the compressions are done too low the newborn's liver or gut could be damaged.

4. Push the sternum down with the thumbs 1–2 cm.
5. Compress smoothly, rhythmically, and evenly. Allow equal time for release and compression.
6. Compress 120 times per minute or twice per second.
7. An assistant should palpate for a femoral, brachial, radial, or carotid pulse during compressions and if possible the newborn should be attached to a cardiac monitor.
8. Stop compressions for 5 seconds every 5 minutes to assess the newborn's spontaneous heart rate.
9. Discontinue compressions when the newborn's spontaneous heart rate is over 80 bpm.
10. Record the events and interventions in the patient's record.

Peripheral Venous Access

Purpose

To establish and maintain a route for the delivery of fluids and medications to a compromised newborn.

Guidelines

1. All newborn IV's should be administered via volumetric infusion pump.
2. Intravenous fluids, tubing, filters, and stopcocks should be replaced every 24 hours, or as indicated by hospital policy.
3. Newborns receiving IV fluids should have accurate intake and output measurements.
4. Heelstick glucose determination should be assessed once every 8 hours or as ordered to rule out hyper- or hypoglycemia while on IV fluids.
5. The IV site should be inspected hourly or more frequently during medication administration.
6. Peripheral IV's that appear infiltrated should be evaluated by another professional and removed.
7. Preferred areas for peripheral venous access in the newborn (see Fig. 33–11) are the scalp veins, veins on the dorsum of the hands and feet, and the superficial veins of forearms (Bean et al., 1978).

Equipment

1. Heat and light source.
2. IV pump, solution ordered, tubing, and filter.
3. Arm board, tape, cotton balls, rubber band.
4. Syringe with sterile flush solution.
5. Preferred needles, i.e. 23 g butterfly, 25 g butterfy, 24 g intercath with T-connector.
6. Razor (if hair removal will be necessary).
7. Alcohol wipes and scissors.

Procedure

1. Set up the infusion pump, purge the tubing, clear the filter, and set the desired infusion rate and volume on the pump.
2. Utilize a heat source to maintain the newborn in

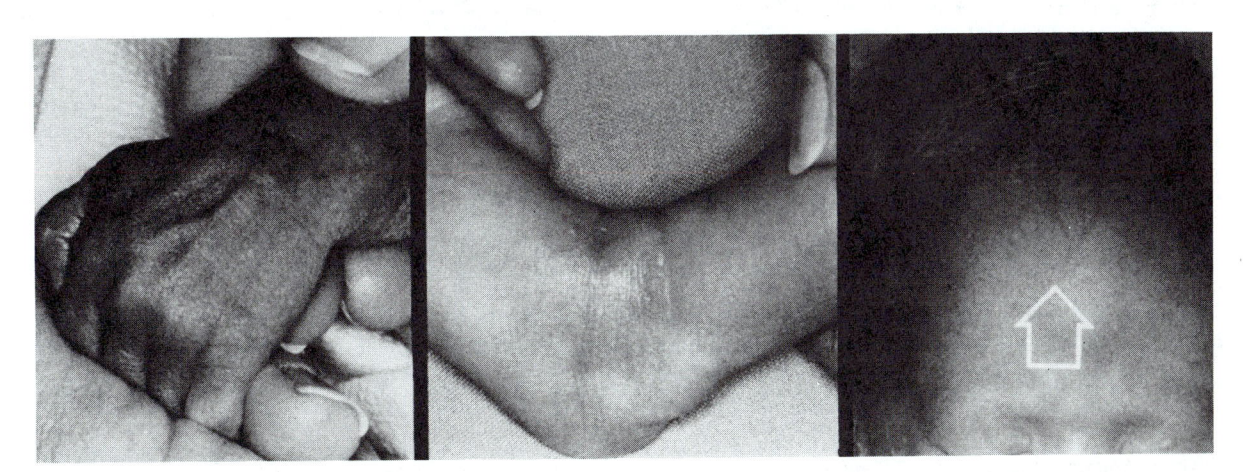

FIGURE 33–11. Preferred IV sites in the neonate.
SOURCE: Bean et al. (1978).

a neutral thermal environment to minimize stress during the procedure.
3. If a scalp vein is used, visualize the vessel to be used by:
   a. parting the hair to expose the vein (use liquid skin barrier to secure the hair in place);
   b. shaving a small area of scalp with a disposable razor (save hair for parents).
      If an extremity is used, secure the extremity to a padded board with tape.
4. Wipe the skin at the IV site with alcohol.
5. Apply pressure above the vein with a rubber band tourniquet or finger.
6. Insert the needle and tape securely to prevent accidental dislodgement. Use cotton to pad and support the needle or extremity as needed.
7. Confirm patency by infusing a small amount of flush solution.
8. Connect the needle tubing to the IV tubing and infuse the solution ordered at the prescribed rate.
9. Record the procedure in the nursing record. Include the size of needle used and the amount and type of flush solution administered.

SUMMARY

Newborn infants have unique physical and physiologic characteristics that make their resuscitative interventions different than adult codes. Most newborn arrests are respiratory rather than cardiac. Newborns have a large surface area to body size ratio and a large head size to body size ratio which makes heat and water loss a major consideration. Newborns have immature organ systems which demand special consideration when choosing therapy and implementing treatments. The newborn's primary airway is nasopharyngeal. Newborns are small, helpless, and lack purposeful movements, and can easily be injured if interventions are too aggressive or rough. Newborn resuscitation can be performed skillfully and calmly if advanced preparations are made. Prepartum, intrapartum, and postpartum conditions can alert us to fetal compromise and the potential need for rescue or resuscitative interventions after birth. Nurses working in the labor and delivery and newborn areas should check and maintain newborn resuscitation equipment and recertify all

TABLE 33-3. *Infant Resuscitation Drugs*

Drug	Strength or dilution	Dose	Route	Frequency	Action
Epinephrine	1:10,000	0.1–0.3 ml/kg 0.01–0.03 mg/kg	i.v. or endotracheal tube	5 min	Stimulates the heart and vasoconstricts
Naloxone hydrochloride	0.02 mg/ml	0.01 mg/kg	i.v., i.m., sub-q, or endotracheal tube	2–3 min	Narcotic antagonist
O-neg. blood (cross matched to mother), normal saline, Ringer's lactate, 5% albumin		10 ml/kg	i.v.	Give over 5–10 min	Volume expansion for hypovolemic shock
Sodium bicarbonate	4.2% 0.5 meq/ml	1–2 meq/kg	i.v.	Give over 5–15 (do not exceed 1 meq/kg per min)	To correct documented metabolic acidosis in prolonged resuscitation

SOURCES: American Medical Association (1986) and American Academy of Pediatrics (1988).

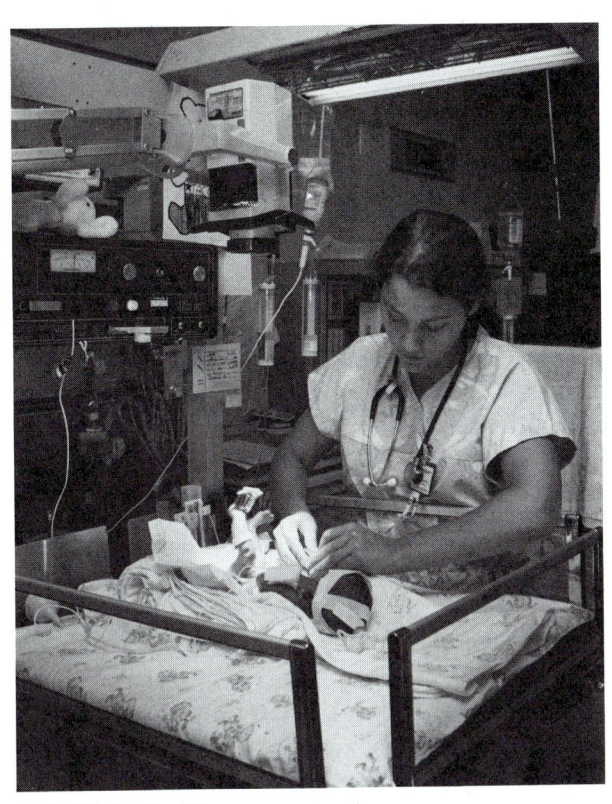

FIGURE 33–12. The nurse caring for the high-risk infant.

personnel to assure competence and success. The Apgar score can be used as criteria for intervention in the delivery room. Skilled observation and vital sign assessment are used as criteria for intervention in the nursery. Resuscitation may follow an ABC approach for ease in recalling steps to take, but is a process when many steps are frequently performed simultaneously. Drugs are infrequently needed in newborn resuscitation but must be readily accessible if requested (see Table 33–3). Hyperthermia and hypothermia place great metabolic stress on the newborn and can be prevented with advanced preparation and environmental control. The nurse as a member of the resuscitation team must create and maintain a safe and therapeutic environment for the tiny patient. Nurses performing or assisting with newborn emergency procedures should be familiar with the equipment needed and steps to follow to assure rapid and successful rescues.

Newborns are resilient and adaptable and most newborn resuscitations are successful. The nurse is a very important member of the health care delivery team and functions in a greatly expanded role in the newborn area (see Fig. 33–12).

REFERENCES

American Academy of Pediatrics, Committee on Drugs. 1988. Emergency drug doses for infants and children. *Pediatrics* 81:3.

American Medical Association. 1986. Standards for CPR and ECC Part IV: Neonatal advanced life support. *JAMA* 255(21):2969–2973.

Avery, G. B., ed. 1987. *Neonatology, pathophysiology and management of the newborn*, 3rd ed. Philadelphia: J. B. Lippincott.

Bean, H.; Harris, T.; and Cornett, J. 1978. *Starting IVs in neonates*. Slide/tape presentation. University of Arizona Biomedical Communications, Tucson, Arizona.

Behrman, R., ed. 1983. *Neonatal–perinatal medicine: Diseases of the fetus and infant*, 3rd ed. St. Louis: C. V. Mosby.

Britton, H. L., and Britton, J. R. 1984. Efficacy of early newborn discharge in a middle-class population. *Am. J. Dis. Children.* 138:1041–1046.

Fletcher, M., and MacDonald, M., ed. 1983. *Atlas of procedures in neonatology*. Philadelphia: J. B. Lippincott.

Graf, H.; Leach, W.; and Arieff, A. I. 1985. Evidence of a detrimental effect of bicarbonate therapy on lactic acidosis. *Science.* 222:756–754.

Klaus, M., and Fanaroff, A. 1979. *Care of the high-risk neonate*, 3rd ed. Philadelphia: W. B. Saunders.

Lindemann, T. 1982. Endotracheal administration of epinephrine during cardiopulmonary resuscitation. *Am. J. Dis. Children.* 136:753–754.

Tochen, M. 1979. Orotracheal intubation in the newborn infant: A method for determining depth of tube insertion. *J. Pediatrics.* 95:6.

34

Maternal and Neonatal Transport

BEHAVIORAL OBJECTIVES

Upon completion of this chapter, the reader should be able to:

- Define neonatal transport.

- Define maternal transport.

- Describe the rationale for developing perinatal transport.

- List the most common clinical indications for perinatal transport.

- List the factors that determine the mode of transport.

- Outline a quality assurance program that monitors the effectiveness of the transport service.

- Describe an overview of the transport process delineating responsibilities of the referral hospital and the perinatal center.

- Outline stabilization procedures for the neonatal and maternal patient by the referral hospital and by the transport team.

- Identify the advantages of return transports.

CONCEPT OF TRANSPORT

In the 1960s, groups of obstetricians and pediatricians in England, Canada, and the United States began to make headway into improving care for high-risk and low-birthweight infants. Special units were identified for neonatal intensive care in an increasing number of hospitals. These units spawned a specialty team of pediatricians and nurses who were trained in the unique needs of the high-risk infant.

The next phase in this evolution of care was to develop a program that ensured availability of such specialty care to all perinatal patients. The National Committee on Perinatal Health, with financial and administrative assistance from the National Foundation–March of Dimes, was formed in 1972. This committee established guidelines for perinatal care that recognized three main goals: quality of care to all pregnant women and newborns, maximal utilization of highly trained perinatal personnel and intensive care facilities, and assurance of reasonable cost effectiveness (Committee on Perinatal Health, 1976).

To accomplish these goals, regions (geographically defined population groups) were identified, and hospitals within each region were categorized according to the complexity of obstetrical and neonatal care provided by each. The three categories were:

1. Level I refers to a hospital which provides primary maternity and neonatal care. Any complicated pregnancy or neonatal course should initiate a transfer of the patient to a hospital that specializes in the provision of more complex care. Level I hospitals should have the necessary equipment and personnel to perform resuscitation and initial stabilization measures prior to the patient's transfer.
2. Level II describes a hospital that provides a moderately complex level of care. This institution needs to transfer those patients who require a highly technical and intensive level of care.
3. Level III describes a tertiary care center where the highest level of technological care is provided. Various subspecialties are represented at such centers to ensure a comprehensive program of care for the mother and/or infant.

The overall goal of regionalization was to reduce perinatal morbidity and mortality. This would be accomplished by providing a well-defined integration of clinical expertise, limited duplication of services, controlled costs, a system of communication, equal accessibility to intensified perinatal care for high-risk pregnancies, a system of transport for high-risk mothers and infants, consultation services, education programs for health professionals and the general public, and a follow-up program to monitor the high-risk infant during the first year of life.

For this system to work, the communication and coordination among the three levels of hospitals needed to be prioritized. Health professionals had to assume the responsibility of recognizing when a pregnant woman needed more intensive care and then referring them to the appropriate hospital (center). The responsibility of providing access to critical care services is usually assumed by the regional tertiary care center. This is done through a highly specialized team of personnel – the transport team. It is their role in the provision of perinatal care that will be reviewed in this chapter.

THE TRANSPORT SYSTEM

Neonatal Transport

The transport of the sick newborn to the tertiary care center was a necessary consequence of regionalization. Such a system is based on the premise that the specialized care at the regional center will lower infant mortality and improve outcome. Traditionally, this system is represented by the "two-way" transport. The tertiary center sends a team of highly trained staff members to the referral hospital to stabilize the infant. The goal is to bring the services of the neonatal intensive care unit to the referral hospital and to provide this level of service throughout the transport process.

Some regions have elected to implement the "one-way" transport. The referral hospital stabilizes the infant and then transports the infant to a Level II or Level III hospital. This type of system has shown to be effective in certain situations (Sumners et al., 1980). The success of such a system depends on the effective triaging of patients to appropriate Level II and Level III hospitals and the ability of the referral center to provide care for the infant *en route*. Careful monitoring of this system by the regional center is necessary to ensure that optimal health care is afforded all infants in a timely manner.

The two-way transport remains the most widely utilized system at present. It is this type of system that will be addressed.

The regional center demonstrates its commitment to offering highly specialized care to all infants by providing a transport program that mobilizes a team in an efficient manner and sends them to the referral hospital to stabilize and transport the infant to the neonatal intensive care unit. While it is understood that the success of a transport is based on the initial care given by the referral hospital, the transport team brings a high level of expertise that builds on the initial stabilization efforts and improves the infant's outcome.

This type of care has become a subspecialty over the years as smaller infants are born and survive, as more knowledge of the disease process is learned in these fragile patients, and as equipment that can be adapted to the transport environment becomes available. Transport is not without its own unique challenges. It relies heavily on:

1. The ability of the referral hospital to identify the infant at risk and provide effective transitional care.
2. The ability to mobilize the team in a reasonable amount of time.
3. The training and experience of the team members who must demonstrate a high level of care in an unfamiliar environment with somewhat limited resources.
4. The dependability of battery-powered equipment that is continually exposed to vibration and abuse as it travels countless miles in aircraft and ground vehicles.
5. The communication between referral hospital staff and perinatal center staff, between air and ground ambulance operators, and among team members.
6. The ability of the transport personnel to pull together effectively as a team, utilizing each team member to his or her maximum so that the necessary care can be provided effectively and efficiently.

Indications for Transport

The following conditions are general indications for neonatal transport:

1. Low birthweight (below 1500 g) or preterm (less than 34 weeks).
2. A need for respiratory assistance.
3. A need for continuous physician attendance or a high degree of nursing care (e.g. apnea and bradycardia, temperature instability, feeding problems).
4. A need for surgery, especially when intensive postoperative care will be required.
5. Suspected cardiac disorder.
6. Seizure disorders.
7. Persistent fetal circulation.
8. Asphyxia.

Indications for transport will range from subtle signs of sepsis (e.g. temperature instability and occasional apnea) to life-threatening surgical emergencies (diaphragmatic hernia). Complimentary to the availability of transport is the easy access to consultation. Calls from referral hospital personnel are diverted to the neonatologist and, based on the information given on the infant's status, a decision is then made on the need to transport.

Maternal Transport

The correlation between the development of neonatal intensive care units and transport systems and the subsequent reduction in neonatal morbidity and mortality has been well documented in the literature (Feldman and Sauve, 1976; Meyer, Harris, and Daily, 1973; Pettett et al., 1975; Swyer, 1970). As this evidence became more widely known, some centers began to take this approach of increased accessibility of specialized perinatal care one step further. If a reduction in neonatal morbidity and mortality could be seen when an infant is transported to the tertiary care center within the first several hours of life, would the mortality rate be further reduced if the high-risk infant was born at the tertiary care center?

It has always been generally accepted that the best transport vehicle is the mother's uterus. Transporting the mother and fetus provides this optimal vehicle and allows for specialized care of the infant immediately at the time of birth. This can be a notable factor in neonatal outcome, because insults suffered in the first few hours of life before a transport team arrives can exact a heavy toll on the infant's developmental sequelae.

With this factor in mind, centers developed high-risk maternal transport systems to compliment already well-established newborn transport and intensive care systems. This broadened the scope of patients to whom neonatal intensive care was offered and resulted in an even further reduced neonatal morbidity and mortality in various regions (Anderson et al., 1981; Cordero, Backes, and Zuspan, 1982; Harris, Isaman, and Giles, 1978; Miller, Densberger, and Krogman, 1983).

Several options are available through such a

comprehensive program. A telephone consultation may be all that is necessary. It may be beneficial to transport the mother with her own physician or with a team from the perinatal center. The mother's condition may be such that the consultant may travel to the referral hospital to assist with the delivery. If the labor is too far advanced or other reasons outweigh the benefits of a maternal transport, the neonatal transport team may be sent prior to the delivery to assist with initial stabilization efforts and facilitate an early transport to the tertiary care center.

Indications for Transport

The following conditions are indications for a maternal transport:

1. Care immediately available to the patient is not adequate to manage the anticipated obstetrical, medical, or surgical complications.
2. The patient needs to be monitored and attended by personnel who are skilled in managing a suspected or confirmed condition, and such personnel are not available at the referral hospital.
3. It is anticipated that the infant will require access to a neonatal intensive care unit.
4. The initial referral hospital is a long distance away from the perinatal center and possible maternal–fetal complications are suspected.
5. There is premature rupture of membranes (less than 36 weeks gestation or fetal weight estimated at less than 2000 g).
6. There is premature labor (less than 36 weeks gestation or with fetal weight estimated at less than 2000 g).
7. There is presence of any condition that may result in a premature delivery:
   a. preeclampsia;
   b. multiple gestation;
   c. metabolic disorders (e.g. diabetes);
   d. intrauterine growth retardation;
   e. signs of fetal distress (e.g. abnormal estriol values, positive oxytocin challenge test, meconium-stained amniotic fluid, etc.);
   f. third trimester bleeding;
   g. Rh sensitization;
   h. premature dilatation of the cervix.
8. There are maternal infections which may result in premature delivery.
9. There is severe organic heart disease.
10. Renal disease is present.
11. There is evidence of drug abuse.
12. Trauma requiring surgical interventions beyond the capabilities of the referral hospital is present.
13. There are nonobstetrical acute surgical emergencies.
14. There are antenatally diagnosed fetal conditions that will require immediate access to neonatal intensive care (Committee on Practice of the Nurses Association of the American College of Obstetricians and Gynecologists, 1983).

The decision on whether to initiate a maternal transport is dependent on the reliability of information given by the referral hospital. The accurate assessment of the mother's condition will allow the referral hospital and the perinatal center to make the best decision concerning transport options.

Organization

Transport programs were a natural evolution of regionalization. Each program is designed to bring the skills of the intensive care unit to the referral hospital as represented in a specially trained team of health professionals. The number of team members may vary in programs depending upon the resources and philosophy of the perinatal center. A growing trend is for transport services to be a separate department instead of being a part of the respective intensive care unit. The system is usually managed by both a medical director and a transport coordinator (usually a registered nurse). While the medical director develops policies regarding the medical care of transport, the transport coordinator manages the day-to-day activities of the system. This person will be responsible for the development and implementation of transport protocols, a quality assurance program, training of personnel, monitoring of equipment reliability and repairs, and establishment of adequate documentation standards. A transport system requires a multidisciplined approach to the delivery of care, so the transport coordinator usually liasons with several department representatives as well as with outside ambulance carriers. The coordinator's role is quite simply to keep everyone working together to provide a team that will render a highly skilled service to any hospital within a defined region, and to provide reliable and effective equipment to allow for the delivery of critical care medicine from the time the team arrives at the referral hospital until the time the team arrives back at the tertiary care center.

Depending upon the size of the transport program, other organizational components may include a dispatch center, a business manager, a data analyst, and assistant management personnel. The challenge is to establish a program that provides the desired level of care and, at the same time, be financially solvent.

One other component that is integral to the organization is outreach education. Regionalization defines certain responsibilities for all three levels of hospitals. It is the responsibility of the regional center (perinatal center) to provide education to the community hospitals that will facilitate the early recognition of a high-risk perinatal patient, the timely referral when a transport is needed, and the delivery of adequate stabilization procedures prior to team arrival.

Communication

Dispatch Center

These types of centers may either be representative of the hospital or the region. A hospital that has a multiservice transport department may have a dispatch center that handles all initial referral calls and diverts them accordingly. This may include linking the call with the appropriate consultant, verifying bed availability, and mobilizing team members and ambulance carriers. There may be one dispatch center for a large geographical location that includes several regions. This center will be regularly updated on bed availability at the tertiary care centers. When a referral call comes in, the dispatch center can then refer that call to the closest regional center.

Such a dispatch center may also be a source of data collection. In northern California, one perinatal dispatch center performs this service for five regions. Based on data that is sent to the center by all of the transport systems, reports are generated quarterly that reflect referral patterns, clinical management at the referral hospital, and clinical management by the transport team.

In the absence of a dispatch center, the provision of one phone number, often a toll-free number, must be provided that allows the referral hospital a direct link with the tertiary center staff. This phone number must be well publicized so that the referral hospital does not waste precious time searching for this information when a consultative call is needed.

Two-way communication is often possible between the transport team and the tertiary center when the team is in the ground or air ambulance. This allows for immediate consultative accessibility, accurate updates on the patient's condition, and more reliable reports on estimated times of arrival.

Referral Patterns

The main objective of a regional dispatch center is to increase the number of transports to the nearest appropriate facility. By doing so, regionalization is promoted, relationships between the community hospitals and the tertiary care center are established, and more direct referral patterns are the result. One main component in the establishment of strong referral patterns is the effective communication between the tertiary center and the community hospital. Referring physicians must be assured of consultative accessibility at any hour of the day. They must also receive timely follow-up on the transported patient's condition from the consultant. Nursing staff at the referral hospital also rely on periodic updates of the transported patient's condition. There is a strong identity with the patient by the referring staff who participated in the initial stabilization process. Getting periodic reports from the tertiary center on the patient's progress recognizes the referral staff's contribution to the health care plan. Since recovering infants are often transported back to the referral hospital before final discharge, these updates prepare the staff for the specialized needs of the infant, thus promoting continuity of care.

The establishment of strong referral patterns allows for the observance of regionalization as it was intended. Referral hospitals and the regional center become familiar with each other's capabilities. Educational needs of the referral hospital can be easily identified and provided by the tertiary center. The bond between the two in the provision of the best care possible to the community becomes the basis for standards of practice in perinatal medicine.

The Team

In the best situation, early identification of the high-risk mother, followed by appropriate consultation and possible transfer to a regional perinatal center, will result in the efficient provision of optimal care to both mother and infant. When such a transfer cannot occur, the transport of the ill newborn to the neonatal intensive care unit becomes necessary. Both of these situations require the provision of a highly specialized type of care.

Several studies have shown that the provision of specially trained teams to accommodate such transfers can reduce maternal and neonatal morbidity and mortality rates (Anderson et al., 1981; Harris, Isaman, and Giles, 1978; Hood et al., 1983; Thompson, 1980).

The composition of these teams will vary and is based on the philosophy and resources of a particular institution. The team is usually led by either a physician or a nurse who has been trained in an expanded role. Other possible team members are respiratory therapists, paramedics, and emergency medical technicians. Whatever the composition, the team must be able to demonstrate collectively the skills and knowledge necessary to provide the level of care that is indicated by the clinical needs of the patient.

Delineation of roles is essential if the team is to function effectively. The medical director of the unit from which the transport is initiated is ultimately responsible for ensuring that team members have received appropriate clinical training and for the medical care of the patient during the transport. The team leader may either be a physician or a nurse. This role coordinates the medical plan provided by the team. Studies have shown that nurse-supervised and physician-supervised transports can result in the same quality of care (Cook and Kattwinkel, 1983; Reedy et al., 1984).

Team members must meet specific requirements for clinical experience as designated by the hospital. In addition to clinical skills, they must demonstrate an evolution of leadership abilities, consistent organization and prioritization of care, ability to deal with the stress of emergency situations in the clinical setting, and the ability to communicate effectively with the health care team and with the patient's family. A transport team member must be willing to accept the challenge of the unpredictable situation. What can happen in the field cannot always be anticipated. Team members learn to rely on each other to such an extent that they feel confident in the team's ability to handle any situation that might occur. Since some transport centers cover areas that are in rugged terrain and must recognize the possibility of being stranded due to ambulance failure, survival training may be incorporated into the educational requirements.

Availability of team members is an essential component of transport. A team must be available 24 hours a day. In those centers where a substantial number of transports are done, the need for team availability is often met by having a crew of team members whose only role is to fulfill the transport needs of the institution. Having a "dedicated team" requires an on-call system. Other centers will pull transport personnel directly from the unit where they are in a staff assignment. Whichever method is used, the goal is to provide team mobilization that is conducive to the emergency status of the situation.

Training programs will vary depending on role expectations. All personnel must be adequately prepared for their transport responsibilities through orientation to the transport system by means of an initial didactic course and ongoing continuing education classes.

The initial training program must be approved by the medical director responsible for patient transport and must provide team members with sufficient information to facilitate effective transport of the perinatal patient. Annual evaluations and recertification of team members are often incorporated into programs to ensure the competency of personnel.

In addition to topics on medical management, team members should also be trained in the management of aeromedical emergencies. They need to know how the aeromedical environment will affect their patient and how it may affect team members.

Because of the type of activity demanded of the transport team, it is necessary to provide adequate insurance coverage for each member. While every effort is made to ensure the safety of the team and the patient, the mere nature of transporting a patient via ground ambulance, fixed-wing aircraft, or helicopter, puts the team members at increased risk during the course of performing their duties. Many hospitals have accident and life insurance policies specific to transport personnel.

Equipment

The type of equipment that is provided by a transport center will depend on the type of patients transported. In a two-way transport system, the perinatal center provides transport equipment that makes intensive care possible for the patient during the entire transport process.

Overall, transport equipment should be designated for the sole purpose of the team's use. It needs to be routinely tested and maintained so that it is always available for an emergency call. It is designed with the realities of the transport environment in mind. Equipment needs to be portable, lightweight, and easy to troubleshoot. It must be adequately shielded so that it does not interfere with navigational instruments in the aircraft or with radios in the ground or air ambulance. It must have the capability of being secured or tied-down in any ambulance vehicle. It should have the ability to function on its own battery source for a period of 2 hours. Both the aircraft and the ground ambulance should provide a power source with a heavy-duty, high-quality inverter that is tested regularly. In the most ideal of circumstances, the power source in the transport equipment should only be needed for short periods, since equiment is usually run off the wall current at the referral hospital and via the inverter in the ground or air ambulance. Reality is such, however, that if an inverter does not function during the course of the transport, the battery capability of the equipment itself must be relied on to provide the power source for the remainder of the journey. Transport equipment must be able to endure the frequent abuse of vibration and exposure to the environment.

A gurney with appropraite restraints and safety belt is provided for a maternal transport. The neonate requires an incubator or isolette that has been specifically designed for and tested in the transport environment (see Fig. 34–1). This isolette should be a completely self-contained unit that provides clear visibility of the patient, has adequate internal lighting, is easy to clean and service, and provides the necessary heat to keep the infant warm despite the weather to which it is exposed. The incubator should be able to maintain a temperature of 38.4°C if needed (Harris and Belcher, 1982).

Other features of the transport isolette give it highly technical capabilities. A ventilator that has proven itself reliable in the transport environment, is compact and lightweight, and is battery-powered, is attached to the isolette. Before such instruments were available, teams had to hand-bag infants enroute back to the tertiary center. The ventilator allows for the continuous and accurate provision of positive pressure ventilation during the transport course.

Monitors accompanying the patient must be capable of measuring heart rate, respirations, blood pressure, and temperature. They are usually mounted on the isolette where they are easy to view.

Air and oxygen is routinely taken on transport and the capability of blending air and oxygen to provide a precise oxygen concentration for at least 1 hour is a basic necessity. A good rule is to always have twice as much oxygen and air as is anticipated. Most medical air and ground ambulances provide oxygen and air sources as alternative sources. Portable suction machines should be available, either built into the isolette itself or carried as a separate unit. Infusion pumps must be small, lightweight, and battery-powered. Certain pumps presently available have a battery-life of up to 5 days if fully charged and can deliver a volume as low as 0.1 cc/hour. The pump must be able to provide a programmed volume that is not affected by altitude, movement of the patient, aircraft or ground ambulance, or intravascular pressure.

Transcutaneous oxygen monitors have become available in the past few years for transport. They are small in size and can easily be mounted on a transport isolette. This equipment has proven useful on transport by allowing the continuous observance of an infant's response to the respiratory management. Even when an infant's paO$_2$ is within an acceptable physiologic range, episodes of hypoxia and hyperoxia may occur in response to environmental stimuli. The use of a transcutaneous monitor during the transport allows for needed changes in respiratory therapy while en route back to the neonatal intensive care unit (Miller et al., 1980; Clarke et al., 1980). Since hyperoxia, even for periods as short as 30 min, has been associated with retrolental fibroplasia and also as a contributing factor in the development of bronchopulmonary dysplasia, avoidance of such an occurrence is a primary goal of the transport team (Clarke et al., 1980). Some transport programs are using pulse oximetry in lieu of transcutaneous oxygen monitors. While the goal is the same for the use of this equipment, its reliability in

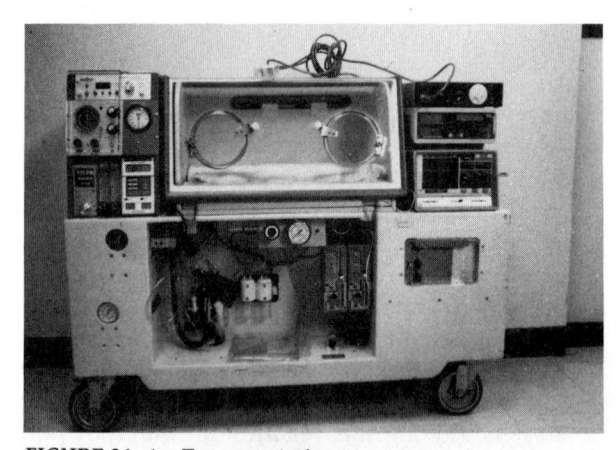

FIGURE 34–1. Transport isolette.

the transport environment needs to be documented.

Equipment/Supplies: Maternal Transport

If screening is done appropriately, supplies are limited in maternal transport compared with neonatal transport. This is not the case, however, if it cannot be assured that delivery will not occur *en route*. If the latter is the case, supplies for the transfer of both mother and infant must be provided.

Basic equipment for maternal transports provide for emergency resuscitation, the delivery of oxygen, suction, intravenous therapy, medications, pelvic examinations, and monitoring vital signs of the mother and fetus. A list of the equipment and supplies used by one maternal–fetal transport service is illustrated in Table 34–1.

Equipment/Supplies: Neonatal Transport

The supplies needed are often extensive because the infant is critically ill and requires immediate intensive care. The capability of the transport isolette has been discussed. The isolette pictured in Fig. 34–1 provides heat by means of convective and conductive sources. A fan circulates the heat that is generated in two heater plates beneath the mattress. In addition, the top heater plate warms the thermal gel mattress. Due to its chemical composition, the mattress is able to passively retain its warm temperature during the transport. The respiratory equipment on the left side of the isolette can provide ventilatory assistance either in the form of continuous positive airway pressure (CPAP) or intermittent positive pressure ventilation (IPPV) along with a blend of oxygen and air. Oxygen and air tanks are nestled within the bottom of the unit. The battery pack is also secured within the frame that is constructed of a strong but

TABLE 34–1. Maternal Transport Equipment List

Medications		Syringes, plastic:	
Pitocin 10 U/L ml	4 ampules	3 ml	4
Methergine 0.2 mg/1 ml	2 ampules	6 ml	4
Ephedrine sulfate 0.05 g	2 ampules	12 ml	2
Epinephrine 1 ml, 1:1000	2 ampules	20 ml	2
Sodium luminal 2 gr/1 ml	2 ampules	60 ml	2
Sodium amytal 250 mg	2 ampules	Tubex syringes	2
Apresoline 20 mg/1 ml	2 ampules	Needles 18G, 20G, 22G	4
Diazepam 10 mg	2 syringes	Alcohol sponges	10
Sodium bicarbonate 50 mEq	4 syringes	Adhesive tapes 0.5", 1", 2"	1
Magnesium sulfate 50%, 5 g/10 ml	4 syringes	Bandaids	6
Magnesium sulfate 10%, 2 g/20 ml	4 ampules	Doptone stethoscope	1
Calcium gluconate 10 ml	2 ampules	Ultrasound gel	1
Compazine 10 mg/2 ml	2 ampules	B/P cuff with stethoscope	1
Benedryl 50 mg/1 ml	2 tubexes	Reflex hammer	1
Naloxone (Narcan) 0.4 mg/1 ml	2 ampules	Padded tongue blade	2
Xylocaine 1%	1 vial (20 ml)	Rubber airway	2
Dramamine 50 mg	6 tablets	Ambu bag, adult size	1
Aromatic ammonia	2 vaporoles	Grocery bags with plastic liner	2
Sterile H_2O for injection 10 ml	2 ampules	Chix wipes (box)	1
		Sterile gloves, pairs	
Equipment and supplies		size $6\frac{1}{2}$	2
IV solutions and tubing			
Dextrose 5% lactated ringers	500 ml	size $7\frac{1}{2}$	2
Dextrose 5% water	500 ml	Sterile gloves, singles	
Plasma	250 ml	size small	4
IV tubing – Y type blood	1	size medium	4
IV tubing – standard	1	Redtop Vacutainer tubes	2
		Purpletop Vacutainer tubes	1
Miscellaneous supplies		Money, dimes (for telephone)	40c
Angiocaths 18G, 16G, 14G	3	Penlight flashlight	1
Tourniquet, elastic	2	Pen	1
		Forms and paper supplies	2

SOURCE: Giles (1979).

lightweight combination of styrofoam and fiberglass. Intravenous therapy is provided by three syringe-pumps, all small and lightweight and programmed to deliver as little as 0.1 cc/hour. Suction is provided in two capacities, one for oral or endotracheal tube suctioning and one for chest tube suctioning. Vital sign monitoring is viewed on the screen on the right side of the unit. It provides the capability to monitor heart rate, respirations, blood pressure, isolette ambient temperature, and infant temperature. A transcutaneous oxygen monitor is mounted on top of the cardiorespiratory monitor and provides a continuous readout of paO_2 and $paCO_2$ values. A pulse oximeter is secured on top of this monitor and gives arterial oxygen saturation values. Overall, the isolette provides the same capabilities as a neonatal intensive care unit. The main difference is that this mobile intensive care must subject itself to the unpredictable variables of the moving environment.

Supplies are carried in two customized bags (see Fig. 34–2) and provide for emergency resuscitation, and the delivery of oxygen, suction, intravenous therapy, medications, diagnostic and monitoring procedures, and specific treatment procedures. A list of the equipment and supplies used by one neonatal transport service is illustrated in Table 34–2.

Administrative Aspects

Quality Assurance Program

Quality is an elusive and difficult concept to measure. In order for quality to be put into measurable terms, the philosophy of the system which is being evaluated must be clear. The purpose of the quality assurance program is for a transport program to provide a mechanism for continual evaluation of that system's operation. The goal of such an evaluation is to ensure the provision of effective critical care to the patient requiring transport and to help define and support the relationship between the transport center and the community hospitals in the provision of such care.

To assure that this goal is continuously pursued, designated personnel must be granted the authority to review and evaluate all operational and clinical issues of the transport system. This is usually done by the transport coordinator who reviews all transports, trains transport personnel, develops and implements policies and procedures, conducts meetings specific to transport issues, and documents all transport-related problems, specific follow-up to each, and outcome of such follow-up.

Clearly defined expectations, roles of the team members, policies and procedures specific to transport issues, standards of care, and administrative personnel with authority to manage the system responsibly must be in place for effective quality assurance to be attainable. The complexity of coordinating a multidisciplined system dictates the need for a strong quality assurance program. The nature of the patient who is transported, the number of personnel who participate as team members, and the external agencies involved in the process make standards of practice imperative. The perinatal transport system needs continual evaluation and improvement to ensure the safe and efficient transfer of patients to the appropriate institution.

Data Collection

A specific tool that allows for the continual evaluation of the transport system is a database program. This not only verifies the status of patients

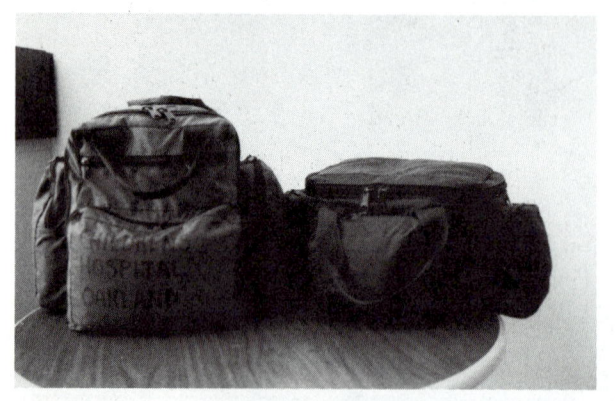

FIGURE 34–2. Customized bags to carry transport supplies.

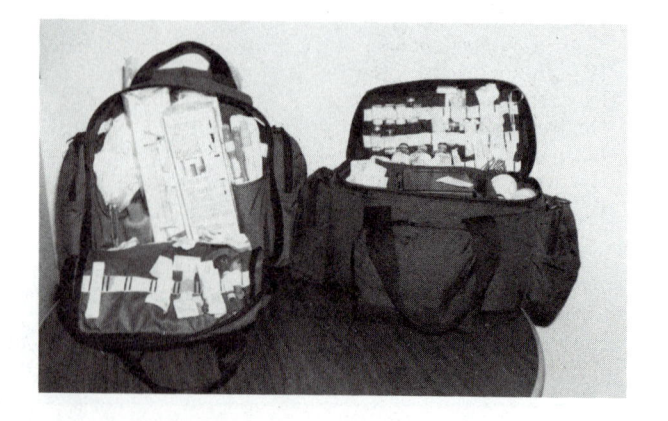

TABLE 34–2. Neonatal Transport Equipment List

Medications		Syringes, nos:	
Atropine 1 ml, 400 µg/ml	2	20 cc	2
Aquamephyton 1 ml, 10 ml/ml	1	10 cc	10
Decadron	1	5 cc	10
Digoxin 1 ml, 0.1 mg/ml	2	3 cc w/needles	10
Dramamine	6	3 cc plain	10
D10W 3 ml	3	tuberculin	10
Epinephrine 1 ml, 1 mg/ml	2	Luerlock stopcocks	6
Gentamicin 20 mg/2 ml	2	NG tubes, nos 5, 8	3
Heparin 1 ml, 1000 units/ml	4	Pressure tubing	2
Inderal 1 mg/ml	2	Suction catheters nos 5, $6\frac{1}{2}$, 8, 10	3
Isuprel 5 ml, 1 mg/ml	2	Transducer kit	3
Lasix 2 ml, 20 mg/2 ml	2	IV tubing	3
Narcan 2 ml, 0.02 mg/ml	1	Adhesive tape	3
Neostigmine	1	D5W, 250 cc	1
Phenobarbital 6 mg/ml	2	D10W, 500 cc	2
Priscoline 10 ml, 25 mg/ml	1	Micropore tape	3
Lidocaine 2 ml, 10 mg/ml	2	Ringers lactate 500 cc	1
Dilantin 2 ml, 100 mg/ml	1	Blood culture bottles	2
Ampicillin 125 mg	2	Oxygen masks, nos 1, 2, 3, 4	2
Ampicillin 250 mg	1	Foil	
Calcium chloride 10%, 10 ml, 1 g/10 ml	1	Saran wrap	
Calcium gluconate 10%, 10 ml	1	2×2's	
Potassium chloride 10 ml, 2 meq/ml	1	4×4's	
Albumin 5%, 50 ml	1	BP cuffs, nos 1, 2, 3, 4	2
D50 50 ml	1	Bulb syringe	1
Dopamine 5 ml, 200 mg/5 ml	1	Limb restraints	2 sets
Mannitol 50 ml	1	Tube connectors, misc. sizes	
Sodium bicarbonate 50 ml	1	ECG pads	8
Abbojects:		Hollihesive	3
epinephrine 10 ml, 1:10,000	2	Lead wires	3 packs
atropine 5 ml, 0.05 mg/ml	2	Gelfoam	2
sodium bicarbonate 10 ml, 1 meq/ml	2	Sterile drap	
		Sterile scissors	
		Umbilical catheters, nos $3\frac{1}{2}$, 5	3
Equipment and supplies		Batteries "C"	2
Alcohol wipes		ET tubes, nos $2\frac{1}{2}$, 3, $3\frac{1}{2}$	3
Betadine swabs		Laryngoscopes	2
Capillary tubes	1 Bottle	Laryngoscope blades, nos 0, 1	2
Chemstrips	1 Bottle	Chest tubes, nos 8, 10, 12	2
Lancets		Heimlich valves	2
Arm boards	3	Vaseline gauze	1
Syringe pump tubing	3	Betadine	1 bottle
Scalp vein butterfly needles, nos 23, 25	10	Specimen tubes:	
Cotton balls		red top	3
T Connectors	4	purple top	3
Injection caps		green top	1
Insyte catheters, nos 22, 24	10	Measuring tape	4
Jelco catheters, nos 22, 24	10	Scalpels	4
Line boards		Suture 4-0 silk	4
Op-site		Transducer cable	1
Normal saline 10 ml	8	Umbilical tie (sterile)	2
Saline flushes for ETT	10	Volutrols	3
Sterile H$_2$O 10 ml	8	Cutdown tray	1
Hemostats	1	EZ drape isolation bag	1
Intramedics, nos 18, 20	4	Knitted caps	3
Logan's bows	4	Lubafax	
Needles, nos 18, 20	8	Pacifiers	
Needles (filter)	6	Porta-warm pediatric mattress	2
Olive tips	2	Replogyle suction catheter no. 10	2
Razor	1	Tylenol	8
Rubberbands		Pleurevac	1
Safety pins		Bubble paper	1
Scissors		Sterile gloves (all sizes)	2

SOURCE: Used with the permission of the Children's Hospital, Oakland.

transferred, but also documents the effectiveness of care by the referral hospital and by the transport team. Such data can then be used to justify the need for education of referral staff and/or team members, revision in transport policies, and need for more transport team personnel or equipment. It documents the type of patients transferred within the region, the level of expertise of staff at the referral hospital, the timeliness of the referral call by the community hospital and the response time of the team, and the effectiveness of team intervention.

Financial Solvency

This continues to be a topic of considerable controversy among transport systems. The definition of financial solvency differs widely among transport programs. Some may only be interested in recovering the cost of the system, some view the program as supportive of inpatient services and are disinterested in the financial aspects of the system itself, whereas some view transport as part of the overall marketability of the hospital and are not as concerned with the cost of the system as with the additional patient revenue it brings into the hospital. With the health care industry being severely affected by the realities of DRG's and reduced third-party reimbursement, the concepts of reducing costs and maximizing reimbursement have become the major theme of hospital administrators.

The potential for financial solvency of any transport program is directly linked to the volume of transports done. Simply put, the more transports done, the lower the running costs of the system. The costs fall into three general areas: transport vehicle, transport team, and equipment and supplies. Each program must decide on a mechanism for charging and tracking costs that has been proven to maximize the reimbursement for each third-party payer. The mode of transport must not only be appropriate for the medical status of the patient, but must also be the most cost-effective (e.g. a fixed-wing aircraft will cost less than a helicopter for long-distance transports). Transport vehicles can be shared with other institutions to decrease expenses. Some aircraft and ambulance operators bill the patient directly instead of the hospital and, thus, absolve the hospital of incurring cost liability. Team composition and on-call systems can notably affect the cost of the program. Some programs have removed the physician from transport, because the cost of such a team member is high and the quality of care with the specially trained nurse/nurse, nurse/ respiratory therapist, or nurse/paramedic team has shown to be comparable (Cook and Kattwinkel, 1983; Thompson, 1980). For an institution that does a high volume of transport, an on-call system for team members may ensure a higher potential for acceptance of the transport. On-call systems are extremely expensive, so the high number of transports must be linked to the increased availability of on-call team members to justify the cost. Other programs may pull team members who are already working in specialty areas of the hospital. While such a method is less costly, the loss of transport admissions due to unavailability of team members must be monitored continuously.

During these challenging times in the health care industry, when both the public and third-party payers are questioning all costs of hospitalization, it is imperative that each hospital that develops and maintains a transport program understands the significance of effective cost accounting. It is not possible to minimize the costs of a program unless these costs can be identified and monitored. The institution must invest the time to study the specifics of the transport phase of hospitalization, identify the costs of the program, support the contribution of the program to the institution's mission, and explore the reimbursement potential for this phase of hospitalization.

Medicolegal Aspects

The unique aspects of perinatal transport, namely the critical status of the patient, the shared responsibility of the transport team and the referring hospital, and the reality of providing care in an unfamiliar environment, often bring questions of liability to the forefront. In order to assess the legal responsibility of the transport team, it is important to evaluate three legal principles.

The first legal principle is that of *respondent superior*, or "let the master answer". The employer assumes responsibility for the actions of employees acting within the scope and course of their employment (Brimhall, 1987). If the hospital has a perinatal transport program, it must legally protect those individuals who function in the role of transport team members. The hospital minimizes its liability by authorizing the system that has been implemented, namely the composition of the team, team member requirements, team training, team member roles, and standards of practice.

The second principle requires that the team functions under the direction of a qualified physician. Since the team is performing various patient care activities in an environment other than its home-base hospital, it needs to be supervised by a designated physician. Transport programs provide this supervision whether by direct phone communication between transport team leader and the attending physician in the Neonatal Intensive Care Unit (NICU) or by preapproved written standardized procedures.

The third principle involves individual liability. Each individual assumes professional accountability for his or her own actions. Even though the employer offers legal protection to its employees, the individual must exercise competent judgment in the performance of his or her own role and must display conduct that is within the scope of practice as defined by the institution and the state.

To minimize the risk of liability, the following aspects of a transport program should be observed:

1. The transport team should be effectively trained to deliver the required care.
2. Ongoing evaluation of the team member's performance must be maintained. Recertification of a team member's acceptable performance should be done at stated intervals.
3. Protocols for patient care management should be approved by the medical director of the transport program.
4. There must be specific policies on how the transport program is structured and managed. This should be approved by the perinatal unit administration and by the hospital administration.
5. Informed consent must be obtained from the patient, parents, or legal guardians at the time of the transport.
6. Communication between the referral hospital, the transport team, and the perinatal center needs to be collaborative and respectful. Each should value the contribution of the other so that a trusting atmosphere is created.

Brimhall (1987) states: "In today's litigious society, there are few if any actions that can reduce litigation aside from effective communication, safe practice, and common sense public relations." This is demanded in the transport environment.

THE TRANSPORT PROCESS

Outreach

An important aspect of establishing an effective transport system is to simultaneously implement a comprehensive outreach program. The referral call and the initial stabilization effort is initiated by the community hospital. It is, therefore, essential that the community hospital have a well-established relationship with the perinatal center. This relationship should be one of mutual trust and dedication toward providing optimal perinatal care. The community hospital staff is the patient's initial link with regional care. The staff need to be able to recognize early signs of clinical problems with patients so that appropriate referrals can be made. The staff further need to know how to provide initial stabilization in emergency situations until the team arrives. This type of education, a fundamental aspect of the transport program, is provided by the perinatal center and is often referred to as the outreach education program. Education is provided in a variety of ways which include didactic classes, skills labs, attendance by tertiary care center staff at community hospital meetings where clinical cases are discussed, and informal feedback to the community hospital staff on stabilization efforts. In some centers it is also a function of the outreach program to keep community staff updated on the clinical status of their patients who have been transported (see Table 34–3).

The Referral Call

The community hospital must have ready access to consultative services at the perinatal center. The decision to transport is made jointly by the referring and receiving physicians based on the clinical status of the patient, the availability of bed space and nursing staff to accommodate the admission, and the availability of a team to respond to the transport call. Once the acceptance of the admission is confirmed, the receiving physician maintains phone contact with the referral facility so that recommendations for stabilization can be made and updated until the team arrives. Having a referral hospital directory that specifies the capabilities of each hospital allows the receiving physician to make realistic recommendations for patient care. Also, having a checklist for the referral hospital that outlines information that will be needed by the receiving physician can facilitate the exchange of accurate information that will affect recommendations for therapy (see Fig. 34–3).

Before Team Departs Receiving Hospital

At the Receiving Hospital
The team must assemble within a specified time frame and prepare all necessary equipment for

TABLE 34–3. Preparation for Neonatal Transport

Material given to community hospitals through the Outreach Education Program.

Once the decision has been made to transfer a child to Children's Hospital, the following guidelines are recommended:

Call the neonatologist handling the transport regarding any problems: (415) 428-1054

Provide 1:1 nursing care for the infant

Keep infant warm
Place on prewarmed radiant warmer, and attach temperature probe.
Be certain infant is well dried and lying on a dry surface.
Keep sides of table up.
Consider use of Porta-warm mattress, heating lamp, warm water-filled gloves (covered with a linen), and aluminum foil on sides of table for small infants with hypothermia.

Oxygenate and ventilate as needed
Assess for improved color, breath sounds, chest movement, and heart rate.
Pass oral gastric tube for decompression.
Have an oxygen blender available so that oxygen can be weaned as color improves.
Monitor FIO_2 with an oxygen analyzer. Check that analyzer is calibrated.
Chart all changes in oxygen concentration, pressure, and rate.

Intubation
Have laryngoscope and endotracheal tube at bedside.
Make sure bulb in laryngoscope is bright and tight.
ETT size guidelines:

Infant weight	Recommended tube size
>4000 g	4.0
>2500 g	3.5
>1000 g	3.0
<1000 g	2.5

Distance to advance ETT:

Infant weight	cm in from lip*
1 kg	7
2 kg	8
3 kg	9
4 kg	10

*Oral: add 1 cm in for nasal.

Once intubated, listen in axillary line for equal breath sounds bilaterally.
Use hollihesive, tape, and Logan's bow to secure tube.
Obtain chest x-ray as soon as possible. Be sure head is turned to side, and neck is not flexed or hyperextended.
ETT should be at the level of T_1 to T_2.

Monitor vital signs
Place infant on cardiac, respiratory, and blood pressure monitors.
Place electrodes along axillary lines.
Monitor vital signs every 15–30 min.
Normal range of vital signs:
   Temperature: axillary: 97.8–98.6°F (preferred);
                  rectal: 98–99°F.
   Heart rate: 120–160 beats/min.
   Respiratory rate: 30–60 per min.

TABLE 34-3. Continued

Material given to community hospitals through the Outreach Education Program.

Blood pressure: acceptable systolic pressures:

750 g	34–54
1000 g	37–59
1500 g	40–62
2000 g	43–66
2500 g	46–70
3000 g	51–75

For hypotension: May give albumin 0.5–1 g/kg slowly over 10–30 min. If using 25% albumin, dilute to 5% with NS, and give 10 cc/kg over 10–30 min. If indicated, may give PRBC's 10 cc/kg over 10–30 min. IV, UV, UA.

Monitor blood gases
Prefer arterial, otherwise, warmed heelstick.
Place transcutaneous monitor (TCM) on right upper chest.
Obtain blood gas to correlate TCM.
Obtain blood gas with any change in baby's color or condition.
Obtain blood gas 15 min. after any FIO_2, pressure or rate change.
Obtain blood gas 15 min. after sodium bicarbonate is given.
Chart all blood gas results.
Recommended values for most disease entities:

pO_2:	55–70 (arterial), 40–50 (heelstick),
pCO_2:	35–45,
pH:	7.35–7.45,
B.E.:	−5–+5.

Recommended values if persistence of fetal circulation suspected:

pO_2:	100–150 (preductal arterial) if full-term,
pO_2:	80–90 (preductal arterial) if premature,
pCO_2:	20–30,
pH:	7.55–7.60.

If any values are not within the recommended range, consult the physician.
If pO_2 low: may increase FIO_2, pressure, or rate.
If pO_2 high: may decrease FIO_2, pressure, or rate.
If pCO_2 low: may decrease rate or pressure.
If pCO_2 high: may increase rate or pressure.
If base deficit: may give sodium bicarbonate 2–3 meq/kg always diluted 1:1 with sterile water or D_{10}.
Give slowly, preferably over 15–30 min., never faster than 5 min.
$NaHCO_3$ not recommended if $pCO_2 > 50$.

Monitor Dextrostix
Check every 15–30 min until stable; then every hour and prn.
Maintain Dextrostix between 45 and 130.
If the Dextrostix is a weak 45 or lower, obtain a STAT serum glucose. Do *not* wait more than 10 min. for the lab to draw this.
Do *not* wait for results to come back before treating.
Treat with 10% glucose, 5 cc/kg, preferably IV, UV, or UA.
If no line available, may give po if clinically indicated.
Continue to monitor Dextrostix.
Repeat 10% glucose prn.

Check Hct
Prefer central; otherwise, warmed heelstick.
If less than 45%, may administer blood: PRBC's 10 cc/kg.
Before giving blood, obtain a type and cross, state screen, and if it is a baby who will need chromosomes drawn, this should be drawn before blood is transfused.

Continued

TABLE 34-3. Continued

Material given to community hospitals through the Outreach Education Program.

Repeat Hct after 1 hour and prn.
O Negative PRBC's can be given unmatched in emergency, with M.D.'s OK.
If the central Hct is greater than 65%, a partial exchange may be indicated. May use normal saline or 5% albuminated normal saline.

Fluid administration
Recommended fluid administration rates:
Infants with RDS, asphyxia, and sepsis:
  D10W 50–65 cc/kg per day (approx. 2–3 cc/kg per hour)
  Example: 1000-g infant (2 lb, 3 oz) = 2–3 cc/hour;
  Example: 2000-g infant (4 lb, 7 oz) = 5–6 cc/hour;
  Example: 3000-g infant (6 lb, 10 oz) = 8–9 cc/hour.
  Begin with 10% glucose.
  If needed, may increase glucose concentration to 12.5%.
  To increase glucose: In volutrol, mix 93.8 cc of D10W with 6.2 cc of D50 to make 100 cc of D12.5W.
Infants with abdominal wall defects:
  150 cc/kg per day (approx. 6 cc/kg per hour)
  Example: 1000-g infant (2 lb, 3 oz) = 6 cc/hour;
  Example: 2000-g infant (4 lb, 7 oz) = 12 cc/hour;
  Example: 3000-g infant (6 lb, 10 oz) = 18 cc/hour.

Administer antibiotics
Draw blood cultures and begin antibiotics on any infant with symptoms of respiratory distress, suspected sepsis, or meningitis.
Recommended doses:
  Ampicillin:
    100 mg/kg per day − divided q12 if infant < 7 days old;
                      − divided q8 if infant > 7 days old.
    300 mg/kg per day − divided q6 if treating meningitis.
    IV, UV, UA preferred; may give i.m.
  Gentamicin:

	<1 week of age	>1 week of age
Preterm		
<1000 g	2.5 mg/kg q24 hours	2 mg/kg q12 hours
>1000 g	2 mg/kg q12 hours	2 mg/kg q12 hours
Term		
>37 weeks	2 mg/kg q12 hours	2.5 mg/kg q8 hours

Using a two-syringe method, dilute with 1 cc of sterile water. Give over at least 20 min, IV, UV, or UA.

Paper work
We will need the following items sent with the transport team:
  xeroxed copies of the infant's and mother's chart;
  infant's x-rays (these will be returned);
  10 cc of cord blood in a clot tube;
  10 cc of mother's blood in a clot tube.

Parents
Please remind parents that they are welcome to call and visit the nursery at Children's at any time of the day or night.
If the mother is planning to breastfeed, provide her with breastfeeding information and encourage her to pump her breasts.
All breast milk should be collected in a sterile container (we use Gerber bags and then double bag for the freezer).
Label all containers with the name, date and time collected.
The milk should be frozen immediately.

TABLE 34-3. Continued

Material given to community hospitals through the Outreach Education Program.

Report
When the transport team from Children's arrives, we will need your report on the infant's history and condition since birth, and your assistance with stabilization for transport. If the shift changes before the transport team arrives, please give a complete report to your relief nurse.

Special circumstances
For *all* infants, closely monitor temperature and Dextrostix.

Asphyxia
Monitor blood gases if in oxygen.
Fluid restrict to 50 cc/kg per day.
Do baseline neuro and head exam.
Observe closely for seizure activity.
Keep a high index of suspicion for persistence of fetal circulation.

Persistence of fetal circulation (PFC or pulmonary hypertension)
Suspect PFC in any infant who has suffered asphyxia and whose oxygenation fluctuates greatly with small changes in FIO_2, whose hypoxemia seems to be out of proportion to the degree of lung disease, and who shows marked improvement with 100% oxygen.
Goal of therapy: vasodilate pulmonary arterioles, maintain BP, and prevent hypoxia and acidosis.
Monitor blood gases.
May obtain simultaneous gases: UA & Rt Radial to determine presence of a right to left shunt through PDA.
Keep well oxygenated: pO_2 100-150 in term, pO_2 80-90 in preterm.
Keep pCO_2 20-30.
Keep alkalotic: pH 7.55-7.60.
Wean *very* gradually (1-2% at a time), and with caution.
Maintain systemic blood pressure.
Minimize stresses to baby to prevent hypoxia and vasoconstriction of pulmonary vessels.

Seizures
Suction stomach contents ASAP.
Phenobarbitol 5-10 mg/kg. May repeat up to a loading dose of 20 mg/kg per day. Maintenance dose = 3-7 mg/kg per day.
Phenobarbitol doses must be double checked.
Phenobarbitol may cause respiratory depression or hypotension.
Watch respiratory effort: Have bag and mask ready.
Monitor blood pressure closely: have albumin available.
Monitor Dextrostix!

Tracheo-esophageal fistula (TEF)
Elevate HOB.
Keep NPO. Maintain IV.
Nos 8 or 10 feeding tube to blind pouch on low intermittent suction.
Keep infant from crying to prevent distension.
Frequent oral-pharyngeal suctioning.
Use positive pressure ventilation only if absolutely necessary to avoid forcing air through the fistula into the GI tract where it can not be vented.

Omphalocele/Gastroschisis
Cover the defect with warm, sterile, normal saline moistened lap pads and wrap with saran wrap. Support defect so that there is no torque, kinking, or drying of the bowel.
If possible place baby in a plastic bag to neck or nipple line.
Keep NPO
IV: keep well hydrated: D5 1/3 NS 150 cc/kg per day.
N/G tube to low intermittent suction for G.I. decompression.
Maintain temperature!

Continued

TABLE 34–3. Continued

Material given to community hospitals through the Outreach Education Program.

G.I. obstruction/abdominal distension
Keep NPO.
Maintain IV.
N/G tube to low intermittent suction.
Elevate HOB.

Diaphragmatic hernia
Do *not* mask bag if possible.
If assisted ventilation is required, intubate immediately and ventilate rapidly and gently to prevent pneumothorax.
Be sure the ETT is not below the carina.
N/G tube to low intermittent suction for G.I. decompression.

Myelomeningocele
Cover defect with warm, sterile, normal saline soak and wrap in saran wrap, chuck, or diaper.
If possible, place baby in a plastic bag to include area above defect.
Keep infant on stomach.
Maintain temperature!

Cardiac
Administer oxygen as needed.
Monitor blood gases.
Prevent crying for maximum pulmonary blood flow.
Assess pulses, perfusion, BP, HR, murmur, precordial activity.
Minimize stresses that will lead to hypoxia.

Pulmonary air leak
Assess for equal breath sounds, chest excursion, PMI.
Chest x-ray as soon as possible.
Have pneumo kit for needling chest (alcohol wipe, no. 20 jelco, T connector, stopcock, 20-cc syringe).
If chest needled, continue to evacuate air until chest tube is placed.
Chest tube placement: Have chest tray, nos 8, 10, 12, or 14 feeding tube with water seal and suction setup.

SOURCE: Courtesy Children's Hospital, Oakland.

---

transport. In addition to the incubator and supplies discussed earlier, additional equipment might be necessary for the neonatal transport, e.g. blood for a transfusion, special drugs like prostaglandin E and narcotics, a Polaroid camera, and bubble paper or saran wrap. All equipment must be checked for readiness and reliability. An update on the patient's condition should be given to the team by the receiving physician just prior to team departure. When the team is *enroute* they can discuss the patient's status and formulate a plan for assessment and therapy. Medication calculations can be made so that the appropriate drugs can be readily drawn up if needed.

At the Referral Hospital

The staff will follow the recommendations of the perinatal center until the transport team arrives. For the maternal patient, this usually consists of continuing therapy to control labor if it is in progress and to provide psychosocial support for the patient and her family.

For the neonatal patient, once delivery room care, including establishing and maintaining an airway, drying the infant and providing radiant heat at all times, and providing any resuscitation measures that are necessary, is completed, the infant is transported to the nursery where the same basic care is continued. Providing a neutral thermal environment, maintaining the infant's airway and providing adequate oxygenation and ventilation, providing adequate hydration per intravenous therapy, preventing hypoglycemia, monitoring vital signs, and administering antibiotics are basic stabilization procedures that should be initiated as necessary by the referral hospital. Recommended guidelines from the perinatal cen-

Neonatal Transport Checklist

To initiate a neonatal transport, call (415) 428-1054 and ask for the neonatologist on call. The following information will be requested by the neonatologist:

Infant

Name _____ Sex _____ Gest. Age _____

Date of Birth _____/_____/_____ Time: _____ Weight _____ Gm.

Apgars 1 _____ 5" _____ C/S _____ Vaginal Birth _____

Single/Multiple Birth _____

Referral Diagnosis _____

Birth History _____

Antibiotics: _____ Blood Cultures _____

Vit K _____ Eye Treatment _____ X-Ray _____

Other Medications _____

Temp _____ HR _____ Resp _____ BP _____ Dextro _____

Hct _____ (central / heel) IA _____

Ventilatory support _____

1st gas: pO2 _____ pCO2 _____ pH _____ BE _____

(A/V/C)

Ventilatory support _____

Latest gas: pO2 _____ pCO2 _____ pH _____ BE _____

(A/V/C)

Maternal

Age _____ E/D/C _____/_____/_____ Gravida _____ Para _____

Prenatal Care: _____ yes _____ no Date started _____

Maternal Diagnosis/Risk Factors: _____

Rupture of Membranes: # hours ruptured _____

Recommendations by neonatologist:

This can be filled out by referral M.D. or R.N. & should be used as a worksheet.

FIGURE 34–3. Neonatal transport checklist for use by the referral hospital.
SOURCE: Courtesy Children's Hospital, Oakland.

ter that pertain to the stabilization of all neonates and more comprehensive guidelines for specific diagnoses can contribute to a successful attempt by the referral hospital to initiate needed therapy in a timely manner (see Table 34–3). The effectiveness of this early intervention will clearly affect the patient's prognosis and the degree of stabilization that will be required by the transport team.

Care After the Team Arrives at Referral Hospital

Once the team has arrived, both the maternal and fetal patients are assessed. The control of labor through tocolysis may be initiated and modified as needed. The mother will be transported via a gurney, and bed rest will be maintained. Fetal well-being will be monitored throughout the transport process. Hydration will be provided via intravenous therapy. Documented assessment will include the following: verification of maternal history; vital signs; hand grasp; reflexes; nature of uterine contractions (frequency, intensity, and duration); and patient response to all therapy. If the team concludes that the patient's status is stable enough for transport, the departure for the perinatal center is initiated. If the patient's status indicates that delivery is imminent, the decision may be made to deliver the patient at the community hospital with the likelihood of the need for subsequent dispatch of a neonatal transport team. The goal of neonatal transport is to provide enough stabilization at the referral hospital so that further emergency interventions will not be necessary *en route* to the regional center. On arrival of the team, assessment and documentation of the patient includes the following: verification of maternal history; vital signs; a central hematocrit; an arterial or capillary blood gas if indicated for respiratory distress; a chemstrip to monitor the glucose level; a complete physical assessment; verification of the infant's intake and output; verification of all medications, blood products, and therapy received prior to team arrival; and review of all lab tests done and x-rays taken (see Fig. 34–4). If therapy has been initiated by the referral hospital, its effectiveness must be evaluated by the transport team which has now assumed a major role in the infant's management. Alterations in management, based upon this initial and comprehensive assessment, can then be implemented.

Three areas warrant specific review due to their inherent necessity in the transport situation. These include temperature regulation, fluid therapy, and oxygenation and ventilation.

Temperature Regulation

One of the most basic interventions that will reduce the transported infant's morbidity and mortality is to prevent cold stress. An infant who becomes cold stressed increases oxygen consumption and increases the rate of glucose consumption, leading to metabolic acidosis. The production of surfactant may also be inhibited, thus worsening the infant's respiratory status. Providing a neutral thermal environment in the transport setting can be one of the biggest challenges to the team since weather and the length and mode of transport can affect the temperature within the incubator.

To emphasize the importance of temperature regulation, certain interventions have become standard practice in the transport setting. They include the following:

1. Use a radiant warmer at the referral hospital if it is available. Frequent access to the infant makes the maintenance of a neutral thermal environment impossible in an isolette.
2. Always verify if the radiant warmer is being used correctly by the referral hospital. The temperature probe should be placed correctly, and the warmer should be turned on and set to servo-controlled, and the dial on the warmer should be set at a good starting point (e.g. 97.5°F).
3. Remove all wet linens and make sure the infant's skin is dry to prevent evaporative heat loss. If the infant has a defect that is covered with wet soaks, redress the defect with warm soaks and wrap the defect in saran wrap to prevent evaporative heat loss.
4. Line the sides of the radiant warmer and the transport incubator with aluminum foil. The aluminum foil will reflect the heat back to the infant. Keep the sides of the radiant warmer up as much as possible to reduce drafts.
5. If the radiant warmer is near a doorway, close the door or move the warmer to further reduce the likelihood of drafts.
6. Use a portawarm mattress. These are available as a single-use disposable item that chemically heats to 104°F and retains heat for approximately 4 hours.
7. Prewarm the transport incubator to the infant's neutral thermal environment plus 4 degrees. The extra degrees provide a margin of safety to compensate for heat loss when the infant is placed inside the incubator (see Table 34–4).
8. An infant of very low birthweight (1000 g or less) should be covered with bubble paper, saran, or a heat shield in the transport incubator.
9. Prewarm the ambulance and the aircraft on cold days before the incubator is moved from the referral hospital.
10. Cover the plexiglass of the transport incubator with a blanket before going outside on a cold day to reduce heat loss through the plexiglass.
11. At the referral hospital use additional warming lights near the radiant warmer or cloth-wrapped warm water gloves surrounding the

Children's Hospital Medical Center

NEONATAL TRANSPORT NOTES

RESPONSE TIME

Call Received ______________ am/pm
Transport accepted ______________ am/pm
Ambulance Called ______________ am/pm
Ambulance Arrived ______________ am/pm
RN __________ Ready ________ am/pm
MD __________ Ready ________ am/pm
RT __________ Ready ________ am/pm
EMT __________ Ready ________ am/pm
Left CHMC ______________ am/pm
Arrived Ref. Hosp. ______________ am/pm
Left Ref. Hosp. ______________ am/pm
Arrived CHMC ______________ am/pm

Mode of Transport

☐ Ground ☐ Fixed Wing Aircraft ☐ Helicopter

INTAKE DATA

INFANT	Name:				Sex ☐ M ☐ F		
DOB / /	Time:		Wt. gm.		G.A.		
Apgars 1" 5"	☐ C. Sect. ☐ Vaginal		☐ Single ☐ Mult. Birth				
Referral Diagnosis:							
Birth History:					☐ **STATE SCREEN**		
Antibiotics: ☐ Blood Cultures	Other Meds ☐ Vit K ☐ Eye Care				X-ray		
Hct central/heel	T.	HR	RR	BP	Dextro	IA	
Vent. Support #1 gas	PO_2	PCO_2	pH	BE	A V C		
Vent. Support Last gas	PO_2	PCO_2	pH	BE	A V C		
MATERNAL	Age	EDC / /	Gravida Para	Prenatal Care: ☐ yes ☐ no			
Maternal Diagnosis/Risk Factors:				R.O.M. (hours ruptured):			

TRANSPORT INFORMATION

Date of Transport: ____________
Ref. Hospital: ____________
Ref. O.B.: ____________
Ref. Ped.: ____________
Maternal Transport: ☐ yes ☐ no
Ref. Hospital: ____________
Ref. O.B.: ____________
Neonatologist: ____________
Charge Nurse: ____________
Recommendations by Neonatologist:

TIME	Temp.		Vital Signs			Ventilator		Blood Gases				TCM	Medications (Add volume if > than 1 cc)	INTAKE		OUTPUT		X-Ray Hct Dextro Lab	COMMENTS
	I	Ax	BP	HR	RR	FiO2	Press	P02	PC02	pH	B.E.	02 / C02		Type	Amount	Type	Amount		Color, Tone, Activity, Procedures, Treatments, etc.
Admission Time	I	Ax	BP	HR	RR	FiO2	Press	P02	PC02	pH	B.E.	TCM	Total Meds:	TOTAL IN (on transport):		TOTAL OUT (on transport):		ADMISSION	
													Total Flush:	Total since 12 A.M. (à transport):		Total since 12 A.M. (à transport):		Hct / Dextro	TRANSPORT NURSE: Parent has been phoned / Nursery has been phoned

FIGURE 34–4. Neonatal transport notes document initial information on patient's condition, team response time, mode of transport, and transport activities.

SOURCE: Courtesy Children's Hospital, Oakland.

776 HIGH RISK MOTHER, INFANT AND FAMILY

TABLE 34-4. *Neutral Thermal Environment Chart (Incubator Air Temperatures, First 24 Hours)*

Birthweight (gr)	Temperature Median and Range °C		°F
500	35.5	0.5	95.5
1000	34.9	0.5	95.0
1500	34.0	0.5	94.0
2000	33.5	0.5	92.5
2500	33.2	0.8	92.0
3000	33.0	1.0	91.5
3500	32.8	1.2	
4000	32.6	1.4	

infant's body to provide additional warmth. Caution must be observed when using warm water-filled gloves around the body of a low-birthweight infant since this source of heat can cause second- and third-degree burns. These gloves *must* be covered with linen to control the degree of heat to which the infant's skin is exposed.

12. Once in the transport incubator, the infant should only be accessed when necessary and only through the portholes of the incubator to minimize the loss of warmed air.

Fluid Therapy

Since most infants will be fluid restricted on transport, it is important to pay strict attention to the amount of fluid the infant has already received and the amount given on transport. Intravenous therapy must be administered via an infusion pump that is designed to deliver consistent, accurate, low rates. It often becomes necessary on transport to insert an umbilical arterial or an umbilical venous line. Such vascular access allows for ready collection of blood specimens to monitor blood gases, which is the most accurate way of verifying oxygenation.

Oxygenation/Ventilation

The transport team has the capability of providing respiratory management of the infant comparable to what is offered at the regional center. An umbilical arterial line to monitor blood gases is usually placed so that accurate reflections of the arterial oxygen and carbon dioxide levels will determine the course of respiratory treatment. The infant may require oxygen per hood or nasal CPAP, or may require intubation and support on a ventilator. Equipment to provide such management along with the equipment to monitor the infant's continued response to it (e.g. TCM and pulse oximeter) are routine transport capabilities. The goal is to stabilize respiratory status so as to allow for a safe transport to the regional center. Common parameters that are reflective of adequate oxygenation and ventilation are a paO_2 of 50–70 torr and a $paCO_2$ of 30–40 torr.

Documentation

Since the team is functioning as agents of the perinatal center at a referral institution, the activity of the team, the assessment of the infant, the interventions attempted, and the infant's response to therapy must be comprehensively documented. Parameters to include in the transport nurse's record are vital signs, central hematocrit, arterial blood gases and corresponding pulse oximeter and/or transcutaneous monitor values, medications, blood glucose, intake and output, laboratory specimens and results, x-rays, endotracheal tube and umbilical line placement, and clinical observations of the infant's appearance and response to therapy.

Before Departure from Referral Hospital

To ensure additional safety during the transport, a nasogastric tube is inserted and the stomach is emptied of its contents. The nasogastric tube is taped in place and left open to gravity to allow for accumulated air to escape.

Supplies that might be utilized in transit to the perinatal center should be set aside so that the team has easy access to them when needed. Before leaving the referral hospital, the following items and documents are assembled: a copy of the mother's chart, a copy of the infant's chart, x-rays, signed consent forms, and properly labeled specimens.

A call back to the perinatal center is then made to alert the receiving staff of the infant's condition and the present therapy being used. This allows the receiving hospital to assemble whatever equipment will be necessary to allow for a smooth transmission of care from the transport team to the neonatal intensive care unit.

Parental Contact

The last stop that is made prior to departure is in the mother's room. There, the family is encouraged to briefly interact with the infant. Prior to this, the physician should have visited with the family to explain the therapy that has been initiated and to obtain a written consent for transport. The parents need to be prepared for what they will see when the infant is brought into the mother's room by the team. Numerous tubes attached to electronic devices are common sights to the team, but need to be explained carefully to the parents.

This is a time of extreme anxiety for the parents. Because they are in crisis, they may ask the team the same questions repeatedly. This is the infant that the couple may have planned and eagerly awaited. Now they find that the infant is not the perfect child they dreamed about, may not live, or may have a questionable future. There are more questions that the team will *not* be able to answer and this will only increase the parents' anxiety.

Leaving two Polaroid pictures of the infant will help the parents see that the infant they had, and who was so swiftly whisked away from them, is very real. The team should try to focus the parents on the present, giving them explanations for the treatment that is presently being utilized. The parents will also benefit from being told about the neonatal intensive care unit. It is helpful if the team can leave a brochure with the parents that includes information on the neonatal intensive care unit and the regional center (e.g. map, visiting hours, phone numbers, places to stay, places to eat, and other support services).

This visit with the family only requires about 10 minutes and can be so essential to facilitating the attachment between parents and their infant. Parents should be encouraged to touch their infant before the team departs. The transport nurse can further decrease the mother's anxiety by assuring her that she will be called as soon as the team arrives at the perinatal center. Mothers have often expressed relief at just knowing when the team has arrived safely.

Management en route

Close monitoring of the patient (maternal–fetal or neonatal) is the priority of management *en route* to the perinatal center. Since auscultation of respirations and heart rate become impossible due to vibration and noise in the transport vehicle, vital sign parameters are usually available via digital readouts. Turbulence and sudden stops can add to the fatiguing nature of the transport situation. All equipment must be secured and the patient and team members require the use of seat belts. The respiratory status of the patient can be evaluated by specific monitors and by observing the patient's color and the quality of respiration. Oxygen and ventilator parameters must be continuously monitored and adjusted based upon the patient's condition.

If the transport includes a flight, various aspects of aeromedical physiology must be considered. Simplistically, problems with the expansion of air within the patient can jeopardize patient safety when traveling in an unpressurized cabin at a high altitude. An infant may experience abdominal distention sufficient to cause respiratory distress. Additionally, oxygenation requirements may be increased at altitude. Team members who participate in aeromedical transport must be knowledgeable on how changes in atmospheric pressure can affect both patients and team members.

If an emergency arises during the journey back to the regional center, the team must be ready to intervene immediately. All equipment must be readily accessible. Team members must be located in close proximity to the patient to constantly observe for signs of problems and to intervene appropriately.

Transition of Care at the Perinatal Center

An ETA (estimated time of arrival) is usually given by the ambulance when the team is 10–15 minutes away from the receiving hospital. All should be ready at this point to accept the admission. When the team arrives at the appropriate unit, the receiving staff will start assuming care of the patient. The team will give a complete report and will remain in the unit to answer questions that arise. Documentation will then be completed, equipment will be cleaned, and supplies restocked. Communication with the referral hospital is also completed, both with the mother of the transported infant and with the maternal or neonatal staff at the referral hospital. A copy of the transport record should be mailed back to the referral hospital so that they have a record of the team's activities and interventions. Periodic calls are then made by the receiving physician and nurses to referral physicians and nurses to update them on the status of the patient. Such communication emphasizes and supports the concept of teamwork that is so basic to a network referral system (Dunn, 1982).

MODES OF TRANSPORT

Various factors must be considered when choosing the optimal mode of transport: (1) distance to the referral hospital, (2) clinical condition of the patient, (3) ability of the referral hospital to stabilize the patient, (4) availability of personnel and vehicle, (5) the region's geography, (6) weather and traffic conditions, and (7) cost of the vehicle (Committee on Hospital Care, 1986).

If a transport program is comprehensive and services a large region, it usually offers the capability of responding to a transport call via ground ambulance, fixed-wing aircraft, or helicopter.

Ground Ambulance

This vehicle has the advantage of availability and readily serves as a mobile intensive care unit (see Fig. 34–5). It provides an environment that is spacious and well-equipped so that interventions with the patient can be done relatively easily. If a patient requires emergency procedures to be done *en route* to the tertiary center, the ambulance can pull off to the side of the road to allow for a more stable environment. Most ambulances keep within the speed limit during a transport unless the patient's condition warrants immediate access to the perinatal center. The disadvantages of the ground ambulance are its limitations in heavy traffic or when the distance to the referral hospital is extensive. Long distances impact negatively on response time and minimize the advantage of cost-effectiveness, since the vehicle is usually billed per mile traveled.

Fixed-wing Aircraft

This vehicle is advantageous when the distance to the referral hospital is extensive, usually over 100 miles. It provides a vehicle that can cover long distances in a short period of time. It can be used in marginal weather as it can fly above or around weather systems that would restrict the use of a helicopter. It usually provides an environment that is spacious enough and well-equipped enough to allow for emergency stabilization of the patient. It should provide a pressurized cabin so that the respiratory status of the patient is not adversely affected.

The disadvantage to such a vehicle is that it requires a number of ground ambulances – an ambulance to take the team to the airport, an ambulance to meet the team at the destination airport, an ambulance to take the team and the patient back to the airport, and an ambulance to meet the team and return them and the patient to the perinatal center. Such a transport involves effective communication and cooperation among carriers. Cabin space may be limited in some aircraft making it a less than conducive environment in which to actually intervene with the patient. Turbulence may be experienced during marginal or even clear weather, making team members and the patient prone to motion sickness. Since maintenance costs of a fixed-wing aircraft are high, the cost to the patient is also considerable.

Helicopter

The main advantage of this vehicle is its ability to respond quickly to a call and to be able to land in a variety of places. In interhospital transports, however, it needs a designated area to land. If no landing pad is present at the hospital, then landing at a nearby airport and using a ground ambulance to accommodate that leg of the transport is necessary. Cabin space may be limited, but many of the newer models provide a well-lit and spacious environment to accommodate the patient and the team. Noise and vibration and a non-pressurized cabin are inherent characteristics of helicopters. Weather conditions that are acceptable for a flight are more restrictive than with a fixed-wing aircraft. The maintenance costs are very high, as is

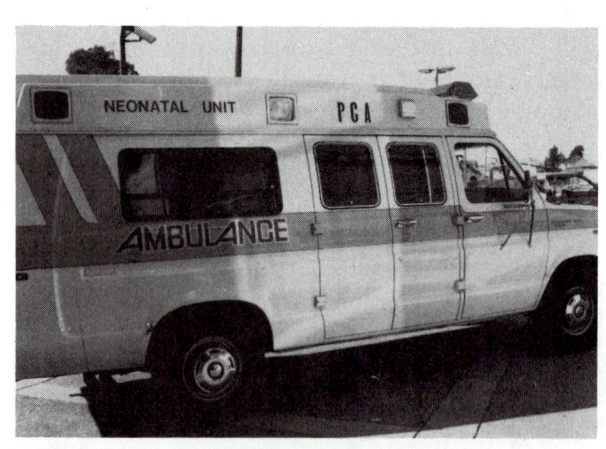

FIGURE 34–5. Ground ambulance.

the cost to the patient. The safety record of helicopters has come under close scrutiny by the federal government. The helicopter industry has responded aggressively by formalizing safety standards that call for comprehensive monitoring of the aircraft, flight crews, and operations of emergency medical service helicopter programs.

RETURN TRANSPORTS

In order to provide the most efficient use of the neonatal intensive care unit, the return transport has become an integral part of transport programs. When such a transport is necessary, it completes the circle: high-risk mother or critically ill infant is transported, intensive care is made available to the patient at the perinatal center, then a convalescing infant is transferred to the referring hospital where care can be administered at a lower cost to the family.

The advantages of such a system are many, and depend on the identified level of care of the hospital to which the infant is returned. The perinatal center's outreach education program provides the community hospitals with perceived educational needs. Due to the resulting relationship and familiarity with community hospital resources, return transports can easily be arranged and continuity of care provided.

Return transports increase the availability of bed space for critically ill infants at the tertiary center. They further maximize bed usage at the Level I and Level II nurseries. They promote a relationship of trust between the referral center and the tertiary center as both become integral to the patient's and family's recovery. They allow for more frequent visiting by the family since traveling needs are reduced. They allow for early involvement of the family pediatrician with the infant's care. They also reduce the cost of hospitalization for the family.

While return transports are not always optimal for the transported infant, as when hospitalization is brief or when the convalescing and discharge needs of the patient are too extensive, they provide an optimal approach to regionalized care.

SUMMARY

In an effort to provide optimal perinatal care to a designated area, regional programs have been implemented. The concept of this program recognizes the efficient utilization and concentration of resources at various hospitals. The most highly skilled care is provided at the perinatal center of the region. Variations of skill level are provided at the community hospitals.

When a maternal patient has been identified as experiencing problems with her fetus, a referral call to the perinatal center is made. At this center, consultation is accessible and a mutual decision to initiate a maternal transport may be reached. The perinatologist must decide, based upon the information given by the referral physician, if the mother should be transported to the perinatal center before delivery. If a maternal transport is initiated, the team must be prepared to handle all aspects of care for the high-risk mother, including possible delivery and stabilization of the newborn during the transport.

If the infant is born at a community hospital, the health care team must have the ability to recognize those problems that categorize the infant as being at risk. A referral call can then be made for consultative services or for the initiation of a transport. The neonatal transport team must have the ability to respond to the call quickly and provide intensive care to the infant as soon as the team arrives. This care must then be provided *en route* to the perinatal center where a smooth transition of care can occur.

For a successful maternal or neonatal transport to occur, a well-coordinated system must be established. This system recognizes and facilitates the efforts and resources of the perinatal center, the referral hospital, and the transport carriers in making maternal and neonatal transport an integral part of regionalized care. It is only in working collaboratively that the goal of reducing perinatal morbidity and mortality can be achieved.

REFERENCES

Anderson, C.: Aladjem, S.; Ayuste, O.; Caldwell, C.; and Ismail, M. 1981. An analysis of maternal transport within a suburban metropolitan region. *Am. J. Obstet. Gynecol.* 140:499–504.

Brimhall, D. 1987. Medicolegal aspects of neonatal transport. *J. Perinatal Neonatal Nurs.* 1:77–82.

Clarke, T.; Zmora, E.; Chen, J.; Reddy, G.; and Merritt, T. 1980. Transcutaneous oxygen monitoring during neonatal transport. *Pediatrics.* 65:884–886.

Committee on Hospital Care, American Academy of Pediatrics. 1986. Guidelines for air and ground transportation of pediatric patients. *Pediatrics.* 78:943–950.

Committee on Perinatal Health. 1976. *Toward improving the outcome of pregnancy*. White Plains: The National Foundation–March of Dimes.

Committee on Practice of the Nurses Association of the American College of Obstetricians and Gynecologists. 1983. *OGN nursing practice resource: Maternal–neonatal transport.* Washington, D.C.: NAACOG.

Cook, L., and Kattwinkel, J. 1983. A prospective study of nurse-supervised versus physician-supervised neonatal transports. *J. Obstet. Gynecol. Neonatal Nurs.* 12:371–376.

Cordero, L.; Backes, C.; and Zuspan, F. 1982. Very low-birth weight infant. *Am. J. Obstet. Gynecol.* 143:533–537.

Dunn, N. 1982. Fostering good interhospital relationships through neonatal transport. *Neonatal Network.* 1:20–27.

Feldman, B. H., and Sauve, R. S. 1976. The infant transport service. *Clin. Perinatology.* 3:469–477.

Giles, H. 1979. Maternal transport. *Clin. Obstet. Gynecol.* 6:206–207.

Harris, B., and Belcher, J. 1982. Equipment and planning for neonatal air transport. *Medical Instrumentation* 16:253–255.

Harris, T. R.; Isaman, J.; and Giles, H. 1978. Improved neonatal survival through maternal transport. *Obstet. Gynecol.* 52:294–300.

Hood, J.; Cross, A.; Hulka, B.; and Lawson, E. 1983. Effectiveness of the neonatal transport team. *Critical Care Med.* 11:419–423.

Meyer, H. B. P.; Harris, T. R.; and Daily, W. J. R. 1973. Statewide reduction of neonatal mortality through effective regionalization of newborn intensive care. *Pediatric Res.* 7:404.

Miller, C.; Clyman, R.; Roth, R.; Sniderman, S.; Ballard, R.; Henning, D.; Riedel, P.; Rosen, A.; and Burden, L. 1980. Control of oxygenation during the transport of sick neonates. *Pediatrics.* 66:117–119.

Miller, T. C.; Densberger, M.; and Krogman, J. 1983. Maternal transport and the perinatal denominator. *Am. J. Obstet. Gynecol.* 147:19–24.

Pettett, G.; Merenstein, G. B.; Battaglia, F. C.; Butterfield, L. J., and Efird, R. 1975. An analysis of air transport results in the sick newborn infant: Part I. The transport team. *Pediatrics.* 55:774–782.

Reedy, N.; Alonso, B.; Bozzelli, J.; and Depp, R. 1984. Maternal–fetal transport: A nurse team. *J. Obstet. Gynecol. Neonatal Nurs.* March/April:91–100.

Sumners, J.; Harris, H.; Jones, B.; Cassady, G.; and Wirtschafter, D. 1980. Regional neonatal transport: Impact of an integrated community/center system. *Pediatrics.* 65:910–916.

Swyer, P. R. 1970. The regional organization of special care for the neonate. *Pediatric Clin. N. Am.* 17:761–776.

Thompson, T. 1980. Neonatal transport nurses: An analysis of their role in the transport of newborn infants. *Pediatrics.* 65:887–892.

35

Care of the High-Risk Family: Strategies for Mobilizing Families in Perinatal Crisis

BEHAVIORAL OBJECTIVES

Upon completion of this chapter, the reader should be able to:

- Understand how problems in the perinatal period can be manifested.

- Recognize some of the ways in which families might benefit from intervention.

- Identify opportunities for intervention in the context of the hospital setting.

- Learn about some commonly used, successful forms of intervention.

- Identify ways in which families can maintain psychological integration and sense of control.

In most areas of the United States, high-risk pregnancies and seriously ill (largely preterm) infants are treated in regional centers (hospitals). As a result, families are separated, sometimes hundreds of miles from one another: from their sick infant and from the supportive environment of their homes and communities.

For example, a pregnant mother who is concerned about back pains in the morning may visit her obstetrician and by nightfall find herself transported by plane to a distant city, to a regional center she has never heard of, to await the birth of an endangered infant who was not due for another 3 months. If the infant is delivered, parents who were joyously anticipating the birth of their first baby only hours before, watch in horror as their newborn is placed in an incubator, intubated, and whisked off by doctors they have only just met.

Dramas like these are enacted every day. Families, sometimes without warning, find themselves in an environment that is totally foreign to them: a world of tests, blood gases, monitors, and sounds that one father likened to arriving at another planet. The intimacy and magic of pregnancy becomes, in an instant for some, a medical emergency shared with strangers.

Because regional centers are so often teaching hospitals, parents encounter caregivers at differing levels of training and expertise, whose communication skills are varied. More important is the sheer number of new people to whom a family must entrust their lives.

For example, a woman in preterm labor who delivers a baby who requires intensive care may encounter, in her first 48 hours in the hospital, a full complement of obstetricians, neonatologists and anesthesiologists, six shifts of nurses, plus technicians, clerical staff, and others. Perhaps as many as 20 or more care providers are involved, with countless more to come. Mercifully, for many, the worry and crisis are brief. For others, those whose babies have anomalies or are very preterm, the crisis is protracted over months.

The demands on a family in the midst of a perinatal crisis are incalculable. The tumult is unimaginable for those who have not experienced it. The resources and strengths that families need to call upon are often unknown. How nurses can help families find and marshall resources to cope with a perinatal crisis is the focus of this chapter.

THE HIGH-RISK FAMILY

For purposes of this chapter, "high-risk family" refers to a family trying to cope with the problems of pregnancy. When a woman's pregnancy is not normal, possibilities exist for fetal abnormality, neonatal illness, and even death. When such a circumstance exists, normal living patterns and relationships are disrupted within the family and its extended community. Frequently, hospitalization is required. The following discussion is directed toward identifying ways the nurse can support a hospitalized patient during the hours or weeks of her perinatal stay.

In a time of perinatal crisis, parents who have previously experienced the birth of a normal child and those presented with their first childbirth experience frequently have no role models on which to base coping behaviors. They find themselves in a foreign environment, where they do not know how to contribute to, or participate in, what is happening to them. They are intermittently overcome with concerns about work, home, family, finances, siblings, and grandparents. They are fearful and anxious about their unborn child, and they are worried about the health of the pregnant mother. They are dependent upon people they do not know to treat them for problems they may understand poorly. Parents vary widely in their responses to this lack of control. They struggle to find a role to play in this alien environment.

Whether their struggle goes on for 3 weeks while efforts are made to stave off preterm labor or for 3 hours to prepare for the birth of a sick preterm baby, the hospital team has goals for families that remain relatively constant and transcend the medical particulars. These goals include helping them adapt, cope, and ultimately assume responsibility for their own and their infant's care.

For this progression to happen successfully, health care providers need to empower and enable families to develop coping mechanisms. There are a number of ways this can be facilitated. Essential elements include communicating information, supporting the family, and developing approaches to problem solving.

In an ideal perinatal center, health care team members from numerous disciplines and perspectives meet different aspects of a family's needs (Miles, 1979). Nurses, and in particular bedside nurses, are the team members who remain closest to the family. They are available for extended periods of time, and they have opportunities to intervene at different times during the day (Baird, 1979).

Nurses can help decrease a family's stress in a number of concrete ways. It is the nurse, for example, who can best recognize the magnitude of a family's disruption and the positive strengths individual family members bring to the crisis (Miles, 1979). Once helped to identify and mobilize its strengths, the family regains its sense of control and begins to cope with the disruption it faces.

Nurses can help parents assess problems and identify solutions and choices, whether it is the need to visit with a 2-year-old at home or tour the nursery where the preterm infant will be cared for. The nurse has the opportunity to develop ideas and interventions to alleviate short- and long-term stress.

Parents, often isolated from friends and families,

rely on members of the health care team for primary support. It is the nurse to whom the family looks first for help. The relationship developed between nurse and family is often a function of "chemistry" and timing. The primary nurse, especially, becomes the pivotal person in determining the success with which the family's needs are identified and appropriate plans made to meet them.

The antepartum high-risk mother who has been hospitalized is treated as ill and requiring "special" care (Gyves, 1985). She is most distressed by separation from home and family, health concerns for herself and her baby, and her changing self-image (White and Ritchie, 1984). Family members can increase her level of stress and conflict if they fail to understand her illness or the risk to her baby (Gyves, 1985).

The task for the nurse in caring for high-risk antepartum mothers is "promoting adaptation to decrease stress and preparing the mother for labor, delivery, and parenting while recognizing the risks for mother and fetus" (White and Ritchie, 1984, p. 47). Information must be presented and reinforced.

Case Presentation 1

This case presentation highlights some of the stresses that confront a mother with a high-risk pregnancy. Some of the opportunities and approaches for intervention are noted. The nurse may want to consider areas that he or she may want to pursue with the family.

Antepartum mothers are often thrust into the hospital and out of the mainstream in what seems to them an instant. For example, one mother, Mrs. K, anticipated leaving her job a month before the birth of her baby. She planned to use this part of her maternity leave to get herself, her spouse, home, and 2-year-old toddler "ready" for the new baby. Instead, almost 3 months early (30 weeks gestation), Mrs. K's membranes ruptured while she was at work. After she phoned her obstetrician, she went to the emergency room to be evaluated. Five hours later, she found herself a "high-risk OB patient" in a perinatal center 300 miles from home.

Now, she is on strict bedrest, receiving IV medication to stop her early and unwanted contractions. The medication makes her breathless and weepy. While she longs for the company of her husband, they both agree that their toddler son needs his father at home until arrangements can be made for her mother, some 3000 miles away, to leave her own husband and job to care for her grandson. She worries, too, about her unfinished tasks at work.

Mrs. K worries most about her toddler. Her concerns about how his adjustment to a new sibling are replaced with worries of how he will react to the added stress of her absence. Her anxiety is heightened by many phone calls from members of her family and extended community. Shocked by the upheaval in her life and distracted by her medication, Mrs. K begins to contemplate what is in store for the baby she carries.

Whether Mrs. K proceeds on with her pregnancy for hours, days, or even weeks longer, she needs new information. She needs to learn new language and to understand its meaning, so that she can participate in decisions that will affect her own health and well-being and her unborn child's. Mrs. K will undergo numerous procedures, ranging from a sonogram to assess fetal age and size to amniocentesis. The latter, performed to determine fetal lung maturity and the presence or absence of amnionitis, is painful and intrusive. If the baby's lungs are immature, medication will be given to accelerate their maturation and prevent or reduce respiratory distress syndrome after birth. There may be discussions about experimental drugs. She will experience fear and anxiety about her baby's chances for survival or life-long problems.

Possible Nursing Approaches

The primary nurse can help orient Mrs. K to the hospital, its changing shifts and related events, and facilitate communications and relationships with the cast of characters. The nurse can talk with Mrs. K to assess her level of understanding of the medical facts and review with her the plan for her care. She can interpret and reinforce the goals of the treatment plan.

Mrs. K will receive, integrate, and interpret new data for herself and will feel responsible for conveying this information to her family. The offer of a phone call to extended family members can relieve Mrs. K of this pressure.

Mrs. K's family will need to prepare for a number of possible courses. In this case, bedrest in the hospital and its consequent separation from home may continue for a week or more. More likely, Mrs. K's baby will be born prematurely and possibly quite ill. Because her membranes have been ruptured for a relatively long time, there is a risk of complicating, serious infection.

Orientation to the intensive care nursery, while

a bit overwhelming, is generally appreciated by families. A verbal overview, a look at some photos, written information and, when appropriate, a tour of the unit help desensitize the family to what is ahead. Frequently, parents are able to prepare better if they can visualize the situation. Various team members can offer their varied perspectives and present the family with an idea of what to expect of them. Some repetition and review helps families integrate this new information and feel more comfortable with it.

If Mrs. K is unable to leave her bed to see the nursery, her husband and mother can visit and bring back reassuring news. In this case, Mrs. K's baby was more mature than had been predicted. Baby girl K had responded well to the drugs her mother had received before her birth, and she did not suffer from serious respiratory disease. She showed no signs of infection. She required transient help from a respirator and breathed unassisted 48 hours after birth.

Despite the need for Baby girl K to be admitted to the intensive care nursery, Mrs. K and her family were reassured. They had seen the nursery and other babies on respirators, and they felt prepared for problems. Although they were limited in their ability to care for their baby, Mrs. K and her family were encouraged to visit. The baby's nurse presents the parents with tasks, such as axillary temperature-taking and changing diapers. Mrs. K is encouraged to pump her breasts to provide milk for feedings, and is helped to understand that this is an important contribution to her baby's care.

Before discharge from the postpartum unit, Mrs. K and her family meet with members of the baby's health care team. General expectations about the baby's course after leaving the intensive care nursery are discussed. Baby K, still a growing premie, will be transferred to her local community hospital until she is medically ready to to go home. While Mrs. K likes the idea of her baby being nearby, she is concerned about whether the local hospital can meet the baby's needs. She is worried about making another transition.

Mrs. K's baby has survived preterm birth. With another 3 weeks of hospital care anticipated and a normal outcome expectation, Mrs. K dreads her own discharge from the hospital and is overwhelmed. When she is alone with her primary nurse, with whom she has developed a trusting relationship, she confesses her fears about leaving her baby "alone" in the hospital. Simultaneously, she experiences conflict regarding leaving her husband and toddler. Once she leaves for home, she knows she must face all of her unfinished business there and at work. With a sympathetic listener, Mrs. K reveals her feelings of guilt about delivering her baby early and her sadness at disappointing her family. She feels that she has "let her husband down", and she worries that her 2-year-old feels abandoned. She hadn't really planned to get pregnant so soon, and sometimes wonders if she is being punished for having regretted getting pregnant. Finally, Mrs. K is sad to leave the community of care providers who understand what she has experienced and whom she trusts to meet her needs. A skillful nurse can help Mrs. K focus her concerns. Together, they can identify some specific short-term problems and options for dealing with them.

Case Presentation 2

The family who experiences the birth of a preterm infant frequently feels unprepared and inadequate. It is common for parents to be fearful, angry, and guilty about their baby's being born sick or premature. While some families have time to prepare, others are caught totally offguard. The speed of events leaves them disoriented. In this state of numbing disequilibrium, they must adapt to the normal stress of the postpartum period and the new and added stress that accompanies having their baby in the intensive care nursery. For many families, this stress is further exacerbated if the baby must be transferred to another hospital. This may be as close as the next county or hundreds of miles away.

Mrs. D has had an entirely normal first pregnancy, and looks forward to a natural childbirth experience in April. In the first week of January, she feels back pain and experiences a leaking of amniotic fluid. She calls her obstetrician and then, with her husband, goes to the hospital. An hour later, she gives birth to a 2-lb infant, 12 weeks before term. She sees her son, Daniel, only briefly before he is transported to an intensive care nursery across the city.

Mrs. D becomes fearful and teary. Although she and her husband are given information about the baby, she has difficulty comprehending what the doctors tell her. Mr. D wants to comfort and support her, to call family members to let them know what had happened. They agree, however, that he should follow the ambulance to the intensive care nursery to be with the baby. Mr. D feels bad about leaving his wife, unsure of what to tell the family, and confused and worried about his baby.

When he arrives at the Intensive Care Nursery, he finds himself in a brightly lighted beehive of activity. Surrounded by machines, monitors, and staff is his son, who seems even smaller and more fragile than he remembers.

Mr. D, exhausted from the events of the past 4 hours, unready and unprepared, nonetheless begins his orientation to the nursery and his premature son. In the hours and days that follow, he and his wife learn about the language and the environment of neonatal medicine. They learn about the development of the premature infant and about how to care for their baby and themselves. They prepare themselves for the choices and decisions that need to be made.

NEEDS OF THE HIGH-RISK FAMILY

One of the major challenges for the health care team is to support families through a perinatal crisis. Each family brings its own personal combination of coping skills, mechanisms, and style to the problems it confronts.

The physiologic changes during normal pregnancy and birth are well documented. Families stretch to adapt and to accommodate to the birth of a new baby. When a pregnancy becomes high-risk (when there is a possibility of fetal death, abnormality, or serious illness in the antepartum or newborn period), normal adaptation is disrupted (Penticuff, 1982).

Maladaptation leads to family stress and increased risk of both short-term and long-lasting problems in the relationship between the parents, and between the mother and infant. The possibilities for guilt and blame abound. While once a personal and intimate experience, the pregnancy becomes a time shared with health care "teams". Even when the care providers are well trained, skilled, and sensitive, they are nonetheless strangers with whom parents must share an intrinsically private experience.

Often, nurses and physicians know more about a family's pregnancy than the family members themselves. This is a fact of life for the hospitalized high-risk mother and a phenomenon that heightens parents' feelings of alienation and loss of control. In the transition from normal to high-risk pregnancy, adaptation depends on understanding the degree of risk to the mother, fetus, or newborn, the available support systems, problem-solving skills, and ultimately on the resolution of the high-risk situation (Penticuff, 1982).

A basic strategy of adaptation to a threatening event is to understand it. Concrete information is crucial to the ability of parents in the midst of a perinatal crisis to begin the adaptation process. Information about obstetrical and neonatal problems is often technical and complicated, and the parents are often fearful, medicated, or ill. Communication, although vital to adaptation, easily becomes confused and confounding to the fragile family. Important information about a pregnancy or baby's status should be conveyed *as soon as judiciously possible* to family members.

Usually, parents want to hear news together. Sometimes they want a close friend or extended family member with them. The primary physician, nurse, or social worker should be present, so that when information is reviewed later, it will be consistent with the first presentation. With some insight into the family's dynamics, the primary support person can answer their questions and provide reassurance in the most appropriate and effective way.

Ideally, conferences with families should be held away from the busyness and interruptions of patient care areas. An office space or meeting room with ample seating is optimal. Visual aids, diagrams, photographs, and even printouts on a particular issue can be helpful to nervous parents who are trying to follow what is being said.

Preparation for surgery or imminent delivery is made easier when the nurse or physician verbally describes the process of the next few hours or days, so that the parents can anticipate events. If one can first gently elicit from a family their understanding of what is happening, incomplete information can be supplemented, misunderstandings can be corrected, and emphasis added where needed. Parents will often then be able to focus on the area of greatest concern and organize their thoughts more concretely.

Preparing the Antepartum Family for the Birth of a Preterm Infant

Although the prospect of preterm delivery may have already been discussed as a possibility, the reality of the imminent birth of a baby 2–3 months prematurely can be terrifying. Desensitizing family members to some of the most unsettling aspects of the newborn period can be helpful.

After the high-risk obstetrical concerns have been addressed, attention needs to be focused on the premature infant and neonatal care. A brief overview of prematurity and how the baby's various organ systems may not yet be able to function independently at a given gestational age helps parents understand the need for specialized technical intervention. For example, parents may benefit from a description of ventilatory support (using some of the new language they have been learning) if a 30-week gestation baby with immature lungs is anticipated. The fact that their baby will not eat with a nipple until he is closer to term is information that they can comprehend and will help shape the vision of what is to come. A picture of a small baby on a respirator or a book or brochure about intensive care nurseries might enhance this. Finally, whenever possible, parents and the extended family need an opportunity to tour the intensive care unit. Once they have heard its sounds and experienced its energy, the nursery becomes less threatening. Once they have seen premature babies and understand what is happening to them, their own prospective experience seems less frightening.

Family Meetings

Whatever the particulars of the medical data presented, meeting with a family is a critical opportunity to familiarize them with the hospital's environment and its language. Taking a few moments with a family to assess their level of understanding and identify areas of needed education is a major step in helping them focus their attention, mobilize their coping strengths, and adapt to their situation. With increasing mastery of the medical information, parents can better advocate for themselves and their infant. They can become active participants in decision making about the infant's care and feel a sense of control over events. When feelings of alienation are thus reduced or overcome, parents can project themselves beyond the present circumstances and begin to adapt and plan. They can begin to prepare themselves for a pregnancy that may require weeks or months of bedrest for the mother. They can ready themselves to accept an abnormal baby or brace themselves for their infant's impending death.

The advantages gained by presenting medical information with several team members together are great. There is a large amount of information to be conveyed. When the patient is a sick preterm infant, his or her condition is constantly changing. When parents receive piecemeal information from various caregivers, each with a different vantage point, they perceive different and sometimes seemingly conflicting reports.

Family meetings become a time for everyone to come together at a fixed point in time and clarify what has happened and what can be expected. The meetings provide a perspective for families and for caregivers as well; they offer an opportunity to step back from the technical aspects of blood gas results, ventilator settings, and heart murmurs to gain an overview of the circumstances that will help them foresee oncoming events and support the parents as they look forward.

Family meetings are cumbersome, and finding a time when everyone can come requires effort. Sometimes a physician will stop by a bedside to share information hurriedly with a family about a working diagnosis. Sometimes a nurse who sees parents may decide to share new information gained during report. Although this spontaneous transfer of specific information may be satisfactory, families can become confused, or they may be unable to integrate the new information into the overall picture of what is happening.

When a family member asks, for example, about a baby's status, he or she may want to know whether the baby's condition is better or worse. However, families may also request specific information about details of medical management, such as blood pressures, ventilator settings, or hematocrit. It is always helpful to clarify what information is being sought. One way to get clues is to ask the parent what his or her last information was. Primary nurses are usually the team members who are best equipped to convey ongoing information. They are with the patient most often and, over time, they become most adept at presenting information at the level most suitable for a family's ability to comprehend. In reality, families may come into contact with many different nurses during the 21 shifts each week and not develop the same kind of relationship that is possible with a consistent primary nurse.

Maintaining continuity of communication is not only good medical care but supportive to families. Even when numerous nurses are involved in a baby's care, parents are reassured if they hear that an identified primary nurse has communicated their baby's likes and dislikes or particular behavioral responses to new caregivers. When a father tells a primary nurse that his baby would not have had a setback if the nurse had been there on the weekend, he is conveying a number of things. He is letting her know how much he trusts her care. He is also telling her how fearful he is when his baby is under someone else's care. When he asks a new nurse for information about his baby, he is not only seeking new information but is also testing to be sure she knows and understands his baby. It is important to respond rather than just react. The motivation for the questions asked should be understood so that, along with providing facts, the underlying concern can be addressed.

Telephone Communication

The telephone provides a critical link between family members and their hospitalized newborn, and can provide extended family support to parents far from home with their sick baby. However, telephone communication of medical information can sometimes be hazardous. Most obviously lacking is the ability to assess the nonverbal cues that signal that a parent or family member is or is not understanding the information given. Again, asking what the latest information the person received not only facilitates continuity and accurate response, but provides direction for the most satisfactory level of communication at which the response is needed.

For example, when Mrs. J called the nursery to inquire about her baby's recovery after surgery, she was told that her baby's nurse was too busy to come to the telephone. The nurse taking the call, who was totally unfamiliar with Mrs. J, said that "the IV in the baby's head had blown", and efforts were in progress to find a site and start a new line. She also said that the nurse would call back when she had time.

Mrs. J was so fearful that she left home and drove 3 hours in the middle of the night to see her baby. She thought the IV fluids had spilled into the baby's brain. Referring to a scalp vein i.v. as "in the head" is verbal shorthand. In a busy intensive care nursery setting, a special language exists that abbreviates verbal communication among team members. However, it can confuse and mislead families. In the case of Mrs. J, it was alarming.

When medical personnel speak directly with an antepartum mother or anxious family member, misunderstood communication may be revealed by a blank look or furrowed brow. When communicating by telephone, nurses should be prudent in their choice of words, keep sentences simple, and elicit periodic feedback to assess understanding by the caller. If a baby's nurse cannot come to the telephone, family members assume the reason is some crisis related to their infant. Anxiety can be allayed if the family can be told that the baby's condition is stable and an approximate time given when the baby's own nurse (or doctor) can call back.

Changes in Status

If the status of a patient's condition changes abruptly, communication with families should be initiated by a member of the team with all due speed. Expressing the information about the change within the context of the patient's overall course is helpful. Family members need to be told how worrisome a change is for the recovery process. Is this a setback? Does this change alter the anticipated outcome? Is this a life-threatening event? Inability to grasp the significance of bad news is a common form of unconscious denial, and prevents the hearer from integrating what is being said. Providing an opportunity for questions and making a follow-up call after the family member has had an opportunity to process the new information, or the offer of a meeting, can leave communication open and present coping choices for the family.

It is helpful to discuss medical changes within the context of other babies' or mothers' experience in similar circumstances. Being told whether a change is usual or unexpected helps families comprehend and adjust to the change. If a change is worrisome, families need to be informed. The cumulative effect of communication with families determines how realistically they perceive events and how well prepared they are for subsequent ones. With information and guided understanding, families can participate more confidently in decision making. Even in the case of seriously ill infants, parents can begin to assume an advocacy role and undertake parenting tasks, and tolerate better the stresses of crises that arise. The parent, at best, becomes a participating member of the health care team rather than a passive observer.

SUPPORTING THE FAMILY

The family's process through crisis toward resolution is continuous. The health care professional, and in particular the nurse, must determine (sometimes in the course of a single shift) just how far the family has progressed in understanding and accepting the medical situation, what their needs for support are, and how to help effectively. The following are some guidelines and ideas on which to develop nursing involvement and helpful support.

There are various aspects and approaches for providing support for families during a perinatal crisis. Gentle warmth, empathy, compassion, and understanding are critical components. How families manifest stress also varies. The nurse, by refraining from judgment, allows a family to respond within the context of their own lives. There is no "appropriate" behavior or set of norms for response to crisis. A description of behavior as "inappropriate" usually means that a response differs from the observer's personal concepts of the "right" way to respond. If care providers bring to their interaction with families a preconceived set of behavioral expectations, the establishment of a trusting and communicative relationship is impaired. Limits should not be set on responsive behaviors, other than on those that disrupt staff, the functioning of the unit, or disturb other patients.

Facilitating adaptation to the perinatal crisis is the main goal of supportive care. The family system, once it has accommodated to the birth of a sick newborn or the stress of pregnancy complications, resumes its equilibrium. An unsuccessful crisis resolution is one in which a family functions less well than before the crisis situation (Baird, 1979). The goal, thus, is to help the family reestablish its customary level of mental health.

Frequently, close friends and family members are the most capable resource for helping parents toward this end. The involvement of other significant family and friends can be both comforting and reinforcing. Early intervention from close social contacts can be invaluable in easing the transition from hospital to home.

Sometimes, because of logistics (distance from home, difficulty visiting the hospital, or a degree of social isolation), parents rely on members of the health care team for support and help in solving problems. Nurses have the most contact with family members and are most often called upon to meet these needs.

Counseling Suggestions

Listening well is the crux of counseling. Finding a time and place where distractions are minimal and attention can be undivided is essential.

Families who are under great stress and overwhelmed by circumstances need reinforcement of their coping strengths. The nurse must recognize the magnitude of the disruption the family faces and be able to assess how they have managed matters thus far. This information then enables the nurse to reinforce the family's own coping systems and encourage confidence in their ability to assume control of their lives outside the immediate medical crisis (Baird, 1979).

Counseling or supporting a family in an acute care hospital setting often involves breaking down other problems into definable, time-limited, attainable goals. Once a family defines what is most problematic at a given time, options for solution need consideration. The nurse draws on her experiences with other families in a similar situation. In doing so, parents see that quite different approaches are permissible and acceptable. Families need to find solutions that work best for them.

An example of this is the struggle parents confront in leaving a premature baby in the hospital and going home when the mother is discharged. The postpartum nurse can acknowledge a mother's reluctance about discharge. She can encourage discussion about the baby who must remain in the intensive care nursery. She can help the mother identify her ambivalence about leaving, and she can appreciate the mother's commitment to her baby. The nurse can listen to what the mother is most worried about and assess her understanding of the baby's condition. She can urge a parent to talk with the medical care team to gain reassurance about the baby's status, and she can initiate an opportunity to do so. The postpartum nurse can help find ways for the parents to stay close to the baby if the infant's condition warrants this. Finally, the nurse can give "permission" for parents to leave. Opportunities for contact in the form of visits and phone calls can be affirmed and recommended. Thus, by learning good listening skills, developing her capabilities to provide encouragement (not advice), and recognizing avenues for solution of problems, the nurse is able to become a highly effective provider of supportive patient care.

Intervention can be nonverbal or indirect. Nurses can demonstrate behaviors or communication skills that a family can emulate (Miles, 1979). Parents who are fearful and apprehensive about touching their baby and holding their son or daughter can learn techniques and confidence from the nurse who holds, feeds, talks to, and fondles the infant. She can encourage the developing parent–infant relationship by pointing out their infant's behavioral responses to these actions. By listening carefully and being available, the nurse can provide empathy and solace. The nurse's sympathetic presence itself can be a therapeutic advantage to families in crisis.

Referrals for Long-term Support

The shock and disequilibrium experienced by families in perinatal crisis can sometimes result in depression and inability to function. This is part of the normal process of grieving at the loss of a normal pregnancy and the idealized perfect baby.

Crisis sometimes worsens underlying problems in a marriage. A crisis such as the preterm birth of a baby may cause a parent with fragile mental health to decompensate. Special consideration, in concert with a mental health professional, needs to be given to such families, and referrals for long-term therapy need to be introduced.

In the main, families adjust. Parents are the best ones to judge when and if they need outside intervention to help them deal with their problems. In response to the nurse's eagerness to provide referral to professional mental health counseling resources, the parents may come to think that they are not able to manage themselves. To parents who have experienced a profound sense of loss of control over such central events as pregnancy and childbirth, this can be a discouraging message. Instead, information about resources, ranging from parent support groups to psychiatrists, needs to be made known to families. Parents can then seek out the appropriate kind of support or help when they themselves deem this type of intervention is warranted.

PREPARATION FOR DISCHARGE

Often, families who have adapted to an infant's need for intensive neonatal care, again experience disequilibrium at the prospect of leaving the hospital. Implicit in the process of discharging an infant from the intensive care nursery is the transferrence of care from the medical team back to the parents and family. Some units have identified discharge planners who work with families to assure that planning and coordination of resources for the infant and the family are accomplished and continuity of care maintained. In others units, discharge planning may be coordinated by a primary care nurse.

Since discharge from the medical setting is a transition from dependence on the medical care team to independence from it, parents need to formulate a plan for discharge that works well for them. Families differ in their need to resume their independence and privacy as they vary in their feelings of confidence and competence. Parents may resent the intrusion of a community health nurse coming to their home and may prefer to take their baby to their doctor's office for more frequent check-ups. Others may be overwhelmed at the prospect of repeated visits to the doctor and welcome the convenience and privacy of having follow-up home visits. In any case, whenever possible, choices should be presented.

The most complete and competent discharge plan may fail if it is arranged without sufficient discussion and approval by the family. The conscientious nurse who feels the need to enroll a family for every resource that might be helpful may overwhelm the family in transition. One single contact in the home community at the time of discharge may be quite sufficient. A capable public health nurse, in concert with the family's physician, can assess needs over time and introduce resources gradually as the need for them becomes apparent to the care providers and the family.

Fortunately, a vast array of resources are available throughout the United States. Parents are effective in finding resources in their communities with the help of friends, relatives, and contact with others in similar situations. Parent-to-parent support groups are often the resource of choice, although the timing of this and other kinds of referrals differs.

Parents, at the time of discharge, may be amenable to meeting others in early labor or who are at home with a preterm infant. Some are eager for this kind of contact early in the crisis. As with other forms of help, parents need to know it is available. It is the parent who must decide how much help is needed and acceptable.

There are exceptions, of course, such as cases in which drug or alcohol abuse and apparent dysfunction threaten the health and safety of an infant. These situations (by law in most case) should be referred to the local child protection agency, and should be managed by a social worker. Assessment of the home and family here is of paramount importance. When problems such as these are contributing causes of preterm labor and birth, sickness, or even drug withdrawal of the newborn, interaction with families becomes strained.

SUMMARY

High-risk families are those whose pregnancies and childbirth experiences are not normal. Nurses and other health care providers can help to minimize stress for families during this period of crisis. With the use of clear communication, both in conveying information and supportive listening, nurses can help families maintain or regain their equilibrium. When this is successful, families can become active participants in the health care process rather than passive recipients. By helping families to identify and solve problems, nurses can support them in facing the painful realities of perinatal crisis situations. When families can make informed decisions about their lives, their ability to assume control and maintain the family's integrity is enhanced.

REFERENCES

Baird, S. F. 1979. Crisis intervention strategies. In *High risk parenting: Nursing assessment and strategies for assessment*, ed. S. H. Johnson, Philadelphia: J. P. Lippincott.

Consolvo, C. A. 1986. Relieving parental anxiety in the care-by-parent unit. *J. Obstet. Gynecol. Neonatal Nurs.* 15:154–159.

Cox, C. L.; Sullivan, J. A.; and Roghmann, K. J. 1983. A conceptual explanation of risk-reduction behavior and intervention development. *Nurs. Res.* 33:168–173.

Crnic, K. A.; Greenberg, M. T.; Ragozin, A. S.; Robinson, N. M., and Basham, R. B. 1983. Effects of stress and social support on mothers and premature and full-term infants. *Child Dev.* 54:209–217.

Cronenwett, L. R. 1985. Network structure, social support, and psychological outcomes of pregnancy. *Nurs. Res.* 34:93–99.

Cutrona, C. E. 1983. Causal attributions and perinatal depression. *J. Abnorm. Psychol.* 92:161–172.

Georgas, J.; Giakoumaki, E.; Georgoulias, N.; Koumandakis, E.; and Kaskarelis, D. 1984. Psychosocial stress and its relation to obstetrical complications. *Psychother. Psychosom.* 41:200–206.

Goodman, J. R., and Sauve, R. S. 1985. High risk infant: Concerns of the mother after discharge. *Birth.* 12:235–242.

Gorsuch, R. L., and Key, M. K. 1974. Abnormalities of pregnancy as a function of anxiety and life stress. *Psychom. Med.* 36:352–362.

Gyves, M. T. 1985. The psychosocial impact of high risk pregnancy. *Adv. Psychosom. Med.* 12:71–80.

Johnson, S. H. 1979. Behavior modification strategies. In *High risk parenting: Nursing assessment and strategies for assessment*, ed. S. H. Johnson. Philadelphia: J. P. Lippincott.

Kemp, V. H., and Page, D. K. 1987. Maternal prenatal attachment in normal and high-risk pregnancies. *J. Obstet. Gynecol. Neonatal Nurs.* 16:179–184.

Leander, K., and Pettett, G. 1986. Parental response to the birth of a high-risk neonate: Dynamics and management. *Physical & Occupational Therapy in Pediatrics.* 6:205–16.

Mercer, R. T.; May, K.; Ferketich, S.; and DeJoseph, J. 1986. Theoretical models for studying the effect of antepartum stress on the family. *Nurs. Res.* 35:339–346.

Miles, S. M. 1979. Counseling strategies. In *Risk parenting: Nursing assessment and strategies for assessment*, ed. S. H. Johnson. Philadelphia: J. P. Lippincott.

Miller, B. C., and Sollie, D. L. 1980. Normal stresses during the transition to parenthood. *Family Relations.* Oct.: 459–465.

Minde, K. K. 1984. The impact of prematurity on the later behavior of children and their families. *Clin. Perinatol.* 11:227–244.

Mitchell, K., and Mills, N. M. 1983: Is the sensitive period in parent–infant bonding overrated? *Pediatr. Nurs.* Mar–Apr: 9(2) 91–94.

Orkow, B. 1985. Implementation of a family stress checklist. *Child Abuse Negl.* 9:405–410.

Penticuff, J. H. 1982. Psychologic implications in high-risk pregnancy. *Nurs. Clin. Nth Am.* 17:69–78.

Peterson, E. R.; Bento, S.; and Chance, G. W.; 1987. Maternal emotional responses to preterm birth. *Am. J. Orthopsychiatry.* 57:15–21.

Petrick, J. M. 1984. Postpartum depression: Identification of high-risk mothers. *J. Obstet. Gynecol. Neonatal Nurs.* 13:37–40.

Sims-Jones, N. 1986. Back to the theories: Another way to view mothers of prematures. *Maternal Child Nurs.* 11:394–397.

White, M., and Ritchie, J. 1984. Psychological stressors in antepartum hospitalization: Reports from pregnant women. *Maternal–Child Nurs. J.* 13:47–56.

Wohlreich, M. M. 1986. Psychiatric aspects of high-risk pregnancy. *Psychiatr. Clin. Nth Am.* 10:53–68.

Zeskind, P. S., and Iacino, R. 1984. Effects of maternal visitation to preterm infants in the neonatal intensive care unit. *Child Dev.* 55:1887–1893.

36
Perinatal Loss

BEHAVIORAL OBJECTIVES

Upon completion of this chapter, the reader should be able to:

- Identify the major causes of fetal and neonatal death.

- Discuss the immediate and long-term reactions of parents after a perinatal loss.

- Identify some of the differences in reactions of parents and family members.

- Discuss appropriate tools that facilitate good communication between staff and parents.

- Discuss the rationale for self-help group referrals.

Both before and after confirmation of a pregnancy, plans, dreams, and future hopes are formulated. When a perinatal loss occurs, all future plans and dreams are dashed along with the innocence that accompanies anticipatory expectations. This influences and compounds the loss.

At present, one in five pregnancies ends in miscarriage, and approximately 1 percent of infants die within the first few days of life. These losses are categorized as *perinatal losses*. These statistics, though much improved, require that health care professionals be knowledgeable about the psychologic and physiologic processes that occur and how they affect the families enduring the loss.

COPING WITH LOSS

Adaptation to experiences such as death is influenced by previous similar experiences, expected outcomes, and peripheral support systems. Since most couples are fairly young during the childbearing period they may not have had prior exposure to death. Couples with previous experience in dealing with grief may be able to cope somewhat better than those that have had none (Schneider and Daniel, 1979). This should not imply that the event is less painful, but rather perhaps less frightening.

The maturational level of the parents needs to be considered in evaluating the type of intervention that will be the most beneficial. A 39-year-old woman may exhibit a much profound response to the loss compared with a 16-year-old.

Individual Reactions

Families need to know that the pain associated with perinatal loss diminishes slowly with time. Each member of the family may respond differently. A supportive environment which invites individuals to verbalize how they are feeling about the loss should be encouraged.

Mothers' Reactions

Being unable to bring a pregnancy to term, or being unable to prevent the death of one's own infant, causes mothers to feel like failures. They frequently report that they resent their own bodies, and do not feel in control. Mothers search for reasons to explain why it is they who have been singled out or why they are being punished. Not being able to fulfill a basic biological process, and the uncertainty of the future, creates a very unstable period for the mother. This period may be heightened for some and lessened for others depending on a number of variables, including age, attachment, multiple loss, and predicted prognosis.

Fathers' Reactions

Frequently, fathers are placed in the position of being a care provider and support person rather than afforded support themselves. Situations like this often arise because of the need to return to work, or to care for other children. Traditional roles may also interfere with a father's expression over the loss.

Acknowledgement, and offering support to the father, is especially valuable. It helps him clarify his role and identifies some of his needs. The depth for which he might experience the loss is frequently dependent upon his expectations, attachment, and the duration of the pregnancy.

Siblings' Reactions

Depending upon the age of the surviving children, their reaction may be one of reacting to a disruption in a family routine, or one of fear, guilt, and anger. Brief, honest information geared to their level of understanding should be given. Support and encouragement regarding their own well-being is extremely valuable. Reassurance about their mother's absence and her condition will lessen the anxiety during the crisis period.

Teachers or day care providers should be informed of the situation, and report any change in behavior. Children should be encouraged to express their feelings verbally, artistically, or through play.

Grandparents' Reactions

Grandparents usually respond to the pain and suffering their own children are enduring more so than to the loss of their grandchild. This response frequently causes their children to resent their focus or feel as though the perinatal loss is not being acknowledged properly. Grandparents report that this is sometimes done deliberately, to try and minimize the pain their son or daughter is experiencing. This needs to be communicated to the parents.

Grandparents should be offered support, and their personal loss as a grandparent should be acknowledged.

PHYSIOLOGY OF PERINATAL LOSS

Miscarriage/First Trimester Loss

Miscarriage is the loss of a pregnancy in the first trimester. It is often difficult to establish the etiology, but research has shown that most miscarriages occur as a result of genetically or anatomically defective embryos (Chez et al., 1978). Bright red bleeding with an open cervix is the true sign of a miscarriage, and in most cases perinatal loss is unavoidable. If there is some bleeding but the cervix is closed, bedrest may be the treatment of choice, and the pregnancy may be continued. Tissue cultures may also be carried out to rule out infection or chromosomal anomalies as the cause for the miscarriage. The major tool for diagnosis is ultrasound (see Chapter 13). The gestational sac with the embryonic echo is present at 4–7 weeks gestation. A flattened sac may be normal within the first 2–3 weeks, but it is always considered abnormal beyond 7 weeks gestation (Chez et al., 1978). The real-time scan shows no movement and no heartbeat if the fetus is dead. With the Doppler beaming on the sac, the heartbeat can be heard 40–60 percent of the time from 7 to 8 weeks gestation (Hutson and Fox, 1982). The method of choice for termination once the diagnosis of miscarriage is confirmed is dilation and curettage (D&C). This procedure is considered safe until 12 weeks gestation.

Abortion

An *abortion* is a perinatal loss before 20 weeks gestation. Most abortions occur with fetuses weighing less than 500 g. The etiology for this perinatal loss is not always known, but it may be due to bacterial or viral infection; diabetes; hypertension; premature rupture of the membranes, and the chorioamnionitis that may occur concomitantly; congenital abnormalities; abruptio placentae; or incompetent cervix (Chez et al., 1978). The major diagnostic test is ultrasound, which shows no heart movement (Hutson and Fox, 1982). Termination of pregnancy, if it is not spontaneous, may be done by dilation and evacuation (D&E), by prostaglandin suppositories to induce labor and delivery, or by a pitocin induction. Pitocin induction is slower and usually reserved if one of the other two procedures is contraindicated. D&E can be performed in the outpatient department. Prostaglandin-induced abortion requires admission into the hospital, and it can take up to 24 hours or more for the delivery of the infant, and the mother experiences a long, hard labor.

There are risks and benefits to each procedure. If a D&E is performed, no viewing of the body is available. Sometimes the exact cause of death, e.g. from a cord accident, is not possible to detect, because during the evacuation procedure, the fetus is not always removed intact. The procedure for a D&E is done rapidly. Mothers recover quickly from the procedure with minimum residual physical effects. The induction time-frames of pitocin and prostaglandin are unpredictable. Prostaglandins have many side-effects – nearly 50 percent of women experience vomiting, 36 percent diarrhea, 10 percent headaches, 17 percent chills, and 34 percent transient pyrexia (Southern and Gutknecht, 1976). Prostaglandins are very effective in the induction of labor during the second trimester of pregnancy.

Antepartum Fetal Death

The term *antepartum fetal death* refers to the death of a baby after 20 weeks gestation but before the onset of labor. As with abortion, the etiology is unknown, but death may be due to various maternal or fetal causes. Once the diagnosis of fetal death is confirmed, termination of the pregnancy is by D&E, which is safe up to 26 weeks gestation, by prostaglandin suppository, or by oxytocin induction. If the fetal death occurs late in the pregnancy, the physician may choose to allow the mother to go into labor spontaneously. In about 75 percent of cases spontaneous labor will occur within 2 weeks of the death; in about 90 percent of cases within 3 weeks (Chez et al., 1978).

Genetic Abortion

Genetic abortions are abortions performed after a diagnostic procedure or test to confirm that the developing fetus is imperfect. Tests used in making the diagnosis include ultrasound, alpha feto protein serum test, amniocentesis and, the newest procedure, the chorionic villi sampling test (CVS). The mother and her partner are counseled as to the test results and their predictive value, and they may select the method of termination with the lowest risk and the highest benefit.

Stillbirth

Stillbirth is the term used for an infant not born alive. Stillbirth may be differentiated from antepartum fetal death, since stillbirth refers to an infant who might have been potentially viable (after 26 weeks). However, both stillbirth and antepartum fetal death can and are used interchangeably. If the infant is of full-term gestation, stillbirth is an unexpected event to the parents. The majority of stillbirths are of unknown etiology. Delivery of the infant is accomplished by induction or spontaneous labor. As with any antepartum fetal death, in

75 percent of cases spontaneous labor occurs within 2 weeks of the death, 90 percent within 3 weeks (Chez et al., 1978). Careful monitoring of the mother's condition is necessary to prevent the mother from developing septicemia if the pregnancy is allowed to await spontaneous labor. Induction may also be encouraged so that autopsy and tissue sampling can proceed and possibly help determine the cause of death.

Neonatal Death

Neonatal death is death that occurs after birth but before 28 days of life. This type of death usually results from premature birth, birth defects incompatible with life, or neonatal asphyxia.

THE PSYCHOLOGY OF PERINATAL LOSS

In order for the staff, physicians, nurses, and social workers to be able to present appropriate information and to understand the needs of families experiencing perinatal loss, they need to be aware of their own feelings and attitudes. They should have resources within the community to draw upon, and have policies or guidelines to help them intervene with the family in crisis.

First Trimester

Mothers who have lost a pregnancy in the first trimester report that they were given very little support from family, friends, and health care workers. They generally complain that their loss being so common, was generally dismissed. For some women and their partners an early miscarriage is not a traumatic ordeal, but for others it represents a profound loss. Here, as in other situations, the nurse should assess how each individual is responding to a miscarriage. Open-ended questions facilitate good communication. The nurse should also be aware of nonverbal responses. For example:

1. Ask directly: "What are you feeling, how are you feeling?"
2. Acknowledge and give feedback to responses to your questions (nodding of the head, eye contact, asking for further explanations).
3. Acknowledge their loss. A simple "I'm sorry about what happened to you" is sufficient if time is a limiting factor, or if you cannot think of what to say.

Second Trimester

Having passed the first trimester, parents in this group often express relief and a sense of false security. A lot of guilt plagues these parents. If an infection is associated with the fetal death, mothers in particular feel responsible.

Many parents in this group choose to see their small babies and are quite surprised as to how developed they are. Unfortunately, few of their friends or family are given this opportunity, and mistakenly refer to the loss in terms that are upsetting to the parents.

Third Trimester

Commonly, parents report that after having reached the third trimester, their concerns were more focused on labor, delivery, and parenting issues, and that when a loss occurs they feel totally out of control and overwhelmed.

If the infant dies because of anomalies, the parents must grieve the baby they expected and indeed the baby that was delivered. If the death occurs during the laboring process or after postdates, the parents frequently fear that death could have been prevented.

Neonatal Death

The death of a neonate, especially when unexpected, is extremely sad and difficult. The shock that accompanies this event may interfere with the family's ability to exert their preferences. The staff need to be sensitive and realize that parents are often unsure as to what is available to them or even what their role or expected behavior is. Offering them the opportunity to express their individual needs and concerns is extremely important.

Genetic Abortion

Probably the hardest thing a couple will ever encounter is the news received, most often over the telephone, that all is not genetically correct with their unborn child. Others find out this information while undergoing ultrasound evaluation. Although parents receive counseling before genetic screening tests, they never think they will be the ones faced with the news that something is wrong.

Isolation often surrounds the parents going through a genetic abortion. Many times they choose to tell family members and friends that the pregnancy terminated spontaneously. Fear of disapproval prevents them from disclosing the facts surrounding their loss. Though parents actively participate in the decision to terminate the pregnancy, for most it is the hardest decision they will ever have to make.

Subsequent Pregnancies

After a family has gone through a pregnancy and it has terminated unsuccessfully, they are naturally a little apprehensive about considering and then proceeding with another pregnancy. Many variables, e.g. medical risk factors, length of pregnancy, support, and predictive prognosis, influence the decision to get pregnant again. Parents need a great deal of support and information to help identify risk factors and complications from anxiety-induced symptoms during subsequent pregnancies.

Some of the concerns and feelings are expressed in the following story:

A Portrait of Emily

I vividly remember the first year after Emily was born. It seemed like 5 years packed into one. In 1 year I had felt and experienced so many emotions that were new to me. I was a different person, perhaps forever. All of this in one short year following Emily's birth and death just a few short hours later.

As the months went by I did not cry as much as I had in the beginning. I made it through days even weeks without tears. Sleep was easier and more restful. Lovemaking returned to my life; however, not with all the passion as had been there before. Many times our closest moments ended with tears. We did not speak, we just held each other closer.

Some things were changing, some never would. It's difficult to pinpoint an exact time but we finally realized we wanted to try again. We wanted a baby. Not Emily, but another child, with his or her own characteristics and future.

In the weeks that followed our decision I became more aware of my body than ever before. I was looking for those first "signs" that follow conception. Were my breasts tender or not? Was I especially tired or was it my imagination? There was such disappointment and "grief" at the onset of my period. Three months later no period. Vague symptoms and yes a positive home pregnancy test. I was pregnant again. Joy and disappointment; fear, uncertainty. It was difficult to sort out my feelings. There were moments I knew I had made a mistake. Then I realized I wanted a baby but I did not want another pregnancy.

My husband and my friends seemed to welcome this pregnancy. I heard over and over how great I looked, and what a great pregnancy this was. I believe this was done to reassure me but it implied Emily had died because things were not as great during my time I had with her. I resented some of their superficial optimism.

I decided to attend a parent support group held locally: a group run by a hospital to put parents in touch with other parents who have experienced the loss of a baby from miscarriage, stillbirth, or genetic abortion. I needed to talk with someone who understood my feelings.

A conscious decision had been made to create a new life but it reminded me so much of the life that was forever gone. It felt good at the meeting to share Emily's story out loud. I could say out loud how much I missed her. I was hopeful that the future would bring a new healthy child, or I would not have become pregnant again. I was also afraid after the birth of a new child Emily would be forgotten. I knew for me she would always be my first, and hold a special spot in my life.

My physician was great. He knew I needed more than monthly visits, even at first. I needed a lot of reassurance that things were proceeding alright.

We had an autopsy done on Emily. I was grateful for that. Though it did not give us all the answers for why she had died, a lot of the information reassured us that we were not at any greater risk for a repeat problem with our subsequent child.

Standing at the checkout stand at the grocery store during my eighth month, the clerk asked me if I was expecting my first child. I chose to say yes. I did not think he cared to hear Emily's story. I know I handled the situation correctly but I felt so guilty. It was though I had denied Emily and her existence.

Labor was particularly stressful. Except for one nurse who apparently "didn't get the word", the staff understood we were not the typical happy, expectant parents to be. It was such a stressful time for us, and we were thankful that they seemed to understand.

Our new daughter Amanda was beautiful. Pink, breathing, crying, and yes she opened her eyes. Dark beautiful eyes through which we could see a future.

Amanda will know of her sister: through this, maybe her life will be enriched.

Experiencing the loss of a baby is probably the worst thing that could happen to a couple. Having supportive medical and nursing staff makes it easier. Peer support groups make life bearable and give hope for the future.

Nursing Intervention

Nursing intervention to a family in crisis is not limited to performing tasks in a skillful manner. It includes being aware of options and choices available to families experiencing perinatal loss and making sure that in a timely fashion these are offered to them.

Choices and options that pertain to seeing and holding the dead infant are included here. Most families are so unprepared and unfamiliar with hospital procedures and the hospital environment that they do not request to see and hold their baby. This omission causes a great deal of regret later on. Therefore, it is important to suggest to a family that they see and hold their infant.

Photographs, a lock of hair, footprints, and any tangible evidence of the infant should be preserved for the family. This should be done even if at first the parents do not request or feel they will want such items. They can be kept with the patient's records should the parents change their minds and request them at a later date.

Figure 36–1 shows a sample checklist developed for use by the nurse to assure that everything is taken care of when a stillborn or neonatal death occurs. Not only is the reminder of the hospital paperwork important, but a reminder of what should be done for the parents is also helpful to the nurse dealing with this difficult situation.

The Health Care Team

Caring for families suffering a perinatal loss can be a difficult yet rewarding assignment. To lessen the burden on the health care worker it is important to keep in mind the following:

1. Being a good listener is sometimes more beneficial than having all the right answers.
2. People are more alike than different.
3. What you don't say probably won't hurt you.
4. Your simple presence and the fact you care is helpful.
5. You cannot fix what has happened, you can only make it easier to bear.

Providing Information

Information provided to families in a clinical setting should be brief, timely, and without ambiguity. Initially the parents are unable to take in a great deal of information. Mothers and fathers at this time may find it difficult to make decisions. They may need to hear from several staff members the same message before being able to grasp the situation. They should be given as much time and privacy as possible to explore options, procedures, and expected outcomes.

Case Presentation

Real-time ultrasound confirmed the fetal demise of Sherry's fetus at 28 weeks gestation. While the machine was being removed the physician told Sherry "the baby's heart has stopped beating". The doctor then asked the nurse to transfer Sherry to labor and delivery. After the doctor left the room Sherry asked the nurse "what will they do to start my baby's heart?"

The information the doctor gave Sherry was not sufficient to convey his findings. Sometimes stress, language barriers, hearing deficits, or unfamiliar terms interfere with communication. It is important to use precise simple terms, and to assess the patient's level of understanding.

Self-help Organizations

Peer support groups following a perinatal death provide a healthy environment to facilitate the grief process (Brezin, 1982). Without such an environment many couples find the disruption in their lives nearly unbearable. A support group may be the bridge to begin the processing of a perinatal loss (see Fig. 36–2).

Feelings can be dealt with in an open and supportive manner. Ideas and suggestions for overcoming obstacles are offered from those individuals who have experienced similar problems and losses. Groups provide an atmosphere which is sensitive and educational (Borg and Lasker, 1981). They are becoming increasingly more common and accepted by lay people and health care professionals (Mereness and Taylor, 1973).

Sharing "the story", and talking about the baby is extremely common. It seems to help process the event, and make it more real. This in turn seems to help incorporate the experience into the individual's life (Kirksey, 1982). Groups encourage the sharing of stories. Writing about the experience also provides a healthy outlet. This is one mothers' story (reprinted with permission):

The Death and Birth of Our Son

Thursday, November 13, 1980, I had an appointment at the hospital for my weekly ultrasound and non-

Place on mother's chart. Not a permanent part of the chart.

CHECKLIST
(Liveborn and Stillborn)

Not a permanent part of the chart.

Did you:	Yes	No
1) Addressograph the Notification of Death with the mother's (or baby's) plate?	☐	☐
2) Note the time and date of death on the Notification of Death?	☐	☐
3) Write "stillborn" in red across the front of the Notification of Death (if stillborn)?	☐	☐
4) Check with the M.D. regarding whether it's a coroner's case?	☐	☐
5) Notify the switchboard operator?	☐	☐
6) Check with the M.D. regarding autopsy?	☐	☐
Does he or she want one?	☐	☐
If so, did you have the parent(s) sign two (2) autopsy permits?	☐	☐
Are the permits on the mother's chart?	☐	☐

If not, where are they? _____
(Baby's chart/Med. Rec./Pathology)

	Yes	No
7) Check with the family regarding the disposition of the remains?	☐	☐
Did you have the parent(s) sign two (2) copies of the Retain and Dispose permits?	☐	☐
If so, are the permits on the mother's chart?	☐	☐

If not, where are they? _____
(Baby's chart/Med. Rec./Pathology)

	Yes	No
Does the family want a private burial?	☐	☐
8) Take a picture of baby? (Use the black and white camera from nursery. Label the picture(s) with the baby's name and date. Offer the pictures to parent(s). If the parent(s) don't want them, save the pictures in an envelope to be added to Fetal Demise file.)	☐	☐
9) Take footprints of the baby? (Place them on the crib card obtained from nursery. Offer them to the parent(s). If the parent(s) don't want them, save the footprints in an envelope to be added to Fetal Demise file.)	☐	☐

Did you:	Yes	No
10) Give the parent(s) a copy of "When HELLO Means Goodbye"? (available in L & D)	☐	☐
11) Give parent(s) a SAND (Support After Neonatal Death) brochure and referral?	☐	☐
12) Allow the parent(s) time alone with infant (if desired)?	☐	☐
13) Call the orderly to remove the body?	☐	☐
Did you give him or her the Notification of Death to take to the nursing office?	☐	☐

If not, where is it? _____

14) Complete these charting tasks?

a) **Stillborn**

	Yes	No
1. Did you note what forms were signed on the Infant Newborn Sheet (N-6)?	☐	☐
2. Did you chart the weight and length of the body?	☐	☐
3. Did you chart whether the parent(s) saw or held the infant?	☐	☐
4. Did you chart when the body was taken to the morgue and by whom?	☐	☐
5. Did you write "stillborn" in red in the Apgar section of N-6?	☐	☐

b) **Liveborn**

	Yes	No
1. Did you note the weight and length of the baby on the Infant Newborn Sheet?	☐	☐
2. In nurse's notes in the Newborn Chart, did you note what forms were signed?	☐	☐
The time of pronouncement of death?	☐	☐
3. Label the body with the crib card? Wrap and tape the body in a baby blanket and label it with another crib card?	☐	☐
4. Note when the body was taken to the morgue and by whom?	☐	☐
5. Send the Newborn Chart to Medical Records?	☐	☐

FIGURE 36–1. Checklist developed to assist nurses to ensure that all requirements are fulfilled.
SOURCE: Obstetrics Department, Alta Bates Hospital, Berkeley, California.

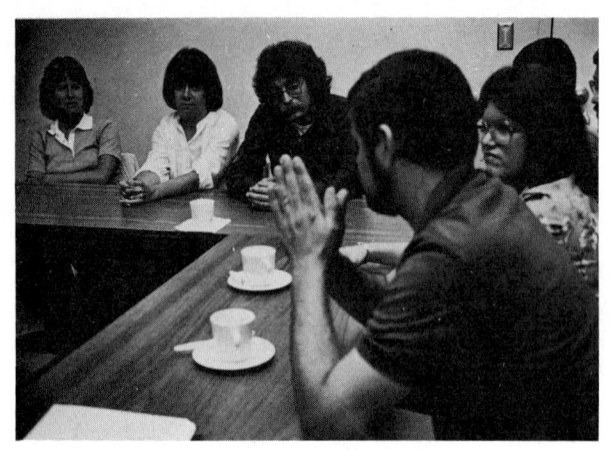

FIGURE 36–2. Parents in support group.

stress tests. The same technician who had done my first two ultrasound tests (at 5 weeks and 8 weeks) was the one who took the pictures. After the technician used the smaller machine, she asked me if I'd felt the baby move recently. I couldn't remember feeling any movement since Wednesday afternoon. I knew right then that something was wrong. The technician told me that she was going to call the doctor. Again, I knew something was seriously wrong. As I waited for the doctor, I think I realized the baby's heart wasn't beating. I knew that the ultrasound equipment showed the baby's heartbeat. The doctor arrived and checked the ultrasound scope. Again, I could see there was no heartbeat.

The doctor sat down next to me and told me that my baby was dead. I remember he said something about deformities probably being the cause of the baby's death. I was horrified by the news and didn't want to believe it. With each week of delay of labor, I had become more and more optimistic about our baby's chances. I was thinking in terms of how long the baby would be in the intensive care nursery, rather than life versus death. The doctor called Jim (my husband) and told him about the baby and also told my mother. My mother came in and said something about it being better that the baby died since it wasn't going to be normal. I didn't feel like it was better. The ultrasound technicians were very sympathetic and allowed me to stay in the ultrasound room until I felt ready to go up to the doctor's office.

My mom and I went upstairs to the doctor's waiting room. My mother talked about everything but the baby. The doctor's receptionist moved us to an examining room. While we were waiting for the doctor, Jim arrived. We held each other and cried for our baby. The doctor came in and gave me a vaginal exam and found I was 4 to 5 cm dilated. He talked to us about inducing labor to which we agreed. I couldn't imagine wanting to continue the pregnancy since the baby was dead. The doctor was too businesslike at a time when our lives were falling apart.

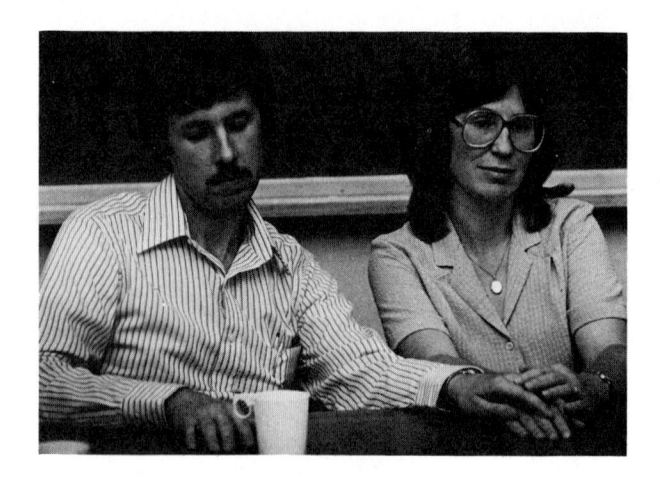

A nurse from labor and delivery (L & D) came upstairs to get me at 12:30. We walked to L & D, and the walk seemed to take forever. We went into labor room 8, which was the same room we used on October 13, the day I was originally hospitalized for premature labor. Jim joined me in the labor room almost immediately. Susie, one of our favorite nurses in L & D, came in and provided us with the comfort of her open arms and a shoulder to cry on. We waited for about an hour for the IV to be started with Pitocin to induce labor. During this time our regular obstetrician called. Jim spoke with him first, and then I spoke with him. As usual he was very sympathetic and supportive. He mentioned how sorry he was that our 5-week ordeal had ended this way. My doctor gave me the option of inducing labor, which I agreed to do. I remember starting to cry again and handing the phone back to Jim. My doctor also said that he would be over to talk with us in about half an hour.

The L & D nurse came in and tried to start my IV. She had the nurse anesthetist start the IV after I screamed because her probing hurt. I remember my doctor coming into the labor room around 2:00 P.M. He told us that the baby probably had something wrong with it. We also discussed what would happen to the baby after the delivery and autopsy.

In addition, he explained the drugs he would use. He gave me Valium through the IV and then used a kind of plastic probe to break my bag of waters. There was a huge flood of fluid onto the bed, and my stomach noticeably decreased in size. The bed linens had to be changed.

Around 3:00 P.M. the nursing shift changed. Jane came in and cried with us. One of the most comforting things was to have the nurses we had gotten to know so well come in and share our grief. To me it was natural and healing to be held by someone and to cry with them. Unfortunately, our friends at home didn't react this way. Mary and Kathy, two more friends from the L & D staff, also came on duty at 3:00. My contractions began to get stronger and closer together. Jim kept reminding me to relax and breathe deeply. He provided pressure on the small of may back, which really helped. Mary was a wonderfully calming influence as the contractions got closer together. I felt like there was no time between contractions. I began to get frightened, and I remember whimpering. Mary told me to ride each contraction as a wave. The idea of a wave distracted me from the pain and helped for the next few contractions. I remember thinking I couldn't stand the contractions much longer. I felt like there was a huge pressure on my bladder and my bowels. I tried to talk Mary into letting me get up to go to the bathroom. Mary checked my cervix and found that I was 10 cm dilated. I began to feel a tremendous urge to push. Mary and Jim coached me to pant to prevent me from pushing. With one of the next urges to push, I really panicked. Mary had left the room to set up the delivery room I guess. The urge to push was a new sensation for me and it really scared me. Momentarily Mary and Kathy arrived with a gurney to take me to the delivery room. I had dilated from 5 to 10 cm in about 1 hour. I hated moving onto the gurney. I remember feeling anger that I was being forced to move. The bed was rolled across the hall to the delivery room.

In the delivery room I had to move to another bed. Again I felt anger at having to move my body. I was frightened at being in a different room. I remember asking where Jim was and feeling a bit panicky without him. Jane was helping Jim put on scrubs. Jim has since told me that my doctor gave me Demerol through my IV although I don't remember it. I wish that I could remember more of the details. My legs were placed in the leg supports. I was upset that the birth was in the sterile delivery room and that my legs were in the stirrups, because I had planned to have such a different birth, with Jim and me in control. Ironically, nothing really mattered since our baby was dead.

Jim arrived with mask, cap, and green outfit, and I didn't recognize him. I didn't have my glasses on, and the drugs made my doctor seem like a shadowy figure who was about 20 feet away. During my earlier hospital stay, I had placed great importance on having my doctor help us with the birth of our baby. I felt so far away from him that I remember thinking afterwards that it didn't matter who the doctor was. I think I was wrong. I'm sure that having him with us made both Jim and me feel more relaxed and confident about the birth process.

I remember being told to push about four to five times by my doctor. Pushing didn't seem that hard to me, perhaps because of the drugs. I remember this wonderful sliding sensation when the baby's head and body were born. I seemed to have forgotten that the baby was dead. My doctor told us the baby was a boy. I was crying that I didn't want the baby to be dead. Kathy had the baby and showed him to us. His face had a lot of the white vernix on it. He looked so small and cute to me. My doctor delivered the placenta and stitched up my episiotomy. Then he brought our baby over and talked to us about the facial deformities. I had a very hard time concentrating on what he was saying, and I resented the drugs I'd been given. I asked for my glasses, which Kathy got for me. Kathy brought our baby over to us again, and I looked carefully at all the deformities and touched his cheek. I loved him and wanted him to be alive regardless of the deformities. I deeply regret that I turned down Kathy's offer to hold our son.

The next thing I remember is being in labor room 3. My doctor came in and talked with us about the baby. Again the drugs interfered with my ability to concentrate. An autopsy and tissue study would be done. Kathy, Jane, and Mary were all so supportive during our crisis. In addition, Mary made a trip to our house the next day to check on my progress. The nurses in L & D were excellent. It was especially comforting to have three nurses we knew in the delivery room with us. The nicest thing our doctor did was to let me go home that evening at 9 P.M. It would have been terrible to spend the night alone in the hospital. I needed to be with Jim after losing our son.

To Almost Andrew
from His Dad

Little blue baby boy
With the funny face
Somehow our love for you
Seems out of place.

How can we love four pounds of sorrow?
How can we love lost hopes for tomorrow?
How can we love you the way we do?
Lifeless little blue baby boy.

Sleep peacefully, little blue baby boy.

Grief Responses

Grief is a normal response to loss (Kubler-Ross, 1969). Often animals exhibit behavior or mood changes suggestive of remorse, anger, loneliness, or despair. Animals of many species and levels demonstrate their response to grief by refusing to eat or sleep, or by neglecting their personal hygiene. A loss of self-esteem is sometimes exhibited. Humans sometimes turn to alcohol, barbiturates, or other chemical substances to temporarily alter their mood.

Grief is cumulative and very painful. It is helpful to deal with it in an open manner. Some parents experience increased illness and symptomatology.

It is also reported by parents that there is an increase in accidents, ranging from slamming one's finger in the door to car accidents. Colds seem to plague parents who previously had been healthy. Self-help, bereavement support groups are found to be helpful in minimizing some of the emotional and physical sequelae. Parents enduring a perinatal loss need a supportive environment to facilitate their own personal resolution to grief (Kirksey, 1982).

The readjustment period for some parents following a perinatal loss takes approximately 18–24 months (Schwiebert and Kirk, 1986). Families and friends usually expect parents to be "over it" in a few weeks, or certainly just a few short months. If parents feel this type of pressure to comply and heal within others' expectations, the adjustment process can be more difficult and isolating. Communicating information to close friends and families about the "normal" adjustment period can be beneficial for the parents.

Practical Information

1. *Autopsies.* Provide a great deal of information. They do not always, however, determine the cause of death, but they do rule out a number of possibilities when considering future pregnancies. There is no charge at most institutions.
2. *Naming the baby.* The loss of the baby becomes more significant and personal when family and friends use the name of the baby. Names can be placed on fetal death certificates and an amendment, including the name, can be made at any time.
3. *Seeing and holding the baby.* This opportunity should be offered to all families, even when there is a birth anomaly, maceration, or early birth. Wrapping the infant in baby's blankets and presenting the infant to the parents and/or family members in a respectful and tactful manner usually allows the family to cherish the moment. The parents should be prepared beforehand as to the physical appearance, size, and color of the infant. Be sure to point out the "normal" features of the infant.
4. *Photographs/footprints/locks of hair.* It should be stressed that if these and other mementos are not saved for families, they can never be duplicated. Placing or attaching these mementos on a card and offering them to the parents should be standard practice.
5. *Due dates/anniversaries.* If a birth occurred prematurely, the upcoming "due date" may represent a particularly sad period for the parents. The anniversary of the death may also result in increased anxiety. This should be explained to the parents so that they are aware of it. This anxiety, like many other intense feelings, will recede with time.
6. *Twins.* The loss of a twin pregnancy is an extremely difficult thing to come to terms with. To become pregnant with twins again is most unlikely. If one twin survives, there is both joy and grief – feelings which oppose each other – and the parents must feel free to express both.
7. *Funerals/memorials.* Cremations carried out by a hospital are usually done so free of charge. However, there are no ashes that can be obtained. Privately, the cost can range from $100 to $300. Burials can be arranged simply for about $375 to $550. Brief chapel services within a hospital are free. Memorial gifts, wakes, or simple gatherings can also be arranged. Doing something seems to be helpful. Nothing has to be decided upon right away. Options and choices should be presented, and the time-frame for decisions should be left open.
8. *Death announcements.* Getting the word out to people is not always easy. Sending a printed or hand written announcement is helpful. It not only informs a number of people about the loss but it also initiates a response which can be extremely supportive.
9. *Baptism/clergy.* Parents should be given the chance for a pastor or chaplain to visit. Very often they do not think of this until well after the event. A nurse, family member, or member of the clergy may perform the rite of Baptism. If performed, it should be charted in the infant's and mother's record.

SUMMARY

Professional nurses need to be aware of how a perinatal loss can affect a family. It can be a welcome relief if the pregnancy was not wanted, or it can represent the ending of a legacy. Nurses need to equip the individuals in their care with information about the grief process. Options, choices and resources should be provided.

The nurse's role is to provide the highest level of care available to promote the healthiest resolution for individuals and their families. To obtain this, nurses must be equipped with the skills and knowledge to assess, assist, and intervene in areas of perinatal loss.

REFERENCES

Adolf, A., and Pratt, R. 1980. Neonatal death: The family is the patient. *J. Family Practice.* 10(2): 317–321.

Borg, S., and Lasker, J. 1981. *When pregnancy fails: Families coping with miscarriage, stillbirth, and infant death.* Boston: Beacon Press.

Bowlby, J. 1968. *Attachment and loss.* Vol. 1: *Attachment.* New York: Basic Books.

Brezin, N. 1982. *After a loss in pregnancy: Help for families affected by miscarriage, stillbirth or the loss of a newborn.* New York: Simon and Schuster.

Chez, R.; Cefalo, R.; Hobbins, J.; and Schruefer, J. 1978. Dealing with antepartum fetal death. *Contemp. Obstet. Gynecol.* 11:134–184.

Clark, A.; Affonso, D.; and Harris, T. 1979. *Childbearing: A nursing perspective.* 2nd ed. Philadelphia: F. A. Davis.

Clyman, R. Clyman, R.I., Green, C. and Rowe, J. 1980. Issues concerning parents after the death of their newborn. *Crit. Care Med.* 8(4):215–218.

Elliot, B. 1976. Neonatal death: Reflections for parents. *Pediatrics.* 62(1): 100–102.

Enriquez, M. G. 1982. Dealing with neonatal death. *Neonatal Network.* 1(1):23–28.

Harrison, H. 1983. *The premature baby book.* New York: St. Martin's Press.

Hutson, J., and Fox, H. 1982. Real-time ultrasonography for the differential diagnosis of intrapartum fetal death. *Am. J. Obstet. Gynecol.* 142:1057–1059.

Janik-Fendel, M.; Jung, H.; and Friedrich, E. 1980. Importance of ultrasound–echography in early pregnancy in the event of threatened abortion. *Perinatology–Neonatalogy.* 4:16–20.

Kennell, J.; Slyter, H.; and Klaus, M. 1970. The mourning response of parents to the death of a newborn. *New Engl. J. Med.* 283(7):344–349.

Kirksey, J. 1982. S.A.N.D.: Support after neonatal death. *California Nurse.* December: 8–10.

Kirksey, J. 1987. The impact of pregnancy loss on a subsequent pregnancy. In *Pregnancy loss: Medical therapeutics and practical considerations,* eds. J. R. Woods and J. L. Esposito. Boston: Williams and Wilkins.

Klaus, M., and Kennell, J. 1982. *Parent–infant bonding.* St. Louis: C. V. Mosby.

Kubler-Ross, E. 1979. *On death and dying.* New York: Macmillan.

Mereness, C., and Taylor, M. 1978. *Essentials of psychiatric nursing.* St. Louis: C. V. Mosby.

Peppers, L., and Knapp, R. 1980a. Maternal relations to involuntary fetal/infant death. *Psychiatry.* 43:155–159.

Peppers, L., and Knapp, R. 1980b. *Motherhood and mourning: Perinatal death.* New York: Praeger.

Pizer, H., and Palinski, C. O. 1980. *Coping with a miscarriage: Why it happens and how to deal with its impact on you and your family.* New York: Plume Books/New American Library.

Schiff, H. S. 1981. *The bereaved parent.* New York: Penguin Books. Schneider, K., and Daniel, J. 1979. Dealing with perinatal death. *Perinatal Press.* 3:101–105.

Schwiebert, P., and Kirk, P. 1981. *When hello means goodbye.* Portland, Oregon: University of Oregon Health Sciences Center.

Schwiebert, P., and Kirk, P. 1986. *Still to be born.* Portland, Oregon: University of Oregon Health Sciences Center.

Slagle, K. W. 1982. *Living with loss.* Englewood Cliffs, N.J.: Prentice-Hall.

Southern, E., and Gutknecht, G. 1976. Management of intrauterine fetal demise and missed abortion using prostaglandin E, vaginal suppositories. *Obstet. Gynecol.* 47(5):602–606.

Worlow, D. 1978. What do you say when the baby is stillborn. *RN.* 41:74.

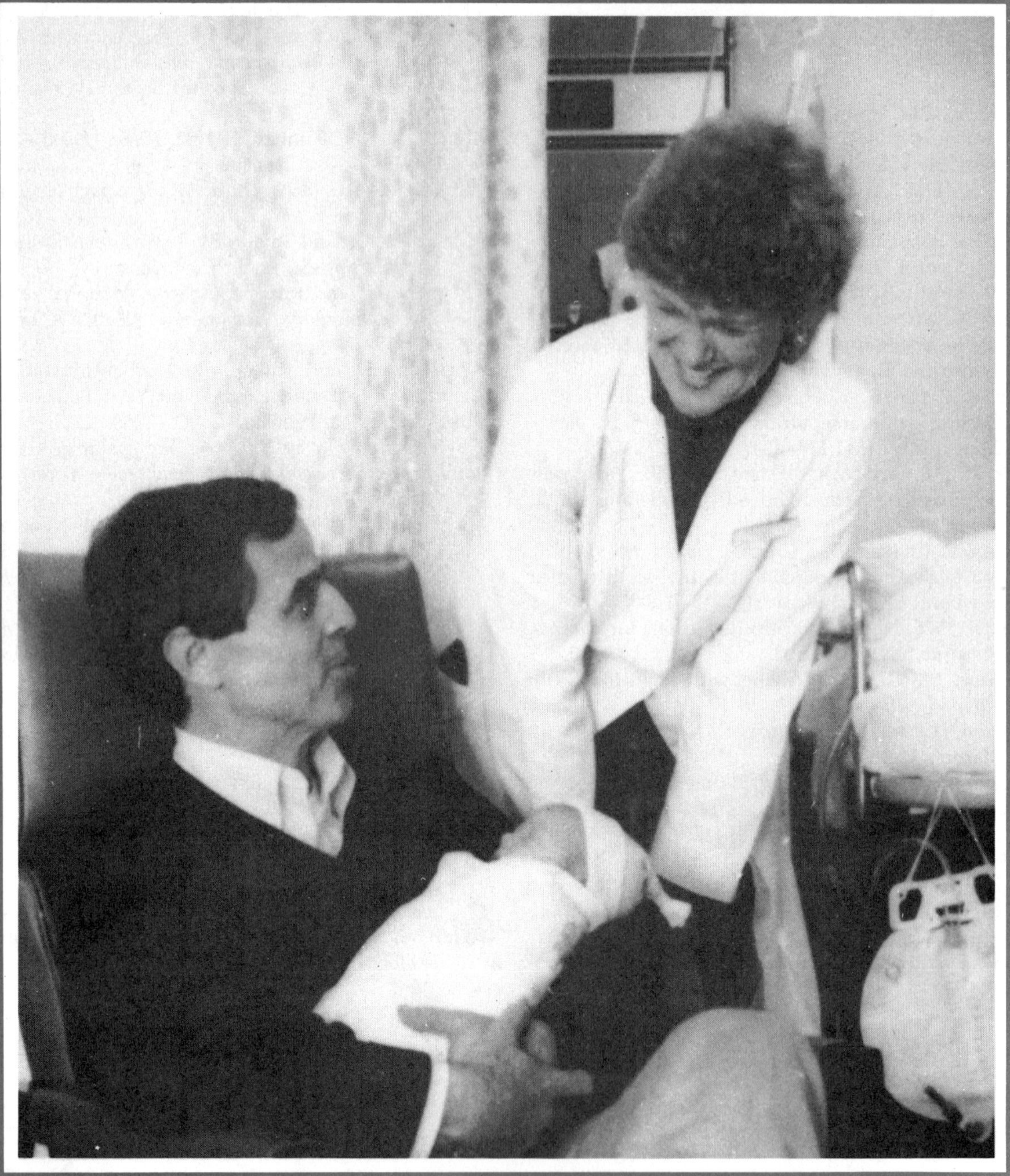

UNIT SEVEN

CHANGE AND VARIATIONS

37

The Father's Role

BEHAVIORAL OBJECTIVES

Upon completion of this chapter, the reader should be able to:

- Discuss the historical foundations of fathers' participation.

- Identify needs and concerns of expectant fathers from conception through the neonatal period.

- Describe benefits to members of the family when the father is included in the childbirth team.

- Utilize specific guidelines for assisting the father in being supportive.

Birth is a transition, a change, and working with the mother and father during this significant change is one of the most dynamic roles of the nurse. The nurse is able to sensitize the father, even if he is lacking in formal prenatal classes, to the needs of the laboring woman and the newborn.

The time immediately before and after delivery is characterized by a state of dependency for the mother. The cooperative relationship between mother and father at this time facilitates a natural assistance by the father. Even before the assistance by women specially trained to meet the needs of the laboring woman, fathers were actively involved in the supportive care of their mates. As more births began to occur in hospitals, midwives who had been trained to deliver in the home were not needed as often and, more importantly, fathers were not allowed in the hospital labor and delivery room. Separation of the baby from mother and father during hospitalization for normal childbirth became the usual practice. Where fathers were once seen as "unnecessary sources of infection", today, in modern hospitals, they are viewed as "essential sources of affection" (Kunst-Wilson and Cronenwett, 1981). While there are some health care providers who continue to separate the family members for the benefit of hospital routine, in general an effort is made to keep the mother, father, and baby together during the immediate postdelivery period. The father is being recognized as a person in need of intimacy with the mother and infant, and the mother and infant as persons with needs that the father might meet. The interaction of the father and baby and the father and mother after birth assists nurses in planning care for the mother–infant dyad and for the total family unit.

In primitive societies, couvade was practiced by the father, an activity intended to draw away evil spirits from the laboring mate. It was also a means of sympathizing with her, because the actions simulated the pain of childbirth, among other things. Both *couvade ritual* (the father actually exhibiting symptoms of labor pains during the mate's labor) and *couvade syndrome* (symptoms of the father which are reactions to his wife's pregnancy) are currently understood as *couvade*. Today, however, the concept describes the equivalent of the syndrome, not the ritual, once seen in primitive cultures (Heggenhougen, 1980; Trethowen, 1972). The ritual of passing out cigars or gum after the birth of a baby is analogous to this primitive activity, but the actual labor pains are not seen. Rather, symptomatology resulting from a reaction to the pregnancy and the pregnant woman's symptoms are seen, and have been described in the literature.

The men who are most likely to experience couvade symptoms tend to show some of the following characteristics:

1. Highly involved in the pregnancy.
2. A member of an ethnic minority.
3. Already fathered children.
4. A member of a lower socioeconomic group.
5. Past experience with ill health just prior to the period of the pregnancy (Clinton, 1986; Wolkind, 1981).

The array of symptoms experienced by expectant fathers are found to be primarily alimentary and mimicry in nature. Colds, weight gain, gastrointestinal disturbances, irritability, nervousness, inability to concentrate, headache, toothache (as well as other aches and pains), restlessness, fatigue, and insomnia have been found in men during their mate's pregnancy and postpartum period. Body image changes similar to those of the mother are reported also (Clinton, 1985; Trethowen and Conlon, 1965; Fawcett, 1978).

Similarities in paternal behavior which can be observed across cultures offer clues to biological influences, as in the case of hormonal influences. The cultural differences are important, in that they help us understand the effects of social adaptation (Rypma, 1976). Strickland (1987) studied couvade symptoms over each trimester and discovered differences that were apparently due to cultural orientation. Early pregnancy symptoms were more frequent for black expectant fathers, with a decrease in frequency as pregnancy progressed. White expectant fathers, on the other hand, experienced more symptoms over time. Anxiety was a significant predictor of couvade in this study. A positive relationship of emotional stress to overt signs of pregnancy-related symptoms suggests, therefore, an explanation for this phenomenon in our society.

THE MEANING OF PREGNANCY FOR FATHERS

The father plays a unique role in pregnancy, labor, delivery, and the early postpartum. His presence accomplishes goals for patient care of the mother and baby because he is so actively involved in the relationships of this developmental phase of the family. Further, he can play a significant and productive part in the process when he is prepared to offer the specific kinds of help his wife and baby need. Patterns of interaction between father and mother and between father and newborn are significant for the family system and for the development of the new family member. The focus on the neonate as the recipient of interaction and on the father as generator of this interaction, for example, is intriguing. A father's self-esteem and marital satisfaction increase with an active father–infant relationship (Lamb and Lamb, 1976). Research has shown that human events such as birth and postpartum can be measured for quality and quantity of specific behaviors. This chapter focuses on change in family members during pregnancy and birth, particularly on the impact of birth on the father.

In recent Western society fathers have not been socialized to take on the father role through a formal structure such as baby showers. However, the type of parenting the father received does play a part in his anticipation and acceptance of the pregnancy cycle in his adult life. Like his wife, the father responds to the pregnancy in phases, beginning with confirmation of the fact that there is indeed a baby on the way. Fetal movements and the evidence of the enlarged abdomen trigger an awareness of the approaching parenthood role.

The important aspects of pregnancy for the father do not end with the delivery. The developmental crisis the family experiences continues to progress toward resolution until the new member of the family is integrated into the system. But for the first-time father, important antecedents to the father role are pregnancy confirmation, fetal movement, and uterine growth (Phillips and Anzalone, 1982).

THE FATHER'S PARTICIPATION IN LABOR AND BIRTH

The traditional male role is specifically placed in the category of *instrumental,* in contrast to the maternal *expressive* role function. *He* is responsible for the family's economic and social position. *She* is responsible for domestic and nurturing activities for the family. This extreme role differentiation led many authors to propose tasks for the expectant father and new father that supported the mother, but fell short of his direct participation in the events of pregnancy, delivery, and care of the neonate (Parsons and Bates, 1954).

Early writers such as Bowlby (1969) tended to place the father in a secondary position of assisting his wife throughout pregnancy without a meaningful role during the labor and delivery experience. Emotional support was considered to be important as a masculine activity during the pregnancy but was not considered a legitimate function in labor and delivery, because most births occurred in hospitals (Bowlby, 1969).

Today, the father's sharing with his wife during labor and delivery are accepted as important contributors to successful coping for the laboring mother. The father's involvement is behavioral involvement, such as attendance at prenatal classes to prepare for the labor and delivery experience. The role of coach for his wife is accepted and encouraged by many hospitals. Campbell and Worthington (1982) contributed to the father's role in labor by suggesting ways to teach expectant fathers how to be better childbirth coaches. Fathers were encouraged to meet together to discover ways to alleviate concerns and to learn how to deal with anxieties about the approaching labor and delivery. The leader of such a group was a father who had participated in childbirth education classes and who had successfully coached during his wife's labor. Included in this teaching were: (1) a discouragement/motivation routine; (2) a panic routine; and, (3) the conflict routine for the coach. The three remedies for his wife's discouragement, for example, were to give a lot of attention, to support her verbally and physically, and to remain calm and controlled. Lamaze breathing techniques were used as an illustration in this teaching session, but fathers could also coach their wives toward relaxation and control with other types of childbirth preparation. The key to successful coaching, according to this approach, is for the father and his expectant wife to practice before coming into the hospital. As the events of the laboring process unfold, the husband/coach becomes an advocate. The father is the ideal person to assist the woman in labor, since he is aware of what medication and comfort measures she desires to use or avoid.

For fathers who do not wish to be involved in labor and delivery, there may be some negative effects when they know the benefits of this experience. When a study of fathers was carried out to determine the effects of *not* being present at the birth of their children, compensation behavior, such as quilt-like action, was observed on follow-up 5 months later (Palkovitz, 1980, 1982).

The question of whether a reluctant father should be urged to participate in the labor, delivery, and postpartum experience is appropriate in decision making on the maternity unit. A relaxed atmosphere which promotes healthy family relationships is beneficial to the developing mother–father–infant relationship. A method of care of the family which suggests that all fathers participate actively, including observing the delivery, must include the adjustment potential of *not* including fathers when cultural, personal, or other factors increase the likelihood of problems (Palkovitz, 1986).

Why wouldn't every father want to be involved? In Wolkind's (1981) study, the husband's involvement was greater in proportion to the length of time the couple were married. The fathers who chose less than average involvement during pregnancy were those marrying after the conception and those married for less than 1 year at the time of conception.

BENEFITS OF FATHER PARTICIPATION TO THE MOTHER

Emotional Support

Fathers present during labor who are actively involved in physical and emotional caregiving activities offer a quality of care different in comparison to the nurse. Verbal support between mother and nurse is predominant, whereas the "most helpful" husbands, as viewed by patients, were observed to talk less than those husbands who were rated as "less helpful". Even when husbands simply sat in a chair through the process of labor, several women in the study reported their presence being very helpful. The attachment of husband and wife facilitates positive coping abilities when they are together through a crisis. Touching adds to this positive influence, but is not always necessary. The mere presence of a significant person with whom the mother has a fond relationship appears to facilitate coping, in terms of the mother's perception of the labor event (Klein et al., 1981).

Mothers have described their labor and delivery experiences as enjoyable when the father participated in a continuous manner (Block and Block, 1975; Block et al., 1981). *Rapturous* is a term some mothers have used to express this feeling. Intangible effects of the husband's presence can be observed indirectly but seem to be impossible to capture for measurement.

In relating the birth experience to others, mothers describe the presence of the father in such ways as, "I couldn't have done it without him." The word *intimate* is used to describe the atmosphere in the labor and delivery area when the father is actively participating with the laboring woman.

Both complicated and uncomplicated maternity events require coping skills that are facilitated by the father's presence. When a stress is added to the laboring experience, presence of the father has shown to be a factor affecting a more positive emotional outcome (see Fig. 37–1). Fear counter-

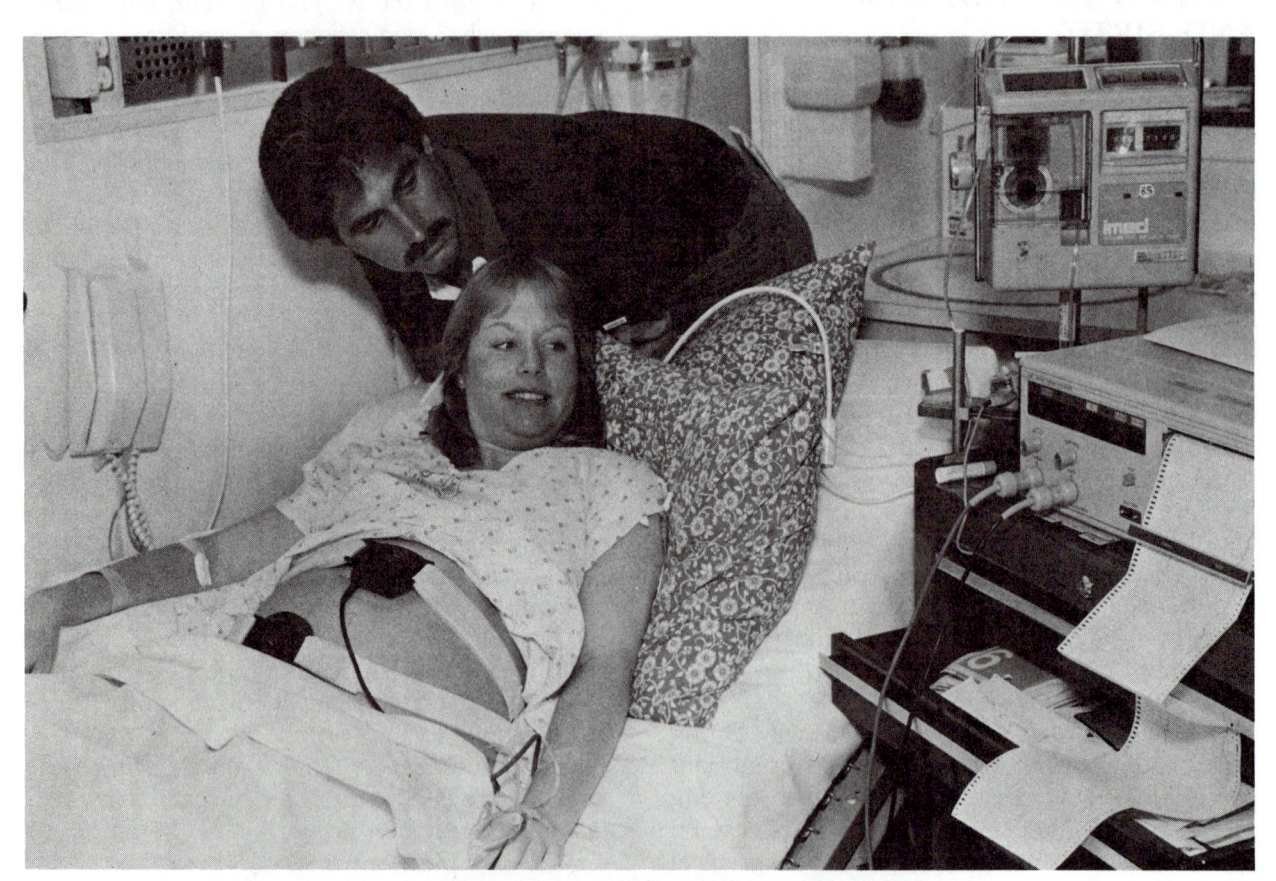

FIGURE 37–1. The father provides a comforting presence to the laboring woman.

acts the preparation mothers make for labor. Not only do fear and anxiety lessen the chances for pain control, but more severe effects have been seen during labor when emotional support does not balance feelings of fear and anxiety. The father can provide this kind of emotional support.

The father's involvement in labor and delivery brightens the mood of his mate, which encourages her participation in the family system as mate and mother. The positive participation and involvement of the father through pregnancy and labor and delivery results in a more self-confident mother after delivery. This is particularly evident in the interaction patterns with the newborn (Liebenberg, 1974; Blair et al., 1970). This good outcome was seen as therapeutic for a group of newly delivered women with severe childhood trauma (Blake-Cohen, 1966).

The Gatekeeper Function

Studies of family interaction and development have focused on the *gatekeeping* functions of the male. These consist of offering support to the woman by giving approval and creating an environment conducive to the development of her maternal skills. The willingness of the pregnant woman to attend childbirth classes has been found to depend on her mate's willingness to accompany her. The type of class she chooses to attend is also found to be determined by her husband's preference. The usefulness to fathers of the content in childbirth preparation classes has been helpful in encouraging them to participate in the experience. When physical comfort measures are omitted from a given type of class, the father's support during labor becomes a gatekeeping function for effective pain control (Block et al., 1975).

The father's participation in prenatal classes is one reliable predictor of the effectiveness of his participation in labor and delivery. However, the lack of attendance of a father in prenatal classes should not be the primary criterion for forbidding his presence in the entire process. He offers a unique and consistent support that cannot be duplicated by hospital personnel, regardless of their skills.

Another gatekeeper function of the father relates to the mother's postpartal maternal skills. When the father is supportive of the mother in her infant care activities by showing approval, she becomes more effective in caregiving activities such as feeding the baby, which enhances her self-esteem. If, on the other hand, the father produces a high-tension environment during the mother's infant feeding activity, she may appear more inept. Approval or disapproval by the father has been shown to modify the childbearing and postpartal experience for the woman (Parke, 1979).

Pain Control

Less need for medication for pain during labor and delivery has been attributed to the father's influence, both direct and indirect. The woman attends birth preparation classes in response to the gatekeeping function of the father, and her attendance may be a factor in decreasing the need for pain medication at the time of labor and birth (Enkin et al., 1972). More directly, the father is viewed as the person in the laboring woman's environment who can help the woman to cope with her pain, which can result in less dependence on medication (Block et al., 1975).

According to studies, preparation for parenthood and the presence of the father in the delivery room contribute to the mother's comfort in delivery (Davenport-Slack and Boylan, 1974; Henneborn and Cogan, 1975). Other studies support the principle of decreasing pain perception. The presence of a supportive companion, even one unknown by the woman, has been shown to be effective in decreasing the anxiety associated with pain (Sosa et al., 1980).

Research has revealed specific ways that fathers have assisted laboring women to decrease pain. Less pain medication is required and less pain is experienced when the father is not only present but also providing comfort measures. These comfort measures constitute a functional approach, and the father's presence provides a psychologic boost. In comparing the practical with the psychologic nature of pain control, the transition period between labor and delivery is perceived as a time when practical help is more beneficial (Henneborn and Cogan, 1975; Block and Block, 1975; Allen et al., 1978). In comparison with the nurse or the doctor, the father has been listed five times more often as the person most helpful during transition (Smith, Priore, and Stein, 1973).

A husband who is taking an active role in the labor process is likely to time contractions, give massages and back rubs, support the lower back during active labor, assist with patterned breathing, and support his wife's posture to facilitate second-stage coping. The husband's support in both vaginal deliveries and cesarean deliveries is associated with a more satisfactory postpartal outcome. The postoperative pain associated with cesarean deliveries is less apparent for those who view the birth experience as satisfactory, and the father's presence has been found to be the most important factor influencing the woman's perception of cesarean birth as satisfactory.

The Father's Influence on Mother–Infant Bonding

Mothers have been found to smile more at their newborn and to explore it more when the father is present than when he is not. A mother who perceives her relationship with the baby's father as "good" has been found to spend significantly more time in eye-to-eye contact with the baby (en face) than a mother who does not view the relationship as such. The quality of the relationship determines whether the father attends the childbirth or not, and women spend more time en face when the father has attended the childbirth (Trevathan, 1983).

Research supports the principle that events prior to birth affect the bonding experience for the mother and that a mother's expectations during labor and delivery affect the process of bonding. The father's presence and active participation create a positive childbirth experience conducive to positive maternal attitudes toward her infant (Bibring et al., 1961; Peterson and Mehl, 1978). The nurse should keep in mind the father's influence on the mother's postpartal self-concept and the maternal–infant bonding experience.

BENEFITS OF FATHER PARTICIPATION TO THE FATHER

Labor is a stressful time for the father. Observation of the father's role in labor and delivery has revealed that the excitement and positive outcomes for the father who participates bring personal benefits to him. Attachment to the baby begins during pregnancy. The father and mother become more aware of the implications of the birthing experience for the health and welfare of their baby. Fathers want to have a part in the experience. During pregnancy and childbearing the father gains an understanding of the process occurring in the body of his mate.

The father's efforts directed toward assisting his mate through her stressful time appear to be beneficial for both partners. Fears, anxieties, and a sense of helplessness have plagued fathers who have not been part of the labor experience.

When information is given prior to a stressful experience, the stress is reduced. Whether the father has attended classes to prepare him for handling the stress of labor, or whether he is given "on location" instructions in the hospital, his attendance can be an ego-building experience. The emotionally nourishing encounter with the reality of childbirth is a bright contrast to the former "waiting room" feelings of weakness, uselessness, and being a general nuisance. An example of the latter is described by a father discussing the attitude of the hospital staff as they hurriedly took his wife away: "They looked at me as though to say, 'You got her into this, we'll get her out'" (Wonnell, 1971).

When a woman focuses on her husband rather than the obstetrician as the nurturing one in the childbearing cycle, the outcome for the father is more positive. Since he has been there every day of her pregnancy, observing and sharing her physical and emotional changes, he seems to be the logical one to share in the culmination of the experience. As he moves forward with her through each stage of the events of pregnancy, labor, and delivery, he begins to take on the fatherhood role (see Fig. 37–2).

Father's statements about their experiences tell more about the positive influence on their lives than merely looking at outcomes of studies. For example, fathers are quoted as saying after participating in labor and delivery:

"What a great experience! I was there the whole time. It was the best experience of my whole life, something I'll never forget."

"I can't even express the joy I felt watching my

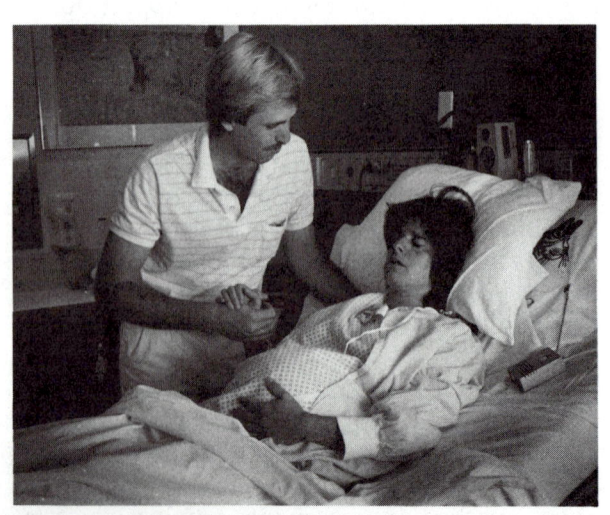

FIGURE 37–2. The father's presence is beneficial to both parents during labor.

daughter be born. What a miracle – to see what two people can create."

"Sharing this birth experience had to be the highlight of my life. When I saw Johnny's head come out, I suddenly realized that I was a father."

Fathers have made the statement that seeing their wives work so hard produced sympathy pains, that they have felt closer to their wives and had a deeper understanding for their situation as a result of being with them during labor and delivery.

The focus of the father's attention changes during the labor process. During the first stage of labor he is extremely interested in the progress of labor and how he can relieve the discomfort. As delivery begins, the father becomes concerned about the baby, noting the appearance. Most fathers do not recall what happened to their mate during delivery, and few can give accurate information about the woman's initial reactions to their newborn. The father's new role becomes real at delivery.

BENEFITS OF FATHER PARTICIPATION TO THE INFANT

The importance of a father's involvement during the early hours and days of the newborn is no less than that of the mother, in terms of the child's development. This statement is based on the position that the father is an important member of the childbearing and childrearing family in all of its stages of growth and development. Early studies indicated this through the negative effects of deprivation of the father's influence (Goldfarb, 1945). The role of stimulation on children's intellectual achievements has been adequately presented in the literature showing bad effects of unstimulating environments. Rocking, looking, touching, and walking – all related to the young child's mental abilities – and the timing of these activities are important. *Responsive* stimulation rather than that performed randomly produces a better quality of infant growth and development, in that the child sees him- or herself as important enough to cause an effect. Pederson, Rubinstein, and Yarrow (1979) demonstrated that fathers' input affects their infants' cognitive development. The father in the home from birth is shown to enhance a baby's quality of life (see Fig. 37–3).

Newborns begin the bonding experience at birth, when they are alert and seeking contact.

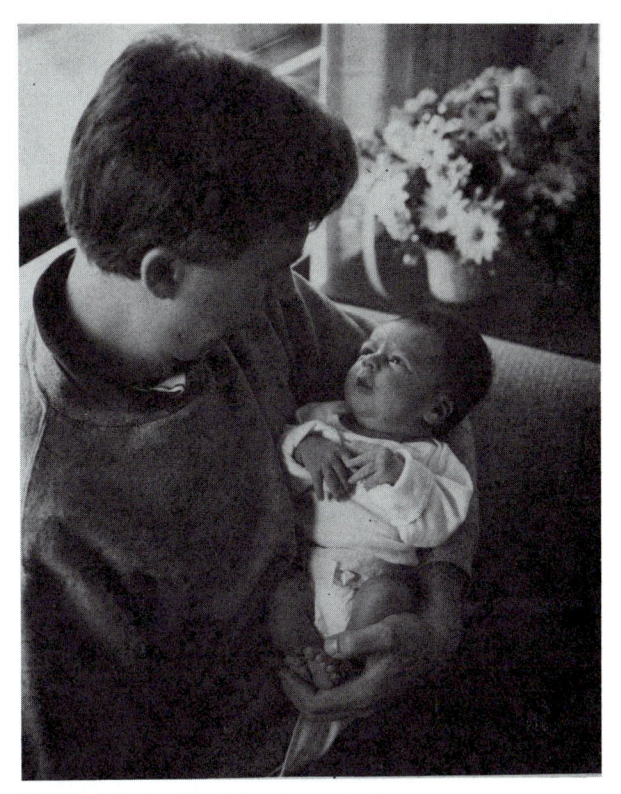

FIGURE 37–3. The father is involved early in attachment with the newborn infant.

Early and mutual attachment occurs between baby and those who take time for interaction. Infants are "uniquely" attached to both parents because of the early bonding experiences with them. Mother, father, and baby influence each other at this time. This early interaction remains consistent – babies tend to direct more affiliative behaviors to their fathers as early as 8 months of age. The cause is presumed to be that at this age babies are fun to interact with (Klaus and Kennell, 1982).

When the father has been an active member of the labor and delivery team, all phases of the childbearing experience, including newborn interaction, are perceived by the mother as more satisfying. The attachment process with her newborn is also enhanced. The mother displays more positive behaviors toward the newborn when the father is present, particularly more smiling behavior (Parke, 1978).

Maternal–infant interactions that have been shown to be affected by the presence of the father include feeding skills, general appearance of the infant during caretaking activities, and the alertness and motor maturity of the infant (Pederson, Yarrow, and Strain, 1975).

The events of labor and delivery are more important than the prenatal attitude of the father in predicting the father's involvement with his newborn. A homelike atmosphere for the birth encourages freedom of expression for the father and has resulted in more significant attachment behaviors by the father toward his newborn (Peterson, Mehl, and Leiderman, 1979).

Just as maternal attachment behaviors are altered by the father's presence, so the father's behaviors toward the newborn are different when the mother is present. Fathers smile and explore their newborn more in the presence of their mates than when alone. This triadic situation offers the infant a unique adventure in learning called *paired stimulus comparisons*. The infant begins early to learn the difference between mother's and father's voice quality, visual image, extent of behaviors in interaction, and responsiveness. Fathers communicate in a different way with their infants than mothers do. In newborn interactions, fathers touch, gaze, vocalize, and kiss in frequency equal to the mothers. Fathers actually exhibit more nurturant behavior in the triadic context than mothers and an equal amount when alone with the baby. There is only one nurturant behavior, smiling, in which the mother surpasses the father (Pederson, Yarrow, and Strain, 1975).

Newborns have been found to react differently in interactions with each parent. The mother's softspoken voice tends to allow the newborn to set the pace in communication. The newborn's face tends to brighten, the arms and legs reach out toward her in a gentle manner, the back curls in a type of rhythmic motion. Throughout this interaction the baby appears relaxed (see Chapter 29). The father tends to approach his newborn with clipped tones, then proceeds to poke or jiggle the baby while interacting. As the baby gets excited, one can observe that the baby's shoulders take on a hunched posture, the eyes widen as if in anticipation, and facial movements cease as the baby waits for the next event in the interaction. Jerky movements and increased respiration characterize the excited state of the baby (Brazelton, 1981).

Fathers treat babies differently even in the newborn period, depending on the appearance and the sex of the baby. Attractive infants are stimulated more through caressing and kissing than less attractive infants. However, when a baby is irritable and crying, the father will persist longer in his effort to form a relationship with a male offspring than with a female (Redina and Dickerscheid, 1976). Male babies receive more vocalization and touching than female babies. While fathers tend to hold female babies more closely and snugly for greater lengths of time, mothers tend to hold male babies more closely and more often. Visual and tactile interaction are more frequent between fathers and male babies, while these behaviors are seen more often between mother and female babies. Since parents seem to stimulate their same-sex infants more and to hold opposite-sex infants more, they complement each other, which is of greatest benefit to the infant in the early bonding experience (Parke and Sawin, 1977; Lamb, 1975).

Engrossment

Some cultures appear to encourage direct early interaction between father and newborn. The present trend in the United States is to encourage the father to become a more direct and powerful influence in infant care than in the past. The old stereotype of the distant father was perhaps acceptable when extended family members were more accessible to help when the newborn came home from the hospital. Women's concerns about career and other out-of-the-home activities have also encouraged a more direct relationship between father and infant. Fathers in our nuclear family structure are being seen more in prenatal classes, in labor and delivery rooms, and in the newborn's immediate caretaking activities. Rather than influencing the newborn only indirectly through the mother, the father is establishing his own unique relationship with the baby.

Engrossment refers to the involvement of the father with his newborn infant. The term was coined in current literature by Greenberg and Morris (1974) and signifies a sense of absorption and a preoccupation and interest in the infant. A bond between fathers and infants begins sometime during the first 3 days after birth, and very early contact seems to be the deciding factor in releasing engrossment behaviors in the father. The potential for engrossment has been presented as inborn in all males (see Fig. 37–4).

As in the mother–infant relationship, there is a sensitive period when the father's contribution to the relationship is vital. Some have found that there is a problem in the father's showing affection for children when the father have been absent in the early months (Stolz, 1954). Mothers comment on the difference in the closeness of the relationships between the father and those children he was with at birth and those whom he was not with until later. This difference in closeness has not been validated by research to date. Observable

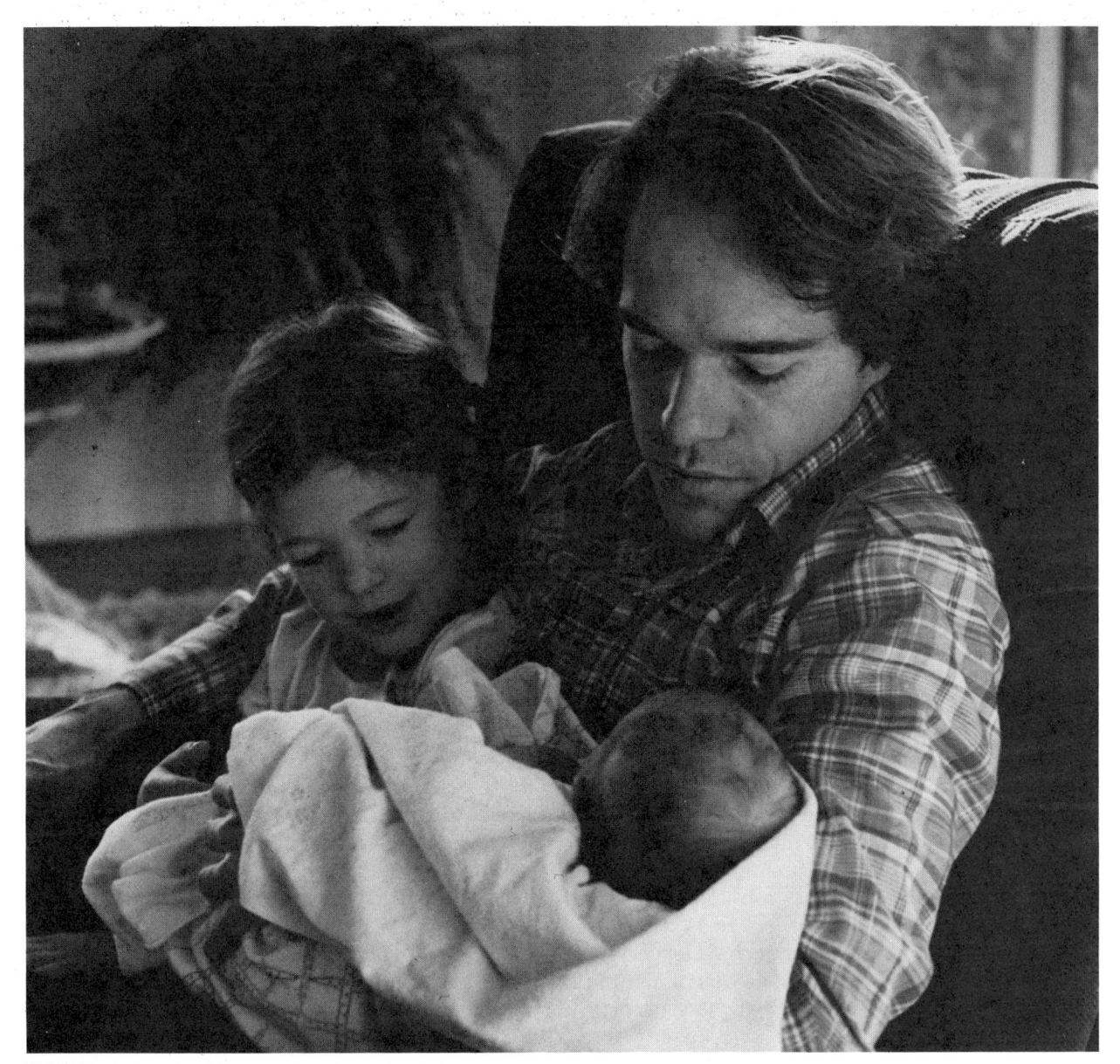

FIGURE 37-4. The father's early attachment to the infant influences later parent-infant relationships.
SOURCE: Jeff Weisman, courtesy of Alta Bates Hospital.

indications of engrossment by the new father are (Greenberg and Morris, 1974):

1. *Visual awareness.* He prefers to look at his own newborn rather than anything else in the environment.
2. *Tactile awareness.* He seeks skin contact with the newborn. He experiences pleasure in holding, caressing, and kissing the infant.
3. *Awareness of distinct characteristics.* He distinguishes his own newborn from others. He sees his own likeness in the baby.
4. *Perception of the infant as perfect.* The baby is described as beautiful and perfect even if it is not.
5. *Development of strong feelings of attraction.* He excludes others, seeking a relationship only with the newborn.
6. *Experience of extreme elation.* He describes this feeling as a "high" lasting for days.
7. *Increased sense of self-esteem.* He feels proud and delighted when he sees the baby. He is pleased to show the baby to others, and he derives satisfaction from others' reactions to "his" baby.

Engrossment is a stimulus for social interaction. Social stimulation activities such as verbalizing and playing between adults and infants encourages attachment, as does the responsiveness of the infant to the adult's attention. Father–infant attachments have been measured in relation to specific activities. Frequency of caretaking activities, such as diaper changes, has been directly related to the degree of attachment. Intense play activities tend to increase attachment behaviors in infants. The amounts and types of activities vary according to the sex of the infant. Male infants about 2 years of age have been shown to prefer fathers over mothers during play activities (Pederson and Robson, 1969).

Illness and Death of the Newborn

Adjustment on the part of the family is a real part of the birthing environment when the newborn is ill or dies. A problem results when there is lack of support for the mother or father when this occurs. Fathers should be encouraged to remain with an ill newborn who is being transported to another hospital for care. The father should travel to the unit and remain several hours with his ill newborn. He can get acquainted with the baby, staff, and physicians and can then serve as an intermediary between mother and infant. He can offer psychologic comfort for the mother at this time by giving her details of the baby's condition and care (see Chapter 36).

Following a complicated labor and delivery, a father will tend to do better in the caretaking role after the baby gets home than if there have been no complications. The family is a system, and the additional requirements of a crisis result in caring for other members as the need demands (Grossman, Eichler, and Winickoff, 1980).

Studies of premature infants indicate an abnormally high rate of abuse of these children and a risk for parenting disorders. An important finding involves the father's influence on the mother's interaction with her baby. Low-interacting mothers consistently reported poor relationships with the father, while high-interacting mothers had more satisfying relationships (Minde, 1980).

Early in the newborn period the father has the opportunity to interact with the new baby who is placed in the premature or intensive care nursery. As a group, fathers of these infants continue to be more involved with their babies at home than fathers of full-term infants. Mothers and fathers initiate more interaction with their premature babies than with full-term babies.

Most fathers prefer to be present during the birth of a defective or dead baby and to be given an opportunity to view the baby. Since the father is to be the one to offer initial support to the mother when the time of grieving begins, the father needs to be included in the events of the birth process (Leonard, 1977), see Chapter 36.

PREPARATION OF FATHERS

Terms women use to describe the father's assistance are those of comfort, helpfulness, supportiveness, and understanding. Nurses need to support the father in his unique and comprehensive contribution to the care of the woman. The father is also a client in the sense that the goals of family stability and emotional health for the family members can be better attained when nurses include him as an active member of the health care team.

Culture

Biologic and cultural factors affect fathers' involvement in the birth process. Cultural responses are those learned as social adaptations. Paternal behavior that tends to be similar across cultures, however, is viewed as biologic in source (Rypma, 1976).

In the United States, the role of the father is equated with responsibility. However, one cannot equate the role of the father only with the responsibility as the breadwinner for the family. During the childbearing phase, the role includes attending childbirth preparation classes, coaching for the woman in labor, attending at delivery, and serving as co-worker in childcare activities. Subcultures within Western society still expect mothers to be the primary caretakers of infants and fathers to be the providers of the financial needs of the family. Recognizing the constraints imposed on the parent–infant relationship when the father is not present and active during infancy, compels health care professionals to work with the cultural expectations of couples to reconcile what is expected of the couple and what they, in their unique culture, expect of the health care system (see Chapters 6 and 11).

Social support and fatherhood is a topic that needs analysis, since the mother turns to the father for support, and if the mother has been the primary support for him, to whom now does he turn for assistance to cope successfully? Unless his male peers have experienced this process, they will tend to undervalue the importance of it for the father. Lein (1979) discovered that peers offer low-esteem communications to men who are involved in what has traditionally been women's role responsibilities.

Fathers have few formal or informal support sources to encourage early and active involvement in pregnancy, delivery, and child care activities. Nurturant parenting is seen as the mothering role in the traditional home, but today's families are looking to a more satisfying relationship between all members of the family than was usual in the stereotypical family, which viewed the father as simply an indirect support and primarily the wage earner. Clark-Stewart (1978) found mothers filling the caretaking role in the home with a newborn. However, in the context of knowing how to perform these activities, and feeling that the fathering role includes this, activities may not be so much mother-specific, but mother-skilled. If father were skilled, and peers accepted the activities, the father may be equally likely to perform these procedures.

There is less infant-related anxiety observed in fathers who share child care activities, and there is a more satisfying relationship with the mother in the area of childrearing (Fein, 1978).

Attitudes of Nurses

To encourage father participation in labor and delivery, a nurse must be committed to family-centered maternity care. The nurse must understand the importance of the father's presence during the intrapartal period. Nurses are responsible for determining hospital guidelines for fathers' admittance into labor and delivery and, therefore, must understand that the father's active participation is important. The rationale for withholding permission for a father to attend delivery when he has not been able to attend prenatal classes should be examined. Fathers not attending formal classes but attending delivery have been found to have more positive attitudes toward childbirth than fathers who have not attended delivery, whether prepared by classes or not (Cronenwett and Newmark, 1974).

Fathers who initially had negative expectations have made statements such as: "Seeing what my wife and I and God produced together was a great experience. We like to be together in things, and we wanted to be together in this, too."

Nurses who experience these interactions recognize the importance of family unity at the time of delivery. Family strengths are enhanced when such enthusiasm is evidenced at birth (Gabel, 1982).

The nurse has been rated by fathers as the "most helpful person" to them and their mate during labor and delivery. They described the nurses positively, as friendly, kind, cheerful, thoughtful, and interested (Leonard, 1977). The fathers tend to feel that acceptance of their presence by nurses reflects these helpful attitudes.

The emerging family requires information for decision making in the childbearing and childrearing stages of development. Fathers should be included in a wide range of educational offerings. Fathers who attend prenatal classes with their mates look for guidelines to alert them to the fathering role. The findings on the benefits of father participation are important, since a higher self-concept and a greater degree of pleasure in the father–infant interaction can be predicted when the father views his role as a positive influence for the mother and the baby. It is necessary to teach the father actual child care skills prior to delivery to attain the best effects of the early father–infant bonding process. This includes diapering, feeding, holding, and bathing the baby (Wieser and Castiglia, 1984).

The nurse assesses the infant's capacity to maintain an alert state prior to encouraging initial interaction of the baby and the father. The best time for bonding with the baby is within the first hour while the baby is awake, since the reciprocal behaviors of father and infant encourage interaction and formation of a relationship. The ability of the father (or other caretaker) to quieten the infant is also a very important aspect of interacting in a positive manner. The father is encouraged to repeat the participation activity if the baby responds to this efforts.

An important aspect of nursing care is the assessment of the father's expectations prior to labor and delivery. If the nurse is sensitive to promoting the role of the father through this process, his choices are known and respected. The level of involvement that a father finds comfortable is the correct amount. The nursing care plan should reflect the rationale for any lack of enthusiasm for involvement, when observed. The perceptions of the fathering role differ from culture to culture, and from individual to individual. Meeting the father's individual needs in relation to the family system is the nurse's primary goal. The nurse continues to encourage the father's involvement when applicable, and prepares for future births in that family. More prenatal fathering classes are encouraged for those fathers who are assessed as lacking pertinent information for correct decision making. Time spent in the postpartum period watching self-care and baby-care videos, which also include the benefits of the involvement of the father in the process, will encourage reluctant fathers for future childbearing.

The strategies which nurses can use to support fathers in their involvement in the pregnancy and birth of the baby are shown in Table 37–1. Interventions are included which encourage healthy family relationships, which is the purpose of the father's active participation throughout this crisis event in the family unit.

Nursing strategies need to be assessed, and clinical nursing research needs to be on-going to evaluate the effects of specific nursing intervention methods properly (audiovisual material, baby bath demonstrations, supervised infant care in the mother's room, etc.).

One of the ways to evaluate the fathering role after delivery is to assess his active participation by using a tool, such as the one developed by Wieser and Castiglia (1984) (Fig. 37–5). This too was utilized by the authors for a time-series evaluation, beginning at birth, and continuing through the day of discharge. If the aim is to strengthen father–infant interaction, use of this tool can confirm a nursing intervention as positive, or can indicate its lack of usefulness for the hospital experience.

The least well understood feature of family dynamics at birth is the stress related to fatherhood. In research findings, fathers state that they want to participate more than they actually do after the baby arrives. To increase father-infant activity after birth, one must find, therefore, another intervention over and above motivation. It is necessary to teach the father the importance of the relationship, in that it is different from the mother's, and equally as important. The infant's social competence will be enhanced by the sensory input of the father's playful and stimulating activities with the baby. This type of interaction, seen mainly in fathers, is highly rewarding for the baby

---

TABLE 37–1. *Strategies to Support and Promote the Role of the Father, by Stages of Pregnancy*

Antepartum	Intrapartum	Postpartum
1. Include the father in initial antepartum visit and encourage his participation in all subsequent visits	1. Encourage the father's presence during labor and delivery. Support his planned role in labor, if appropriate	1. Encourage the father to come to follow-up pediatric visits
2. Encourage the father's involvement in birthing and parenting classes	2. Allow time for the father to hold and fondle the newborn	2. Conduct postpartum classes for both parents to discuss infant care and related issues
3. Include educational material that portray "active" father and joint-parental involvement in infant care	3. Allow time for the father and mother to be alone with the newborn after delivery	3. Raise specific questions about difficulties experienced in sharing infant care responsibilities. Offer to help parents renegotiate a plan for sharing infant care, if appropriate
4. Raise questions directly related to concerns fathers are likely to experience around childbirth and infant care	4. Encourage the father to "room in" with the mother during hospitalization, if appropriate	4. Support the formation of father-, mother-, or joint-postpartum lay support groups. Offer to provide consultation to the support group or to the individuals, as needed
5. Host one session for fathers only. Invite "highly involved" fathers to come and discuss parenting issues	5. Support the father's active involvement with the infant during hospitalization (feeding, holding, changing the infant, etc.)	
6. Encourage parents to negotiate parenting "roles" and infant care issues. Offer to serve as a facilitator of those discussions		

SOURCE: Kunst-Wilson and Cronenwett (1981) p. 208.

NURSING INVENTORY FOR ASSESSING EARLY FATHER-INFANT INTERACTION						
Frequency of contact						
Observation number						
Postpartum day						
Time						

Paternal behavior	Observation 1	2	3	4	5	6	7
Inspection							
Looks at infant							
En face							
Smiles at infant							
Expresses awareness of distinct characteristics of infant							
Truns away from infant							
Verbalization							
Vocalizes to infant							
Calls baby by name; uses affectionate terms							
Tactile contact							
Touches with fingertips							
Touches with whole hand							
Rocks infant							
Kisses infant							
Holds infant							
Refuses to hold infant							

	Observation 1	2	3	4	5	6	7
Caretaking							
Feeds infant							
Burps infant							
Cleanses infant							
Diapers infant							
Responds to infant's cues							
Infant's state							
Active							
Alert inactivity							
Waking activity							
Passive							
Sleeping							
Periodic crying							
Almost continuous crying							
Vocalizing							
Urinating, stooling, or spitting							
Wrapped in blanket or covered							
Unwrapped in shirt and diaper							
Undressed, with loose diaper or no diaper							
Maternal/other influences							
Father alone with infant							
Father with mother and infant							
Mother/other verbally encourages father-infant activity							

FIGURE 37–5. Nursing inventory for assessing early father-infant interaction.
SOURCE: Tool for Evaluation of the Father Role. Wieser and Castiglia (1984) p. 105.

(Pederson and Robson, 1969). The ability of the baby to discriminate between these two significant persons in his life will encourage a lower frustration level when interacting with others later in life (Kunst-Wilson and Cronenwett, 1981).

GUIDELINES FOR FATHER PARTICIPATION

All fathers should be encouraged to participate in the childbearing experience, whether prepared or not (MacLaughlin and Taubenheim, 1983). The following guidelines should offer direction for nurse intervention in encouraging father participation:

1. *Preparation (prior to admission if possible).* Offer a tour of the labor and delivery area. Specifically point out the area for changing into scrub clothes. Show him the location of the admission office and encourage him to preadmit his mate so that he can remain with her on admission. Indicate where the parking area is and remind him of parking policies. Show him all eating areas in the hospital and encourage him to bring a snack with him and a book for slow times.
2. *On admission.* Encourage the father to express his views about whether he wants to remain with his wife during the admission procedures (if allowed). If the father leaves during admission, find out where he is going and when he will be back. Greet the couple warmly to allay anxiety. Explain each procedure and policy simply, quickly, and in advance to encourage relaxation.
3. *Early labor.* Support the father's right to be

present by treating him as a member of the team. Assist him in his coaching functions. If the father does not want to participate actively, encourage him to remain with his wife as much as he wants, and support his decision. Explain where he can obtain nourishment as needed, and insist on his taking breaks while the nurse relieves him. Have playing cards and magazines available for couples who are in very early labor. The father is the ideal companion for the mother during a long wait. Health teaching is an important part of the early stage of labor and may tend to relax the father. Remind the father to offer praise occasionally. The nurse may also praise him for his supportive efforts.

4. *Active labor*. The father should be taught to count contractions if he does not already know how. Giving him a pencil and paper to keep accurate records will help him to feel useful.

   Demonstrate the need for a calm, quiet atmosphere by being quiet and dimming the lights. Avoid loud laughter and talking at the nurses' station.

   When leaving the room, let him know where he may find a nurse and when you will return. Nurses should return at predictable time intervals.

   The father should assist the woman through physical comfort measures. Teach him to offer a comfortable position, ice chips, and a wet cloth. Teach him to place his fist at the woman's lower sacrum for counterpressure when back pain becomes a problem.

   Controlled breathing techniques for prepared couples offer assistance at this time. If the father has been preparing for this, he should coach the mother. His voice carries a familiar sound, and he uses commands to which she has become accustomed.

5. *Transitional phase*. The father can change into scrub clothes at 7 cm cervical dilation so that he will not have to interrupt his involvement during transition. Teach the couple about the relatively short time span of this part of labor so that the severity of contractions will not seem so ominous. The nurse should be present during transition. A controlled nurse will serve as a role model to the father, helping him to deal with difficult behaviors in the laboring woman.

   Assist the father-coach with pant-blow breathing if the couple is prepared. Too rapid breathing at this time is common. The father may be the best channel for direct commands given during transition. The father can be a strong influence in helping his mate regain control.

6. *Delivery*. The father can help the mother maintain the upright position during pushing efforts.

   As the woman is wheeled into the delivery room, the father is offered shoe covers and face mask. The place of delivery will vary with the hospital, but usually the father is encouraged to remain near the head of the table and away from the sterile field as much as possible. A chair is placed near the head, and the mirror is situated so that both father and mother can view the birth of the baby.

7. *After delivery*. The new parents should be congratulated on their success. If the baby is not too premature or ill, the father should be allowed to hold it.

   The father can change into his regular clothing after the delivery. During episiotomy repair is a good time to call relatives and friends. He can then put on a cover gown and return to the recovery room for a get-acquainted time with his new baby.

SUMMARY

The father who is encouraged to participate actively in the process of labor and delivery will respond by being less isolated from his family and new baby. The fright and sense of helplessness that once accompanied the father through the waiting room experience are being replaced by feelings of exhilaration and self-confidence. Active involvement of the father results in a better relationship with the newborn as well as a better mother–infant relationship through offering the mother needed emotional support through the crisis of pregnancy, labor and delivery, and the immediate newborn period. The father can be prepared to coach his mate through labor. Even the unprepared father can feel that he is special and can be taught ways to meet his mate's needs. Benefits to the mother include the decreased need for pain medication. Benefits to the baby include an initial bonding experience.

The nurse should employ guidelines that utilize the resources of the father to meet the needs of the laboring woman. The nurse can promote a smoother transition into parenthood by encouraging the father's participation during the intrapartal period.

REFERENCES

Allen, C.; Noor, K.; Block, C.; Meyering, S.; and Meyers, E. 1978. Obstetric and psychological effects of psychoprophylactic preparation for childbirth. *Am. J. Obstet. Gynecol.* 131(1):44–52.

Bibring, G.; Dwyer, T.; Huntington, D.; and Valenstein, A. 1961. A study of the psychological processes in pregnancy and of the earliest mother–child relationship: I. Some propositions and comments. *Psychoanal. Study Child.* 16:9–29.

Blair, R.; Gilmore, J.; Playfair, H.; Tidall, M.; and O'Shea, C. 1970. Puerperal depression. *J. Roy. Coll. Gen. Practit.* 19:22–25.

Blake-Cohen, M. 1966. Personal identity and sexual identity. *Psychiatry.* 29:1–14.

Block, C., and Block, R. 1975. The effect of support of the husband and obstetrician on pain perception and control in childbirth. *Birth Fam. J.* 2:43–50.

Block, C., and Block, R. 1981. Husband gatekeeping in childbirth. *Family Relations.* 30:197–204.

Bowlby, J. 1969. *Attachment and loss.* New York: Basic Books.

Brazelton, T. B. 1981. *On becoming a family.* New York: Delacorte.

Campbell, A., and Worthington, E. 1982. Teaching expectant fathers how to be better childbirth coaches. *MCN.* 6(1):28–32.

Campbell, S., and Taylor, P. 1980. Bonding and attachment: Theoretical views. In *Parent–infant relationships,* ed. P. Taylor, New York: Grune & Stratton.

Clark-Stewart, K. 1978. And daddy makes three: The father's impact on mother and young child. *Child Devel.* 49:466–478.

Clinton, J. 1985. Couvade: Patterns, predictors, and nursing management. *Western J. Western Res.* 7:221–243.

Clinton, J. 1986. Expectant fathers at risk for couvade. *Nurs. Res.* 35(5):290–295.

Cohen, L., and Campos, J. 1974. Father, mother, and stranger as elicitors of attachment behaviors in infancy. *Dev. Psychol.* 10:146–154.

Cronenwett, L., and Newmark, L. 1974. Fathers' responses to childbirth. *Nurs. Res.* 23(3):210–216.

Davenport-Slack, B., and Boylan, C. 1974. Psychological correlates of childbirth pain. *Psychosom. Med.* 36:215–223.

Enkin, M.; Smith, S.; Dermer, S.; and Emmett, J. 1972. An adequately controlled study of the effectiveness of PPM training. In *Psychosomatic medicine in obstetrics and gynecology,* 3rd International Congress, ed. N. Morris. London: Basal.

Fawcett, J. 1978. Body image and the pregnant couple. *Am. J. Mat. and Child Nurs.* 3:227–233.

Fein, R. 1978. Research on fathering: Social policy and an emergent perspective. *J. Soc. Issues.* 34:122–135.

Fishbein, E. 1981. The couvade: A review. *J. Obstet. Gynecol. Neonatal Nurs.* 10(5):356–359.

Gabel, H. 1982. Childbirth experiences of unprepared fathers. *J. Nurse-Midwifery.* 27:5–8.

Goldfarb, W. 1945. Effects of psychological deprivation in infancy and subsequent adjustment. *Am. J. Orthopsychiatry.* 15:247–255.

Greenberg, M., and Morris, N. 1974. Engrossment: The newborn's impact upon the father. *Am. J. Orthopsychiatry.* 44:520–531.

Greenberg, M.; Rosenberg, I.; and Lind, J. 1973. First mothers rooming-in with their newborns: Its impact upon the mother. *Am. J. Orthopsychiatry.* 43:783–788.

Grossman, F.; Eichler, L.; and Winickoff, S. 1980. *Pregnancy, birth and parenthood.* San Francisco: Jossey-Bass.

Heggenhougen, H. K. 1980. Father and childbirth: An anthropological perspective. *J. Nurse-Midwifery.* 6:21–26.

Henneborn, W., and Cogan, R. 1975. The effect of husband participation in reported pain and the probability of medication during labor and birth. *J. Psychosomatic Res.* 19:215–222.

Klaus, M., and Kennell, J. 1982. *Parent–infant bonding.* 2nd ed. St. Louis: Mosby.

Klein, R.; Gist, N.; Nicholson, J.; and Standley, K. 1981. A study of father and nurse support during labor. *Birth Fam. J.* 8(3):161–164.

Kunst-Wilson, W., and Cronenwett, L. 1981. Nursing care for the emerging family: Promoting paternal behavior. *Res. Nurs. Health.* 4:201–211.

Lamb, M. 1975. Fathers: Forgotten contributors to child development. *Human Development.* 18:245–266.

Lamb, M., and Lamb, J. 1976. The nature and importance of the father–infant relationship. *Fam. Coord.* 25:379–383.

Lein, L. 1979. Male participation in home life: Impact of social support and breadwinner responsibility on the allocation of tasks. *Fam. Coord.* 28:489–495.

Leonard, L. 1977. The father's side, a different perspective on childbirth. *Canad. Nurse.* 73:16–20.

Liebenberg, B. 1974. Expectant fathers. *Am. J. Orthopsychiatry.* 37:358–359.

MacLaughlin, S., and Taubenheim, A. 1983. A comparison of prepared and unprepared first-time fathers' needs during the childbirth experience. *J. Nurse-Midwifery.* 28:9–16.

Maxwell, J. 1976. The keeping fathers of America. *Fam. Coord.* 27(4):387–392.

Minde, K. 1980. Bonding of parents to premature infants: Theory and practice. In *Parent–infant relationships,* ed. P. Taylor. New York: Grune & Stratton.

Palkovitz, R. 1980. Predictors of involvement in first-time fathers. *Dissertaton Abstract International.* 40:3603B–3604B (Univ. Microfilms No. 705-801).

Palkovitz, R. 1982. Father's birth attendance, early extended contact and father–infant interaction at five months postpartum. *Birth: Issues in Perinatal Care and Education.* 9(3) 173–177.

Palkovitz, R. 1986. Laypersons' beliefs about the 'critical' nature of father–infant bonding: Implications for childbirth educators. *Maternal–Child Nurs. J.* 15(1):39–46.

Parke, R. 1978. The father's role in infancy: A reevaluation. *Birth and the family.* 5:211–213.

Parke, R. 1979. Perspectives on father–infant interaction. In *Handbook of infant development,* ed. J. Osofsky. New York: John Wiley & Sons.

Parke, R., and Sawin, D. 1977. The family in early infancy: social interactional and attitudinal analyses. Paper presented to the Society for Research in Child Development. New Orleans, March.

Parsons, T., and Bates, R. 1954. *Family, socialization and interaction process.* Glencoe, Ill.: Free Press.

Pederson, F., and Robson, K. 1969. Father participation in infancy. *Am. J. Orthopsychiatry.* 39:466–472.

Pederson, F.; Yarrow, L.; and Strain, B. 1975. Conceptualization of father influences and its implication for an observational methodology. Paper presented in Guildford, England, July.

Pederson, F.; Rubenstein, J.; and Yarrow, L. 1979. Infant development in father–absent families. *J. Genetic Psych.* 135:51–61.

Peterson, G., and Mehl, L. 1978. Some determinants of maternal attachment. *Am. J. Psychiatry.* 135: 1168–1173.

Peterson, G.; Mehl, L.; and Leiderman, P. 1979. The role of some birth-related variables in father attachment. *Am. J. Orthopsychiatry.* 49(2):330–338.

Phillips, C. R., and Anzalone, J. T. 1982. *Fathering: Participation in birth.* 2nd ed. St. Louis: C. V. Mosby.

Redina, E., and Dickerscheid, J. 1976. Father involvement with first-born infants. *Fam. Coord.* 25: 373–379.

Rypma, C. 1976. Biological bases of the paternal response. *Fam. Coord.* 27(4):335–339.

Smith, B.; Priore, R.; and Stein, M. 1973. The transition phase of labor. *Am. J. Nurs.* 73:448–450.

Sosa, R.; Kennell, J.; Klaus, M.; Robertson, S.; and Urrutia, J. 1980. The effect of a supportive companion on perinatal problems, length of labor, and mother–infant interaction. *New Engl. J. Med.* 303:597–600.

Stolz, L. 1954. *Father relations of war-born children.* Stanford, Calif.: Stanford University Press.

Strickland, O. 1987. The occurrence of symptoms in expectant fathers. *Nurs. Res.* 36(3):184–189.

Trethowen, W. H. 1972. The couvade syndrome. In *Modern perspectives in psycho-obstetrics,* ed. J. G. Howells. Edinburgh: Oliver & Boyd.

Trethowen, W., and Conlon, C. 1965. The couvade syndrome. *Brit. J. Psychiatry.* 3:57–66.

Trevathan, W. 1983. Maternal "en face" orientation during the first hour after birth. *Am. J. Orthopsychiatry.* 53:92–98.

Wieser, M., and Castiglia, P. 1984. Assessing early father–infant attachment. *MCN.* 9:104–106.

Wolkind, S. 1981. Fathers. In *Pregnancy: A psychological and social study.* eds. S. Wolking and E. Zajicek. New York: Grune and Stratton.

Wonnell, E. 1971. The education of the expectant father for childbirth. *Nurs. Clin. N. Amer.* 6:591–603.

38
Adolescent Pregnancy

BEHAVIORAL OBJECTIVES

Upon completion of this chapter, the reader should be able to:

- Discuss why adolescent pregnancy is considered primarily a socioeconomic problem and not a psychologic or medical problem.

- Identify the complex factors that account for the increased number of adolescent pregnancies.

- Discuss the crucial role of comprehensive sex education.

- Identify the medical risks involved in adolescent childbearing, particularly when prenatal care is inadequate.

- Identify the medical risks involved in adolescent childbearing, particularly when prenatal care is inadequate.

- Identify the behavior and reactions particular to the adolescent patient during the antepartum, labor and delivery, and postpartum periods.

- Discuss the importance of involving the adolescent father in all aspects of adolescent pregnancy.

- Identify the major resources available for adolescent parents and how and when to utilize them.

- List the different levels on which the problem of adolescent pregnancy must be approached.

Adolescent pregnancy is primarily a socioeconomic problem with medical consequences. Although pregnancy in the middle-class, white adolescent population is on the increase, the birth rate for the poor and nonwhite teenager remains statistically far ahead. Teenage lifestyle, vulnerability to complications, and lack of or poor prenatal care predispose the adolescent population to change that results in a less favorable outcome. Approximately 50 percent of poor and nonwhite pregnant teenagers do not receive prenatal care during the first trimester, and 20 percent do not receive it in the second trimester (Smith and Mumford, 1980). This chapter explores the scope of the problem of adolescent pregnancy and the reasons behind it. The chapter's main objective is to provide the health practitioner with an understanding of the complexity of the problem and specific suggestions for more effective intervention at each critical stage.

Adolescent pregnancy has reached epidemic proportions, but it is by no means a new problem. It has its roots in the post-Second World War baby boom. As the problem has become more visible and the statistics more staggering, concern has become widespread. Researchers unanimously agree that adolescent childbearing results in more adverse consequences for society and the individual than it does positive effects. These consequences have been described as the "syndrome of failure" (Fig. 38–1). For the adolescent in this syndrome, education is often interrupted or permanently abandoned. This curtailment of education limits employment opportunities, which results in either a reliance on the welfare system or a marginal existence. This, in turn, tends to fragmented family life and compromised ambition. Children born into this situation do not escape

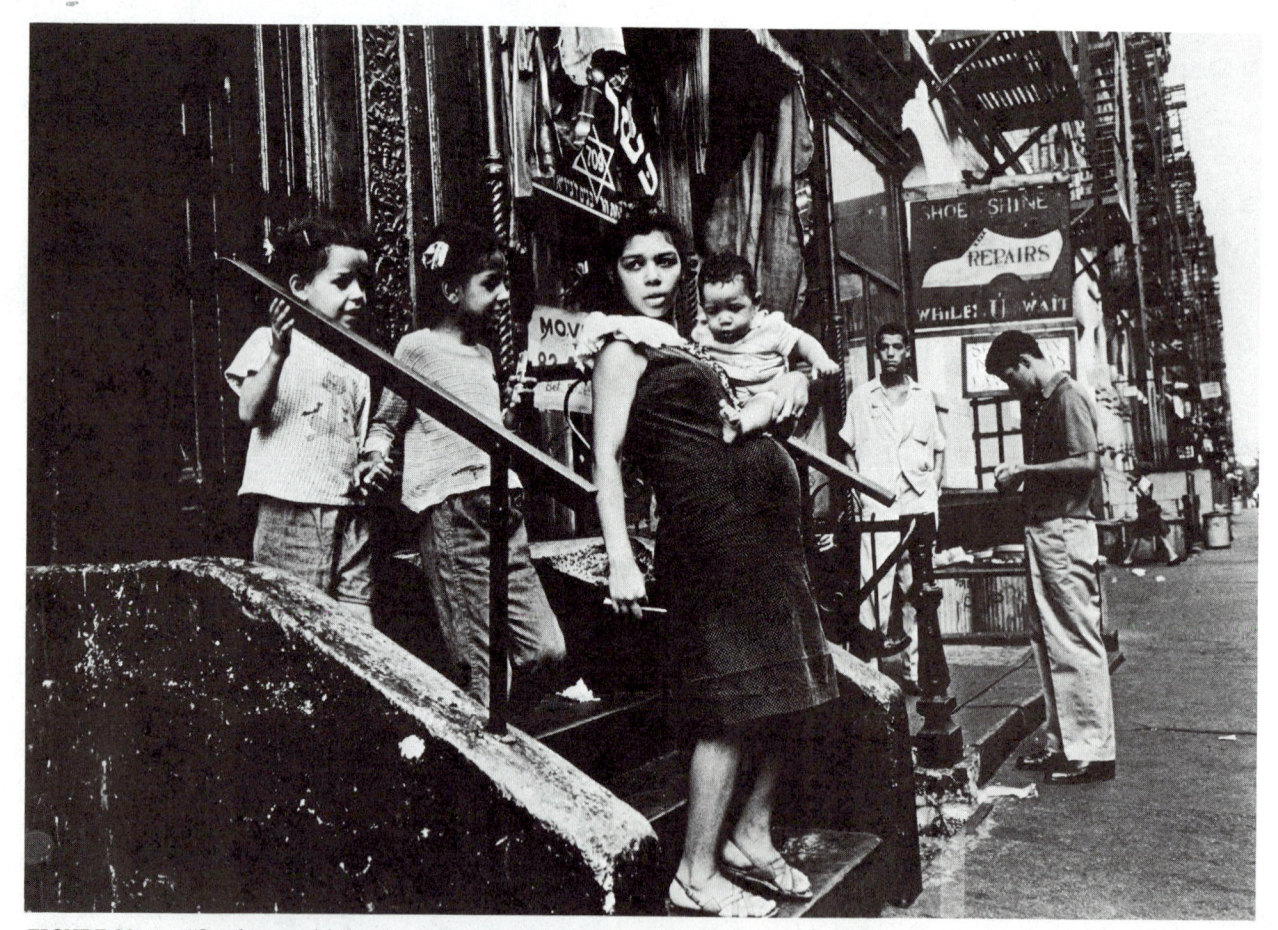

FIGURE 38–1. "Syndrome of failure": adolescent with multiple children.
SOURCE: Courtesy Ken Wittenberg.

unscathed. They show a much higher incidence of poor school adjustment and impaired intellectual functioning. Repetition of this negative cycle is well documented. Nearly 25 percent of teenage mothers and 50 percent of teenage fathers have had at least one teenage parent (*Teenage Pregnancy*, 1981).

STATISTICS

In 1978 it was documented that:

> Today's 14-year-old, by the age of 20 (1984), will discover the following: 21 percent of her peer group will have experienced at least one live birth, 15 percent will have obtained at least one legal abortion, and 6 percent will have had one miscarriage or stillbirth (Tietze, 1978).

This projection is based on statistics from 1978, when there were approximately 29 million adolescents in the United States. It is estimated that 12 million were sexually active (7 million males and 5 million females). Figures from Planned Parenthood record 1,142,000 pregnancies, 300,000 therapeutic abortions, 150,000 spontaneous abortions, 362,000 births to the unmarried female, and 192,000 births to the married female. A further breakdown shows us that 375,000 girls between the ages of 13 and 14 were sexually active, and in this age group we find 30,000 pregnancies with 13,000 live births. This figure is among the highest of all Western nations, with only Romania, New Zealand, Bulgaria, and East Germany surpassing these numbers. It is also important to note that approximately 70–80 percent of these pregnancies were unintended. In summary, approximately 10 percent of adolescent females got pregnant and approximately 6 percent gave birth in 1978. In terms of teenage pregnancies, recent data indicates the number is decreasing except for those under the age of 15 at the time of pregnancy:

18–19 years	Decrease of 23 percent
15–17 years	Decrease of 1 percent
Under 15 years	Increase of 30 percent

95 per 1000 teenagers (still approximately 10 percent) (Hollingsworth and Felice, 1986).

In the last decade two other important changes have emerged: (1) the pregnancy rate to girls between 16 and 19 has declined, with a simultaneous increase in pregnancies to females under the age of 15; and (2) the pregnancy rate among minority group members has remained more or less constant, whereas pregnancy among white, middle-class females has noticeably increased.

ISSUES INVOLVED IN THE INCREASE IN ADOLESCENT PREGNANCY

Planned Parenthood has found that in the course of the 1970s sexual activity among unmarried women between the ages of 15 and 19 rose by two-thirds. In addition, in 1978, 20 percent of the 8 million 13- to 14-year-olds had had sexual intercourse. The most obvious reason for the high absolute numbers of teenage pregnancies is that we have a numerical pool of many more teenagers today than in prior decades. Another reason for the increase is that sexual activity is beginning at a younger age and is occurring among more of these teenagers.

There are also both physiologic and sociologic reasons for this change. In 1900 the average age of menarche was 14.2 years. In 1980 the average age was 12.5 for whites and 11.8 for blacks. Marriage is delayed in our culture, but heavy sexual messages pervade our society on every level. With increased peer pressure, sexual involvement becomes difficult to avoid. The breakdown in the double standard also contributes to increased sexual involvement. We are told, with the advent of women's liberation, that it is acceptable and even healthy for young women, as well as young men, to explore their sexuality outside of marriage.

Unfortunately, society has not been able to keep up with the increased sexuality of its young people. We fall far short of even a marginal adequacy in two critical areas: (1) sexual education and responsibility, and (2) the availability and appropriateness of birth control resources and methods. A short discussion of both of these subjects is necessary in order to both understand and begin to correct this overwhelming problem.

Sex Education and the Adolescent

It has been shown repeatedly that effective sex education does not lead to increased sexual activity but rather to more responsibility and awareness of the consequences of sexual involvement. When sex education includes "plumbing and morals", a detailed discussion of the relative safety and efficacy of all birth control methods, resources in the community where birth control devices can be obtained, and a realistic picture of early parenthood, the incidence of contraceptive use increases dramatically, with a corresponding decrease in pregnancy rate (Zelnik and Young, 1982; see Fig. 38–2).

Sex education must begin early, before experimentation begins. Parents often feel that they should assume this emotion-laden responsibility themselves, but they often find it difficult to know the right approach. Ideally, parents should be given the opportunity to learn to communicate relevant information. In some communities, schools or family-planning clinics offer classes directed at parents for this purpose. Presently, however, few children learn the accurate facts and objective information they need from their parents. Instead, they obtain their information, sketchy and often erroneous, from their peers, or they remain totally ignorant. For example, 40 percent of the student body of a large urban high school had no understanding of the relationship between the menstrual cycle and the time of ovulation. They were under the mistaken impression that midcycle was the "safe time".

The issue regarding sex education and whether or not it should be mandatory in school systems is controversial. The issues regarding sex education and whether or not it should be mandatory in the school system is presently being closely scrutinized. This, in part, is a consequence of the fact that the AIDS epidemic is filtering down into the adolescent population. The Surgeon General of the United States has come out strongly in favor of indepth discussion within the school system of such critical issues as the modes of transmission of this lethal disease and ways to protect oneself and avoid exposure. Open and direct information is now nationally available on the benefits of condom use as a main source of prevention of this and other sexually transmitted diseases. Condom ads are now almost commonplace on TV and in other media sources which reach large numbers of teenagers. We are indeed witnessing a minor revolution in the availability of information on issues previously considered "private", "adult", and certainly controversial. In addition, the options of delaying sexual involvement and abstinence are discussed with more frequency in sex education and health classes. It is still too early to assess the impact of these new developments on teenage pregnancy rates.

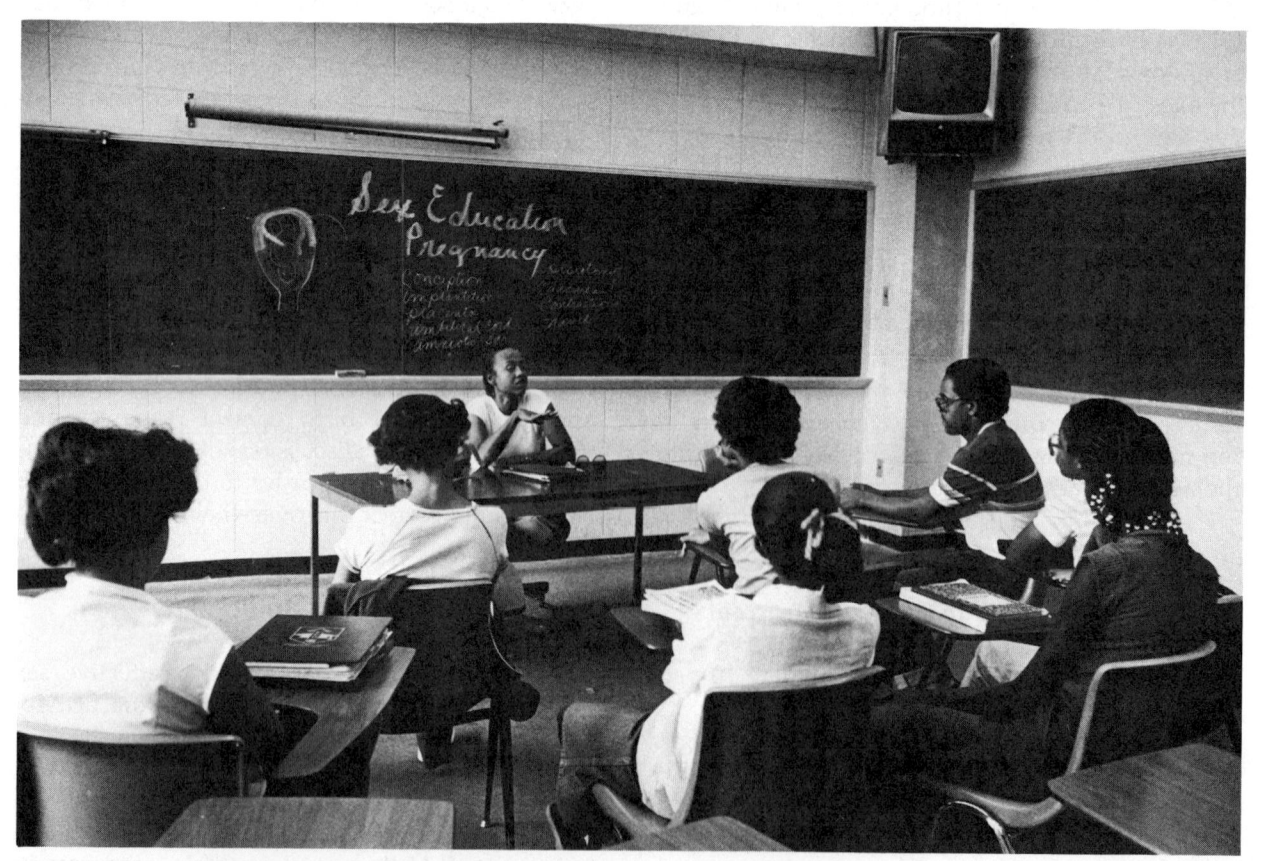

FIGURE 38–2. Adolescents in sex education class.
SOURCE: Courtesy Sybil Shelton/Peter Arnold Inc.

Contraception and the Adolescent

It is no wonder, in light of the information presented here, that only 4 out of 10 sexually active teenagers seek out birth control. Nearly two-thirds of all unwed teenagers never use birth control or use it inconsistently. Teenagers come to family-planning clinics (on the average) 1 year after they begin sexual intercourse. This is of particular concern because 50 percent of all initial adolescent pregnancies occur in the first 6 months of their involvement. If intercourse first takes place at age 15 or under, these young women are twice as likely to get pregnant in the first 6 months as those who wait until they are over 18 (Zelnik and Young, 1982).

When the relationship between pregnancy and contraceptive use is reviewed, we recognize the need to increase accessibility and availability of family-planning clinics. Of teenage pregnancies, 62 percent occur among those who never use a birth control method, 30 percent occur when a method is used inconsistently, 14 percent occur when a method (often withdrawal or a nonprescription method) is always used, and 7 percent occur when a medically prescribed method is consistently used (*Teenage Pregnancy*, 1981).

Several major complications prevent family-planning clinics from offering a complete solution to our dilemma. Presently, the birth control methods available are inappropriate or unreliable for the adolescent population. We must also look at the stages of adolescent psychologic development to understand why, even when birth control is available, it is often not used. It should be noted that with the accessibility of abortion more teenagers unfortunately simply do not worry about pregnancy as much, and they feel they could, if necessary, escape the consequences through abortion of an unwanted birth. Many adolescents see abortion as an option for birth control.

Our present methods of birth control all have imperfections. It is difficult enough for the older and more mature sexually active woman to find a comfortable and reliable method, and the problems are compounded for adolescents. In the last decade the Pill has become less popular. Our society and its young people have become more health conscious. Using hormones, especially when sexual activity may be rare and sporadic, is often looked at with disfavor by both doctor and teenager. Ironically, teenagers are most influenced by the adverse publicity on the Pill but, according to research, are the least likely to suffer from complications (Zelnik and Young, 1982).

In 1978 there were fewer teenagers using the Pill than in 1971 (*Teenage Pregnancy*, 1981). The IUD has not been available since the early 1980s. Drug companies, in response to the litigation stemming from health problems related to the Dalkon Shield, removed all IUDs from the market. Increased incidence of pelvic inflammatory disease and ectopic pregnancies has been noted with this method, which is waning in popularity. The diaphragm is often considered impractical for the adolescent because it runs contrary to her vision of spontaneity and lack of premeditation in regard to sexual involvement. Many teenagers are squeamish about touching their genitals, which, of course, is necessary if a diaphragm is used. If chosen as a birth control method, the diaphragm all too often remains in the drawer or purse.

Although less effective than some other methods of birth control, condoms are gaining new popularity. Many recommendations have been made to increase the popularity and accessibility of birth control. These include media promotion (especially advertisements by teen "idols"), hotlines (because of their anonymity), and outreach through schools, public health departments, and community and recreation centers. A study done by Planned Parenthood found that teenagers were more likely to choose a clinic if it provided confidentiality, a sympathetic attitude toward this age group, proximity, and good, prompt, free or low-cost service. They recommend, wherever possible, open displays and easy availability of nonprescription contraceptives. They argue that it would make more sense for vending machines to carry condoms than cigarettes. They have found that if adolescents begin with a nonmedical method, they are more likely to switch to a medically prescribed method after being exposed to educational material and after feeling comfortable and welcome in a clinic environment.

Clinics should provide sensitive counseling to both young men and young women to help them understand the many aspects of contraceptive use. They need to share feelings, gain reassurance, and acquire communication tools to be used in their sexual relationship. For example, they need to know how to actually say to their partner, "Are you using any birth control?" They need to know how responsibility can be shared. Sex education should focus more on the adolescent male population. Females have traditionally been held more responsible for taking precautions. This only undermines the couple's sense of responsibility as copartners and can have negative ramifications in the future by setting the stage for less involvement of the male in other experiences that should be shared, such as pregnancy and parenthood.

In summary, appropriate family-planning resources are a critical component in the solution to the problem of increased incidence of adolescent pregnancy. Planned Parenthood has calculated that between 1971 and 1979, with a sevenfold increase in clinic populations, 2.6 million teenagers were helped to prevent unintended pregnancy (Forrest, Hermalin, and Henshaw, 1981). As noted earlier, many teenagers will not benefit from these services because of the underlying dynamics of adolescence, which may undermine their ability to accept responsibility for their reproductive potential. Some common reasons stated for not using birth control include: "I just didn't get around to it", "I didn't think I'd get caught", and "I was afraid my parents would find out". In addition to fear of the exam that precedes prescription and the birth control methods themselves, more subtle reasons exist. To understand what these reasons may be we need to explore some of the changes that take place during the adolescent period.

THE STAGE OF ADOLESCENCE IN RELATION TO ADOLESCENT PREGNANCY

Adolescence is the time one establishes one's own identity. It has often been characterized as a period of "confusion, intense emotions, excess energy, dogmatism, conformity, and togetherness" (Kandell, 1979). Old ties with parents are altered, to be replaced by ties with peers in a process of separation and change. But often a lingering and complicated dependency remains. A teenager can thus feel both dependent and independent at the same time. This may lead to acting-out behavior and risk taking in an effort to explore one's boundaries. This risk taking can extend to acts with long-term consequences, such as unprotected sexual intercourse. Adolescents also tend to be romantic and to have many fantasies. This is especially true in the middle-class adolescent population. Birth control becomes too mundane and disruptive an issue to worry about at the moment. Premeditated sex may cause underlying conflicts to surface, such as the longstanding traditional belief that being a virgin when one marries is a good thing.

Much has been written on the preexisting psychologic differences between teenagers who become pregnant and those who do not. It is generally agreed that there is no psychologic "type" that becomes pregnant. Certain personality traits may be more apparent in the young woman who gets "caught", but a more disturbed or defined psychiatric disorder is not evident. In summing up the literature on this subject, Furstenberg (1981) writes that:

> A major tendency has been to search for psychological or characterological factors which motivate adolescents to enter parenthood prematurely, such as the need for affection, the quest for adult status, resolution of the Oedipal conflict, the desire to escape parental control, or the inability to foresee a more gratifying future. No doubt some of these reasons apply in some instances. Most studies show that only a small minority of adolescents become parents because they want to have a child (at least at the time of conception). Most become pregnant unwillingly, and many are reluctant to terminate the pregnancy by abortion once conception occurs.

Contrary to another often-heard misconception, teenagers do not seem to be as promiscuous as we are led to believe. The available data show that only 10 percent engage in numerous casual relationships, as compared to 90 percent who have one steady partner (Chilman, 1979).

Peer pressure is strong during adolescence. In addition, the competing interests of young males and females in heterosexual interaction and their underlying insecurities often create an atmosphere in which communication is unclear or lacking. Males, to get much-needed respect from their peers, want to "score", and females, in fear of losing much-desired masculine attention, will not demand their rights within a relationship and will hesitate to bring up a potentially alienating subject such as responsibility. Denial and adolescent idealism replace realistic planning. Parents often contribute by not facing up to their intuitive feelings that their children may be sexually active. Mistrust and avoidance may characterize their inability to know how to communicate their concern, and they are able to offer little practical or supportive assistance.

THE PREGNANT ADOLESCENT

Psychologic Characteristics and Risk Factors

Although we do not see blatant psychopathologic differences in the young pregnant versus nonpregnant population, we can identify a complex of psychosocial (and related socioeconomic) dynamics that clearly make a young woman more likely to become pregnant. These factors will continue to affect her throughout her pregnancy and parenthood and are thus important for us to understand. A comprehensive discussion of this subject would necessitate breaking down our adolescent population into early (ages 13–14), middle (15–17), and late (18–19) stages of development. Although psychosocial development does not always parallel chronologic age, there are, for example, clear differences between 13-year-old and 19-year-old pregnant adolescents. There are also sharp differences between socioeconomic groups – for example, between the inner-city black adolescent and the white adolescent from a wealthy suburb.

Low self-esteem and limited educational achievement are two traits commonly seen in the pregnant adolescent of a limited socioeconomic background. These traits can pervade one's outlook, lifestyle, and goals. It is obvious that being of lower socioeconomic status in the United States seriously hampers one's opportunities:

> This translates into a tendency to live for today with less emphasis on education and training, as one expects a lesser degree of material success. As a result there is a reduced need to set aside time for education and training, which leads directly into a sequence of events in which dating and intimate relationships are entered more quickly (Furstenberg, 1981).

Thus the cycle begins. A sexual relationship leads to direct and immediate primary rewards such as attention, new clothes, and places to go. It also represents a form of pseudointimacy to which a lonely or insecure adolescent is particularly vulnerable.

Absence of family support, especially from a mother, appears to predispose the adolescent to much higher risk. Often these girls are from single-parent homes and are in competition with other siblings for parenting. Pregnancy does provide a transient increase in attention. For some adolescents it may be seen (often subconsciously) as a way to provide a change of future direction, negative as the new direction may be.

The data on such areas as educational attainment, marital history, and economic status illustrate just how negative this direction proves to be. Eight in ten pregnant teenagers under the age of 17 do not finish high school. Four in ten under the age of 15 do not finish eighth grade. Teenage fathers are 40 percent less likely to finish high school than nonfathers. Marriage in the 14- to 17-year-old age range has an accompanying divorce rate of 72 percent, and in the 18- to 19-year-old range the rate is 46 percent. These young marriages are frequently based on bonds only newly formed, and they typically would not occur but for the early pregnancy. Furthermore, it has been suggested that any advantages that these early marriages may have, such as legitimizing the birth, are undermined by the tendency for the newly married adolescent to drop out of school because of the demands of the marriage itself. When these relationships break up, the unmarried adolescent mother is at a disadvantage in that she is even less prepared for the responsibilities of single parenting than she might have been if she had not married. Fifteen percent of adolescent mothers are pregnant again within 1 year of the birth of their first child, and two-thirds of them are on public assistance for at least 5 years after their infants are born (*Teenage Pregnancy*, 1981).

Pregnancy during adolescence superimposes a situational crisis on the developmental crisis of adolescence, and the pregnancy places increasing demands on the individual who may not even have the capacity to meet the challenges of adolescence (Dickerson and Ovellette, 1982). Pregnancy fosters dependency and loss of self-direction and thus interrupts and undermines the normal maturational process of adolescence. The adolescent mother is left at a distinct disadvantage relative to her nonpregnant peer.

Physical Characteristics and Medical Risks

Studies indicate that adolescents receiving adequate prenatal care overall do not have a greater incidence of medical complications than older women. It has been suspected that problems arise more from the impact of poverty than from age (Hutchins, Kendall, and Rubino, 1979).

> Under optimal conditions, the medical risk to the child and mother does not differ appreciably from that of the population as a whole, but the availability of such optimal conditions is rare, because the early teenage mother is generally poor (note that two-thirds of teen mothers in 1978 had incomes in the lower one-third of distribution), black, and medically and nutritionally unsophisticated (Dott and Fort, 1976).

One exception to this may be the very young 13- to 15-year-old, who can still be physiologically immature or underdeveloped. However, some researchers question the inevitability of complications even in this group. It has been demonstrated that the unique medical problems associated with early teenage pregnancy are controllable and that the outcome of the pregnancy should not differ appreciably from that among the older population. However, the young adolescent uses prenatal services much less than older women do, and the consequences of nonuse are often detrimental to the mother and infant (Briggs, Herren, and Thompson, 1962). Whether unavoidable risk factors exist in this group remains controversial. However, this relatively small group (under 15), plus the large number of pregnant teenagers who receive inadequate, late, or no prenatal care, account for a statistically high rate of mortality and morbidity for the adolescent group as a whole.

Maternal mortality rates are 18 out of 100,000 for the adolescent under age 15, 2.5 times higher than they are for women in the 20- to 24-year age range. Teenagers between 15 and 19 are twice as likely to die from pregnancy-associated hemorrhage or miscarriage as are women 20–24. Toxemia and anemia are 3.5 times as likely in those under 15 and 1.5 times as likely in the 15–19 age range (*Teenage Pregnancy*, 1981). Pregnancy-induced hypertension, or preeclampsia, is the most consistently encountered high-risk complication. Only 1 percent of the nonpregnant adolescent population at large suffers from hypertension, compared to 7–30 percent of pregnant adolescents. In general, for all maternity patients the rate is 7 percent. It appears that the incidence of toxemia diminishes with age, with adequate prenatal care, and with increasing socioeconomic status. The incidence of abruptio placentae is also greater in the young adolescent because of its relationship to toxemia. Conversely, placenta previa occurs less often among adolescents because of its relationship to multiparity. Cephalopelvic disproportion due to pelvic immaturity appears to be a problem primarily for girls under 15 years of age. Although cesarean section rates are lower in the adolescent than in the adult population they tend to be higher in the lower age range than in older teenagers. Anemia, a very common complication of pregnancy, is undoubtedly largely due to the notoriously poor nutritional habits characteristic of this population (Dott and Fort, 1976).

Regarding gestational outcome, Dott and Fort (1976) write that "the burden of young motherhood falls mostly heavily upon the offspring of these mothers. Increased fetal wastage, infant morbidity (prematurity, neurological deficits), and infant death are the greatest medical risks associated with teenage pregnancy." Indeed, 25 percent of all postneonatal infant deaths are to infants of adolescent mothers, who represent only 16 percent of the maternal population. The overall infant mortality rate in the United States is approximately 13 in 1000 births. For adolescents between the ages of 16 and 19, it rises to 31 in 1000, and for mothers under 15 years of age it is 44 in 1000. Complications in these infants stem largely from the high percentage (26 percent) that are born prematurely or suffer from intrauterine growth retardation (IUGR). Poor nutrition and underdeveloped vasculature of the uterus in the young primiparous adolescent are suggested as the medical factors responsible for these complications. Many of these infants have a marked and persistent disadvantage long after birth. Again, social and environmental factors contribute heavily to these problems. Emphasis on preventive prenatal care is the critical first step needed to interrupt this pattern of both short- and long-term morbidity.

THE ADOLESCENT PATIENT IN THE ANTEPARTUM PERIOD

Early Intervention: Making Choices and Assessing Needs

Once an adolescent is aware of her pregnancy, and if the gap between suspicion and confirmation is not too long, she has four choices. She can get married and begin her family, or she can remain unmarried and do so. She can consider having an abortion, or she can decide to give her infant up for adoption. The decision is rarely totally acceptable and is almost always a difficult one to make, and it is made even more difficult by the scarcity of appropriate and objective counseling services. Adolescents are often incapable of realistically assessing the implications of being pregnant or of predicting the impact that alternative decisions will have on their life (Peterson, Sripada, and Barlow, 1982). The young adolescent is rarely mature enough to fully comprehend the commitment that parenthood should entail.

The adolescent pregnancy is often confirmed late, when not all options remain open, and decisions are often made of necessity rather than by choice. Although 3 in 10 pregnant adolescents do choose abortion, more might do so if it were not for delay and other obstacles. The poor adolescent, according to Planned Parenthood, is only 40 percent as likely to obtain an abortion as her white middle-class counterpart. Aside from late confirmation, distance (8 in 10 counties have no government-sponsored health facilities for abortion), cost, parental consent requirements, and lack of familiarity with the medical system thwart the adolescent who might otherwise choose to terminate an unintended pregnancy. Adoption is an increasingly unpopular option in the adolescent culture, perhaps because single motherhood is not as stigmatized today as it once was. Presently, 90 percent of white adolescents keep their infants, and almost a full 100 percent of black adolescents keep theirs (*Teenage Pregnancy*, 1981).

Seventy percent of pregnant adolescents continue their pregnancies. Health practitioners are familiar with the young adolescent who may not remove her bulky winter jacket all day long or who employs other elaborate measures to conceal a growing abdomen. Denial frequently characterizes the early weeks and months of an adolescent's pregnancy and can occasionally be present until close to term. This is particularly true in the young adolescent whose menstrual cycle may be irregular and who is still gaining weight from the addition of fatty tissue as part of the normal maturational process. Denial can be conscious or unconscious. It can be accompanied by distortions of the somatic sensations and bodily changes that occur during the early stages of pregnancy (Furstenberg, 1981). Weight gain and enlarged girth are often thought to be from eating too much, and early fetal movement is "gas". Denial is the major contributing factor in obtaining prenatal care.

After the initial shock of discovery, the adolescent's familiar world is in continuing disequilibrium from the resulting change in her biologic, social, and interpersonal situation. She needs counseling and care, but having never been on her own in regard to making her own appointments and obtaining her own medical care, she may not know where to turn for help. She must deal with her fear and anxiety, her family, peers, the father of the infant, school, and her new physical changes and discomforts. Her ability to cope will depend on many factors. Most crucial will be the following (Chilman, 1979):

1. Her stage of ego development and her use of ego defense mechanisms.
2. Her stage in adolescence in terms of dependence–independence conflicts.
3. Her values.
4. Her relationship to her parents and their cultural norms and personalities.
5. Her relationship to her boyfriend and his reaction.
6. Her physical condition.
7. The kinds of material and community resources available to her.

Each pregnant adolescent is as different from all the others as the older maternity patient is from her peers. Each must be assessed individually by the first health practitioner she comes in contact with. It is likely that early intervention will be provided by a school nurse or health practitioner in a family-planning or prenatal clinic where the young adolescent may have gone for a pregnancy test.

Ideally, each patient should be followed closely by one or two health practitioners (such as a clinical nurse specialist and a medical social worker) throughout her pregnancy and into early parenthood. It has been found that a strong and trusting individual relationship may be critical in gaining the willingness of the adolescent to use other beneficial services. The adolescent has the tendency to view the well-meaning adult as not having much to offer and the probing interview as an invasion of her privacy. Therefore, it is recommended that offers of concrete help be given early. There is a greater call for active involvement with these than with other patients, and the relationship should allow for greater initial dependency before the adolescent separates out and is encouraged to stand on her own. If she is forced too early to obtain services on her own, the pregnant adolescent is more likely to fail and become discouraged. Room must be made for both child and adult behavior. Trust is essential. The adolescent may demand expressions of caring through repeated testing. The health practitioner must continue to show genuine interest, even through missed appointments, noncompliance with treatment, and demands for individual attention. A sensitive approach is most effective. In the beginning an educational or relaxed advice-giving approach often works best, as it is nonthreatening and helpful.

A most important initial intervention will be to evaluate areas in which the adolescent patient is deficient or lacking in familial and other resources (social, financial, and medical). Every effort should be made to help the adolescent to find and use services to fill in these gaps.

Family support is of critical significance both during the pregnancy and after delivery. Initially, family support is often compromised by underlying disappointment or by outright anger. It is a common mistake of the middle-class health practitioner to assume that because pregnancy occurs more frequently in the lower socioeconomic groups and because infants are invariably enveloped into the fold of extended families, there is not profound disappointment when a daughter becomes pregnant. The pregnancy may be looked upon symbolically as an event that signifies failed aspirations for a whole family, and it can indeed catapult the entire family into crisis. Counseling must be offered to the conflicted or rejecting family. If the family is basically a well-functioning unit, it can offer strength and comfort to the pregnant adolescent.

Conflict within a dysfunctional family does not usually occur over one incident or event. If a family reacts to a pregnancy as a confirmation of its negative expectations for a particular child, this can signify a long-term nonsupportive environment and it indicates the need for continuing counseling. On the other hand, if the pregnancy is viewed as a one-time traumatic event, causing initial shock and negative reactions, short-term crisis intervention is indicated as the treatment method of choice.

In these situations patient care management should be directive, active, and highly focused on a limited number of behavioral changes or changes in the immediate environment. For example, encouraging the young pregnant adolescent to demonstrate her incentive to remain in school may reassure a disappointed parent, or deciding with the family that the teenager should temporarily move into a relative's less crowded home may help to minimize stress. The goal of intervention should be to increase communication, reestablish self-esteem within the disrupted family, and educate the entire family regarding the adolescent's condition and needs (Bolton, 1980). It is hoped that the family would then be able to offer support and to participate in helping the young patient to manage her pregnancy.

If family support is not forthcoming, it is necessary for the health practitioner to identify at least one responsible adult who will function as primary support in the difficult months ahead. This may be the father of the baby or a friend, minister, social worker, or nurse. It should be kept in mind that this traumatic time can be a period when, with proper guidance, positive changes can be made. Kandell (1979) writes that "understanding the unconscious motivation and the powerful forces of unmet needs in the pregnant adolescent, the nurse (or other supportive health practitioner) can perhaps open eyes, ears, and hearts; indeed she may pivot a crisis into growth".

In addition to ensuring adult support, early intervention should include the following: convincing the young adolescent of the long-term importance of continuing school and helping her to explore ways in which this can be accomplished; linking the adolescent to suitable and convenient ongoing medical care; and encouraging and providing for the involvement of the father of the infant in all aspects of the pregnancy and ensuing parenthood. We will explore the importance of each in turn.

Continuation of Education

Some believe that school represents society's best chance to improve the outcome of adolescent pregnancy – through early detection, counseling, and other services – because medical institutions often do not see the pregnant adolescent until late in the pregnancy. Others feel that schools have been unfairly burdened with the responsibility for solving society's problems, to the detriment of their primary task, which should be academic training. Special school programs as they now exist are uneven in many respects, and there is much disagreement about the "best" approach. This is a complex and controversial issue that is beyond the scope of this chapter, but health practitioners who work with pregnant adolescents need to be aware of some of the problems involved.

In 1972, Title IX of the Education Amendment provided that teenagers who are pregnant or who have a child, regardless of their marital status, are entitled to the same rights as other students; they cannot be barred from any program, course, or extracurricular activity on account of pregnancy or parenthood. The law allows for the separation of educational programs for pregnant teenagers, but the programs must be both voluntary and comparable in quality to regular classes (Zellman, 1982).

Research has shown that most educational programs lack administrative support and have serious academic weaknesses. Most school districts neither seek nor want an active role in dealing with pregnant students. They are passive and uncommitted, primarily because of financial concerns and other priorities. Special programs, as they now exist, might actually have negative effects, because, although they often provide information on pregnancy, child development, and parenthood, they are academically inferior and perhaps contribute to further stigmatizing the pregnant adolescent by virtue of being a short-lived and inadequate response to her needs. Schools might do better to integrate or main-stream pregnant students with the student body as a whole, while providing special individual counseling to assist the young woman to know her needs, schedule a realistic and attainable course load, and utilize existing and ongoing community services, some of which may overlap or duplicate school programs. In the late 1980s, school-based programs have taken on a new importance. This, in part, is a result of the failure of the "comprehensive program" to meet their more global aims. Innovative new approaches, discussed at the end of this chapter, are giving new vitality to school-based programs.

Academic opportunities should remain equal even if study is interrupted or prolonged. It should remain the school district's responsibility to establish a follow-up process to ensure that girls reenter school as scheduled. Contact should be maintained during the first crucial year after delivery to provide needed support and encouragement, and greater effort should be given to helping school officials, teachers, and counselors understand the problems and needs of pregnant and returning school-age mothers (Zellman, 1982).

Educational success can be the key to change. We must keep in mind that the problems that contribute to the etiology of the pregnancy also make educational achievement unlikely. Hosts of problems can make school continuation difficult for even the most highly motivated teenager; for those who are less motivated, such difficulties might make it almost impossible. On an optimistic note, however, the 1972 amendment has had a noticeably positive effect on the number of pregnant and parenting adolescents who do remain in school.

Regardless of whether appropriate programs exist in a particular community, the health practitioner's responsibility must be to encourage consistently the continuation of education. She or he must help the young adolescent explore and utilize all personal and community resources that will allow her (and the adolescent father) to remain in school both during her pregnancy and into parenthood. It should be stressed that in the long term she is being a better and more concerned parent to consider her own future, and that seemingly interrupted goals are still attainable. This important message is well stated by Conger (1973): "What remains as a task is convincing the pregnant adolescent that the position that she finds herself within at the moment is time-limited. The adolescent must be provided the message that her current choices and behaviors need not automatically mandate a life characterized by on-going dysfunction."

Prenatal Care

Pregnant adolescents receive less prenatal care than older women – they have fewer prenatal visits and these start later in pregnancy. The American College of Obstetrics and Gynecology recommends one medical visit every 4 weeks for the first 28 weeks of pregnancy, one visit every 2 weeks for the next 8 weeks, and one visit per week thereafter until term. In 1978, 79 percent of older women received this care, compared to 70 percent of adolescents. The younger adolescent is even less likely or able to comply with these recommendations. Thirty-eight percent of those under 15 years of age and 32 percent of 16- to 17-year-olds receive inadequate care (Zelnik and Young, 1982).

Several explanations have been suggested for why this occurs, including: (1) denial of pregnancy; (2) ignorance of the need for care; (3) a casual attitude toward the importance of proper care for both mother and infant; (4) nonavailability of services; and (5) inappropriate methods of service delivery.

In our society, health care delivery, particularly that directed at the lower socioeconomic group, is presently oriented more toward emergency care than preventive care. This approach results in a particular way that these groups then utilize health care. Doctors and clinics are for conditions of sickness, not wellness. In addition, we see that in what is frequently a crisis-oriented lifestyle, there is an immediacy of survival needs that often overrides any decision to seek out preventive care. Prenatal care is no exception. Since pregnancy is not viewed as a sickness or as a condition that necessarily warrants a doctor's intervention, care is often put off until a complication develops or delivery is approaching. The value of prenatal care may simply not be appreciated. If we add to this the fact that clinics may not be convenient and that logistics of obtaining care may be time-consuming and complicated, reluctance to seek out care becomes easier to understand.

The adolescent population has different needs than older maternity patients. Treatment programs must be specialized with this in mind. The presence of fear, anxiety, and ignorance is more common in the young and must be addressed through sensitive management:

> Long waits in crowded clinics located at distances from home, perfunctory inquiries, a constant changing of the staff, lack of privacy, and the like do not offer effective counterinfluences to indifferences, whether the indifferences relate to real difficulties or intrapsychic or cultural factors. The conduct of the examination can also deter girls from continuing care. Despite the sexual laxity which their out-of-wedlock pregnancy may imply, many of them possess a large measure of modesty. They can be fearful and highly vulnerable to slights, real or fancied, and frequently need the reassurance which comes with sensitive handling in the atmosphere of privacy. (Dott and Fort, 1976).

Recognizing the critical necessity of comprehensive prenatal care, we cannot overemphasize the need for clinic programs that are appropriate to the unique problems of the adolescent patient. Intensive medical, nursing, psychologic, and social services must be offered. Unfortunately, many gaps in service continue as community efforts become bogged down in red tape and as government commitment wanes with the return of a more conservative political atmosphere.

Physicians in clinics that treat pregnant adolescents should recognize that because it is common for teenagers to develop special feelings toward their doctor (as do many older maternity patients), the physician is in a unique position to have a positive influence. If the physician treats the young patient with utmost sensitivity and tenderness, compliance with treatment increases dramatically. Dread of the pelvic exam, which contributes to a high dropout rate and a high number of missed appointments, can be reduced. As mentioned earlier, special alliance with a particular nurse or social worker also leads to greater compliance with treatment.

Teenagers are very concerned about their physical appearance and body image. Many, being in this stage of normal narcissism, dread the changes in their bodies that pregnancy brings, especially the weight gain. These feelings and a common underlying ignorance about nutrition often lead to irresponsible or improper eating habits – for example, continued dieting or an imbalanced intake. There is often much to be unlearned or worked through. Nutritional education that includes active participation in the preparation of healthful meals and snacks should be a primary component of any prenatal program. Group discussions in which concerns about body changes and somatic complaints can be shared are of great help (see Chapter 11).

Groups provide an excellent educational as well as supportive function. Adolescents do not tolerate lectures well, but they enjoy active participation in learning. Peer groups, in which friends share a common experience, can provide an atmosphere in which relaxed learning can take place and can be practiced and reinforced. Communication is shared and on an understandable level. Relationships started in these groups often outlive the prenatal period. Groups also provide an "observational arena" for health practitioners to identify the needier patients for more in-depth emotional support and counseling. Peer groups should be an integral part of any prenatal program, as their effectiveness is well documented (Bolton, 1980; Fig. 38–3).

Anxiety grows as delivery approaches. Preparation for childbirth should include resources similar to those used for all maternity patients – for example, classes, films, and a tour of the delivery

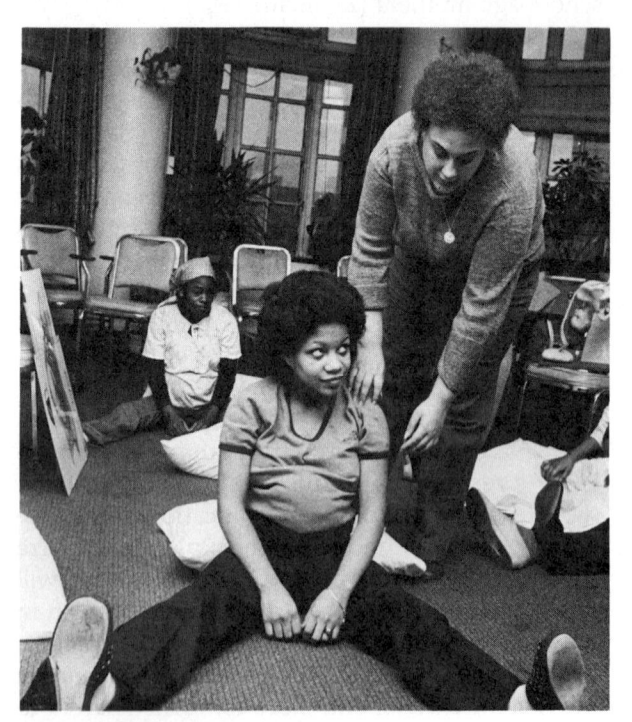

FIGURE 38–3. Adolescents in preparation for labor and delivery class.

SOURCE: Courtesy Erika Stone/Photo Researchers Inc.

suite and maternity unit in which the patient will be hospitalized. This visit is often neglected, but it can be most useful both to defuse fantasies about childbirth and to introduce the young patient to the unfamiliar environment of the hospital. Premature labor and delivery are proven risks for adolescents. Teaching the adolescent to recognize the symptoms of early labor and helping her to feel at ease in the health care delivery system are absolute necessities.

Many adolescents, especially the very young, may differ from adult women in the way they relate psychologically to the fetus. In a recent study by R. Klue, the evidence indicates that:

> Many pregnant adolescents seemed neither to form mental representations of their unborn child, nor to bond with them. The teenagers in the study did not appear to respond to physical clues emanating from the fetus and seemed only distantly connected to their unborn children. Many of the girls in the study evidently did not clearly differentiate fetal movement from self-sensation, which may have accounted for their sparse and disaffected comments about the fetuses (Peterson, Sripada, and Barlow, 1982).

If, indeed, this detachment occurs consistently, it can have damaging consequences for later mother–infant attachment. It suggests the need to focus more on the unborn by encouraging the mother-to-be to talk more about her baby and to direct her attention to its stage of development. She might be encouraged to choose names, discuss desired sex, and participate in listening to fetal heart tones and identifying fetal position and parts. Realistic planning for the infant's future should begin early, as it has been found that the young adolescent tends to present a pattern of overcompensating – making unrealistic plans for her baby, with little inclination to think about what she really wants or expects from motherhood.

The health practitioner in the prenatal clinic should pay close attention to the potential development or exacerbation of emotional problems during this stressful time. Double jeopardy exists: pregnancy adds a situational crisis to a normal developmental crisis (adolescence) for these young women, who may be more likely to have underlying psychologic frailties to begin with. Family conflicts and boyfriend troubles frequently erupt during this time. Tension and depression have been found to be far more common in the pregnant adolescent than in the older pregnant patient. The suicide rate, increasing for all adolescents, is seven times higher in this specific group (Peterson, Sripada, and Barlow, 1982).

Involving the Adolescent Father

Ironically, in the reams of literature on adolescent pregnancy one finds relatively little mention of the adolescent father. Perhaps this is because he is not affected as directly or obviously. Or perhaps he is simply more elusive, and social scientists have difficulty pinning him down for controlled studies. Whatever the reasons, we must begin to focus more concern his way, as his contribution to the problem is undeniable and his own future, like that of the young adolescent mother, is jeopardized.

Chilman (1979) writes that "age-old cultural norms tend to cast the young man as the villain in the piece. He is seen as irresponsible, exploitative, and promiscuous." The few studies that are available contradict this and show that many of these young men would like to marry their partners and want to give their pregnant girlfriends what financial, social, and psychologic support they can. Unfortunately, the young adolescent male usually comes from the same deprived background as his girlfriend and is unable to offer what he would like to. He is subject to the same syndrome of failure she is. This is demonstrated in the fact that he is 40 percent as likely to finish high school as his nonparenting peer.

In 1978 there were approximately 150,000 live births with fathers under 20. Estimates are difficult to make, but it appears that between 45 and 65 percent of these fathers maintained contact with their offspring. From the same sample, the father's contact with the infant's mother occurred as follows: after 1 year, 23 percent of adolescent mothers had married the fathers of their infant; 23 percent were still seeing the father regularly; 18 percent were seeing him periodically; and 35 percent never saw the father of their infant (Panzarine and Elster, 1982).

Health practitioners find it difficult to reach and work with young fathers. There may be several reasons for this. Few programs are organized to offer any concrete services to young male adolescents. Less than 50 percent of the present clinics that care for the adolescent mother include the father in their treatment plans (Panzarine and Elster, 1982). In part, this occurs because our society as a whole does not have any guidelines for preparation for fatherhood. In addition, a young man's own ambivalent reaction to his situation, and his internal conflicts regarding his role, may interfere with his desire and ability to participate. The young man who chooses to remain single may be particularly acutely affected.

The adolescent father-to-be may be conflicted with feelings of self-doubt regarding his capabilities as a father, since many low-income families are single-parent households with minimal or no paternal contact. He is thus provided with a negative or absent role model to imitate. He will undoubtedly have financial concerns and fears of "getting trapped". Consider that he may feel coerced to demonstrate commitment to an unplanned and often tenuous relationship that may take time away from his peer culture, which he still needs and wants. His girlfriend's family may be covertly or overtly angry and accusatory, and his own family, disappointed. If he remains committed, his relationship with his girlfriend will undergo a transition. He will also have to deal with her changing body image and mood swings. He is probably ignorant about the medical aspects of pregnancy and harbors fears about his girlfriend's health and anxiety about labor and delivery. If he is frequently left out, his role will remain undefined during the pregnancy and into parenthood.

Our young male adolescents need to be treated with far more enlightened and sensitive understanding. They need to be included whenever possible as an integral part of a couple and a future family. What is implied here, of course, is a need for restructuring or changing our societal outlook, which perpetuates a myth about the value of the tough, self-sufficient, aggressive male and neglects and negates, to everyone's disadvantage, the gentle and nurturing side that, in many young men, yearns for an outlet.

Specifically, intervention should include health education, guidance, and participatory experiences that give the young man a chance to feel a part of the pregnancy (Fig. 38–4). He should be included in hearing fetal heart tones, feeling movement, identifying fetal parts, and participating in childbirth and child care classes. Ideally, clinics would provide rap sessions and support groups for fathers-to-be to share their fears and anxieties in a nonthreatening atmosphere. Clinics are making more of an effort to hire male counselors, as it has been demonstrated that they often act as positive role models and can be more effective in reaching the young adolescent father than a female counterpart. As with the adolescent girl, counseling should include broader issues such as continued education, sources of financial support, and information on job training.

In summary, including the adolescent father in all aspects of the pregnancy and addressing his specific needs can only positively affect the long-term outcome. In addition, studies suggest that an adolescent father's involvement in his partner's pregnancy boosts the young mother's sense of confidence in her nurturing skills, increases her sense of security postdelivery and, similarly, raises the father's self-esteem (Sander and Rosen, 1987). By accepting responsibility and planning, he will become a better companion and father and will enrich his own life.

THE ADOLESCENT PATIENT DURING LABOR AND DELIVERY

All maternity patients have their individual, often unpredictable reactions to labor and delivery. This is true for the young adolescent patient as well, but certain specific responses are far more common among this group. Hospital staff should be cognizant of what to expect.

Childbirth for the middle-class mature woman with a planned pregnancy and good preparation is often an ultimately joyful and positive experience. This is not the case for the young adolescent patient, who is, more than likely, terrified by the thought of having pain and may have a much lower threshold to begin with. The adolescent will have more difficulty separating pain from outcome and may view the entire ordeal as a punishment. The increased incidence of prolonged labor, technologic interference of monitoring, cephalopelvic disproportion, and cesarean sections only aggravates anxiety and creates more apprehension. It is not unusual to see regression to a more childish stage and an increase in dependency. Modesty and the need to feel in control are two characteristics of adolescence. Embarrassment, indeed mortification, about being so exposed and even about viewing one's own genitals is common. Feeling helpless and not in control can lead to poor cooperation. During labor and delivery, poor pushing, for example, is a manifestation of this.

Intervention should be geared toward assisting the young adolescent woman to feel that she can indeed have some control over her labor. The

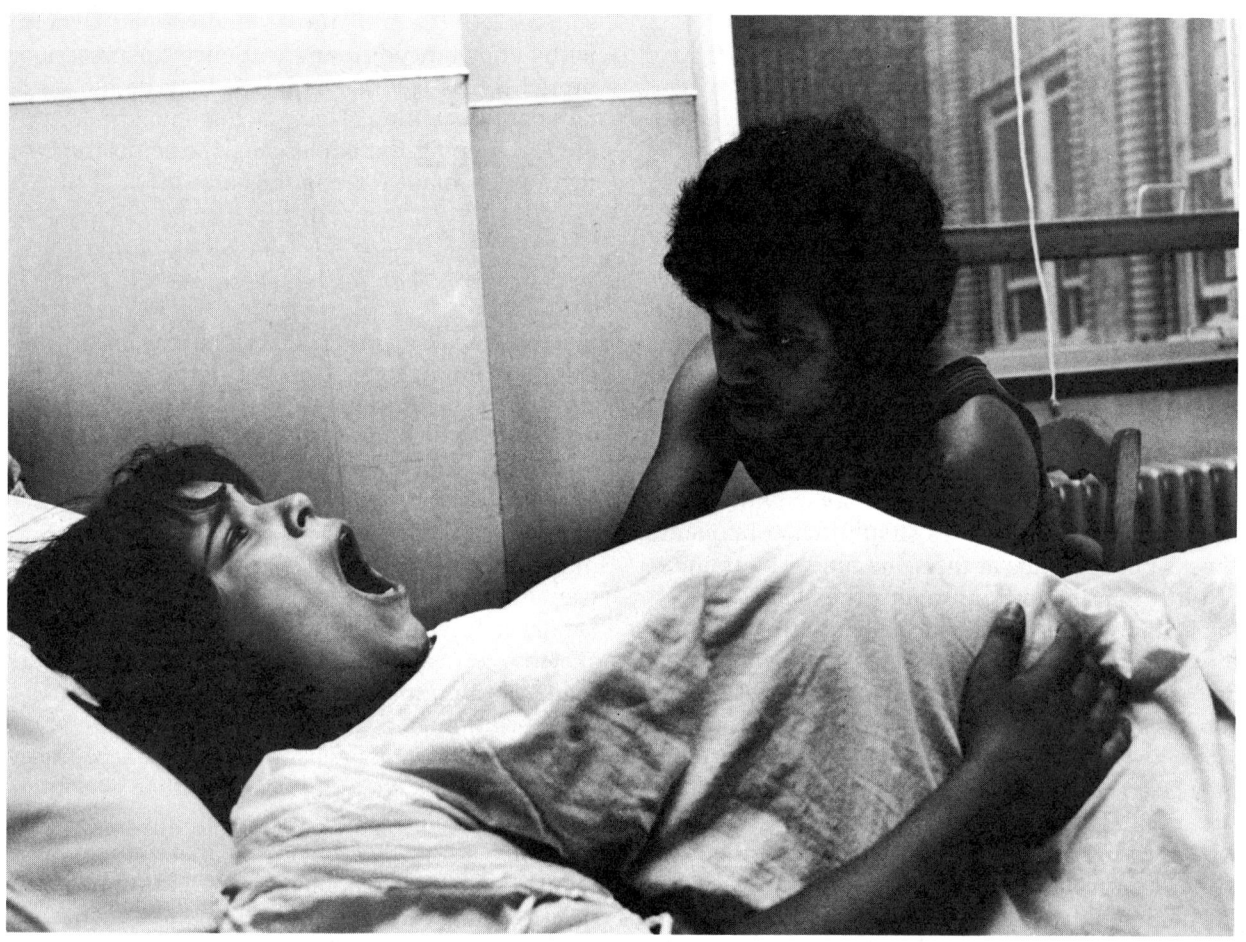

FIGURE 38-4. Adolescent mother in labor with adolescent father supporting her.
SOURCE: Courtesy Mary Ellen Mark.

approach should be relaxed and directive, while at the same time supportive and reassuring. Much repetition may be needed, and as little change in personnel as possible is recommended. Protecting the teenager's modesty during labor can be difficult, but it may of major concern to her. Careful draping and nonverbal communication of understanding helps protect some of her integrity. Working closely with the patient's family or primary support system is crucial. During labor, conflicts in her support system may come to the surface, with mother and boyfriend competing for the spotlight. Staff may need to intervene to help the young patient decide who would be most helpful to her and to provide her with suggestions for handling the conflict diplomatically.

With the possibility of cesarean section, the teenager will undoubtedly be concerned about disfigurement and her postpartum appearance. Explaining the reason for the cesarean section delivery, how long it will last, and why and where the incision will be made will help the teenager cope better. Much of her previous information may have come from sources highly dramatic and inaccurate, such as friends, television, or motion pictures. Most teenagers like to know the reasons why procedures are done, and they can detect honest communication. They do not like to be talked down to, as if they were young children. We need to remember they are adolescents caught up in an adult situation and they need special care to cope (Foote, 1981).

The operating room nurse or delivery room nurse can play a key role in helping the adolescent with gentle, reassuring support and communication. The hospital environment is also important. Liberal visiting hours and flexibility are necessary. Few adolescents have had prior hospitalization. Friendly, cheerful staff help to minimize feelings of anxiety and alienation.

THE ADOLESCENT IN THE POSTPARTUM PERIOD

The Hospital Stay

Teenagers tend to have a lower pain threshold than older patients and as a result may complain more about physical discomfort following delivery. After-birth pains, pain from incisional healing and episiotomy, and breast engorgement can together or separately cause misery. Regressive behavior surfaces, such as not wanting to move, get up, or do anything for oneself or simply wanting and needing to be babied. Homesickness and loneliness (it may be the first time away from family) can lead to demanding behavior with much need for attention. Nurses should make frequent checks but set limits at the same time. The trauma of birth may linger or produce the *amnesia effect*, the inability to recall what actually occurred during the birth. Often, young patients will continually distract themselves through watching television or constant use of the telephone. Perhaps this behavior is just another symptom of immaturity, or it may be an attempt to avoid facing the reality of the situation. This can be a real frustration to the nurse who is trying to engage the adolescent in the care of her newborn infant.

The immediate postpartum period is not an appropriate time to begin childcare teaching, even though we may feel the urgency to do so. The practicalities of having an infant may not be felt or realized while the young patient is in the hospital. Aside from having 24-hour nursing assistance, the young adolescent will probably be busy enjoying the short-lived flood of attention that she may be receiving from family, staff, and others during these few days in the hospital. If the young mother seems open and receptive to instruction, then of course it should be provided. Some adolescent mothers demonstrate competency from the start, usually because they have had infant-care experience. For the nurse to assume, however, that because education is provided it will necessarily be absorbed can be doing a disservice to the new mother and her infant. Individual assessment is always needed.

Breastfeeding is becoming more popular among teenage mothers. It has been found that if young mothers-to-be are introduced to the benefits of breastfeeding as part of their prenatal education, they are more likely to give it a try. On the other hand, for teenagers planning to return to school shortly after birth it may be unrealistic to place this extra demand on their already overextended resources. For the immature or deprived adolescent, with her own needs for dependency still present or unmet, breastfeeding an infant may be too emotionally threatening. These factors must be considered in helping the adolescent decide on the best method of infant feeding for her.

Follow-up Needs and Assessment

Hospital health practitioners, in particular discharge planning nurses and obstetric social workers, have insufficient time and an inaccurate setting in which to assess the competence and maternicity of the new adolescent mother. Studies suggest that immediately after birth the young mother's attitudes are likely to be transitory. The nurse must listen closely to the messages from teenage mothers and take into account several factors in the evaluation. An evaluation, even if sketchy, is necessary to ensure that at least rudimentary support services are provided from the very beginning. Since needs vary considerably, individual assessment is of the utmost importance.

By definition, the adolescent mother is at high risk. Bolton (1980), after reviewing much research and data, drew the conclusion that the environment of the typical adolescent parent and that of the parent at risk for child maltreatment are virtually interchangeable. Both the demographic and psychosocial dynamics are parallel. In both groups of parents, for example, there is a high potential for crisis that pervades all aspects of life and brings with it relationship stresses. Educational and occupational deficiencies lead to lower life expectations, frustration, and financial insecurity. In abusing families, one sees children born in close succession to young, single mothers. These mothers often have unrealistic expectations for their initially unwanted children. In addition, they are ignorant of child development and care, and they have both low self-esteem and a negative role model on which to pattern their own parenting behavior. High risk is further established with the presence of prematurity, which has been found to lead to a higher incidence of child abuse, probably because of early separation and interruption of bonding (Bolton, 1980).

Although statistically teenage mothers are at high risk, any attempt to describe individual human behavior before there are facts to evaluate is both unjust and risky. To derive a realistic perspective on potential parenting patterns, we must look carefully at both the short-term and long-term factors and their implications in our assessment. We can by no means assume that parenting problems are inevitable in this group. To the contrary, evidence exists that a large number of adolescent parents are, in fact, competent, resourceful, and loving, even if their parenting patterns may not be typical (Fig. 38–5).

Short-term factors, observed in the days following birth, can give an initially distorted impression. A difficult or prolonged labor may cause a new or immature mother to feel temporarily angry at her infant for putting her through a traumatic ordeal. She may have wanted a son for the father of the baby and be worried about his reactions to a daughter. Feeling tired, sore, and frightened in the hospital may overshadow motherly feelings that will surface later. Adolescent jargon and slang can also give a distorted impression in that communication that sounds negative ("this is a 'bad' baby", for example) may in fact mean the opposite. Professional judgment and evaluation must be based on less superficial criteria than observable behavior in the hospital. Initial reactions may give hints of future dysfunction, but alone they are insufficient grounds for grave concern, unless, of course, behavior is obviously extreme or pathologic.

For an assessment to be accurate and useful, certain variables in the adolescent's psychosocial makeup must be evaluated. Ideally, a patient's follow-up needs would be evaluated by the per-

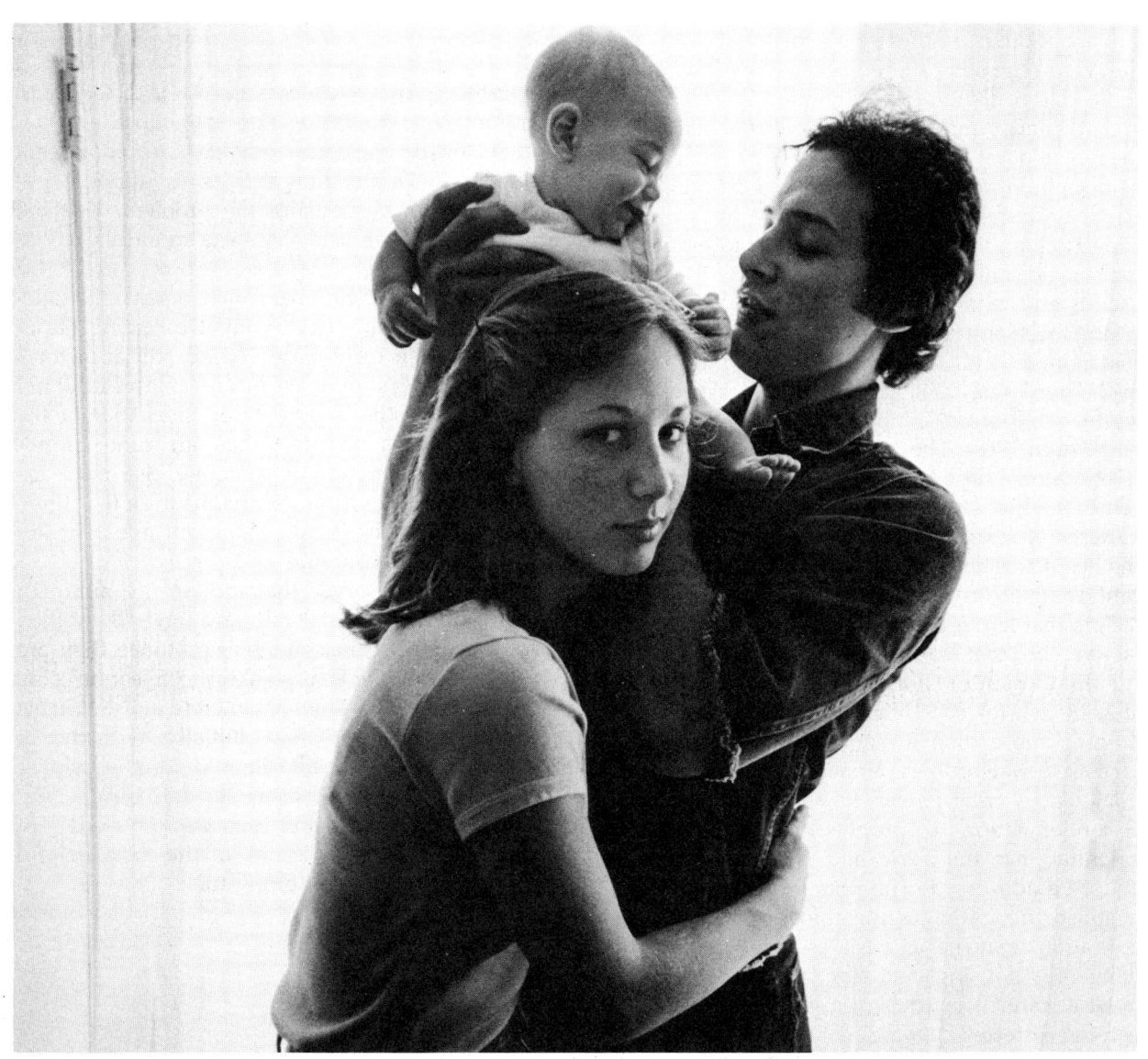

FIGURE 38–5. Adolescent father with his young family.
SOURCE: Courtesy Mary Ellen Mark.

sonnel who provided her prenatal care, as they should be familiar with her ongoing situation, and either their involvement would continue or appropriate continuity of care would be established before delivery. If this has not been done, meaningful evaluation may fall to the public health nurse, who should have the time to spend in the patient's environment during the initial home visits. The variables to be explored are the following: the adolescent's support system, the involvement of the father in the care of the infant, the mother's past experiences with childcare, the mother's intellectual level of functioning, the mother's level of maturity, and peer pressure.

There are several dysfunctional dynamics that are often unpredictable before the postpartum period but that may surface after delivery. It is not uncommon for new mothers to feel let-down or sinking feelings in the weeks following birth. In the young patient these feelings may be more acute. The validation and attention received during pregnancy may come to an abrupt halt once the new mother is home with her baby. There may be disappointment regarding unmet expectations. Life may be the same as it was before, but with the added demands of an infant who has not provided that magic solution. As the lack of interest (from friends and family and perhaps the father of the infant) becomes more apparent and the parental role more difficult, adolescent mothers may return to the pervasive passivity and powerlessness that led them into the role initially (Barglow, Bornstein, and Exum, 1968). The cyclic nature of the problem has its roots in the fact that these mothers usually return to the same environment, partners, and patterns of sexual behavior that they left to enter the hospital. The vast majority of recurrent adolescent pregnancies are generated through the same factors that led to the initial pregnancy. It is these factors, too, that lead to potential child abuse.

Identification of the adolescent parent as being at high risk for child abuse should be viewed as nothing more than a signaling of the need for increased watchfulness and for offering help in immediately critical areas. It should not be seen as a condemnation or prophecy. It is absolutely essential that the basic and concrete issues in abuse be addressed. The primary stressor factors in abuse, in addition to unemployment and undereducation, may be as basic as inadequate food, dangerous housing, and lack of transportation to medical care. It is vital to understand that intervention directed toward concrete services (for example, providing nutritional education, establishing voucher eligibility, or obtaining occupational training) is as important as, if not more

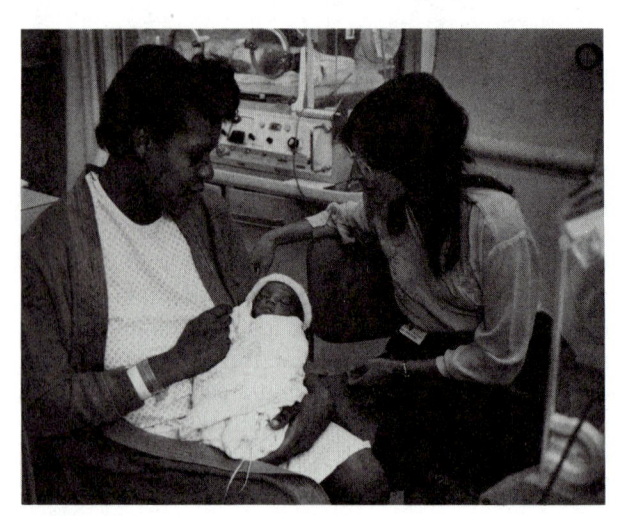

FIGURE 38–6. Adolescent mother with her infant.

important than, psychodynamically directed intervention (Bolton, 1980). This statement is a reminder of the socioeconomic basis for adolescent pregnancy. Deprivation results in a poor self-image, which perpetuates the problem. It is not the other way around, as some moralists would like us to believe.

The health practitioner must assess the adequacy of the home environment carefully. He or she must then focus on a second crucial factor – again, ongoing support from a reliable adult. If not the young mother's parents or the father of the infant (if he is mature), then an aunt, grandmother, close friend, or someone else must assume this role. In the rare circumstance that there is no one, very close and consistent public health follow-up must continue.

It has been observed that adolescents, although slow to obtain prenatal care, are more likely than older women to seek out services once they are mothers. They are also quickest to reject ongoing help if it does not provide concrete and workable solutions to their problems initially. With this in mind, health practitioners should adopt a helping style that is practical, concrete, and caring (Fig. 38–6). A thorough and current knowledge of community resources is one of the most helpful and necessary tools for doing this.

RESOURCES AND REFERRALS

The young adolescent who is not involved in an ongoing perinatal program needs the public health nurse to serve as a link in the transition from hospital to home adjustment. Most hospital discharge planning staffs rely heavily on this beneficial resource for new mothers. In addition to being familiar with the concrete services available in the community, public health nurses offer support, supervision, and continued childcare education (and reinforcement of basic skills, such as making formula, bathing the baby, and so on), and they can act as a much-needed liaison between the mother and physician and the mother and the community. Many health departments have a specialized protocol that allows for more visiting and greater flexibility in the nursing role with adolescent mothers because of their designation as high risk.

Help with concrete services is a logical and necessary first step that should ideally accomplish two goals: it should minimize immediate stress regarding basic life maintenance, and it should assist in keeping the young mother involved in services that ultimately offer more substantial and positive alternatives to her present situation. Indeed, providing certain concrete services, such as arranging for adequate infant care, will offer both short- and long-term benefits.

Minimal follow-up services should provide the following range of resources:

1. *Ongoing medical care.* This must include both maternal care and childcare. Too often young women skip their 6-week postpartum checkup and once again neglect or delay obtaining contraception. Planned Parenthood has shown that persistent and appropriate intervention at this particular time can increase birth control use dramatically. For the healthy infant, an appointment must be made either with a convenient pediatrician or at a local well-baby clinic. If the infant has medical problems, appropriate specialized care should be initiated and assistance given to ensure that the mother is able to follow through on treatment recommendations.

2. *Nutritional services.* Women and Infant Care (WIC) is a supplemental food program specifically aimed at women, infants, and children. It provides nutrition education and supplemental high-protein foods, and it should be offered to all eligible mothers. The program, which starts in the prenatal period, continues for the mother for up to 6 months after birth if she is not breastfeeding and for 1 year if she is. Supplemental food, including formula, is provided until the child's fifth birthday. If nutritional problems continue, the program can be extended. Another important advantage of this program is that to maintain eligibility, proof of ongoing medical care for the infants and children involved must be demonstrated.

3. *Financial support.* If the patient is not on public assistance and expresses anxiety over financial matters, a determination of eligibility for financial aid should be initiated. Additional subsidy services, such as food stamps, unemployment benefits, and state disability, should also be explored. The young adolescent may need assistance with filling out application forms and with transportation to various offices.

4. *Subsidized transportation.* Lack of funds or inadequate funds for transportation can interfere with otherwise good motivation to follow through on obtaining necessary services or complying with medical follow-up. When available, vouchers for subsidized transportation (bus or taxi) should be obtained. Other resources, such as community volunteer bureaus or the Red Cross, will also provide transportation for doctor or clinic appointments.

5. *Parenting services.* Services are necessarily broad in scope and range from continued public health supervision to the involvement of children's protective services and dependency investigation if it is determined that a mother is incompetent to care for her child. As mentioned earlier, careful assessment of mother–infant bonding and interaction over an extended period of time is essential as a basis from which to suggest or initiate intervention, unless, of course, the infant is clearly in jeopardy (Fig. 38–6). Hasty negative judgments about parenting at this time can interfere with and damage the early and often fragile bonding process. At the same time, the infant's well-being must be ensured. As health practitioners, if we observe neglect or abuse we are legally responsible to report our findings to the proper agency. Parenting training, suggestions for disciplinary alternatives, and parental stress organizations are some options that should be provided for the immature and stressed young parent. In many communities parental stress organizations have a 24-hour hotline and can offer respite care (out-of-home overnight babysitting) when a potentially explosive situation warrants it. Parent support groups and childcare services should also be explored.

6. *Childcare services.* Infant care programs, daycare centers for older children, and nurseries adjoining public schools are all available to some degree in most communities. In addition, in some counties public assistance will reimburse the parent for individual babysitting,

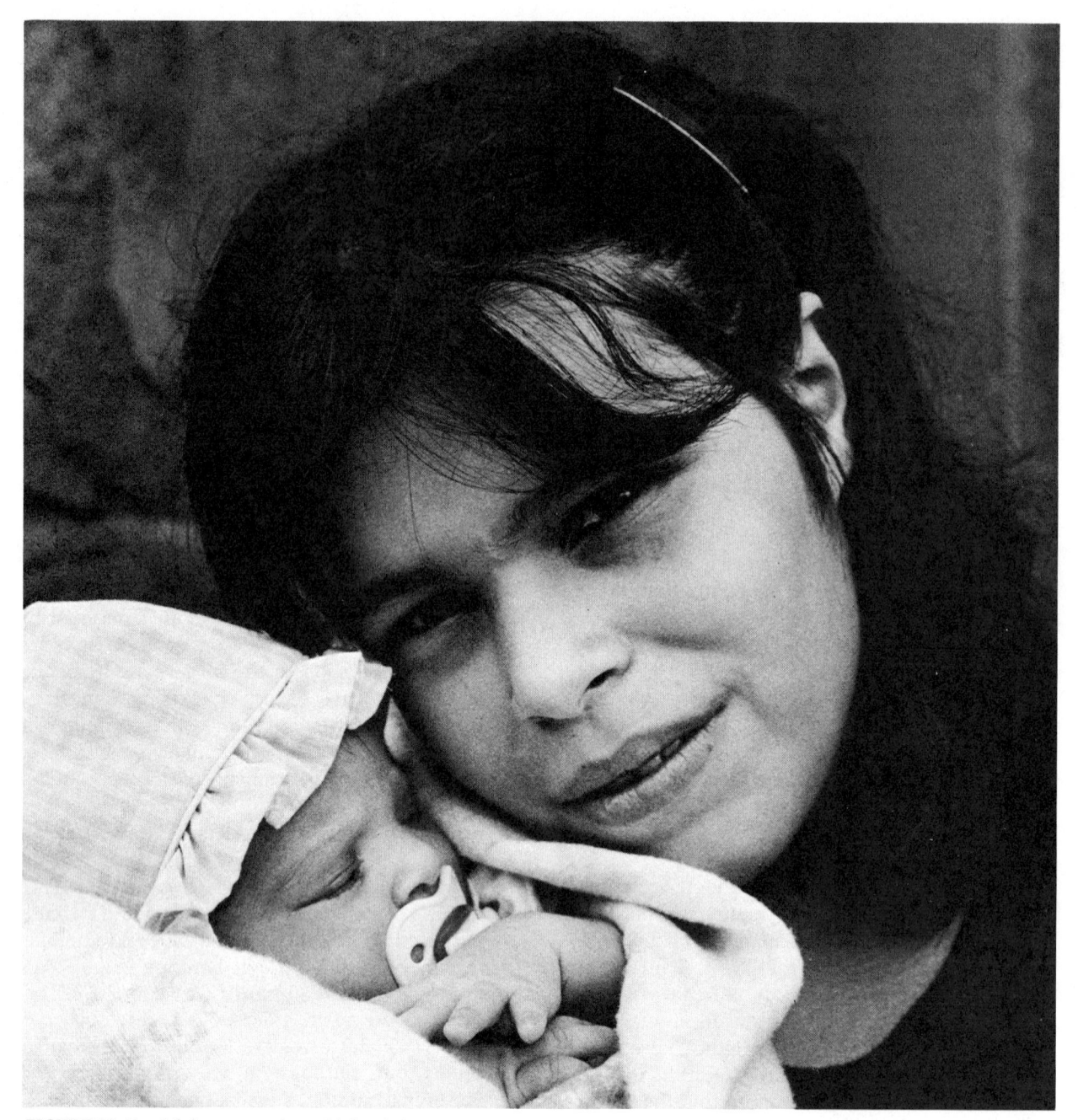

FIGURE 38–7. Adolescent mother with her infant.

albeit on a low wage scale. Sometimes, however, being able to hire an aunt or friend, even for a small amount of money, relieves the parent's feeling that she is using or taking advantage of this person and will then allow the young parent to continue school with less guilt and ambivalence. Lack of childcare is the primary reason, and excuse, for not pursuing educational and occupational goals. Recognizing this fact, more enlightened and committed communities are establishing infant and childcare centers within the confines of the high school, which allows the parent to see and interact with the child but still attend classes. Ongoing childcare education is also usually included. This is the ideal arrangement, but it is still not available in most communities. Helping a young parent obtain childcare is perhaps the most valuable service we can provide (after basic needs are met), and thus it is a goal that should be pursued until a satisfactory arrangement is found.

7. *Career counseling.* Once again, emphasis must

be placed on the possibilities of a young parent obtaining a more fulfilling future than he or she may deem likely. Young parents must be helped to plan for the future in such a manner that small, realistic, achievable goals are met on a regular basis. It might mean, for example, helping the young mother find tutoring to assist her in passing the GED or high school equivalency test, or assisting the young father to enroll in an apprenticeship program. It will entail discussing all career interests and options and directing young parents to resources that will help them pursue their individual goals. Schools with career counseling services should make a special effort to meet the needs of the young mother and father. Too often this group is short-changed, and priority is given to the needs of the unburdened or college-bound student.

NEW APPROACHES AND PROGRAMS

"Services to pregnant and parenting adolescents are too shallow, too uncaring, too removed and too short for too long" (Bolton, 1980). Bolton and other professionals in the field point out repeatedly the need to approach this problem on many levels if we are to see change in the present trends. Funding is poor. What monies exist go into public assistance programs or isolated community efforts that deal exclusively with a single element of the problem. The Guttmacher Institute found, for example, that:

> Too often support for maternal and child health is traded off against preventive efforts such as family planning and abortion, or research into a new contraceptive method is given low priority because of the long lead time needed for its development. (*Teenage Pregnancy*, 1981).

Prevention *and* dealing with the realities of the present are both crucial.

What we have learned is that intervention must be very broad if any long-term impact is to be accomplished. We need a "consistent attack over time" (Bolton, 1980) upon all contributing factors – prevention through sex education and contraception, crisis intervention at the point of discovery, prenatal care and education during pregnancy, and ongoing community resource utilization after the birth of the infant.

By the mid 1980s it became increasingly apparent that the "Comprehensive Programs" envisioned in the 1970s, because of their inherent problems, were not the magic bullet. The underlying assumption of the comprehensive program presupposed that the core components of the program, such as hospitals, clinics, schools, and welfare programs, already existed within each community and simply needed to be linked together. This became not only unwieldy but impossible, as many programs and institutions had their funding cut quite dramatically and developed internal problems within their organizations. Outside funding, needed to develop and sustain services, has not been available. Adolescent pregnancy competes with a host of equally worthy claimants such as the homeless, the hungry, and the abused, for the limited funding available. It must be remembered that teenagers are not strong advocates for themselves. "The adolescents themselves are without political resources and their parents have little to gain by calling attention to what some would consider a failure of parental supervision" (Hollingsworth and Felice, 1986). The comprehensive model, in summary, presented over-optimistic goals in order to secure political and material support; most have fallen short of meeting even modest goals, let alone are they the solution to such a complex problem.

Perhaps as a response to the failure of these programs, some promising new trends are beginning to be seen which, although more modest in their goals, could contribute some positive and fundamental changes. It has been demonstrated that programs with the clearest statistical evidence of success are health clinics located in or within close proximity of high schools. There are approximately 75 high school-based clinics in the United States with 50 percent of these distributing birth control *with* parental consent. Several programs claim to have cut their pregnancy rates by 50 percent (Levine, 1987). Other programs within the school system deal with the crucial underlying problems of peer pressure, specifically in relation to postponing early sexual involvement and/or taking responsibility for birth control in a relationship. Other topics of discussion involve self-esteem issues, future plans, and the realities that young parenthood, devoid of its romantic aura, truly entails. In one San Francisco health education class, teenagers are assigned 5-lb "babies" (in actuality, dressed-up bags of flour). They are solely responsible for their "babies" 24 hours a day over several weeks, which involves not being able to leave them unattended and being accountable for the condition of their "infants" (a clever dose of reality therapy). In some classes teenagers are asked to envisage what they want for themselves in the future and are helped to focus on making long-term goals which are tangible. This often involves job training as part of the school curriculum. Another new approach is to engage teenagers, after being trained, to teach their peers about birth control and other important health issues. This variation on the effectiveness of the self-help therapy movement benefits both teacher and student. In summary, more programs are being designed to creatively educate the adolescent population with the long-term goal of substantially decreasing, through prevention, the numbers of pregnancies that would otherwise occur.

It is an unfortunate assumption made by those responsible for funding that at the time the adolescent pregnancy situation becomes the adolescent parenting situation, the intense need for services is reduced. In fact, it remains the same or becomes more intense (Osofsky and Osofsky, 1978). We must remember that when these mothers leave a program for pregnant adolescents, they are still adolescents and still subject to the same pressures and difficulties that contributed to their becoming pregnant in the first place. Programs must be broad in scope, beginning long before the problem reaches crisis proportions, and they must be continuous in their availability or extend long after the immediate crisis has been resolved.

To establish successful programs, our society must be educated and redirected to recognize that the problem is on the rise as a direct result of social conditions rather than as a result of some innate flaw within those individuals who are trapped by circumstances that we know to be so difficult to transcend. Planned Parenthood suggests that with this corrected attitude acknowledged, we do indeed have the resources to solve much of the problem. The issue is one of national concern. It is important to consider the allocation or redirection of funds from other less critical areas into an eight-point program that would include:

1. Realistic sex education;
2. An expanded network of preventive family-planning services.
3. Unbiased pregnancy counseling services.
4. Equal availability and accessibility of legal abortion services.
5. Adequate prenatal, obstetric, and pediatric care for teenage mothers and their children.
6. Educational, employment, and social services for adolescent parents.
7. Coverage by national health insurance of *all* health services related to teenage pregnancy and childbearing.
8. Expansion of biomedical research to develop new, safe, and effective contraceptives more appropriate to the needs of young people.

We need to recognize that the cost of such services would be insignificant when compared to the huge price already being paid by individuals and society for adolescent pregnancy and childbirth (*Teenage Pregnancy*, 1981).

SUMMARY

As dedicated health practitioners working directly with adolescent patients, we are given the difficult task of keeping our focus both broad and narrow. We need to work to accomplish the larger goals, but we also need to concentrate on meeting the needs of our individual young patients at every step along the way. It is easy to feel frustrated, given the overwhelming nature of the problem and the present lack of resources. During these times of frustration we must look to our individual small successes, such as the young mother who does finish high school, in part because of our efforts, or the healthy and bright 3-year-old child of an 18-year-old mother whose presence in prenatal clinic we were able to maintain consistently.

We must keep in mind that the most successful programs have involved a single individual who builds a relationship with the adolescent early. With sensitive understanding of both the broad and specific issues involved, nurses can have a significant and valuable impact on pregnant adolescent patients and on their relationship with their infants.

REFERENCES

Barglow, P.; Bornstein, M.; and Exum, D. 1968. Some psychiatric aspects of illegitimate pregnancy in early adolescence. *Am. J. Orthopsychiatry.* 38:672–687.

Bolton, F. 1980. *The pregnant adolescent: Problems of premature parenthood.* Beverly Hills, Calif.: Sage Library of Social Research.

Briggs, R. M; Herren, R. R.; and Thompson, W. B. 1962. Pregnancy in the young adolescent. *Am. J. Obstet. Gynecol.* 84:436–440.

Chilman, C. 1979. *Adolescent sexuality in a changing American society: Social and psychological perspectives.* Bethesda, Md.: DHEW Public Health Service, National Institute of Health (No. NIH 79-1429).

Conger, J. J. 1973. *Adolescence and youth: Psychological development in a changing world.* New York: Harper & Row.

Daniels, A. M. 1969. Reaching unwed teenage mothers. *Am. J. Nurs.* 69:332–335.

Dickason, E., and Schult, M. 1979. *Maternal and infant care.* New York: McGraw-Hill.

Dickerson, P., and Ovellette, M. 1982. Prenatal education for adolescents in a delinquent youth facility. *J. Obstet. Gynecol. Neonatal Nurs.* 11(1):39–44.

Dott, A., and Fort, A. 1976. Medical and social factors affecting early teenage pregnancy. *Am. J. Obstet. Gynecol.* 125:532–535.

Foote, J. 1981. Special needs of teenage cesarean section patients. *AORN J.* 43:855–858.

Forrest, J.; Hermalin, A.; and Henshaw, S. 1981. Impact of family planning clinic programs on adolescent pregnancy. *Fam. Plan. Perspect.* 13(3):109–116.

Furstenberg, F. F., ed. 1981. *Teenage sexuality, pregnancy and childbearing.* Philadelphia: University of Pennsylvania Press.

Hardy, J. B.; Welcher, D. W.; Stanley, J.; and Dallas, J. R. 1978. Long-range outcome of adolescent pregnancy. *Clin. Obstet. Gynecol.* 21:1215–1235.

Hollingsworth, D. M., and Felice, M. 1986. Teenage pregnancy: A multi-racial sociologic problem. *Am. J. Obstet. Gynecol.* 155:741–746.

Hutchins, F.; Kendall, N.; and Rubino, J. 1979. Experience with teenage pregnancy. *Obstet. Gynecol.* 54(1):1–5.

Kandell, N. 1979. The unwed adolescent pregnancy: An accident? *Am. J. Nurs.* 79:2112–2114.

Levine, A. 1987. Taking on teenage pregnancy. *U.S. News and World Report.* March 23.

Lorenzi, M. 1977. Marital outcomes of adolescent pregnancy. *Adolescence.* 12:13–22.

Makinson, C. 1985. The health consequences of teenage fertility. *Fam. Plan. Perspect.* 17:132–139.

Mercer, R. 1980. Teenage motherhood: The first year. *J. Obstet. Gynecol. Neonatal Nurs.* 9:16–27.

Osofsky, J., and Osofsky, H. 1978. Teenage pregnancy: Psychosocial considerations. *Clin. Obstet. Gynecol.* 21:1161–1172.

Panzarine, S., and Elster, A. 1982. Prospective adolescent fathers: Stresses during pregnancy and implications for nursing intervention. *J. Psychosoc. Nurs.* 20:21–24.

Peoples, M. 1979. A model for the delivery of health care to pregnant adolescents. *J. Obstet. Gynecol. Neonatal Nurs.* 6:339–345.

Peterson, C.; Sripada, B.; and Barlow, P. 1982. Psychiatric aspects of adolescent pregnancy. *Psychosomatics.* 23(7):723–733.

Ryan, G., and Schneider, J. 1980. Teenage obstetrical complications. *Clin. Obstet. Gynecol.* 21:1191–1197.

Sander, J. H., and Rosen, J. L. 1987. Teenage fathers: Working with the neglected partner. *Fam. Plan. Perspect.* 19:107–110.

Smith P.; and Mumford, D., eds. 1980. *Adolescent pregnancy: Perspectives for health professionals.* Boston: G. K. Hall.

Smith P.; Mumford, D.; and Hamner, E. 1979. Childrearing attitudes of single teenage mothers. *Am. J. Nurs.* 79:2115–2116.

Tatelbaum, R., et al. 1978. Management of teenage pregnancies in three different health care settings. *Adolescence.* 8(52):713–728.

Teenage pregnancy: The problem that hasn't gone away. 1980. New York: Alan Guttmacher Institute.

Thornburg, H. 1979. *Teenage pregnancy: Have they reached epidemic proportions?* Phoenix: Governor's Council on Children, Youth, and Families.

Tietze, C. 1978. Teenage pregnancy: Looking ahead to 1984. *Fam. Plan. Perspect.* 10:205–207.

Tyrer, L.; Mazlen, R.; and Bradshaw, L. 1978. Meeting the special needs of pregnant teenagers. *Clin. Obstet. Gynecol.* 21:1200–1213.

Weatherley, R. A.; Perlman, S. B.; Levine, M. H.; and Klerman, L. V. 1986. Comprehensive programs for pregnant teenagers and teenage parents: How successful have they been? *Fam. Plan. Perspect.* 18:73–78.

Zabin, L., and Clark, S. 1981. Why teens delay getting birth control help. *Fam. Plan. Perspect.* 13(5):205–217.

Zellman, G. 1982. Assessing public school programs for pregnant adolescents. *Fam. Plan. Perspect.* 14(1):15–21.

Zelnik, M., and Young, K. 1982. Sex education and its association with teenage sexual activity, pregnancy, and contraceptive use. *Fam. Plan. Perspect.* 14(3):117–126.

39

The Parent with a Physical Disability

BEHAVIORAL OBJECTIVES

Upon completion of this chapter, the reader should be able to:

- Identify various disabilities in women that can affect pregnancy.

- List available community resources that can be utilized to help disabled parents.

- Discuss various considerations for meeting the needs of parents with the following disabilities: hearing impairment, visual impairment, spinal cord injury, multiple sclerosis.

- Discuss the nurse's role in providing antepartal, intrapartal, and postpartal care to a physically disabled pregnant woman.

- Identify special accommodations that can be made for the blind, deaf, and other disabled women in a hospital's obstetric department.

- Develop a nursing care plan based on the assessment of the spinal-cord-injured woman.

One of the most striking aspects of disability in this country is the incredible discrepancy between the size of the population with disabilities and the amount of information about them. The difficulty of getting accurate statistics is itself a reflection of this paucity of information. One of the more dramatic estimates is found in the 1980 Carnegie study, which estimated that 10 percent of all children are disabled, 20 percent of all adults are disabled, and at least 50 percent of all able-bodied adults have a disabled spouse, child, parent, or close friend (Gliedman and Roth, 1980). Other government-based statistics estimate the overall disabled population to be 1 in 11 people, or somewhere close to 36 million persons nationally. This is far greater than any ethnic minority within the United States. But outside of a few isolated sections of the country where the disabled independent-living movement is strong, one can travel extensively and never see a disabled person. So the question arises, "Where are they?" All too often they are still in institutions or in the back bedrooms of family homes. This invisibility vividly points out the segregation, the ignoring, the denial – indeed the physical, social, and emotional containment – of disability within the majority able-bodied culture.

Being an oppressed minority – as frequently pitied as despised – disabled people are doubly isolated. They have not only been isolated from the mainstream of society, denied access to housing, schools, jobs, social services, and transportation, they have also been isolated from one another. Disability crosses all ethnic, religious, and sexual barriers. But unlike ethnic minorities whose communities and families provide some sort of pride and identity that helps compensate for the overall stigmatization and oppression, the overwhelming majority of disabled people have no such group culture. The only exceptions are the deaf community and "little people's" groups. Otherwise, disabled persons groupings have traditionally been defined in terms of able-bodied professionals' disease and disability categories (MS Society, United Cerebral Palsy, and so on). Initially defined by pathologies, only later, if ever, are the disabled seen as complete human beings who happened to have disabilities. Even the achievements of disabled people are portrayed as exceptions, overcompensations, and inspirations.

This perspective helps one understand the development of the disabled independent-living movement – the civil rights movement for people with disabilities. In the early 1970s, first in college and then in consumer-based service settings, disabled people began to organize around common social needs. As a result, disabled communities – a sense of a culture – began to emerge.

It is important for the health care professional to realize that the disabled movement was partly a reaction to the degree to which the disabled person's life is defined by the patient role. This is reflected by some of the issues in the movement:

1. The emphasis on crossing medically defined disability lines to enhance power and to learn from one another (seen in the varied population of disabled community organizations).
2. The emphasis on independence, empowerment, and respect for the disabled person as a fully participating adult member of society rather than as dependent.
3. The emphasis on the disabled person as an expert on his or her disability.
4. The emphasis on the disabled person as a provider, not just a recipient, of services.

Deinstitutionalization, getting out of parental homes, moving into independent living, and mainstreaming have also been tied to the recognition of the sexuality of the disabled adult. As a result, research and services on disability and sexuality have been flourishing for the past 15 years.

The focus of the work on sexuality has been on the provision of birth control. In this field, the general message has been that disabled people should not have children. Yet the fact is that the social changes taking place among disabled persons – the move to independent living, the demand for a fuller life, the formation of relationships, more active sexuality – are increasingly leading to pregnancy and parenthood (see Fig. 39–1).

The problems faced by disabled parents indicate that the majority culture has not yet adapted to this new development, either attitudinally or in terms of its institutions' provision of support services. Funding is needed, particularly for low-income, severely disabled parents' adaptive equipment and in-home babycare assistance. Parenting by disabled people demands mainstreaming – integration beyond the disabled community into all kinds of new areas. Access is needed to parenting-related services such as obstetricians, maternity departments, schools, pediatricians, social services, and recreation. Disabled parents report a multitude of problems: A stranger tells a disabled woman "You can't be pregnant" 1 month from delivery; a newly developed disabled housing project makes no provision for parents; a maternity floor in a major urban hospital has no accessible bathrooms, so a disabled mother has to be taken to a rehabilitation floor.

One of the most striking aspects of this problem

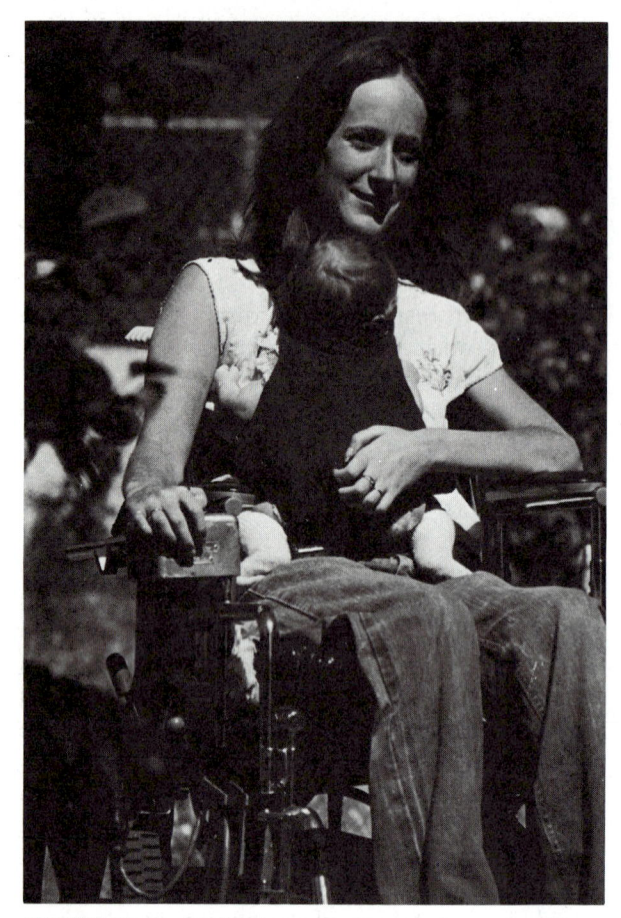

FIGURE 39–1. Disabled women are mothers too.

– both for the disabled parent and for the nurse working with the disabled parent – has been the amazing lack of information on disabled parenting. Locating information about specific disabilities and obstetric concerns or on specific parenting issues is difficult. This seems partially a reflection of cultural attitudes – a message that parenting by disabled people is and should be nonexistent.

This chapter represents an effort to change this situation. It is compiled from a review of scattered and insufficient literature, as well as from interviews with professionals and disabled parents. The chapter focuses on parents with four major disabilities: (1) deafness, (2) blindness, (3) spinal cord injuries, and (4) multiple sclerosis. The specific disability focus should not obscure the fact that disabled parents have many common issues and needs that cross disability lines. It should also not obscure the fact that parents with disabilities are, above all, parents. It is hoped that this chapter will offer support for nurses and disabled parents in their work together.

THE DEAF PARENT

One out of every 16 Americans has a hearing problem, and 1 in every 100 cannot hear enough to understand spoken messages (Schein and Schreiber, 1978). American Sign Language (ASL), used by the deaf culture, is the fourth most used language in the United States.

Just as with other cultural groups, it is essential for nursing professionals to begin learning about the deaf culture so that they can be sensitive to the client's potential strengths as well as the potential problem areas.

When considering deaf parents, the central issue is, of course, the need for full and reciprocal communication between the deaf patient and the hearing health care professional. Like all expectant or new parents, deaf parents have a tremendous need for information and planning to make the transition to parenthood.

Potential problems in the relationship of medical personnel and deaf patients are suggested by research indicating that many deaf people feel there is a deficiency in the doctor–patient relationship – that is, that their questions are not fully or clearly answered, insufficient information is offered, an incomplete medical history is obtained, complaints are not thoroughly explored, and exams are not complete (Nemon, 1980).

Professionals who are competent to deal with other problems and disabilities seem to lose their competence when dealing with deaf people, exhibiting "shock–withdrawal–paralysis", or an inability to handle the situation. Negative attitudes apparently impede communication (Schlesinger and Meadow, 1972). The invisibility of the disability tends to be disorienting. Unmet expectations about communication lead to frustration, embarrassment, feelings of inadequacy, and the desire of the health care professional to terminate contact with the deaf person quickly (Garrett and Levine, 1962).

The hearing impaired rely on both hearing communication devices (TTY) and sign language (ASL) for communication. American Sign Language (also called Ameslan) is different in structure from English, and English does not translate directly into Ameslan. The following excerpt addresses the communication problem both in form and content. It was written by a deaf mother on a TTY and utilizes ASL syntax. Hearing professionals often misinterpret such language as implying lack of intelligence.

> The problem I noticed the most during my Dr. visits was the patience of and understanding for the need of patient about questions and answers. . . . But I kept demanding to write down what he tried to tell me. Often I find that Dr. intend to say "Don't worry" after being asked some questions. I prefer to see them answer the questions no matter if they are silly and stupid or good. After my first baby was born I felt anxious about how to breastfeed my baby and taking care of my breasts while staying in the hospital. I felt the nurses were little helpful as they kept to say "Don't worry". . . . I felt so frustrated because of wanting to know more.

This placating and avoiding of deaf parents is a recurring motif; its impact is at best patronizing and undermining of parents' essential learning and coping processes. Its effect on this particular resourceful and sophisticated mother (who subsequently received help from the La Leche League) was less serious than is the effect on "low verbal language and education" mothers, whom she was concerned about. She became aware of the needs of such mothers when they sought help from her and apparently had no idea about community parenting resources.

Generally speaking, deaf parents are at a disadvantage in retrieving information from the predominantly hearing culture. Many services and resources are still not accessible to them. Also, deaf education is still insufficient in many respects. One inherent source of difficulty is the fact that for the hearing it is said that 90 percent of what we learn is overheard. It seems that this might be particularly true in the folk wisdom–rich area of childbirth and parenting. The same deaf mother comments:

> I asked my (hearing) roommate in our maternity room if she knew about breastfeeding, although she had had her first experience of having baby. She said she heard and heard and picked up some information and then asked the nurses. Maybe that tells the difference between hearing and deaf. Deaf couldn't hear so can't think of questions they should ask. So I think with deaf patients the nurses and doctors should go ahead giving information no matter if deaf patients haven't asked question. They couldn't think of anything to ask until they face problems.

It is fairly common for deaf people to nod or otherwise pretend comprehension of what hearing people say, in order to avoid or withdraw from uncomfortable interactions. When this behavior is combined with the health care professional's lack of communication ability, quality and consistency of health care can certainly suffer.

The Heterogeneity of Deaf Culture

In general, it is common for hearing professionals to underestimate the intelligence of deaf people. It is also often assumed that deaf culture is homogeneous; however, it is, in fact, heterogeneous. Not only do deaf persons vary in intelligence, socioeconomic status, personality, and other areas of individuality, they also vary widely in the manner and ease with which the communicate with hearing people. The following three distinctions may be helpful in considering this variety.

1. *Prelingual or congenital deafness.* When deafness has been present from birth or prior to speech development, the person usually relies on signs (ASL) for communication. English remains a second and foreign language. Prelingually deaf people's speech, if present, tends to be difficult to understand. Written communication may be limited because of low English vocabulary and poor reading skills. The average deaf high school graduate scores on a fourth or fifth grade level on reading tests.

    Deaf people's intelligence and sophistication is frequently underestimated because of these problems with written communications. One common source of confusion is a lack of awareness of the fact that, when writing, many deaf people tend to transcribe ASL, with its distinct grammatical structure. For instance, the English "I fell down the stairs, hurt my back, and think my legs are paralyzed because I have no feeling in them" might be transcribed from ASL as "I fell stairs, pain back, legs nothing" (What if your patient is also deaf?, 1976).

    People in the prelingual deaf category are sometimes called the "low verbal" or "low verbal language" deaf. This is not a reflection on their intelligence or linguistic sophistication in ASL. Furthermore, not all prelingually deaf are "low verbal". Prelingually deaf born to hearing parents are at the greatest risk developmentally.

2. *Postlingual deafness.* When deafness occurs after the development of speech and language, the degree of English verbal skills depends partly on the age and degree of education at

which the person became deaf. Some postlingual deaf will be able to lip-read – perhaps 10 percent well. These individuals tend to be more "cross-culturally adept" and are more likely to be considered "high verbal" or "high verbal language" deaf.

3. *Adult-onset deafness.* If deafness happens suddenly to hearing adults, they have speech and writing skills but, at least initially, no sign language, no lipreading skills, and no deaf culture support system.

Differences among deaf persons also depend on educational and family background, which can affect the degree of identification with deaf culture. People who went to oralist schools, with their emphasis on speaking and lip-reading and disdain for signing, may contrast with those educated in schools more affirming of sign language and deaf culture. People from multi-generational deaf families may not consider themselves disabled. Others, perhaps more educated in the oralist tradition, may not consider themselves thoroughly a part of the deaf culture. And, of course, deaf people come from all different ethnic and socioeconomic groups and vary in a multitude of other ways.

Because of this heterogeneity, it is crucial not to make assumptions about deaf people's needs. Rather, a more reasonable approach is to *ask* about preferences of communication modes, to *elicit* needs, and to *offer* information. Setting aside biases that screen perception and acknowledging that communication may take more patience than that between hearing people, the nurse can be attentive and can pragmatically assess the situation. Working out the communication process with the deaf patient can be both challenging and creative.

Most deaf parents will be polymodal communicators, depending on the circumstances as well as their own preferences (see Table 39–1). For example, when one deaf woman's obstetrician was impatient with her communicating in writing, the woman brought in an interpreter (although she preferred more privacy). When the doctor was still uncomfortable with the communication, she chose to switch doctors.

The Role of Planning

Deaf parents stress the importance of planning ahead for the birth so that their preferences for care and communication can be respected. Sometimes this means a frustrating search for medical personnel who will be sensitive to their communication difficulties and needs. Developing trust, rapport, and a workable communication arrangement with medical personnel can be a satisfying process.

Personal considerations enter into communication strategies chosen for the birth itself. Couples vary as to their comfort about having an interpreter present at birth, their preference for a female interpreter, and their ideas about whether the interpreter should be a friend or family member or someone with whom they have a formal relationship. Some couples prefer no interpreter in this intimate setting and are satisfied with the use of lip-reading, gesturing, signals, and writing. Others use written communication throughout prenatal visits but use and recommend an interpreter for the intense time of delivery.

Some of the most satisfying birth experiences have involved interpreters who developed a relationship with the couple beginning with prenatal visits or childbirth classes and continuing throughout delivery and postpartum. In one case, the couple had two interpreters, who worked in shifts through a long labor.

Even the most thorough preparations may be upset by unexpected personnel changes or crises. One sophisticated and involved deaf/hearing couple, planning for a natural delivery, had carefully established a relationship with an obstetrician, had arranged for an interpreter, and had even brought a hearing communication device (TTY) to the hospital. Yet during the labor they ended up having to educate four different back-up physicians about the role of interpreters before their regular physician arrived. And even worse, during a long and difficult labor they had a replacement nurse who reportedly:

> wouldn't tolerate the interpreter being in the room. She tried to physically block the communication by standing between us. It was difficult for her because he was a male interpreter. She seemed to feel he was an intruder. . . . She didn't like it that everything she said was interpreted, thought she was being talked about . . . [or] he was advising interfering with treatment. She also complained there were too many people there, but there were just the two of us, the interpreter and her. . . . We hadn't had time to educate her beforehand.

Later the nurse did not allow the deaf father to go with the hearing mother to the shower during transition, saying she could *call him* if she needed him.

These difficulties indicate the need for nursing

TABLE 39-1. *Guidelines for Communicating with Deaf Parents*

Mode of Communication	Guidelines
Sign language	Learning some signs is usually appreciated as an indication of respect and good will. However, misunderstanding and disappointment might result if your amateur status is not made clear at the outset. Avoid restricting the patient's hands – for example, IVs in both arms. Keep the preferred signing hand free.
Interpreters	Always speak to the patient directly, not to the interpreter. Do not say, "Tell the patient. . .," as the interpreter will interpret each word you say. Slow down your speech to allow for fingerspelling time. The interpreter should be slightly behind you and to either side, without a strong light behind, so the patient can see both you and the interpreter simultaneously. It is improper for hospitals to make use of friends or family members as interpreters without the consent of the deaf patient. In particular, avoid using hearing children of deaf parents as interpreters, particularly in emotionally charged situations.
Lip-reading/speech-reading	Only about 10 percent of deaf people are proficient at this skill. Face the patient and avoid standing in front of bright light. Speak slowly and naturally and avoid shouting, since that distorts your mouth. Don't obstruct your mouth or turn away. If the patient doesn't understand, repeat the thought using different words. Utilize context and visual aids to clarify – for example, "time" and "dime" look the same as spoken, but you can indicate the former by pointing to a watch. Adjust for use of face masks.
Written communication	Deaf people may use ASL syntax in writing. If necessary, use simple vocabulary and avoid idioms.
Speech	If the patient has some speech ability, words may be pronounced as if English obeyed strict phonetic transcription rules; speech rhythms will be changed.
The visual dimension	Because deaf people are visually oriented, nursing care is compromised by restricting or eliminating the visual mode. A night light is suggested, as is a room in visual contact with the nurse's station. Avoid annoying light changes – flashing lights are like an alarm clock buzzing. Visual aids, such as videotapes with captions, are helpful, as is written material. Indicate your presence before interventions. Make use of nonverbal communication – body language, facial expression, eye contact.

SOURCE: Sabatino (1976).

staff to be sensitive to the care of the deaf patient and to be flexible in adapting to deaf parents' needs. Some suggestions are (1) assigning the same nurse each shift so that rapport and communication can be established; (2) bending hospital rules concerning visitors and rooming-in; and (3) opening emergency treatment, recovery room, and intensive care units to interpreters.

In crises, many communication modes may not be practical. If a patient is groggy from medications or anesthesia or is absorbed in the labor or delivery process, any lip-reading or writing ability may become unusable. Surgical masks may be a big problem. The possible avoidance of masks should be discussed with the physician beforehand. A hearing mother giving birth is hardly the best interpreter for her deaf husband, as she will probably lapse into speaking, not signing. In such situations the role of interpreters becomes essential. The more under stress, the more information the deaf parent will need to allay anxiety and permit involvement in crucial decisions. When a baby is taken out of the delivery room suddenly after birth, telling a deaf parent not to worry will not suffice.

The use of an interpreter during crisis can mean a positive emotional outcome, as in this example reported by a deaf father:

I was able to share in all the joy and all of the knowledge and decisions (which is unusual for me because I've always felt like I've only known *in part* what was going on or found out *later* what was going on), and to be fully and immediately aware of everything – of all the events . . .

Even in the absence of interpreters, sensitivity to the deaf parent's needs can result in beautiful and long-remembered gestures. A deaf mother, separated from her baby after birth, grew anxious and wrote:

"Where's my baby?" Right then, before I could go see him the nurse brought me a picture. The nurses and I wrote back and forth and they brought more pictures until I could get up and see my baby. When we left they put many pictures on a birthday card and said he was the most beautiful baby in the nursery. I was so touched.

Focusing on One Cultural Issue: Will the Baby Be Deaf?

A particularly sensitive cultural issue is whether the parents prefer their baby to be deaf or hearing. Some deaf parents will say that they want their child to be hearing. If this preference indicates a desire for an easier life for their child as an able-bodied person, this is a healthy parental concern. But if it is because "The child will be able to be an interpreter for me, help me understand and navigate the hearing world, be a buddy and companion," there is reason for concern.

Many deaf parents will say that they hope their child will be deaf. This might indicate, "I want my child to be the same as I am, and if my experiences with my hearing parents were not good [early communication may have been severely limited], then I don't want to be on the other end of that with my hearing children." The parents' preference may also be primarily a cultural issue – a desire of parents to share their culture with their child – as well as a desire for ease of communication (Berman, personal communication).

Health care professionals may initially blunder and offend by assuming that genetic counseling and avoidance of a deaf baby is a goal. Although 10 percent of deafness is inherited, deaf parents in general are not terribly concerned with genetic counseling. This lack of concern stems in part from a sense of cultural pride. With the issue of the baby's hearing or deafness such a sensitive one within deaf culture, a negative attitude on the part of health care professionals can complicate the situation, particularly during the vulnerable period of labor and birth.

Audiologic testing at birth can be extremely offensive and inappropriate. The parents' autonomy and the timing of nurse intervention should be considered when testing the baby's hearing.

My sister's deaf, too, and when she had a baby girl . . . the nurse was so insensitive that she had to see the baby and quickly did a hearing test – clapped her hands in the baby's ears and the baby cried. My sister was so upset – screamed at the nurse to leave her alone. "I'll decide when to give her a test – not you!" That's such a cruel test for a newborn anyway. And then the other nurse brought all this audiological equipment into the delivery room.

In the midst of the intimate greeting and celebration of the birth of the baby, immediate hearing tests may be seen as a pathologically minded and culturally insensitive assault. A deaf father recalled:

We learned from my sister – we had it all over the chart that we didn't want any hearing tests – that was something we wanted control of. We trusted so little I went with the baby everywhere – I knew they were curious whether the baby could hear.

Respect for and awareness of the cultural issues surrounding whether a baby will be deaf or hearing can have meaning and repercussions far beyond the time of birth. Permitting and encouraging a deaf man married to a hearing woman to be actively involved throughout birth may set an important precedent. It may suggest a strategy for dealing with his concerns about being left out or too uninvolved in the ongoing communication process if his baby turns out to be hearing. This may have been the case for the deaf father whose interpreter was resented and interferred with so much by an unfamiliar nurse. The father's drive to remain involved was fiercely persistent; he overcame many obstacles in the process and later formed a deep attachment to his hearing baby.

The majority of deaf expectant parents, recognizing the complexity of the issue, express that whether their child is deaf or hearing they will face the situation lovingly, and in their own way. It is hoped that nurses and other health care personnel will increasingly facilitate the process.

THE BLIND PARENT

Visually disabled persons form a varied and seemingly small group, but their needs and right to caring and informed service should not be ignored. In particular, women with visual disabilities have special needs and characteristics during pregnancy, labor and delivery, and the postpartum period.

Identifying the Visually Disabled Person

There are dozens of conditions as well as accidental injuries to the eye that can result in severe visual disability. Visually disabled women are not all the same type of woman, any more than blonde women are all the same. One generalization that *can* be made is that a visually disabled woman is a person whose sense of sight has a limitation that directly affects her major life functions.

The word "blind" will sometimes be used here for the purpose of brevity, but even the word itself is sometimes misleading. "Legal blindness" refers to having a measured visuality acuity of 20/200 or lower in the better eye with the best normal correction possible, or a field of vision less than 20 degrees (Mehr and Fried, 1975). This means that the person who is legally blind has 10 percent or less of normal visual acuity. Estimated over the past 20 years in this country, between 60 and 80 percent of persons categorized in government figures as legally blind have some usable, residual vision.

A more accurate and meaningful term for discussing the majority of visually disabled persons is "low vision". Persons with low vision may be defined as having reduced central acuity or visual field loss that even with the best optical correction provided by regular lenses still results in significant visual impairment (Mehr and Fried, 1975). What one person can or cannot see is highly individual and not necessarily elucidated by ophthalmologic findings. Factors such as environment, intelligence, emotional state, concentration level, light levels, and contrast determine actual visual functioning. Thus, two women with the same vision condition and acuity may function quite differently. A meaningful understanding of the visual functioning of the particular woman is best approached by the nurse via repeated contact and observation and the development of rapport sufficient to allow open communication about the issue.

Blindness is considered to be a "low-incidence" disability in this society, meaning that it occurs in 5 percent or less of the total population. However, both the National Society for the Prevention of Blindness and the U.S. Department of Health and Human Services note that the data are inadequate at best and probably do not account for many legally blind persons or others who do not fall into the typical groups from which statistics are drawn. Some recent anecdotal data would indicate an increase in the rate of congenital blindness directly related to the success of neonatal care facilities. That is, more infants are living who would have died prior to recent advances in neonatal treatment, and these infants are so young and small that the visual centers in the brain and the optic nerves may not be adequately developed for seeing properly.

The Attitudinal Problem

Many of the attitudes about disabled persons in general apply equally to the blind. However, there are certain attitudes that seem to apply primarily to the blind person as viewed by the sighted culture. Many popular expressions, for example, create negative associations to blindness that can exist in our unconscious minds and provide input to attitudes. Some of these expressions include blind faith, blind drunk, blind to the truth, wandered blindly, robbed blind, the blind leading the blind, and blind man's buff. These and other such expressions promote the notion directly or indirectly that blindness carries with it such negative qualities as ignorance, stupidity, foolishness, incompetence, and disgrace. Persons with visual disabilities are often repulsed and righteously angered by the impact they feel from the type of stereotyping done through these linguistic patterns. Furthermore, blind women frequently report such sterotypes expressed in negative reactions to their pregnancy and parenting.

The Effect of Blindness on a Pregnant Woman

In many cases the changes that occur in the body during pregnancy have little or no physiologic effect on the visual disability. However, in most cases the pregnancy does affect the disability as it relates to the psychologic make-up of the woman, including her self-esteem, body image, and confidence. The periods of elation and excitement that many pregnant women feel are sometimes diminished in the blind woman. The responses of family, friends, and even strangers can affect her sense of well-being. A 32-year-old low-vision mother in her first pregnancy recalled:

> I always felt very glad that I was pregnant. My child had been planned for four years. The problem was when I would be on the bus or walking down the street. People would say things and shake their heads in disgust as they watched me walk down the street pregnant and using the cane.

At times it becomes almost impossible to separate the influence of the external messages from the internal ones. Whatever the source of beliefs and attitudes, the blind woman, like all pregnant women, is highly emotional and sensitive. A 32-year-old mother of two contrasted her first pregnancy 12 years ago to their second pregnancy only 2 years ago:

> When I was carrying my first daughter, I was amazed at how my body and my attitude about myself changed. I did not believe that I would really be normal even though I was going to college, married and doing those seemingly normal things until I became pregnant. I thought that I looked good pregnant, and this was the first time in my life that I can remember thinking that my body was attractive in any way. I felt that I had finally found the thing in my life that I knew that I could do well and like.
> My husband supported my feelings of confidence. However, others such as my in-laws and family muttered quietly at family gatherings about their fears for my child and gentle chastisements for my husband for letting this happen.
> During my second pregnancy, I felt much less amazement, renewed confidence based on ten years' performance as a parent, and the same public response as the first time. Although I was far from my family, the strangers on the street and acquaintances timidly voiced concerns, fears, and questions. Even with my own confidence and knowledge, I sometimes felt lonely, alienated, and angry.

As the pregnant body changes in shape and center of gravity, the blind woman must sometimes make mobility and other adjustments. If she uses a cane she must sometimes practice a bit to regain the perspective of the point at which the cane touches the surface. Women who have some residual vision lack depth perception or a clear sense of their "new" body's position in space. Again, practice and understanding of what is happening solve this type of minor problem quite satisfactorily. Occasionally, the dizziness common to vision problems, including nystagmus, will aggravate the nausea and dizziness associated with pregnancy. This is usually a temporary and minor problem. Some women who have had this problem report that they could lessen the discomfort by just sitting still for a short time without focusing on anything in particular. Soon the feeling would pass.

The Effect of the Childbearing Process on Blindness

With some visual conditions, pregnancy, labor, delivery, and postpartum have no consequences on the disabling condition or on the level of functioning of the woman. With others there may be varying degrees of consequences. Information about complications of disability due to childbearing is primarily based on limited case studies and reported experiences. Well-designed empirical research on the subject is lacking and much needed.

Retinal Detachment

There are several conditions that are known as retinal detachment. The most common condition occurs in persons who are myopic (nearsighted). Because in myopia the retina is stretched and becomes thinner, a tear or a hole can occur in the retina, allowing fluid to escape from the vitreous humor of the eye into the subretinal or the potential space between the rod and cone layer in the pigment epithelium. Such retinal detachment tends to happen when people are repeatedly exposed to trauma or surgery on the eye. Surgery is the commonly used treatment for this condition. However, the surgery is considered successful if an acuity of 20/200 with a good field (legal blindness) is obtained (Schut, 1974). If a woman is at risk for retinal detachment, it is often recommended that she refrain from any activity that could cause trauma to the eye, including the act of pushing in the delivery room.

Glaucoma

Approximately 15 percent of blindness in American adults is attributed to glaucoma. In this condition the intraocular pressure rises to a dangerous level. The optic nerve is highly vulnerable to increased pressure, resulting in loss of vision (Schut, 1974). One woman with congenital glaucoma reported that she experienced a noticeable loss of residual vision immediately after giving birth. When she saw her ophthalmologist about 4 weeks later, he diagnosed increased pressure in her eye. He attributed this sudden increase in pressure and the subsequent loss of vision to the process of labor. On the basis of this situation, she was placed on medication that only partially returned her newly lost vision. She was further advised by her physician that any subsequent pregnancies could produce additional vision loss.

Nystagmus

The dancing eye syndrome, as nystagmus is called, is associated with several disabling conditions and occasionally occurs independently in its congenital type. It is a poorly understood neuromuscular dysfunction in which involuntary movements of the eye preclude focusing well and prevent the development of acuity when it occurs in young children. It is associated with such visual disabilities as congenital cataracts and albinism. Although this condition is not deteriorated by pregnancy and childbirth, it is affected by these processes. A mother with congenital nystagmus discussed her own experiences with these effects:

> I did note during both my pregnancies that I had a greater tendency toward nausea during the times when I would get dizzy. Getting dizzy is common with my vision problem. It could best be described as the condition wherein everything around is moving all the time at very different rates. You have to keep trying to focus on moving things. It does make you dizzy at times. During the active parts of my labors, I temporarily lost significant vision because of the strain of labor on my entire body. Also, my blood pressure rose dramatically during labor, which has always affected how well I could see. The condition did go back to normal as soon as my blood pressure did.

The three conditions just described are only a few of those that may be found in the visually impaired. A fourth that has a direct and critical role in pregnancy is diabetic retinopathy (see Chapter 14).

Other visual disabilities are transmitted genetically, but their hereditary nature does not in and of itself influence the pregnancy. On a psychologic level, however, the hereditary nature of certain visual disabilities plays a definite role in the pregnancy process. Women who are otherwise genuinely happy about the prospect of parenting may experience great anxiety and fear about the prospects of giving birth to a blind infant or an infant who may become blind later in life. Others may feel quite resolute that being blind is not a tragic consequence at all. These women may be much more interested in other aspects of their pregnancies. The point is that it is unwise for the professional to assume that the mother or father is viewing his or her prospects of producing a blind infant as negative. Further, parental reactions on this issue may be expected to be intense at times. As in many areas of work with the disabled, the patient may be the best authority on the appropriate areas of concern and consideration.

Care and Treatment Issues

There are certain considerations in the care and the treatment of the blind pregnant woman that she may not be knowledgeable about or experienced with. Women educated in segregated programs for the blind are likely to have little accurate knowledge of anatomy and physiology, sexuality, and reproductive processes. Those educated in a mainstreamed situation often lack appropriate books and other learning materials to provide them with the same information that sighted people get about the subject matter. In addition, health and family planning education and services are usually inaccessible to the visually disabled. Professionals in these fields know little about blindness, and the materials are seldom adapted into forms accessible to the visually disabled. Furthermore, the attitudes of service providers tend to reflect the negative societal attitude about blind persons having families. As a result of all these factors, blind women tend to lack knowledge about what is happening in their pregnant body. And what little information they do have may be sketchy and sometimes false.

This lack of correct information is sometimes difficult for the professional to recognize. This is due to a phenomenon known as "verbalism in the blind": the ability of the blind person to use words accurately at a complex or sophisticated level for which she lacks concrete experiential or conceptual knowledge. For instance, the woman may use terms such as *uterus* or *cervix* but have no idea of the relationship of these words to actual parts of her body. She may even be able to verbally describe the location of the uterus but be unsuccessful in pointing to the area of her abdomen where it is located. This verbalism does not mean that she is intellectually inferior; it is simply a measure of her lack of opportunity for concrete experience as compared with her opportunity for verbal experience.

Unplanned pregnancies seem to arise out of a lack of information about birth control and lack of education and familiarity with the functioning of the reproductive system. Many blind women have been saddened and bewildered by the negative way they have been treated upon seeking diagnosis and intervention in such situations. Rather than being given complete and impartial counseling, they have been hastily advised to have abortions. They have been made to feel that the primary reason for the abortion is their blindness. In addition, they have not been given necessary information about the psychological consequences of abortion and have subsequently suffered depression and loss, complicated by confusion and a sense of having nowhere to turn for support within the medical community.

Blind women, like all women, need conscientious and caring prenatal counseling that acknowledges the normal human need to procreate as it exists in the blind as well as in the sighted.

Techniques to Enrich and Improve Obstetric Care for the Blind Parent

The nurse can enrich and improve the experience for the blind parent in three areas: (1) prenatal care, (2) labor and delivery, and (3) postpartum.

Prenatal Care

The blind woman should be given an individual guided tour of the clinic or office setting so that she can become oriented and feel more comfortable. This tour should allow her to move slowly through areas where her treatment will take place and, when possible, should include laboratory areas that the sighted patient would be able to perceive visually. Care providers should introduce themselves by name. When entering the room, they should always speak to her, acknowledging her presence, as they would give a simple nod to the sighted patient. The woman should be offered assistance with filling out forms. As the patient is weighed, she should be told the weight as a part of the routine. The same applies to her blood pressure readings. She should also be allowed to tactually or at close visual range examine all instruments to be included in her examinations.

Efforts should be made to locate and use high-contrast large diagrams of the pelvis, or in the case of the totally blind person, tactile models. These aids will provide her with important information about anatomy and physiology and the progress of pregnancy. In advance of the delivery date, a tour of the delivery area should be scheduled for the blind mother as well as the father, especially if he is blind.

Labor and Delivery

The needs of the blind patient tend to be more immediate and urgent in labor and delivery. Some of the techniques used to make the woman more comfortable in the prenatal care situation may distress her here. For instance, prenatal care is enhanced by increased tactual interaction and exploration of the woman's body, but during the transition period of the labor, she may not wish to be touched at all and may react strongly if she is touched. She should be assisted to feel totally at ease and in control of her environment. All interactions should be verbal. No one should enter or leave her room without informing her. Activities that are outside her visual range should be described to her by the nurse or her supportive others. Support persons should remain close to her so that she will not need to expend energy on difficult visual searching tasks.

In an alternative birthing situation, the blind couple, like other couples, may choose to be alone for a while as the labor progresses. An auditory signal should be devised so that staff can be present when needed and the couple can still have the privacy they wish. In this situation, the blind father must receive the same adaptive considerations as the blind mother.

Postpartum

The postpartum period is a new experience for the blind parent. There is much to learn about recovery and about parenting. A rule of thumb is that most things that can be accomplished visually can also be accomplished nonvisually. A second rule of thumb is that, for individuals with low vision, most things that can be accomplished at a visual distance of 14 inches can also be accomplished at a visual distance of 4 inches or less. It is often a good idea to have an experienced visually impaired parent visit with the new parents to share information and experiences. The nurse can also be supportive by being patient and by promoting confidence, giving the blind parent an opportunity to experiment.

As the nurse and the parents begin to work as a team, whose goal it is to promote a successful and fulfilling parent–child relationship, many of the anticipated obstacles will seem to fall away. The parents can have a positive experience with the medical profession that leaves them willing to seek help when needed without fear of humiliation or frustration. Meanwhile, the nurse can gain satisfaction through genuinely caring for the blind parent.

THE PARENT WITH A SPINAL CORD INJURY

The most common complaint expressed by spinal-cord-injured mothers regarding health care professionals is their lack of information. Women with spinal cord injuries also often complain about not being believed or respected by the health care team regarding their disability. Yet the spinal-cord-injured woman is usually the best authority on her own situation, particularly in regard to self-care and prevention – independent living skills, bowel, bladder, and skin care, and autonomic dysreflexia.

Information presented in this chapter can be used as a basis for exploring the application of the woman's past disability experience to the changes involved in pregnancy. It can serve the planning process that is so crucial to empowerment, and it should be used sensitively to avoid unnecessary anxiety. Given the desire of parents for deliveries to be as natural as possible, and given the preliminary stage of perinatal disability research, the health care professional should be particularly alert to issues of overtreatment.

Issues in Maternal and Infant Well-being

Drugs

It is typical for spinal-cord-injured patients, particularly with high injuries, to be given drugs such as Mandelamine (often with vitamin C) to raise urine acidity, antibiotics in case of urinary tract infections, and antispastic drugs such as Valium, Dantrium, and Lioresal (Ohry et al., 1978). The teratogenicity of such drugs should be considered – if possible before pregnancy – in an attempt to eliminate or substitute for any medication that may affect the developing fetus.

The nurse should be alert for substance abuse, in particular prescription drugs such as Valium, which is frequently overprescribed by physicians for disabled people, with resultant dependencies (Hepner, Kirshbaum, and Landes, 1980/81).

Diet, Weight Gain, and Infant Growth

In addition to the usual dietary concerns during pregnancy, it is particularly important that the diet contains sufficient fiber and bulk and that the woman's bowel program continue. Also, attention to the inclusion of iron-rich foods is important in preventing anemia, a common problem exacerbated by pregnancy. Dietary sources of iron may preclude taking oral iron supplements that can contribute to constipation. Increased fluids are important because bladder infections are more common during pregnancy.

"The calcium balance is disturbed in these patients. It is not known, however, whether the growth of the fetus deprives the paraplegic mother of calcium enough to worsen the osteoporosis usually affecting bones below the injury" (Ohry et al., 1978). One article cautions about balancing sufficient calcium intake needed for fetal development with the need not to have more ash than the mother can handle (Robinault, 1978).

The pressure of the growing fetus has been reported to sometimes make an adequate diet or optimal weight gain difficult, particularly when associated with ongoing nausea.

Such problems as scoliosis may alter the positioning of the baby and make intrauterine growth difficult to estimate without intermittent sonograms. L/S ratios and P/G levels in the amniotic fluid are sometimes used to estimate gestational maturity.

Anemia

Anemia and hypoproteinemia are common in spinal cord injuries, and the problem may be worsened by pregnancy. Anemia increases fatigue and the tendency for bladder or kidney infection and pressure sores due to decreased tissue resistance. Taking of temperature and of blood for serum protein, and Hgb—Hct tests is recommended (Ohry et al., 1978). In addition to dietary prevention through iron-rich foods, suggestions for restoring blood count include blood transfusion and parenteral iron or oral iron therapy in conjunction with stool softeners (Young, Katz, and Klein, 1983).

Bladder or Bowel Programs: Bladder Infections

Bladder and blowel programs may be disrupted and need to be adjusted during the pregnancy. A high-fiber, high-bulk diet combined with stool softeners or suppositories may be helpful in preventing the constipation that may be increased during pregnancy, particularly as a result of oral iron intake. Fecal impaction may cause autonomic dysreflexia (to be discussed later in this chapter). Women with spinal cord injuries have reported the occurrence of bowel accidents late in pregnancy, thought to be due to pressure from the developing baby as well as lack of normal tone in rectal muscles.

In assessing the effect of pregnancy on the bladder program, the nurse needs to consider the completeness of the injury and whether or not the woman is aware when her bladder is full. Distention of the bladder may cause autonomic dysreflexia. A survey of 19 spinal-cord-injured pregnant women showed a wide variety of bladder management choices, including ileo conduit, indwelling catheter, and intermittent catheterizations. Most women which controlled voiding had injuries below T-6 (Verduyn, 1983).

> In women with upper motor neuron lesion the muscle tonus is generally spastic and the bladder "automatic". This causes incontinence, so that diapers or pads have to be worn and frequently changed. In lower motor neuron lesion the bladder must be emptied often, either by trigger or by pressing the bladder area, and diapers must also be worn. . . . Despite poor bladder control during pregnancy, permanent catheterization is to be avoided, except when there is considerable residual urine and infections. Catheterization itself may cause sepsis and endangers the upper urinary tract – this must be particularly remembered during early pregnancy, when the range of safe antibiotics is limited (Ohry et al., 1978).

The usual susceptibility of pregnant women to bladder infection is increased for spinal-cord-injured women, who, due to the bladder paralysis and the use of a catheter, are prone to bladder infections when not pregnant. Chronic infection of the urinary tract is not a contraindication to pregnancy, provided renal function is preserved (Young, Katz, and Klein, 1983). Of the 19 women in Verduyn's (1983) study, 10 had urinary tract infections during their pregnancies that were attributed to the presence of Foley catheters.

Preventive interventions include increasing the fluid intake, meticulous catheter care and hygiene, and emptying the bladder before and after intercourse:

> If the patient manages her bladder by stimulating reflex voiding several times a day, she normally may have a limited fluid intake to avoid incontinence. She will need support and guidance to alter her routine and increase her fluid intake. Methenamine mandelate, a commonly used urinary antibacterial drug, requires an acidic urine to be effective. Therefore, the client should drink a large volume of cranberry, plum, or prune juice, or take oral vitamin C by tablet. She can easily be taught to check her urine pH with Nitrazine paper, as well as test for infection either with a dipstick for bacteria or a home culture kit (Johnston, 1982).

Contractures or Spasms

Increasing spasticity may occur during pregnancy. As one C5-6 quadriplegic put it, "It felt like I was turning inside out sometimes in my lower abdomen – very uncomfortable – painful, though it didn't interfere with my mobility much. Relaxing in a warm bath helped." Positioning during labor and delivery may need to be adjusted in response to contractures, although the increased leg and perineal spasms that occur during delivery have not been found by obstetricians to hinder vaginal delivery or episiotomy and repair (Young, Katz, and Klein, 1983).

Independent Living Skills and Balance

The woman's present level of functioning in self-care and mobility should be assessed. The nurse may offer anticipatory guidance in regard to the use of new adaptive equipment and the possibility of services such as attendant care. In addition to problems caused by increased spasticity, if sitting balance or transfer balance is difficult before the pregnancy, the weight of the fetus in the uterus will tend to worsen balance (Mooney, Cole, and Chilgen, 1975). As the pregnancy proceeds, self-catheterization may become increasingly difficult.

Circulation: Thrombophlebitis

Parapelgic and quadriplegic women have complained about swelling in their ankles and legs during pregnancy. One woman stated:

I was sitting a lot and as my stomach swelled I think it affected the blood flow. I used to notice vaginal swelling. Propping my feet up helped. Also, I began spending more and more time lying down. I'd been told after the 30th week it wasn't a good idea to lie on my back – supposedly for blood flow. So I lay on one side or the other.

Thrombophlebitis is reported to be more frequent during pregnancy because of the pressure of the growing uterus on venous return. With the limitations on mobility in spinal-cord-injured women, there is stasis in the veins of the pelvis and the lower extremities (Ohry et al., 1978). In cases where there are frequent spontaneous muscle spasms in the lower extremities, thrombophlebitis would not be anticipated as a significant hazard (Geiger, 1977).

One of the main problems is that a woman with a spinal cord injury would be unlikely to be aware of the earliest sign of thrombophlebitis – pain in the calf or the thigh. She therefore needs to be advised to examine her legs regularly and to watch for redness or swelling. She should also be aware of a change in range of motion. Prompt mobilization and physiotherapy are recommended to avoid thrombophlebitis after delivery.

Respiratory Function
Able-bodied pregnant women experience shortness of breath when the enlarging uterus presses against the internal organs and the diaphragm, and this difficulty may be increased to different degrees in the spinal-cord-injured woman. The extent of the problem depends on the level of injury and on which respiratory muscles can still be used. For instance, a quadriplegic may only be able to use the diaphragm for breathing. Increased pressure of the uterus on the diaphragm could make breathing more difficult, which could lead to the accumulation of secretions that may cause bronchopneumonia (Ohry et al., 1978). Severe respiratory compromise could affect the fetus because of a decreased oxygen supply (Morrison et al., 1978).

Although this complication should be noted and dealt with, it is important to maintain the perspective provided by the generally positive outcome for infants of spinal-cord-injured women. In addition,

the patient can be taught deep breathing and coughing to prevent the pooling of secretions. Breathing exercises, such as blowing noise-makers and musical instruments, and use of simple equipment such as blowbottles can help maintain or increase her breathing capacity. Respiratory status should be monitored throughout the pregnancy, usually with vital capacity measurement. The patient should be well-informed of the signs and symptoms of upper respiratory infections and encouraged to report them promptly (Johnston, 1982).

Skin Care
Decubitus ulcers are always a potential problem in patients with spinal-cord injuries. They are more common during pregnancy because of increased pressure on weight-bearing areas and because of fatigue. During pregnancy, there is even less mobility than usual; weight shifts, and push-ups from the chair become more difficult and relieve the pressure less effectively (Ohry et al., 1978). As mentioned previously, skin problems may also be exacerbated by anemia.

Because of the increased risk of skin breakdown, padding and cushioning of contact surfaces should be reevaluated. The woman should be instructed to check for red spots daily, to avoid pressure on questionable areas, and to keep the area dry and clean. Some women use massage and lotions such as vitamin E and Aloe Vera. Bedrest may be required to alleviate pressure.

Contact with harsh, rough, stiff equipment and surfaces should be avoided during medical interventions throughout the perinatal period. Nurses should become familiar with advances in protective materials used in rehabilitation, such as synthetic skin-like silicone fabrics. Stirrups can be covered with posey heel cups, and examining or delivery tables can be carefully padded, with the use of sheepskins. Sanitary belts, leg straps on delivery tables, and fetal monitoring straps can be a problem, especially if the patient is spastic. Several specialists recommend delivery in bed, still with proper padding and sheepskin. Women have complained of being left too long on hard x-ray tables, resulting in much discomfort during labor. Repositioning every 2 hours, using pillows for support, is essential.

Skin vulnerability must be taken seriously, not only because of possible medical complications from decubitus ulcers, but also because the postpartum experience could be compromised unnecessarily by health problems resulting in enforced bedrest.

Breastfeeding
Generally, breastfeeding is unaffected by spinal cord injury, even with cervical leisons, other than

the considerations of positioning (Sandowski, 1976).

Experience of Premature Labor

The literature suggests that spinal-cord-injured women may have a problem with premature labor (Ohry et al., 1978). Premature labor is said to be more common when leisons are above the level of T-11 (Tsoutsoplides, 1982).

One potential problem is that women with higher injuries may not feel the onset of labor and may be unaware of it, particularly if it begins during sleep (Geiger, 1977; Ohry et al., 1978). The problem may be compounded by stronger, more prolonged, and more frequent contractions than are usually seen during labor (Young, Katz, and Klein, 1983). Early hospital admission or repeated sterile cervical exams to detect dilation and effacement during weeks 28–32 are recommended, particularly for multigravidas. Hopefully, preterm labor monitors with alarms will be developed that can be used during sleep to signal the onset of labor.

One childbirth educator used the following approach with a woman she described as a C-7 quadriplegic:

> Since my patient would not be able to feel her labor contractions, I told her to watch for loss of the mucous plug, a bloody show, and leakage of amniotic fluid from her vagina. I also described how the uterus contracts during labor, making her abdomen appear heard and boardlike. At rhythmical intervals she could expect to see her abdomen tighten for some 20 to 60 seconds, gradually soften, then tighten again several minutes later. Even if she could not feel her contractions, she could observe them (Asrael and Kesselman, 1983).

Some women are aware of either Braxton Hicks or labor contractions when they have autonomic dysreflexia symptoms. A T-6 paraplegic reported the feeling of "heating up and flushing" on her face and neck, similar to how she felt when her bladder was full. A C-7 quadriplegic was reported to anticipate a contraction during labor when she started to experience an upward pressure, a feeling in her throat like "the baby is coming up" (Asrael and Kesselman, 1983). A T-12 paraplegic with dulled senation in the pelvic area reported feeling "hardening" during contractions and phantom hip pains during active labor; an incomplete quadriplegic felt "tightening". As previously discussed, spasticity may increase.

Autonomic Dysreflexia or Hyperreflexia

A serious complication of spinal cord injury is *dysreflexia*, which is quite common during labor contractions when the level of paralysis is T-6 and above. In Verduyn's (1983) survey, 12 out of 16 deliveries in the category of T-6 and above involved autonomic dysreflexia. According to Johnson (1982):

> A lesion at this level deprives the body of hypothalamic control over sympathetic spinal reflexes. Stimuli which trigger this "mass reflex" response include visceral distention or contraction including contraction of a pregnant uterus, stimulation of pain receptors, and stimulation of the skin. The afferent impulses from these stimuli ascend the spinal cord and result in an autonomic reflex response which originates from the lateral horn cells. This reflex produces vasoconstriction and resultant hypertension. In response to the hypertension, the vagus nerve produces bradycardia, but the spinal cord lesion blocks impulses which would normally produce vasodilation and a lowered blood pressure. The symptoms persist in the form of systolic blood pressure readings as high as 250 mm Hg and diastolic of 50 mm Hg.

Other symptoms include severe headaches, "gooseflesh", flushing above the level of the lesion, sweating, nasal stuffiness, tingling, severe anxiety, and in some cases bradycardia, tachycardia, or cardiac arrhythmias. Infrequently, blurred vision or dilation of the pupils occurs. The symptoms can occur in any combination or degree of severity. If untreated, the syndrome can cause cerebrovascular accidents, brain damage, or death. It is crucial to distinguish autonomic dysreflexia from preeclampsia, with which it is often confused and which is actually more unusual in the spinal-cord-injured woman (Young, Katz, and Klein, 1983).

Long-term prevention of dysreflexia includes optimal skin care and management of bladder infections. Because distention of the bladder or rectum can cause or exacerbate dysreflexia, especially when combined with a distended uterus, keeping these organs emptied during labor may help control the problem. Enemas should be avoided, since they cause distention and are reported to precipitate dysreflexia in the nonpregnant spinal-cord-injured woman (Chui and Bhatt, 1983). Topical anesthetics are recommended when inserting a urinary catheter or doing a rectal or cervical examination (Johnston, 1982). A sitting position or having the head of the bed elevated to

30–45 degrees is recommended to reduce intracranial pressure and blood flow (Johnston, 1982; Chui and Bhatt, 1983). The use of a birthing chair might be considered. However, one of the best approaches to prevention is to assess whether the woman has ever had autonomic dysreflexia, what her particularly early warning signals are, and how she usually manages it.

A variety of drugs are recommended to control dysreflexia. They act promptly, either by vasodilation or by counteracting the passive sympathetic outflow, as with intravenous hydralazine infusion (Young, Katz, and Klein, 1983). Amyl nitrate, Arfonad, and nitroprusside have also been recommended (Verduyn, 1983). Epidural anesthesia is sometimes used. However, there may be difficulty with a lumbar puncture and adequate monitoring of the level of the block in spinal-cord-injured women (Chui and Bhatt, 1983).

In general, the dysreflexia problem seems to be resolved by the birth of the infant and delivery of the placenta. The following report was given by a woman who was an incomplete C5-6 quadriplegic:

> I had dysreflexia in labor both times. It was worse when I was lying down – sitting up made the headache better. With the first baby they gave me a spinal. It made me sick for days with chills and dizziness and I couldn't enjoy my baby then. It took time to get back to my normal level of mobility. With the second baby they said natural childbirth wasn't possible so it didn't make sense to take birthing classes. They planned an epidural. After I got a headache, before my water broke, the anesthesiologist insisted on it. But I got relief from the dysreflexia as soon as I had a bowel movement – even before the baby was crowning. And the baby came so fast it was born naturally in the labor room. Everything was fine and the anesthesiologist couldn't believe it! I felt wonderful after that baby – my mobility was the same as usual, and I could take care of him right away.

It should be remembered that the strategies for handling dysreflexia are still being developed; because of the seriousness of the condition, there may be a tendency toward overtreatment.

Delivery

In the past, cesarean sections were commonly recommended for women with injuries of T-10 and above. Although a number of women are still being given this information, vaginal deliveries may be encouraged unless there are complications such as deformities of the spine or pelvis, other obstetric indications, or uncontrolled autonomic dysreflexias (Ohry et al., 1978).

The literature is unclear about the ability of the spinal-cord-injured woman to assist in birthing her infant. This vagueness is probably due to lack of specificity about levels of injury and completeness or incompleteness of lesions. For instance, one source says that the second stage of labor may be prolonged by an inability to bear down in cases where the abdominal muscles innervated by T-10, T-11, and T-12 vertebras are affected by the lesion (Tsoutsoplides, 1982). However, another source maintains that a woman with a low lesion can assist, while for a woman with a high lesion spasms or cramps in the pelvic muscles may cause difficulties beyond the inability to push (Heslinga, Schellen, and Verkuvl, 1974). The following example describes a C-7 quadriplegic assisting with pushing while using a birthing chair. Note that the fundal pressure described may not be considered safe.

> The woman was told to start pushing whenever she felt the pressure of a contraction in her throat and neck. As a contraction came, she filled her lungs, pulled up with her arms, and pushed as hard as she could At the same time the nurse applied constant fundal pressure to her uterus. With three pushes the baby crowned (Asrael and Kesselman, 1983).

A birthing chair uses gravity to compensate for muscular weakness or paralysis.

Outcome: The Baby

A study of 187 pregnancies found that fetal malformations occurred only in babies whose mothers were injured during their pregnancies (Goller and Paeslack, 1972). Despite potential complications, spinal-cord-injured mothers have the same proportion of healthy babies as able-bodied mothers do (Griffith and Trieschmann, 1975; Sandowski, 1976; Verduyn, 1983).

There have also been numerous cases of uncomplicated pregnancy and vaginal delivery of women with spinal-cord injury (Comarr and Gunderson, 1975; Dickinson, 1977; Hardy and Warrell, 1965; Robertson, 1979; Verduyn, 1983).

Much information needs to be assimilated in order to provide appropriate care for the spinal-cord-injured woman. Information can serve the coping process of the disabled woman, as described in the following report by a T-6 paraplegic who discovered that she was pregnant at 4 months. She had received her spinal-cord injury

NURSING CARE PLAN:

THE SPINAL-CORD-INJURED MOTHER

Nursing Diagnosis	Expected Outcome	Nursing Orders
LABOR		
1. Potential impairment of skin integrity related to decreased sensation/mobility	1. Skin will remain intact and without pressure areas	1a. Confer with doctor and delete perineal prep if possible b. Turn side to side every 2 hours using extra pillows for support c. When positioned on back elevate the head of the bed to a 45° angle d. Observe skin under fetal monitoring straps and devices every 2 hours for the development of pressure areas
2. Potential alterations in patterns of urinary elimination related to pressure on bladder or changes in fluid intake	2. Previous voiding patterns will be maintained; bladder distention will be absent	2a. Confer with client and follow established voiding pattern b. Obtain an order and insert a no. 16 Foley with 5-ml bag if intermittent catheter necessary more than every 3 hours, or if distention occurs in 2 hours c. If catheter is inserted, remove when dilation is complete d. Catheterize after delivery and send C&S of urine if indwelling Foley is used e. If i.v. is necessary, maintain a maximum infusion rate of 100 ml/hour
3. Potential alterations in patterns of bowel elimination (constipation, diarrhea, incontinence) related to fetal pressure on the bowel	3. Previous patterns of elimination will be resumed after delivery	3a. Confer with doctor and delete admission enema if possible b. Suggest the use of a Fleet's biscodyl enema 1.25 oz size if an enema is necessary c. Plan bowel evacuation depending on mobility or stage of labor, i.e. ruptured membranes, quadriplegic, paraplegic d. Do not use bed pan; plan evacuation on a chux or bedside commode
4. Potential development of dysreflexia related to bowel or bladder distention or fetal pressure on the perineum (second stage of labor)	4. Blood pressure will remain at the baseline level; there will be no headache	4a. Monitor blood pressure every hour – an increase is probably due to dysreflexia not toxemia b. Check blood pressure immediately if patient complains of headache c. Check bladder and bowel for fullness if blood pressure increases and headache present d. Notify doctor of symptoms of dysreflexia e. Have Apresoline and saddle block tray available
DELIVERY		
5. Impaired physical mobility related to paralysis	5. Patient will be able to identify assistance needed in transfers	5a. Have extra people or mechanical device available for transfer from labor bed to delivery table and from delivery table to a recovery room bed

NURSING CARE PLAN: Continued

THE SPINAL-CORD-INJURED MOTHER

Nursing Diagnosis	Expected Outcome	Nursing Orders
		b. Have extra people available to help position patient if saddle block is necessary
6. Potential impairment of skin integrity related to decreased sensation	6. Skin will remain intact without the development of pressure areas	6a. Place extra padding on stirrups and under straps b. Make sure perineal area is clean and dry after delivery c. Do not apply sanitary belt after delivery – it can cause a sacral pressure area
POSTPARTUM 7. Potential alterations in patterns of urinary elimination related to possible urethral edema	7. Bladder will not become distended; input and output will be balanced	7a. Begin intermittent catheterization in recovery room every 1–2 hours b. Reinsert Foley catheter if not on an intermittent catheterization program c. Determine previous intermittent catheter program and reestablish it as soon as possible d. Allow patient to do self-catheterization when she is able to do so e. Accurately measure I&O
8. Potential alterations in patterns of bowel elimination: constipation related to decreased bowel mobility	8. Patient will be able to maintain or reestablish previous bowel program	8a. Determine previous bowel program and consult with doctor relative to continuation of the same medications b. Maintain bowel program at established time c. Obtain a bedside commode or assist patient to bathroom d. Suggest that drugs containing codeine be avoided due to their constipating effect
9. Actual impairment of skin integrity related to episiotomy	9. Episiotomy site will be clean and without evidence of infection	9a. Inspect perineum QID for signs of irritation, chafing, hematoma, infection, or skin breakdown, especially from peripads b. Due to decreased sensation, do not use peri lights or sitz bath treatments to episiotomy site; *use tepid compresses if necessary* c. Cleanse area after each voiding with tepid water
10. Potential impairment of skin integrity related to decreased mobility and sensation	10. Skin will remain intact and without pressure areas	10a. Change position every 2 hours b. Provide extra pillows as necessary to assist with position changes c. Initiate proning as soon as possible after delivery; allow patient to prone as tolerated d. Do not use sanitary belt e. Check boney prominences BID for signs of pressure areas

SOURCE: Craig (1983).

1½ years prior to the pregnancy. The only information she could find at the beginning of her pregnancy was that spinal-cord-injured women could get pregnant:

> When I visited the hospital and looked in the delivery room it reminded me of the room I was put in before surgery. I had to remind myself that this is a positive situation – not like my injury when so much was unknown. The unknown is what's scary. I want to know lots of detail and plan ahead as much as I can.

Maternity nurses caring for the spinal-cord-injured woman need to assimilate and offer extensive disability information without overfocusing on the disability rather than on the particular woman who is their patient. In this way they can help facilitate the positive developmental process of becoming a parent.

THE PARENT WITH MULTIPLE SCLEROSIS

Multiple sclerosis (MS) is a progressive neurologic disorder known for its unpredictability and the variability of its prognosis and symptoms, which may include weakness or fatigue, incoordination, sensation changes, speech and visual problems, some incontinence, and paralysis. It is now generally accepted that as many as one-third of the cases of MS tend to remain mild and relatively stable. Most MS patients will never need to use a wheelchair – in fact, one study indicated that after 25 years, two-thirds were still ambulatory (Wasserman, 1978). It is typical for MS to become symptomatic during the childbearing years, from 20 to 40. Its cause remains unknown; epidemiologic studies have suggested a wide variety of causal theories.

The Genetic Issue

Researchers have long noted that the occurrence of MS in the same family is slightly higher than might be expected by sheer chance. However, a number of studies (MacKay and Myrianthopoulos, 1966; Leibowitz and Alter, 1973) have failed to demonstrate a direct genetic mechanism for the disease.

The risk of a family having more than one member with MS is comparable to the risk of a family having more than one member with paralytic poliomyelitis. This suggests a strong role for common exposure to an environmental factor (Poskanzer, Schapira, and Miller, 1966). However, since the incidence of MS is also higher among second- and third-degree relatives who are not in the same household, simple exposure is not an adequate explanation.

Researchers theorize that there is a genetic "predisposition" to develop the disease under the appropriate environmental conditions. The environmental factor seems to be dominant or somehow far more important, since the overwhelming majority of cases are the only ones in their families and there have been a few cases when only one of monozygotic twins has MS (Poskanzer, Schapira, and Miller, 1966; Berry, 1969; McAlpine, Lundsen, and Acheson, 1972; Leibowitz and Alter, 1973).

Given the lack of specific knowledge about the disease mechanism, it is helpful to look at empirical data. A recent study of nearly 8000 persons suggests that the risk for first-degree relatives, such as children, is 0.5–1.0 percent greater than for the general population (Sadovnick and Macleod, 1981). The overall incidence of MS in the United States is from 25 to 30 out of 100,000 (Kurtzke, 1980). This places the genetic risk factor in perspective and provides the sort of material that will be important to use in allaying the considerable anxieties of parents on this subject. It may be useful to add that MS has no influence on the incidence of fetal abnormalities (Janz, 1978) or of spontaneous abortion (Poser, Wikstrom, and Bauer, 1979).

MS and Pregnancy Research

A correlation between the onset or relapse of MS and pregnancy has been noted in the literature for at least 70 years. Early researchers even recommended therapeutic abortion. However, more recent studies have found no detrimental effect of pregnancy on the overall course of the disease (Ghezzi and Caputo, 1981). Because the time when MS usually becomes active and is diagnosed corresponds to the childbearing years, the chances that onset and relapse occur around pregnancy are heightened. Some researchers suggest that this coincidence explains the observed association. Leibowitz and Alter (1973) have suggested that pregnancy, particularly in the 1–2 years prior to neurologic symptoms, may have a precipitating effect; that is, it may cause the disease to become manifest more quickly, but it is not a cause of the disease itself. A precipitating factor is not of etiologic significance.

In women who already have MS, the exacerbation rate increases during the three postpartum months but not during the pregnancy itself (Schapira, Poskanzer, and Miller, 1966). A deterioration in neurologic conditions has been seen during postpartum, but this has not been the rule and is generally temporary; on the other hand, pregnancy and the postpregnancy year generally produce a favorable effect on the disease course so that the long-term prognosis remains the same (Ghezzi and Caputo, 1981).

Information and Its Communication

Patients with MS complain that they are not informed about recent research on pregnancy and MS. For the most part women with MS are still advised against having children and are warned of exacerbations associated with pregnancy. If they are not made aware of statistics about overall prognosis and they experience such an exacerbation, they tend to assume it means a permanent worsening of their condition.

Information and how it is conveyed can have a particularly powerful impact in alleviating or increasing stress. The nurse should therefore avoid describing disastrous cases. One MS mother told of how vividly she had remembered the cases of exacerbated MS due to pregnancy described to her 20 years before to dissuade her from more childbearing; these descriptions had caused her a great deal of stress through her birthing year.

Avoidance and denial on the part of health care professionals can also be problematic. Another woman resented her obstetrician for not having dealt with her worries and strategies regarding possible postnatal exacerbations. He just kept saying, "You're going to be all right," and after she delivered and had an exacerbation, he still did not want to acknowledge it.

Because of the role of stress in MS, it is extremely important that information be accurate and current so that unnecessary anxiety will not be produced. Information should not be withheld or distorted because of attitudes about disability. One woman felt that her pregnancy was more stressful because so many of her care providers were both ignorant and alarmed about MS. They were

> . . . asking me things that showed they didn't even know it had to do with the nervous system. This did *not* inspire confidence. When they heard I had MS they immediately freaked out and put me in a high-risk category, which meant more frequent office visits. I was exhausted from doctor's appointments.

> When the slightest thing happened (I almost passed out, had palpitations once) they acted hysterical. Or they'd get very serious and ask how does the MS affect you. All of this made me tense and nervous.

When professionals try to dissuade a woman with MS from having children, it is usually because they are concerned that if she progresses to the point of severe disability she will not be capable of parenting – particularly as a single mother. This attitude ignores the impact of the disabled independent-living movement, in which people with progressive ilnesses have learned a great deal about survival strategies and maintaining quality and fullness of life from those who have stable but severe disabilities.

The Role of Planning

Information serves the crucial processes of decision making and strategizing. Given the relative unpredictability of MS, it is even more important than usual to help the patient build resilience and adaptability into her plans. Self-care and a support system that works for the individual are important. Because MS exacerbations may occur no matter what the patient does, the nurse should encourage her to avoid self-blame if they occur.

MS is so varied and uncertain in its course that there may be some problems during pregnancy. With mild MS the problems may primarily be fatigue and balance difficulties. Women with more advanced MS may have problems with bladder infections, incontinence, increased spasticity or temors, skin care, thrombophlebitis, or regaining independent-living skills. A long strenuous labor might create problems resulting from muscular weakness and fatigue, and there may be poor expulsive efforts during delivery.

One woman reported pospartum difficulties she attributed to having had spinal anesthesia. Whether physically or emotionally based, the paralysis of her legs and subsequent exacerbation presented avoidable difficulties for her. It is suggested by one neurologist that when anesthesia is required, an epidural or general might be preferable, since it is better to avoid introducing foreign substances into the spine.

In general, however, as research indicates, most women do well during their pregnancies, sometimes actually feeling better than usual. The irony of well-being during pregnancy becoming problematic later was expressed by one woman: "I felt so good it almost fooled me. It made me feel like I'd gotten better – the MS had gone away. I had such a tremendous amount of energy!"

Her physicians had differed in their approaches to MS and pregnancy. While one had tended to alarm the patient about the negative long-term results of pregnancy, the other had tended to deny any problems. Both forms of paternalism had a detrimental effect. Because of the first doctor's approach, the woman was anxious about a change in long-term prognosis when she did in fact have a postnatal exacerbation. The second doctor's approach undermined her planning and self-care strategies, since feeling so good during pregnancy resulted in underestimating the degree of support needed after delivery:

> I was nursing every $2\frac{1}{2}$ hours around the clock, I was totally exhausted. Also I had insomnia and sometimes couldn't get back to sleep after nursing. . . . I had a bad exacerbation and my doctor prescribed a nurse that took care of both of us for 2 months. After that I used a babysitter, and now daycare. I've recovered but I'm still more fatigued than before my pregnancy. . . . If I could do it again I wouldn't have put such a heavy pressure on myself about nursing with no supplements. I'd introduce supplements from the beginning. And I would have gotten more household help. I was expecting too much from myself.

Another mother described her first birth, when there had been stress from a recent move, a great deal of anxiety because of her physician's horror stories about the results of pregnancy, and insufficient household support afterward. At that time she had a serious exacerbation, which subsided. With the second baby she had much less anxiety, less stress, more support, and no exacerbation.

Sometimes new fathers with MS also experience exacerbation around the time of birth. Often their ablebodied pregnant wives have been apprehensive about just this possibility, and the actual exacerbation has created a great deal of stress for the couple. For these reasons it is advisable for any couple dealing with MS to consider postnatal family support.

Social and Emotional Considerations When Plans Go Awry

Sometimes unexpected developments confound a patient's plans, and the insufficiency of social institutions becomes clear. The situation may seem overwhelming for parents and nurses. One woman who had an unusually difficult pregnancy, full of nausea, fatigue, and exacerbations, told a long story replete with bureaucratic inefficiency and unresponsiveness. The unexpected pregnancy and postpartum complications, and a family crisis, had upset her plans:

> I had to stop working at three months so I lost my medical insurance. I was on state employment disability so I was told I couldn't get MediCal. I was too ill to go to a social service agency and deal with all this. . . . I wasn't told about the public maternity program until my fifth month. The care was quite poor there. . . . My state employment disability ran out sooner than I had expected. When I was seven or eight months' pregnant I had no income, no government assistance for medical care, no food. Welfare wouldn't send out a worker because of cutbacks. So I threatened them with a suit and within the next day I had a worker at the house, some medical coverage and food stamps in 2 weeks. . . . I'd expected my partner to help but his son was dying of leukemia, and he had to be with him. . . . So much pressure was on my daughter to help she got pneumonia and was home sick for months. I had inefficient labor for days – couldn't sleep, was totally wiped out. . . . Pitocin didn't work. . . . Finally I had a C-section. . . . I had a bad exacerbation after the birth and also a uterine infection from the C-section. . . . I applied for unemployment insurance and choremaker money . . . their doctor said I didn't meet their criteria for disability. I was terrified I was going to whip myself into a more serious exacerbation out of worry I'd have to temporarily place the baby. I couldn't get out of bed myself. My friend's attendant helped me for free and I got through all of this.

At the point where her need and exhaustion were the greatest, there seemed to be incredible bureaucratic problems:

> I needed to be nurtured then – I needed to be taken care of myself so I could take care of my baby and I had to go deal with this inhuman bureaucracy. . . . On top of that I was dealing with being severely disabled for the first time. . . . I was grieving over my dream of being independent.

As her situation stabilized and her exacerbation subsided, she had the emotional energy to realize that her fears of future disability progression and dependence could motivate her to start developing a strategy for adapting to the situation. Her resilience may seem incredible and even somewhat intimidating. Yet one of the advantages of being a parent with MS is the enhancement of resilience and survival skills prior to parenting.

PARENTING ISSUES

There is a paucity of information about disabled parents, and most of the existing studies are strikingly poor in quality. The most popular opinion reflected in both the designs of the studies (that is, the choice of hypotheses) and in the conclusions asserted (whether or not supported by the data) is that "disabled parents have maladjusted children".

It is natural for research design to grow out of our underlying cultural biases and beliefs. And since the attitudes of the able-bodied are so negative toward people with disabilities (English, 1977), it is not surprising that this is reflected in most of the hypotheses of the limited existing research. Nevertheless, the better-designed studies (Olgas, 1974; Buck, 1980) are contradicting the expectation of negative outcome. For instance, Buck's comprehensive research on spinal-cord-injured fathers has found their parenting to be completely sufficient and even superior to that of normal fathers in some respects. Extensive and careful research is finding normal attachment patterns between deaf parents and infants (Meadow, Greenberg, and Erting, 1983). The prelingually deaf children of hearing parents are actually more at risk. Eighty-eight percent of deaf parents have hearing children whose existence in two cultures is both advantageous and problematic (Bunde, 1979). Longitudinal descriptive data is beginning to emerge from the first research and demonstration projects concerning physically disabled parents and their able-bodied infants. This work documents the ingenuity of disabled parents and remarkably early adaptation of their infants during basic baby-care activities. It suggests that good parenting outcomes can be expected even where the parent is severely disabled, as long as psychosocial functioning is not problematical (Kirshbaum, 1988) (Fig. 39-2). In general there is a tremendous need for carefully controlled, in-depth, and longitudinal studies of a wide range of disabled parents — studies that consider repercussions, strengths, and weaknesses.

Parenting Anxieties

Some interventions by professionals imply that disabled parents totally lack concern, knowledge, or strategies around childcare and parenting and they are oblivious to their own physical limitation. For instance, most deaf parents interviewed had been asked such questions as, "But how will you hear your baby cry?" or "How will your baby learn to talk?" The mixture of irritation, amusement, and incomprehension in deaf parents' responses to these questions is a reaction to the negative attitudes behind the questions and reflects the degree of cultural insensitivity and ignorance of the interviewers.

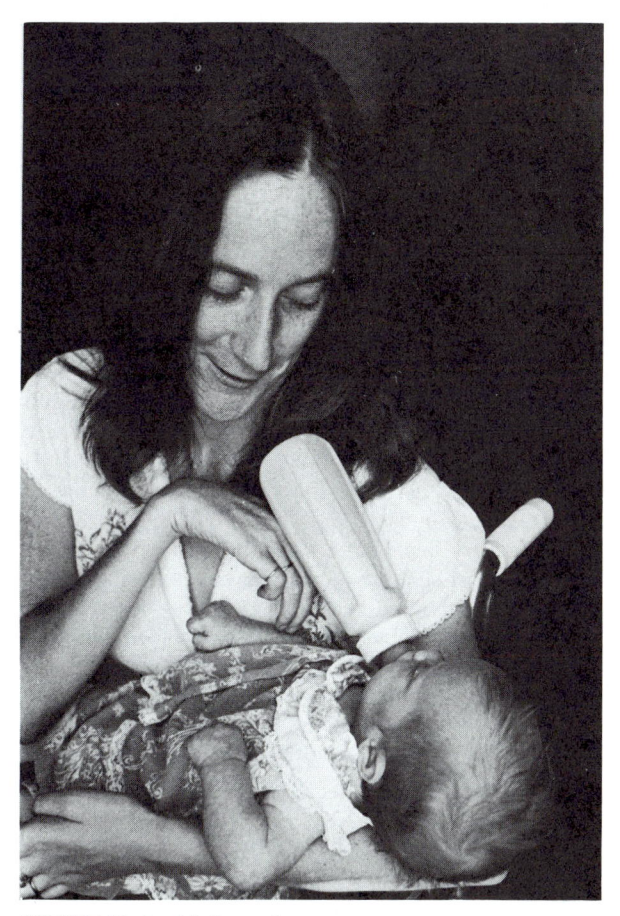

FIGURE 39-2. Mother using compensatory strategy to feed newborn.

Most disabled parents have usually considered the potential and actual difficulties and are aware of social attitudes about their having children. One father with severe cerebral palsy stated:

> I worry about being seen as incompetent. There's the issue in people's minds, I think, of how can an individual who is dependent be responsible for the dependence of their offspring? If able-bodied people are afraid of the loss of control over their own bodies, I'm sure they assume that people who don't have control over theirs can't be responsible for their children.

The anxieties of disabled parents about their ability to care for their baby are like those of all expectant or new parents. However, these anxieties are often intensified by lack of information, lack of role models, and lack of community support services. Negative attitudes from the community, family, friends, and the disabled person himself or herself may serve as obstacles to asking questions, acknowledging difficulties, and experimenting with methods of dealing with specific situations. One legally blind mother stated:

> When my . . . daughter was born, I bit my lip and tried new things when no one was looking. I often made excuses to myself and pretended that I did not need special help simply because there was nowhere that such help was available. To let myself ask for it would have just made me feel more frustrated and inadequate. I knew that I loved my child and would do the very best that I could do. If I asked seeing parents for help with a task, they would just do it for me rather than help me develop a way of doing it for myself. I just did not know any other women who had visual disabilities. My child was five before I met another blind mother.

For some people who have been disabled from birth or childhood, the thought or the reality of having a baby brings up memories of early disability experiences, childhood lack of self-esteem, or early trauma around parenting. As disabled babies or children, some of these mothers experienced lengthy hospitalization or institutionalization, and many had parents who were under stress, grieving, or depressed because of their disability.

Women may be anxious about the functioning of their bodies during pregnancy and may have fantasies that a disabled body cannot give birth to a healthy child. These anxieties may be without any genetic basis, as in the case of a women with mild cerebral palsy who said:

> During my pregnancy I had a neurosis about crushing the infant with my spasticity. . . . Around the seventh month I got all upset about forceps damage, since that's what had caused my C.P.

Because a sensitive and supportive nurse elicited this concern, the mother was able to discharge it and move on to a smooth and beautiful delivery.

Planning

Most parents with disabilities deal with their anxieties and realistic concerns by planning and strategizing prior to the birth of their children. This is a way of mastering anxiety and of pragmatically empowering themselves:

> I got all the literature and information that I could while I was pregnant and even before. I was very clear with my friends and those who were providing my prenatal care that I was in charge! I made it clear that they were there to help make having my daughter as beautiful and successful an experience for us both as possible. However, after she was born, I found that old fears and feelings of being inadequate from my own early childhood as a blind child came up as I would face new situations for the first time as a mother. Had I not spent much time doing research and surrounding myself with very supportive people that believed I could do it, I am sure that my experience would have been very unhappy.

Support for disabled parents is still seriously lacking in society, aside from high-risk obstetric programs, public health nurses, and some role models located through disabled community-based programs. Therefore, over the years, disabled parents have sought support from a wide variety of places. Extended families have been supportive for some parents but have had negative impact on others. Deaf parents appear to have more of a source for role models and support within deaf culture, although sometimes relationships with hearing grandparents are problematic. Able-bodied partners play an important role when present. Household and babysitting support are sought, and attendant work tends to be increased when possible. There is a critical lack of public funding for low-income severely disabled parents who need expanded in-home assistance during pregnancy and parenting.

It is important that support facilitate and not detract from the disabled parent's full parental role. One father with severe cerebral palsy did a great deal of planning to maximize his involvement, including attending birthing classes (see Fig. 39–3). He also "assumed the position of pillow" for this partner during birth:

> When my baby was young I felt bad I couldn't handle him that much because of my disability. That myth of fathers breaking newborns has even more reality in my situation because any minute I could go into a spasm. I was afraid of my own strength. . . . I was always trying to catch up to the physical contact with my son by whatever means I had. My wife could cuddle him and nurse him but I could tickle him on the ear to kind of let him know there was a physical connection between the two of us. . . . Because my mouth is one of my most controlled areas, I would suck his toes and I'd rub my cheeks against his stomach. . . . Now I put the infant seat on my lap and my wife buckles it in and he and I go out for

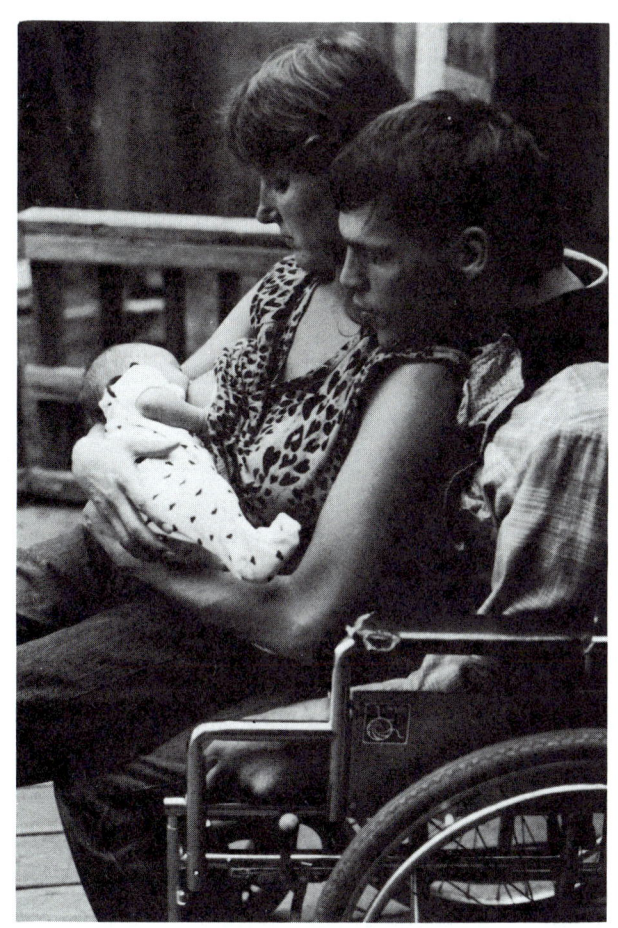

FIGURE 39–3. Father with cerebral palsy participating in care of newborn.
SOURCE: Andre.

walks in the power chair. I have it turned so we keep eye contact.

Another father with postpolio high-level quadriplegia recalls:

> We went to hospitals to make arrangements for the birth. . . . I wanted to be there in my iron lung or with a portable respirator. . . . The hospital staff was afraid like a lot of people I'd met before. They said it might cause sparks or noise or disruption – that was all bullshit. They saw me as terrifically dependent, though I said I would being an attendant. . . . So we took charge of the process and chose home birth, though our doctor was under pressure from his colleagues not to do it. But I've lived in hospitals. I truly think they're very dangerous places – full of infections and staph. We had a doctor and a nurse-midwife, a back-up ambulance and oxygen and resuscitation equipment. I checked D's dilation during the early labor. I was in an iron lung during the birth. . . . I cried the first time I had him close to me. . . . Later we fastened a baby seat on the arm of my chair so he could be over my lap and next to my chest . . . or he would lie across my lap and sleep. . . . there were problems cuddling when I was in the iron lung, but we made the most of our opportunities to get close.

This father maintained control and power in his parenting partly by orchestrating the care of his baby – that is, by verbally directing and thus maintaining his participation, while attendants carried out the actual physical care. The difficulty of making physical contact led to more depth and intensity in the moments of physical contact.

Nurses should remember that pregnancy or post-partum problems may make the earliest period of the parent–child relationship highly stressful. Adequate support of the disabled parent means support for the attachment between parent and child. Perhaps this role will seem less overwhelming if the nurse considers the natural determination of the stressed disabled parent to connect with his or her baby. For instance, parents faced with separations from their infant may pack much more quality of bonding into the times together. This was the case for one mother whose disability was triggered by pregnancy, beginning with an "undiagnosed dermatitis". She was kept separated from her baby for a month after birth, and family members did her nursing care since it was feared she was contagious. During that time she had only two glimpses of her infant:

> I cherished those so much – it really kept me going. . . . I felt like we had a kind of bond. It was as if when we had looked at one another right at birth it had left an imprint on my mind . . .

Through the next 6 years they had a great many separations when her condition exacerbated. But building on the model of maintaining that first bond, they learned to pack a great deal of love, connection, and *joie de vivre* into the times they had together. They are presently working out the complexities of the mother–daughter relationship in adolescence, utilizing a great deal of mutual respect and openness of communication.

Parenting Strategies

Specific details about adaptive equipment and compensatory strategies are best worked out in a way that is responsive to the individual situation. Again, the goal is maximizing the parenting role for the disabled parent, thereby enhancing the well-being of the infant. An example of the problems and solutions for blind parents results from the inability to read a visual thermometer (an adaptive thermometer had been prohibitively expensive until recently):

> I feared that my child would have a high fever and I would not be able to take the appropriate action. Finally after 14 months, she developed her first fever. I was immediately aware when I went to her crib to respond to her crying. She was very warm to my touch. Her skin felt clammy. I am not totally blind, so when I held her close to my face, I could see that her face was redder than usual. Although I was very concerned, I was also relieved. My fear that I would not be able to respond properly when she was sick was somewhat lessened.

Many blind parents worry also about losing track of their child's location:

> One mother, who had four little children at home, bought four bells with different tones, so her skill as a child-chaser was more refined. With the twins, I found bells distracting. Nothing on earth moves as much as toddler feet, and when there are so many feet, the noise can be awesome. Instead, I learned to know the sound of every object in the house, and to listen became automatic (Cranston, 1982, p. 26).

Deaf parents use various methods to be responsive to their baby's crying. Most use "baby cry alarms" that flash and visually alert the parent. Others sleep with the baby's face near theirs, use dogs, or rely on a hearing person in the household. Parents usually are very aware of their child's language (sign and speech) development and consider how it might be enhanced.

A mother who is a postpolio paraplegic solved her problems lifting and retrieving her crawling baby from the floor by making a wide canvas belt fastened with long strips of Velcro, which she combined with a "reacher". Other parents in wheelchairs with some upper-body strength have used harnesses for the same purpose. Changing tables, cribs, and so on are adapted to a wheelchair or to suit the degree of fine motor ability. Rooms are arranged to minimize walking and maximize support for those who are ambulatory but unstable. The baby and equipment may be kept next to the parent's bed at night. A bassinet or portacrib on rollers may be used for moving the baby around, or the baby may be held in a front pack, on an attached infant seat or tray, or in the lap. Nursing is often recommended for convenience; thorough childproofing is emphasized.

The variety of solutions is endless and ingenious. Occupational therapists, rehabilitation engineering departments, but most of all other disabled parents can be helpful in developing such strategies. Videotapes documenting adaptive strategies of other disabled parents are extremely effective for stimulating the individual's unique process of adaptation during baby care (Kirshbaum, 1988). An increasing amount of published material is available.

SUMMARY

Nurses can facilitate disabled people's effectiveness as parents by intervening in a respectful and empowering manner throughout the childbearing period. During the natural unfolding process of interaction between infant and parent, there is a reciprocal adaptation around the parent's disability. A cooperative, reciprocal, and mutually respectful relationship frequently emerges.

Disabled parents are not immune to the problems of other parents. Disabled people are, after all, an oppressed minority, often have a low income, may have had poor education, may be isolated and have poor social skills, and may have had a traumatic childhood, including abandonment, institutionalization, rejection, or multiple medical crises and separation. For people who become disabled or more disabled during pregnancy or postnatally, separations, grieving, and depression over body image alterations may complicate the formation of the parent–infant bond. Yet the cultural stereotype that equates a physical disability with psychological disability is not valid. In general, disabled people are survivors; they tend to apply their survival skills to overcoming the considerable obstacles to parenthood (Fig. 39–4).

The developmental transition to parenthood is demanding, and for the disabled parent it means a reworking and reconfronting of disability issues in a new and particularly vulnerable context. The disabled parent comes to the obstetric care situation with an extensive disability-related medical history. The medical setting may be associated with and may trigger cumulative negative feelings. Because of this charged history of medical issues, a positive experience with the health care professional is especially important during the transition to parenthood.

Sometimes the cumulative experiences of the past and the stressful, inadequately supported circumstances of the present combine to exhaust

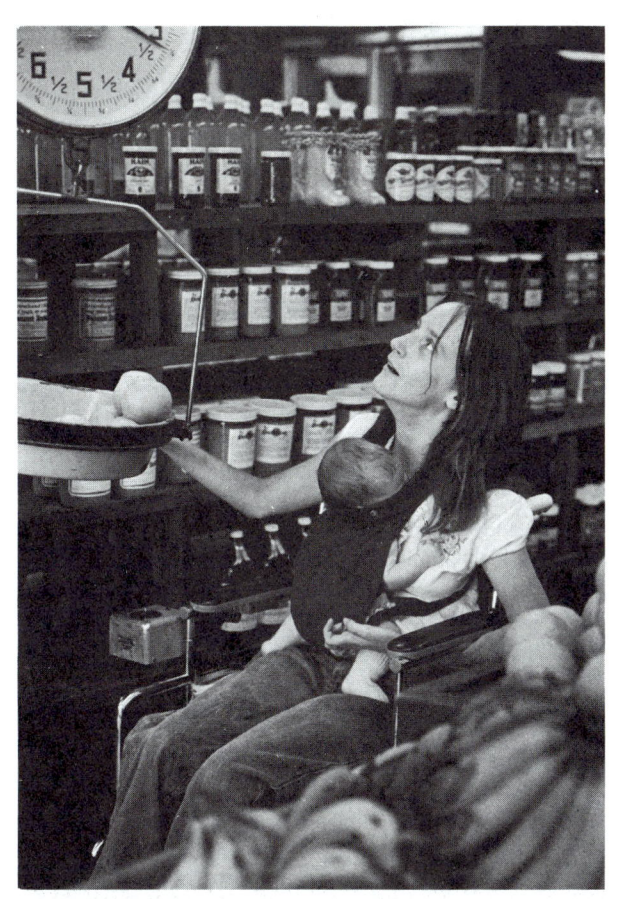

FIGURE 39–4. Quadriplegic mother grocery shopping with baby.

the disabled parent's coping skills. During hospitalization for birth, such a parent may experience a combination of pain, anger, and ambivalence about dependency. Thus, particular attention should be paid to the patient's history and to the social and emotional context of the parental behavior. Nursing care may be sabotaged; the double message may be: "Help me. You can't help me." It is hoped that the work of nursing staff in such a situation can be informed by a consideration of the issues presented in this chapter.

But most disabled parents seem to deal with their feelings about medical settings by carefully strategizing and planning, attempting to empower themselves during the birthing period. By facilitating or cooperating with the parents' planning process and by exploring strategies together, nursing staff can begin the process of developing rapport with the disabled parent.

It is easy to feel overwhelmed by the need for education about disability; the need to be sensitive to the disabled client's history; the need to confront one's own negative attitudes or fears about physical vulnerability, mortality, or that which cannot be cured or fixed; and the need for social change around disability. Upon encountering her first disabled patient the nurse may be expected to be fully knowledgeable about the disability itself, the ramifications of the problem in the life of the person, and the full spectrum of the patient's emotional needs. This situation can produce feelings of inadequacy, frustration, guilt, alienation, and even repulsion. Professional codes of conduct discourage acknowledgment of these feelings, but the reality of the feelings may be shared unconsciously with the patient. Also, the nurse is likely to have known disabled people only in the medical setting, in a sick role, with all the overtones from the cumulative history discussed earlier. An awareness of disabled people in their diverse roles in the community would better serve the functioning of the nurse during the disabled parents' process of birthing. Whether from such broadening of nonpathological experiences with disabled people, from drawing on disabled community support services, from using rehabilitation nurses' expertise, or from personal emotional work, it is wise for the maternity nurse to be well supported as she initially confronts disabled parenting situations.

The essential needs of disabled parents are simple and human. As one disabled mother said, "I'm a mother, too, and I need what other mothers get – the caring attention you would want yourself in that position." Over and over disabled parents stress that what they want from the nurse is respectful eliciting of their needs, acknowledgement of their expertise about their own disability, and facilitation or cooperation with their attempts to maintain autonomy.

Disability and its medical effects need to be dealt with thoughtfully and realistically, but they must not subsume the dimension of human celebration of birth. The essential need is easy to state: the formation of a mutually compassionate working relationship between the nurse and patient that serves the normal developmental transition to parenthood.

REFERENCES

Anthony, E. 1970. The mutative impact of serious mental and physical illness in a parent on family life. In *The child in his family, I*, eds. E. Anthony and C. Koupernick. New York: John Wiley & Sons.

Asrael, W., and Kesselman, S. 1983. Classes for the disabled. *Childbirth Educator*. Winter:18–21.

Berman, H. 1984. Personal Communication.

Berry, R. J. 1969. Genetical factors in the aetiology of multiple sclerosis. *Acta Neurol. Scand.* 45:471–483.

Buck, F. 1980. *The influence of parental disability on children: An exploratory investigation of the adult children of spinal-cord-injured fathers.* Unpublished doctoral dissertation, University of Arizona.

Buck, F., and Hohemann, G. 1983. Parental disability and children's adjustment. In *Annual review of rehabilitation, III,* eds. E. L. Pan, T. E. Backer, and C. L. Vash. New York: Springer-Verlag.

Bunde, L. T. 1979. *Deaf parents – Hearing children.* Washington, D.C.: Registry of Interpreters for the Deaf.

Carroll, J. 1971. Our set of circumstances. *New Outlook for the Blind.* 65:174–180.

Castro de la Mata, R.; Gingas, G.; and Wittower, E. 1960. Impact of sudden, severe disablement of the father upon the family. *Canad. Med. Assoc. J.* 82:1015–1020.

Catanzaro, M. 1977. Multiple sclerosis: Exploding myths that compromise patient care. *RN.* 40:42–46.

Chui, L., and Bhatt, K. 1983. Autonomic dysreflexia. *Rehab. Nurs.* 8(2):16–19.

Cole, T. 1975. Sexuality and physical disabilities. *Arch. Sex. Behav.* 4(4):389–403.

Comarr, A. E., and Gunderson, B. B. 1975. Sexual functioning in traumatic paraplegia and quadriplegia. *Am. J. Nurs.* 75(2):230–255.

Conine, T. 1987. *Aids and adaptations for disabled parents.* Vancouver, BC: University of British Columbia.

Craig, D. I. 1983. Nursing care plan for a pregnant spinal-cord-injured patient. *Rehab. Nurs.* 8(2):26–28.

Cranston, R. 1982. *Parenting without vision in 1000 easy lessons.* Berkeley, Calif.: Bananas Child Care Service.

Dean, G. 1975. Epidemiology: What is new and what remains to be done. *Multiple sclerosis research.* London: Her Majesty's Stationary Office.

DiCaprio, N. S. 1971. Factors affecting child's evaluation of the visually handicapped parent. *New Outlet for the Blind.* 65(6):181–186.

Dickinson, F. T. 1977. Paraplegia in pregnancy and labor: Report of case and review of literature. *J. Am. Osteop. Assoc.* 76:537–539.

Duffy, Y. 1981. *All things are possible.* Ann Arbor, Mich.: Gavin & Associates.

English, R. 1977. Correlates of stigma toward physically disabled persons. In *The psychological and social impact of physical disability,* eds. R. Marinelli and A. Dell Orto. New York: Springer-Verlag.

Fitz-Gerald, D. 1977. Deaf people are sexual too! *Siecas Report.* 6(2):13–15.

Garrett, J. F., and Levine, E. S. 1962. *Psychological practices with the physically disabled.* New York: Columbia University Press.

Ghezzi, A., and Caputo, D. 1981. Pregnancy: A factor influencing the course of multiple sclerosis? *Europ. Neurol.* 20(2):115–117.

Geiger, R. C. 1977. Sexual implications of spinal cord injury. In *Physical medicine and rehabilitation approaches in spinal cord injury,* eds. J. Cull and R. Hardy. Springfield, Ill.: Charles C. Thomas.

Gleidman, J., and Roth, W. 1980. *The unexpected minority.* New York: Harcourt Brace Jovanovich.

Goller, H., and Paeslack, V. 1972. Prenancy damage and birth complications in the children of paraplegic women. *Arch. Sex. Behav.* 7:213–217.

Greenberg, M. T., and Marvin, R. 1979. Attachment pattern in profoundly deaf preschool children. *Merrill-Palmer Quarterly.* 25(4):265–279.

Griffith, E. R., and Trieschmann, R. B. 1975. Sexual functioning in women with spinal cord injury. *Arch. Phys. Med. Rehab.* 56(1):18–21.

Hardy, A. G., and Warrell, D. W. 1965. Pregnancy and labour in complete tetraplegia. *Paraplegia.* 3:182–188.

Hepner, R.; Kirshbaum, H.; and Landes, D. 1980/81. Counseling substance abusers with additional disabilities: The Center for Independent Living. *Alcohol Health and Research World.* 5(2):11–15.

Heslinga, K.; Schellen, A.; and Verkuvl, A. 1974. *Not made of stone: The sexual problems of handicapped people.* Springfield, Ill.: Charles C. Thomas.

Janz, D. 1978. Haben antiepileptica eise teratogene wirkungbeim. Mensechen? *Deutsche Medizinische Wochenschrift.* 103:485–487.

Johnston, B. 1982. Pregnancy and childbirth in women with spinal cord injuries: A review of the literature. *MCN.* 2(1):41–46.

Kennedy, K. M., and Bush, D. F. 1979. Counseling the children of handicapped parents. *Personnel and Guidance Journal.* 58:267–270.

Kirshbaum, M. 1988. Parents with disabilities and their babies. *Zero to Three.* VIII(3):

Kurtzke, J. F. 1980. Epidemiological contributions to multiple sclerosis: An overview. *Neurology.* 30(2):61–79.

Leibowitz, U., and Alter, M. 1973. *Multiple sclerosis: Clues to its cause.* New York: Elsevier.

McAlpine, D.; Lundsen, L. E.; and Acheson, E. D. 1972. *Multiple sclerosis: A reappraisal.* 2nd ed. Baltimore: Williams & Wilkins.

MacKay, R. P., and Myrianthopoulos, N. C. 1966. Multiple sclerosis in twins and their relatives. *Arch. Neurol.* 15:449–462.

Meadow, K. 1976. Personality and social development of deaf persons. In *Psychology of deafness for rehabilitation counselors,* ed. B. Bolton. Baltimore: University Park Press.

Meadow, K. 1980. *Deafness and childhood development.* Berkeley: University of California Press.

Meadow, K.; Greenberg, M.; and Erting, C. 1983. Attachment behavior of deaf children with deaf parents. *J. Am. Acad. Child Psych.* 22(1):23–28.

Mehr, E. B., and Freid, A. N. 1975. *Low vision care.* Chicago: The Professional Press.

Mooney, T. O.; Cole, T.; and Chilgen, R., 1975. *Sexual*

options for paraplegics and quadriplegics. New York: Little, Brown.

Morrison, J.; Chang, A.; Thearle, M. J.; Tabett, D. G.; and Teoh, G. 1978. Acute traumatic tetraplegia during pregnancy. *Australia–N. Zealand J. Obstet. Gynecol.* 18:82–85.

Nemon, A. 1980. Deaf persons and their doctors. *J. Rehab. of the Deaf.* 4(2):1719–1723.

Ohry, A.; Pelig, D.; Goldman, J.; David, H.; and Rozin, R. 1978. Sexual function, pregnancy, and delivery in spinal cord injured women. *Gynecol. Obstet. Invest.* 9:281–291.

Olgas, M. 1974. The relationship between parents' health status and body-image of their children. *Nurs. Res.* 23:319–324.

Parks, S. 1984. *HELP: When the parent is handicapped.* Palo Alto, Calif.: VORT Corporation.

Pavlou, M. 1979. *Variety and possibility in multiple sclerosis.* Chicago: BioService Corp.

Poser, S.; Wikstrom, J.; and Bauer, H. 1979. *J. Neurolog. Sci.* 40:159–168.

Poskanzer, D. C.; Schapira, K.; and Miller, H. 1966. Multiple sclerosis and poliomyelitis. *Acta Neurolog. Scand.* 42 (Suppl. 19):85–90.

Robertson, D. N. 1972. Pregnancy and labor in the paraplegic. *Paraplegia.* 10:209–210.

Robinault, I. P. 1978. *Sex, society, and the disabled: Developmental inquiry into roles, reactions, and responsibilities.* New York: Harper & Row.

Rutter, M. 1966. *Children of sick parents: An environmental and psychiatric study.* London: Oxford University Press.

Sabatino, L. 1976. Dos and don'ts of deaf-patient care. *RN.* 39(6):64–68.

Sadovnick, A. D., and Macleod, P. M. J. 1981. The familial nature of multiple sclerosis: Empiric recurrence risks for first-, second-, and third-degree relatives of patients. *Neurology.* 31:1039–1041.

Sandowski, C. L. 1976. Sexuality and the paraplegic. *Rehab. Lit.* 11-12:322–327.

Schapira, K.; Poskanzer, D. C.; and Miller, H. C. 1963. Familial and conjugal MS. *Brain.* 86:315–332.

Schein, J., and Schreiber. F. 1978. Communicating with hearing-impaired patients: A training manual for hospitals. Unpublished.

Schlesinger, H., and Meadow, K. 1973. *Sound and sign: Childhood deafness and mental health.* Berkeley: University of California Press.

Schut, A. L. 1974. *Anatomy and physiology of the human eye.* Kalamazoo: Western Michigan University Press.

Thurman, S. K. 1985. *Children of handicapped parents: Research and clinical perspectives.* London and San Diego: Academic Press.

Tsoutsoplides, G. C. 1982. Pregnancy in paraplegia: A case report. *Int. J. Gynecol. Obstet.* 20:79–83.

Verduyn, W. H. 1983. Spinal-cord-injured women: Pregnancy and delivery. Unpublished.

Wasserman, L. 1978. *Living with MS: A practical guide.* Boston: National Multiple Sclerosis Society.

Ware, M. A., and Schwab, L. O. 1971. The blind mother providing care for the infant. *New Outlook for the Blind.* 65(6):181–186.

What if your patient is also deaf? 1976. *RN.* 39(6):59–63.

Wright, B. 1960. *Physical disability: A psychological approach.* New York: Harper & Row.

Young, B.; Katz, M.; and Klein, S. A. 1983. Pregnancy after spinal cord injury: Altered maternal and fetal responses to labor. *Obstet. Gynecol.* 62(1):59–63.

Zola, I. K., ed. 1982, *Ordinary lives.* Cambridge/Wathertown: Applewood Books.

40
Substance Abuse

BEHAVIORAL OBJECTS

Upon completion of this chapter, the reader should be able to:

- Discuss the incidence of drug abuse in the United States.

- Define the physiologic, psychologic, and sociologic aspects of drug use and abuse.

- Describe the effects of the use of drugs and alcohol on the fetus.

- Assess the infant for signs of fetal alcohol syndrome and drug withdrawal.

- Discuss the risks associated with maternal smoking and use of caffeine during pregnancy.

- List the potential dangers to the fetus associated with maternal use of prescribed and over-the-counter drugs.

- Define the nurse's role in caring for drug-using pregnant women and for infants affected by drug use and abuse during pregnancy.

Drug use and abuse has become a topic of considerable national concern over the past decade. In particular, drug abuse among teenagers and young adults is a major public health problem. During the twentieth century in the United States, the health of every age segment of the population has improved from decade to decade except teenagers and young adults age 15–24. These young people are dying at a rate 16 percent greater than in 1960, and they are dying primarily as a result of motor vehicle accidents, suicides, and homicides. It is believed that many of these deaths are related to drug abuse (Dupont, 1981).

Drug abuse among young people is reaching epidemic proportions. In 1962 only 1 percent of American adolescents 12–17 years old used marijuana. By 1979, 33 percent of the nation's 12- to 17-year-olds had used the drug. In 1980, 60 percent of high school seniors had used marijuana at least once, and 40 percent were regular users. Statistics reveal that 9 percent of high school seniors were smoking an average of 3.5 joints per day each. American teenagers drop out of high school at a rate of 20 percent, and research has shown that dropouts have a considerably higher rate of drug abuse than teenagers who stay in school (Dupont, 1981).

Although marijuana is by far the most widely used illicit drug, it is not the only substance being abused. In 1962 less than 1 percent of young people 12–17 years old had ever used hallucinogens, cocaine, or heroin. By 1979 the proportion trying these drugs had increased to 9 percent. Among those between 18 and 25 years of age, 33 percent had used hallucinogens, cocaine, or heroin, compared to 3 percent in 1962. Alcohol use and abuse among teenagers has also increased greatly. This epidemic is a relatively new phenomenon in American society, but it is showing no signs of going away (Dupont, 1981). An all-out effort to reduce drug abuse is essential, and health professionals as well as concerned citizens must become involved.

The purpose of this chapter is to give the health care provider information regarding abuse of both illicit drugs and prescribed and over-the-counter medications during pregnancy. In addition, the use of tobacco, caffeine, and alcohol during pregnancy are discussed. Finally, the role of the nurse in dealing with pregnant clients who may use drugs during pregnancy is examined.

DEFINITIONS OF DRUG TERMS

Before discussing drug use and abuse, we should define some basic drug terms (Wilson and Kneisal, 1983).

Substance abuse refers to the overuse or misuse of any chemical substance, which may include illicit drugs as well as prescribed or over-the-counter medications, alcohol, tobacco, or caffeine.

Drug use is the ingestion in any manner of a chemical that has an effect on the body. This includes taking an aspirin for a headache or using nasal spray for an allergy.

Drug abuse is a state of chronic intoxication, detrimental to the individual, that is produced by repeated ingestion of a drug. Characteristics of drug abuse include:

1. An overwhelming desire to take the drug despite legal, social, or medical problems.
2. A willingness to obtain the drug by any means, including illegal methods.
3. A tendency to desire increasing doses of a drug.
4. Physical dependence on the drug.

Drug dependence occurs when:

1. The body requires the drug to keep functioning.
2. The body develops a *tolerance* for the drug so the dose must be increased to obtain the same effect.
3. Physical *withdrawal symptoms* are present if the drug is stopped.
4. The person believes it is impossible to live without the drug.

Drug abuse is a general term which includes any substance taken legally or illegally, such as alcohol, coffee, tobacco, prescription drugs, LSD, marijuana, or cocaine. Regardless of the recognized therapeutic uses of certain compounds, they are frequently utilized in a non-therapeutic manner for their mood-altering effects or pleasurable purposes (Brande et al., 1987).

CHARACTERISTICS OF DRUG ABUSERS

The causes of drug abuse, including alcoholism, are complex. Multiple factors are usually involved. The problem has physiologic, psychologic, and sociologic aspects that are not well understood by health care professionals. Some classify drug abuse as an illness, while others consider it from a specific psychologic, sociologic, or legal point of view. Regardless of the specific causes of the problem, certain predisposing factors tend to influence the development of drug abuse behaviors.

The drug-dependent lifestyle is often thought to result from a particular social role – that is, the attitudes and behaviors that characterize this lifestyle may be learned from the members of a particular group or culture. It was previously believed that socioeconomically deprived individuals were most likely to become drug abusers. It has become obvious, however, that the problem crosses all socioeconomic levels and cultural barriers. In fact, the number of addicts from middle- and upper-middle-class families has increased steadily, indicating that the problem is not limited to the poor and underprivileged.

Certain personality traits are associated with drug abuse. These characteristics include:

1. Dominating and critical behavior, with underlying self-doubts and passivity.
2. Personal insecurity.
3. Problems with sexual identity.
4. Rebellious attitudes toward authority.
5. Marked narcissistic trends, with absence of a strong superego.
6. A lack of the ability to form close and lasting relationships.

There is disagreement as to the role personality traits play in drug abuse, but it is thought that many individuals use drugs to suppress anxiety and to relieve conflicts related to their own personality structure (Wilson and Kneisal, 1983).

The incidence of drug and alcohol abuse among adolescents is at an all-time high. Because adolescence is a period when peer group influence is very important, many young people take drugs to be one of the crowd. There is a love of risk-taking during this age and a feeling of unlimited power leading to the belief that "I'll never get hooked." This belief is a myth, and far too many young people become either psychologically or physically dependent on drugs or alcohol. Drug use among girls is also correlated with sexual promiscuity, which often leads to an unplanned pregnancy. Promiscuous adolescents also increase the risk of contracting sexually transmitted diseases and other pelvic infections that are detrimental not only to them but to their offspring.

DRUG ABUSE DURING PREGNANCY

The age group identified as having the highest incidence of drug abuse (ages 18–24) is also the group with the highest pregnancy rate. Epidemiologic data gathered in recent years indicate an increase in the rate of substance abuse for females that is rapidly approaching the higher rates for males (Brande et al., 1987). Because most drugs in the maternal system will reach the fetus to some extent, there is a great deal of concern regarding the potential effect of drug use and abuse on the unborn baby. In addition to illicit drugs, the use of alcohol, one of the most widely abused legal drugs, has been linked to serious problems in the fetus.

There is also cause for concern in the number of prescribed and over-the-counter drugs consumed by pregnant women. A recent study found that they typically take an average of 11 different drugs during pregnancy (Kaplin and Kolesari, 1982). In another study of 2500 pregnancies, 23 percent of the women were given narcotic-containing drugs, 13 percent consumed psychotropic drugs, and 6.2 percent took tetracycline, which is contraindicated in pregnancy. Some of the agents taken by pregnant women are prescribed by physicians, but many are over-the-counter medications that are not perceived to be harmful (Kaplin and Kolesari, 1982).

The nutritional intake of women who abuse drugs is often inadequate to meet their own needs, much less the increased demands of pregnancy. In addition, the drug abuser may enter pregnancy in a debilitated state of health, which predisposes her to infections and other complications of pregnancy. Often she is unable to assume responsibility for her own care or that of her baby. And even though the pregnant woman may be concerned about her baby's well-being, it is usually difficult to get her to comply with the health care regimen.

When a drug abuser becomes pregnant, she places herself and her baby in jeopardy. If the pregnancy does not end in spontaneous abortion or result in a stillbirth, the baby may be born seriously handicapped, either mentally or physically, or both. The infant of a drug-addicted mother may also experience the effects of drug withdrawal after birth.

To further complicate matters, many pregnant drug abusers have become alienated from their family and friends and lack any real support systems to help them during pregnancy. There has often been a disintegration of the family unit. The pregnant woman with a drug-abuse problem may not know where to turn for help. And because she lacks financial resources, she is likely to delay seeking prenatal care.

FETAL EFFECTS OF MATERNAL SUBSTANCE USE AND ABUSE

It has been confirmed that any drug that has ready access to the central nervous system (CNS) is also easily transferred across the placenta to the fetus. Studies of cord blood obtained at delivery have confirmed the presence of all drugs of abuse studied to date. Less understood are the factors governing the rate and extent of fetal exposure to different drugs and the relationship between the pharmacodynamic effects on the fetus and the extent of fetal drug exposure (Brande et al., 1987).

Chemical Teratogenesis

Teratogenesis is the process by which chemical agents interfere with embryologic development, producing defects in one or another organ system. Each step in the embryonic process is dependent on a previous one, and the development of many organs and systems takes place at a precise stage of gestation. Thus, timing of exposure to a chemical substance is critical in its teratogenic effects (Hahn et al., 1982).

Although the Federal Drug Administration (FDA) attempts to determine the safety of drugs during pregnancy, very little is actually known. In fact, no drug in use today can be considered completely harmless. In many cases, drugs once considered harmless to the fetus have been found to cause abnormalities later on – thalidomide and its effects on the extremities is a notable example. Most studies on the effects of drugs on the fetus have been conducted in animals, and the results cannot always be applied to humans.

In determining the potential effects of drug use during pregnancy, gestation may be divided into three major periods, the preembryonic, embryonic, and fetal:

1. *The preembryonic period.* This period begins with fertilization and ends with the third week after fertilization. It may also be calculated from the date of the last menstruation to the fifth week after the last menstrual period. This stage of development is characterized by rapid cell division, which provides the cells for organ building. During the preembryonic period the developing baby is *least sensitive* to the action of drugs (Kaplin and Kolesari, 1982). If large doses of teratogens are given, the embryo may be aborted, but if it survives it usually develops into a normal infant.
2. *The embryonic period.* This period begins with the sixth week after the last menstruation (fourth week after fertilization) and lasts until the tenth week after the last menstrual period (eighth week following fertilization). This is the *most sensitive* period for the developing embryo. It is the time of organogenesis, when organs are forming, and each organ system may easily be malformed (Kaplin and Kolesari, 1982).
3. *The fetal period.* This period is from the ninth week following fertilization or the eleventh week after the last menstruation until the birth of the baby. It is a time of rapid growth; the organ systems are already developed and are undergoing rapid expansion in volume and weight. During this stage the fetus becomes increasingly resistant to the effects of teratogens, although there is never a period of complete resistance. Therefore, caution must be used when taking any type of drug during pregnancy, whether prescribed, over-the-counter, or recreational (Kaplin and Kolesari, 1982).

Table 40–1 presents a list of antimicrobial agents and their effects when used during pregnancy (The Medical Letter, 1987). Table 40–2 presents chemical substances that are known or suspected to have teratogenic effects on the fetus. Table 40–3 presents a list of drugs often used and their effects on the fetus and neonate. It is essential to remember that this table is not all inclusive, and many drugs that are believed to be safe today, may later be found to have adverse effects. Therefore, no drug should ever be considered absolutely safe for use during pregnancy.

Alcohol

The effects of maternal alcohol ingestion on the developing fetus was described as early as the eighteenth century. It has been considered as the single most common cause of infant mental retardation.

The adverse effects of maternal alcohol consumption on the mental development of the offspring includes a group of disorders ranging from cerebral palsy and mental retardation to children with normal intelligence suffering from attention deficit syndrome (Gal and Sharpless, 1984; Streissgerth, 1986).

TABLE 40–1. Antimicrobial Agents in Pregnancy

Drug	Toxicity in Pregnancy	Recommendation
Antibacterial		
Aminoglycosides [a]	Possible 8th-nerve toxicity in fetus	Caution*
Aztreonam (Azactam)	None known	Probably safe
Cephalosporins [b]	None known	Probably safe
Chloramphenicol (Chloromycetin; and others)	Unknown – gray syndrome in newborn	Caution*, especially at term
Cinoxacin (Cinobac)	Arthropathy in immature animals	Contraindicated
Clindamycin (Cleocin)	None known	Caution*
Dapsone (Avlosulfon; and others)	None known; carcinogenic in rats and mice; hemolytic reactions in neonates	Caution*, especially at term
Erythromycin estolate (Ilosone; and others)	Risk of cholestatic hepatitis appears to be increased in pregnant women	Contraindicated
Erythromycins, other	None known	Probably safe
Imipenem-cilastatin (Primaxin)	Toxic in some pregnant animals	Caution*
Methenamine mandelate (Mandelamine; and others)	Unknown	Probably safe
Metronidazole (Flagyl; and others)	None known – carcinogenic in rats and mice	Caution*
Nalidixic acid (NegGram; and others)	Unknown – arthropathy in immature animals; increased intracranial pressure in newborn	Contraindicated
Nitrofurantoin (Furadantin; and others)	Hemolytic anemia in newborn	Caution*; contraindicated at term
Norfloxacin (Noroxin)	Anthropathy in immature animals	Contraindicated
Penicillins [c]	None known	Probably safe
Spectinomycin (Trobicin)	Unknown	Probably safe
Sulfonamides	Hemolysis in newborn with G6PD deficiency; increased risk of kernicterus in newborn; teratogenic in some animal studies	Caution*; contraindicated at term
Tetracyclines	Tooth discoloration and dysplasia, inhibition of bone growth in fetus; hepatic toxicity and azotemia with IV use in pregnant patients with decreased renal function or with overdosage	Contraindicated
Trimethoprim (Proloprim; and others)	Folate antagonism; teratogenic in rats	Caution*
Trimethroprim-sulfamethoxazole (Bactrim; and others)	Same as sulfonamides and trimethoprim	Caution*; contraindicated at term
Vancomycin (Vancocin; and others)	Unknown – possible auditory and renal toxicity in fetus	Caution*
Antituberculosis		
Capreomycin (Capastat)	None known	Caution*
Cycloserine (Seromycin; and others)	Unknown	Caution*
Ethambutol (Myambutol)	None known – teratogenic in animals	Caution*
Ethionamide (Trecator-SC)	Teratogenic in animals	Caution*
Isoniazid (INH; and others)	Embryocidal in some animals	Caution*
Pyrazinamide	Unknown	Caution*
Rifampin (Rifadin; Rimactane)	Tetratogenic in animals	Caution*
Streptomycin	Possible 8th-nerve toxicity in fetus	Caution*
Antifungal, systemic		
Amphotericin B (Fungizone; and others)	None known	Caution*
Flucytosine (Ancobon)	Teratogenic in rats	Caution*
Griseofulvin (Fulvicin P/G; and others)	Embryotoxic and teratogenic in animals; carcinogenic in rodents	Contraindicated
Ketoconazole (Nizoral)	Teratogenic and embryotoxic in rats	Caution
Miconazole (Monistat IV)	None known	Caution*
Nystatin (Mycostatin)	None reported	Probably safe
Antiviral, systemic		
Acyclovir (Zovirax)	None known	Caution*
Amantadine (Symmetrel; and others)	Teratogenic and embryotoxic in rats	Contraindicated

TABLE 40–1. Continued

Drug	Toxicity in Pregnancy	Recommendation
Ribavirin (Virazole)	Mutagenic, teratogenic, embryolethal in nearly all species, and possibly carcinogenic in animals	Contraindicated
Vidarabine (Vira-A)	Teratogenic in rats and rabbits	Caution*
Zidovudine (Retrovir)	Unknown – mutagenic in vitro	Caution*
Antiparasitic		
Chloroquine (Aralen; and others)	None known with doses recommended for malaria prophylaxis	Probably safe in low doses
Crotamitron (Eurax)	Unknown	Caution*
Dehydroemetine	Not established, but known to be cardiotoxic	Contraindicated
Diloxanide (Furamide)	Safety not established	Caution*
Emetine	Not established, but known to be cardiotoxic	Contraindicated
Furazolidone (Furoxone)	None known; carcinogenic in rodents; hemolysis with G6PD deficiency in newborn	Caution*; contraindicated at term
Hydroxychloroquine (Plaquenil)	None known with doses recommended for malaria prophylaxis	Probably safe in low doses
Iodoquinol (Yodoxin)	Unknown	Caution*
Lindane (Kwell; and others)	Absorbed from the skin; potential CNS toxicity in fetus	Contraindicated
Mebendazole (Vermox)	Teratogenic and embryotoxic in rats	Caution*
Metronidazole (Flagyl; and others)	None known – carcinogenic in rats and mice	Caution*
Niclosamide (Niclocide)	Not absorbed; no known toxicity in fetus	Probably safe
Oxamniquine (Vansil)	Embryocidal in animals	Contraindicated
Paromomycin (Humatin)	Poorly absorbed; toxicity in fetus unknown	Probably safe
Pentamidine (Pentam 300)	Safety not established	Caution*
Permethrin (Nix 1% Creme Rinse)	Poorly absorbed; no known toxicity in fetus	Probably safe
Piperazine (Antepar; and others)	Unknown	Caution*
Praziquantel (Biltricide)	None known	Probably safe
Primaquine	Hemolysis in G6PD deficiency	Contraindicated
Pyrantel pamoate (Antiminth)	Absorbed in small amounts; no known toxicity in fetus	Probably safe
Pyrethrins and piperonyl butoxide (RID; and others)	Poorly absorbed; no known toxicity in fetus	Probably safe
Pryimethamine (Daraprim)	Teratogenic in animals	Caution*
Pyrimethamine-sulfadoxine (Fansidar)	Teratogenic in animals; increased risk of kernicterus in newborn	Caution*, especially at term
Quinacrine (Atabrine)	Safety not established	Caution
Quinine	Large doses can cause abortion; auditory nerve hypoplasia, deafness in fetus; visual changes, limb anomalies, visceral defects also reported	Caution*
Suramin sodium (Germanin)	Teratogenic in mice	Caution*
Thiabendazole (Mintezol)	None known	Caution*

[a] Amikacin (*Amikin*), gentamicin (*Garamycin;* and others), kanamycin (*Kantrex;* and others), netilmicin (*Netromycin*), streptomycin, tobramycin (*Nebcin*)

[b] Cefaclor (*Ceclor*), cefadroxil (*Duricef; Ultracef*), cefamandole (*Mandol*), cefazolin (*Ancef;* and others), cefonicid (*Monocid*), cefoperazone (*Cefobid*), ceforanide (*Precef*), cefotaxime (*Claforan*), cefotetan (*Cefotan*), cefoxitin (*Mefoxin*); ceftazidime (*Fortaz; Tazidime; Tazicef*), ceftizoxime (*Cefizox*), ceftriaxone (*Rocephin*), cefuroxime (*Kefurox; Zinacef*), cephalexin (*Keflex;* and others), cephalothin (*Keflin;* and others), cephapirin (*Cefadyl;* and others), cephradine (*Anspor;* and others), moxalactam (*Moxam*)

[c] Amdinocillin (*Coactin*), amoxicillin (*Amoxil;* and others), amoxicillin-clavulanic acid (*Augmentin*), ampicillin (*Polycillin;* and others), azlocillin (*Azlin*), bacampicillin (*Spectrobid*), carbenicillin (*Geocillin; Geopen; Pyopen*), cloxacillin (*Tegopen;* and others), cyclacillin (*Cyclapoen-W*), dicloxacillin (*Dycill;* and others), hetacillin (*Versapen*), methicillin (*Staphcillin*), mezlocillin (*Mezlin*), nafcillin (*Nafcil; Unipen*), oxacillin (*Prostaphlin;* and others), penicillin G, penicillin V, piperacillin (*Pipracil*), ticarcillin (*Ticar*), ticarcillin-clavulanic acid (*Timentin*)

SOURCE: The Medical Letter (1987).

TABLE 40-2. *Drugs with Known or Suspected Teratogenic Effects*

Drug	Effect	Drug	Suspected Effect

Anticonvulsants
  Trimethadione
  Phenytoin
	Facial dysmorphogenesis, mild mental retardation, growth retardation	Alkylating agents
		Hormones
		  Oral contraceptives
		  Progestins
			Abortion, anomalies
			
			Limb and cardiac defects
			Limb and cardiac defects

Anticoagulants Coumadin and congeners	Nasal hypoplasia, epiphyseal stippling, optic atrophy	Lithium carbonate Nicotine	Ebstein's anomaly Growth retardation
Alcohol (ethanol)	FAS – growth retardation, mental retardation, increase in anomalies	Sulfonylureas Tranquilizers	Anomalies Facial clefts, cardiovascular defects

Folic acid antagonists
  Methotrexate
  Aminopterin
	Abortion, multiple malformations		

Hormones Diethylstilbestrol	Vaginal adenosis, carcinogenesis, uterine anomalies, epididymal anomalies		
Androgens	Masculinization of female fetus		
Methyl mercury	CNS damage, growth retardation		
Thalidomide	Phocomelia		

SOURCE: Rayburn and Zuspan (1980).

TABLE 40-3. *Drugs in Pregnancy*

	Effects on the Fetus and Neonate	
Medication	First Trimester	Second and Third Trimesters, Labor, and Delivery
Alcohol	Fetal alcohol syndrome: Mental retardation, microcephaly, craniofacial abnormalities, intrauterine growth retardation, cardiac anomalies (usually atrial-septal defect), limb deformities, retardation	Increased risk of spontaneous abortions
Analgesics Narcotics		Central nervous system and respiratory depression; withdrawal syndrome following prolonged intrauterine exposure

TABLE 40-3. Continued

Medication	Effects on the Fetus and Neonate	
	First Trimester	Second and Third Trimesters, Labor, and Delivery
Nonsteroidal anti-inflammatory agents		Abnormal platelet function; closure of ductus arteriosus *in utero*, leading to persistent pulmonary hypertension in the newborn
Salicylates	Conflicting data; may be associated with cleft palate and lip, hypospadias, and other congenital anomalies	
Anesthesia	Women working in operating rooms exposed to inhalation agents may have increased incidence of spontaneous abortion and congenital malformations; nitrous oxide inhibits activity of B_{12} and may be causative	Central nervous system depression, bradycardia, apnea, hypotonia, seizure *Note:* Problems are more common after paracervical block
Anticoagulants	Fetal warfarin syndrome: nasal hypoplasia, chondrodysplasia punctata	Fetal warfarin syndrome: optic atrophy, microcephaly, mental retardation, fetal and neonatal hemorrhage
	Note: Heparin is preferred for prevention of thromboembolic disease, except in patients with prosthetic valves, with whom benefits of warfarin outweigh risks. Heparin should be used in all patients who need anticoagulants during last three weeks of pregnancy.	
Anticonvulsants	In general, infants of women taking anticonvulsants have increased incidence of congenital malformations that include cleft palate and lip, cardiac anomalies, and skeletal defects	Coagulation disturbances
Carbamazepine (Tegretol)	No data	No data
Phenobarbital	Digital and facial anomalies, congenital heart lesions	Hypocalcemia in the newborn due to vitamin D deficiency; symptoms of drug withdrawal follow long-term exposure *in utero*; administer vitamin K at birth
Phenytoin (Dilantin)	Fetal hydantoin syndrome – Craniofacial anomalies: low, broad nasal bridge; epicanthal folds; hypertelorism; ptosis; strabismus. Limb defects: hypoplasia of the distal phalanges, fingerlike thumbs, alteration of the palmar crease. Intrauterine growth retardation, mental retardation, congenital heart disease	Administer vitamin K at birth
Primidone (Mysoline)	See phenobarbital	See phenobarbital
Trimethadione (Tridione)	V-shaped eyebrows, low-set ears, palate abnormalities, developmental delay, speech disturbances, cardiac anomalies, intrauterine growth retardation, ocular defects, simian creases, hypospadias, microcephaly	
Valproic acid (Depakene)	Risk of spina bifida	No data

Continued

TABLE 40-3. *Continued*

	Effects on the Fetus and Neonate	
Medication	*First Trimester*	*Second and Third Trimesters, Labor, and Delivery*
Antimicrobial agents		
Aminoglycosides	May cause auditory impairment due to damage to eighth nerve; streptomycin should not be used to treat tuberculosis during pregnancy, unless other first-line agents are ineffective	
Chloramphenicol (Chloromycetin)		Risk of gray-baby syndrome if used during labor
Chloroquine (Aralen)	Conflicting data: May be associated with congenital deafness; nonetheless, it is drug of choice for treating malaria in pregnancy	
Pyrimethamine (Daraprim)	Theoretical risk of congenital abnormalities	
Quinine	At high doses, associated with hypoplasia of optic nerve and congenital deafness	
Rifampin (Rifadin)		Risk of hypoprothrombinemia and bleeding; continues to be used in treating tuberculosis, if a third drug is needed
Sulfonamides		Avoid use in G6PD deficient patients; theoretical risk of hyperbilirubinemia
Tetracycline	Tooth discoloration and enamel hypoplasia	
Trimethoprim	Theoretical risk of congenital abnormalities	
Cardiovascular medications		
Magnesium sulfate		Side effects may occur if used close to delivery: respiratory depression, hypotonia, convulsions, ileus
Propranolol (Inderal)		Intrauterine growth retardation, bradycardia, hypoglycemia
Thiazide diuretics		Thrombocytopenia (one case reported); theoretical risk of hypoglycemia
Cytotoxic agents	All cytotoxic agents should be avoided if possible during first trimester	
Alkylating agents	Multiple congenital abnormalities	Intrauterine growth retardation
Folate antagonists	Cleft palate, cranial dysostoses, ear anomalies, skeletal defects, spontaneous abortion	
Diphenhydramine	May be associated with cleft palate	
Endocrine therapy		
Androgens	Masculinization of female fetus, involving clitoral enlargement and fusion of labia with scrotal folds	
Diethylstilbestrol	Vaginal adenocarcinoma of female offspring, vaginal adenosis, uterine abnormalities, urogenital tract abnormalities in male offspring	

TABLE 40–3. Continued

| | Effects on the Fetus and Neonate ||
Medication	First Trimester	Second and Third Trimesters, Labor, and Delivery
Estrogens	Masculinization of female fetus	
Glucocorticoids	Risk of cleft palate with high doses; intrauterine growth retardation	Monitor newborn for adrenal insufficiency
Oral contraceptives (combination of estrogen and progesterone)	Small risk of congenital anomalies – VACTREL syndrome: anomalies of the vertebrae, anus, cardiovascular system, trachea, renal tract, esophagus, and limbs	
Oral hypoglycemic agents		Neonatal hypoglycemia
Progesterone, ethisterone, norethisterone, nor-ethynodrel (Enovid)	Masculinization of female fetus	
Psychotherapy		
Chlordiazepoxide		Withdrawal syndrome in the newborn following long-term exposure *in utero*
Diazepam (Valium)	Conflicting data; may be associated with an increased risk of cleft palate	Withdrawal syndrome after long-term exposure *in utero*; administration prior to delivery may cause hypotonia, sedation, and poor feeding in the newborn; doses > 30 mg during labor are associated with hypothermia and low Apgar score
Haloperidol (Haldol)	Limb deformities (two cases reported)	
Lithium	Cardiovascular anomalies	Toxic levels may produce hypotonia and cyanosis; goiter, transient hypothyroidism, and nephrogenic diabetes insipidus have been reported
Phenothiazines	Risk of limb deformities	Extrapyramidal reactions in the newborn
Thyroid therapy Antithyroid medications: carbimazole, methimazole (Tapazole), propylthiouracil	Risk of goiter and hypothyroidism; propylthiouracil is agent of choice in pregnancy	
Iodides	Contraindicated in pregnancy; risk of goiter, thyroid enlargement, hypothyroidism, and mental retardation *Caution:* Over-the-counter cough medications containing iodides should be avoided	
Tobacco	Intrauterine growth retardation, possible risk of spontaneous abortion, developmental delays	

SOURCE: Stile, Hegyi, and Hiatt (1984).

It is well known that alcohol crosses the placenta and affects the fetus, and there is little disagreement regarding the risks of excessive maternal drinking during pregnancy. There is, however, some controversy regarding the dangers associated with even a moderate intake of alcohol during pregnancy. It is essential that health care professionals become informed regarding the research being done on the effect of alcohol use during pregnancy so that they can assist women in making informed decisions.

The Surgeon General of the United States issued an advisory on drinking during pregnancy in July 1981. This report recommended that every patient be told about the risks of alcohol consumption during pregnancy. The warning states that pregnant women should not drink alcoholic beverages and should also be made aware of the alcoholic content of foods and drugs (Fetal effects of maternal alcohol use, 1983).

Fetal Alcohol Syndrome
Findings indicate decrements in the birth weight of infants whose mother's average intake of absolute alcohol was as little as 30 ml (1 oz) per day. There also appears to be an increased risk of spontaneous abortion with the ingestion of 30 ml of alcohol per week. In comparing 1 oz of absolute alcohol to other beverages, this amount would be less than two beers, or less than two 4-oz glasses of wine, or less than two 80-proof drinks of hard liquor. (One 12-oz can of beer, 4 oz of wine, or one and a half drinks of 80-proof liquor equals 0.6 oz of absolute alcohol.)

In addition, studies have found an increased incidence of major deformities and impairments, characterized as *fetal alcohol syndrome* (FAS), in infants of some women who drank small amounts of alcohol during pregnancy. Fetal alcohol syndrome is usually associated with heavy maternal drinking. However, a number of reports regarding both heavy and moderate drinking confirm a relationship between maternal alcohol consumption and the risk of fetal abnormalities (Fetal effects of maternal alcohol use, 1983).

Although the association between alcohol abuse during pregnancy and fetal abnormalities has been of medical concern for over 250 years, the disorder FAS was not named until 1973 by Jones and Smith, who found FAS in 11 newborns. Since then, several hundred cases have been reported in the literature. The incidence of FAS ranges from 1 in 300 to 1 in 2000 live births, depending on the population being studied. Thirty to forty percent of infants of alcoholic mothers are affected (Fetal effects of maternal alcohol use, 1983).

FAS is characterized by abnormal facial characteristics; prenatal and postnatal growth deficiency in height, weight, and head circumference; and central nervous system involvement, including mental retardation. Abnormalities in other organ systems have also been found. A 50 percent increase in facial abnormalities has been found in infants of mothers consuming 3 oz of absolute alcohol (6 drinks) during early pregnancy. Drinking 3–4 drinks at a time significantly places the baby at increased risk.

Children with FAS have also exhibited impaired immunologic function and appear to be predisposed to carcinoma. Psychomotor developmental impairment is also significantly increased in FAS (Gal and Sharpless, 1984). Table 40–4 provides a summary of the characteristics associated with FAS.

A study by Rosett et al. (1983) revealed that women who were heavy drinkers early in pregnancy and who reduced consumption before the third trimester had a decreased incidence of growth retardation. Their infants did, however, exhibit more congenital anomalies than those of women who did not consume large amounts of alcohol in the first trimester. Women who continued heavy drinking throughout pregnancy had both retarded fetal growth rates and increased infant abnormalities.

Acute alcohol toxicity in the neonate results in withdrawal symptoms lasting up to 72 hours, followed by lethargy for 24–48 hours. The symptoms include agitation, hyperactivity, tremors, and seizures. Alcohol may be detected on the infant's breath soon after birth.

There is no known safe level of alcohol consumption during pregnancy. A comparative study was made of children from middle-class, well-educated families whose mothers consumed moderate or small amounts of alcohol and offspring of mothers who drank little or no alcohol during pregnancy. The results revealed that 4-year-olds of mothers who drank moderate amounts of alcohol had diminished uninterrupted attention span compared to children whose mothers consumed little or no alcohol during pregnancy (Gal and Sharpless, 1984). Ideally, women of childbearing age who wish to have a baby should stop drinking prior to becoming pregnant. Certainly once a woman knows she is pregnant it is imperative that she be encouraged to abstain from alcohol. Preventive education regarding the effects of alcohol on the fetus is essential (Hill, 1984).

TABLE 40-4. Characteristics of Fetal Alcohol Syndrome

Area	Characteristics
Growth deficiency	
Prenatal	Less than 3% for weight and length
Postnatal	Less than 3% for both weight and height
	Failure to thrive
	Diminished or disproportionate adipose tissue
Facial characteristics	
Eyes	Short palpebral fissures (small eye openings)
	Myopia, strabismus, ptosis
Nose	Short and upturned
	Flat or absent groove above upper lip (hypoplastic philtrum)
Mouth	Thinned upper lip (vermillion)
	Receding jaw in infancy (retrognathia)
Central nervous system	
Intellectual	Mild to moderate mental retardation, learning disability
	Microcephaly
Neurologic	Poor coordination
	Decreased muscle tone
Behavioral	Irritability in infancy
	Hyperactivity in childhood
Other abnormalities	
Cardiac	Murmurs, atrial septal defects, ventricular septal defects, tetralogy of Fallot, great vessel anomalies
Skeletal	Limited joint movements, primarily fingers, elbows, and hip dislocations
	Aberrant palmar creases
	Pectus excavatum
Renal	Kidney defects
Genital	Labial hypoplasia
Cutaneous	Hemangiomas

SOURCES: Clarren and Smith (1978); McCarthy (1983).

If a pregnant woman chooses to continue drinking during pregnancy, she should be advised to limit her consumption to one and never more than two drinks on any one occasion. In addition, drinks should be spaced at least 2 hours apart and the woman should be encouraged to eat along with the alcohol, which will allow the body to metabolize the alcohol at a faster rate and keep the maternal blood alcohol levels lower, resulting in less fetal exposure. Daily drinking should be avoided. Fetal alcohol syndrome and other alcohol-related birth defects can be completely prevented by abstaining from alcohol during pregnancy.

The Nurse's Role

The nurse must be supportive when dealing with patients who have difficulty abstaining from alcohol during pregnancy, especially if they are psychologically or physiologically dependent on alcohol. It is essential that an accurate assessment be made of the client's use of alcoholic beverages. The quantity and frequency of drinking as well as the type of alcohol consumed should be determined. Questions must be asked tactfully if honest answers are to be elicited. Information regarding the presence of alcohol-related birth defects or FAS in siblings should also be obtained.

It is important for the nurse to be understanding as well as supportive in order to prevent undue anxiety and to gain the woman's cooperation. If the client becomes defensive, she may hide the amount of alcohol she is using or even delay obtaining prenatal care.

Many times the pregnant woman wishes to stop drinking but is unable to do so without professional counseling and medical help. If detoxification is needed, hospitalization is essential in order to monitor the effects of alcohol withdrawal on the fetus as well as the mother. When medications are used to alleviate maternal withdrawal symptoms, the possibility of placental transfer must be considered. Some drugs used for the treatment of alcoholism are carcinogenic or teratogenic. A study of maternal barbiturate sedation has indicated that it may increase the child's risk of developing cancer later (Spencer and Nicholas, 1983). Librium and Valium, often used in alcohol detoxification, are contraindicated because of possible teratogenic effects. Antabuse, which is sometimes helpful in treating alcoholism, is also unsafe for use in pregnancy because it inhibits enzyme action (Spencer and Nichols, 1983).

The mother who has used alcohol during pregnancy may also experience feelings of guilt at the time of birth because of the effect the drinking may have had on her infant. The nurse must be available to provide emotional support and to assist her with the grieving process if the child is affected by the use of alcohol in pregnancy.

The nurse must assume an active role in the education of the public regarding the potential harmful effects of alcohol use during pregnancy.

One reason many women continue to drink during pregnancy is that they are unaware of the potential risks to their baby. Explaining that the baby's immature liver metabolizes alcohol slowly and that the kidneys are unable to excrete alcohol as quickly as in the mother may encourage women to stop drinking. Alcohol enters the bloodstream of the fetus in the same concentration as it enters the mother's, and the infant's blood alcohol level remains high long after the mother has had her last drink (McCarthy, 1983). Teaching patients this type of information could help to prevent many alcohol-related problems.

Marijuana

Marijuana is now the most widely used illicit drug in the United States, with more than 50 million people having used it at least once (Reynolds, 1983). Marijuana is a drug derived from the leaves, stems, fruiting tops, and resin of the hemp plant, *Cannabis sativa*. The active ingredient is tetrahydrocannabinol (THC). Marijuana is metabolized at a much slower rate than alcohol, and the psychoactive components of the drug remain in the body for a long time. It is believed that the THC and its metabolites from one marijuana cigarette may last in the body for as long as 3 weeks.

A 1982 report by the National Academy of Science revealed a number of potential serious health hazards associated with the use of marijuana. Marijuana impairs motor coordination and affects tracking ability and sensory and perceptual functioning. It also causes feelings of euphoria and mood changes with periods of anxiety, confusion, and even psychosis-like episodes. Smoking marijuana usually causes acute changes in the heart and circulation. It increases the workload of the heart by raising the heart rate and sometimes the blood pressure (Reynolds, 1983). This rise in cardiac workload poses a considerable threat to pregnant women, whose cardiac workload is already increased by pregnancy.

Acute exposure to marijuana smoke causes bronchodilation, and chronic use may result in inflammation and preneoplastic changes in the lungs. These changes suggest that prolonged marijuana use may lead to lung cancer and serious impairment of lung function. It has been found that in terms of lung damage, smoking five joints is equivalent to smoking six packs of cigarettes. The THC readily crosses the placenta.

Studies are limited regarding the effects of marijuana on the human reproductive system and chromosomes. There is evidence that the drug has a moderate suppressive effect on sperm production and that it lowers testosterone levels in men. Women users of marijuana have been found to have anovulatory menstrual cycles or a shortened fertility period. Animal studies indicate that levels of estrogen, progesterone, and pituitary growth hormones are altered by marijuana use. This suggests that there may be a higher level of infertility among marijuana smokers (National Institute of Drug Abuse, 1980; Reynolds, 1983). In humans, marijuana use has been associated with an increased prevalence of abnormal sperm cells (Nahas, 1986).

The chemicals in marijuana readily cross the placenta and have the potential for teratogenicity. Animal studies confirm that birth defects occur when high doses of marijuana are given. Extracts of marijuana smoke have also caused dose-related mutations in bacteria and have affected chromosome segregation during cell division, resulting in an abnormal number of chromosomes in daughter cells (Reynolds, 1983).

A study by Gal and Sharpless (1984) of infants exposed to marijuana revealed the following: the infants were: (1) less responsive to light that was repeatedly directed at their eyes; (2) less successful at self-quieting than controls; and, (3) more easily startled and showed increased levels of tremors. One-third of the babies also had a high-pitched cry similar to those undergoing narcotics withdrawal. These symptoms were noted in the babies of regular marijuana users.

Another study by Greenland et al. (1982) identified the primary problem observed in the infants of marijuana users as a significantly higher incidence of meconium staining (57 *vs* 31 percent in nonusers). Meconium staining is frequently associated with fetal hypoxia and stress, occurring most often in SGA babies who are term or post-term (Gal and Sharpless, 1984).

The use of marijuana is definitely contraindicated in pregnancy because of the potential dangers to both the mother and her offspring. Animal studies reveal that THC from marijuana can be transmitted to the baby through the mother's breast milk. Furthermore, traces of the chemical can be found in the urine and feces of nursing infants whose mothers smoke marijuana (National Institute of Drug Abuse, 1980; Nahos, 1986).

While much study is still needed to explain many of the unanswered questions regarding the effects of marijuana, we do know enough to discourage its use, especially in pregnant women. There is also concern about the potential effects on offspring of marijuana use by the father. What little is known about marijuana justifies national concern.

Some people falsely believe that marijuana is less harmful than alcohol; however, evidence does not confirm this. Marijuana remains in the system much longer than alcohol, which might suggest that the effect on the fetus may last much longer than that of alcohol. Marijuana's circulation time from lung to brain is 14 seconds, which is much faster than ingested alcohol reaches the brain. The potential risks to both mother and fetus are great, and all women should be encouraged to abstain from using marijuana during pregnancy. Ideally, both parents should stop using marijuana long before a pregnancy takes place. This would require at least 3–6 months abstinence from marijuana use because THC lasts so long in the body. It is not known what permanent effects may remain from long-term marijuana use.

The nurse plays an important role in obtaining the history of marijuana use by the pregnant woman and by the baby's father. Once such information is obtained, the client should be encouraged not to use marijuana during pregnancy. Appropriate referrals should be made for counseling or hospitalization if needed. There is disagreement regarding whether marijuana causes physiologic withdrawal symptoms, but there is agreement that psychologic withdrawal occurs.

Long-term cannabis smokers are difficult to treat because of their denial of the progressive negative effects of their dependency and the lack of severe physical after-effects such as those associated with alcohol or other narcotic drugs. Treatment should employ methods that encourage abstinence from the drug and to foster a drug-free lifestyle (Nahas, 1986).

The pregnant woman may experience guilt and the nurse should provide understanding and support. In addition, nurses should be encouraged to become involved in research concerning the effects of marijuana use during pregnancy. The nurse can also join with other health care professionals to provide educational programs for the public regarding the dangers of marijuana use.

Narcotics

Heroin and morphine are considered to be among the most dangerous drugs for pregnant women. An increased incidence of spontaneous abortion, prematurity, and stillbirths is found in pregnancies of narcotics addicts. Those infants who live are prone to many neonatal complications. The respiratory system in the fetus may be depressed, and a decreased responsiveness is often found in the newborn. The neonate's psychophysiologic functioning is depressed and drug withdrawal occurs. Signs of withdrawal include:

1. Hyperactivity or jitteriness.
2. Shrill, persistent crying.
3. Frequent yawning or sneezing.
4. Decreased Moro reflex.
5. Increased tendon reflexes.

The symptoms may begin within 24 hours after birth. In some cases the baby may appear to be normal at birth, with withdrawal symptoms beginning as early as 72 hours to as long as 2 weeks after birth. Symptoms may be mild to severe, continuous or transitory, or intermittent with periods of apparent recovery (Phillips, 1986). If the condition is left untreated, vomiting, diarrhea, fever, convulsions, apnea, and death may result. Treatment of withdrawal consists of the administration of phenobarbital or paregoric. The choice of treatment depends on whether symptoms are related to the gastrointestinal system, the central nervous system, or both. The dosage is gradually decreased over a 2-week period or until withdrawal signs subside.

Babies born to narcotic-dependent women often show intrauterine growth retardation. Approximately 40 percent are small for gestational age, and 60 percent are premature (Korones, 1981). It is uncertain whether growth impairment is due to the narcotic itself or to the adverse socioeconomic and health conditions found among addicts. It is possible that the growth retardation results from multiple factors.

When methadone maintenance programs have been instituted, some of the adverse factors associated with drug addiction appear to be reduced and intrauterine growth retardation is improved. Other research suggests that the growth retardation associated with heroin addiction differs from that associated with malnutrition (Naeye et al., 1973; Phillips, 1986).

The use of cocaine has become exceedingly popular. An estimated 10 million Americans have used cocaine at least once, with 5 million using it on a regular basis. It is therefore probable that a large number of women who are pregnant have used cocaine (Chasnoff et al., 1985; Madden et al., 1986).

In studies of pregnant women using cocaine, there was a higher incidence of spontaneous abortion than in those who used heroin during previous pregnancies. Cocaine acts to inhibit nerve conduction and prevent norepinephrine uptake at nerve terminals producing increased norepinephrine levels with subsequent vasoconstriction tachycardia and an abrupt rise in blood pressure. In addition, placental vasoconstriction occurs, thereby decreasing blood flow to the fetus. The increased norepinephrine levels may also increase uterine contractability. There is also an increase in abruptio placentae immediately following self-injection of cocaine. The Brazelton Neonatal Behavioral Assessment Scale revealed infants exposed to cocaine showed significant depression to interactive behavior and poor organizational response to environmental stimuli (state organization) (Chasnoff et al., 1985).

Long-term follow-up of infants born to cocaine-using mothers is necessary to identify accurately all of the potential problems which may be encountered in these babies.

When caring for narcotic-dependent pregnant women, the nurse should use an understanding and supportive approach. The woman must feel accepted as a human being. She should be recognized and acknowledged for her decision to seek medical care. A careful assessment of the client's drug use is essential. The nurse should attempt to determine what kinds of drugs are being used, how much, and how often. The pregnant woman must be placed under appropriate medical and nursing care as soon as contact is made. The heroin and morphine addict must gradually withdraw from the drug in order to prevent premature labor or intrauterine death of the fetus. Hospitalization is often required for this withdrawal process. Maintenance doses of methadone are often administered on a daily basis. Some authorities prefer to avoid detoxification during pregnancy (Rosner, Keith, and Chasnoff, 1982). Psychologic counseling is needed to help clients and their families deal with the many problems associated with narcotic addiction and pregnancy. The nurse should provide emotional support and education throughout the pregnancy.

Careful observation of the neonate for signs of drug withdrawal is essential, and prompt treatment is needed to ensure the infant's well-being. The mother may be worried and may experience guilt feelings because of the effect her addiction may have had on her baby. She should be kept informed of the infant's condition and involved in the care of the child if possible. Maternal–infant bonding should be encouraged. If the father is present, he should be included in the plan whenever possible. If he is also an addict, appropriate referrals for his treatment are needed. Drug-addicted parents may be alienated from family and friends and may lack any real support systems. If family members or friends are available and able to provide support, their help should be encouraged.

When the mother and baby are discharged, follow-up care is essential. Referral to appropriate social service agencies is needed in order to provide continued support and to monitor the infant's care. The progress of the mother's treatment of her addiction should also be followed. Infants of narcotics addicts may be neglected or abused because of the lifestyle of their parents; thus, the importance of close follow-up care cannot be over-emphasized. An infant may need to be placed in foster care while the mother receives treatment for addiction and is unable to care safely for her baby.

Caffeine

Caffeine is a xanthine alkaloid found in coffee, tea, cocoa, colas, and other carbonated beverages. It is also present in many over-the-counter medications, including cold and allergy preparations and appetite suppressants. The majority of over-the-counter medications contain approximately 200 mg of caffeine. There are no recorded deaths specifically related to caffeine overdose, although it is believed that the fatal dose in humans is 10 g (Roberts and Weigle, 1983).

In 1983 the Food and Drug Administration issued a warning regarding the potential dangers of caffeine to the developing fetus. Human studies of these effects have been limited; however, the information provided by animal studies resulted in the FDA's removal of caffeine from the Generally Recognized as Safe list (FDA Drug Bulletin, 1980).

Caffeine is rapidly absorbed from the gastrointestinal tract. In the adult the biologic half-life of caffeine is approximately 3.5 hours. Most of the ingested caffeine is excreted by the kidneys. Metabolic derivatives such as monoethyl, dimethyl xanthines, and uric acid are excreted in the urine. Caffeine is distributed in the tissues in proportion to their water content; thus, the greatest amount is found in skeletal muscles. Caffeine readily passes across the blood–brain barrier and the placenta (Roberts and Weigle, 1983).

Caffeine and its metabolites excreted by the fetus have been found in the amniotic fluid. If the maternal plasma caffeine levels and fetal levels are high, high concentrations of caffeine are also found in the amniotic fluid. Because the fetus ingests amniotic fluid during the third trimester, the amount of caffeine to which the baby is exposed may be equivalent to several milligrams a day. The fetal brain is able to accumulate caffeine, which could cause abnormal development of the nervous system. Caffeine is excreted largely unchanged in fetal urine for 1-3 days after birth (Roberts and Weigle, 1983).

Caffeine may act as a mutagen because of its chemical structure as a purine, one of the constituents of DNA. Some animal studies suggest that caffeine can alter genes and break chromosomes. Caffeine increases circulating levels of catecholamines, which causes vasoconstriction that could alter uterine and placental circulatory patterns. In animals, increased catecholamine levels have caused congenital abnormalities such as aortic arch anomalies, cleft palate, and digital defects (Roberts and Weigle, 1983).

A study of the effects of caffeine intake during pregnancy correlated with increased central apnea in infants. This effect was not expected because caffeine is a central nervous system stimulant. In mice, chronic caffeine treatment was found to increase the number of adenosine receptors in the brainstem. Adenosine is a purine base produced during severe hypoxia, and its analogs induce respiratory depression in fetal and newborn animals. It is possible that infants exposed to caffeine on a regular basis experience increased sensitivity to hypoxia (Toubas et al., 1986).

Studies of the risk of caffeine use on the human fetus are limited and reports are inconclusive. Some experts believe that caffeine is harmless, while other suggest that high levels of consumption can cause adverse fetal consequences. In a study now in progress, babies of heavy coffee drinkers are showing lower activity levels than infants of noncoffee drinkers (Roberts and Weigle, 1983).

Some women decrease their use of coffee during pregnancy because of nausea or a dislike for the smell. Perhaps such reactions have played a role in reducing pregnancy-related complications associated with caffeine use.

The primary role of the nurse is to educate pregnant women regarding the potential teratogenic effects of caffeine. Informing them of the sources of caffeine in food and medications is also helpful. Although there is no conclusive proof linking caffeine to birth defects, pregnant women should be advised to limit their caffeine intake.

Cigarette Smoking

For over 20 years the Surgeon General has warned of the harmful effects of smoking. Smoking is known to be linked to lung cancer, heart disease, and emphysema. Despite overwhelming evidence of the health hazards associated with smoking, many individuals, including pregnant women, continue to smoke cigarettes.

The effects of smoking during pregnancy have been documented for several years. Babies born to mothers who smoke are usually smaller in both weight and length than those born to nonsmokers (Matsuto et al., 1984). There is also an increased incidence of spontaneous abortion and premature delivery among smoking women. Other complications that have been linked to smoking include increased bleeding during pregnancy, abruptio placentae, placenta previa, and prolonged rupture of membranes. Research has also found an increased incidence of anencephaly, cleft palate, cleft lip, and congenital heart defects in infants of smoking mothers (Chernick, Childiaeva, and Ioffe, 1983). Several studies show that maternal smoking is significantly related to signs of poor physical, neurological, and intellectual status in school-aged children. A decrease in both gross and fine motor development has been seen in children of smoking mothers. Long-term studies suggest that slight delays in neurological development persist in the school-aged child and into adolescence. Delays in reading comprehension in children of smoking mothers have been observed at 7, 11, and 16 years of age (Gusella and Fried, 1984; Naeye and Peters, 1984).

Cigarette smoke contains carbon monoxide (CO), which readily crosses the placenta. There is normally a 50 percent increase in CO production during pregnancy, and smoking increases maternal levels even more, thus interfering with oxygenation of fetal tissue. Carbon monoxide poisoning can develop, and the infant may exhibit neurologic problems (Spencer and Nichols, 1983; Cahan, 1987).

Two other components of cigarette smoke, tar and nicotine, are currently being investigated for carcinogenicity and teratogenicity in the fetus. Nicotine increases body heat production by 15 percent. Following ovulation, basal body temperature increases 0.3°C to 0.6°C, and this increase is maintained until halfway through pregnancy, when the temperature returns to normal. In the smoking woman the temperature may remain elevated, and the excessive heat could have adverse effects on the fetus (Spencer and Nichols, 1983).

Ericksen and Marsal (1987) found that with mothers who only smoked one cigarette a day, there was still a significant increase in FHR, together with a change in the aortic velocity waveform, indicating an increase in myocardial contractability and an unchanged peripheral resistance. Another study by Magnusson (1986) found an association between cigarette smoking during pregnancy and an increased risk of subsequent infant allergies developing before 18 months of age.

Nurses and health care professionals should be aware of the effects of smoking on both the mother and her baby. Setting an example by not smoking would be most beneficial. Providing education to the public, especially pregnant women and their families, may encourage them to stop smoking during pregnancy. If a woman is unable to stop smoking completely during pregnancy, she should be encouraged to reduce the amount she smokes. Nonsmokers who breathe cigarette smoke may also be adversely affected. A nonsmoking pregnant woman living with a husband who smokes inhales the noxious elements from his cigarette smoking. Therefore, all family members should be encouraged to quit or at least reduce the amount they smoke – for their own health as well as that of the baby.

It has been suggested that adults who smoke may inflict serious damage upon the developing child, beginning with its embryonal life and continuing throughout the formative years. Nicotine may also be found in breast milk. Cahan (1987) has suggested that smoking during pregnancy and around children is a form of child abuse.

It is essential for the nurse to provide encouragement and support for any efforts made to quit or reduce the amount of smoking. Because many people smoke due to stress, anxiety, or nervousness, the nurse should explore alternate coping mechanisms with the pregnant woman and her family.

Prescribed and Over-the-Counter Medications

As mentioned earlier, pregnant women frequently take a number of medications during pregnancy. This is potentially dangerous because of the effects such drugs may have on the fetus. Increased maternal blood and plasma volumes during pregnancy cause a decrease in the concentration of maternal serum protein. This results in a lower capacity of protein to bind *any* drugs in the maternal system. The lower the molecular weight of a substance, the greater its chance of crossing the placenta (Spencer and Nichols, 1983).

Many women take over-the-counter drugs without realizing they can be harmful. The drugs are assumed to be safe because they can be bought without a prescription. This assumption is in error, however – many commonly used nonprescription medications can be very harmful to the fetus. For example, aspirin is a drug used almost universally, yet according to unconfirmed reports, it may cause congenital anomalies when taken during the first trimester, as well as increased hemorrhagic tendencies and inhibited platelet aggregation in the newborn. It may also cause prolonged pregnancy as a result of prostaglandin biosynthesis and salicylate poisoning (Hahn et al., 1982).

Because of the potential dangers associated with maternal use of any medication, it is essential that nurses and other health care providers conduct a public education campaign to provide parents with appropriate information regarding the use of drugs during pregnancy. Ideally, such a program would encourage women to stop taking medications prior to becoming pregnant.

Any woman who suspects she may be pregnant should avoid self-medication. In addition, she should inform her physician that she is or might be pregnant so that the pregnancy can be taken into consideration prior to prescribing medications. Routinely asking women of childbearing age whether they might be pregnant prior to prescribing a medication could prevent errors in giving a fetotoxic agent. If a woman is unsure whether she is pregnant, a pregnancy test can be done.

An assessment of the drugs a pregnant woman has used or is using should be made at the first prenatal visit. A woman who is taking medications will often willingly stop once she has been informed of the potential dangers to her baby. Because the woman may be anxious about having taken a drug that might harm her infant, she should receive understanding and support from the nurse. Undue fright should be avoided. If the woman is seen early in pregnancy, it is possible that the drug was taken during the preembryonic period of development. As mentioned previously, there is less risk at this time than during the embryonic period. Patients who must take medications for health reasons should be under close medical and nursing supervision. Every effort should be made to use drugs that have no known fetotoxic or teratogenic effects.

SUMMARY

The nurse's role in the management of drug use and abuse during pregnancy has been discussed throughout this chapter. It is essential for nurses to keep up to date regarding the effects of drugs on the fetus. It must be emphasized to the pregnant woman that no drug can be considered absolutely safe for use during pregnancy.

The major aspects of the nurse's role include:

1. Using an understanding, supportive approach when dealing with the pregnant woman and her family.
2. Providing education and information to the public regarding the potential effects of drug use during pregnancy.
3. Encouraging all women who wish to become pregnant to stop using chemical substances prior to pregnancy and to seek prenatal care early.
4. Making a careful assessment of all pregnant women regarding their use of any chemical substances.
5. Involving the pregnant woman and her family in setting up a realistic plan of care in order to gain their cooperation in dealing with the problem associated with drug use and abuse during pregnancy.
6. Providing appropriate nursing care for the mother and her baby, cooperating in implementing the therapeutic medical plan of care, and observing the neonate carefully for signs of drug or alcohol withdrawal.
7. Making appropriate community referrals for rehabilitation as well as continued follow-up care after delivery.

REFERENCES

Brande, M. C. et al. 1987. Prenatal drugs of abuse. *Fed. Proc.* 46:2446–2453.

Cahan, W. J. 1987. Abusing children by smoking. *Cancer J. Clin.* 37(1):31–32.

Chasnoff, I. et al. 1985. Cocaine use in pregnancy. *New Engl. J. Med.* 313(11).

Chernick, V.; Childiaeva, R.; and Ioffe, S. 1983. Effects of maternal alcohol intake and smoking on neonatal electroencephalogram and anthropometric measurements. *Am. J. Obstet. Gynecol.* 146:41–47.

Clarren, S. K., and Smith, D. W. 1978. The fetal alcohol syndrome. *New Engl. J. Med.* 298:1063–1067.

Dupont, R. L. 1981. First annual awareness banquet speech. October 17.

Eriksen, P. S., and Marsal, K. 1987. Circulatory changes in the fetal aorta after maternal smoking. *Br. J. Obstet. Gynecol.* 94:301–305.

FDA Drug Bulletin. 1980. Caffeine and pregnancy. 10(3):19–20.

Fetal effects of maternal alcohol use. 1983. *JAMA*. pp. 2517–2521.

Gal, P., and Sharpless, M. K. 1984. Fetal drug exposure – behavioral teratogenesis. *Drug Intelligence Clin. Pharm.* 18(3):186–201.

Gusella, J. L., and Fried, P. A. 1984. Effects of maternal drinking and smoking on offspring at 13 months. *Neurobehav. Toxicol. Teratol.* 6(1):13–17.

Hahn, A. B.; Bergersen, B. S.; Barkin, R. S.; and Destreich, S. J. K. 1982. *Pharmacology in nursing*. St. Louis: C. V. Mosby.

Hill, L. M., and Klanberg, F. 1984. The effects of drugs and chemicals on the fetus and newborn: Part 2. *Mayo Clin. Proc.* 59:755–765.

Kaplin, S., and Kolesari, G. L. 1982. Drugs and pregnancy. *Fam. Pract. Recert.* 4(9):103–108.

Korones, S. R. 1981. *High-risk newborn infants: The basis for intensive nursing care*. St. Louis: C. V. Mosby.

Madden, J. D. et al. 1986. Maternal cocaine abuse and effect on the newborn. *Pediatrics*. 77(2).

Magnusson, C. J. 1986. Maternal smoking influences serum IgE and IgD levels and increases the risk for subsequent infant allergy. *J. Allergy Clin. Immunol.* Nov.:898–904.

Matsuto, M. et al. 1985. Mechanism of fetal growth retardation caused by smoking during pregnancy. *Acta Physiologica Hungaria.* 65(3):295–304.

McCarthy, P. A. 1983. Fetal alcohol syndrome and other related birth defects. *Nurse Practitioner*. 8:33–37.

Naeye, R. L., and Peters, E. C. 1984. Mental development of children whose mothers smoked during pregnancy. *Am. J. Obstet. Gynecol.* 64(5):601–607.

Naeye, R. L.; Blanc, W.; LeBlanc, W.; and Khatamee, M. A. 1973. Fetal complications of maternal heroin addiction: Abnormal growth, infections, and episodes of stress. *J. Pediatrics*. 83:1055.

Nahas, G. J. 1986. Cannabis: Toxicological properties and epidemiological aspects. *Med. J. Australia*. 145:82–87.

National Institute of Drug Abuse. 1980. For parents only: What you need to know about marijuana. Washington, D.C.: U.S. Department of Health and Human Services.

Phillips, K. 1986. Neonatal drug addicts. *Nursing Times*. 82(12):36–38.

Rayburn, W. F., and Zuspan, F. P. 1980. Drug use during pregnancy. *Perinatal Press*. 4(134):115–117.

Reynolds, E. S. 1983. Marijuana and health. *Texas Medicine*. 79:42–44.

Roberts, B. W., and Weigle, A. 1983. Caffeine and pregnancy outcome. *J. Obstet. Gynecol. Neonatal Nurs.* 12:21–24.

Rosett, H. L., et al. 1983. Patterns of alcohol consumption and fetal development. *Obstet. Gynecol.* 61(5):539–546.

Rosner, M.; Keith, L.; and Chasnoff, I. 1982. The Northwestern University Drug Dependence Program: The impact of intensive prenatal care on labor and delivery outcomes. *Am. J. Obstet. Gynecol.* 144:23–27.

Spencer, R. T., and Nichols, L. W. 1983. *Clinical pharmacology and nursing management.* Philadelphia: J. B. Lippincott.

Stile, I. L.; Hegyi, T.; and Hiatt, I. M. 1984. *Drugs used with neonates and during pregnancy.* 2nd ed. Oradell, N.J.: Medical Economics Books.

Streissgerth, A. P. et al. 1986. Attention, distraction, and reaction time at age 7 years and prenatal alcohol exposure. *Neurobehav. Toxicol. Teratol.* 8(6):717–725.

Toubas, P. L. et al. 1986. Effect of maternal smoking and caffeine habits on infantile apnea: A retrospective study. *Pediatrics.* 78(1):159–163.

The Medical Letter on drugs and therapeutics. 1987. Antimicrobial drugs in pregnancy. 29:61–63.

Wilson, H., and Kneisal, C. 1983. *Psychiatric nursing.* Reading, Mass.: Addison-Wesley.

41

Sexually Transmitted Diseases: Impact on Perinatal Infections

BEHAVIORAL OBJECTIVES

Upon completion of this chapter, the reader should be able to:

- Identify common sexually transmitted diseases and discuss theories as to their incidence and reoccurrence as a Public Health Problem(s) today.

- Identify common pathways of maternal–newborn disease transmission for the following infections: *Chlamydia*, herpes simplex, CMV, hepatitis B, human immunodeficiency virus, syphilis, and gonorrhea.

- Identify and discuss appropriate measures for prevention of sexually transmitted diseases.

- Discuss nursing roles and responsibilities by identifying appropriate interventions in caring for perinatal (maternal–newborn) patients at risk because of a sexually transmitted disease.

- Identify and discuss universal infection control precautions that would be appropriate for the perinatal area.

Sexually transmitted diseases (STDs) are those that are caused by organisms that truly enjoy a protective medium in which to thrive and have fairly rigid requirements about transmission. We are extremely concerned about these diseases simply because of their rapidly escalating numbers, consequences, and complications. The 1960s "flower power" generation ushered in the "free love" era and the "easy sex" generation of the 1970s. The numbers of all the historically identified sexually transmitted diseases are resurging with the looming threat of the "AIDS" generation in the 1980s. Certainly, by totally immobilizing the immune system, as the HIV (Human Immunodeficiency Virus) is capable of, we will see a proliferation of other sexually transmitted diseases. The genital region is attractive to organisms because of pH, temperature, moisture, and hormonal influences. Most of the organisms do not thrive well outside of a narrow thermal or pH range or without nutritive support. Thus, the amount of inoculum, supportive mediums, and methods of transmission are crucial issues for the successful growth of an organism labeled an STD.

Pregnant women have special concerns regarding STDs. The amount of fetal wastage, and maternal morbidity from pelvic infections has increased by 50 percent in the last 10 years. Gonorrhea, *Chlamydia*, herpes, and other organisms have been isolated as being responsible for repeated abortions, premature rupture of membranes, premature labor, chorioamniotis, as well as neonatal sepsis.

Perhaps the growth in sexually transmitted diseases is related to the progressive change in our sanitation and economic systems in the United States. With other diseases such as polio, the improved socioeconomic conditions prevented early exposures to various pathogens. Many infections were acquired in early childhood and thus immunity was already developed against infections for the adult years. Herpes simplex, type 1 was very prevalent 25 years ago, as at least 90 percent of the population had immunity to it during their childhood years. Evidently, this provided some protection against HSV-2, to which the adult population is now more vulnerable. Organisms were more readily transmitted by secretion transmission, from mother to infant, child to child, and during sexual activity. When childhood disease acquisition is delayed because of social improvements, running water, good hygiene practices, sewers, and garbage collections, sexual activity seems to become a major method of exposure. Methods of exposure are certainly important to consider in looking at the incidence patterns of *Chlamydia*, herpes simplex and hepatitis B virus.

Sexually transmitted diseases in women are more difficult to identify and not obvious. Frequently, they are asymptomatic, yet the complications for women are greater. Genital herpes can be very painful for women. Pelvic inflammatory disease (PID) with salpingitis as a complication is very serious for women, because it causes increased infertility and ectopic pregnancy. These complications have shown a three-fold increase with an epidemic of pelvic inflammatory disease. Cervical carcinomas are thought to be related to increased incidences of STDs, particularly HSV-2 and human papilloma virus in women.

In understanding sexually transmitted diseases and their impact on the perinatal unit (the mother and the infant), it is helpful to consider some facts about the human immune system. These facts would include basic disease information as well as transmission methods and incidence.

When diseases are acquired *in utero*, infections can result in the destruction of the embryo, abortion, childbirth dysfunction, intrauterine growth retardation, prematurity, or significant neonatal disease. Infections that are acquired during the birth process may lead to long-term chronic disease such as hepatitis B, or onset of neonatal respiratory disease syndrome such as *Chlamydia*, which may precipitate an early death. Perinatal morbidity and mortality from the effects of sexually transmitted microorganisms present challenging medical and nursing management problems, as well as significant challenges for world health.

GONORRHEA

Organism: Neisseria gonorrhoeae are small Gram-negative cocci that grow in pairs (bacteria).

Epidemiology and Incidence

Gonorrhea occurs most frequently in young adults aged 15–24 years. It is extremely communicable as long as the organism is present. The incidence of new cases each year is approximately 1 million. There are probably a total of 3 million cases, as not all are reported. Many cases in females are not reported as they are usually asymptomatic. The tissue fluid and secretions of infected mucus surfaces most readily transmit the organism from the cervix, pharynx, urethra, or rectum. The period of time from exposure to symptomatic infection is 2–7 days. Gonorrhea is an important cause of pelvic inflammatory disease (PID). The goals of the U.S. Public Health Department include the reduction of the numbers of cases from

380 per 100,000 in 1986 to 280 per 100,000 in 1990 (Center for Disease Control, 1987).

Maternal Issues

Infections during pregnancy are usually subclinical or mild because of the blockage of the normal routes of the organism to the fallopian tubes. Colonization by gonorrhea of the cervix can cause inflammation and weakening of the fetal membranes and cause early rupture. Unfortunately, probably 50 percent of these cervical infections in women are asymptomatic in the early stages. Chorioamnionitis can occur in the antepartum period, labor, and delivery, as well as an increased risk of postpartum endometritis.

Dessiminated gonococcal infection is possible if a person is colonized and asymptomatic for a long time. This may present during pregnancy as arthritis, tendonitis, general aching, fever, and malaise. Risk for premature labor and delivery is high, as well as prolonged second-stage labor due to infection. Treatment of gonorrhea during pregnancy includes either 4.8 million units of penicillin, or 3.5 g ampicillin with 1.0 g probenicid orally. These infections are often accompanied by *Chlamydia*, which requires treatment with erythromycin 500 mg four times a day orally for 7 days (Eshenbach, 1987). Penicillin-resistant gonococci should be treated with 2.0 g spectinomycin.

Any past history of gonorrhea presents a strong possibility that it may reoccur during pregnancy. Partners need to be screened and treated, as the incidence of reinfection after treatment is common.

Newborn Issues

Historically, there has been concern for gonococcal ophthalmia, transmitted to the newborn while traveling down the birth canal. A silver nitrate 1% solution at birth has been the treatment of choice, and more recently erythromycin ointment has been recommended for prophylaxis to include prevention of *Chlamydia* transmission.

Fetal scalp electrodes have been identified as a source for the transmission of infection from mother to infant. Newborn gonorrhea has been isolated from fetal scalp abscesses. Thus, evaluation of the risks of infection migration via fetal monitoring is an important assessment to make if there is a known presence of any sexually transmitted infection.

N. gonorrhoeae has been isolated in gastric aspirates, conjunctival aspirates, and other locations from about 30 percent of infected newborns. Because of the maternal and neonatal risks, testing for gonorrhea is important during pregnancy. Populations of low socioeconomic status have been identified as being at higher risk. Consequently, these populations have higher rates of premature labor, premature rupture of membranes, premature births, and infectious complications (Tuomala, 1986). When cultures are positive, both mother and baby require treatment with IV penicillin.

SYPHILIS

Organism: Treponema pallidum –Thin, mobile spirochete (bacteria).

Epidemiology and Incidence

Contact with ulcerative lesions that shed spirochetes, or mucus membranes of infected people spread syphilis. Sexual transmission between male and female, or female to male is the common method of transmission. Male to male sexual contact is documented in 50 percent of cases. Syphilis is a very common disease transmitted among sexually active adolescents. Indigent women who do not seek prenatal care have a high incidence of congenital syphilis.

Infective ulcerative lesions have been known to appear as late as 1 year after exposure. If people do not receive treatment for syphilis, recurrent lesions have been known to appear on and off for up to 4 years.

The evidence of acquired syphilis is currently estimated to be approximately 50 million people worldwide, with the CDC estimating the U.S. population at 400,000.

Maternal Issues

Transplacental transmission of *Treponema pallidum* from mother to fetus was first described in the early 1600s. Transmission of congenital syphilis results in death in 40 percent of cases. Often the mother is without any symptoms, yet infected. Penicillin as a treatment for primary and secondary syphilis was hoped to alleviate congenital syphilis. In 1986, 365 cases of congenital syphilis were reported to the Center for Disease Control, the largest increase in 15 years (Center for Disease

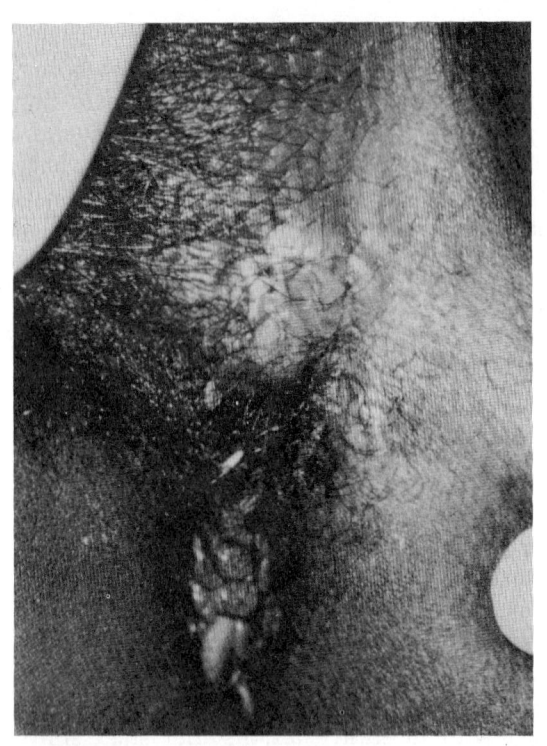

FIGURE 41–1. Primary chancre of syphilis. Note that ulcers appear clean with erythematous base.

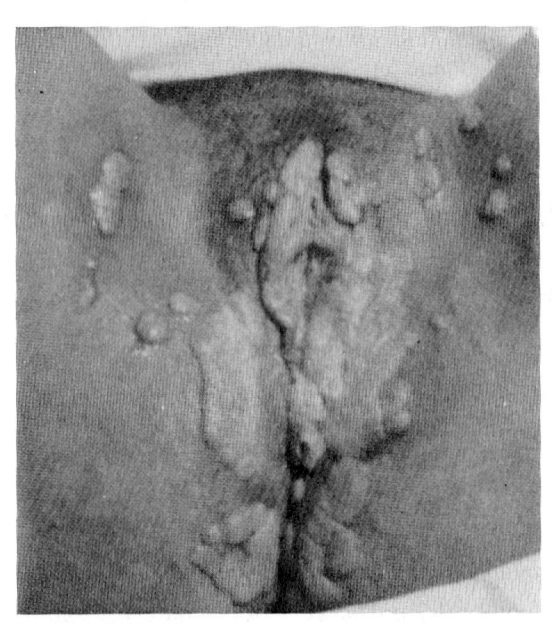

FIGURE 41–2. Secondary syphilis: anogenital condylomata.

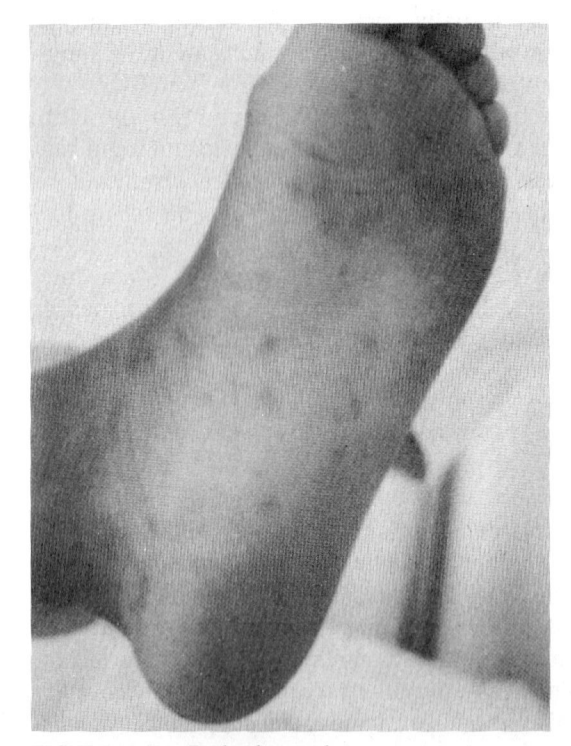

FIGURE 41–3. Rash of secondary syphilis: papular rash on sole of foot.

Control, 1987). Thus, approximately 1 in 10,000 live-born infants had congenital syphilis in the United States. Undoubtedly, this organism is responsible for many stillbirths and spontaneous abortions.

Syphilis has been described in three stages: primary, secondary, and tertiary. Early primary acquired syphilis demonstrates itself as ulcerative lesions of the skin and mucous membranes, usually in the genitalia (see Fig. 41–1). Intimate contact with these lesions will spread the disease. Secondary syphilis, which might evolve 6 weeks later, includes generalized malaise, aching, lymph node enlargement, enlarged spleen, and fever (see Figs. 41–2 and 41–3). Tertiary syphilis would include late onset of systemic exacerbations, including neurologic, cardiac, and other organs. Transmission to the fetus is of grave concern in untreated women, and though it may be transmitted at any time, it usually occurs during the first year after exposure. Bacterial shedding is stopped after 24 hours if appropriate treatment and intervention have begun. Unfortunately, the period between exposure and onset of disease symptoms for primary syphilis can be anywhere from 10 to 90 days.

Syphilis can be identified by dark-field examination of a direct smear of a moist lesion, placenta, or umbilical cord, or aspiration of a lymph node. Screening mechanisms include serological tests for nontreponemal reagin antibody, the Veneral Disease Research Laboratory (VDRL) test, and the rapid plasma reagin (RPR) test. In pregnancy, non-treponemal antibody tests may not respond appropriately and, therefore, antibody titers need to be evaluated. A four-fold decrease in titer ratios demonstrates adequate treatment, whereas a four-fold increase indicates reinfection or relapse. Any positive nontreponemal test should be confirmed by one of the treponemal tests.

The fluorescent treponemal antibody absorbtion (FTA-ABS) test is an excellent confirmatory test. It remains positive for life despite treatment. False positives are possible with both (nontreponemal and confirmatory) tests. Yet the probability of syphilis remains high in a patient whose screen is reactive to both types of diagnostic test.

All pregnant women should be tested early in pregnancy for syphilis. With high-risk categories of women, e.g. adolescents in urban areas with previous sexually transmitted diseases, should be tested again with a VDRL or RPR in the third (28 weeks) trimester. Patients with reactive RPRs should make immediate plans to initiate treatment, for their sexual partner to be referred, and for adequate prenatal care. Serologic nontreponemal tests should be provided for the remainder of the pregnancy if the woman is treated early. If a pregnant woman shows a four-fold increase in titer, or does not show a four-fold decrease within 3 months, she should be retreated. Testing should be repeated with VDRL or RPR 1 month after treatment for STD during pregnancy.

Treatment

According to the Center for Disease Control, the effectiveness of any treatment is variable depending on the stage of maternal infection and the stage of pregnancy. Treatment is considered to fail if congenital syphilis occurs in an infant whose mother was treated. Penicillin is the treatment of choice for syphilis during pregnancy. If pregnant women are allergic to penicillin they should be tested via skin tests and, if positive, the patient should be desensitized and then given standard dosages of the antibiotic. Desensitization is a process by which a patient is given increasing oral or IV doses of penicillin over a 3–4 hour period with careful observation for reactions. This process is accomplished more efficiently in a hospital environment with easy access to an expert consultant and emergency equipment. Tetracycline is known to cause damage to fetal dental development and thus is not recommended during pregnancy for treatment of syphilis. Erythromycin treatment is now generally discouraged due to inacceptable high failure rates (Center for Disease Control, 1987).

Newborn Issues

Newborns should be screened with both nontreponemal and confirmatory tests. Umbilical cord blood may produce false positive results. Serial evaluations are important to compare newborn titers after delivery. The placenta or umbilical cord may be useful culture or smear sites for dark-field microscopy.

All infants delivered to women with a reactive syphilis screening test who were not treated prior to 20 weeks need to be evaluated. This would include an examination for any lesions and an x-ray of the long bones for boney matrix changes (see Fig. 41–4).

Newborn cerebrospinal fluid (CSF) should be evaluated if the infant shows any signs of congenital syphilis, including multisystem failure, liver damage, pneumonitis, and hemorrhage. Late syphilis includes problems with CNS, bone, teeth, skin, and other connective tissues.

Therapy for newborns infected with congenital syphilis includes 10 days of either crystalline or procaine penicillin, 100,000 units/kg IM or IV, if the CSF is infected. Otherwise, a single dose of 50,000 units/kg IM or IV is sufficient.

Nursing Issues

Providing preventive education and resources related to sexual disease identification, clinical treatment, and follow-up are important nursing rules. Families need to be educated about the implications of transmissibility of infections from mother to fetus and the serious ramifications. The nurse is in an important position to attempt to educate and influence patient behaviors and choices related to sexual activities. Patients need to be educated about the early signs of syphilis lesion infections, and appropriate interventions. Women in particular need to be advised of the possibilities of

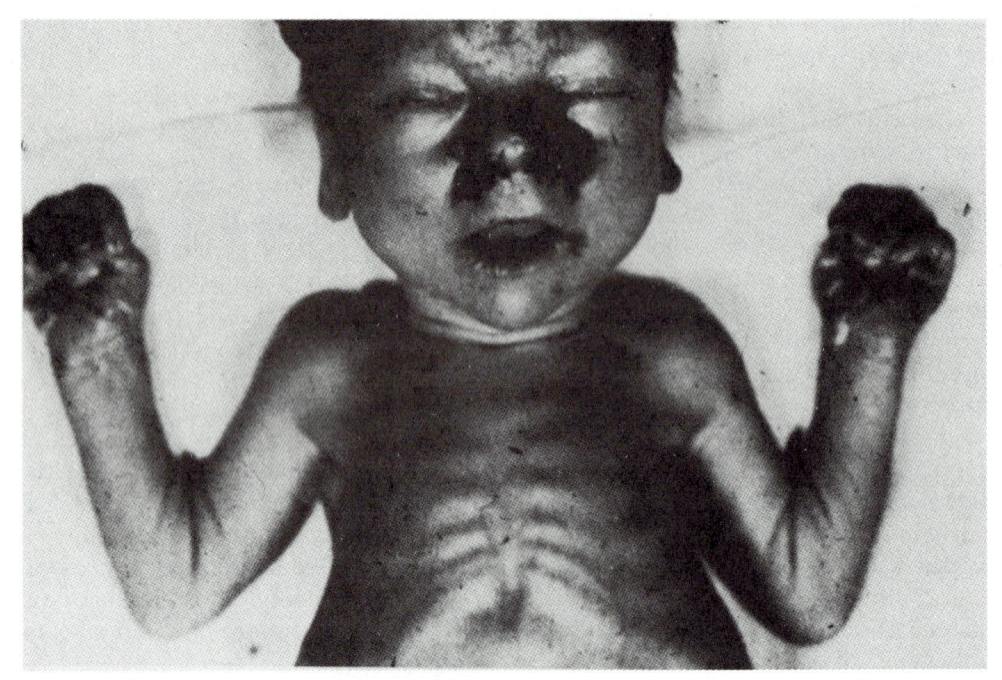

FIGURE 41–4. This infant with congenital syphilis demonstrates hepatosplenomegaly, rhinitis, or "snuffles," and pemphigus syphiliticus, a disseminated vesicular bullous eruption of the palms.

asymptomatic infection, of considering one sexual partner, and of considering testing prior to pregnancy. This is a serious congenital disease, and its resurgence in recent years is confusing given the accessible treatment now available nationwide in STD clinics and Planned Parenthood clinics. Treatment and follow-up screening must be encouraged.

CHLAMYDIA

Organism: Chlamydia is an intracellular bacteria that functions between cells. Thus, it is relatively antibiotic-resistant. Its growth cycle differentiates it from other microbes. There are 15 serotypes, including the ocular organism causing trachoma, frequently found in Africa, and *C. psittaci* causing psittocosis in birds. The serotypes that are most commonly sexually transmitted are *C. trachomatis* D–K.

Epidemiology and Transmission

Chlamydia trachomatis is a very common pathogen that is transmitted sexually. Current estimates are that there are about 2 million cases of *Chlamydia* a year, of which 50 percent are probably women in their productive childbearing years, i.e. between the ages of 14 and 45. A more specific, high-risk group is adolescent, single mothers, who have been identified as having a 20–38 percent incidence of *Chlamydia* in prospective screening studies (Eschenbach, 1987). The infection is often asymptomatic, not clinically apparent, often presenting as cervicitis, salpingitis, urethritis, and pelvic inflammatory diseases. Pelvic inflammatory disease is becoming increasingly worrisome, for it has been associated with increased numbers of ectopic pregnancies, primary tubal infertility, and chronic pain in women. The infection can remain in the genital tract from months to years (Bourcier and Seidler, 1987).

Maternal Issues

A pregnant women infected with a chlamydial infection of the cervix has a 60–70 percent risk of infecting her newborn during the passage through the birth canal. There is a 20–50 percent chance of conjunctivitis and a 20 percent chance of pneumonia (Martin et al., 1982). If the membranes have ruptured prematurely or internal fetal scalp monitoring is used, then the risk of migratory infection from the birth canal is significantly increased. Colonization with *Chlamydia* can easily lead to pelvic infection after an abortion, wound infection after cesarean section, and a late 4–6 week syndrome of endometritis after delivery (Osborne, Ng, and Pratson, 1984).

Symptoms of *Chlamydia* infection can include vaginal discharges, painful urination, and frequency. "Honeymoon cystitis" has often been associated with *Chlamydia* infections. Treatment of sexual partners is extremely important, because estimates of partners of women with nongonococcal urethritis range from 50 to 60 percent (Reem, 1987). Chronic endometritis has also been related to *Chlamydia* infection, demonstrated by abdominal bleeding and uterine tenderness (Eshenbach, 1987).

Newborn Issues

Chlamydia conjunctivitis is identified by a watery discharge from the eyes which progresses to thick and purulent exudate with swollen eyelids. It is most common in the first month of life. This can be eliminated by switching from routine use of silver nitrate drops to erythromycin ointment for ocular prophylaxis against gonococcal opthalmia neonatorium. Erythromycin is effective against gonococcus infection as well as *Chlamydia* and is less irritating to the eye than silver nitrate drops.

Pneumonia can occur in newborns with or without conjunctivitis and subsequent treatment. The incubation period is anywhere from 5 days to 3–4 months. This type of respiratory problem usually occurs later in the newborn period. The newborn typically has a rapid respiratory rate, barreled chest, and increased oxygen requirements. The child may have interstitial infiltrates, palpable liver and spleen, and increased numbers of eosinophils. Typically, titers of IgM and IgG are elevated. Appropriate treatment of this problem will include erythromycin 40 mg/kg per day in divided doses for 3 weeks, possibly including an aminoglycoside.

Screening

Confirmation of maternal *Chlamydia* in the genital tract dictates that she and her partner be treated. If pregnant, erythromycin is the drug of choice, otherwise tetracycline 500 mg orally four times a day for 7 days is preferred. These infections can persist for years, and repeated perinatal transmission has been known to occur if mother or partner are left untreated.

Schachter et al. (1979) have looked at the cost-effectiveness of screening pregnant women prenatally to prevent disease in their offspring. The cost of *Chlamydia* cultures are expensive, approximately $35–45, but compared to the costs of treating newborn cases of conjunctivitis and pneumonia, it becomes extremely cost-effective when, in certain populations, rates of infection are over 6 percent. Additionally, decreasing the cost of postpartum PID, endometritis and other complications will contribute to cost-effectiveness. Thus, in certain high-risk populations, particularly sexually active teenagers, it is extremely cost-effective to implement a screening program.

Rapid diagnosis and screening is now available with the use of monoclonal antibodies. Some states are currently offering *Chlamydia* tests, called Chlamydiazyme. Positive tests indicate need for treatment, although negative tests may need re-screening.

Nursing Issues

Education and counseling are extremely important roles of the nurse. Initial discussions regarding transmission and the ubiquitous nature of the disease should occur. A description of the elusive slow growth pattern between host cells should be given to ensure that clients complete the entire recommended regime of antibiotics. The organism is not deterred with partial treatment. In order to prevent the transmission of the organism sexually, condoms must be used for insertive intercourse. Encourage treatment of all sexual contacts. A discussion of all the possible complications due to the organism, including pelvic inflammatory disease, future ectopic pregnancies, and endometritis, is important. Screening and prevention of newborn sequelae is important.

CYTOMEGALOVIRUS

Organism: Cytomegalovirus (CMV) is one of the most common perinatal infections in humans. It is a member of the Herpes family. It is an enveloped DNA virus that grows very slowly in tissue culture.

Epidemiology and Transmission

Most people in the United States have been infected with this virus, and thus already have antibodies against it. Infected secretions, including breast milk, cervical mucus, semen, saliva, or urine are the reservoirs of this disease. It is easily contracted with intimate contact after organ transplant or blood transfusions.

Certain populations have a higher incidence of CMV infection – e.g. poor black children, of whom 40–60 percent are antibody positive. By the age of 25, 100 percent are positive. Thirty percent of females in middle-class, white populations are positive by age 20 and 60 percent by age 40. In general, men are at less risk. This is probably because women are more likely to handle infants and toddlers who shed the virus in their urine. Interestingly enough, male homosexuals have been found to be CMV positive by age 20 (Knox, 1983). Differences in social status, crowding, and hygiene probably account for the differences between black and white populations.

CMV is defined as a sexually transmitted disease, because viral shedding is only observed in 5 percent of young women with stable relationships, but in 25 percent who have multiple partners (Nelson and Grossman, 1986). The presence of the virus in semen has also been noted. CMV persists as a latent infection and can easily reoccur with immunosuppression, such as that caused by HIV virus in AIDS patients.

Maternal Issues

CMV can present with an infectious mononucleosis-like syndrome with general malaise, liver involvement, extended fever, and fatigue, Transmission to the fetus can occur within 3 days, by transplacental infection of the maternal blood. Contact between the fetus and the virus via the maternal birth canal can cause infection. CMV-infected breast milk can also transmit the virus to the newborn. Studies demonstrate a 60 percent transmission rate from mother to baby with breastfeeding (Nelson and Grossman, 1986).

Maternal cervical infection is very common, and thus many newborns acquire the CMV virus perinatally. Yet those infants that acquire the infection during a primary infection as opposed to a recurrent lesion, seem to have a higher incidence of mental retardation and/or sensory deafness. Severe complications at birth is seen in 5 percent of congenital infections.

Good personal hygiene is important during pregnancy, including frequent handwashing, particularly in any situation when repeated close contacts with toddlers and infants occur.

Newborn Issues

Infants born after recurrent maternal infection seem to have partial antibody protection. In one study (American Academy of Pediatrics, 1986), approximately 5–10 percent had hearing loss, 2 percent had choreoretinitis, and less than 1 percent were mentally retarded. On the other hand, 10–15 percent of infants who were born during a primary infection had intrauterine growth retardation (IUGR), microcephaly, periventricular calcifications, sensorineural deafness, blindness with choreoretinitis, profound mental retardation, hepatosplenomegaly, and jaundice. Of these, 26 percent will die.

Treatment methods are not very clear for this disease. A recently developed investigational drug (DHPG or BW759U) appears beneficial in the treatment of acquired CMV. Good handwashing and appropriate barrier methods of infection control are important for protection from body fluids. Pregnant personnel who may be in contact with CMV-infected patients may need more support and encouragement regarding appropriate barrier protection and handwashing.

Approximately 3 percent of infants in newborn nurseries may be excreting CMV virus (American Academy of Pediatrics, 1986). It is important that these infants are not exposed to severely immunocompromised patients. Transmission of CMV by blood transfusion to premature infants or others is virtually eliminated by the use of CMV-negative donors. CMV hyperimmune globulin has been developed for prophylaxis of the disease in bone marrow transplant patients, and is being considered for newborn infants.

HUMAN PAPILLOMA VIRUS

Organism: Human papilloma virus (HPV) causes genital warts. HPVs are members of the Papovaviridae family. HPV is a double-strand DNA virus. The virus thrives in moist tissues, like the tongue, penis, urethra, perianal skin, cervix, and vagina. *Condyloma acumata* has been identified with two strains of this virus that cause venereal warts.

Epidemiology and Transmission

Genital HPV is a sexually transmitted disease, the incidence of which has increased rapidly over the last 5 years. This rapid elevation parallels the rise in other sexually transmitted diseases. Time from exposure to infection can be anywhere from 1 to 6 months (Bennett, 1987).

Maternal Issues

The presence of warty growths on the vagina, cervix, vulva, perineum, buttocks, or inner thigh are symptoms of HPV. No culture technique is currently available to confirm the virus, only clinical assessment. The presence of these warts during pregnancy is extremely uncomfortable and they can easily obstruct vaginal delivery. Treatment involves different types of electrocautery, cryocautery, or surgical removal. Laser treatment is currently being investigated. Various chemicals and cytotoxic solutions are not appropriate treatment during pregnancy. Careful application of Podophyllin (a cytotoxic chemical preparation) to small lesions is appropriate, but not in large amounts because this chemical is associated with increased fetal disease and preterm labor (Bourcier and Seidler, 1987). Continued application has resulted in maternal neuropathy, seizures, hypotension, and bradycardia. These lesions are very vascular, especially in pregnancy, thus close observation for bleeding is important. Examination and treatment of sexual partners is an important part of the treatment, because 50 percent are infected (Bourcier and Seidler, 1987). Large cauliflower lesions that blossom in the vulva, labia, or vagina often require a cesearian section (see Fig. 41–5).

Newborn Issues

There is significant concern that transmission of HPV to the newborn will result in laryngeal papillomatosis. This causes newborns to have a "weak cry" or hoarseness. Recent estimates suggest that 1.5 percent of women have HPV, thus exposing approximately 45,000 infants per year. There were approximately 3000 cases of confirmed laryngeal papillomatosis in 1987. Thus, many investigators are suggesting that cesarean sections will prevent the transmission of the virus to the newborn (American Academy of Pediatrics, 1986).

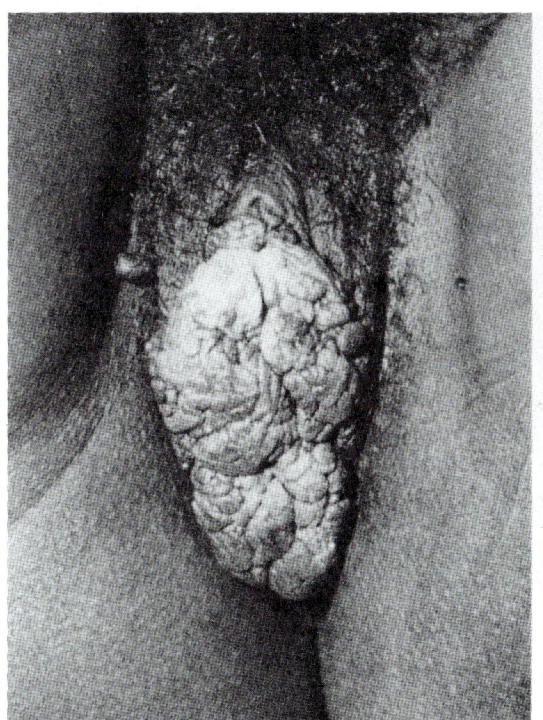

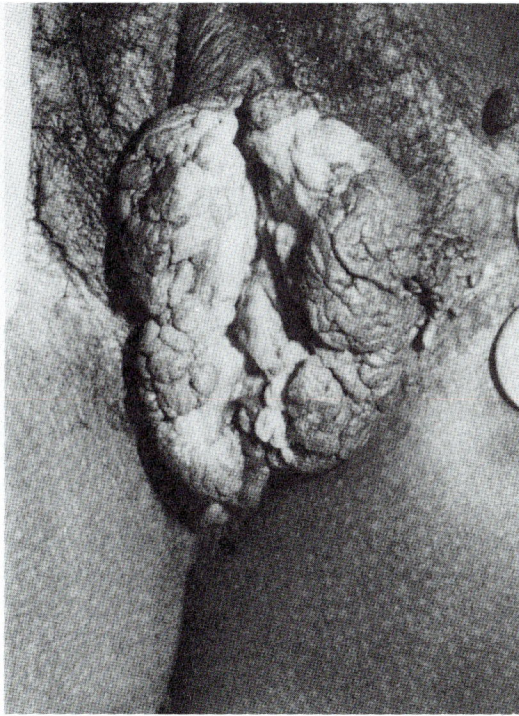

FIGURE 41–5. Condyloma acuminatum lesions have replaced the labia. This patient was delivered by cesarean section.

Nursing Issues

Nursing concerns for this disease focus on the need for education and counseling. Women need to be instructed that human papilloma virus is sexually transmitted and that condoms need to be worn until all lesions are resolved. Instruction should be given regarding good hygienic practices, i.e. washing the genital area and keeping it as dry as possible. All sexual contacts should be encouraged to seek evaluation and treatment if necessary. If the woman has other vaginal infections, treatment should be obtained as concomitant infections can exacerbate the size of genital warts. Emotional support is crucial because it can be very painful and demoralizing to have a venereal disease. Unfortunately these lesions are chronic and have a recurrence rate of 70 percent. Inquiring investigators are predicting a relationship between HPV and cancer of the cervix and vulva (Bennett, 1987).

HERPES SIMPLEX VIRUS

Organism: Herpes simplex virus (HSV) is a large DNA-containing organism. The Herpes family contains CMV (cytomegalovirus), Epstein Barr virus, and Varicilla-Zoster virus which causes chicken pox and shingles. There are two types, HSV-1, which is usually found on the face and skin above the waist, and HSV-2, involving the genitals and skin below the waist. Location has not proven to be an effective way of differentiating the types as there is much cross-contact between oral and genital secretions. Maternal transmission rates are 75 percent to newborns who are HSV-2 and 25 percent who are HSV-1 (American Academy of Pediatrics, 1980).

Epidemiology and Transmission

HSV is a sexually transmitted disease passed on by secretions and/or skin to skin contact during sexual activity. There has been a significant increase in the numbers of cases per year, estimated by the Center for Disease Control to be 300,000–500,000. Because of the recurrent nature of the virus, it is estimated that anywhere from 5 to 25 million Americans may harbor the virus.

A primary infection with HSV has been identified to cause the highest risk to the newborn. The clinical signs would include burning, itching, or tingling at the site of a potential lesion. Within 1–2 days, a fluid-filled blister will appear at the site. Over the next 2 weeks the blister will break and a scab will form, i.e. the lesion will "crust over". These lesions (HSV-1) commonly occur on the eyes, mouth, or other parts of the face. HSV-2 or genital lesions can occur on the penis, vagina, vulva, or cervix (see Fig. 41–6). The majority of genital infections on the cervix or vaginal vault are asymptomatic and difficult to recognize. Thus, a pregnant woman may not know that her infant is in jeopardy.

Recurrent infections are generally less severe and less painful than primary ones. The latent virus uses the sensory nerves to travel back and forth to outbreak sites. Exacerbation of herpes outbreaks are thought to be related to heat, cold, stress, and sunshine.

Maternal Issues

Infection with HSV during pregnancy may be associated with spontaneous abortion, prematurity or, perhaps, congenital anomalies. Viral shedding from a primary or recurrent lesion at the cervix or birth canal may provide easy access for transmission via any open break in the skin, eyes, ears, or mouth. Women with recurrent infections or primary infections during pregnancy, or whose partners have active lesions, should be monitored during pregnancy. Sexual contact should be discouraged during the last several months of pregnancy.

Maternal infection with HSV has serious implications for the newborn. If transmission occurs, neonatal mortality is approximately 60 percent, with significant morbidity including seizures, blindness, and mental retardation if the child lives.

PAP smears are able to screen approximately 75 percent of virus-positive women, but viral cultures are more accurate. Delivery can occur vaginally if the woman has been virus-free for two examinations, one at least 1 week prior to delivery. Otherwise, a cesarian section is recommended in order to prevent infection of the newborn when traveling through the maternal birth canal.

The status of fetal membranes at delivery is an important issue. Internal fetal monitoring is discouraged as it provides access for the virus via an open scalp lesion. If the membranes are intact and the woman has a positive virus culture, or if rupture has been less than 4–6 hours, then cesarean section is recommended. Cesarean-section is not recommended if the membranes have been ruptured 12 hours or more.

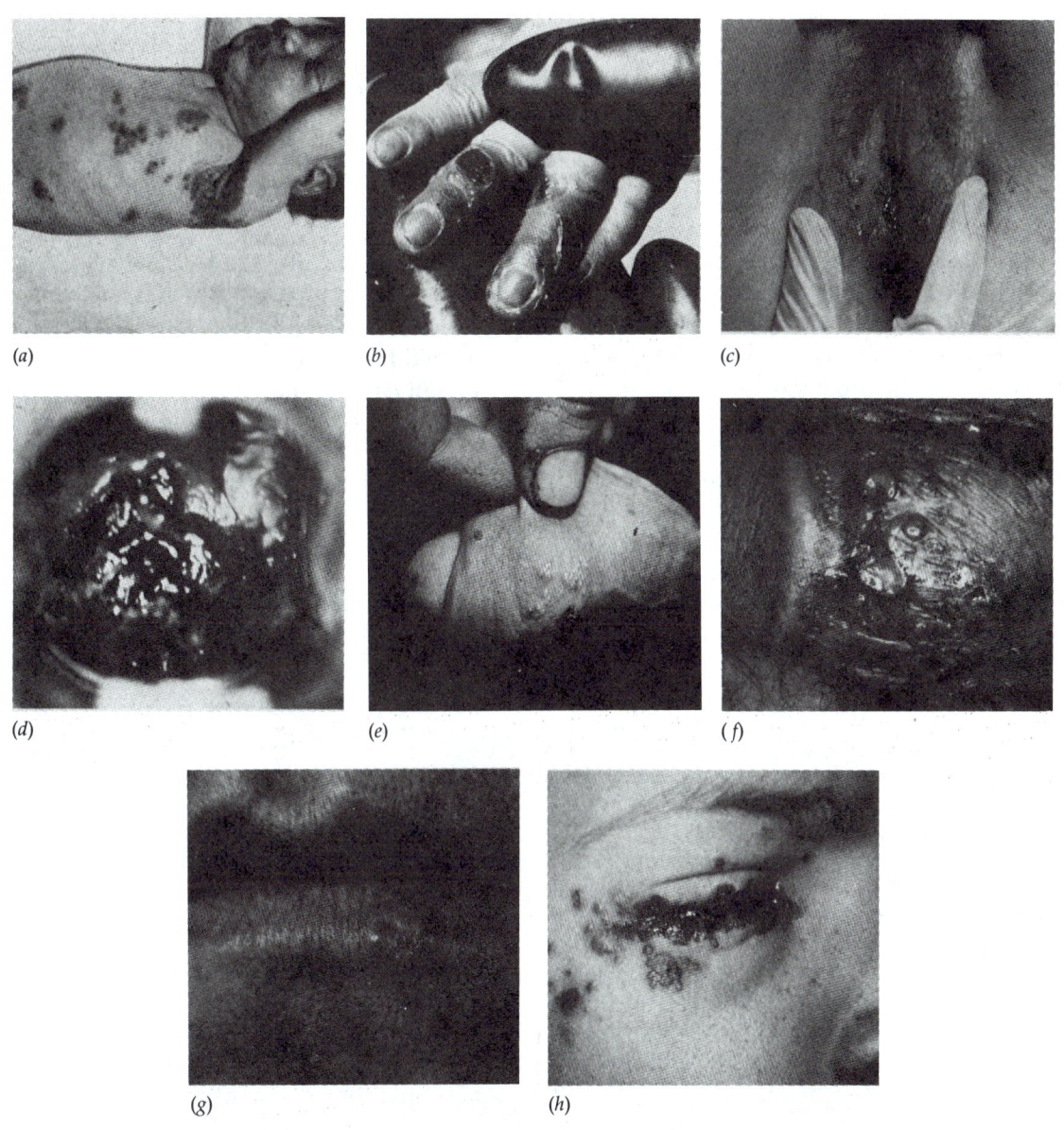

FIGURE 41–6. (a, b) Infections of the labia and cervix. If an outbreak occurs in a pregnant woman at term, a cesarean section may be indicated to protect the infant. (c, d) Papules can appear on the penis or foreskin, but most lesions under the foreskin generally take longer to heal. (e, f) The danger of autoinoculation of such sites as eyes and lips can be minimized by using appropriate barriers and careful personal hygiene. (g, h) The neonate can begin to exhibit HSV disease at any time during the first month; average onset is within 10–16 days of delivery.

Newborn Issues

HSV infections will cause generalized systemic infections in newborns, involving the liver, central nervous system, and other organisms. Local infection may involve the skin, eyes, and mouth (see Fig. 41–6). Eye infections can include conjunctivitis, choreoretinitis, and cataracts. Infants may have significant respiratory distress, sepsis, and convulsions. This disseminated disease may occur at any time from birth to 1 month of age. Increased risks of prematurity and low birth weight accompany infants infected with HSV.

Infants should be followed closely for lesions after a vaginal delivery if the woman has an active lesion. Serial viral cultures and close nursing scrutiny for lesions is important. Circumcisions are discouraged or delayed to lower the risk of viral transmission via a surgical wound (American Academy of Pediatrics, 1980).

Treatment and Prevention

Current treatment recommendations for nonpregnant women suffering from genital herpes includes the drug Acyclovir. It decreases both the painful symptoms and viral shedding. Oral Acyclovir started within 6 days of the onset of the disease will shorten the duration of the exacerbation. Intravenous Acyclovir is used for primary lesions which are severe and require hospitalization. Topical Acyclovir is thought to decrease symptoms and is palatable in nature. Oral Acyclovir given to women who suffer chronic recurrent infections has been shown to decrease the number of outbreaks and shorten the periods of time when there is active viral shedding (Davis, 1987).

Maternal Issues

Mother–infant rooming-in would be highly recommended for the care of an infected perinatal couple. The mother should be instructed in good hygiene procedures, including good handwashing techniques (see Table 41–1). Breastfeeding is acceptable if there are no lesions in the area and active lesions are covered. Until all lesions are crusted and dried, all family members should be instructed in good hygiene techniques and discouraged from contact with lesions.

Recent studies have shown that a woman's history is not necessarily helpful as to whether they are active shedders of the virus. Shedding of the herpes virus is common during pregnancy and all antibody-positive women are at high risk during pregnancy. Apparently, asymptomatic viral shedders, are at highest risk for transmission to the newborn (Thompson, 1987).

Other studies indicate that viral shedding is frequent in about 47 percent of women that attend

---

TABLE 41–1. *Parent Information: Herpes Simplex*

Background Information

Herpes simplex is a virus which can cause sores around the mouth (cold sores, fever blisters) or sores in the genital area. Once a person has had the sores they are likely to get the sores repeatedly. Whenever the sores break out, there is a possibility that the virus may be transferred to others in close personal contact (by kissing, having sex, etc.). Certain precautions should be taken when handling newborn babies if a parent or friend has herpes sores.

Precautions when Sores are Present on Face or Mouth
1. Wash hands with soap for 30 sec before touching or holding baby.
2. Cover sore if possible with bandaid or gauze dressing.
3. Do not kiss or nuzzle baby close to face.
4. Do not touch face while holding baby.
5. Mother can breastfeed baby using these precautions.

Precautions when Genital Lesions Present
1. Wash hands with soap for 30 sec.
2. Do not touch genital area while holding infant.
3. Wash hands after each contact with genital area.
4. Do not bathe in same tub with infant.

Some people who have repeated outbreaks of herpes sores may shed the virus when there are no obvious sores. However, the greatest risk for transmission occurs when lesions are just developing and in the blister stage. When the sore is dry, crusted and healed over, there is very little risk for transmission. Those women who have repeated genital sores should always wash their hands carefully after touching the genital area *and* before handling newborn infants.

SOURCE: Barrett, Trish. Alta Bates Hospital 1988.

sexually transmitted disease clinics (Kotsky, 1987). A careful clinical examination is necessary along with routine PAP smears in order to detect cases of HSV.

Herpes has been identified as an organism that may break down skin barriers and provide access for the transmission of another serious sexually transmitted virus, HIV Human Immunodeficiency Virus (HIV). Thus, condoms are recommended for protection during sexual activity. If either partner has open or shedding lesions, sexual activity should be discouraged (Holmberg, 1987).

Newborn Issues

All newborns born from mothers with active lesions regardless of route of delivery should be observed carefully at 7–10 days postdelivery for signs of active lesions. Treatment of a symptomatic newborn includes the use of the antivirals Vicarabine or Acyclovir. Recent data suggest that adenine arabinoside (Vicarabine) improves the grave outcome of CNS HSV infections in newborns. Tertiary care centers can usually care for the complex needs of these critically ill newborns more adequately.

Nursing Issues

Nursing care is generally supportive for pregnant women with HSV. Keeping lesions clean and dry to prevent secondary bacterial infections is important. The pain, particularly with primary infections, may be alleviated with systemic analgesia or local anesthetics. Cool sitz baths three to four times a day may be helpful and comforting. Urinary retention and dysuria are commonly reported in women suffering with HSV lesions.

Primary nursing responsibilities include HSV education and counseling support. HSV education should include information about the direct mode of transmission, i.e. skin to skin contact with an infected lesion. Clearing up misinformation and myths about disease transmission is important, as is emotional support during repeated exacerbations of a painful genital sore. Reassurance and emotional support are imperative when a mother faces the dilemma of HSV transmission to her newborn infant.

Many women who are infected with HSV are significantly preoccupied with the disease. It is only treatable and not curable. The psychological impact on women who had had more than 13 outbreaks in a year was found to be extremely debilitating. With a long-term chronic disease women become emotionally depressed, even though their physical pain may decrease with recurrent infections (Mertz, 1987).

The implementation of universal precautions (Captain, 1988) as a method of hospital-based infection control methods makes protection for HSV simple. Thus barrier methods of protection – grown, gloves, and masks – if necessary, will minimize transmission by direct contact with viral lesions or secretions.

The American Academy of Pediatrics recommends that nursery and other perinatal personnel who have active HSV infections such as cold sores should have limited patient contact. Proper instruction of barrier methods of infection control are important. Gloves should be worn with hand infections such as herpetic whitlows (see Fig. 41–7). Personnel should not be allowed in the nursery or to have other infant contact until exposed lesions are dry and crusted over.

HEPATITIS B

Organism: Hepatitis B virus (HBV) is a DNA-containing double-strand virus. It is fairly large, approximately 42 mm in diameter.

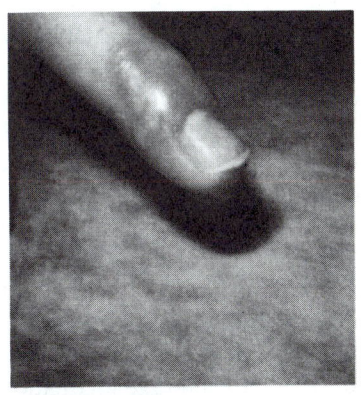

FIGURE 41–7. Herapetic whitlow, an HSV infection of the fingers, is a recognized hazard among ICU nurses, surgeons, anesthesiologists, and dentists.

Epidemiology and Transmission

Contact with infected blood or body secretions, the percutaneous introduction of blood, or the administration of certain blood products are the major ways in which this virus is transmitted. Contamination of mucous membranes during the birth process or during sexual intercourse is another method of transmission. The contamination of wounds or contact with wound serous drainage can transmit infection. The virus is large and strong enough to live on inanimate objects, although exact rates of transmission are unknown.

This virus produces systemic illness, with general overall malaise, jaundice, anorexia, and nausea. Early stages of the disease may present with a rash and sore joints. A chronic carrier state of HBV will precipitate severe chronic liver disease. In Africa, southeastern Asia, and the Pacific Rim, carrier rates are estimated at 35 percent. Perinatal transmission has been identified as the cause of 40 percent of all chronic HBV carriers (Gabbe, Niebyl, and Simpson, 1986).

TABLE 41–2. Women for Whom Prenatal HBsAg Screening is Recommended

1. Women of Asian, Pacific island, or Alaskan Eskimo descent, whether born in the United States or immigrants
2. Women born in Haiti or sub-Saharan Africa

Women with histories of:

3. Acute or chronic liver disease
4. Work or treatment in a hemodialysis unit
5. Work or residence in an institution for the mentally retarded
6. Rejection as a blood donor
7. Blood transfusion on repeated occasions
8. Frequent occupational exposure to blood in medical-dental settings
9. Household contact with an HBV carrier or hemodialysis patient
10. Multiple episodes of venereal disease
11. Percutaneous use of illicit drugs

Maternal Issues

Perinatal transmission is of significant concern in pregnant women who are hepatitis B surface antigen positive (HBsAg), especially if they are also hepatitis B antigen positive (HBeAg). Those women most at risk of transmitting hepatitis B to their offspring have been identified as women of Asian, Pacific island, or Alaskan Eskimo descent, whether born in the United States or not, and women born in Haiti or sub-Saharan Africa (see Table 41–2).

Young women often develop subclinical infections and can easily develop a chronic carrier state. They may be asymptomatic or have overt liver disease. Consequently, they have a significant risk of developing hepatocellular carcinoma in later life. For the duration of their carrier state they are considered infectious. The sharing of bodily secretions during sexual intercourse can easily result in disease transmission. Hepatitis B has a long incubation period, from 50 days to a possible 190 days after exposure with possible onset of symptoms such as jaundice. The average incubation period is 90 days. Serologic testing for HBsAg and antibody to the surface antigen (anti-HBs) is useful. The best indicator of infectiousness is the presence of HBeAg in the blood.

Thus, it is recommended that pregnant women in high-risk categories or engaging in sexual contact with persons suffering from acute hepatitis B be screened so that appropriate follow-up can be provided. Screening also provides additional information about HBsAg status and it is essential for the protection of those who are exposed to antigen-positive blood.

Current hospital infection control policies include a universal precautions approach (see Table 41–3), whereby health workers should assume that all blood and other body fluids – urine, saliva, feces, and wound drainage – are potentially infectious and therefore, barrier protection is required. The treatment for exposures is listed in Table 41–4.

Vaccination is recommended after pregnancy for individuals who are most at risk for exposure to HBV. Intravenous drug users, people with large numbers of heterosexual partners, health care workers, and those in contact with carriers should receive 0.06 ml/kg of the Hepatitis B Immune Globulin (HBIG) vaccine as soon as possible after exposure. HBV vaccine should be offered as well. A 20 ml/kg dose of HBsAg protein is administered to the deltoid muscle immediately, and again at 1 and 6 months.

TABLE 41-3. DO's and DON'Ts Based on CDC Guidelines

1. Do use appropriate barrier precautions routinely to prevent skin and mucous-membrane exposure when contact with blood or other body fluids of any patient is anticipated.
2. Do wear gloves for touching blood and body fluids, mucous membranes, or non-intact skin of all patients, for handling items of surfaces soiled with blood or body fluids, and for performing venipuncture and other vascular access procedures. Gloves should be changed after contact with each patient.
3. Do wear masks and protective eyewear during procedures which are likely to generate droplets of blood or other body fluids to prevent exposure of mucous membranes of the mouth, nose, and eyes. Gowns should be worn during procedures that are likely to generate splashes of blood or other body fluids.
4. Do wash hands and other skin surfaces immediately and thoroughly if contaminated with blood or other body fluids. Hands should be washed immediately after gloves are removed.
5. Do take precautions to prevent injuries caused by needles, scalpels, and other sharp instruments. To prevent needlestick injuries, needles should not be recapped, purposely bent or broken by hand, removed from disposable syringes, or otherwise manipulated by hand. After they are used, all sharp instruments should be placed in a puncture-resistant container for disposal, located as close as possible to the use area.
6. Although saliva has not been implicated in HIV transmission, to minimize the need for emergency mouth to mouth resuscitation, mouth pieces, resuscitation bags, or other ventilation devices should be available for use in areas where the need of resuscitation is predictable.
7. Although pregnant nurses are not known to be at greater risk of contracting HIV infection during pregnancy, the infant is at risk of infection resulting from perinatal transmission. Because of this risk, pregnant nurses should be especially familiar with and adhere strictly to precautions to minimize risks.
8. Do check your hands for any cuts, abrasions, or breaks in the skin and cover with water-proof dressing. Health-care workers who have exudative lesions or weeping dermatitis should refrain from all direct patient care and from handling patient care equipment until the condition resolves.

Newborn Issues

Infants born to mothers who are HBsAg positive should receive HBIG within 48 hours after birth. The proper identification of HBsAg positive women in the perinatal period is very important for adequate follow-up of the newborn. HBV vaccine is given to infants at birth, followed by further doses at 1 and 6 months. Newborns are given half the adult dose or 10 µg (0.5 cc). It is possible to delay administration of the vaccine for up to 3 months if another dose of HBIG is given, but HBIG should be given immediately at birth. Table 41-4 describes details on HBV vaccine administration. All infants should have pediatric follow-up including repeat screening for HBsAg to determine chronic carriers. Much debate worldwide has surrounded the issue of breastfeeding by HBsAg positive mothers, but the current approach of the American Academy of Pediatrics is that the studies in Taiwan and England are not conclusive about breast milk transmission. Thus, breastfeeding is allowed.

Newborns should be handled expectantly using universal infection control precautions, including the wearing of gloves while handling the infant prior to the first bath. Bathing can occur as soon as the newborn temperature is stable. Isolation is not necessary, but again, as with other patients, appropriate barrier methods must be used to prevent exposure to infected blood and body fluids.

Prevention

Proper cleaning and sterilization of instruments contaminated with blood is an important factor in decreasing the amount of HBV transmission. The use of disposable equipment whenever possible is highly recommended.

Currently, all blood products are screened for HBsAg, yet there remains a slight risk of transmission. Thus, the clinical necessity of transfusions and alternative products, e.g. synthetic serum albumin administration for volume expansion, should be considered when trying to prevent the transmission of the hepatitis B and HIV viruses.

Accidental needlesticks present as a significant risk for the transmission of the hepatitis B virus. Approximately 10–20 percent of people who accidentally stick themselves become HBsAg positive. Exposures should be treated with 0.06 ml/kg HBIG as soon as possible, with hepatitis B vaccine

TABLE 41-4. Hepatitis B Virus Postexposure Recommendations[a]

Exposure	HBIG Dose	HBIG Recommended timing	Vaccine Dose	Vaccine Recommended timing
Perinatal	0.5 ml, IM	As soon as possible after birth (within 12 hours of birth)	0.5 ml (10 μg), IM	Within 7 days;[b] repeat at 1 and 6 months
Percutaneous	0.06 ml/kg (maximum, 5 ml), IM	Single dose within 24 hours	1.0 ml (20 μg), IM[c]	Within 7 days;[c] repeat at 1 and 6 months
		or[d]		
	0.06 ml/kg (maximum, 5 ml), IM	within 24 hours; and repeat dose 1 month later	—	—
Sexual	0.06 ml/kg (maximum, 5 ml), IM	Single dose within 14 days of sexual contact	[e]	—

[a] From postexposure prophylaxis of hepatitis B, Morb. Mort. Weekly Rep., 1984;33:285, and Recommendations for protection against viral hepatitis, Morb. Mort. Weekly Rep., 1985;34:313.
[b] The first dose can be given the same time as the HBIG dose but at a different site and with a different syringe.
[c] For patients less than 10 years old, use 0.5 ml (10μg).
[d] For those who choose not to receive HB vaccine.
[e] Vaccine is recommended for homosexually active males and for regular sexual contacts of chronic HBV carriers.

follow-up. Immune Globulin (IG) can be substituted for HBIG. Those individuals most at risk of contracting Hepatitis B, for example, people working in dialysis units or institutions for the mentally retarded or Down's Syndrome patients, those frequently exposed to blood products, people of Asian descent, IV drug users, and heterosexuals with a number of sexual contacts – should consider vaccination (see Fig. 41-8).

HUMAN IMMUNODEFICIENCY VIRUS

Organism: Human Immunodeficiency Virus (HIV) is an RNA transcriptase virus with a protein coat envelope.

Epidemiology and Transmission

AIDS is one of the greatest public health problems the world has ever faced. It has been compared to the plagues in Europe in the 1500s. As of March 1988 there were 56,000 cases reported to the Center for Disease Control. The disease is transmitted via blood, through sexual activity, and perinatally. HIV virus has been recovered from many different body fluids including blood, semen, CSF, saliva, urine, feces, amniotic fluid, breast milk, and vaginal secretions. The virus is fragile and is easily killed with heat or a 1:10 dilution of bleach and water. HIV virus attacks the immune system of a healthy person and immobilizes the helper T-cells, an important subgroup of lymphocytes.

In 1981 the first cases of AIDS were identified, though cases have now been found to have occurred in the 1970s. Those most at risk include homosexual/bisexual men, i.v. drug users, hemophiliacs, the sexual partners of members of high-risk groups, and recipients of blood transfusions or blood products from 1979 to 1985.

Thus, HIV is transmitted through blood and body secretions, most commonly through sexual contact between gay men, bisexual partners, or heterosexual partners. Intravenous drug users who share needles or syringes are likely to become

Comfort for the AIDS Victim

By Venessia R. Poe, CNA

5:10 P.M. Ten minutes late for work. I'm a C.N.A. *(Certified Nurse's Aide)*, working on a medical surgical unit. As I arrived, the place seemed as busy as usual: lights on, nurses with medical carts getting pain medication, doing all the normal things nurses do. I put my things away and went to the head nurse for assignments and reports.

What's this? Something jumped out at me, demanding my attention. According to the patients' information list, the man in Room 133 was marked for "wound and skin precaution," also as "blood and secretion precaution," but the list did not include a diagnosis.

"What is 133's diagnosis?" I inquired of the nurse in charge. She replied with one word, "AIDS." Immediately my head began to spin. I searched my mind for information. *What had I heard on TV? What had I read in the newspaper? What had I seen in pamphlets?* Then fear engulfed me. *I have to take care of this patient? What if I catch AIDS? There's no cure . . .*

Rounding the corner to Room 133, I hesitated. Gloves and gowns were on the cart outside the door. Gloves and gowns? This seemed strange to me. Even though this 64-year-old man suffered from a disease which, for the moment at least, is fatal—still, I knew he deserved as much care and compassion as other patients. Reluctantly, I donned the gloves and gowns, opened the door, and went in—still feeling unprotected.

First, I introduced myself. A man, pale in color and weighing only 115 pounds, looked at me and then turned his face toward the wall. After speaking first, I paused. There was no response. As I proceeded to take his vital signs, he just lay there motionless, with no reaction to my touch. After thanking him for his cooperation, I left the room, removing the gloves and gowns. A deep sadness came over me. For the first time since entering the nursing profession, I felt helpless and unable to perform my job.

Continuing my work during the shift, I couldn't get "Mr. Smith" in Room 133 off my mind. All I could think of was how to reach him and show him I care. Not many people came to see him. He was aware of things around him; he knew what day it was, what time it was, and where he was. But he suffered from incontinency. After reading his chart, I discovered he had acquired this disease through a blood transfusion six years earlier while having open heart surgery. Was there any wonder this man was bitter? He came to the hospital to have his life saved; instead, he acquired something during this emergency that would result in his death.

Two days later, Mr. Smith looked at me for fifteen minutes. *Uninterrupted eye contact?* Three days later, he said, "Hi" and spoke my name. As the days passed, he seemed more comfortable making conversation. He told me he was a contractor. He spoke of his three sons. I also have three sons. The eye contact grew stronger. He faced me. He sipped from the straw for the first time.

As a nurse, I feel the warmth of my touch is an important step toward helping the patient. Mr. Smith was denied this. I had not been able to touch him because of the gowns, mask, and gloves. Yet, my eyes began the human "touching process." I began to realize that, even while there may be very little hope for those with chronic disease, still, I can give comfort. I knew that giving my time, allowing my eyes to come into contact with my patient's—even something as seemingly insignificant as a backrub—are essential.

After being off for two days, I went in to see Mr. Smith. "Hi! I missed you" he said. *Did I imagine the glimmer of a smile? Two days later he looked much weaker.* He did not eat or drink anything. "Don't give up!" I cried. "Tomorrow could be the day they find the cure." But tomorrow didn't come for Mr. Smith.

Some months have passed since Mr. Smith died, and yet I think of him often, reflecting on what he taught me. All this time, I felt it was *I* who needed protection. But it was *he* who had no immune system. There was no way for him to protect himself from me or others like me, whose fear of the unknown produced so much anxiety.

If you should be assigned to care for an AIDS patient, remember: you know how to protect yourself. They don't. If the human touch doesn't seem to work, then use *eye contact*. It's the only other tool you have.

This is dedicated to Judy Black, my mental health instructor, who taught me that getting in someone's space, giving them your undivided attention with good eye contact, works.

FIGURE 41–8. HBV vs HIV.

---

infected. Women who are unknowingly infected prior to pregnancy can easily transmit HIV to their offspring.

Antibody screening is carried out to determine exposure to the HIV virus. When a person is viremic, i.e. initially infected with the antigen, there is a 6–12 week period before the antibody is formed. Thus, if antibody screening is carried out during this time, it will be negative, yet the person will be infected. The presence of the antibody not only indicates prior exposure to the virus but means the person can transmit the disease. Thus, people who are antibody positive have potentially infectious blood and body secretions and need to take appropriate steps to insure the protection of others, i.e. use condoms with all sexual activity, and do not share needles or drugs.

Maternal Issues

Women compose 7 percent of the cases of AIDS in the United States today. Approximately 80 percent of these women are of childbearing age, i.e. between 15 and 49. These women are mostly black

> TABLE 41–5. **Women in the United States with AIDS/HIV Infection, January 1988**
>
> 1. Women make up 7 percent of the total number of cases of AIDS
> 2. More than 70 percent are black or Latina
> 3. Almost 80 percent are between the ages of 13 and 39
> 4. It is estimated that 70,000–140,000 women in the United States are infected with HIV
>
> SOURCE: Courtesy of R. Farnher.

and Latina. The distribution geographically is similar to AIDS in general, with a higher incidence in large urban cities – New York, Newark, and Miami (see Table 41–5).

Early reports suggested worrisome outcomes for infected women who subsequently became pregnant. The problems of AIDS related to the physiological process of pregnancy seemed to be exaggerated. Women who were antibody positive were progressing to AIDS Related Complex (ARC), and from ARC to AIDS with pregnancy. More recent prospective studies indicate that more women are able to maintain their pregnancies, give birth, and not necessarily suffer severe exacerbations of opportunistic infections or death (Willoughby et al., 1987).

Approximately 55 percent of HIV-positive women are IV drug users. The second largest group of women were infected sexually, from men with AIDS. The other large group of infected women are those who have received infected blood or blood products. It is an extremely painful experience for women who are unaware of their own HIV status until they give birth to an infected child. Women engaging in high-risk behavior, i.e. IV drug users, women with multiple sex partners (more than five per year), recipients of blood transfusions between 1979 and 1985, and sexual partners of IV drugs users or bisexual men, should consider antibody testing (see Appendix).

The symptoms of AIDS in women include (1) persistent fatigue, (2) fever, chills, and night sweats, (3) severe diarrhea, (4) sudden unexplained weight loss, (5) swelling lymph nodes/glands, (6) shortness of breath or a dry cough, (7) pink or purple spots on the skin, and (8) persistent yeast infections. Most people infected with AIDS feel no symptoms in the beginning. The latency of the virus from 5 to 10 years may delay to onset of symptoms. Women wanting confirmation of their antibody status should seek confidential antibody testing with appropriate counseling. Appropriate interventions should be provided as necessary. Pregnant women who test positive early in pregnancy should be followed carefully. Antibody testing should also be repeated later in pregnancy if initially negative, but risk behaviors continue to be an issue.

Newborn Issues

Maternal transmission of HIV to unborn children is estimated to be between 40 and 60 percent (see Table 41–6). Knowledge of maternal antibody status is important, particularly for arranging appropriate follow-up for the infant. Infants are thought to become infected transplacentally via infected maternal serum, or from exposure to the organism in the genital track. Cesarean section has not proven to be an effective way of eliminating newborn infection. Cases have been reported of infants becoming infected from the breast milk of a woman who became HIV positive after receiving an infected blood transfusion in the postpartum period. Therefore, breastfeeding is discouraged if women are known to be HIV positive.

Passive transmission of maternal antibody at birth to an infant means that there may be a 5–10 month initial period when the infant demonstrates only maternal antibody. Mothers who are identified as HIV positive need to have their infants successively screened to determine if the antibody is lost, thus indicating that they are not infected.

> TABLE 41–6. **Children in the United States with AIDS/HIV Infection, January 1988**
>
> 1. Children make up 1.4 percent of the total number of cases of AIDS
> 2. Almost 80 percent are black or Latina
> 3. Almost 80 percent had a parent with or at risk for AIDS
> 4. 30–70 percent of infants born to HIV-infected mothers are infected
> 5. Most perinatally infected infants become ill within 4–6 months, and most die before the age of 2
> 6. It is estimated that by 1991 at least 3000 children will have AIDS; many more will be HIV infected
>
> SOURCE: Courtesy of R. Farnher.

Infected infants have difficulties with repeated viral and bacterial infections and often die before they are 2 years old. A newborn is already a compromised host, and further destruction of the immune system by the HIV virus is grave. Many babies may show no symptoms initially but then may suffer from similar symptoms to adults, such as (1) failure to thrive or gain weight, (2) enlarged lymph glands, (3) fever, (4) diarrhea, (5) yeast thrush infections, (6) pneumonia, and (7) enlarged liver or spleen. Circumcision is a theoretical risk to HIV-positive newborns and is thus discouraged.

Nursing Issues

All sexually active adults need to be educated to reduce the risk of HIV transmission. Currently, the United States Public Health Department is conducting a household campaign regarding general information about AIDS and its transmission. Instructions for safe sex include how to apply a latex condom and the importance of always using one, and that spermicidal jelly or foam that contains non-oxynol 9 will kill the HIV virus. Women using IV drugs should be encouraged to join a treatment program, should not share needles, and should be shown how to clean them properly with water and bleach. Intercourse or any sexual activity that creates cuts in the skin and might allow the virus to enter the bloodstream should be discouraged. Any high-risk behavior, e.g. unprotected sex with an IV drug user or bisexual man, or multiple sex partners of unknown antibody status, should be discouraged.

The fear of AIDS is a very difficult and complex issue (see Table 41–7). It is the role of the nurse to support and clarify the patient's fears as well as dealing with their own fears as a health care worker. There is a worldwide epidemic and there has been a lot of hysterical media coverage. Because the disease is fatal, fears about transmission are real, and it is important to deal with this honestly and openly. There was an early precedent for extensive precautions. More recently, it is understood that precautions necessary are those similar for other blood-borne viral infections such as hepatitis B.

Prevention issues are very important for perinatal health care workers who may inadvertently be exposed to the HIV virus. Universal blood and body secretion precautions should be considered as an infection control policy for hospital settings (see Table 41–3). Sample perinatal guidelines for an inpatient hospital unit are included in the Appendix.

SUMMARY

Each of these sexually transmitted organisms has serious implications for the perinatal unit, the mother, and infant. A primary responsibility of the perinatal nurse is clear and concise education about the signs and transmission of the disease. General principles regarding transmission are helpful in providing this patient education.

Some infections may be more virulent during pregnancy, though often the general physiological changes of pregnancy and the theorized decreased immunity may predispose the pregnant woman to inadequate host defenses. Maternal infection which causes intrauterine infections is often asymptomatic. Antibody titers have thus become an important method of screening for the presence of the organism. Primary infections, i.e. herpes simplex or hepatitis B and CMV, affect the fetus more severely.

The major routes of perinatal acquisition or transmission include:

1. Infections present in the maternal bloodstream with transplacental passage.
2. Invasion from the genital tract allowing for (a) exposure and direct contact with organisms, or (b) ascending infections into the amniotic sac via intact or ruptured membranes (see Table 41–8).

Therefore, sexually transmitted infections can affect pregnancy significantly. There is a potential for an increased incidence in spontaneous abortion, preterm labor, premature rupture of membranes (PROM), prematurity, intrauterine growth retardation, intrauterine devices, or exaggerated maternal disease (see Table 41–9).

TABLE 41–7. Fear of Disease

1. New disease, worldwide epidemic
2. Fatal outcome
3. Hysteria promoted by media
4. Early precedent for excessive precautions
5. Transmission similar to other blood-borne viral infections
6. Low, but not zero, risk of occupational exposure

SOURCE: Courtesy of R. Farnher

TABLE 41–8. Routes of STD Infection
1. Organisms present in maternal blood stream: transplacental passage.
2. Organisms present in the lower genital tract:
a. Direct exposure during birth process;
b. Ascending infections up genital tract to amniotic membranes (intact or ruptured).
3. Organisms present in breast milk: direct exposure.

The effects of these infections in perinatal patients are varied but some general principles are important. Prematurity has remained a constant problem in the world and its incidence has remained at approximately 10 percent of all deliveries. Researchers have discovered that the incidence of prematurity is intrinsically related to premature rupture of membranes, because 25–45 percent of all cases of prematurity are complicated by PROM. There is an increased incidence of prematurity and preterm labor in lower socioeconomic groups (Tuomalo, 1986).

Fetal effects would most certainly depend on the gestational age and the timing of the exposure of the organism. When organs are developing, i.e. during the first trimester, it is a vulnerable time for teratogenic effects. Major organ systems can be interrupted and damaged by significant infections present in the first few months of pregnancy.

Other infections simply cause destruction to already developed body tissues and organ systems, usually by inflammation. We observe congenital syndromes such as CMV, neonatal diseases (e.g. Chlamydial pneumonia), and/or chronic infections and delayed effects with untreated hepatitis B virus in the newborn. On the other hand, we also see infants who, for what ever reason, are unaffected by perinatal infections.

The control of perinatal infections is an important issue for both patients and staff. Fortunately, the implementation of universal blood and body secretion precautions in all perinatal units is increasing. Health care workers are thus instructed that all blood and body fluids, including saliva, urine, feces, wound drainage, and amniotic fluid, require a barrier, whether it be gloves, mask, clear glasses, or a gown.

Also, one major nursing role in the care of perinatal patients is education regarding appropriate methods of birth control and disease prevention. A demonstration of the use of condoms with spermicidal jelly is important for the prevention of sexually transmitted diseases, as the condom acts as a barrier against infection. Increasing numbers of sexually transmitted diseases, particularly the identification of the fatal HIV infection, has encouraged more media attention and education about transmission. Abstinence and monogamy have become attractive options in the battle against these hazardous infections (see Table 41–10).

Counseling and support are also important nursing roles. For example, the herpes virus, with its unique pattern of recurrent exacerbations and painful outbreaks, demands psychological support and understanding. There is a lot of guilt and anger generated over the unknown transmission of disease between sexual partners, and its impact on an unborn child. Women may be unknowingly infected with *Chlamydia* or gonorrhea, and transmit it to their child. HIV infection in a woman may

TABLE 41–9. Implications of Sexually Transmitted Infections for Mother and Newborn

Effects on Pregnancy	Effects on Fetus/Newborn
Preterm labor	Prematurity
PROM	Congenital anomalies
Chorioamniotitis	Intrauterine growth retardation
Spontaneous abortion	Neonatal disease
Intrauterine demise	Chronic infections and delayed effects
Exaggerated maternal disease	Early newborn death

TABLE 41–10. Key Nursing Roles when Caring for the Infected Perinatal Patient

Education
1. Disease identification;
2. Disease transmission;
3. Disease prevention.

Counseling and support
1. Recurrent infections;
2. Long-term sequelae;
3. Fear of unknown;
4. Complications, often painful;
5. Impact on family unit/lifestyle;
6. Anger/guilt over unknown disease transmission.

only be discovered after a child is found to be antibody positive. A woman may not know her risk factors for HIV infection, and only discover perhaps that her partner was bisexual or an IV drug user after perinatal transmission. Repeated infections during pregnancy may require a lifestyle change, and considerations may need to be made for the entire family unit.

REFERENCES

American Academy of Pediatrics. 1980. Committee on the Fetus and Newborn, Committee on Infectious Diseases. Perinatal herpes simplex virus infections. *Pediatrics.* 66(1):147–149.

American Academy of Pediatrics. 1986. Report of the Committee on Infectious Diseases. *The Red Book.*

Barrett, T. 1988. Parent Information: Herpes Simplex, Alta Bates Hospital, Infection Control Manual, Berkeley, CA.

Bennett, E. C. 1987. Sexually transmitted diseases. *NAACOG Newsletter.* 14(8).

Bourcier, K. M., and Seidler, A. J. 1987. *Chlamydia* and *Condylomata acuminata:* An update for the nurse practitioner. *J. Obstet. Gynecol. Nurs.* 16(1):17–22.

Captain, J. 1988. Universal precautions: AIDS and other infectious diseases. *California Nurs. Rev.* May/June:29–34.

Center for Disease Control. 1987. Progress toward achieving the National 1988 Objectives for sexually transmitted diseases. *Morbidity and Mortality Weekly Report.* 36(12):

Davis, G. 1987. Update on genital herpes from Physicians' Radio Network. Summary of 1987 International Society for STD Research.

Eshenbach, D. 1987. Sexually transmitted diseases: Clinical Practices. *Obstet. Gynecol. Audio Digest Foundation.* 34(17):

Gabbe, S. E.; Niebyl, J. R.; and Simpson, J. L. eds. 1986. *Obstetrics: Normal and problem pregnancies.* New York: Churchill Livingstone.

Holmberg, D. 1987. Update on genital herpes from Physicians' Radio Network. Summary of 1987 International Society for STD Research.

Knox, G. 1985. Cytomegalovirus: Impact on sexual transmission. *Clin. Obstet. Gynecol.* 26:145.

Kotsky, C. 1987. Update on genital herpes from Physicians' Radio Network. Summary of 1987 International Society for STD Research.

Martin, D. H.; Koutsky, L.; Eschenbach, D. A. et al. 1982. Prematurity and perinatal mortality in pregnancies complicated by maternal *Chlamydia trachomatis* infection. *JAMA.* 247:1585–1588.

Mertz, G. 1987. Update on genital herpes from Physicians' Radio Network. Summary of 1987 International Society for STD Research.

Nahmias, A. J., Keyeserling, H. L., and Kerrick, G. M. 1983. *Herpes Simplex.* In Remington, J. S., and Klein, J. P. Infectious Diseases of the Fetus and Newborn Infant, Philadelphia. W. B. Saunders Co.

Nelson, B. I., and Grossman, J., III. 1986. Perinatal infections. In *Obstetrics: Normal and problem pregnancies.* eds. S. E. Gabbe, J. R. Niebyl, and J. L. Simpson. New York: Churchill Livingstone.

Osborne, Newton G; Ng, L; and Pratson, C. 1984. Sexually transmitted diseases and pregnancy. *J. Obstet. Gynecol. Neonatal Nurs.* 13(8):9–12.

Reim, M. F. Educational Audiotape. Family Practice Audio Digest Foundation. Vol. 35 #28, July 27, 1987. "The Ubiquitous Chlamydial Organism."

Schachter, J.; Holt, J.; Goodner, E.; Grossman, M.; Sweet, R.; and Mills, J. 1979. Prospective study of chlamydial infections in neonates. *Lancet.* 2(8/39):377–380.

Thompson, S. 1987. Update on genital herpes from Physicians' Radio Network. Summary of 1987 International Society for STD Research.

Tuomala, R. 1986. Relationship of genital tract infection during pregnancy and prematurity. Infectious problems in obstetrics. What's here and ahead in Ob./Gyn. In *Infectious problems in obstetrics,* Vol. II. Audio Digest Foundation.

Willoughby, A.; Mendez, H.; Minkoff, H.; Holman, S.; Goedert, J.; Landesman, S. 1987. Human immune deficiency virus in pregnant women and their offspring. Paper presented at the Third International Conference on Acquired Immunodeficiency Syndrome (AIDS), June 1–5, Washington, D.C.

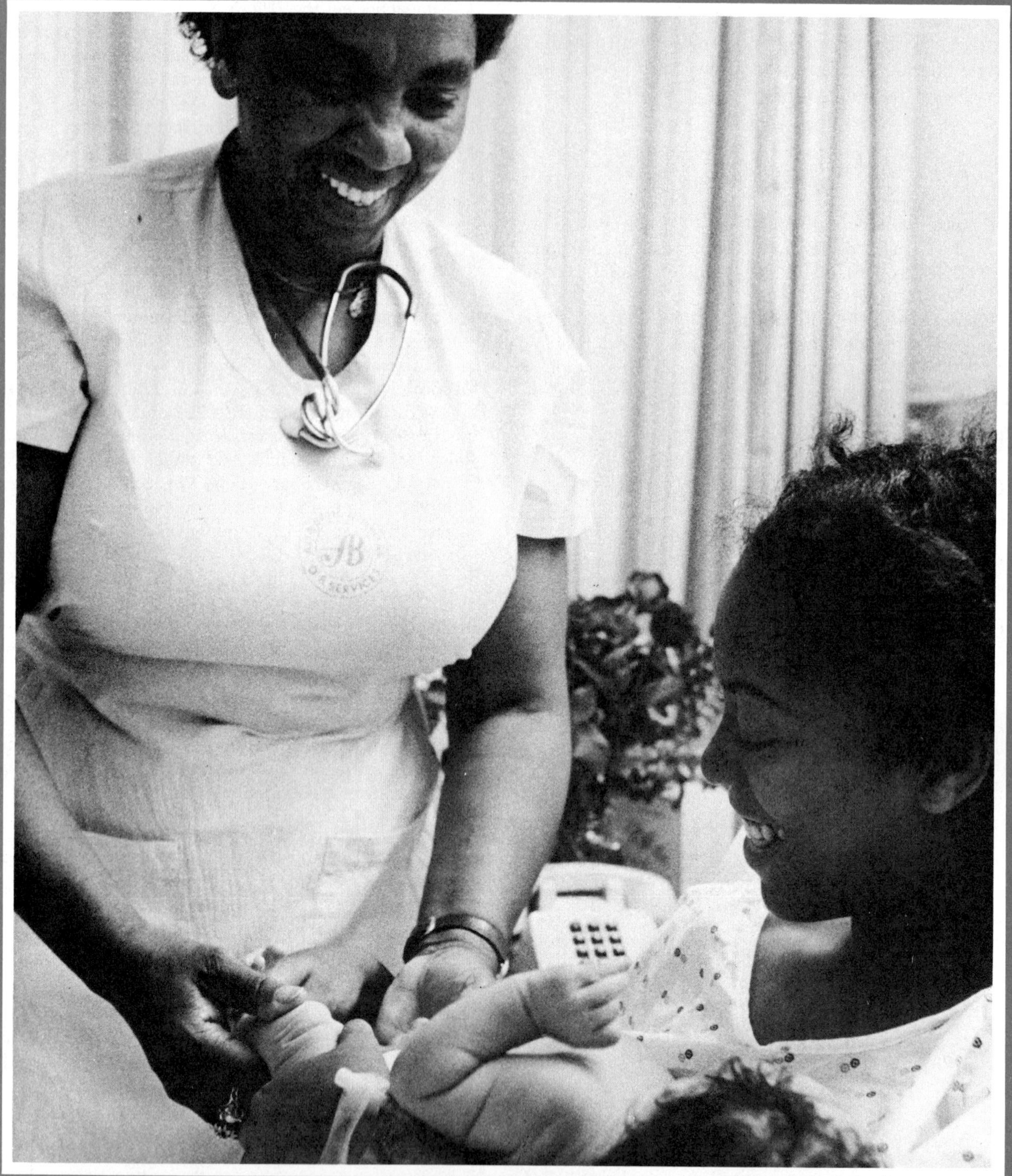

UNIT EIGHT
IMPLEMENTING CHANGE

42

Alternative Birthing Methods

BEHAVIORAL OBJECTIVES

Upon completion of this chapter, the reader should be able to:

- Identify factors contributing to the present consumerism in client care for childbearing.

- Compare and contrast the philosophies of various alternative birth centers (birthing center in hospital, birthing center out of hospital, home birth, family-centered maternity care units) and traditional maternity care units.

- Analyze advantages and disadvantages of various methods of alternative birthing.

- Develop a personal philosophy of the essential components of family-centered maternity care.

- Analyze the physiologic and psychosocial considerations important to the family planning a vaginal birth after a prior cesarean birth.

- Develop a nursing care plan for the unique needs of clients choosing alternative birthing settings and practices for childbearing.

- Develop an understanding for the nurse's role in the alternative centers and in the change process.

Most births occurred at home 40 years ago, but most births today happen in hospitals. Over the years, the process of childbirth has changed; it has moved from a natural, fact-of-life experience to an illness-focused event. Most pregnant clients today deliver in hospitals because of the perception that giving birth to a child may be life-threatening to both mother and baby. However, the belief that the hospital is the only safe place for childbirth has not always been prevalent. For centuries women labored wherever and however they were comfortable and received little medical intervention in their labors. Perhaps the higher infant and maternal morbidity and mortality rates of the nineteenth and early twentieth centuries encouraged consumers to deliver in hospitals, where emergency equipment would be available if problems occurred in childbirth. Even with today's lower infant and maternal death and illness rates, many childbearing couples still want the safety of the hospital environment. Peer pressure also encourages couples to accept hospital birth. Additionally, both lack of knowledge and client perception that hospital routines can be altered if couples speak about their needs have also directed couples to greater acceptance of the hospital as a delivering environment (Gillespie, 1981). The challenge of the 1980s has been to provide humanistic care to a variety of families with different financial and social support needs (Flanagan, 1986).

HISTORICAL OVERVIEW OF CHILDBEARING BELIEFS

Primitive women were ideally suited for childbirth since they ate nourishing, uncomplicated diets, worked hard, and had appropriate pelvic dimensions. Unlike primitive women, who often labored in the field, women of the sixteenth century used a birthing chair to provide anatomic support for labor and delivery. They were fully clothed to protect their modesty and appearance while a midwife consistently applied genital manipulation to aid in childbirth. The chairs worked well in utilizing gravity to shorten the length of labor (Findley, 1934). However, midwife manipulations of the genitals often caused hematomas, infections, fistulas, and badly torn perineums.

The birthing chair was used until Louis XIV's time. Louis initiated a profound change in childbirth practices when he ordered his court physician to deliver Louis's mistress in the supine position so that Louis could see the birth of his child. Even today, many clients deliver in the supine position because of tradition and because physicians can more readily assess the perineum in labor and delivery in the back-lying position. Louis's use of the court physician to deliver his mistress created another change in maternity practices, since up to that time most women were delivered by midwives, who were women. After Louis's time, pregnancy became more illness-focused, and physicians became predominant in providing most obstetric care (Lieberman, 1976).

With the use of anesthesia increasing in the twentieth century, more frequent use of forceps and surgical intervention was needed to ensure a safer hospital delivery. Now medicine has achieved more control over fetal and maternal morbidity and mortality, but many of these surgical interventions and high-risk client-monitoring techniques have remained, even for uncomplicated deliveries. In fact, many of today's consumers have been taught to believe that in order to have a safe and satisfying delivery, hospitalization with complicated devices and medications is necessary (Gillespie, 1981).

There can be no doubt that sufficient staffing often exists in hospitals to take care of unforeseen emergencies in childbirth. In addition, hospital delivery can provide a restful time for a new mother and also provide guidance to new parents in their educational and psychosocial needs. However, many consumers are now clamoring for a more natural, family-centered birth experience without the routines of the hospital. The request for an alternative birth experience (one other than the traditional hospital setting with intravenous infusion, enema, and monitor, for example) skyrocketed in the 1970s and remains a childbirth choice for many couples today. With the popularity of the Lamaze, Dick-Read, and Bradley methods of childbirth preparation, consumers have fueled the natural childbirth movement and the concept of control with their labor and delivery. Increasingly, clients are requesting not to have routine IVs, suprapubic preps, and enemas. Clients are also resisting laboring and delivering in different rooms, and also being separated from family members while laboring and while recovering from labor and delivery.

Various factors may have influenced the rise of the natural childbirth movement. The feminist movement encouraged greater self-reliance, autonomy, control, and responsibility for the health of the individual and the couple. The effects of this change toward greater individual responsibility for education and health can be seen in the increased number of hospitals allowing fathers in the delivery room for the birth of their child (Gillespie, 1981). The feminist movement also stressed control over women's bodies, a central theme in natural childbirth. From the 1950s through the present, a consumer movement in medicine has begun to evolve. There is now a strong self-help movement, as evidenced by the increasing number of individuals taking charge of their health, education, and well-being. This can be contrasted to the time when people relied on health professionals to educate and treat them on health-related matters.

The alternative birthing center concept became a popular one in the 1970s. The enthusiasm for alternative birth centers has continued from that time, and the American College of Obstetricians and Gynecologists (1981) notes the existence of many alternative birth centers, most of them located in hospitals. Actually, the philosophy of alternative birth centers was implemented in 1925 by Mary Breckenridge, when she founded the Frontier Nursing Service in Hyden, Kentucky (see Chap. 2). The service provided to poor pregnant women by the Frontier Nursing Service lowered the maternal mortality rate during the period from 1925 to 1951 to 9.1 per 10,000 births. This can be contrasted with 34 per 10,000 live births for the rest of Kentucky and the United States for the same period.

Today there is a need for alternative birth centers that can provide safe but effective family-focused care. Alternative birth centers can provide an informed choice between methods of birthing at a reasonable cost to the consumer. Many traditional maternity services are astronomical in cost. For example, over the past decade, the cost of anesthesia has risen as much as 233 percent, a cesarean birth 200 percent, and basic obstetric fees 140 percent.

The cost of physician liability insurance is relevant to increased consumer costs for services. Although the annual premium for some New York obstetricians in 1982 was estimated at $25,000 (Dorman, 1982), rates in 1987 are far higher due to recent litigation activity. In fact, many obstetricians have simply been unable to practice due to the high liability insurance rates. In 1989 these rates have increased to an excess of $40,000.

Almost two-thirds of obstetricians and gynecologists have been sued, and this has created a significant problem in determining which medical practitioners can provide quality maternity care (NAACOG, 1987). Even nurses in expanded roles (nurse-midwifery, for example) have recently been denied liability coverage due to their "high-risk" status in the provision of care to childbearing families. At present, the insurance industry, health care agencies, nursing professional groups, and the legal system are collaborating on ideas and practices which will help alleviate the liability insurance crisis.

The use of expanded role providers such as nurse-midwives and alternative birthing areas such as birthing centers may well decrease the cost of childbearing. In 1983, the average hospital cost for an uncomplicated birth was approximately $2572 (Lubic, 1983). A comparable hospital cost in 1989 would be more than $3,000. However, the cost could have been decreased to $1375 (about 40 percent less than in a hospital) by delivering in a birthing center. The above mentioned expenses are usually for a 3-day stay. A childbearing center of the Maternity Center Association can usually decrease the cost because care is delivered in a residential center rather than in a hospital (Lubic, 1983). Nurse-midwives, rather than physicians, usually deliver in birthing centers, which can also decrease costs. There is a minimum of expensive equipment at the alternative birth centers, and staff costs are usually less because practitioner liability costs are lower when compared to liability fees of obstetricians. Additionally, family members help provide client care, which also decreases staff salary charges. These combined factors help decrease the cost of delivery and allow a closer family involvement—two goals of couples experiencing childbirth.

FAMILY-CENTERED MATERNITY CARE

Current Practices

When asked to define their most important goal in Lamaze classes, couples respond that they want a healthy baby and minimum pain with labor and delivery. Increasingly, however, consumers want more than just a healthy baby and a tolerable labor and delivery. Many childbirth educators and nurses are finding that couples feel they have the right to spend time with their baby after delivery and to practice parenting skills in a supportive environment (see The Pregnant Patient's Bill of Rights in Appendix E). Increased time after delivery can also be used by couples to work on their goals of reestablishing intimacy and adapting to the changed concept of family.

Overall, couples who accept hospital birth as the best setting for childbirth also want greater humanization of care in the hospital environment. This type of care can be provided in many hospitals that practice family-centered maternity care, with the focus on safe physical and psychosocial care of the entire family and on child bearing as a socially significant process relevant to family growth. An attempt is made in family-centered maternity care to individualize client care to meet unique needs of the client. For example, parents may be offered options for their childbirth experience (rooming-in, type of anesthesia, attendance at classes) to best meet their special needs. Also, some hospitals provide special dinners for the couple to help them celebrate the birth of their infant (see Fig. 42–1).

A family-centered maternity care approach that visualizes each member of the family as an individual with specific needs and desires to be met by the nursing process is favored. In order to ensure family-centered maternity care, nursing must change its attitudes. The profession must be willing to listen and to explore what consumers want, and then work with consumers to see that optimal health care is delivered (Gillespie, 1981).

Improvements in Family-Centered Maternity Care

Family-centered maternity care can be a viable approach to caring for the needs of the new family. For example, if health care professionals could meet consumer demands to make the experience more family focused and natural, greater client satisfaction could result. Fathers and other family members should be encouraged to participate actively in the preparation and management of birth so that greater family closeness may develop (see Fig. 42–2). Early rooming-in policies, child-care classes, early discharge programs, and use of a *montrice* (childbirth coach) should meet couples' demands for greater support in their childbearing needs. Additionally, the practice of primary nursing for each mother–baby dyad should allow

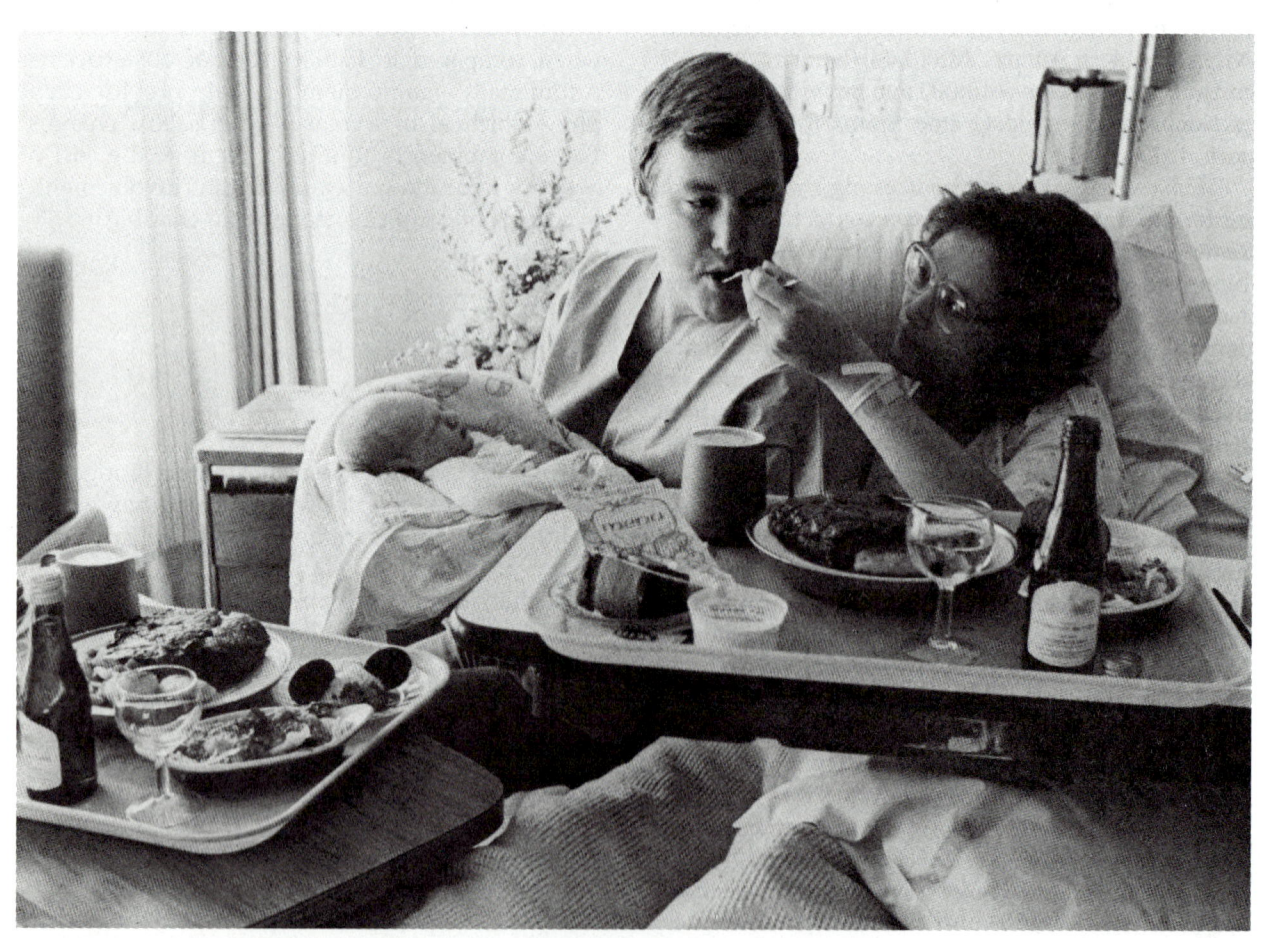

FIGURE 42–1. Couple enjoying special dinner after delivery.

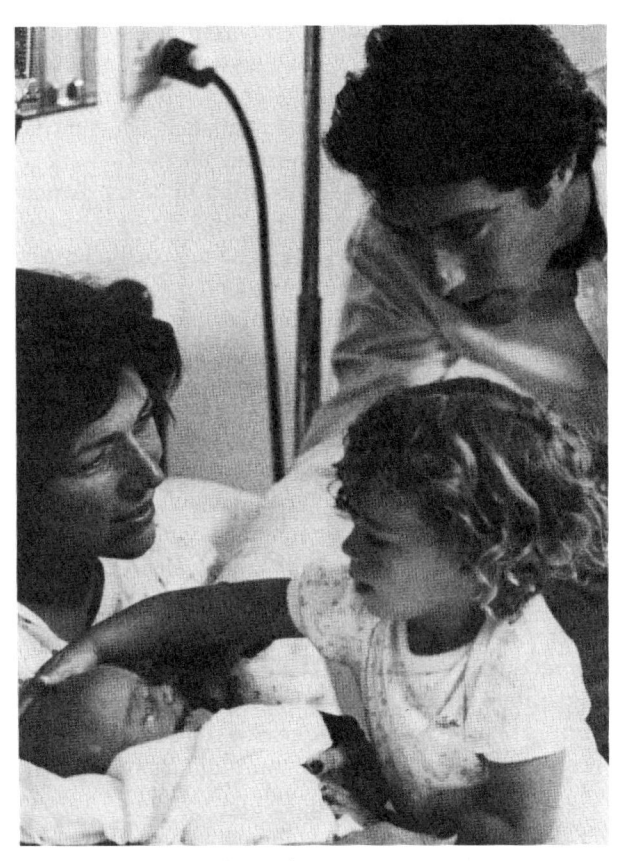

FIGURE 42-2. Family involvement in the birth process.

increased trust and rapport between client and caretaker. Greater maternal confidence in parenting might also result from mutual goal setting by client and caretaker for more satisfactory parenting.

Although not widely used in this country, montrices may prove to be an effective asset to support clients' needs during labor and thus to meet the criteria for family-centered maternity care. In some areas, montrices can provide backup support for fathers who need guidance or relief during labor and delivery. In addition to providing physical and emotional support, after birth the montrice can provide parenting education and skill training. Frequently, the montrice can provide this support in the early postpartum period by preventing separation of the family (Carlson and Summer, 1976).

Some birthing centers employ montrices to assist laboring couples who have had prenatal Lamaze or Bradley classes. In these programs, montrices have worked with couples in seeking assistance from hospital staff in a nonantagonistic manner. Montrices can be of great service in assisting couples in communicating their needs to health care providers (Gillespie, 1981). Frequently, parents approach providers as adversaries, and that hinders the establishment of a working relationship between client and provider. Ultimately, care and safety suffer when a satisfactory rapport cannot be gained between practitioner and consumer in the process of health care delivery.

Many family-centered maternity care childbearing units encourage support by a significant other during pregnancy, labor and delivery, and the postpartum stay. Couples who have had childbirth preparation classes do not seem to need as much analgesic support with labor and delivery as couples not prepared in classes. The presence of a supportive other (husband, boyfriend, montrice, mother) may also decrease the amount of medication needed by a client to be comfortable with the childbearing process. The decrease in required medication results in a decrease in potential side-effects that can have an impact on perinatal outcome. If couples can pass through labor and delivery with little medication but with optimal interpersonal support, both mother and baby seem to fare better. If a physician routinely prescribes medications in varying amounts, clients need to be encouraged to discuss with their physician the need for medication, possible side-effects, and how the medication will affect the labor and delivery participants.

Likewise, clients need to discuss with their physicians their ideas on when the use of a cesarean birth, forceps, and fetal heart monitoring is necessary. None of these procedures will negate family-centered maternity care but any of them can affect the degree of participation by the mother and her support person. For example, if a cesarean birth is performed, rooming-in with the baby will be delayed until the mother feels well enough to ambulate and care for the baby's needs. The necessity for fetal heart monitoring should also be discussed by consumer and physician, because many doctors consider fetal heart monitoring to be routine obstetric care. The client needs to express any fears or concerns about various labor and delivery procedures to prevent later unacceptable feelings and misunderstandings about the procedure. Particularly in the case of cesarean birth, clients need to be encouraged to discuss with their physicians whether a vaginal birth can be performed after a previous cesarean. Increasing numbers of women are able to have a vaginal birth after having had a cesarean, provided no indications exist for a repeat cesarean birth (see Chap. 31).

The Role of the Nurse-Midwife

Basically, the philosophy of nurse-midwifery includes a family focus that views birth as a highly emotional and significant group event. Nurse-midwives by most state laws and philosophy care for "uncomplicated" pregnancies. If a client develops any high-risk factors while under nurse-midwifery care in the prenatal period, that client is generally referred to a physician or is seen jointly by a nurse-midwife and a physician (Melson, 1983). The philosophy of midwifery includes the right of the family to be in control of its labor and delivery (Lichtman, 1983).

It is the belief of midwives that once clients are educated about the processes of pregnancy and labor and delivery, these clients should determine their delivery based on full realization of the impact of their decisions. During labor, pain medications can be given should clients desire; but, generally, regional medications (epidurals) and other interventions are avoided by nurse-midwives. A midwife serves a dual function—as an educator as well as a caregiver. Most midwives hold a holistic client focus and intervene in promoting an entire family's health during pregnancy. They do "careful watching" of a client's labor and delivery (Lichtman, 1983). The role of the nurse-midwife in giving emotional and physical support in this "careful watching" is of immeasurable value in achieving a satisfactory labor and delivery. Additionally, the use of a primary nurse (one who can take care of all the needs of the client) from the start of a pregnancy to its end can do much to reach client-defined goals for pregnancy. Frequently, with a primary-caretaker approach, a close interpersonal relationship between nurse-midwife or nurse and client can be attained, since both parties are aware of one another's needs and goals (Asby and Roebuck, 1979).

Family-Centered Maternity Care in Hospitals

The setting in which a delivery takes place often determines its cost. Although nurse-midwives stay with a client for lengthy, continuous periods of time during a labor, the cost of a nurse-midwife is often less than that of a physician in a traditional labor and delivery in a hospital. Unfortunately, not all states have licensed nurse-midwives to practice delivery of uncomplicated pregnancy cases. Lack of licensure may be tied to the problem of a few states that have third-party reimbursement of insurance coverage for deliveries and pregnancies monitored by a nurse-midwife.

In response to consumer demands for alternative birth centers, the American Nurses' Association (ANA), the Nurses' Association of the American College of Obstetricians and Gynecologists (NAACOG), the American Academy of Pediatrics (AAP), and the American College of Nurse-Midwives (ACNM) collaborated and later published, in 1978, the *Joint position statement on the development of family-centered maternity/newborn care in hospitals* (see Appendix H). This statement was later endorsed by the American Hospital Association and has now been implemented in many maternity units to provide better family-centered maternity care. The ability of the five groups to work together on the position paper demonstrates that all these professional groups are concerned with meeting consumer demands for more family-focused maternity care. The community of practicing nurses is now called upon to demonstrate its support of consumer demands for a flexible, noninterventionistic, and humanitarian type of client care in childbearing (Hogan, 1980).

HOME BIRTH

In accordance with the philosophy that childbirth is a natural and family event, many couples are now seeking home births (see Fig. 42-3). Home births are acceptable for low-risk women (Patterson and Peterson, 1980). Many families select the home for a delivering environment because it is more comfortable, familiar, and natural, and family support is available. Home-birth mothers feel a sense of harmony and nostalgia with the family in the home during birth. These feelings often cannot be experienced in the impersonal surroundings of the hospital (Anderson, Bauwens, and Warner, 1978). Being in her own home increases the mother's sense of peace and tranquility (White, 1983). Overall, the benefit and safety of home birth to the mother and fetus must be considered in evaluating the morality of home birth.

Advantages of Home Birth

Some couples elect to deliver at home because they do not want excessive intervention in a process they consider to be a highly natural and personal event. Most home-birth couples choose to deliver

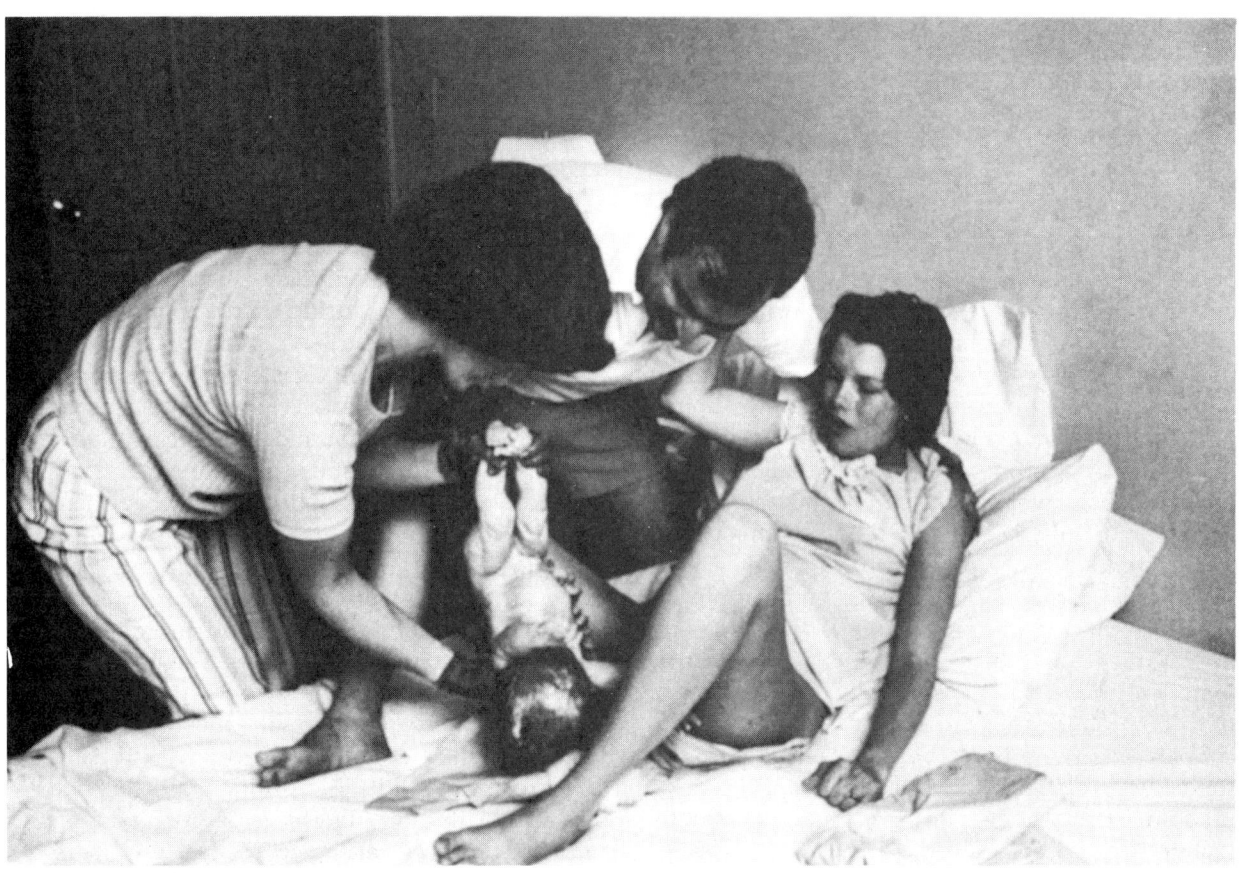

FIGURE 42–3. Couple experiencing home birth.

at home because of their philosophy that childbirth should occur in the family focus (Richie and Swanson, 1976). Others may choose to deliver at home because it is cheaper than a hospital or birthing center. At-home delivery may not be less expensive though. Physician fees may be higher, because extra time and equipment are required and because a small group takes responsibility for the home birth (White, 1983).

Couples who deliver at home may distrust the health care profession. These couples may have previously been unable to work with physicians and nurses in determining and meeting their needs with labor and delivery (Anderson, Bauwens, and Warner, 1978). In fact, as parity increases, home births may become more popular among childbearing couples (Shy, Frost, and Ullom, 1980). Some couples may also feel they can handle the personal responsibility of childbirth as well as many health care practitioners but without the restrictive environment of a hospital. Often the type of environment they are trying to avoid may contain limited visiting hours for partner and family, lack of sibling visitation, and little nursing support for breastfeeding or post-partum physiological and psychosocial discomforts.

Various studies of couples who seek home births show that the majority are white, married, and well-educated. Many home-birth couples live in urban areas, have had a previous child in the hospital, have taken childbirth preparation classes, and have placed a high priority on keeping the family intact (Herman, Miller-Klein, and Ventre, 1979; Schneider, 1986). Home-delivery couples frequently do not fear physiologic dangers of childbirth outside the hospital as much as they favor the psychologic advantages to the family that a home birth provides. In the home, supportive caregivers are consistently available. A client can also be more in control due to an active decision-making role in her labor; she may be able to choose a variety of positions for labor with supportive family members nearby. Parent–infant bonding may be enhanced since the baby is never separated from its parents. Home-birth proponents also point out that with less medical intervention during labor and delivery, fewer problems such as infection (maternal and fetal) result from a home birth.

Disadvantages of Home Birth

Couples who elect to deliver at home must be aware of the dangers of not delivering in a hospital and not having skilled personnel available for emergencies of childbirth. The Association of Childbirth at Home International estimates that approximately 40 percent of United States home births are unattended by health care professionals (Sieden, 1981). In one Arizona county, 56 percent of home births were attended only by the baby's father, and only 17 percent of the home births were attended by a physician (Anderson, Bauwens, and Warner, 1978). The reason most physicians do not attend home births is that they are inconvenient and also not sanctioned by the majority of the medical community. Overall, home birth attendants are hard to find; so, frequently, couples wanting a home birth are "forced" to do the delivery alone. Without skilled help, the risks inherent with home birth increase markedly (White, 1983).

If there are complications in the labor or delivery of a home birth, infant or maternal death or illness may result without immediate health care attention. Particularly if the couple has no health care professional available for assistance, they may have access to few back-up services such as a hospital or clinic. In Holland, where home births are more widely accepted than in the United States, "flying squads" are available to provide supplies and to transfer clients in need of childbearing assistance. No such sophisticated back-up exists in most parts of the United States (Lichtman, 1983). Home births are disapproved of by many health care professionals, and sometimes these professionals refuse aid to couples who have chosen home delivery (Gillespie, 1981).

Another disadvantage of home birth is the need to perhaps transfer to a hospital at the time when labor discomfort is the greatest. Couples planning a home birth need to discuss how they will best meet their needs if transfer is necessary. Plans should also be made before the beginning of labor about routes to take to the nearest hospital should transfer be necessary.

The ACOG has issued various statements against home births. The organization has stated that neonatal deaths are greater in home births than in the hospital. However, many women who choose home delivery are older, are multiparous, and may have multiple gestation or low-birth weight high-risk factors (Shy, Frost, and Ullom, 1980). Thus, these clients are already at high risk and may contribute to a greater neonatal mortality rate with home births than hospital births. In addition, the frequent claims of higher neonatal deaths occurring during home births may be inaccurate, because a large percentage of complicated home births are registered, whereas normal births may not be. Also, many physicians report that mortality and morbidity of both infant and mother have diminished markedly over the past half century, when hospital delivery became more routine. But mortality and morbidity have declined in the past decades because of improved sanitation, better nutrition, and better education of the public, rather than because of improvement in hospital practices for childbirth. The hospital environment may not be more safe than the home—low infant and maternal mortality and morbidity rates exist in the Netherlands, where home birth is popular (Devitt, 1977). Additionally, the present lower death and illness rates for infants and mothers may be related to the fact that there are now fewer women giving birth at the extreme ages of childbearing, fewer babies spaced further apart, and fewer low-birth weight babies (Estes, 1978).

There have been a few well-controlled research studies to delineate the positive and negative outcomes of home birth (Shy, Frost, and Ullom, 1980). For example, in one survey in England, a higher rate of episiotomy, perineal tears, and Apgar scores lower than 7 were found in hospital-delivered women as compared to women who delivered at home (Shearer, 1985). With the interventions routinely applied in traditional labors, there are potential risks and adverse effects to both mother and baby. Thus, hospital deliveries cannot be without risks. Many studies of the risks of home birth include mortality and morbidity for all out-of-hospital births. These studies do not differentiate the planned from the unplanned home births, nor do they indicate whether the deliveries occurred in a doctor's office or the home.

One would imagine that unplanned home births would be more consistent with higher mortality and morbidity rates than planned home births, although additional research needs to be done to support that belief. In one study, most deaths from home births resulted from untrained or poorly trained birth attendants or in cases where an infant weighing less than 1500 g was delivered in an unplanned home birth. This study showed that in planned home births attended by physicians, certified nurse-midwives, or state recognized midwives, there was no significant difference in observed and expected deaths between home births and hospital births (Schramm, Barnes, and Bakewell, 1987). Additionally, one study has shown that unplanned home births do have a high mortality, whereas planned home births have a relatively low mortality (Campbell et al., 1984).

A Back-up System for Home Birth

The chance of complications with home birth is about 10 to 15 percent. Without professional birth attendants, the risks are greater (Melson, 1983). However, back-up services for home births may be expensive to maintain and frequently do not provide the best use of manpower in the health care system (Gillespie, 1981).

The Nurse-Midwife's Role in Home Birth

If a nurse-midwife contracts with a couple for a home birth, the nurse usually visits the couple at approximately the 37th week of pregnancy to assess for present or potential problems with the labor and delivery. It is expected that the client will have had prenatal care with a health care professional during most of her pregnancy. The nurse-midwife answers any questions the couple may have about the home birth. This visit often increases trust and confidence in both parties for the home delivery. Many nurse-midwives will recommend that couples attend childbirth preparation classes together, prepare other children for the event, and have sufficient equipment and support systems at home to decrease the risks of home delivery (see Table 42–1). All home-birth mothers should be encouraged to breast-feed to avoid postpartum uterine atony (White, 1983). A visit by the nurse-midwife at the 37th week of pregnancy also gives the nurse and the couple a chance to

---

TABLE 42–1. Equipment and Drugs for Home Delivery

Resuscitation Equipment	Obstetric Equipment	Drugs
Ambu bag and mask (adult, pediatric)	Fetoscope	Sodium bicarbonate (adult, pediatric)
Dual airways	Ultrasound fetal stethoscope (Doptone)	Epinephrine (adult, pediatric)
Endotracheal tubes (adult, pediatric)	Lubricating jelly, sterile	Calcium gluconate
Disposable De Lee traps	Tape measure	Oxytocin
Laryngoscope (adult, pediatric)	Kelly clamps, cord scissors	Methylergonovine (Methergine)
Stylette for ET tube	Needle holder, tissue forceps	Isuprel
IV solutions, tubing, needles	Episiotomy scissors	Lavophed
Dextrose LR	Allis clamps	Dopamine
Dextran	Sponge forceps	Hydralazine (Apresoline)
Bulb syringe	Retractor, long russian forceps	Dextrose 50%
Blood pressure cuff	Amniotone	Xylocaine
Stethoscope (adult, pediatric)	Outlet forceps	Silver nitrate
Umbilical artery catheterization set-up	Nitrazine paper	Aquamephyton
Tourniquet	Urine dipstick	Portable oxygen with delivery system
Syringes and needles	Sterile disposables (sponges, gloves, sterile towels, swabs, suture material)	Sterile water and saline
Dextrostix	Urinary catheter	
	Scale	
	Light source	
	Culturettes	
	Vacutainers	

SOURCE: Estes (1978).

check over the list of equipment for the birth and to plan for arrangements for transfer to a hospital if that becomes necessary. Continued prenatal care with either a physician or nurse-midwife for the duration of pregnancy is also to be encouraged.

Workers in an alternative birth center should know their legal basis for practice and the amount of support in their community for a nontraditional birthing environment (see Chapter 8). In the state of New Mexico, a state-licensed nurse-midwife can deliver a baby in the home; however, in Massachusetts only a physician can legally assist in home births (Melson, 1983). In some states, birth centers need the approval of state boards of health; without such approval, the centers can be shut down. Nurses in alternative birth centers should be advised to carry adequate liability insurance to avoid problems with coverage later. In stituations in which a nurse-midwife has contracted with a client for a home birth and specified terms of delivery, payment, and other significant matters, questions of liability probably will not arise.

Since the risks of an unattended home birth are greater than those of an attended birth, prepared nursing professionals could make an impact on family life by offering their services to unattended couples. Nursing has an obligation to establish standards of safe care, education, and practice in the area of maternity nursing. In the process of establishing standards, nurses could also enhance their collegial relationships with physicians. With increased communication between nurses, physicians, and other health care professionals, research could be carried out on optimal birthing practices. Perhaps policies and procedures could be changed to more adequately meet consumer demands for a more natural and caring delivery setting. In both research and practice areas, nurses could serve consumers well in the role of client advocate.

OUT-OF-HOSPITAL BIRTHING CENTERS

The childbearing option of having birth occur outside a hospital but in a safe environment with health care professionals readily available pleases many couples. At present, there are at least 12 birthing centers in the United States that are located outside the hospital environment. The philosophy of these centers is very much like that of the home-birth movement–birth is a uniquely personal event meant to be shared in a family's life history.

Advantages of Out-of-Hospital Birthing Centers

In a birthing center, significant others have the right to participate in the birth and to share the wonderful experience of the childbearing event if the couple so desires. Gillespie (1981) explains that many clients who use the Maternity Center Association's Childbearing Center have a distrust of traditional hospital practices that may be used routinely, even in uncomplicated labors. Birthing-center couples also want to decrease hospital costs for the delivery and want a private birth experience without student observation. Furthermore, many couples want to avoid moving from a labor room to a delivery room when all their concentration is needed at labor's end. With use of a birthing room, labor and delivery can occur in the same room, with loved ones available for the event.

Clients who use a birthing center are usually screened closely for use of the facility. Criteria for use of many out-of-hospital centers are: (1) clients must be defined as low risk; (2) they must have prenatal care starting by the 20th week of pregnancy; (3) they must have attended prenatal classes as part of their prenatal care; and (4) they must be motivated to deliver in a birthing center. With these criteria met, couples can use the center, provided no emergency situation arises with the mother or infant. Some emergency resuscitation equipment is usually available. Should the nurse-midwife or doctor determine that hospitalization is necessary to stabilize mother or baby, backup services are available in a hospital close to the birthing center.

The philosophy of birthing centers dictates that the family be left intact throughout the labor and delivery. To further encourage family cohesiveness, new mothers often go home within 12 hours of delivery. Many can be discharged as early as 2–3 hours after birth. Birth centers outside a hospital provide follow-up services by visiting nurses every few days after birth. The visiting nurse may check on the mother and infant on the day of birth, the day after birth, and then every other day for a week to ensure optimal postpartum adaptation. Most clients find the visiting nurse service to be quite helpful and supportive for the 6 weeks after delivery (Kieffer, 1980). The continuity of care provided by the birthing center staff also allows enough time to identify family needs and strengths. Staff support also aids the couple in coping with their new roles as parents.

Out-of-hospital birthing centers are primarily

staffed with nurse-midwives, although some obstetricians may also be involved. These practitioners can provide continuity of care during labor and delivery, either working alone or in collaboration with a physician. Frequently, nurse-midwives serve as administrators of the centers in addition to fulfilling educator and practitioner roles in the intrapartal and postpartal periods. Even though nurse-midwives provide a more continuous presence in the childbearing process than physicians do, nurse-midwife care in a birthing center is generally less expensive than the cost of prenatal care and delivery in a traditional hospital. Lower costs of birthing center services may result from lower liability insurance costs of nurse-midwives and also their lower salary (as compared to that of physicians). Nurse-midwives work in a center that is generally not equipped with the expensive, invasive machinery used in high-risk pregnancies (Melson, 1983). Frequently, a birthing bed is the most expensive piece of equipment found in the birthing center.

Disadvantages of Out-of-Hospital Birthing Centers

Many clients feel the psychologic benefits of the birthing center outweigh the potential risks of transfer to a hospital. However, clients of a center need to be aware that, should transfer be necessary, traveling to the hospital will be more uncomfortable in later stages of labor than if done in early labor. Criteria for transfer vary from birthing center to birthing center.

Many insurance policies cover births and baby care only if they occur in hospitals, not out-of-hospital birthing centers. Thus, the cost of having a baby in a nonhospital environment may ultimately be more expensive than a hospital birth.

Childbearing Centers

The Childbearing Center of the Maternity Center Association in New York is perhaps the best known out-of-hospital birthing center. The center was established in 1975 and is quickly becoming a model for other birthing centers in the United States. In fact, the enthusiasm for birthing centers is so great that in 1983 the National Association of Childbearing Centers was formed. This group writes standards and develops programs for those facililties interested in developing birthing centers.

With consumer satisfaction at a high level in most out-of-hospital birthing centers, nurses often enjoy their work in these centers. Many times these nurses are more independent than nurses who work in traditional labor and delivery units. Since alternative-birth-center nurses are employed relative to their abilities to provide individualized, complete, and caring approaches to clients, creative problem solving is often an expectation for role performance. Alternative-birth-center nurses must also demonstrate the good communication skills necessary to develop mutual trust and respect with their clients. Good communication skills are essential because the alternative-birth-center nurse frequently serves as a client advocate in a consumer's choice of a nontraditional mode of childbearing (Melson, 1983; see Appendix H).

IN-HOSPITAL BIRTHING CENTERS

Clients who choose to use a birthing center connected to a hospital also need to meet criteria to deliver in a nontraditional setting (Gillespie, 1981). Many birthing centers require that the client perceive herself as being healthy and informed, that the pregnancy and birth not be of high risk status, that attendance at prenatal classes be consistent, and that no regional or general anesthesia will be used in the center.

Unlike couples desiring home births, there also appears to be an acceptance of hospital obstetrical authority and the expertise of physicians among couples opting for an in-hospital birthing center experience (Klee, 1986). Figure 42-4 shows an in-hospital birthing room agreement that itemizes criteria for using the room. Part of the reason for these criteria may be that nurse-midwives, who handle only noncomplicated pregnancies, may be the primary caregivers in nontraditional birthing centers. Table 42-2 lists some contraindications for using a birthing room.

Advantages of In-Hospital Birthing Centers

The concept of birthing centers located in hospitals is rapidly gaining favor with consumers. Frequently, the calm and comprehensive approach to family health care taken by the nurse-midwife or nurse is consistent with the "homey", unhurried,

Since we realize that the Birthing Room facility can only be offered to those who are prepared and have a normal pregnancy, we the undersigned agree to the following requirements for acceptance to the Birthing Room program at Georgia Baptist Medical Center:

1. That we have read and understand the Criteria for Admission as stated on the accompanying sheet.
2. That we understand our doctor has final discretionary power as to our candidacy for this type of labor and delivery experience.
3. That the patient must have had adequate prenatal care with a minimum of six prenatal visits.
4. That we must attend Lamaze Prepared Childbirth Classes and must have completed at least four classes. It is preferred that we attend the classes offered by the hospital since they include special instruction regarding the Birthing Room.
5. That the father or one other support person approved by the physician, having attended the minimum required prenatal classes, must accompany the parturient in the Birthing Room.
6. That we agree to accept the use of fetal monitoring equipment if the physician or nurse in charge feels it is indicated.
7. That we agree to any transfer to the delivery room deemed by the doctor as necessary for the safety of mother and/or baby.
8. That the patient must receive minimal medication and be awake, aware and participating in her labor and delivery experience or be transferred to the regular labor unit.
9. That epidural anesthesia rules out delivery in a birthing room.
10. That should complications arise in the infant, this will take precedence over the union of the family and the infant will be removed to the appropriate nursery facility.
11. That visitors will not be allowed at any time in the labor and delivery area.
12. That we, as a family unit, may be transferred to an alternate room if the Birthing Room is needed.
13. That we agree to have our baby seen by a pediatrician within 48 hours.
14. That in order to qualify for early discharge we understand that both mother and baby must be examined and released by a physician.
15. That our hospital bill will be individualized according to services rendered.

Patient_____Date_____

Father_____Time_____

Support Person_____

Witnesses_____Date_____

FIGURE 42–4. An in-hospital birthing room agreement establishing criteria for use of the room.
SOURCE: Averitt (1980).

and intimate atmosphere of a birthing center. Overall, clients who have used birthing centers have perceived the experience as a positive one. Women who have delivered in birthing centers perceive their husbands as more supportive than women who have used the traditional hospital delivery room as the birthing environment (Cohen, 1982). In-hospital birthing centers provide emergency care, and personnel are readily available; this is a definite advantage over the home birth or the out-of-hospital birthing center.

Presently, many in-hospitals birthing rooms or centers exist in the United States. Frequently, these rooms, which have a homey, nonsterile decor, are situated close to a traditional labor and delivery unit. Couples who are in active labor and are not defined as being at high risk through the prenatal period can use the birthing rooms. Although hospitals vary in their definition of high-risk status, some hospitals will allow clients to remain in the birthing room even if they develop complications that would have prevented them from being admitted to the birthing room initially. Some of these complications may be oxytocin augmentation, epidural anesthesia, use of forceps, management of multiple gestation, and preeclampsia and eclampsia. Other hospitals transfer their clients in birthing rooms to traditional labor and delivery rooms as soon as a high-risk factor presents (see Table 42–3). The rate of transfer from the birthing room to a traditional labor and delivery suite can range from 8 to 25 percent (Klein and Westreich, 1983).

In one hospital, only 41 percent of women electing a birthing suite delivery actually delivered there. Transfers to traditional labor and delivery areas occurred due to premature rupture of membranes, pregnancy-induced hypertension, premature labor, postdates, meconium-stained fluid, or fetal heart rate declines (Saldana et al., 1983).

This wide range of rates of transfer from birthing room to traditional labor and delivery exists because different hospitals use different criteria for transfer. Also, in some hospitals, only one birthing

TABLE 42–2.	Contraindications for a Birthing-Room Delivery

Heart disease
Diabetes
Thrombophlebitis
Cephalopelvic disproportion
Rubella in pregnancy
Previous history of uterine surgery including cesarean section
A known history of genetic disorder that may be life threatening
An isoimmunized pregnancy
Anemia
Having a bleeding disorder of pregnancy–suggesive of placenta previa or abruptio placentae
Multiple births
Presentations other than vertex
Blood pressure readings of 140/90 or over in the last month of pregnancy or two consecutive readings more than 24 hours apart with elevations of 15 mm Hg systolic or 20 mm Hg diastolic
Membranes ruptured in excess of 24 hours prior to delivery
Membranes ruptured over 12 hours before onset of labor
Second stage no longer than 2 hours
Failure to progress at normal rate as stipulated in Friedman criteria
   Primigravida–first stage 2.5 cm/2 hours
   Multigravida—first stage 3 cm/2 hours
Premature labor
Postmature fetus as determined by the attending physician
Known drug or alcohol addiction
Smoking in excess of one pack of cigarettes per day
Hydramnios

SOURCE: Gillespie (1981).

TABLE 42–3.	Reasons for Transfer to Delivery Room

Fetal distress
Cord prolapse
Abruptio placentae or any other bleeding problem
Membranes ruptured more than 24 hours prior to delivery
Abnormal progress in labor as determined by Friedman criteria
Retained placenta
Epidural anesthesia
Excessive use of medication rendering parturient unable to participate in her delivery experience
Forceps required for rotation or delivery
Any other condition deemed by the physician to be hazardous to mother or baby

SOURCE: Averitt (1980).

room exists, and low-risk clients are, therefore, entitled to use it more than high-risk clients. However, if the staff consistently adheres to the philosophy of the birthing room, clients who are admitted to the hospital after the birthing room is occupied could be moved to a regular labor suite and still be allowed to deliver according to birthing-room policies. In addition, transfer may relate to staff motivation to use the birthing room. If a separate staff exists for the birthing room, generally that group will be more supportive of continued birthing room experience despite the development of complications. A highly motivated staff can perpetuate the philosophy of the birthing room and center with competent intrapartal monitoring in a standard labor and delivery suite.

The objective of the birthing room (Fig. 42–5) is to provide an atmosphere that meets the emotional needs of the family in labor. If the policies the couple desires are safe, there is no reason for the couple's wishes not to be granted. Although some physicians have resisted using the birthing room for various reasons (for example, the bed is too small or the carpeting on the floor makes the room unsterile), physicians have generally accepted delivery in the birthing room. Consumer response to the birthing room has been positive (Maloni, 1980). Most clients indicate they would repeat the experience if offered the chance. Kieffer (1980) submits that 33 percent of her birthing-center clients would have used home delivery if that option had existed for them. Thus, the birthing room and center concept is providing a safe method of delivery to a large part of the population. Unlike costs associated with home birth, which are generally not covered by insurance, in-hospital birthing-center costs are seen as appropriate for insurance coverage.

Disadvantages of In-Hospital Birthing Centers

Because delivery occurs in a hospital, birthing center births are generally covered by insurance. However, the setting of the birth in a hospital may mean that couples will find unnecessary technological intervention and policies that are used because these interventions and policies are accepted in the hospital environment. Staff in the birthing center may also work in traditional labor and delivery units. This may be a disadvantage, because these workers may not provide a supportive atmosphere consistent with the philosophy of natural, nontraditional childbirth.

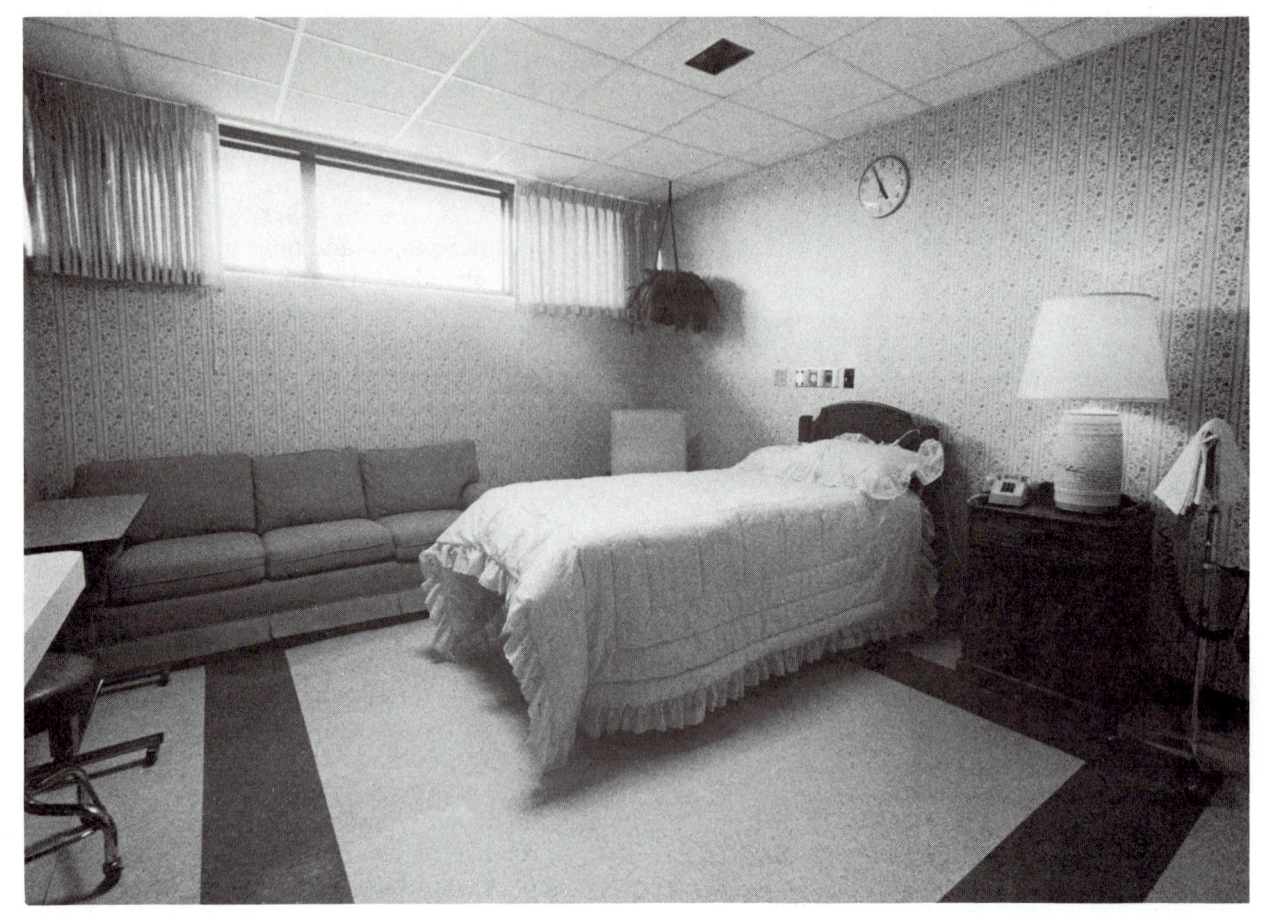

FIGURE 42–5. Alternative birthing room in a hospital.

Preparation for Use of a Birthing Center

Many hospitals schedule an orientation to the birthing center and birthing room for couples planning a delivery in that setting. The philosophy of the room, client consent forms, criteria for use, and transfer to a traditional labor and delivery unit are discussed. Once approved for use of the room, clients frequently have to receive permission from their doctor to use the birthing room. Once permission is received, arrangements can be made for a pediatrician to examine the baby shortly after birth and provide continued follow-up. Many facilities offer a film on birthing-room delivery so couples can plan for their own delivery experience and responses. Consistent attendance at prenatal classes is expected of both parents for birthing-room use, because couples need to be aware of what will happen and must be prepared to intervene effectively during the labor and delivery.

In many cases, couples will be quite independent in meeting and controlling their own physical and emotional needs during labor. In other situations, couples may request frequent nursing and medical assessment to effectively progress through labor. Most nurses in birthing-room environments are flexible and willing to meet each couple's individual needs and approach to their labor and delivery in the birthing room. Usually, a cooperative arrangement between the client and health care staff is evident, so that the experience is mutually satisfying, stimulating, and memorable to both couple and health care practitioner. Since many clients stay in the hospital only 24 hours after delivery, the costs of the birthing-room experience are less than that of a traditional labor and delivery. The professional fee of about $1200 is typical for use of a birthing room. This can be contrasted to the cost of $1700 or more for a typical 12 hour stay after labor and delivery.

Regardless of whether childbirth occurs in a hospital, in a birth center located in or outside a hospital, or at home, consumers need to know both the positive and negative aspects of all birth settings (see Table 42–4). Only with full information can consumers make safe and wise choices in the childbearing process.

TABLE 42-4. *Advantages and Disadvantages of Various Approaches to Childbirth*

Approach	Advantages	Disadvantages
Home birth	1. Mother in a familiar, supportive place—does not have to be moved 2. Avoids unfamiliar and/or unsupportive attendants 3. Family and friends can be present at any point and for any amount of time 4. Least chance of medical intervention 5. Best environment for bonding	1. May require transfer to hospital 2. Medically trained individuals to assist in birth difficult to find 3. Emergency equipment not readily available 4. Insurance eligibility varies
Out-of-hospital birthing center	1. Individualized care 2. Labor and delivery in one room 3. Minimal intervention by staff 4. Parents and baby not separated after birth 5. Early discharge	1. May require transfer to hospital, posing risks for mother and baby 2. Only low-risk patients who remain low-risk can deliver in this setting 3. Unfamiliar environment 4. Insurance coverage uncertain
In-hospital birthing room/center	1. Presence of husband, friend, or relative throughout 2. Emergency care immediately available 3. Opportunity to have a professional stay throughout labor and delivery 4. Labor and delivery in same room 5. Emphasis on normal rather than emergency aspects of care 6. Warm, relaxed atmosphere 7. Comprehensive health insurance coverage	1. Possibility of unnecessary technologic intervention or unwanted hospital routines 2. Care by regular hospital staff who may not share philosophy of birthing-room attendants after birth 3. Risks of in-hospital infections 4. Possible limitations of visiting hours
Traditional (hospital) birth	1. Widely available, traditional, accepted 2. Qualified physicians 3. Equipped to handle high-risk patients and complicated labor and delivery 4. Resuscitation and infant intensive care for newborns 5. Hospital staff give mother physical help, rest, and support 6. Limited visiting hours may keep new mother from becoming overtired 7. Comprehensive insurance coverage	1. Greatest likelihood of routine use of medical intervention 2. Least control over environment 3. No choice on position for delivery 4. Unfamiliar labor attendants 5. Likely to remain in bed 6. Customary separation of mother and baby after birth

SOURCE: Gillespie (1981).

LEBOYER BIRTH

Leboyer delivery is a particular approach to childbirth, rather than a method intentionally at variance from traditional ways of childbearing. In the Leboyer approach, focus is placed on decreasing trauma to the newborn at birth. The newborn perceives excessive stimulation as pain. Newborn trauma is diminished by enhancing the maternal–infant bond and by eliminating adverse environmental stimuli at birth and shortly thereafter (Leboyer, 1975). The essence of the Leboyer approach is a gentle but controlled birth that satisfies the physiologic and emotional needs of both mother and infant (Gimbel and Nocon, 1977).

The labor of a Leboyer birth proceeds much like the labor of any natural birth. Fetal heart monitoring is sometimes used, and frequently there is reliance on the Friedman labor curve, both indices of fetal outcome. The Leboyer approach stresses patience, communication, and understanding. With these personal characteristics of the people involved in the delivery, the infant can be delivered with a minimum of intervention. Qualities such as patience, communication, and understanding can also decrease parental anxiety and increase the potential for a strong parental–infant bond (Gimbel and Nocon, 1977).

Once delivery is imminent, however, the birthing atmosphere is much quieter and calmer than in a usual delivery. For example, the lights in the delivery room are dimmed, and only lighting essential for a safe delivery is used. Forceps are sometimes used and an episiotomy may be performed. The cord is clamped once the pulsations cease. To introduce the infant to the extrauterine world gently, the infant is placed on the mother's abdomen (skin to skin) after birth and is gently stroked by either the doctor or the nurse-midwife. The father may then bathe the baby in a tub of warm water (about 98°F for 3–6 min), to simulate the uterine environment and to replace lost heat. Once bathed, the infant is dried, diapered, and left alone for a time in a quiet, protected place. The timing of Leboyer activities is based on the baby's needs, which are assessed jointly by the obstetrician and the parents. Intervention is applied only when necessary, for maternity complications increase with intervention and force during labor and delivery (Steer, 1950).

Infant responses to the Leboyer approach include less hand tension, less trembling and blinking in the first 15 min of life, and greater alertness, compared to these responses in babies delivered in the traditional mode (Oliver and Oliver, 1978). However, further research on the long-term effects of the Leboyer approach is needed to support the positive aspects of the method. For example, one might ask what effect this approach has on parental–infant attachment and on the child's intellectual abilities and mental health later in life.

VAGINAL BIRTH AFTER CESAREAN BIRTH

The concept of vaginal birth after cesarean birth (VBAC) is relevant to the alternative birthing movement. For many years, the adage "once a section, always a section" has been held by the health care community. Today's concern with liability and maternal and infant mortality and morbidity has further perpetuated this adage. However, many clients and their families now desire a more natural, family-focused delivery if indications are satisfactory for a vaginal delivery.

Research presently supports that the risk of attempting a VBAC is minimal with closely supervised clients (Miller and Sutler, 1985). Additionally, if the condition indicating the first cesarean does not exist, labor is progressing within normal limits, and infant weight is under 4000 g, chances are that the client will be successful in achieving a VBAC (Whiteside, Mahan, and Cook, 1983).

Emphasis is now being placed on the need to reexamine beliefs about when a cesarean is indicated. There has been a great increase in the number of candidates for a trial labor. Today more than 2 percent of all childbearing women are candidates for cesarean due to primiparous breech presentation, labor longer than 24 hours, pregnancy-induced hypertension (PIH), or uterine dysfunction. In fact, many hospitals are reporting cesarean birth rates of 12–15 percent; these rates often reflect primary, low cervical transverse cesarean deliveries. Economic costs also need to be considered–abdominal surgery costs more than vaginal delivery. In many cases, extensive and costly prenatal testing (for example, sonography and amniocentesis) must precede a cesarean birth to validate fetal gestation and a low probability of respiratory distress syndrome. Additionally, the postdelivery costs of a cesarean birth are higher than those for a vaginal delivery. Neonatal intensive care charges must be considered–a scheduled cesarean birth may deliver a premature infant and have considerable impact on a family's psychosocial and economic support systems.

Vaginal birth after cesarean birth is possible because many of today's cesarean births are of the low cervical transverse type, which has less potential for uterine rupture than the classical incision of cesarean birth used many years ago (Gibbs, 1980). Women who have previously delivered by low cervical transverse cesarean can deliver vaginally without complications if they are properly monitored during labor.

The needs of couples who plan a vaginal birth after cesarean birth are much the same as the needs of any couples experiencing pregnancy (Shearer, 1982). Couples who plan a vaginal birth after a previous cesarean birth need to know birthing and relaxation techniques as well as what happens during labor and delivery. They may need to mourn the loss of a previous opportunity for an ideal birth and to understand the reasons for the prior cesarean. Couples also need to understand why a vaginal birth after cesarean birth is now possible. Frequently, a childbirth class can replace the couples' fears and concerns with knowledge. A class instructor who is available to meet couples' unique informational and emotional needs can do much to make the vaginal birth after cesarean birth a success. Often the instructor can help the couple increase trust and confidence in their abilities and their health care practitioner's competency. Couples who are in control of their labor and delivery and who have thought deeply about the personal meaning of the vaginal birth after cesarean birth can communicate their needs to their physician and nurse. This communication makes the experience less anxiety-provoking for everyone involved (Shearer, 1982).

OTHER ALTERNATIVE BIRTHING CONCEPTS

Maternal Position in Labor

Until recently, most women labored in the supine position in bed. The supine position makes it easier to inspect the perineum, to auscultate the fetal heart tones (FHTs), and to maintain asepsis. However, the supine position has been called the worst position that can be used for labor. This position may cause maternal hypotensive syndrome, abnormal fetal presentation, and delayed labor. Various research studies have noted increased fetal acidosis and bradycardia with a maternal supine position during labor (Caldeyro-Barcia, 1975).

More research is being done on maternal positions and their effect on whether labors are more rapid, easier, less dangerous to mother and baby, and more effective. In fact, it may be most effective to vary positions during labor (sitting, walking, lateral position, and standing) at the discretion of the laboring client. Some studies indicate that multigravidas change positions more selectively, particularly in late labor, as compared to primigravidas due to different perceived discomforts of the two groups (Carlson et al., 1986). Contractions may be more intense and effective in dilating the cervix in the standing as compared to the supine position (Mendez-Bauer et al., 1975). Contractions are perceived as less intense in a sitting position than in a lateral position during labor (Roberts, 1979). Although most women still labor on their backs because physicians prefer it, women are being encouraged to rest in lateral or upright positions during labor. Lateral and upright positions have been found to increase venous return to the heart and to increase the effectiveness of uterine contractions, thus shortening the length of labor. The maternal sitting position allows for stronger bearing down pressure and often a shorter stage 2 for many laboring women (Chen, Aizaka, and Kigawa, 1987). Overall, maternal positioning during labor should be based on maternal comfort, uterine contractility, and cardiovascular considerations to ensure an optimal childbirth outcome (Roberts et al., 1984).

Some studies have found that ambulation during labor decreases discomfort and so can decrease the need for maternal analgesia. Pain perception is decreased with ambulation because pain control is easier with the psychologic benefits of ambulation. Ambulant labor mothers have also been found to have shorter labors, less need for labor augmentation, and better infant Apgars than mothers who remained in bed with labor (Flynn et al., 1978).

If ambulant labors are to be encouraged in the future because of potential benefits to mother and baby, radiotelemetry or ambulant fetal heart monitoring must be developed. At the present time, great strides have been made in the science of radiotelemetry. Machines have been developed that allow clients to be monitored in labor while they are up and out of bed. Portable monitoring devices prevent maternal perception of being "hooked up" to a bedside fetal monitoring machine. A bedside machine severely limits a laboring mother's perception of control and of a natural delivery. It is interesting, however, that in some instances, only 45 percent of telemetry clients may elect to be out of bed with their portable devices during labor, and those clients choose to do so only for short periods (Calvert, Newcombe, and Hibbard, 1982).

Maternal Positions for Delivery

Various changes have occurred recently in the delivering positions of clients. Many birthing centers are now encouraging their clients to squat for the second stage of labor. Squatting allows the pelvis to spread. For high-risk mothers, squatting can be considered essential to hasten infant delivery. The sitting, semisitting, and lithotomy positions, with legs flexed to the abdomen, are also advocated in the second stage of labor. These positions provide some of the advantages of squatting, which utilizes the beneficial effect of gravity in improving the efficiency of labor (Myles, 1971). Squatting may also allow gradual stretching of the perineal floor and decrease the incidence of episiotomies in many women. Although factors such as maternal parity, analgesia/anesthesia, and infant weight are considered, maternal position does affect perineal outcome in most women (Nodine and Roberts, 1987).

Some women have positively evaluated delivery of their baby from a birthing chair. Anatomically, the chair allows gravity to assist in the birth; many women feel more comfortable sitting with their labors and indeed find their labor maximized due to the sitting position. Recently, several studies have examined the effect of delivery in the birthing chair. In one sample of primiparous women, there was no significant differences in the average length of the second stage of labor, average duration of bearing down, or the average amount of blood loss in women who delivered in the chair and in the traditional lithotomy position. The rate of episiotomies, forceps, lacerations, and hemorrhoids was similar in both groups, although perineal edema was statistically greater in the birthing chair group (Cottrell and Shannahan, 1986).

Kneeling while leaning forward on the knees can also aid in rotation of the fetal head in the pelvis. The kneeling posture may provide benefits of precultural behavior: kneeling simulates the praying position and may help induce a relaxed but committed state. For preterm deliveries, kneeling may be helpful to decrease oxygen consumption and muscle activity of the client and so increase oxygenation to the fetus (Odent, 1981).

A darkened setting is sometimes favored for labor and delivery. Darkness decreases sensory stimulation and aids labor. Often laboring, and even delivering, in a pool of water is helpful, because water decreases inhibitions, increases dreaming and relaxation, and helps the mother attain altered consciousness. Water may also be a symbol of motherhood and comfort. Many women become so comfortable in their pool of water that they deliver in the water. Recently, several Russian women have delivered in large pools of water with obstetric guidance. This underwater birthing is not currently widely practiced in the United States. However, with the psychologic and perhaps physiologic benefits of in-water birthing, childbearing in that alternative setting may become quite acceptable in the future (Odent, 1981).

SUMMARY

Alternative birthing methods and alternative birth centers have become popular because they have met the needs and desires for a family-centered childbirth experience. In an attempt to more satisfactorily meet childbearing couples' needs and to provide the safety of the hospital environment, more hospitals are establishing family-centered maternity care units. In this age in which the concepts of self, family, natural birth, and control are predominant, health care professionals must creatively provide care attuned to client needs. Nurse-midwives have traditionally offered complete, family-focused maternity care in uncomplicated pregnancies. This family-centered approach taken by nurse-midwives will undoubtedly increase future demand for nurse-midwives by childbearing couples.

In such a significant event as childbearing, consumers have the right to a safe and satisfying experience. By taking creative and individual approaches to their clients, nurses can become leaders in guiding consumers to better meet their own needs.

REFERENCES

American College of Obstetricians and Gynecologists. 1981. *Alternative birthing centers: A survey and bibliography*. Washington, D.C.: American College of Obstetricians and Gynecologists.

Anderson, S.; Bauwens, E.; and Warner, E. 1978. The choice of home birth in a metropolitan county in Arizona. *J. Obstet. Gynecol. Neonatal Nurs.* 7(2):41–45.

Asby, V. A., and Roebuck, R. N. 1979. Considering patient-centered obstetric care: Why and how? *J. Obstet. Gynecol. Neonatal Nurs.* 8:297–301.

Caldeyro-Barcia, R. 1975. Supine called worst position during labor and delivery. *Ob. Gyn. News.* p. 1.

Calvert, J. P.; Newcombe, R. G.; and Hibbard, B. M. 1982. An assessment of radiotelemetry in the monitoring of labor. *Brit. J. Obstet. Gynecol.* 89:285–291.

Campbell, R., et al. 1984. Home births in England and Wales, 1979: Perinatal mortality according to intended place of delivery. *Brit. Med. J.* 289:721–724.

Carlson, B., and Summer, P. 1976. Hospital "at home" delivery: A celebration. *J. Obstet. Gynecol. Neonatal Nurs.* 5(2):22–23.

Carlson, J. M. et al. 1986. Maternal position during parturition in normal labor. *Obstet. Gynecol.* 68(4):443–447.

Chen, S. Z.; Aisaka, K.; and Kigawa, T. 1987. Effects of sitting position on uterine activity during labor. *Obstet. Gynecol.* 69(1):67–73.

Cohen, R. L. 1982. A comparative study of women choosing two different childbirth alternatives. *Birth: Issues in Perinatal Care and Education.* 9:13–19.

Cottrell, B. H., and Shannahan, M. D. 1986. Effect of the birth chair on duration of second stage labor and maternal outcome. *Nurs. Res.* 35(6):364–367.

Devitt, N. 1977. The transition from home to hospital birth in the United States 1930–1960. *Birth Family J.* 4:47–58.

Dingley, E. 1980. The place of birth. *Perinatal Press.* 4:61.

Dorfman, D. 1982. Hey, Mom, babies are a bargain! *New York Daily News.* p. 69.

Ernst, E. 1979. The evolving practice of nurse-midwifery. *Health Law Project Libr. Bull.* 20–23.

Estes, M. 1978. A home obstetric service with expert consultation and backup. *Birth Family J.* 5: 151–157.

Flanagan, J. A. 1986. Childbirth in the eighties: What next? When alternatives become mainstream. *J. Nurse-Midwifery.* 31(4):194–199.

Findley, P. 1934. *The story of childbirth.* New York: Doubleday.

Flynn, A.; Kelly, J.; Hollins, G.; and Lynch, P. F. 1978. Ambulation in labor. *Birt. Med. J.* 2:591–593.

Gibbs, C. E. 1980. Planned vaginal births following cesarean section. *Clin. Obstet. Gynecol.* 23:507–515.

Gillespie, S. A. 1981. Childbirth in the 1980s: What are the options? *Issues Health Care Women* 3:101–128.

Gimbel, J., and Nocon, J. J. 1977. The physiological basis for the Leboyer approach to childbirth. *J. Obstet. Gynecol. Neonatal Nurs.* 6(1):11–15.

Herman, E.; Miller-Klein, V.; and Ventre, F. 1979. A survey of current trends in home birth. In *Compulsory hospitalization or freedom of choice in childbirth,* Vol. 2, eds. D. Stewart and L. Stewart. Marble Hill, Mo.: NAPSAC.

Hogan, K. A. 1980. Home versus hospital delivery: Issues and perspectives. *Issues Health Care Women.* 2(3–4):11–24.

Holt, H. 1982/1983. Debate: Where to give birth. Hospital by doctor. *Childbirth Educator.* 2(2):53–58.

Kieffer, M. J. 1980. The birthing room concept at Phoenix Memorial Hospital. Part II: Consumer satisfaction during one year. *J. Obstet. Gynecol. Neonatal Nurs.* 9:155–159.

Klee, L. 1980. Home away from home: The alternative birth center. *Soc. Sci. Med.* 23(1):9–16.

Klein, M., and Westreich, R. 1983. Birth room transfer and procedure rates—what do they tell about the settings? *Birth: Issues in Pernatal Care and Education.* 10:93–97.

Leboyer, F. 1975. *Birth without violence.* New York: Alfred A. Knopf.

Lichtman, R. 1982/83. Debate: Where to give birth. Hospital by midwife. *Childbirth Educator.* 2(2):53–58.

Lieberman, J. 1976. Childbirth practices: From darkness into light. *J. Obstet. Gynecol. Neonatal Nurs.* 5(3):41–45.

Lubic, R. W. 1983. Childbirthing centers: Delivering more for less. *Am. J. Nurs.* 83:1053–1058.

Maloni, J. A. 1980. The birthing room: Some insights into parents' experiences. *MCN.* 5:314–319.

Melson, J. 1983. The role of the nurse in alternative birth settings. In *Handbook of maternal–newborn nursing,* eds. K. A. Buckley and N. W. Kulb. New York: John Wiley & Sons.

Mendez-Bauer, C., et al. 1975. Effects of standing position on spontaneous uterine contractility and other aspects of labor. *J. Perinatal Med.* 3:89–100.

Miller, C. F., and Sutter, C. S. 1985. Vaginal birth after cesarean. *J. Obstet. Gynecol. Neonatal Nurs.* 14(5): 383–389.

Myles, M. F. 1971. *Textbook for midwives.* 7th ed. London: Churchill Livingston.

NAACOG. 1987. *Professional liability series.* Washington, D.C.: NAACOG.

Nodine, P. M., and Roberts, J. 1987. Factors associated with perineal outcome during childbirth. *J. Nurse-Midwifery.* 32(3):123–130.

Odent, M. 1981. The evolution of obstetrics at Pithiviers. *Birth Family J.* 8:7–15.

Oliver, C., and Oliver, G. M. 1978. Gentle birth: Its safety and its effect on neonatal behavior. *J. Obstet. Gynecol. Neonatal Nurs.* 7(5):35–40.

Patterson, K., and Peterson, V. 1980. The alternative birth centers movement in the San Francisco and Bay area. *J. Nurse-Midwifery.* 25(2):23–27.

Richie, C. A., and Swanson, A. B. 1976. Childbirth outside the hospital: The resurgence of home and clinic deliveries. *MCN.* 1:375–377.

Roberts, J. E. 1979. *The effect of maternal position on labor.* Unpublished doctoral dissertation, University of Illinois.

Roberts, J. E., et al. 1984. Effects of lateral recumbency and sitting on the first stage of labor. *J. Repro. Med.* 29(7):477–481.

Saldana, L. R., et al. 1983. Home birth: Negative implications derived from a hospital-based birthing suite. *Soc. Med. J.* 76(2):170–173.

Samuels, M. 1981. Considering the choices. *Family J.* 1:6–10.

Schneider, D. 1986. Planned out-of-hospital births. New Jersey, 1978–80. *Soc. Sci. Med.* 23(10):1011—1015.

Schramm, W. F.; Barnes, D. E.; and Bakewell, J. M. 1987. Neonatal mortality in Missouri home births 1978–84. *Am. J. Public Health.* 77(8):930–935.

Shearer, E. C. 1982. Education for vaginal birth after cesarean. *Birth: Issues in Perinatal Care and Education.* 9:31–34.

Shearer, J. M. 1985. Five year prospective study of risk of booking for a home birth in Essex. *Brit. Med. J.* 291(6507):1478–1480.

Shy, K. K.; Frost, F.; and Ullom, J. 1980. Out-of-hospital delivery in Washington state, 1975 to 1977. *Am. J. Obstet. Gynecol.* 137:547–552.

Sieden, A. 1981. Alternatives in childbirth. In *Health care of women: A nursing perspective,* eds. C. Fogel and N. Woods. St. Louis: Mosby.

Steer, C. M. 1950. Effect of type of delivery on future childbearing. *Am. J. Obstet. Gynecol.* 60:395–400.

White, G. 1977. A comparison of home and hospital deliveries based on 25 years of experience with both. *J. Repro. Med.* 19:291–292.

White, W. G. 1983. Where to give birth: Out of hospital. *Childbirth Educator.* 2(4):33–34, 36.

Whiteside, D. C.; Mahan, C. S.; and Cook, J. C. 1983. Factors associated with successful vaginal delivery after cesarean section. *J. Repro. Med.* 28(11):785–788.

43

Caring in Perinatal Nursing

BEHAVIORAL OBJECTIVES

Upon completion of this chapter, the reader should be able to:

- Define caring, including the components of empathy and self-understanding.

- Discuss nursing as an art and a science.

- Relate the effects of science and technology to concerns about the dehumanization of the patient as voiced by the consumer.

- Discuss the patient's responsibility in compliance with medical regimen.

- Relate accountability and advocacy to the professional role of the nurse.

Change is a part of life. Change has a way of accummulating around us, sometimes without our even noticing it. There are changes in society, the health care system, and maternity nursing. There is a certain amount of stability in the familiar, a certain amount of security when things stay the same. A situation that does not change yields a sense of knowledge about how to react and how to respond. Change upsets the status quo, interrupts homeostasis, and can lead to disorganization and fear. Therefore, it is within the nature of human beings to resist change rather than to risk an upset in this balance of things as they are.

The period of pregnancy and childbearing is a time of change and adaptation for the patient/client and family. The nurse needs to be an effective change agent. The childbearing couple looks to the nurse for encouragement, support, knowledge, and nurturance. The perinatal patient needs understanding and acceptance and will seek to avoid the nurse who is dominant, harsh, or rigid. The more person-centered the nurse, the more supportive the nurse seems to the patient. An effective change agent understands that the patient's cooperation and participation are needed if change is to be the result.

The nurse can be instrumental in assisting the family to have a stable beginning by being sensitive, warm, and caring. The nurse who seeks to deliver nursing care that conveys concern for the patient as a human being implements caring.

CARING AND NURSING EDUCATION

A goal of nursing education is to teach nursing *care* that centers on the patient as a human being having individual needs. Person-centered nursing care treats another individual, the patient, as the "subject" rather than the "object" of care. *Subject* implies that the patient is the reason for the nurse's being. To consider the patient as subject places the patient and nurse on a horizontal plane and connotes a working with the patient. *Object* is less personal and places nurse and patient on a vertical plane, with the nurse doing *for* rather than *with* in the delivery of care. It is hoped that by the time the student becomes a graduate professional nurse he or she will have internalized and actualized the philosophy of person-centered care in the delivery of nursing care.

There must be a point at which idealism intersects realism. The concept of care in nursing can exist in practice as well as theory. Even in the complex health care system of today, with all of the routine tasks that are necessary to "get the job done", nurses can find ways to develop a closeness with the patient. No one can better close the gap that exists between the philosophic placement of the patient at the center of nursing care and actual practice than nurses themselves.

Direct involvement with the patient is important in any area of nursing, but particularly in perinatal nursing. The nurse's role in prenatal care involves motivating couples to register early for care and guiding them in their selection of doctor and hospital. Helping to make each visit as satisfying as possible for the mother is a nursing opportunity. Acceptance of the parents lays a foundation for the professional nurse–parent relationship from the first contact throughout the childbearing years. Open communication with the couple should be maintained from the beginning of the pregnancy through the postpartum period (Fig. 43–1).

The nurse serves as the link that keeps the chain of communication intact. Skill in communication techniques is essential in obtaining a thorough assessment upon which to develop a plan of care for the patient. To create a climate of trust that will lead to the appropriate planning of care, the nurse must communicate human warmth and caring. This involves the nurse's putting himself or herself in the patient's place. Carl Rogers refers to the need for the health professional to become "psychologically sensitive". He writes: ". . . if I can be sensitively aware, then the likelihood is great that I can form a helping relationship toward another" (Rogers, 1961, p. 51). To be humanistic is to be available with all of one's being to the whole being of the patient during the time spent in direct contact with that particular patient. In this type of relationship, the nurse fosters respect for the dignity and intrinsic worth of the human being.

HISTORICAL PERSPECTIVE

The Paternalistic Focus

Historically, nursing was taught in the hospital as an apprenticeship. Nurses were under the control of doctors, and there was a strong paternalistic focus. Since nurses were in a position of submission to the doctors, they were not expected to make any decisions regarding the patient's care and were, in fact, encouraged not to do so. Emphasis was placed on how to deliver skillful nursing care and not on the underlying reasons why. Nurses were taught primarily diagnosis and treatment of disease by doctors from medical textbooks. The medical focus was on *cure* of the patient, not *care* of the patient. In the paternalistic mode nurses were not encouraged to be creative or independent, and they lacked the power to implement change.

In the United States, nursing education continued to take place in hospital-based diploma nursing programs until the 1940s. At that time a movement to transfer nursing education from the hospital to the university began. In the universities, nurses began to receive a broader education in

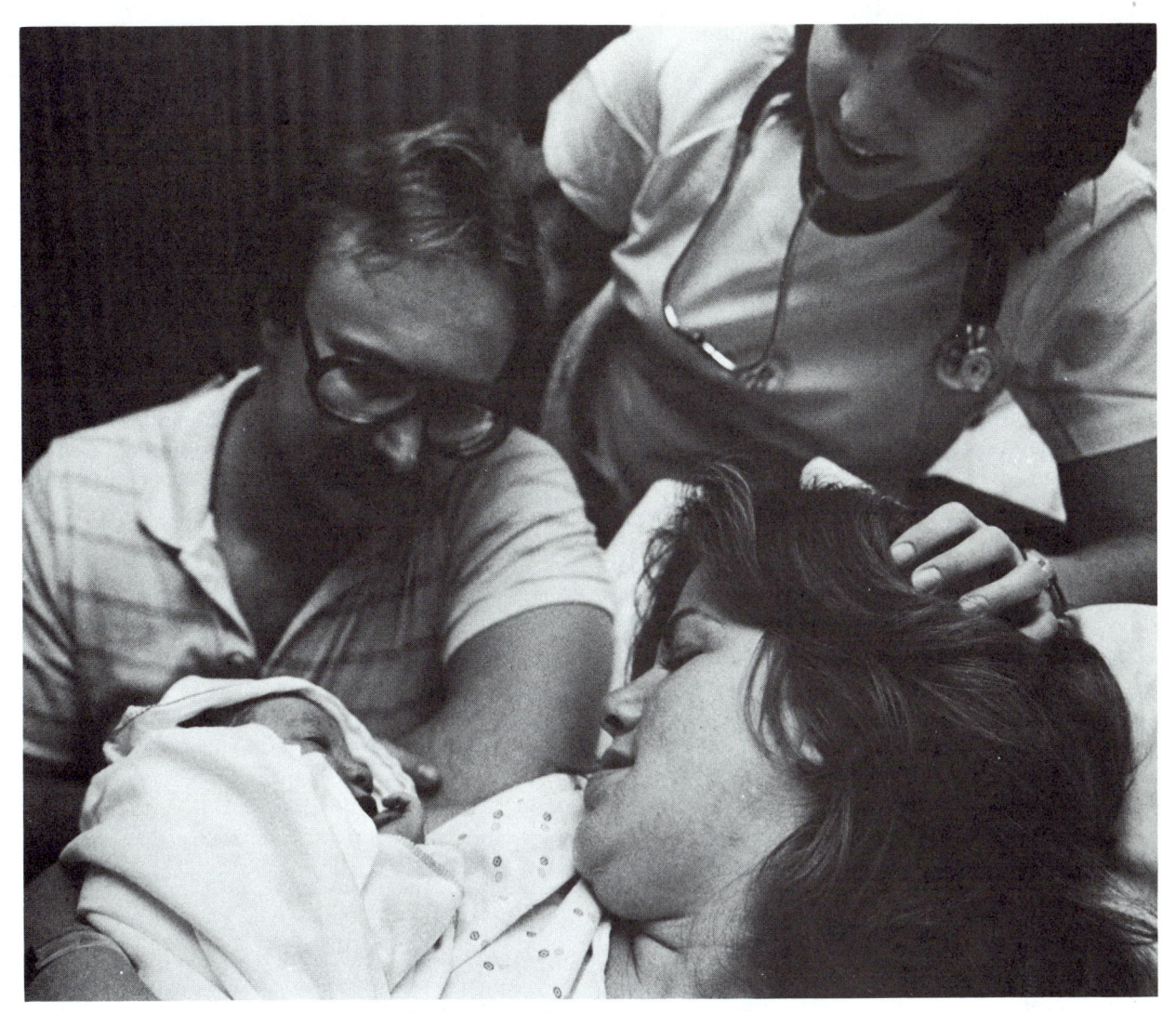

FIGURE 43-1. Nurse with newly delivered mother and father in postpartum recovery room.

the physical, social, and behavioral sciences and in the humanities. Nurse educators, educationally prepared at the graduate level in the sciences and arts, began to replace doctors in the role of teaching student nurses.

Science and Technology

In order to function within a highly technical health care system, nurses are required to take more and more science courses in their college curricula. Today's technology has the nurse engaged in activities that require interactions with instruments and equipment. These technical activities demand time and often seem to take precedence over the patient's personal needs and concerns. Consumers of health care voice complaints that nurses are impersonal in their manner toward them, and the patients feel they are becoming depersonalized within the system.

There are nursing functions that hold the potential to dehumanize patients. Objectivity and specialization have been isolated as two contributing factors. *Objectivity* has been described as a separation of thoughts from feelings, while *specialization* emphasizes a division or fragmentation of labor. These two factors are capable of taking the focus of nursing away from the human dimension of patient care (Pilette, 1980). The nurse's use of objectivity can become a protective defense to deny his or her own humanness, leading to a false, or counterfeit, way of dealing with personal emotions. Specialization may tend to decrease the human quality of wholeness by dividing patients into compartments of organs and disease processes. Nurses need to guard against following any nursing activity to become routine, fragmented, or mechanical.

Technologic advances are influencing the care of perinatal patients. Since the need for electronic monitoring of the state of the mother and fetus is so prevalent, it is important for the nurse to learn how to care for the patient despite the machine (Fig. 43–2). Balancing the technology of care with the human dimension of care is a challenge.

Nursing as an Art and a Science

As early as the 1890s, Florence Nightingale stressed that the patient was to be the central focus of care. She advocated an organized, practical, and scientific base as necessary for the delivery of patient care, but the patient as a human being was to be given primary attention. She conceptualized nursing as a human art form concerned with "living bodies and minds and feelings of both body and mind" (Seymer, 1954, p. 365). Nursing as a science has been derived from empirical research. The art of nursing utilizes this research in service to man (Rogers, 1970). The science of nursing is grounded in theory. The patient receives knowledgeable, safe, competent care from educated nurses. The art of nursing is the manner in which that care is delivered to the patient, making the patient feel cared for in a personal way.

Nurses have the responsibility to be prepared at the highest possible educational level to deliver patient care. "As a university subject, nursing must achieve a delicate balance between scientific knowledge and humanistic practice behaviors" (Watson, 1985, p. 3). The patient should be kept at the center of focus regardless of how technical health care delivery becomes. In addressing the dilemma of providing personable nursing care that is sensitive to human needs while operating in a technologic society, Giuffra (1980, p. 17) writes:

> The human being, the person, must harness technology and not be driven and determined by it. It is not enough to learn what is expected of one, what behaviors one must perform, what chores are attendant to working with this person or this disease or this piece of equipment. If that is all one does, the nurse becomes a robot and in time the machinery

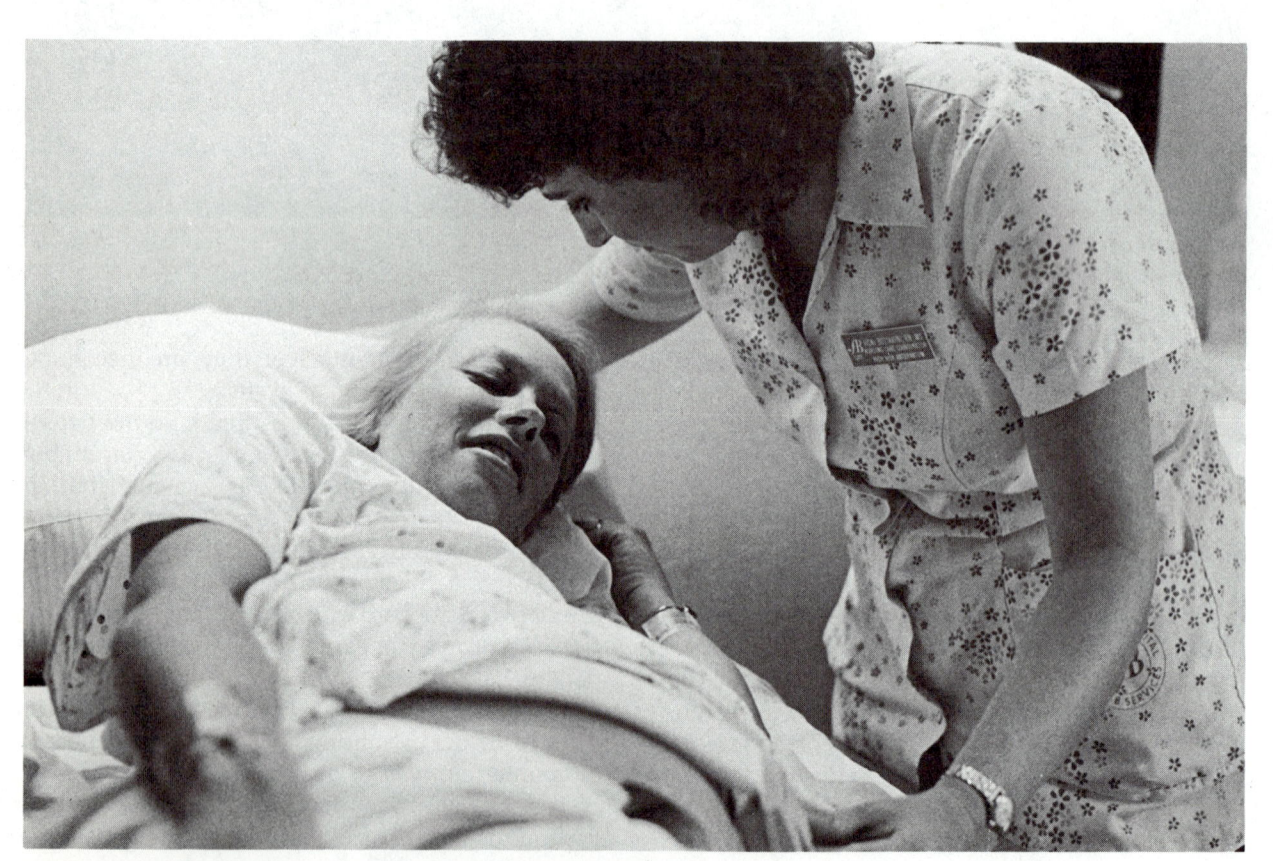

FIGURE 43–2. The nurse is responsible for focusing on the patient despite the machine.

becomes primary, the human is relegated to second or third place.

Caring as Human Sensitivity

Empathy and knowledge of self are two central components in the personalization of health care (see Fig. 43–3). The relationship of the health professional's understanding of self is parallel to the ability to understand and respond to the humanness of the patient.

Empathy is a construct that implies an understanding of the other person, of being able to take the other person's view, of being able to accept the other person as one who is in the process of becoming – one who is changing, not fixed or already shaped by the past.

Empathic understanding in the therapeutic personality is described as the ability to "sense the client's private world as if it were your own, but without ever losing the 'as if' quality" (Rogers, 1957, p. 99). Empathy is expressed by the nurse who understands the effects of long-term hospitalization on the antepartum patient. A sensitive nurse will find "new" projects for this patient or will refer her to occupational therapy so that she can be engaged in appropriate activities. During labor this nurse will spend extra time comforting and being with the patient who is alone. A sensitive nurse caring for a baby in the intensive care nursery will make frequent trips to the mother's room to give her

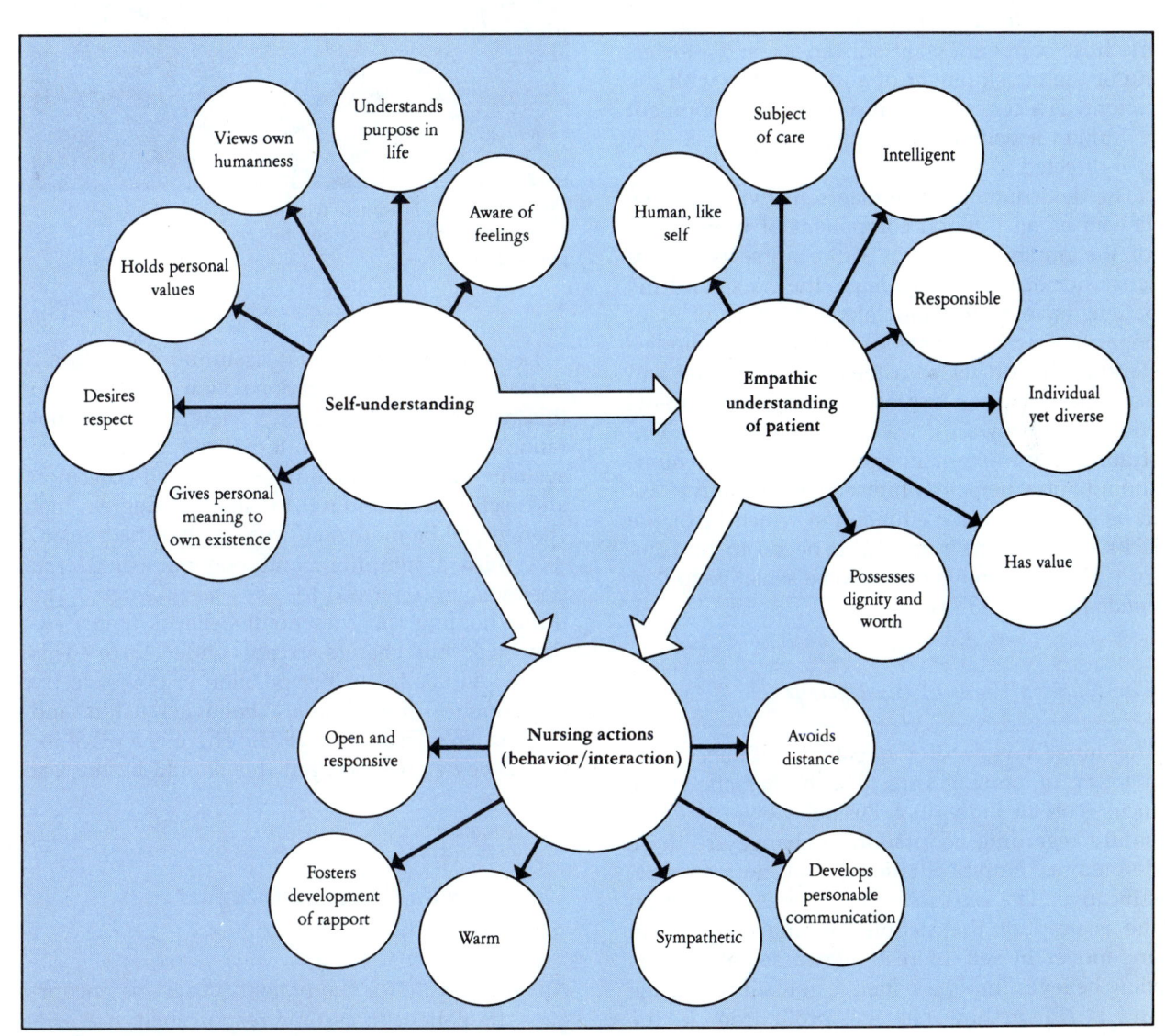

FIGURE 43–3. Characteristics of a caring nurse with resultant nursing actions.

reports about the progress of her sick baby. This nurse is aware of the parents' need to interact with their premature baby and will encourage their participation in the infant's care. If distance prevents the parents from visiting the baby frequently, this nurse will encourage phone calls to the nursery so that they can get current information about the infant's weight gain, feedings, and behavior.

Self-understanding implies an increasing awareness of one's personal values that affect the delivery of patient care. A growing understanding of self affects the nurse's perception of the patient's humanness – that is, the patient's dignity, worth, individuality, and diversity. Empathy can be evidenced by certain behaviors and interactions, such as warmth, responsiveness, understanding, helpfulness, and supportiveness. Interactions that tend to be characteristic of empathy are those of openness, attentiveness, and a fostering of the development of a relationship with the patient. The conceptualization of the development of human sensitivity as depicted in Fig. 43–3 is goal-directed.

The development of human sensitivity must be viewed as an integral component of preparation for the nursing process. "If the nurse is able to sense her or his own feelings, the nurse and the patient have a common reference point of emotional experience" (Watson, 1979, p. 28). In understanding his or her own feelings about grief and loss, the nurse can express sadness with parents when their baby dies. The nurse may cry, demonstrating involvement in the situation. The nurse should know herself or himself well enough to ask to be excused from a situation in which he or she lacks control. The nurse who needs to be comforted by the parents ceases to be sensitive to *their* needs (see Fig. 43–4).

The Nurse's View of the Patient

The nurse's view of the patient influences the delivery of nursing care. The humanistic nurse focuses on the individual. Positive views of human nature regarding adaptation to change are those defined as empirical-rational and normative-reeducative. The *empirical-rational* view is based on the assumption that people are guided by reason and moved by self-interest. The nurse holding this view believes that if a patient can justify a change and is shown how she will profit from it, the patient will incorporate the change into her lifestyle.

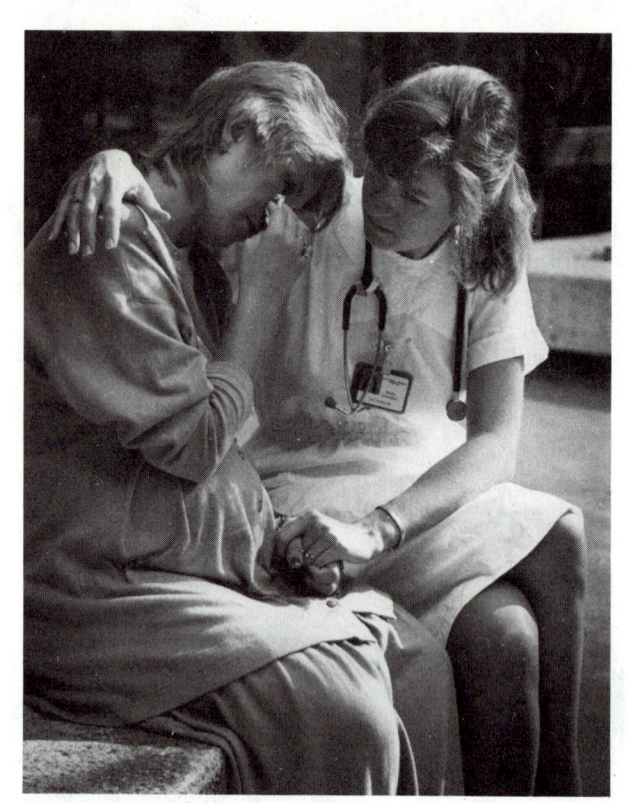

FIGURE 43–4. The nurse who has self-understanding can comfort the grieving mother.

The *normative-reeducative* assumption is closely related to the empirical-rational view. According to this assumption, a person's viewpoints are not rational alone but are internalized into a value system. Reeducation strengthens self-education and self-understanding to such a degree that change will be motivated from within the person.

A third assumption, and one not considered positive, is referred to as *power-coercive*. The nurse holding this viewpoint believes that a patient will not change except under force. This nurse will use his or her position of power to try to influence the patient's behavior (Chin and Benne, 1969; Fischman, 1973). There is a place for use of power coercion but this should be the last choice.

The Patient's Responsibility for Self-Care

As an advocate for the patient, the nurse encourages the patient to assume responsibility for self-care and supports the patient's decisions. The nurse is responsible for clarifying to the patient both alternatives and consequences of a particular situation. Once the patient is clearly informed, the patient makes the decision. The previously more common tendency of nurses to be domineering and controlling, to attempt to make decisions for the patient, is being superseded by increased interest in society regarding the rights of the individual (see Appendix D). In the current view the patient has autonomy and is able to make decisions for his or her own care. If the patient is kept dependent and passive and does not engage in self-change, the work of the health professional should be questioned.

The nurse's role is to accept the patient's decision unless it may produce harmful results. The decision-making process involves the planning of care with the patient, but the actual implementation of care must be in part due to the patient's internal motivation. The nurse is responsible to convey to the perinatal patient that it is legitimate for her to participate in the planning and setting of goals, that she has the expertise needed to make decisions for her own care because she knows her lifestyle best. In this way the patient is given responsibility for self-care.

The Patient's Compliance to Medical Regimen

Patients are often given a regimen to follow that overloads them, and they simply decide they cannot follow it. "Compliance with a treatment regimen is necessary for any patient because of the need to stop or reverse any harmful condition or disease process. However, it is very difficult to follow a regimen that requires making changes in one's lifestyle" (Moughton, 1982). For example, the patient with pregnancy-induced hypertension has other goals in life besides maintaining a blood pressure within some normal range. The nurse needs to complete a thorough assessment in order to more fully understand the limits of the patient and to know at what point the patient views the regimen as not worth the cost in other areas of her life.

The patient needs to understand the changes that result from complying with a medical regimen. There is a human tendency for nurses to assume that if patients are told to do something, they automatically do it; but this is not always true. Many times patients fail to follow a regimen because they never clearly understood it. The humanistic nurse is willing to invest the time and effort necessary to ensure that the patient fully understands what is expected of her. People do have some capacity for taking responsibility for their own lives. "If we as professionals err, it is probably in the area of not giving people enough room for responsibility" (Dr. Carl Thoresen, personal communication 1978).

Patient contracts have been used successfully to improve patient adherence to medical regimens (Steckel, 1980). A contract is an agreement between two or more persons to do something. Contracts between patient and nurse can be written so that positive reinforcement is used to elicit desired behavior. The patient can receive rewards, agreed upon by patient and nurse, as small steps are taken. In this way the nurse can reinforce the patient's efforts toward self-care (Steckel, 1980). Patients can be encouraged to set goals that have intrinsic rewards, such as becoming competent in a skill, which leads to increased self-esteem.

Nurses, through developing contracts with patients that emphasize positive reinforcement, encourage the patients' participation in self-care activities and promote a movement toward a higher level of health.

THE NURSE AS A PROFESSIONAL

Nurses are being encouraged to exercise their educational preparation and leadership abilities to improve health care. Several dimensions of professional nursing can be emphasized to produce more patient-centered care.

Accountability

Accountability and responsibility are clearly aligned in the delivery of patient care. Being accountable connotes being ready or willing to answer to someone else for one's own actions. The nurse answers not only to someone else but also to himself or herself. The perinatal nurse must exercise self-management and self-direction. Personal health of the nurse is an important factor in working with mothers and babies. Nurses must be aware of the susceptibility of babies, in particular, to infections. The nurse who is a known carrier of staphylococci or intermittent herpes simplex virus should not work in a perinatal setting. Even though this may be the area of choice for the nurse, the risks to the infant are too great. The nurse who realizes that he or she is a carrier of illness and also is accountable for his or her own actions will make responsible decisions and will take sick leave until the condition subsides.

Accountability involves prompt reporting. Any change in the course of the patient's condition, any information volunteered by the patient that requires further attention, and any error in medication or treatment should be reported.

Advocacy

Advocate is a word which primarily often carries legal connotations and may imply a formal, impersonal connection. *Advocacy*, according to one dictionary definition, suggests a person pleading "for or on behalf of another" and thus has a broader applicability. Further, it indicates a personal relationship – "another". From this perspective it could be said that advocacy reflects a humanistic approach.

Kohnke (1982) has introduced advocacy as a nursing career specialty. Her view is that advocacy involves a delicate balance between providing information in an unbiased way and, at the same time, giving support to the patient's/client's decision. An essential component in this interpersonal process is a consideration of the risks involved for the nurse in overstepping these bounds.

For example, a hidden bias in the selection or the omission of certain information may be a subtle persuasive influence in determining the ultimate decision by the other person. In a "yes" or "no" ballot decision, adequate information may not be provided on one or other of the options and the decision is thus skewed. In such a case, the advocate may not be fully aware of this imbalance of information as it is received by the patient/client. But whether intentional or inadvertent, the effect may be the same in terms of the client's decision.

Similarly, there is always the temptation for the "expert" or "specialist" to become impatient with the process of decision making. This process may be uninitiated and unconscious, and might push the client into a premature choice or into one which the advocate favors. Thus the advocate becomes the decision maker.

Part of the professional discipline for the nurse/advocate is from the humanistic standpoint. Therefore, the advocate's role is to be open to viable, available options, even when they run counter to personal biases. This is the case both when providing information and in supporting the decisions of the patient/client. To be perfectly "impartial" is, of course, humanly impossible. But the discipline of striving for impartiality, even when acting as a "partial" advocate, is part of the dialectical tension of what it means to be a "professional".

There are specific steps which can be taken to insure that the advocacy role can be carried out in a professional manner (see Fig. 43–5). A model structure of such an advocacy arrangement might be:

1. Establishing a supportive relationship.
2. Identifying the problem.
3. Formulating a written agreement based on the identification.
4. Agreeing on a plan with the client.
5. Implementing the process toward resolution.
6. Concluding the plan with evaluation (Brower, 1980).

The distinguishing feature seems to be the mutual effort by the nurse/advocate and patient/client to write down the steps whereby the plan can be met.

This concept of mutual goal-setting with and for the client to seek their best interests can be illuminated by referring to Erikson's (1963) delineation of "identity" as one of the eight stages in his epigenetic schematization of human growth and development. Although the "identity crisis" is highlighted in the young adult stage in his developmental chart, it is a continuing element throughout life from early childhood into aging and maturing in the later stages. He explains how this is articulated in a family context:

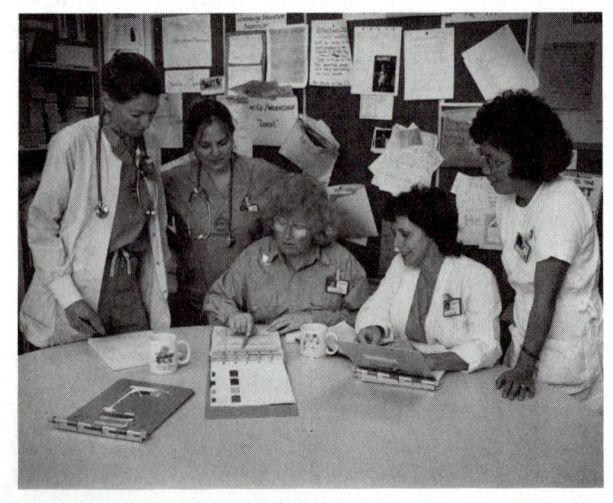

FIGURE 43–5. Advocacy involves a team approach to problem solving.

My whole being receives in them a hospitality for the way in which my inner world is ordered and includes them, which makes me, in turn, hospitable to the way in which they order their world and include me – a mutual affirmation, then, which can be depended upon to activate my being as I can be depended upon to activate theirs. To this, at any rate, I would restrict the term mutuality, which is the secret of love (Erikson, 1968, p. 219).

This enlargement of the meaning of the term *hospitality* to incorporate mutuality and love is worthy of special note considering the setting in which much of the nurse's advocacy work is to be carried out.

Another conceptual framework helpful in giving the idea of advocacy deeper meaning is provided by Kohlberg's stages of moral development. The last stage in his outline is "post conventional". In this stage of moral development, decision making arises out of one's beliefs and values about what is right, just, and humanistically possible. This is beyond the "preconventional" level in which one's own personal needs or wishes are determinative, as well as the "conventional" stage in which rules, roles, and regulations (of the workplace and/or society) are rigidly decisive (Kohlberg and Gilligan, 1971). Measuring one's own instincts and actions against this developmental schema may be helpful in disclosing inner dynamics operating in oneself and affecting decisions regarding the disclosure or withholding of information from the patient/client (Bridston, 1986). It could also be important for the mutuality of the advocacy relationship to be sensitive to the client's level of moral reasoning in so far as that can be discerned.

From a more holistic, sociological approach, Strauss (1984) discusses the deficiencies as well as the assets of the present health care system. From a humanistic perspective, he challenges the status quo as an advocate of the chronically ill, the disabled, the handicapped. For instance, for many young pregnant mothers with small children there is no classification in the system which would include them as "handicapped", i.e. having difficulty in getting to a prenatal clinic during pregnancy. Yet, according to Strauss, *access* to a health care system should be a top priority. Availability is an essential aspect of a system intended to meet human needs. Strauss indicates other guidelines for providing holistic, humanistic health care:

1. Respect for and self-respect by health professionals.
2. Active listening to clients without imposition of health professional biases.
3. Intelligent transactions between the client, the professional and the family (or families).

The qualities of mutuality and respect are central in making such transactions both humane and effective. This broader dimension of advocacy needs sensitive consideration by nurses.

Awareness of the personal and the societal, the psychological and the institutional dimensions of advocacy, may make it appear overly complex and intimidating, and thus discourage nurses from assuming the advocacy role. But again this is what professionalism is about. For example, let us take a simple operation such as circumcision. The permit for circumcision is often signed simply because it appears to the patient/client to be taken for granted by the hospital staff. No presentation of pros and cons are generally provided for early consideration by the parents. Is it so self-evident what the proper decision ought to be? What are the infant's interests and who may best represent them? (Konner, 1988). In addition in this case, circumcision often evokes deep symbolic and mythical reverberations even when it is not a specific religious ritual in their tradition.

The very complexity of such a case, with its cross-currents of personal and societal forces, does not argue against nurse advocacy. In fact, it may be a dramatic demonstration of the need for the advocacy services of one who is not simply attentive to the physical components of the case but is also aware of the other factors which need to be taken into consideration in making the decision. There may be no one who is in a better position than the nurse to serve in this capacity as a kind of ombudsman to represent the variety of interests involved.

In any case, the need for advocacy is going to be an increasingly urgent need in health care for no other reason than contemporary society is becoming ever more culturally diverse, linguistically mixed, and religiously pluralistic (Selby, 1988). Patients with exotic languages, deeply-rooted "alien" traditions, and cultural and religious taboos are no longer exceptional. Western philosophical assumptions and moral codes can no longer be taken for granted. The recent influx of opium through postal packages, not for drug use but for religious ceremonies of recent immigrants from Southeast Asia, is but one example of the phenomenon of the globalization of American society. How is one to provide humanistic health care to patients who cannot express themselves in the lingua franca of American health care systems and its dominant institutions? And how is a

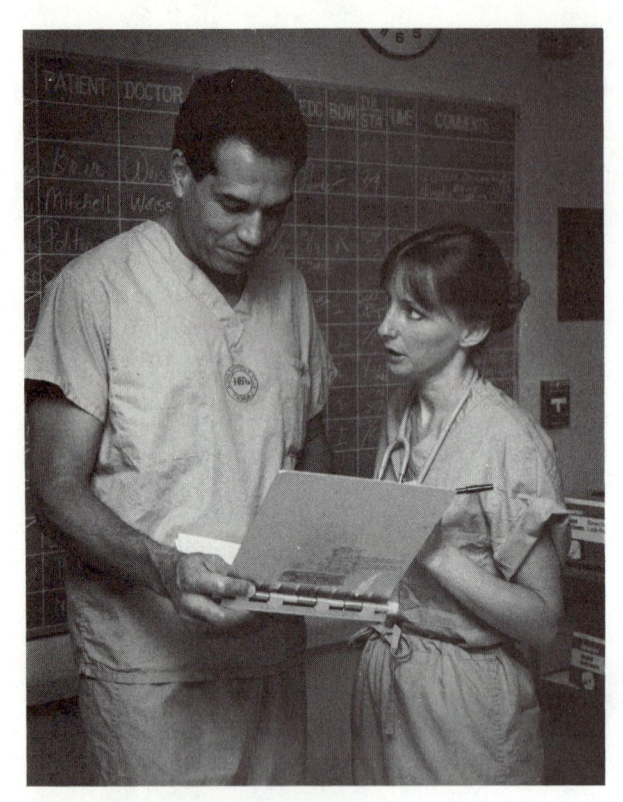

FIGURE 43–6. The nurse as patient-advocate takes time to consult with the doctor on behalf of the patient.

"modern" health care worker to come to terms with "primitive" cures and remedies that such non-Western patients may wish to utilize, and who may have no confidence in any other? The increasing appreciation of the virtues of acupuncture by formerly hostile and suspicious Western medical personnel may be an important parable of the need for humility and the need for a spirit of mutuality in dealing with such multicultural interchange. Again, the nurse advocate may be peculiarly fitted to perform an intermediary function in the health care field which no other professional group can legitimately claim as its own, either by tradition or by training.

As a patient advocate the nurse is encouraged to utilize independent thinking and to be assertive for the patient's benefit. Nurses should consider the need of the mother to be with her newborn. Often babies are fed by the nursing staff and not taken to the postpartum unit because it is inconvenient for the nurses. Change of shift or lack of adequate staff may be factors that place an additional burden on the nurse's time in transporting a baby to the mother. Engaging nursing personnel in creative problem solving to meet these needs is supportive of the mother's concerns.

SUMMARY

Caring in nursing considers the patient as a human being. The nurse who understands that she or he is a person with human needs is able to put herself or himself in the patient's place. The caring nurse is one who is involved in the role of patient advocate, taking time as well as risks to intercede on behalf of the patient (Fig. 43–6). The patient is viewed as ultimately responsible for self-care. The nurse seeks to work *with* the patient through use of positive reinforcement to meet mutually agreed-upon goals. The caring nurse views the patient, not the nurse, as being in control of and responsible for the betterment of personal health.

REFERENCES

American Academy of Pediatrics, American College of Obstetricians and Gynecologists. 1983. *Guidelines for perinatal care*. Evanston, Ill.: ACOG.

Bridston, E. O. 1986. An educational strategy for enhancement of moral-ethical decision making. In *Ethical issues in nursing*, ed. P. L. Chinn. Rockville, Md.: Aspen.

Brower, T. H. 1980. Advocacy: what is it? *J. Geront. Nurs.* 8:141–143.

Chin, R., and Benne, K. D. 1969. General strategies for effecting changes in human systems. In *The planning of change*, 2nd ed., eds. W. G. Bennis, K. D. Benne, and R. Chin. San Francisco: Holt, Rinehart & Winston.

Conway-Rutkowski, B. 1982. The nurse: Also an educator, patient advocate, and counselor. *Nurs. Clin. N. Amer.* 17(3):455–466.

Curtin, L. L. 1978. Human values in nursing. *Supervisor Nurse*. 9:21–33.

Erikson, E. H. 1963. *Childhood and society*. New York: W. W. Norton.

Erikson, E. H. 1968. *Identity, youth and crisis*. New York: W. W. Norton.

Fischman, S. H. 1973. Change strategies and their application to family planning programs. *Am. J. Nurs.* 73:1771–1774.

Giuffra, M. J. 1980. Humanistic nursing in a technological society. *J. N. Y. State Nurses Assoc.* (March):17–21.

Heidegger, M. 1949. *Existence and being*. Chicago: Henry Regnery.

Henderson, V. A. 1980. Preserving the essence of nursing in a technological age. *J. Adv. Nurs.* 5:245–260.

Kohlberg, L., and Gilligan, C. 1971. The adolescent as a philosopher: The discovery of the self in a postconventional world. *Daedalus*. 100:1072.

Kohnke, M. F. 1982. *Advocacy: risk and reality*. St. Louis: C. V. Mosby.

Koniak-Griffian, D., and Ludington-Hoe, S. M. 1988. Developmental and temperament outcomes of sensory stimulation in healthy infants. *Nurs. Res.* 37:70–75.

Konner, M. 1988. Symbolic wound. *New York Times Magazine.* May 8:58–59.

Moughton, M. 1982. The patient: a partner in the health care process. *Nurs. Clin. N. Amer.* 17(3):467–479.

Pilette, P. C. 1980. Caution: Objectivity and specialization may be hazardous to your humanity. *Am. J. Nurs.* 80:1588–1590.

Rogers, C. R. 1957. The necessary and sufficient conditions of therapeutic personality change. *J. Counseling Psychol.* 31:95–103.

Rogers, C. R. 1961. *On becoming a person.* Boston: Houghton Mifflin.

Rogers, M. E. 1970. *An introduction to the theoretical basis of nursing.* Philadelphia: F. A. Davis.

Selby, T. L. 1988. Nurses excel as advocates for patients. The American nurse. *ANA.* 1:7–8.

Seymer, L. R. 1954. *Selected writings of Florence Nightingale.* New York: Macmillan.

Sherwen, L. N., and Toussie-Weingarten, C. 1983. *Analysis and application of nursing research: Parent–neonate studies.* Monterey, Calif.: Wadsworth.

Siantz, M. L. 1988. Defining informed consent. *MCN.* 13:94.

Silverman, H. J. 1978. Dasein and existential analytic. In *Heidegger's existential ambiguity,* ed. F. Elliston. New York: Mouton.

Steckel, S. B. 1980. Contracting with patient – selected reinforcers. *Am. J. Nurs.* 80:1596–1599.

Strauss, A. L. 1984. *Chronic illness and the quality of life.* St. Louis: C. V. Mosby.

Watson, J. 1979. *Nursing: The philosophy and science of caring.* Boston: Little, Brown.

Watson, J. 1985. *Nursing: The philosophy and science of caring.* Colorado: Associated University Press.

Wilson, H. S. 1974. A case for humanities in professional nursing education. *Nurs. Forum.* 13:406–417.

44
Research for Change

BEHAVIORAL OBJECTIVES

Upon completion of this chapter, the reader should be able to:

- Define the research process.

- Compare and contrast the major research methods and discuss how each method may be applied to clinical nursing research, or why it may not be applied.

- Speculate about what direction perinatal nursing research will take in the future.

- Review research conducted in the field of perinatal nursing.

Research activities are essential to the advancement of all clinical areas of the nursing profession. Research, theory, and practice are the three interrelated components through which nursing will maintain itself as a significant discipline within the health care system. In the future, practitioners of nursing will be accountable for their nursing practice as well as being accountable for the documented functions that make up the practice of nursing.

This chapter focuses on the broad perspective of nursing research and its importance to the advancement of perinatal nursing practice. Research findings are discussed as the foundation for, as well as the substantive means for, the change process. Major types of research and investigative methods are reviewed, and each method's usefulness to the different facets of perinatal nursing is discussed. A review of nursing literature is presented. Finally, focuses of future research are discussed as they pertain to the practice of perinatal nursing.

THE RESEARCH PROCESS AND PERINATAL NURSING

Research can be defined as a systematic scientific study of a problem or area of interest. Basic to research is the underlying conceptual framework – simply stated, the ideas, other than the knowledge of the research process itself, that serve to organize and direct the research activities.

Most sources define research in terms of the research process. Although research may differ in whether its goals are pure or pragmatic, the process is the same. Notter (1974) identifies seven steps of the research process:

1. Problem identification
2. Review of the literature relevant to the problem
3. Hypothesis formulation
4. Design selection
5. Data collection
6. Data analysis
7. Reporting of findings of the study

Other nurse researchers may combine some of these steps, making their list shorter, but the research process they describe is essentially the same.

Much has been written concerning the purpose of research. Whether a discipline has an existing scientific body of knowledge or is in the pretheory stage, research is necessary to validate theory and advance the practical application of the discipline. Research may be done to: (1) organize and categorize "things," or create a typology; (2) predict future events; (3) explain past events; or, (4) provide a sense of understanding about what causes events (Reynolds, 1971).

Nursing as a profession is relatively young and, therefore, does not have an extensive body of scientific knowledge. The four areas presented by Reynolds could be considered as necessary and desirable purposes for research in nursing.

All areas of nursing are dependent upon the research process and the communication of the findings of this process for validation of both nursing actions and the scope of practice. Nurse researchers can explore nursing practice to establish a typology, or a method of classification. As the scientific body of knowledge becomes more sophisticated, the research process can be utilized for prediction, explanation and, eventually, understanding.

The research process has led to beneficial changes in perinatal nursing care as well as all other areas of nursing practice (see Chapter 2). Conclusions communicated from research studies provide the rationale for positive changes in the practice of perinatal nursing. Historically, many changes in perinatal nursing were made because the research data indicated that certain nursing practices were beneficial to the health and life of both mothers and infants.

From the beginning of professional nursing under the leadership of Florence Nightingale to the present, research has preceded advances in the care of clients in the maternity nursing system. Semmelweis, Nightingale, Breckenridge, and others kept records of the benefits of their practices. Palmer (1983) discusses Nightingale's collection of data to demonstrate the effectiveness of her nursing interventions. Kopf (1978) has further lauded Nightingale's statistical approach; she "learned the methods, general aims, and results of qualified inquiry into social facts and forces."

Types of Research

Research can be divided into two distinct categories according to the depth of probing and the general purpose of the research. *Basic*, or *pure*, *research* seeks to investigate the underlying causes and meaning of observed phenomena. Pure research is characterized by the sophistication of its conceptual framework and research design. The other category of research is pragmatic and present oriented. This research has been identified by Leedy (1980) as *applied research, action research*, or *developmental research*.

Research activities can be further grouped according to whether the data collected are *quantitative* or *qualitative*. Research activities that deal with quantitative data are characterized by numbers. Data collection yields precise and exact numerical measurements of variables. An important goal of nurse researchers is to design nursing research studies that involve quantitative data collection, to negate or substantiate theory. However, since the central focus of all facets of nursing practice is the human client, it is sometimes difficult to obtain precise, quantitative data.

Research activities that yield qualitative data are descriptive in nature, relying on narration, or words, as the data. Observations are described in words, and interviews are recorded verbatim. Qualitative data can be converted to quantitative data with the assignment of a number system to observed variables; however, precision, or exactness, is lacking. For example, if a nurse researcher were investigating the concept of bonding, data could be collected through observations of parents in contact with their infants (see Chapter 29). Descriptions of these observations would depend upon the researcher's perception, and a certain amount of subjectivity would be inherent. By contrast, if a nurse researcher designed a study to measure heat loss in newborns, the quantitative data, such as temperature readings, would be far more precise.

Basically, there are two approaches the nurse researcher can utilize in designing a research study's format for data collection. One kind of study involves extensive library review to ascertain what concepts have already been investigated relative to the study question under research consideration. The researcher would seek to synthesize into a conceptual framework the conclusions that other researchers have made, in order to design a present study that will go beyond previous findings (Fig. 44–1).

The other, phenomenologic, approach requires researchers to immerse themselves initially in the research process with only a general perspective on the study area and without a preconceived conceptual framework. The focus of this approach is to describe experience as it exists, as it is lived (Oiler, 1982). Using broad categories for study, the researcher will analyze the phenomena observed to give direction to data collection and, eventually, the conceptual framework will evolve from the data. This approach is explained by Glaser and Strauss (1967) as *grounded theory*. Research activities of this kind are inductive – the construction of theory evolves from the specifics of empirical situations (phenomena) to generalizations about the data.

Investigative Methods

Once the research study question has been fully delineated, the nurse researcher will select an investigative method suitable to collect the data.

Experimental/Quasi-experimental Methods

The *experimental method* is typically considered more scientifically rigorous than other investigative methods. In classic experimental design, the researcher maintains maximum control through

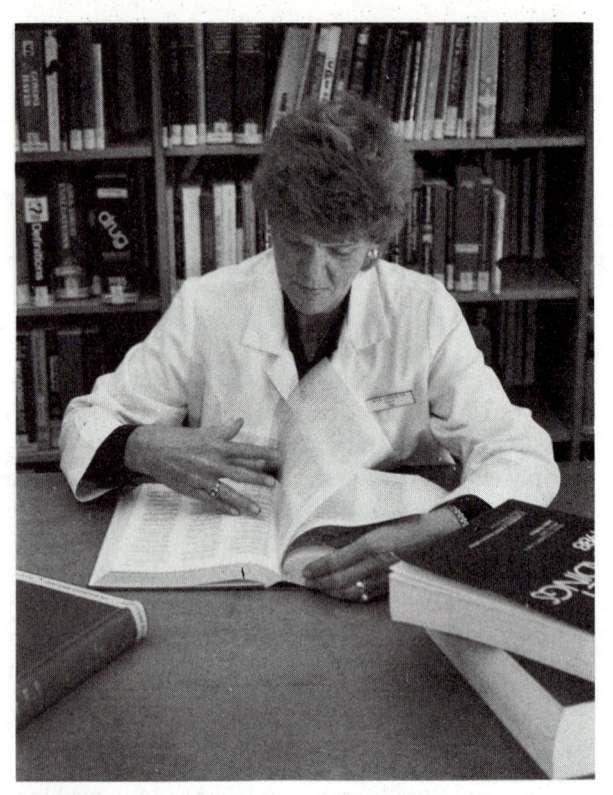

FIGURE 44–1. Extensive library review of the literature is a basis for nursing research.

randomization and manipulation. With this investigative method, the researcher adheres to the principle of *randomization*, which, simply stated, means that each subject or unit of study has an equal chance of being selected for the study sample as well as an equal chance of being in the experimental or control group. *Manipulation* is management by the researcher of the independent variable in order to measure its effect on the dependent variable.

The *quasi-experimental method* is similar, although the researcher does not maintain maximum control. Usually, control is lacking in the area of randomization with the quasi-experimental method – it is not always possible to randomize the study sample. However, as long as the researcher is aware of this, the research study may be conducted as designed, and the results interpreted and reported accordingly.

Descriptive Methods

For many of their research studies nurse researchers use what are called *descriptive methods*. The intent of the research done with descriptive methods is to assemble new information by describing, comparing, contrasting, or classifying phenomena. This can be accomplished through the case study, the survey, and the historical and ethnographic methods.

CASE STUDY. The *case study method* examines a single unit in depth. The unit under investigation can be an individual, group, community, culture, or whatever the researcher defines as the focus of the study. Often the case study approach yields extensive information and insight. This approach is applicable to many different aspects of nursing, such as diagnosis, determination of patterns of health practices, and adherence to a medical regimen. The major advantages of the case study are the exhaustive amount of information that may be secured and the flexibility of the design. The chief disadvantage of the case study method is the question of representativeness: Does the study represent the characteristics of the entire population accurately? Other disadvantages of this method are the extensive amounts of time and materials needed. Does the nurse researcher have the time available for the extensive study necessary, and are materials readily available?

SURVEY. Another descriptive method, the *survey method*, is designed to obtain data in a self-report format from a portion of the population in order to examine the characteristics, attitudes, or opinions of the larger population. Examples of the survey technique include the interview and the questionnaire.

The most effective interview format is the personal interview. Trained interviewers using a precisely designed set of questions interview individuals on a face-to-face basis. This technique is considered the most powerful method for securing extensive data. However, it is very time consuming. The telephone interview is another example of the technique.

The questionnaire format is another self-report technique. Questionnaires are mailed or otherwise distributed to individuals. Questionnaires allow greater flexibility and scope than the interview technique. However, the response rate is not as high.

The major disadvantage of the survey method is the superficiality of data gathered. Although an extremely broad section of the population can be sampled, the individuals surveyed do not provide in-depth information. Also, in a practical sense, the survey method can also prove to be very time consuming and costly for the nurse researcher.

HISTORICAL METHOD. The *historical method* is characterized by the systematic collection and evaluation of data pertaining to the past. An understanding of contemporary issues in nursing can be enhanced by the study of the past. Midwifery is an example of a nursing subject that can be effectively studied using the historical method. Much can be learned from the study of midwives in the past that could be useful in understanding and explaining the expanded roles of nurses in today's realm of perinatal nursing practice.

Research utilizing the historical method is constrained by several factors. Historical research is dependent upon surviving documents and artifacts from the past. Data collection sources include primarily written materials, such as books, periodicals, reports, interviews, letters, diaries, newspaper articles, and legal documents. However, historical research could also include artifacts in the form of objects and visual materials.

The nurse researcher must be cognizant of the biases that may exist in the surviving historical documents. Care must be taken to evaluate each data source critically. Time is another constraint. Locating documents and artifacts requires extensive searches, and the duplication of original sources may pose problems.

ENTHOGRAPHIC METHOD. The *ethnographic method* has been utilized in the social sciences, particularly anthropology, more extensively than in nursing. This method seeks data in an open-ended manner. As data are secured, the researcher incorporates them into the basic design and seeks validation and additional information from the next data source.

Ethnographic research is one type of research used by anthropologists to look at culture. Leninger (1981) emphasizes care as the essence and central focus of nursing. As a nurse-anthropologist, she has investigated cultural care in 30 cultures in order to understand the nature, scope, and function of care relative to nursing. She believes that in nursing, as well as other health disciplines, a cross-cultural focus is needed to gain insight and explain health–illness caring and caring from cultural viewpoints.

A study conducted by Zepeda (1982) examined selected practices of Spanish-speaking women in the postpartum period. The ethnographic method would be necessary to establish baseline data relative to practices of health care in the Spanish-speaking culture in order to design a research study to elect the information sought by Zepeda.

Ethnographic research is particularly important

in perinatal nursing, because culture has an impact on the individual's behavior, coping needs, and childbearing and childrearing practices.

Applicability of Investigative Methods to Perinatal Nursing Research

Each of the previously mentioned investigative methods lends itself to research in perinatal nursing, some methods to a greater degree than others.

Using the Experimental/Quasi-experimental Method

The experimental/quasi-experimental method lends itself to research in perinatal nursing when both experimental and control groups are feasible. This method can be used with human subjects when all ethical and moral criteria for using experimental and control groups have been satisfied. Variables essential to the well-being of clients cannot be studied with the experimental or quasi-experimental method if manipulation of these variables would result in harm (physical or psychologic) to the subjects.

An example of the use of the experimental method is a study reported by Hodnett (1982) on the effects of two types of fetal monitoring systems on patients during labor. Subjects in labor were randomly assigned to either the control group, which received standard monitoring, or the experimental group, which received radiotelemetric monitoring. The major difference between the two fetal monitoring systems is that mobility is possible with radiotelemetry. Immobility of the mother during labor may have a deleterious effect on uterine action as well as negative psychologic effects. The results of the study indicated that those in the experimental group had more positive labor experiences than did the control or standard-electronic-monitoring group. Mothers in the experimental group also demonstrated a higher degree of perceived control and generally had more positive feelings toward fetal monitoring.

An experimental study of infants was conducted by Brown and Grunfield (1980) to determine whether their later preference for sweetened foods is significantly influenced by early feedings. Twenty babies were randomly assigned to both experimental and control groups. The control group infants were fed standard commercial baby food, which contains additional sugar, for 3 months. The experimental group was fed similar food but with no sugar added. The results of the study indicate that neither group was found to prefer one type of food, sweetened or unsweetened, over the other.

These two studies illustrate how the experimental/quasi-experimental method for research can be applied in perinatal nursing. Mothers and infants were randomly assigned to experimental and control groups. Type of fetal monitoring during labor and sweetened/unsweetened foods were the variables manipulated. No harm to human subjects was inherent in either study. Implications of these studies for perinatal nursing are evident; research findings can be applied to management of the labor process and to health education for mothers of infants.

Using Descriptive Methods

Descriptive methods have been widely used in perinatal nursing research. These methods are perhaps the most appropriate for nursing research at the present time. Much can be learned from the new knowledge generated from descriptive research.

CASE STUDIES. The case study approach has not been extensively utilized in perinatal nursing research because of the time involved in securing the data. Although the case study method allows for great depth of information, conclusions for general application to nursing practice cannot be drawn from case studies because of the narrowness of the study focus.

PERSONAL INTERVIEW. Penny (1979) utilized the interview technique in assessing postpartal women's perceptions of touch during labor. Data indicating overall perception of touch during labor were analyzed, as well as data indicating perceptions of touch experiences as positive and negative. Significant differences in relation to whether touch was perceived as positive or negative were reported in the categories of age, race, and marital status. One finding was that touch by the husband was perceived as a positive experience. Therefore, whenever possible, perinatal nurses should provide the opportunity and encouragement for the husband to have physical contact with his wife.

QUESTIONNAIRE. Another descriptive method, the questionnaire, was utilized by Williams and Nikolaisen (1982) in a research study designed to investigate parents' perceptions and responses to loss of their infant through sudden infant death syndrome. Responses differed significantly with sex of the parent as well as marital status; this information can be utilized to individualize counseling at the time of loss and during future pregnancies.

A study reported by Rees (1980) illustrates how a concern in the practice of perinatal nursing can be the stimulus for research. Central to perinatal nursing is the nurse's assessment for the family's ability to cope with the responsibilities of changing roles. This study sought to identify criteria that would be beneficial in predicting, prior to delivery, the nursing assistance a primipara would require in adjusting to and caring for her infant. The researcher developed a way of rating information collected by the self-report descriptive technique to ascertain the primigravida's feelings of motherliness or her perception of the mothering role. The questionnaire consisted of various statements relative to motherliness, conception of the fetus as a person, and fantasies about the baby. The mothers were asked to respond to each question according to six options ranging from "strongly agree" to "strongly disagree."

THE HISTORICAL METHOD. The historical method has not been used widely in nursing research. However, research in nursing is still in an emergent role, and more historical research will probably be conducted in the future. Whether the historical method will prove beneficial as a technique for perinatal nursing research will depend on the existence of appropriate documents and artifacts.

ETHNOGRAPHIC STUDIES. Cultural and ethnic orientation will be a focus of future nursing research. At the present time, the United States is populated by a significant number of Spanish-speaking people as well as increasing numbers of people from other parts of the world. This population trend will have an impact on all clinical areas of nursing. The ethnographic method can prove beneficial in the advancement of nursing research to provide effective nursing to all people.

Choosing a Method

The nature of the proposed research will dictate the methodology used in each study. In clinical nursing research, the descriptive and experimental/quasi-experimental methods have been implemented more extensively than other methods. They have proven effective and efficient for managing research activities as well as for securing information. Both practice and accountability for the practice of perinatal nursing have been improved by the utilization of descriptive and experimental/quasi-experimental methods.

THE RESEARCH PROCESS AND THE CHANGE PROCESS

The research process outlined by Notter (1974) basically proposes a program for the collection and analysis of data to substantiate or validate existing theories. However, it presents certain hazards *vis-à-vis* the change process. As recent studies on scientific method have illustrated, this "textbook" approach to research limits the possibilities of innovative and creative breakthroughs, and thus the possibilities for change.

This recognition raises fundamental philosophical and psychological issues. From the dawn of the modern era, philosophers such as Descartes, Berkeley, and Hume have warned of the relativity of sense perception as a source of truth. As Tennant (1932, p. 188) puts it: "Between the world to be known and knowledge of it stands human nature.... We can perhaps eliminate anthropomorphism, but we can never transcend the anthropic."

Original research, though it is guided by and has respect for traditional theories, also has reservations about them. Facts may not change but our perception and interpretation of them may. Thus the original researcher is open to new concepts and theories which are more adequate to contain and synthesize both old and new or previously neglected data. Such shifts of perspective are not easily attained. In his study of scientific developments from 1300 to 1800, Butterfield, speaking of physiology and circulation of the blood, notes of most scientists in the sixteenth century:

> though they talked of the importance of seeing things with one's own eyes, they still could not observe a tree or a scene in nature without noticing just those things which the classical writers had taught them to observe. Similarly, the historical student, confronted with a mass of documentary material, has a kind of magnet in his mind which, unless he is very careful, will draw out of that material just the things which confirm the shape of the story as he assumed it to be before his researches began (Butterfield, 1956, p. 32).

He continues:

> Until the seventeenth century, therefore, a curious mental rigidity prevented even the leading students

of science from realising essential truths concerning the circulation of the blood, though we might say with considerable justice that they held some of the most significant evidence in their hands.

His general conclusion is: "once again we must wonder both in the past and in the present that the human mind, which goes on collecting facts, is so inelastic, so slow to change its framework of reference" (ibid., p. 41).

It is precisely this psychological phenomenon which Kuhn addresses in analyzing "paradigm shifts" in the history of scientific progress. Coming to a similar conclusion as Butterfield, he suggests that conceptual change is brought about by either "persuasion" by the "translation of good reasons" into language which the holder of the old theories understands, but more likely by a kind of "inscrutable neural reprogramming" which he calls a "conversion experience that I have likened to a gestalt switch." This, Kuhn (1970, p. 205) is convinced, "remains at the heart of the revolutionary process . . . and essential sort of scientific change."

These fundamental structural dynamics of human thought and behavior of course have ramifications far beyond the specificities of research *per se*. An appreciation of them is also relevant to human behavior in general, as well as to professional practice and action in particular. Original research by nurses could be, potentially, a dynamic resource for a variety of change processes which are restricted and inhibited by rigidity in following accepted theories without recognizing their time-bound character and, therefore, their ultimate relativity.

A Boston-based "think-tank" group has explored the whole area of creative capacity. Part of its agenda has been to discover techniques for breaking down the inelasticity, identified by Butterfield and Kuhn, which limits the uncovering of innovative solutions to previously insoluble technological and industrial problems through a process called "Synectics." On the assumption that many of the restrictive mental blocks to innovation lie at the conscious and rational level, they have developed a programmed form of "controlled irrationality."

The reporter of the group, and founder of a consulting firm utilizing its findings, defined the basic approach:

> Synectics theory applies to the integration of diverse individuals into a problem-stating problem-solving group. It is an operational theory for the conscious use of the preconscious psychological mechanisms present in creative activity. The purpose of developing such a theory is to increase the probability of success in problem-stating problem-solving situations. This increase depends on awareness of the mechanisms which must be worked through to arrive at solutions of fundamental novelty (Gordon 1961, pp. 1–3).

Though "the operational mechanics of Synectics are the concrete psychological factors which support and press forward the creative process" (ibid., p. 33), and have been devised out of a "symbiotic relationship with industry" and applied largely in the technological and industrial sector, they are not irrelevant to the problematics of basic research in almost any field including nursing. And since one of the basic motivations of nursing research is to promote and facilitate the change process which is intruding into all aspects of the health care system, understanding the social and psychological dynamics of change—the possibilities it opens as well as the threats it poses—is critical for the nurse, whether as researcher or acting professional in the workplace.

NURSE RESEARCH IN THE PERINATAL FIELD

It has been pointed out that "research, theory, and practice" are the three interrelated components through which nursing will maintain itself as a significant discipline within the health care system. This interrelationship is particularly evident in the perinatal field. The nurse has a unique opportunity through her immediate and continuing contact with the patient/client to exercise functions as researcher, theoretician, and practitioner.

A test of whether this triadic interconnection is maintained in practice is to be found in the literature regarding perinatal nursing (Sherwen and Toussie-Weingarten, 1983). The picture which emerges is encouraging. Since research is a relatively new member of the triad, the increase in nurses' research is a significant clue that a healthy balance is developing.

Several nursing research organizations have come into being. The American Nurses' Association of Nurse Researchers encourages and supports new research, sends out invitations for members to submit abstracts for presentation of results at conferences, and provides opportunities for nurse researchers to meet one another and compare their findings.

The National Institute of Health has established a National Center for Nursing Research (NCNR) as a part of their campus in Bethesda, Maryland, and the NIH budget for nursing research has risen from $18 million to $23 million. A specialist in perinatal nursing, Dr. Dyanne Affonso, who is one of the 12-member NCNR Council, has identified the following as congressional goals: patient care components in health services; interdisciplinary collaboration in research; and the production in the next decade of increased nursing research which is concrete, measurable, and replicable as nursing's major contribution to the nation's health.

The journal, *Nursing Research,* founded in 1952, is dedicated to publishing research studies by nurses in all fields. Several papers reporting on perinatal research have appeared recently. One of the most recent focused on developmental gains achieved through sensory stimulation of healthy infants (Koniak-Griffin and Ludington-Hoe, 1988). A wide variety of other nursing and health-care journals publish research related to perinatal nursing: *Journal of Obstetric, Gynecological, and Neonatal Nursing, American Journal of Maternal-Child Nursing, American Journal of Nursing,* and *Research in Health and Nursing. Nursing Research* reports both quantitative and qualitative improvements in reported nursing research.

Some of the studies represented clearly meet the NIH criteria of concreteness, replicability, and measurability. Articles have included:

1. A new method to quantitatively describe pain behavior in infants
2. Parent coping: A replication
3. Infant behavior, temperament and low birth rate
4. Mother anxiety and infant feeding
5. Sensory stimulation of infants

Although the tendency is toward quantitative analyses, the conceptual approach indicates inclusion of qualitative variables (see Table 44–1).

The clinical setting has increasingly become the primary locus for research arising directly out of the problems faced by nurses in practice in the field. Organized centers for the support of the entire research process have been established, and a research and publication council has been organized. Kissinger and Fraser (1987) describe the process of setting up a council to support research being carried out by nurses. An assistant director of nursing started the council by developing a support group to set goals which could be implemented. This all became a reality when a nurse researcher joined the team. Nationwide conferences centering on nursing research have been held and reflect the emergence of local and regional research networks. For instance, a recent 3-day symposium on clinically based nursing research featured 75 separate presentations of research completed or underway. Nurses also report research work in health, education, and other professional journals. The various professional journals of nursing such as the *Journal of Obstetrics and Gynecological Nursing* and the *Journal of Midwifery,* among others, report developments in the field of perinatology as well as progress reports and results of research in the field (see Table 44–1).

The general impression gained by this activity and the wide exposure of research programs is that nurses' research has attained a recognized standing in the health care community and is acknowledged as not only a critical contribution to more effective nursing practice but also as an indispensible component to be considered by all those engaged in raising the standards and improving the practice in the health care system.

SUMMARY

Research activities are a necessary component for the discipline of nursing in advancing the knowledge base and validating theory. The two major types of research – basic, or pure, and practical – are characterized by the purpose of the research and the level of existing knowledge.

Increasing numbers of research studies are being conducted in the area of perinatal nursing. Several investigative methods can be utilized in maternity nursing. However, the descriptive and experimental/quasi-experimental methods have been more extensively used than others. The future may see nurse researchers using the other methods, particularly the ethnographic method, to advance nursing knowledge about the cultural/ethnic aspects of maternity nursing. Although clinical nursing research is a relatively recent endeavor, much research has been conducted in maternity nursing. Research studies conducted on the physical and psychologic aspects of pregnancy, the labor process, and neonatal care are abundant in the nursing literature. The focus for

TABLE 44-1. *Representative Nursing Research Topics.*

Antepartal
Social support during pregnancy: A unidimensional or multidimensional construct?
Conflicts, satisfactions and attitudes during transition to the maternal role
Spouses' physical and psychological signs and symptoms during pregnancy and postpartum
Antepartum stress and mother's anxiety and feeding of infant
Falling in love: The development of pregnant women's attachment to their unborn children

Intrapartal
Progression of labor pains in primiparas and multiparas
Measurement of maternal anxiety and stress during childbirth
The birthing room: Some insights into parents' experiences
Effects of upright position during labor

Postpartal
Maternal role attainment and identity in postpartum period – Stability and change
Social support, stress and health: A comparison of expectant mothers and fathers
Parent coping, a replication
Spouses' body image changes during and after pregnancy
Return of functional ability after childbirth
Postpartal anxiety

Neonate
A new method to quantitatively describe pain behavior in infants
Infant temperament – Low birth weight
Father of newborn – Interaction effects of social competence and infant state
Developmental progress – Low birth weight
Handling of newborn – Vaginal and cesarean section
Research on sensory stimulation of infants

future research may be directed toward understanding the continued high rate of infant mortality in specific areas and groups.

The research process and change process have similar steps and advantages for professional nursing. The professional nurse can use planned change in a manner similar to the way the nurse researcher conducts research studies. The outcome of each, change or result, should be communicated to nursing practitioners for the advancement of the practice of nursing.

REFERENCES

Brown, M. S., and Grunfield, C. C. 1980. Taste preference of infants for sweetened or unsweetened foods. *Res. Nurs. Health.* 3(1):11–18.
Butterfield, H. 1950. *The origins of modern science.* London: Bell.
Fawcett, 1986. Analysis of research reports. *J. Nurse-Midwife.* 31.
Glaser, B., and Strauss, A. L. 1967. *The discovery of grounded theory.* Chicago: Aldine.
Gordon, W. J. J. 1961. *Synectics the development of creative capacity.* New York: Harper and Row.
Hodnett, E. 1982. Patient control during labor: Effects of two types of fetal monitoring. *J. Obstet. Gynecol. Neonatal Nurs.* 11(2):94–99.
Kissinger, C. D., and Fraser, L. 1987. Development of a research and publication council in a clinical setting. Journal of Pediatric Nursing. 2(2):80–87.
Knafl, 1987. Research activities of clinical nurse researchers. *Nurs. Res.* 36:
Koniak-Griffin, D., and Ludington-Hoe, S. 1988. Developmental and temperament outcomes of sensory stimulation in healthy infants. *Nurs. Res.* 70–76.
Knofpf, E. W. 1978. Florence Nightingale as statistician. *Res. Nurs. Health.* 1(3):93–102.
Kuhn, T. S. 1970. *The structure of scientific revolutions.* Chicago: University of Chicago Press.
Leedy, P. D. 1980. *Practical research.* 2nd ed. New York: Macmillan.
Leininger, M. M. 1981. *Caring: An essential human need.* Proceedings of the Three National Caring Conferences. Thorofare, N.J.: Slack.
L'Esperance, C., and Frantz, K. 1985. Time limitation for early breastfeeding. *J. Obstet. Gynecol. Neonatal Nurs.* March/April: 6–10.

Luckenbill-Brett, J. L. 1987. Use of nursing practice research findings. *Nurs. Res.* 36:344–349.

Notter, L. E. 1974. *Essentials of nursing research.* New York: Springer-Verlag.

Oiler, C. 1982. The phenomenological approach in nursing research. *Nurs. Res.* 31(3):178–181.

Palmer, T. S. 1983. From whence we came. In *The nursing profession: A time to speak,* ed. N. L. Chaska. New York: McGraw-Hill.

Pender, 1987. Collaboration in developing a research program grant. *Image.* 19:

Penny, K. P. 1979. Postpartum perceptions of touch received during labor. *Res. Nurs. Health.* 2(1):9–16.

Rees, B. L. 1980. Measuring identification with the mothering role. *Res. Nurs. Health.* 3(2):49–56.

Reynolds, P. D. 1971. *A primer in theory construction.* New York: Bobbs-Merrill.

Schearer, M H. 1988. Editorial. *Birth.* 15:1–2.

Sherwen, L. N., and Toussie-Weingarten, C. 1983. *Analysis and application of nursing research: Parent–neonate studies.* Monterey: Wadsworth.

Tennant, F. R. 1932. *Philosophy of the sciences.* Cambridge: Cambridge University Press.

Williams, R. A., and Nikolaisen, S. M. 1982. Sudden infant death syndrome: Parents' perceptions and responses to the loss of their infant. *Res. Nurs. Health.* 5(2):55–61.

Zepeda, M. 1982. Selected maternal-infant care practices of Spanish-speaking women. *J. Obstet. Gynecol. Neonatal Nurs.* 12:231–234.

1987. Nursing research center up and running at NIH; new director moves to chart a 5 year course. *Am. J. Nurs.* 87.

Appendixes

APPENDIX A

The Florence Nightingale Pledge

APPENDIX B

Standards for Obstetric, Gynecologic, and Neonatal Nursing

APPENDIX C

Standards of Maternal-Child Health Nursing Practice

APPENDIX D

A Patient's Bill of Rights

APPENDIX E

The Pregnant Patient's Bill of Rights and Responsibilities

APPENDIX F

Resources for Prenatal Educators

APPENDIX G

Resource Organizations Concerned with Parent or Infant Needs

APPENDIX H

The Development of Family-Centered Maternity/Newborn Care in Hospitals

APPENDIX I

Organizations for Alternative Birthing

APPENDIX J

Resources for Parents with Disabilities

APPENDIX K

Instructions for Use of Contraceptives

APPENDIX L

Audiovisuals on Pregnancy, Childbirth and Parenting

APPENDIX M

Infections Representing Potentially Serious Threats During Pregnancy

APPENDIX N

Perinatal HIV Guidelines

APPENDIX O

Testing for HIV-Clinical Diagnosis

APPENDIX P

Preparation for Neonatal Transport

APPENDIX A

The Florence Nightingale Pledge

I solemnly pledge myself before God and in the presence of this assembly to pass my life in purity and to practice my profession faithfully. I will abstain from whatever is deleterious and mischievous, and will not take or knowingly administer any harmful drug. I will do all in my power to maintain and elevate the standard of my profession and will hold in confidence all personal matters commmitted to my keeping and all family affairs coming to my knowledge in the practice of my calling. With loyalty will I endeavor to aid the physician in his work, and devote myself to the welfare of those committed to my care.

Lystra Gretter, 1896

APPENDIX B

Standards for Obstetric, Gynecologic, and Neonatal Nursing

I. NURSING PRACTICE

Standard: Comprehensive obstetric, gynecologic, and neonatal (OGN) nursing care is provided to the individual family and community within the framework of the nursing process.

II. HEALTH EDUCATION

Standard: Health care education for the individual, family and community is an integral part of OGN nursing practice.

III. POLICIES AND PROCEDURES

Standard: The delivery of OGN nursing care is based written policies and procedures.

IV. PROFESSIONAL RESPONSIBILITY AND ACCOUNTABILITY

Standard: The OGN nurse is responsible and accountable for maintaining knowledge and competency in individual nursing practice and for being aware of professional issues.

V. PERSONNEL

Standard: Obstetric, gynecologic, and neonatal nursing staff are provided to meet patient care needs.

APPENDIX C

Standards of Maternal-Child Health Nursing Practice

STANDARD I

Maternal and child health nursing practice is characterized by the continual questioning of assumptions upon which practice is based, retaining those which are valid and searching for and using new knowledge.

STANDARD II

Maternal and child health nursing practice is based upon knowledge of the biophysical and psychosocial development of individuals from conception through the childrearing phase of development and upon knowledge of the basic needs for optimum development.

STANDARD III

The collection of data about the health status of the client/patient is systematic and continuous. The data are accessible, communicated, and recorded.

STANDARD IV

Nursing diagnoses are derived from data about the health status of the client/patient.

STANDARD V

Maternal and child health nursing practice recognizes deviations from expected patterns of physiologic activity and anatomic and psychosocial development.

STANDARD VI

The plan of nursing care includes goals derived from the nursing diagnoses.

STANDARD VII

The plan of nursing care includes priorities and the prescribed nursing approaches or measures to achieve the goals derived from the nursing diagnoses.

STANDARD VIII

Nursing actions provide for client/patient participation in health promotion, maintenance, and restoration.

STANDARD IX

Maternal and child health nursing practice provides for the use and coordination of all services that assist individuals to prepare for responsible sexual roles.

STANDARD X

Nursing actions assist the client/patient to maximize his health capabilities.

STANDARD XI

The client/patient's progress or lack of progress toward goal achievement is determined by the client/patient and the nurse.

STANDARD XII

The client/patient's progress or lack of progress toward goal achievement directs reassessment, reordering of priorities, new goal setting, and revision of the plan of nursing care.

STANDARD XIII

Maternal and child health nursing practice evidences active participation with others in evaluating the availability, accessibility, and acceptability of services for parents and children and cooperating and/or taking leadership in extending and developing needed services in the community.

Source: American Nurse's Association

APPENDIX D

A Patient's Bill of Rights

The American Hospital Association presents a Patient's Bill of Rights with the expectation that observance of these rights will contribute to more effective patient care and greater satisfaction for the patient, his physician, and the hospital organization. Further, the Association presents these rights in the expectation that they will be supported by the hospital on behalf of its patients, as an integral part of the healing process. It is recognized that a personal relationship between the physician and the patient is essential for the provision of proper medical care. The traditional physician-patient relationship takes on a new dimension when care is rendered within an organizational structure. Legal precedent has established that the institution itself also has a responsibility to the patient. It is in recognition of these factors that these rights are affirmed.

1. The patient has the right to considerate and respectful care.
2. The patient has the right to obtain from his physician complete current information concerning his diagnosis, treatment, and prognosis in terms the patient can be reasonably expected to understand. When it is not medically advisable to give such information to the patient, the information should be made available to an appropriate person in his behalf. He has the right to know, by name, the physician responsible for coordinating his care.
3. The patient has the right to receive from his physician information necessary to give informed consent prior to the start of any procedure and/or treatment. Except in emergencies, such information for informed consent should include but not necessarily be limited to the specific procedure and/or treatment, the medically significant risks involved, and the probable duration of incapacitation. Where medically significant alternatives for care or treatment exist, or when the patient requests information concerning medical alternatives, the patient has the

right to such information. The patient also has the right to know the name of the person responsible for the procedures and/or treatment.

4. The patient has the right to refuse treatment to the extent permitted by law and to be informed of the medical consequences of his action.
5. The patient has the right to every consideration of his privacy concerning his own medical care program. Case discussion, consultation, examination, and treatment are confidential and should be conducted discreetly. Those not directly involved in his care must have the permission of the patient to be present.
6. The patient has the right to expect that all communications and records pertaining to his care should be treated as confidential.
7. The patient has the right to expect that within its capacity a hospital must make reasonable response to the request of a patient for services. The hospital must provide evaluation, service, and/or referral as indicated by the urgency of the case. When medically permissible, a patient may be transferred to another facility only after he has received complete information and explanation concerning the needs for and alternatives to such a transfer. The institution to which the patient is to be transferred must first have accepted the patient for transfer.
8. The patient has the right to obtain information as to any relationship of his hospital to other health care and educational institutions insofar as his care is concerned. The patient has the right to obtain information as to the existence of any professional relationships among individuals, by name, who are treating him.
9. The patient has the right to be advised if the hospital proposes to engage in or perform human experimentation affecting his care or treatment. The patient has the right to refuse to participate in such research projects.
10. The patient has the right to expect reasonable continuity of care. He has the right to know in advance what appointment times and physicians are available and where. The patient has the right to expect that the hospital will provide a mechanism whereby he is informed by his physician or a delegate of the physician of the patient's continuing health care requirements following discharge.
11. The patient has the right to examine and receive an explanation of his bill regardless of source of payment.
12. The patient has the right to know what hospital rules and regulations apply to his conduct as a patient.

APPENDIX E

The Pregnant Patient's Bill of Rights and Responsibilities

American parents are becoming increasingly aware that well-intentioned health professionals do not always have scientific data to support common American obstetrical practices and that many of these practices are carried out primarily because they are part of medical and hospital tradition. In the last 40 years many artificial practices have been introduced which have changed childbirth from a physiological event to a very complicated medical procedure in which all kinds of drugs are used and procedures carried out, sometimes unnecessarily, and many of them potentially damaging for the baby and even for the mother. A growing body of research makes it alarmingly clear that every aspect of traditional American hospital care during labor and delivery must now be questioned as to its possible effect on the future well-being of both the obstetric patient and her unborn child.

One in every 35 children born in the United States today will eventually be diagnosed as retarded; in 75 percent of these cases there is no familial or genetic predisposing factor. One in every 10 to 17 children has been found to have some form of brain dysfunction or learning disability requiring special treatment. Such statistics are not confined to the lower socioeconomic group but cut across all segments of American society.

New concerns are being raised by childbearing women because no one knows what degree of oxygen depletion, head compression, or traction by forceps the unborn or newborn infant can tolerate before that child sustains permanent brain damage or dysfunction. The recent findings regarding the cancer-related drug diethylstilbestrol have alerted the public to the fact that neither the approval of a drug by the U.S. Food and Drug Administration nor the fact that a drug is prescribed by a physician serves as a guarantee that a drug or medication is safe for the mother or her unborn child. In fact, the American Academy of Pediatrics' Committee on Drugs has recently stated that there is no drug, whether prescription or over-the-counter remedy, which has been proven safe for the unborn child.

The Pregnant Patient has the right to participate in decisions involving her well-being and that of her unborn child, unless there is a clearcut medical emergency that prevents her participation. In addition to the rights set forth in the American Hospital Association's "Patient's Bill of Rights" (which has also been adopted by the New York City Department of Health), the Pregnant Patient, because she represents *two* patients rather than one, should be recognized as having the following additional rights:

1. *The Pregnant Patient has the right,* prior to the administration of any drug or procedure, to be informed by the health professional caring for her of any potential direct or indirect effects, risks or hazards to herself or her unborn or newborn infant which may result from the use of a drug or procedure prescribed for or administered to her during pregnancy, labor, birth or lactation.

2. *The Pregnant Patient has the right,* prior to the proposed therapy, to be informed, not only of the benefits, risks and hazards of the proposed therapy but also of known alternative therapy, such as available childbirth education classes which could help to prepare the pregnant patient physically and mentally to cope with the discomfort or stress of pregnancy and the experience of childbirth, thereby reducing or eliminating her need for drugs and obstetric intervention. She should be offered such information early in her pregnancy in order that she may make a reasoned decision.

3. *The Pregnant Patient has the right,* prior to the administration of any drug, to be informed by the health professional who is prescribing or administering the drug to her that any drug which she receives during pregnancy, labor and birth, no matter how or when the drug is taken or administered, may adversely affect her unborn baby, directly or indirectly, and that there is no drug or chemical which has been proven safe for the unborn child.

4. *The Pregnant Patient has the right,* if cesarean section is anticipated, to be informed prior to the administration of any drug, and preferably prior to her hospitalization, that minimizing her and, in turn, her baby's intake of nonessential pre-operative medicine will benefit her baby.

5. *The Pregnant Patient has the right,* prior to the administration of a drug or procedure, to be informed of the areas of uncertainty if there is NO properly controlled follow-up research which has established the safety of the drug or procedure with regard to its direct and/or indirect effects on the physiological, mental and neurological development of the child exposed, via the mother, to the drug or procedure during pregnancy, labor, birth or lactation—(this would apply to virtually all drugs and the vast majority of obstetric procedures).

6. *The Pregnant Patient has the right,* prior to the administration of any drug, to be informed of the brand name and generic name of the drug in order that she may advise the health professional of any past adverse reaction to the drug.

7. *The Pregnant Patient has the right* to determine for herself, without pressure from her attendant, whether she will accept the risks inherent in the proposed therapy or refuse a drug or procedure.

8. *The Pregnant Patient has the right* to know the name and qualifications of the individual administering a medication or procedure to her during labor or birth.

9. *The Pregnant Patient has the right* to be informed, prior to the administration of any procedure, whether that procedure is being administered to her for her or her baby's benefit (medically indicated) or as an elective procedure (for convenience, teaching purposes or research).

10. *The Pregnant Patient has the right* to be accompanied during the stress of labor and birth by someone she cares for, and to whom she looks for emotional comfort and encouragement.

11. *The Pregnant Patient has the right* after appropriate medical consultation to choose a position for labor and for birth which is least stressful to her baby and to herself.

12. *The Obstetric Patient has the right* to have her baby cared for at her bedside if her baby is normal, and to feed her baby according to her baby's needs rather than according to the hospital regimen.

13. *The Obstetric Patient has the right* to be informed in writing of the name of the person who actually delivered her baby and the professional qualifications of that person. This information should also be on the birth certificate.

14. *The Obstetric Patient has the right* to be informed if there is any known or indicated aspect of her or her baby's care or condition which may cause her or her baby later difficulty or problems.

15. *The Obstetric Patient has the right* to have her and her baby's hospital medical records complete, accurate and legible and to have their records, including Nurses' Notes, retained by the hospital until the child reaches at least the age of majority, or, alternatively, to have the records offered to her before they are destroyed.

16. *The Obstetric Patient,* both during and after her hospital stay, has the right to have access to her complete hospital medical records, including Nurses' Notes, and to receive a copy upon payment of a reasonable fee and without incurring the expense of retaining an attorney.

It is the obstetric patient and her baby, not the health professional, who must sustain any trauma or injury resulting from the use of a drug or obstetric procedure. The observation of the rights listed above will not only permit the obstetric patient to participate in the decisions involving her and her baby's health care, but will help to protect the health professional and the hospital against litigation arising from resentment or misunderstanding on the part of the mother.

THE PREGNANT PATIENT'S RESPONSIBILITIES

In addition to understanding her rights, the pregnant patient should also understand that she too has certain responsibilities. The pregnant patient's responsibilities include the following:

1. *The pregnant patient is responsible* for learning about the physical and psychological process of labor, birth, and postpartum recovery. The better informed expectant couples are, the better they will be able to participate in decisions concerning the planning of their care.

2. *The pregnant patient is responsible* for learning what comprises good prenatal and intranatal care and for making an effort to obtain the best care possible.

3. *Expectant couples are responsible* for knowing about those hospital policies and regulations that will affect their birth and postpartum experience.

4. *The pregnant patient is responsible* for arranging for a companion or support person (husband, mother, sister, friend, etc.) who will share in her plans for birth and who will accompany her during her labor and birth experience.

5. *The pregnant patient is responsible* for making her preferences known clearly to the health professionals involved in her care in a courteous and cooperative manner and for making mutually agreed-upon arrangements regarding maternity care alternatives with her physician and hospital in advance of labor.

6. *Expectant couples are responsible* for listening to their chosen physician or midwife with an open mind, just as they expect him or her to listen openly to them.

7. Once they have agreed to a course of health care, *expectant couples are responsible,* to the best of their ability, for seeing that the program is carried out in consultation with others with whom they have made the agreement.

8. *The pregnant patient is responsible* for obtaining information in advance regarding the approximate cost of her obstetrical and hospital care.

9. *The pregnant patient* who intends to change her physician or hospital *is responsible* for notifying all concerned, well in advance of the birth if possible, and for informing both of her reasons for changing.

10. In all their interactions with medical and nursing personnel, the expectant couple should behave toward those caring for them with the same respect and consideration they themselves would like.

11. During the mother's hospital stay *the mother is responsible* for learning about her and her baby's continuing care after discharge from the hospital.

12. After birth, the parents should put into writing constructive comments and feelings of satisfaction and/or dissatisfaction with the care (nursing, medical, and personal) they received. Good service to families in the future will be facilitated by those couples who take the time and responsibility to write letters expressing their feelings about the maternity care they received.

All the previous statements assume a normal birth and postpartum experience. Expectant couples should realize that, if complications develop in their cases, there will be an increased need to trust the expertise of the physician and hospital staff they have chosen. However, if problems occur, the childbearing woman still retains her responsibility for making informed decisions about her care or treatment and that of her baby. If she is incapable of assuming that responsibility because of her physical condition, her previously authorized companion or support person should assume responsibility for making informed decisions on her behalf.

Source: American Foundation for Maternal and Child Health and the International Childbirth Education Association, Inc.

APPENDIX F

Resources for Prenatal Educators

American Baby/Childbirth Educator
575 Lexington Avenue
New York, NY 10022

American Academy of Husband-Coached Childbirth
P.O. Box 5224
Sherman Oaks, CA 91413
(Bradley method)

American College of Nurse-Midwives
1012 14th Street NW
Washington, DC 20005

American Society for Psychoprophylaxis in Obstetrics (ASPO)
1840 Wilson Boulevard, Suite 204
Arlington, VA 22201
(Lamaze method)

Cesareans/Support Education and Concern
22 Forest Road
Framingham, MA 01701

Healthy Mothers, Healthy Babies
409 12th Street S.W.
Washington, DC 20024

International Childbirth Education Association, Inc. (ICEA)
P.O. Box 20048
Minneapolis, MN 55480

La Leche League
9616 Minneapolis Avenue
Franklin Park, IL 60131
(Breastfeeding Support Group)

March of Dimes
Birth Defects Foundation
1275 Mamaroneck Avenue
White Plains, NY 10605

Maternity Center Association
48 East 92nd Street
New York, NY 10028

National Association of Parents and Professionals for Safe Alternatives in Childbirth (NAPSAC)
Marble Hill, MO 63764

Nurses Association of the American College of Obstetricians and Gynecologists (NAACOG)
600 Maryland Avenue, Suite 200
Washington, DC 20024

Read Natural Childbirth Foundation, Inc.
1300 S. Eliseo Drive, Suite 102
Greenbrae, CA 94904

APPENDIX G

Resource Organizations Concerned with Parent or Infant Needs

National SIDS Foundation
310 S. Michigan Ave.
Chicago, IL 60604
  Educates the public and professional community on the research of sudden infant death syndrome.

National Organization of Mothers of Twins Club, Inc.
5402 Amberwood Lane
Rockville, MD 20853
  Offers a reading list, compiles research, assists in establishing local clubs for multiple pregnancies.

March of Dimes Birth Defects Foundation
1275 Mamaroneck Ave.
White Plains, NY 10605
  Offers the following publications: Family Medical Record (9-0005), Birth Defects: Tragedy and Hope (9-0026), Your Special Child (9-0239).

Parents of Premature and High Risk International, Inc.
GSUC-CUNY
33 West 42nd St.
New York, NY 10036
  Offers information from other parents, develops materials, increases public awareness, and provides assistance in forming local parent support groups. Publications: Resource Directory, Support Lines.

Parents Without Partners, Inc.
80 Fifth Ave.
New York, NY
  Programs for guidance of parents without partners and their children on their unique problems.

Support After Neonatal Death (SAND)
Alta Bates Hospital
3001 Colby
Berkeley, CA 94750
  Support group for parents who have suffered perinatal loss through miscarriage, genetic abortion, stillbirth, or neonatal death. Also provides assistance to other organizations wanting to start SAND programs.

APPENDIX H

The Development of Family-Centered Maternity/Newborn Care in Hospitals

PREAMBLE

The Interprofessional Task Force on Health Care of Women and Children endorses the concept of family-centered maternity care as an acceptable approach to maternal/newborn care. The Task Force believes it would be beneficial to offer further comment and guidance to facilitate the implementation of such care. To this end, the organizations constituting the Task Force have participated in a multidisciplinary effort to develop a joint statement regarding the rationale behind and the practical implementation of family-centered maternity/newborn care. The effort has resulted in the development of this document, which the parent organizations believe can be helpful to those institutions considering or already implementing such programs. A description of potential components of family-centered maternity/newborn care is presented to assist implementation as judged appropriate at the local level.

DEFINITION: FAMILY-CENTERED MATERNITY/NEWBORN CARE

Family-centered maternity/newborn care can be defined as the delivery of safe, quality health care while recognizing, focusing on, and adapting to both the physical and psychosocial needs of the client-patient, the family, and the newly born. The emphasis is on the provision of maternity/newborn health care which fosters family unity while maintaining physical safety.

POSITION STATEMENT

The Task Force organizations, The American College of Obstetricians and Gynecologists, The American College of Nurse-Midwives, the Nurses Association of The

American College of Obstetricians and Gynecologists, the American Academy of Pediatrics, and the American Nurses' Association, endorse the philosophy of family-centered maternity/newborn care. The development of this conviction is based upon a recognition that health includes not only physical dimensions, but social, economic, and psychologic dimensions as well. Therefore, health care delivery, to be effective and satisfying for providers and the community alike, does well to acknowledge all these dimensions by adhering to the following philosophy:

That the family is the basic unit of society;
That the family is viewed as a whole unit within which each member is an individual enjoying recognition and entitled to consideration;
That childbearing and childrearing are unique and important functions of the family;
That childbearing is an experience that is appropriate and beneficial for the family to share as a unit;
That childbearing is a developmental opportunity and/or a situational crisis, during which the family members benefit from the supporting solidarity of the family unit.

To this end, the family-centered philosophy and delivery of maternal and newborn care is important in assisting families to cope with the childbearing experience and to achieve their own goals within the concept of a high level of wellness, and within the context of the cultural atmosphere of their choosing.

The implementation of family-centered care includes recognition that the provision of maternity/newborn care requires a team effort of the woman and her family, health care providers, and the community. The composition of the team may vary from setting to setting and include obstetricians, pediatricians, family physicians, certified nurse-midwives, nurse practitioners, and other nurses. While physicians are responsible for providing direction for medical management, other team members share appropriately in managing the health care of the family, and each team member must be individually accountable for the performance of his/her facet of care. The team concept includes the cooperative interrelationships of hospitals, health care providers, and the community in an organized system of care so as to provide for the total spectrum of maternity/newborn care within a particular geographic region.

As programs are planned, it is the joint responsibility of all health professionals and their organizations involved with maternity/newborn care, through their assumptions and with input from the community, to establish guidelines for family-centered maternal and newborn care and to assure that such care will be made available to the community regardless of economic status. It is the joint concern and responsibility of the professional organizations to commit themselves to the delivery of maternal and newborn health care in settings where maximum physical safety and psychological well-being for mother and child can be assured. With these requirements met, the hospital setting provides the maximum opportunity for physical safety and for psychological well-being. The development of a family-centered philosophy and implementation of the full range of this family-centered care within innovative and safe hospital settings provides the community/family with the optimum services they desire, request and need.

In view of these insights and convictions, it is recommended that each hospital obstetric, pediatric, and family practice department choosing this approach designate a joint committee on family-centered maternity/newborn care encompassing all recognized and previously stated available team members, including the community. The mission of this committee would be to develop, implement, and regularly evaluate a positive and comprehensive plan for family-centered maternity/newborn care in that hospital.

In addition, it is recommended that all of this be accomplished in the context of joint support for:

The published standards as presented by The American College of Obstetricians and Gynecologists, The American College of Nurse-Midwives, The Nurses' Association of The American College of Obstetricians and Gynecologists, The American Academy of Pediatrics, and the American Nurses' Association.
The implementation of the recommendations for the regional planning of maternal and perinatal health services, as appropriate for each region.
The availability of a family-centered maternity/newborn service at all levels of maternity care within the regional perinatal network.

POTENTIAL COMPONENTS OF FAMILY-CENTERED MATERNITY/NEWBORN CARE

No specific or detailed plan for implementation of family-centered maternity/newborn care is uniformly applicable, although general guidance as to the potential components of such care is commonly sought. The following description is intended to help those who seek such guidance and is not meant to be uniformly recommended for all maternity/newborn hospital units. The attitudes and needs of the community and the providers vary from geographic area to geographic area, and economic constraints may substantially modify the utilization of each component. The detailed implementation in each hospital unit should be left to that hospital's multidisciplinary committee established to deal with such development. In addition to that maternal/newborn health care team, community and hospital administrative input should be assured. In this manner, each hospital unit can best balance community needs within economic reality.

The major change in maternity/newborn units needed in order to make family-centered care work is attitudinal. Nevertheless, a description of the potential physical and functional components of family-centered care is useful. It remains for each hospital unit to implement those components judged feasible for that unit.

I. *Preparation of families:* The unit should provide preparation for childbirth classes taught by appropriately prepared health professionals. Whenever possible, physicians and hospital maternity nurses should participate in such programs so as to maximize cohesion of the team providing education and care. All class approaches should include a bibliography of reading materials. The objectives of these classes are as follows:

A. To increase the community's awareness of their responsibility toward ensuring a healthy outcome for mother and child.

B. To serve as opportunities for the community and providers to match expectations and achieve mutual goals from the childbirth experience.

C. To serve to assist the community to be eligible for participation in the full family-centered program.

D. To include a tour of the hospital's maternity and newborn units. The tour should be offered as an integral part of the preparation for childbirth programs and be available to the community by appointment. The public should be informed of a mechanism for emergency communication with the maternity/newborn unit.

II. *Preparation of hospital staff:* A continuing education program should be conducted on an ongoing basis to educate all levels of hospital personnel who either directly or indirectly come in contact with the family-centered program. This educational program may include:

Content of local preparation for childbirth classes.
Current trends in childbirth practices.
Alternative childbirth practices: safe and unsafe, as they are being practiced.
Needs of childbearing families to share the total experience.
Ways to support those families experiencing less than optimal outcome of pregnancy.
Explanation of term "family" so that it includes any "significant" or "supporting other" individual to the expectant mother.
The advantages to families and to the larger society of establishing the parenting bond immediately after birth.
The responsibilities of the patients toward ensuring a healthy outcome of the childbirth experience.
The potential long-term economic advantage to the hospital for initiating the program and how this could benefit each employee.
The satisfaction to be gained by each employee while assisting families to adjust to the new family member.
How the family-centered program is to function and the role each employee is to perform to ensure its success.

III. *Family-centered program within the maternity/newborn unit:* The husband or "supporting others" can remain with the patient throughout the childbirth process as much as possible. Family-newborn interaction immediately after birth is encouraged.

A. *Family waiting room and early labor lounge*, attractively painted and furnished, should be available in or near the obstetrical suite where:
1. Patients in early labor could walk and visit with children, husbands, and others.
2. The husband or "supporting other" person could go for a "rest break" if necessary.
3. Access to light nourishment should be available for the husband or "supporting other".
4. Reading materials are available.
5. Telephone/intercom connections with the labor area are available.

B. *A diagnostic-admitting room* should be adjacent to or near the family waiting room where:
1. Women could be examined to ascertain their status in labor without being formally admitted if they are in early labor.
2. Any woman patient past 20 weeks' gestation could be evaluated for emergency health problems during pregnancy.

C. *"Birthing room"*
1. A combination labor and delivery room for patient and the husband or "supporting other" during a normal labor and delivery.
2. A brightly and attractively decorated and furnished room designed to enhance a home-like atmosphere. A comfortable lounge chair is useful.
3. Stocked for medical emergencies for mother and infant with equipment concealed behind wall cabinets or drapes, but readily available when needed.
4. Wired for music or intercom as desired.
5. Equipped with a modern labor-delivery bed which can be:
   (a) raised and lowered.
   (b) adjustable to semi-sitting position.
   (c) moved to the delivery room if the need arises.
6. Equipped with a cribbette with warmer and have the capacity for infant resuscitation.
7. Appropriately supplied for a normal spontaneous vaginal delivery and the immediate care of a normal newborn.
8. An environment in which breastfeeding and handling of the baby are encouraged immediately after delivery with due consideration given to maintaining the baby's normal temperature.

D. *Labor rooms:*
1. The husband or "supporting other" can be with a laboring patient whether progress in labor is normal or abnormal.

2. Regulation hospital equipment is available.
3. An emergency delivery can be performed.
4. Attention is given to the surroundings which are attractively furnished and include a comfortable lounge chair.

E. *Delivery rooms* should be properly equipped with standard items but, in addition, should have delivery tables with adjustable backrests. An overhead mirror should be available. The delivery rooms should accommodate breastfeeding and handling of the baby after delivery with due consideration to maintaining the baby's normal temperature.

F. *Recovery room:* Patients may be returned from the delivery room to their original labor rooms, depending upon the demand, or to a recovery room. Such a recovery room should have all the standard equipment but also allow for the following options:

1. The infant should be allowed to be with the mother and father or "supporting other" for a time period after delivery with due consideration given to the infant's physiologic adjustment to extrauterine life. Where feasible, postcesarean section patients may be allowed the same option.
2. The husband or "supporting other" to be allowed to visit with the new mother and baby with some provision for privacy.
3. A "pass" to be given to the father or "supporting other" of the baby to allow for extended visiting privileges on the "new family unit."

G. *The postpartum "New Family Unit"* should:
1. Contain flexible rooming-in with a central nursery to allow:
   a) Optional "rooming in."
   b) Babies to be returned to the central nursery for professional nursing care when desired by the mother.
   c) Maximum desired maternal/infant contact especially during the first 24 hours.
2. Have extended visiting hours for the father or "supporting other" to provide the opportunity to assist with the care and feeding of the baby.
3. Have limited visiting hours for friends since the emphasis of the family-centered approach is on the family.
4. Contain a family room where:
   a) Children can visit with their mother and father.
   b) Professional staff are available to answer questions about parenting and issues regarding adjustments to the enlarged family.
   c) Cafeteria-like meals can be served and eaten restaurant-style by the mothers.
5. Have group and individual instruction provided by appropriately prepared personnel on postpartum care, family planning, infant feeding, infant care and parenting.
6. Allow visiting and feeding by the mothers in the special nurseries such as:
   a) Newborn, intensive care nursery.
   b) Isolation nursery.
7. Allow for breastfeeding/bottle feeding on demand with professional personnel available for assistance.

H. *Discharge planning* should include options for early discharge. If this option is desired, careful attention to continuing medical and/or nursing contact after discharge to ensure maternal and newborn health is important. Potential for utilization of appropriate referral systems should be available.

APPENDIX I

Organizations for Alternative Birthing

These organizations can provide information and support for families and health care professionals interested in alternative birthing methods.

Alliance for Perinatal Research and Services (APRS)
321 South Pitt Street
Alexandria, VA 22314

American College of Home Obstetrics (ACHO)
664 North Michigan Avenue, Suite 600
Chicago, IL 60611

American College of Nurse-Midwives (ACNM)
1522 K Street, Suite 1120
Washington, DC 20005

American College of Obstetricians and Gynecologists (ACOG)
600 Maryland Avenue SW, Suite 300E
Washington, DC 20024

American Foundation for Maternal and Child Health, Inc.
30 Beckman Place
New York, NY 10022

American Society for Psychoprophylaxis in Obstetrics (ASPO)
1411 K Street NW
Washington, DC 20005

Association for Childbirth at Home International
16705 Monte Cristo
Cerritos, CA 90701

Cesarean Birth Council International
P.O. Box 4331
Mountain View, CA 94040

C/SEC
60 Christopher Road
Waltham, MA 02154

Home Oriented Birth Experience (HOME)
511 New York Avenue
Takoma Park
Washington, DC 20012

International Childbirth Education Association (ICEA)
P.O. Box 20048
Minneapolis, MN 55420

International Childbirth Education Association
  Supplies Center
P.O. Box 70258
Seattle, WA 98107

La Leche League International
9616 Minneapolis Avenue
Franklin Park, IL 60131

Manchester Montrices Associates
Manchester Memorial Hospital
71 Haynes Street
Manchester, CT 06040

Maternity Center Association
48 East 92nd Street
New York, NY 10028

National Association for Parents and Professionals for
  Safe Alternatives to Childbirth (NAPSAC)
P.O. Box 267
Marble Hill, MO 63764

Nurses Association of the American College of
  Obstetricians and Gynecologists (NAACOG)
600 Maryland Avenue SW, Suite 200
Washington, DC 20024

APPENDIX J

Resources for Parents with Disabilities

RESOURCES SPECIFICALLY FOR PARENTS WITH DISABILITIES

Written Material

Parenting Without Vision in 1000 Easy Lessons, by Rachel Cranston. Available from Bananas, 6501 Telegraph Ave., Oakland, CA 94609 (in large print and Braille), 1981.

"The Disabled Parent," from *The Source Book for the Disabled*, edited by Gloria Hale. Paddington Press Ltd., New York & London, 1979.

Aids and Adaptations for Disabled Parents by Tali Conine, et al, University of British Columbia, Vancouver, B.C. 1987.

Help: When Parent is Handicapped by S. Parks. Palo Alto, CA: VORT. 1984.

Parents with Disabilities, a national newsletter by Through the Looking Glass, 801 Peralta Ave., Berkeley, CA 94707.

Organizations

Through the Looking Glass
801 Peralta Ave.
Berkeley, CA 94707
(415) 525-8138
    Provides services and information for people with disabilities who are considering pregnancy, are pregnant, or are in the early years of parenting. Also provides adaptive equipment development and information for disabled parents. Consultation and training for professionals, as well as research and assessment of parenting.

American Council of Blind Parents
Route A, Box 78
Franklin, LA 70538
(318) 836-9780
   Produces a quarterly newsletter; networks people in similar situations.

High-risk Ob/Gyn departments, rehabilitation departments, occupational therapists, and public health nurses can also be consulted.

GENERAL DISABILITY RESOURCES

Books

Design for Independent Living: The Environment and Physically Disabled People, by Raymond Lifchez and Barbara Winslow. University of California Press, Berkeley, 1982.

No More Stares, by Ann Cupolo Carillo, Katherine Corbett, and Victoria Lewis. DREDF, 2032 San Pablo Ave., Berkeley, CA 94702, 1982.

Sexuality and Physical Disability, by David Bullard and Susan Knight. C. V. Mosby Co., St. Louis, MO, 1981.

The Unexpected Minority: Handicapped Children in America, by John Gliedman and William Roth. Harcourt Brace Jovanovich, New York, 1980.

Organizations

Center for Independent Living
2539 Telegraph Ave.
Berkeley, CA 94704
(415) 841-4776 (voice)
(415) 848-3101 (TDD)

For other disabled independent living programs, contact the local department of Vocational Rehabilitation or consult the list in *No More Stares* (see above).

Accent on Information
P.O. Box 700
Bloomington, IL 61701
   A computerized retrieval system focused on disability needs.

The American Foundation for the Blind
15 W. 16th Street
New York, NY 10011

Lighthouse for the Blind
(consult phone book for local office)

National Association of the Deaf
814 Thayer Ave.
Silver Spring, MD 20910

National Interpreter Training Consortium
Deafness RT Center
New York University
New York, NY 10003

UCSF Center on Deafness
1474 Fifth Ave.
San Francisco, CA 94143

Regional centers, Easter Seal, and specific disability-focused organizations such as the MS Society, United Cerebral Palsy, and so on can also be consulted.

APPENDIX K

Instructions for Use of Contraceptives

INSTRUCTIONS FOR DIAPHRAGM USERS

Adapted with permission from *Contraceptive Technology, 1984–1985*.

PLAN TO INSERT THE DIAPHRAGM IN PLENTY OF TIME BEFORE INTERCOURSE. YOU CAN PUT IT IN JUST BEFORE INTERCOURSE OR ANYTIME UP TO 6 HOURS BEFOREHAND. ANYTIME IS BETTER THAN NOT AT ALL! YOU MUST USE THE DIAPHRAGM FOR IT TO BE EFFECTIVE. USE THE DIAPHRAGM WHENEVER YOU HAVE INTERCOURSE. DON'T TRY TO GUESS ABOUT YOUR FERTILE TIMES.

Several cases of toxic shock syndrome have been reported in association with use of the diaphragm. For this reason it may be advisable to avoid leaving your diaphragm in place for more than 24 hours, and to avoid using the diaphragm during a menstrual period. While you are using the diaphragm, watch for early symptoms of toxic shock and contact your clinician immediately if you have a danger sign. These are fever above 101° F, diarrhea, vomiting, muscle aches, or a sunburn like rash.

Instructions:

1. To apply contraceptive jelly or cream: Hold the diaphragm with the dome down (like a cup). Squeeze the jelly or cream from the tube into the dome (use about one tablespoon); spread a little bit around the rim of the diaphragm with your finger. If the diaphragm is worn for more than two hours before intercourse, the effectiveness of the spermicide may be diminished. For this reason, a full application of spermicidal jelly, cream, or foam should be placed in the vagina before intercourse in these circumstances. The diaphragm need not be removed for this.

2. To insert your diaphragm: With one hand, hold the diaphragm so that the cup/dome full of spermicide is facing toward your palm. Press the opposite sides of the rim together so that the diaphragm folds, spread the lips of your vagina with your other hand, and insert the folded diaphragm into your vaginal canal. This can be done standing with one foot propped up (on the edge of a bathtub or toilet), squatting, or lying on your back. Push the diaphragm downward and back along the back wall of your vagina as far as it will go. Then tuck the front rim up along the roof of your vagina behind your pubic bone. Once it is in place properly, you should not be able to feel the diaphragm except, of course, with your fingers. If it is uncomfortable or otherwise noticeable, then it is probably not in correct position; take it out and reinsert it.

3. To check the placement of your diaphragm: When it is correctly placed, the back rim of the diaphragm is below and behind the cervix, and the front edge of the rim is tucked up behind the pubic bone. Often it is not possible to feel the back rim. You should check to be sure that you can feel your cervix covered by the soft rubber dome of the diaphragm and that the front rim is snugly in place behind your pubic bone. The spermicidal cream (inside the dome of the diaphragm) should be next to your cervix.

4. Do not use Vaseline or other petroleum products when you are using your diaphragm as these may corrode the diaphragm. If you need extra lubrication, use contraceptive jelly.

5. After intercourse, leave the diaphragm in place at least 6 hours; then remove it as soon as it is convenient for you. If the diaphragm is removed less than six hours after intercourse, it is possible that sperm in the vagina may reach the cervix and swim up into the uterus. Therefore do not douche or remove the diaphragm for at least six hours after intercourse. If you have intercourse more than once, you should try to use an additional application of contraceptive cream, jelly or foam each time.

6. To remove the diaphragm: Place your index finger behind the front rim of the diaphragm and pull down and out. Be careful not to puncture the diaphragm with a fingernail. Even a tiny hole in the dome of the diaphragm will permit sperm to enter. If you find it hard to hook your finger behind the diaphragm, try a squatting position and push downward with your abdominal muscles. In other words, bear down as though you were having a bowel movement. Some women find it easier to remove the diaphragm by inserting a finger between the diaphragm and the pubic bone to break the suction created by the diaphragm in contact with the vaginal wall. Practice inserting, checking the position of, and removing the diaphragm frequently during the first weeks, until you can do so easily and confidently.

7. When you remove the diaphragm, wash it with mild soap and water, rinse it, and dry it with a towel. Store it in its plastic container. Do not use talcum powder or perfumed powder: they may damage the diaphragm or may be harmful to your vagina or cervix.

8. Check your diaphragm for tears or holes each time you use it. Hold it up to the light and stretch the dome slightly with your fingers to check for defects in the rubber.

9. Your diaphragm should not interfere with normal activities. Urination or a bowel movement should not affect its position but you can check its placement afterwards if you wish. It is fine to shower or bathe with the diaphragm in place.

10. Be sure to have your diaphragm checked: 2–3 months after the first fitting, once a year thereafter; if you have trouble inserting or removing it; if it causes discomfort to you or your partner; after you gain or lose more than 20 pounds; after you have a baby or an abortion; or after you have any pelvic surgery (Planned Parenthood, 1986).

YOU SHOULD UNDERSTAND THAT BY FOLLOWING TRADITIONAL USE RULES, YOU CAN EXPECT FAILURE RATES AS LOW AS TWO PERCENT, BUT THAT FLEXIBILITY IN THE RULES IS PREFERABLE TO OMITTING DIAPHRAGM USE IN A PROBLEM SITUATION. IN OTHER WORDS, IN A SITUATION WHEN IT IS IMPOSSIBLE TO FOLLOW THE TIME RULES PRECISELY, IT IS FAR BETTER TO USE THE DIAPHRAGM ANYWAY, THAN TO LEAVE IT IN THE DRAWER.

INSTRUCTIONS FOR USE OF THE CERVICAL CAP

Reprinted with permission from CSUH Student Health Center, 1983.
Instructions:

1. Fill the cervical cap one third to one half full of spermicidal cream or jelly (too much spermicide will prevent the necessary suction from forming). Do not use Vaseline. Because it is petroleum based, it will cause the rubber to deteriorate.

2. To insert the cap, try assuming a squatting or half-reclining position (experiment; every woman has her own way of inserting it). Then separate the labia (vaginal lips) with one hand and with the other grasp the cap between the thumb and forefinger. While squeezing the rim together, slide the cap into the vagina and push along the floor of the vagina as far as it will go. Use your forefinger to press the rim and around the cervix until the dome covers the cervical os (opening).

3. To remove the cap, lift the rim away from the cervix, thus breaking the suction. Then hook your index finger under the rim and withdraw the cap. The

dome can be grasped between the index and middle fingers and pulled outward and down.

4. There is controversy as to how long the cap can remain in place, as well as how long the spermicide remains effective. Women in the 19th and early 20th centuries used to leave the cap in for days or weeks, but current manufacturers say to put the cap in no more than one half hour before intercourse, and to leave it in no more than 24 hours after the last act of intercourse in order for the spermicide to take effect. We know that spermicides are effective for three days after insertion; the cap and spermicide will maintain 98% effectiveness for that period of time. We also know that the cap must remain in place for at least 8 hours after the last act of intercourse in order for the spermicide to take effect.

5. Inflammation or redness of the cervix may be noticed when the cap is removed. This generally subsides if the cap is left off for about 24 hours. If it continues or unusual discharge, pain, or itching are noticed, it may be that a vaginal infection has developed which requires medical followup.

6. Each time the cap is removed, it should be washed with mild soap and water and rinsed. Either refill the cap with spermicide and reinsert, or store until needed. Check for holes before you reinsert it each time by holding it up to a bright light. Sometimes when the cap is removed there may be an unpleasant odor. This can be alleviated by soaking the cap in one cup of water mixed with one tablespoon of cider vinegar or lemon juice for 20 minutes. Another method of eliminating odor is to place one drop of liquid chlorophyll on top of the spermicide before inserting the cap. Chlorophyll is available at most natural food stores. It is not harmful to the body.

7. Some women have reported that their caps become dislodged during intercourse. To be on the safe side, use a condom for the first month of cap use, if you engage in intercourse twice a week. If the intercourse is less frequent, use a condom for the first eight times. Then if the cap does become dislodged due to an improper fit you have a backup method of birth control. If your cap is continually dislodged, you should contact the clinic to have your fit checked. Do not use it again as a contraceptive until that time. Douching while the cap is in place may also cause dislodgement.

8. The cap should not be used as a contraceptive during your period because the menstrual flow may break the suction. However, some women do use the cap to collect menstrual flow. Another method of contraception is recommended at that time.

9. Return for an exam immediately if you miss a menstrual period, if your period is late, or if you experience an unusual flow or bleeding. If you do not experience any of these symptoms, return for a checkup once a year. If you go through childbirth or have an abortion, you should have the size of your cap rechecked for proper fit.

INSTRUCTIONS FOR USE OF CONDOM

Instructions:

1. Condoms come in one size which fits most men. It will say so on the box if they are formed or tighter. Read instructions in condom package and practice putting one on and taking it off well before you plan to use it.

2. A new condom should be used for each act of intercourse as they are not strong enough for reuse. Homemade condoms of saran wrap do not work. A condom should not be tested before use by inflating, stretching or being filled with water. Holes big enough to let sperm through can be too small to detect. The condom may be inadvertently damaged in the checking. Lubricated condoms with reservoir tips are generally the easiest to use. Those lubricated with spermicide are more effective for contraception. The condom must be applied after the penis is erect (hard) and well before ejaculation. Waiting until just before ejaculation can allow drops of preejaculatory fluid containing sperm to enter the vagina. This can lead to pregnancy. Putting it on too early, on the other hand, can lead to problems of the condom tearing from rubbing against sheets, dirt, sand, car seat, etc., or being punctured by a fingernail.

3. Carefully unwrap the package. Most condoms are prerolled in the package. If the condom does not have a reservoir tip, unroll half an inch before placing it on the penis. This leaves space to collect the ejaculate or semen which contains the sperm. For an uncircumcised male, the foreskin must be pulled back from the penis before putting on the condom.

4. As you begin to unroll the condom, squeeze the reservoir end to release air to avoid an air pocket taking up the empty space. Place the condom on the erect penis before any contact with the female's genitals. It should unroll easily all the way down to the base of the penis where the pubic hair is. If it does not unroll easily, it is being unrolled incorrectly. You should start over using another condom. The condom may be placed on the man by the woman as part of lovemaking. You will know the condom is on correctly if there is one half inch of space at the tip end and the rest of the condom fits snugly around the hard penis like a glove on a finger.

5. The condom-covered penis should be withdrawn from the vagina after ejaculation and before the erection is lost. The open end of the condom should be held tightly at the base of the penis so it does not slip or allow any semen to leak out during withdrawal. A soft penis can allow the condom to slip off and leak sperm. The partners must be careful not to spill any semen anywhere near the woman's vagina or genitals. After the condom has been removed, the

penis should not touch any part of the woman's genitals as there may still be sperm on it.
6. If a condom breaks, comes off in the vagina, or leakage occurs for any reason, the woman should immediately insert a spermicidal foam into the vagina. Check the condom before throwing it away for any obvious breaks.
7. If more lubrication is needed, do not use petroleum jelly (Vaseline), cold creams, hand lotions or oil-based lubricants on latex condoms as they may cause the rubber to deteriorate. Acceptable lubricants are K-Y Jelly, saliva or spermicidal creams or jellies. Be sure to have adequate lubrication when using a condom otherwise the rubber may break with vigorous thrusting.
8. Condoms can last for three years if stored in a cool, dry place away from heat (such as body heat from being in a wallet). If a man stores one in a hip pocket, it should be replaced monthly.

Above material adapted from:

1. Nancy E. Dirubbo, N. E. (1987). The Condom Barrier. American Journal of Nursing. Vol. 87, (10): 1306–1309.
2. ACHCSA. (1984). Condom (Rubber). Oakland, California: Division of Communications and Data Services.
3. Sex Education for Disabled People. (1986). Information on the Condom. Oakland, California: Sex Education for Disabled People.
4. Planned Parenthood/Napa. (1985). Condoms. Napa County: Planned Parenthood.

INSTRUCTIONS FOR USE OF CONTRACEPTIVE VAGINAL SUPPOSITORIES

Adapted with permission from Planned Parenthood/Alameda—San Francisco, 1983.
Instructions:

1. Remove the protective wrapper as shown in the instructions just before insertion. This can be difficult to do.
2. No more than thirty minutes before intercourse, insert one suppository as far as possible into your vagina. Be sure it is placed deep into the vagina close to the opening of the uterus (your cervix).
3. IMPORTANT! WAIT TEN MINUTES to make sure the suppository completely dissolves. This is necessary for effective protection. After the suppository has been inserted into your vagina, it gently foams up for about ten minutes and forms a barrier over your cervix to prevent the entrance of sperm. This barrier contains a chemical which destroys sperm on contact. As the suppository foams up, there may be a feeling of warmth; but this should not cause you concern.
4. After the suppository is inserted, remain lying down. If you have to be walking around before intercourse, insert another suppository.
5. Insert a new suppository each time intercourse is repeated, to provide reliable protection.
6. After intercourse, if you need to be up and around before the spermicide is absorbed, a mini pad may be worn to help absorb any fluid that drips out of the vagina.
7. Douching is not necessary. However, if you wish to douche, wait at least 6–8 hours after intercourse.
8. Remember that use of the combination of a condom and the suppository is highly effective in preventing pregnancy. It is much better than the suppository alone.
9. Vaginal suppositories should be stored away from heat. Should a suppository accidentally be exposed to heat, hold it under cold water for two minutes *before* removing the wrapper.
10. Consult your clinic or health care provider if you have a severe allergic reaction to any suppository.
11. Minor burning and/or irritation of the vagina or penis have been reported in some cases. If this happens, try another brand or consult your clinic or health care provider. A suppository may fail to melt completely in the vagina, which can cause increased friction, penile or vaginal irritation, and possibly decreased effectiveness. The result may be a rather gritty effect.
12. Contraceptive suppositories should not be used orally or rectally. They are completely ineffective unless used in the vagina.

INSTRUCTIONS FOR CONTRACEPTIVE FOAM USERS

Adapted with permission from *Contraceptive Technology, 1984–1985*, Hatcher et al.
Instructions:

USE YOUR SPERMICIDE EVERY TIME YOU HAVE INTERCOURSE!
1. Several brands of foam come in preloaded applicators, ready for use.
2. If the foam comes in a separate container from the applicator, the applicator is filled to a designated mark by pressure applied directly onto the top of the container (Emko and Koromex) or by tilting the applicator (Delfen).
3. Shake the can 20 times before using. This insures that there will be plenty of bubbles for the barrier and that the spermicide will be mixed with the foam.
4. At the Emory University Family Planning Program, it is recommended that the woman insert one full

applicator of Emko, Emko Pre-Fil, or Emko Because, or two full applicators of Delfen or Koromex back into the vagina near the cervix each time she has intercourse. Since the bubbles start going flat within a half hour, try to insert the foam just before lovemaking. Placement is usually done while lying on the back with knees slightly raised. It can also be done standing or in any preferred position. After spreading the lips of the vagina apart, insert the applicator as deep as you can, then push the plunger. When you remove the applicator, be careful not to pull the plunger back out or you might suck some foam back into the applicator.

5. Foam protection lasts about 30 minutes so be sure you have inserted foam no more than 30 minutes before intercourse. Use another applicator full of spermicide just before intercourse if more than a half hour has passed. If you have to be up walking around after foam is inserted, use another applicator full before next intercourse. If you have intercourse more than once, insert a new applicator full of foam before every act of intercourse.
6. Douching is not necessary. However, if you want to douche, wait at least 8 hours after your last intercourse.
7. If you need to be up and around before the foam is absorbed after intercourse, you may put in a tampon to absorb it.
8. Wash the applicator with soap and lukewarm water.
9. Keep a spare container of foam on hand. With most brands, there is no way to tell when you are about to run out. Keep foam in a cool place, away from a heat source.
10. The effectiveness of foam in preventing pregnancy can be greatly increased if it is used with another method of birth control, such as condoms.

INSTRUCTIONS FOR USE OF THE CONTRACEPTIVE SPONGE

Detailed instructions for use of the vaginal contraceptive sponge can be found inside each box. This product is available without a prescription at local drugstores or wherever contraceptives are sold.

INSTRUCTIONS FOR USE OF THE ORAL CONTRACEPTIVE PILL

Reprinted with permission from *Contraceptive Technology, 1986–1987*, Hatcher et al.
Instructions:

1. The pill works primarily by stopping ovulation (release of an egg). If there is no egg to meet with the sperm, pregnancy cannot occur. If you follow these directions carefully, the pill is the most effective reversible contraceptive currently available.
2. Choose a backup method of birth control (such as condoms or foam) to use along with your first pack of pills. The pill may not fully protect you from pregnancy during this first month. Keep this backup method handy all the time. Learn to use it well in case you: run out of pills, forget pills, or experience pill danger signals and stop taking pills.
3. There are several ways to start taking your pills. There is no single "right" way to start pills. You should start your pills the way your doctor, nurse, or clinic suggests.

   FIRST APPROACH: Start your first pack of pills on the first day you begin bleeding during your period.

   SECOND APPROACH: Start your first pack on the first Sunday after your period begins.

   THIRD APPROACH: Start your first pack on the fifth day after you start your menstrual period.

   FOURTH APPROACH: Start your pills today if there is absolutely no chance that you could be pregnant. Check with your clinician to see how long to use a backup method.

4. Be sure to read the package insert for the pills you are using. The Food and Drug Administration (FDA) now requires that all family planning clinics, doctors and drugstores give each pill user a copy of an extensive pamphlet to read. The pamphlet is produced by your pill manufacturer and approved by the FDA. It gives you excellent and very detailed information about pill benefits and risks. Instructions for the different birth control pills do vary slightly, so read the pamphlet you receive very carefully.
5. Swallow one pill a day until you finish the pack. Then:
   (a) If you are using a 21-day pack, stop taking pills for one week and then start your new pack. You are protected against pregnancy during the time you are not taking the pills.
   (b) If you are using a 28-day pack, begin a new pack immediately. Skip no days between packages.
6. Try to associate taking your pill with something else that you do at about the same time every day, like going to bed, eating a meal, or brushing your teeth. Establishing a regular routine may make it easier to remember. Pills work best if you take one about the same time every day in order to keep a steady level of hormones in your system.
7. If you have bleeding between periods, try to take your pills at the same time every day. If you have

spotting (light bleeding between periods) for several cycles, you may want to call your clinician. You may need a different pill. Spotting is more likely to occur with the current low-dose birth control pills. From a medical viewpoint, spotting is generally not an ominous sign in young women. If the spotting does not concern you or inconvenience you, it may be managed by your clinician with a "watch and wait" approach. If you suddenly begin to have bleeding between periods, have not previously had this problem, and have not missed pills or taken pills late, consider having your doctor check for infection.

8. Check your pack of birth control pills each morning to make sure you took the pill the day before.
9. If you miss one pill, take the forgotten one (yesterday's pill) as soon as you remember it and take today's pill at the regular time. You probably won't get pregnant. Just to be sure, use your backup method until your next period.
10. If you miss two pills in a row, take two pills as soon as you remember and two the next day. Here is an example: you forget your pills on Saturday and Sunday evenings but remember on Monday morning. What do you do? Take two pills on Monday and two on Tuesday. You may have some spotting. Use your backup method until you get your period. When you have missed pills, despite your "catching up", you may bleed or spot until the next cycle of pills is started.
11. If you miss three or more pills in a row, ask yourself, "Am I a good pill user?" Your ovaries will probably produce an egg (you will ovulate) and then you could get pregnant. In addition, you may get some bleeding. Start your backup method of birth control immediately. Think about switching to a method you can use more consistently, unless you are sure missing pills will not become a habit! If you do want to continue pills, you can either:
    (a) Take two pills a day for three days as shown in the diagram and use your backup method of birth control until you have your next period.
    (b) Stop taking pills from your old pack of pills. Start a new pack of pills the Sunday after you missed three or more pills, even if you are bleeding. Use your second method of birth control while you are off pills AND for the first two weeks that you are on your new pack of pills.
12. If you get sick and have severe diarrhea or vomiting for several days, use your backup method of birth control until your next period. Start using a backup method your first day of diarrhea or vomiting.
13. Periods tend to be short and scanty on pills. You may see no fresh blood at all. If you have only a drop of blood or a brown smudge on your tampon or on your underwear, that counts as being a period.
14. If you have not missed any pills and you miss one period, and you have no signs of pregnancy, you probably don't need to worry too much. You might be pregnant, but it is very unlikely. Many women taking birth control pills miss one period every now and then. If you are worried, call the clinic. You are fairly safe and can start a new package of pills at the regularly scheduled time. A simple indication that you are not pregnant: if your period does not appear during the last few days on pills or during the first three days off pills, take your basal body temperature (BBT); if BBT is below 98° F for three days in a row, you are probably not pregnant so resume next pack of pills on schedule.
15. If you forget one or more pills and miss a period, you should stop taking pills and start another method of birth control. Contact your clinic for a pelvic examination or a sensitive pregnancy test. Ordinary two-minute urine tests will not be positive at this time.
16. If you miss two periods in a row, come to the clinic for a pregnancy test right away, even if you took your pills every day. Bring in your first morning urine in a clean container.
17. If you do become pregnant while taking birth control pills, the most important questions you have to deal with are whether you want to have a child at this time in your life and, alternatively, whether abortion is an option for you. If indeed there is any increased risk, the risk of having a baby with birth defects is only slightly increased by taking pills during the first month or two of pregnancy. The magnitude of this risk is not well defined.
18. If you wish to go off the pill, complete the pill cycle you are presently taking. Be aware that it is a myth that you cannot get pregnant immediately upon discontinuing the pill. Though some women do not have a regular cycle for some months, others return to their normal pre-pill cycle promptly. So, if you are going off the pill and do not wish to become pregnant, start using other methods of birth control as soon as you stop taking the pill (such as foam and condom, available without prescription). If you are going off the pill to become pregnant, it is recommended that you use a barrier method of birth control until you have experienced two regular periods. The reason for this is twofold: 1) There may be a higher incidence of miscarriage among women who become pregnant immediately following pill discontinuance and 2) It makes it difficult for a doctor to determine the date of conception.
19. Anytime you see a clinician for any reason, be sure to mention that you are on birth control pills. This is particularly important if you are admitted to the hospital.
20. If you notice any pronounced mood changes—depression, irritability, change in sex drive—see your clinician. Switching pill brands may help.
21. If you smoke more than 14 cigarettes a day, you should be even more careful to watch out for the pill danger signals and you should probably STOP taking pills at age 35. Better yet, STOP SMOKING.
22. You must learn the pill danger signals. Any one of

these five symptoms may mean that you are in serious trouble. Note that the first letter of each symptom spells out the word "ACHES."

EARLY PILL DANGER SIGNS

CAUTION:
- A—Abdominal pain (severe)
- C—Chest pain (severe), cough, shortness of breath
- H—Headache (severe), dizziness, weakness, numbness
- E—Eye problems (vision loss or blurring), speech problems
- S—Severe leg pain (calf or thigh)

See your clinician if you have any of these problems, or if you develop depression, yellow jaundice or a breast lump.

Which Aches and Pains May Be Warnings of Serious Trouble?

Five Signals	Possible Problem
Abdominal pain (severe)	Gallbladder disease, hepatic adenoma, blood clot, pancreatitis
Chest pain (severe), shortness of breath, or coughing up blood	Blood clot in lungs or myocardial infarction (heart attack)
Headaches (severe)	Stroke or hypertension or migraine headache
Eye problems: blurred vision, flashing lights, or blindness	Stroke or hypertension or temporary vascular problem of many possible sites
Severe leg pain (calf or thigh)	Blood clot in legs

Do not ignore these problems. Do not wait to see if these problems go away. Contact your clinic or doctor right away (that very day) and tell them about your problem. Using birth control pills can be made safer if you get help as soon as problems arise.

INSTRUCTIONS FOR MINI-PILL USERS

Instructions:

1. Mini-Pills contain only one kind of hormone, a progestin, unlike combined birth control pills which contain both an estrogen and a progestin. The amount of progestin in the Mini-Pill is less than the amount of progestin in the combined pill. Progestin-only Pills may have several contraceptive effects including causing a thick cervical mucous which is difficult for sperm to penetrate, inhibiting implantation of the egg and inhibiting ovulation (release of an egg).

2. Mini-Pills may be the initial pill chosen for a patient who:
   (a) is over age 35 (and wants to use birth control pills)
   (b) is over age 30 and smokes more than 14 cigarettes a day
   (c) has a history of headaches, hypertension (high blood pressure), or bad varicose veins
   (d) prefers to initiate Pills immediately postpartum (after having a baby) rather than to wait until 4 to 6 weeks postpartum
   (e) is nursing her baby.
   If a birth control pill is used by a lactating woman, the Mini-Pills are preferred since Mini-Pills seem to increase the length of time during which a woman may successfully nurse her baby. Mini-Pills are preferable to combined Pills which may decrease the flow of breast milk.

3. Very often a patient is provided Mini-Pills after she has a problem using a combined Pill. Headaches, hypertension, and leg pain are the most common side effects of combined Pills which might dictate a switch to Mini-Pills. Just how much safer Mini-Pills are than combined is not known. Many of the undesirable side effects of the combined Pill are caused by its estrogen. Thus the absence of an estrogen should make the Mini-Pill safer.

4. Be sure to read the package insert for your specific brand of Mini-Pills.

5. Start taking Mini-Pills on your first day of menstrual bleeding.

6. Take one pill every single day. You never stop taking Mini-Pills. As soon as you finish one packet of Mini-Pills, go right on to the next packet the very next day. Never miss a day if you are taking Mini-Pills.

7. If you miss one pill, take it as soon as you remember and take your next pill at the regular time. Use a second method of birth control until your next period.

8. If you miss two pills, take two pills as soon as you remember and two the next day. Use a second method of birth control until your next period.

9. If you do not have a period within 45 days of your last one, go to a physician to determine if you are pregnant. Expect changes in the time between periods and in the length of your periods. While on the Mini-Pill, you may experience: spotting between periods, perfectly regular, normal cycles, irregular cycles, or very infrequent periods (one or two per year).

10. To improve the effectiveness of the Mini-Pill, consider using a second method for the first few months and then always during the midcycle. The midcycle is the 8–10 days between two periods when you are most likely to get pregnant. If you have a fairly regular 28-day cycle, your midcycle is from days

10–18 of your cycle (day one is the first day of your period).
11. If you notice any mood changes—depression, irritability, change in sex drive—see your clinician. Switching Mini-Pill brands may help.
12. Watch for the Pill Danger Signals:

EARLY PILL DANGER SIGNS
CAUTION: A—Abdominal pain (severe)
C—Chest pain (severe), cough, shortness of breath
H—Headache (severe), dizziness, weakness, numbness
E—Eye problems (vision loss or blurring), speech problems
S—Severe leg pain (calf or thigh)

See your clinician if you have any of these problems, or if you develop depression, yellow jaundice or a breast lump.

13. Every woman should examine her breasts for lumps or other changes once each month. A good way for you to remember to do a self-breast exam each month is to do the exam when you start a new pack of pills each month.

IMPORTANT INSTRUCTIONS FOR PATIENTS USING AN IUD

Instructions 6, 7, 8, 9 are reprinted with permission of ACHCSA, 1984. The remainder are reprinted with permission from *Contraceptive Technology, 1986–1987,* Hatcher et al.

Instructions:

1. The IUD is a plastic intrauterine device that is produced in various sizes and shapes. Some IUD's contain small amounts of copper or the hormone progesterone, which help the IUD to prevent pregnancy. The most significant mechanism of action of an IUD is to inhibit implantation of a fertilized egg into the wall of the uterus. The presence of an IUD may also dislodge an early implantation.
2. Before you have your IUD inserted, since some women have a fair amount of pain or nausea immediately following the insertion of their IUD, consider the following suggestions:
   (a) If you are going to have to walk a long distance or drive home after your IUD insertion, you may want to come to the clinic with someone who can help you to get home.
   (b) You may have less cramping with IUD insertion if you take a prostaglandin inhibitor (such as Advil or Nuprin, which are available over the counter) before you come to the clinic to have your IUD inserted. Be sure to confirm this suggestion with the person who gives you preinsertion instructions.
3. Always read the package insert for your specific type of IUD.
4. After your IUD has been inserted and before you leave the office or clinic, learn how to feel the IUD string in the back of your vagina.
5. Check for the string frequently during the first months you have your IUD, especially right before intercourse. Then, check after each period or any time you have abnormal cramping whether menstruating or not. You may not be protected by your IUD if: you cannot feel the string, you can feel the plastic part of your IUD, or the string of your IUD gets longer or shorter. If any of these three things occur, use another method of birth control until you can get to the clinic to have your IUD checked. You can expel an IUD without knowing it. Check pads and tampons when you remove them because many expulsions occur during the menstrual period.
6. If at any time after getting an IUD, you have an unexplained fever, pelvic pain or tenderness, severe cramping, or unusual vaginal bleeding or discharge, contact the clinic immediately. These may be signs of infection. Infections with IUD's can be very serious and if untreated can lead to hysterectomy (removal of the uterus) or even death.
7. If you miss a period—call the clinic immediately. If you become pregnant with the IUD in place, you should have it removed because of the danger of infection. Chances are about 25% that removal will cause an abortion, whereas chances are about 50% that spontaneous abortion (miscarriage) will occur if the IUD is left in. To decrease the chance of miscarriage, have your IUD removed before the sixth or seventh week of pregnancy, if at all possible.
8. Do not remove the IUD yourself and do not let your partner pull on the strings. The clinician will have a better idea of the angle at which it went in. It should come out the same way.
9. Get an annual checkup including a Pap smear, breast examination, and a blood test.
10. Special instructions for Copper-7 users if the string of your IUD lengthens:
    (a) Because of the way in which the string of the Copper-7 comes out over the top of the inserter barrel, the excess string may descend down into your vagina (lengthen). It can descend all the way to the opening of your vagina. If this happens, DO NOT PULL ON THE STRING! You should return to your clinician. Use a backup contraceptive such as condoms or foam until you have been seen and evaluated by your clinician.
    (b) This apparent lengthening of the string may mean one of two things: (1) The extra loop of string could have come down into your vagina while the entire IUD has remained right where it

belongs, inside your uterus. In this case you are not at any risk of becoming pregnant. If this turns out to be the case, your physician will probably trim the string of your IUD. (2) Your IUD could be coming out of your uterus (it could be partially expelled) and in this case, you are at increased risk of becoming pregnant. If this is what is happening to your IUD, your physician will remove this IUD.
11. Strongly consider using a backup method of birth control such as foam or condoms for the first three months you have an IUD. For extra protection, some IUD users always add a backup method at midcycle (the 8–10 days between two periods when you are most likely to get pregnant). If you have a fairly regular 28-day cycle, use a second method from days 10–18 of your cycle. Start counting from the first day of your period.
12. Common side effects are increased menstrual flow, menstrual cramping, and spotting. Remember: If you cannot tolerate the IUD, you can always have it removed. Heavier menstrual bleeding may be serious if you are anemic.

EARLY IUD DANGER SIGNS
CAUTION   P—Period late (pregnancy), abnormal spotting or bleeding
           A—Abdominal pain, pain with intercourse
           I —Infection exposure (such as Gonorrhea), abnormal discharge
           N—Not feeling well, fever, chills
           S—String missing, shorter or longer

SPECIAL NOTE OF CAUTION REGARDING SIDE EFFECTS:
Pain, bleeding and discharge in the days or weeks immediately following IUD insertion may be signs of an infection of your uterus and/or Fallopian tubes. This type of an infection may seriously affect your future health. For this reason, pain, bleeding, and discharge in the days and weeks after IUD insertion need to be reported quickly to your clinician to find out whether IUD removal and/or antibiotic treatment is necessary. Infection can occur anytime an IUD is in place but is most likely to develop in the days and weeks immediately following IUD insertion—watch out for these IUD danger signals:
  a. Abdominal pain
  b. Discharge
  c. Bleeding and/or
  d. Fever and chills
13. Iron supplementation is wise for all IUD users two to three days a week and may be wise for all reproductive women.
14. Remember: The Copper-T should be replaced every four years, the Copper-7 should be replaced every three years, and the Progestasert-T every year. The Saf-T-Coil and Lippes Loop can remain in the uterus until menopause as long as you are not having any problems at all.
15. Wait three months after your IUD has been removed before you try to become pregnant. Use another method of birth control for those three months, then begin trying for pregnancy. The policy may protect you from an ectopic (tubal) pregnancy, which is more likely to occur in the months immediately following IUD removal.
16. When you are seen for any medical, surgical, or sexual problem, be sure to tell your clinician that you are currently using a IUD.

INSTRUCTIONS FOR TUBAL LIGATION

(Female Sterilization)

Adapted with permission from *Contraceptive Technology, 1984–1985*, Hatcher et al.
Instructions:

1. Be completely comfortable with your decision to have a tubal ligation: this is crucial! You and your partner MUST BE CERTAIN that you understand (and desire) the permanency of the procedure. You can change your mind at any time prior to the operation.
2. Be prepared for:
  (a) Incisional pain—usually not severe and usually relieved by aspirin.
  (b) Shoulder and chest pain—usually causes the most discomfort of all the side effects but lasts only 24–48 hours. Caused by the anesthesia and by gas in the abdomen
  (c) Occasional pelvic ache or discomfort.
3. Plan to have a flexible schedule for the week following the sterilization. Some women recover less quickly from anesthesia and surgery than others.

INSTRUCTIONS FOR VASECTOMY

(Male Sterilization)

Adapted with permission from *Contraceptive Technology, 1984–1985*, Hatcher et al.
Instructions:

1. Be completely comfortable with your decision to have a vasectomy: this is critical! You and your partner MUST BE CERTAIN that you understand (and desire) the permanency of the procedure. You

can change your mind at any time prior to the operation.
2. Plan to remain quiet for approximately 48 hours following the vasectomy. A 48-hour "rest" period is important in decreasing the risk of complications.
3. Be prepared for some pain and swelling in the scrotal region following the vasectomy. As indicated in your counseling session, there is the possibility of complications, including infection, blood clots, and discomfort.
4. Following surgery, return home and rest for about two days. If possible, you should keep an ice pack on the scrotum for at least 4 hours. This will reduce chances of swelling, bleeding, and discomfort. You may be able to resume your normal activities after two or three days.
5. Avoid strenuous physical exercise for a week. Strenuous exercise means hard physical exertion to which you are normally unaccustomed or lifting or straining that could bring pressure to the groin or scrotum.
6. Wear a scrotal support for 48 hours during both waking and sleeping hours. Thereafter, you may wear it as long as you are more comfortable with it than without it.
7. You may resume sexual intercourse after two or three days if you feel that it would be comfortable, but STOP if it is uncomfortable. Also, avoid putting traction on, rubbing, or otherwise irritating the incision.
8. Remember, you are not sterile immediately. For most men, sperm have not been cleared from the tubes until after at least ten ejaculations. Until then, use another method of birth control to prevent pregnancy. The only certain way of knowing you are sterile is to have the doctor look for sperm under a microscope. Bring your doctor a specimen of your semen for a sperm count after you have had ten ejaculations or whatever number is specified. Two consecutive negative sperm counts are considered adequate proof of sterility.
9. Vasectomy clients should have a post-operative checkup 1–6 weeks after the procedure. The doctor or nurse will simply check the incision area to see that the healing process is proceeding normally.
10. It is important for you to know what is normal and what is abnormal following your surgery. There will probably be some pain and swelling in the scrotal region; the scrotum may be somewhat black and blue (from a small amount of bleeding). This is normal and should not worry you. However, occasionally blood from a tiny blood vessel may escape into the scrotum at the time of surgery and bleeding may continue. Notify your health care provider if you have any of the following danger signals or if you notice any unusual body changes:
    (a) Fever (over 100.4° F)
    (b) Bleeding (from the site of the incision)
    (c) Excessive pain or swelling

INSTRUCTIONS FOR USE OF FERTILITY AWARENESS METHODS

A couple planning to use any combination of these methods of family planning should receive detailed instruction and guidance over time from an instructor specially prepared with this information. Planned Parenthood can give appropriate referrals. The methods are discussed in detail in *Contraceptive Technology, 1984–85*.

INSTRUCTIONS FOR LACTATION AS A CONTRACEPTIVE METHOD

Reprinted with permission from *Contraceptive Technology, 1986–1987*, Hatcher et al.
Instructions:

1. YOU CAN BECOME PREGNANT WHILE NURSING YOUR CHILD!!! Breastfeeding does not give you enough birth control protection to count on.
2. Breast-feeding is a convenient, inexpensive, and nutritious way to feed your baby and it helps to protect the baby against infection. However, breast-feeding only offers PARTIAL CONTRACEPTIVE PROTECTION, which is not effective for most women.
3. If you choose to rely on breast-feeding as protection against pregnancy, you must feed your baby "on demand" for maximum effectiveness. Your baby may demand to be fed once an hour or more when awake, as well as several times during the night. Once you begin to give your baby formula or any other food, your protection against pregnancy is reduced even if you continue some breast-feeding.
4. YOU CAN BECOME PREGNANT BEFORE YOUR FIRST MENSTRUAL PERIOD AFTER CHILDBIRTH because ovulation can begin before menstruation.
5. MENSTRUATION DOES NOT AFFECT EITHER THE QUALITY OR THE QUANTITY OF YOUR BREAST MILK. You don't need to stop breast-feeding because you start your period.
6. Use a method of birth control if you decide to have sexual intercourse before your six-week postpartum visit.
7. Lubricants such as K-Y jelly, birth control foam, or saliva may make intercourse easier after childbirth because decreased estrogen production during breast-feeding causes your vagina to lubricate itself more slowly.

INSTRUCTIONS FOR COITUS INTERRUPTUS

Reprinted with permission from *Contraceptive Technology, 1986–1987*, Hatcher et al.

Instructions:

1. Before intercourse, the fluid at the tip of the penis should be wiped completely off. Millions of sperm may be contained in this drop of liquid.
2. When the man feels that he is about to ejaculate, he should remove his penis from inside the vagina, making sure that ejaculation occurs away from the entrance to the vagina.
3. Withdrawal is not a good birth control method if the couple intends to have repeated acts of intercourse because semen may be retained in the clear fluid at the tip of the erect penis.
4. Withdrawal is not a good birth control method if the man has trouble predicting when he is going to ejaculate.
5. Withdrawal is most appropriate for men who have no seepage of pre-ejaculatory fluid. If pre-ejaculatory seepage usually occurs, a condom should be worn during all coital play to avoid the risk of pregnancy.
6. The couple should try to have a supply of birth control foam or some type of spermicide available in case of an accident. Despite the seeming optimism of this suggestion, if ejaculation does occur, it is probably too late to stop some sperm from swimming up into the uterus.
7. Withdrawal is a considerably better method of contraception than no method at all.

APPENDIX L

Audiovisuals on Pregnancy, Childbirth and Parenting

1. Available through Polymorph Films, Inc
   118 South Street
   Boston, MA 02111
   (617) 542-2004
   A. New Baby Care—23 minutes
   B. New Mother Care—23 minutes
   C. Drugs, Smoking and Alcohol During Pregnancy—20 minutes
   D. Beginning Breastfeeding—23 minutes
   E. Having a Section is Having a Baby—28 minutes
   F. Amazing Newborn—25 minutes
   G. Prematurely Yours—15 minutes
   H. To Have and Not to Hold—21 minutes
   I. Your Baby's First Days—21 minutes
   J. Death of a Newborn—33 minutes

2. Available through University of California
   Extension Media Center
   2176 Shattuck Avenue
   Berkeley, CA 94704
   A. Some Babies Die—54 minutes

3. Available through American Journal of Nursing Co.
   Educational Services Division
   Dept E. 399
   555 West 57 Street
   New York, NY 10019-2961
   A. The Family and the Premature Infant—30 minutes
   B. Death of the High Risk Infant—30 minutes

APPENDIX M

Infections Representing Potentially Serious Threats During Pregnancy

Organisms	General Mode of Transmission	Mode of Congenital Transmission	Associated Congenital Defects	Incidence of Infection	Occurrence of Fetal/Neonatal Infection With Primary Versus Recurrent Infection
Toxoplasmosis	Ingestion of oocysts in raw meats or ingestion of oocysts from hands contaminated by cat feces or soil	Maternal bloodstream *via* placenta	Microcephaly, hydrocephaly, cerebral calcifications, and choreoretinitis	One study indicated that laboratory evidence of congenital infection was present in three of 4048 neonates; but only one of these newborns was symptomatic.	Primary infection
Cytomegalovirus (CMV)	Intimate and/or oral genital contact	Maternal bloodstream *via* placenta	Microcephaly, cerebral calcifications, hepatosplenomegaly, jaundice and seizures	Average incidence is one percent of all births but neonatal infection is most often clinically inapparent. Of this one percent, approximately five percent to 10% have the more virulent form of the disease and either develop serious late complications (hepatosplenomegaly, jaundice, and petechiae) or die. Another 10% of those born with subclinical congenital infection subsequently manifest perceptual, psychomotor, neurologic, or behavioral complications during the preschool period.	Primary and recurrent infection (primary infection is thought to be more serious)
Rubella	Droplet infection *via* respiratory tract	Maternal bloodstream *via* placenta	Heart, blood vessel defects — deafness, cataracts, and glaucoma	Approximately 10% to 15% of women in the childbearing years are estimated to be	Primary infection

Continued

TABLE Continued

Organisms	General Mode of Transmission	Mode of Congenital Transmission	Associated Congenital Defects	Incidence of Infection	Occurrence of Fetal/Neonatal Infection With Primary Versus Recurrent Infection
				susceptible. Percentage of infected fetuses per infected mothers varies according to gestational age. It is estimated to be as high as 54% during the first eight weeks and as low as 10% between 13 and 24 weeks.	
Herpes virus (HSV)	Direct contact with lesions or discharge and sexually transmissible	Rarely *via* placenta — nearly always *via* direct contact with vaginal secretions during delivery or ascending infection after prolonged membrane rupture	Incidence of congenital malformation is rare as HSV infection is usually a neonatal, not a congenital problem	Nahamias *et al.*, indicate that 1/1000–1/1500 private obstetric patients have genital herpes. Incidence is thought to be much higher in lower socio-economic groups. Risk of neonatal infection is about 60% with exposure at delivery to active maternal infections. Amstey estimates this risk at 25% to 30%.	Primary and recurrent infection (primary infection is thought to be more serious)

APPENDIX N

Perinatal HIV Guidelines

BACKGROUND

The guidelines presented here are based on the assumption that all caregivers are familiar with, and adhere to policies and practices as outlined in BODY SUBSTANCE ISOLATION (BSI). BSI focuses on isolating body substances (blood, feces, urine, wound drainage, vaginal secretions, oral secretions, etc.) from the hands of personnel, primarily by increased glove use and handwashing. The appropriate use of other barriers is also described. This system of infection control eliminates many of the ritualistic practices of traditional diagnosis-driven isolation systems, while increasing the use of barriers for all contacts with body substances.

This guideline for care focuses on specific perinatal practices and situations which arise when HIV infection is a concern.

GENERAL COMMENTS

Blood, vaginal secretions, amniotic fluid, placenta, and membranes should all be handled as potentially infectious body substances. Routine practices outlined in BSI in addition to aseptic technique and confine and contain practices carried out during C-Sections and deliveries will prevent transmission of the HIV virus to health care workers and to patients.

Handwashing

Wash hands frequently for at least 10 seconds, paying particular attention to around and under fingernails and between fingers. Always wash hands before and after every patient contact and after removing soiled gloves.

Protective Apparel

A. GLOVES when procedures may involve contact with body substances.

1. Starting IV's or drawing blood
2. Drawing/running cord blood gases
3. Weighing or handling placenta or umbilical cord
4. Handling baby prior to first bath
5. Handling bloody dressings, pads, or linens
6. Contact with meconium stools

Sterile gloves should be worn for

1. Scalp electrode placement and removal
2. Fetal blood sampling
3. Placement of intrauterine pressure monitor

For removal of retained placenta, an extra surgical sleeve secured by a sterile glove will provide an extra length of barrier for the arm and wrist.

Remove soiled gloves carefully by grasping cuff of glove and pulling it off over the fingers, turning it inside out and containing the soiled surface inside the clean surface. Take precautions not to snap glove fingers and create aerosols of blood when removing gloves.

B. GOWNS/SCRUBS for situations where body substances may splash on clothing. Caregivers should change their scrubs or gowns as soon as possible if soiled with body substances. Labor coaches and siblings are not required to wear special attire. However, they should be offered cover gowns or scrubs if they so desire to protect their clothing.

C. MASKS AND EYE PROTECTION when there is a possibility that body substances will be splashed in the face. Splashes to the face are often unpredictable. Care givers involved in the following may wish to wear eye protection routinely:

1. Artificial rupture of membranes
2. Drawing cord blood gasses
3. Delivery/surgical procedures

Safety glasses with prescription or clear glass lenses provide better visual acuity than plastic goggles.

LABOR AND DELIVERY

1. Use gloves for handling baby until after the first bath. Do initial bath as soon as the baby's temperature is stable.
2. Umbilical cords and placentas from known or suspected HIV-infected women should be handled with gloves, disposed of as specified in BSI procedures, and not used for studies or demonstrations.
3. Every effort should be made to confine and contain blood and birth fluids during vaginal deliveries. Disposable paper products and/or reusable linens should be used liberally to soak up fluids. Blood soaked linen should be carefully bagged into plastic linen bags. Use two bags if necessary to prevent leaking. Blood soaked trash should be placed in red infectious waste bags. Use two bags if necessary to prevent leaking.

Special drapes with pockets to contain birth fluids should be used during C-sections and vaginal deliveries to prevent excessive fluid contamination of the floor.
4. For removal of retained placenta, an extra surgical sleeve secured by a sterile glove will provide an extra length of barrier protection for the arm and wrist.
5. Instruments from vaginal deliveries and surgical procedures should be wiped with gauze dampened with saline during or immediately following the procedure to prevent drying of secretions. Gloves should be worn. The instruments should be placed in clear biohazard decontamination bags, and placed in the soiled utility area for removal to Central Processing. (This applies to all instruments, not just those used for HIV infected patients).
6. Do not use Dee Lee suction. Direct mechanical suction of the trachea is recommended with the use of a meconium trap if necessary.
7. Post mortem care for fetal demise should include removal of blood and body fluids.

NURSERY

1. Use gloves for handling baby until after the first bath. Do initial bath as soon as the baby's temperature is stable.
2. Circumcisions are not recommended for confirmed HIV infected infants.
3. Breast feeding is not recommended for known HIV infected women or women known to have engaged in high-risk behavior. If a woman wishes to breast feed, and her HIV status is unknown, she could express and freeze breast milk which could then be used in the event that her antibody test comes back negative.
4. Every effort should be made to provide the usual nuturing and stimulation to a baby born to an HIV infected mother.
5. Follow ACIP guidelines for immunization recommendations for HIV infected infants.
6. Alcohol to umbilical stump with every diaper change to facilitate drying. (For all infants, not only HIV infected infants)

ANTEPARTUM AND POST PARTUM

1. Private room placement is not necessary to prevent transmission of HIV between roommates if routine BSI procedures are followed. In some cases the privacy of the infected patient and/or the psycholog-

ical comfort of the roommate can be controlled in a private room setting. This is basically a social decision and is not an infection control issue. Private room placement is at the discretion of the attending M.D. and the nurse in charge of the unit and is dependent on private room availability.
2. There are no restrictions on mother-baby contact unless the mother has active pulmonary tuberculosis.
3. Portable sitzbath units should be used.
4. Clean blood spills following BSI procedures.
5. Encourage rooming in for interested mothers.
6. Use gloves, masks, and eye protection when assisting with rupturing of membranes. Be prepared to contain fluids with disposable paper products and/or linen. (This should be standard practice, not just for HIV-infected women.)

HIV ANTIBODY TESTING AND RELEASE OF INFORMATION

1. Refer to the attached table for women who should be screened in the perinatal period.
2. Two consents should be signed when testing is initiated in the hospital:
AUTHORIZATION FOR DISCLOSURE OF THE RESULTS OF A BLOOD TEST TO DETECT ANTIBODIES TO THE CAUSATIVE AGENT OF AQUIRED IMMUNE DEFICIENCY SYNDROME
VERIFICATION OF CONSENT FOR TESTING BLOOD TO ANTIBODIES TO THE HUMAN IMMUNODEFICIENCY VIRUS

In all instances, it is expected that the physician will have discussed and obtained consent from the patient/patient representative prior to obtaining the signature on the forms.

Once these consents have been signed, the physician may release the results to those healthcare professionals responsible for the care and treatment of the patient.

Like all aspects of the patient's medical information, this result should be treated with the utmost confidentiality because of the severe emotional, social, and financial consequences which can occur with unauthorized release of the information.

After proper consents have been obtained, this information may be shared in adoptive, foster, or emergency shelter placements.

DISCHARGE PLANNING

1. Women with confirmed HIV infection or at risk for HIV infection should be encouraged to have continued medical follow-up for medical assessment, risk reduction counseling, and future pregnancy counseling.
2. Infants born to HIV infected women should be referred to a program which specializes in the care of HIV infected infants.
3. Family members or home care givers should be instructed in the potential modes of transmission and appropriate infection control precautions.

EMPLOYEE HEALTH

1. Refer to the Employee Health section of the Infection Control Manual for complete guidelines for employee health.
2. Report any needle puncture, sharp object injury, or mucous membrane splash with body substances to the Employee Health Department.

REFERENCES

"Guidelines for the Control of Perinatally Transmitted Human Immunodeficiency Virus Infection and Care of Infected Mothers, Infants, and Children." Rutherford et al. The Western Journal of Medicine, July 1987 pp 104–110

"CDC: Recommendations for assisting in the prevention of perinatal transmission or human T-lymphotropic virus type III/lymphadenopathy-associated virus and acquired immunodeficiency syndrome." MMWR 1985; 34:721–726, 731–732

APPENDIX O

Testing for HIV: Clinical Diagnosis

Testing for Clinical Diagnosis

When a physician has a clinical suspicion that the child patient has a disease suggestive of ARC or AIDS, the antibody test to HIV should be recommended for diagnostic purposes and performed with parental consent observing the necessary confidentiality guidelines. As indicated in the earlier issue of this newsletter, a positive ELISA test cannot be considered definitive until confirmed by the Western Blot or immunofluorescence techniques.

Testing for Early Diagnosis

Because some benefit may accrue to the child as the result of early diagnosis and treatment of HIV infection, testing of children at high risk of having been exposed to HIV should be considered. However, as the prevalence of HIV infection varies from risk group to risk group, the actual risk of perinatal, sexual, or parenteral exposure to HIV also varies. Your local Health Department can help you locally to assess these risks.

The issue of which population might be tested is addressed in the following table.

I.	"High-Risk" Women*	Preconceptual	Yes	
		Prenatal	Yes	1st and 3rd trimester testing recommended.
II.	All Pregnant Women		No	Not reasonable or cost-effective.
III.	Newborn of "high risk"			
		Mother tested	No	Infant antibodies same as mother, follow infant staying with mother carefully.
		Mother not tested	Yes	Positive infant requires careful follow-up
	Foster care		Yes	If mother not tested or does not wish to divulge results.
	Adoption		Yes	Adoptive parents need to know.
IV.	All Newborns		No	Not necessary or cost effective.
V.	Hemophiliac who received blood factors before May 1985		Yes	
VI.	Recipient of blood 1979–March 1985		Yes	If treated with multiple units in high-risk area. The real intent of screening adult blood recipients is to prevent sexual transmission; this is usually not a consideration.
VII.	Clinically suspect HIV infection		Yes	
VIII.	Sexually abused		No	Current data do not warrant routine testing. Testing might be indicated if the perpetrator is thought to be at risk.
IX.	Adolescent "at risk" in custody or institution		No	No positive result of testing can be anticipated from routine testing. Test may be clinically indicated.
X.	Pregnant adolescent "at risk"		Yes	Same as pregnant adult.

*Women "at risk" includes IV drug users; sexual contacts of men known to be infected as well as men potentially at risk of infection including gay and bisexual men, men who are IV drug users, men who are hemophiliacs who have received blood products, transfusion recipients, as well as men from Haiti or Central Africa. It also includes women who have received blood or blood products as noted above. Each woman seen in this setting should assess her own risk.

It is important to note that the whole issue of who should be tested will change radically as soon as a drug becomes available which has a positive influence on the clinical course of HIV infection. It is possible that in the future early testing would confer real treatment benefits. This is not the case at the present time.

We include recommendations about testing women because pediatricians deal with adolescents at risk of infection and pregnancy and because mothers often use the pediatrician as a health adviser.

Moses Grossman, M.D.

APPENDIX P

Preparation for Neonatal Transport

Provide 1:1 Nursing Care for the Infant

Keep infant warm
Place on prewarmed radiant warmer, and attach temperature probe.
Be certain infant is well dried and lying on a dry surface.
Keep sides of table up.
Consider use of Porta-warm mattress, heating lamp, warm water-filled gloves (covered with a linen), and aluminum foil on sides of table for small infants with hypothermia.

Oxygenate and Ventilate as Needed

Assess for improved color, breath sounds, chest movement, and heart rate.
Pass oral gastric tube for decompression.
Have an oxygen blender available so that oxygen can be weaned as color improves.
Monitor FIO_2 with an oxygen analyzer. Check that analyzer is calibrated.
Chart all changes in oxygen concentration, pressure, and rate.

Intubation

Have laryngoscope and endotracheal tube at bedside.
Make sure bulb in laryngoscope is bright and tight.
ETT size guidelines:

Infant weight	Recommended tube size
>4000 g	4.0
>2500 g	3.5
>1000 g	3.0
<1000 g	2.5

Distance to advance ETT:

Infant weight	cm in from lip*
1 kg	7
2 kg	8
3 kg	9
4 kg	10

*Oral: add 1 cm in for nasal.

Once intubated, listen in axillary line for equal breath sounds bilaterally.
Use hollihesive, tape, and Logan's bow to secure tube.
Obtain chest x-ray as soon as possible. Be sure head is turned to side, and neck is not flexed or hyperextended.
ETT should be at the level of T_1 to T_2.

Monitor Vital Signs

Place infant on cardiac, respiratory, and blood pressure monitors.
Place electrodes along axillary lines.
Monitor vital signs every 15–30 minutes.
Normal range of vital signs:
Temperature: axillary: 97.8–98.6F (preferred)
rectal: 98–99F
Heart Rate: 120–160 beats per minute
Respiratory Rate: 30–60 per minute
Blood Pressure: acceptable systolic pressures

750 grams	34–54
1000 grams	37–59
1500 grams	40–62
2000 grams	43–66
2500 grams	46–70
3000 grams	51–75

For hypotension: May give Albumin 0.5–1 gram/kg slowly over 10–30". If using 25% Albumin, dilute to 5% with NS, and give 10 cc/kg over 10–30". If indicated, may give PRBC's 10 cc/kg over 10–30 minutes. IV, UV, UA.

Monitor Blood Gases

Prefer arterial; otherwise, warmed heelstick.
Place transcutaneous monitor (TCM) on right upper chest.
Obtain blood gas to correlate TCM.
Obtain blood gas with any change in baby's color or condition.
Obtain blood gas 15" after any FIO_2, pressure or rate change.
Obtain blood gas 15" after Sodium Bicarbonate is given.
Chart all blood gas results.

Recommended values for most disease entities:
pO2: 55 to 70 (arterial) 40 to 50 (heelstick)
pCO2: 35 to 45
pH: 7.35 to 7.45
B.E.: −5 to +5
Recommended values if persistence of fetal circulation suspected:
pO2: 100 to 150 (pre-ductal arterial) if full-term
pO2: 80 to 90 (pre-ductal arterial) if premature
pCO2: 20 to 30
pH: 7.55 to 7.60
If any values are not within the recommended range, consult the physician.
If pO2 low: may increase FIO_2, pressure, or rate
If pO2 high: may decrease FIO_2, pressure, or rate
If pCO2 low: may decrease rate or pressure
If pCO2 high: may increase rate or pressure
If Base Deficit: may give Sodium Bicarbonate 2–3 meq/kg
always diluted 1:1 with Sterile Water or D10
Give slowly, preferably over 15–30 minutes, never faster than 5 minutes
NaHCO3 not recommended if pCO2 > 50

Monitor Dextrostix

Check every 15–30 minutes until stable; then every hour and prn.
Maintain Dextrostix between 45 and 130.
If the Dextrostix is a weak 45 or lower, obtain a STAT serum glucose. Do *not* wait more than 10" for the lab to draw this.
Do *not* wait for results to come back before treating.
Treat with 10% Glucose, 5 cc/kg, preferably IV, UV, or UA.
If no line available, may give PO if clinically indicated.
Continue to monitor Dextrostix.
Repeat 10% Glucose prn.

Check Hct

Prefer central; otherwise, warmed heelstick.
If less than 45%, may administer blood: PRBC's 10 cc/kg.
Before giving blood, obtain a type and cross, stat screen, and if it is a baby who will need chromosomes drawn, this should be drawn before blood is transfused.
Repeat Hct after 1 hour and prn.
O Negative PRBC's can be given unmatched in emergency, with M.D.'s OK.
If the central Hct is greater than 65%, a partial exchange may be indicated. May use Normal Saline or 5% Albuminated Normal Saline.

Fluid Administration

Recommended fluid administration rates:
Infants with R.D.S., asphyxia, and sepsis:
D10W 50–65 cc/kg/day (approx. 2–3 cc/kg/hr)
example: 1000 gram infant (2 lbs., 3 oz.) = 2–3 cc/hr
example: 2000 gram infant (4 lbs., 7 oz.) = 5–6 cc/hr
example: 3000 gram infant (6 lbs., 10 oz.) = 8–9 cc/hr
Begin with 10% Glucose.
If needed, may increase glucose concentration to 12.5%.
To increase glucose: In volutrol, mix 93.8 cc of D10W with 6.2 cc of D50 to make 100 cc of D12.5W.
Infants with Abdominal Wall Defects:
150 cc/kg/day (approx. 6 cc/kg/hr)
example: 1000 gram infant (2 lbs., 3 oz.) = 6 cc/hr
example: 2000 gram infant (4 lbs., 7 oz.) = 12 cc/hr
example: 3000 gram infant (6 lbs., 10 oz.) = 18 cc/hr

Administer Antibiotics

Draw blood cultures and begin antibiotics on any infant with symptoms of respiratory distress, suspected sepsis, or meningitis.
Recommended doses:
Ampicillin: 100 mg/kg/day – divided q12 if infant < 7 days old
– divided q8 if infant > 7 days old
300 mg/kg/day – divided q6 if treating meningitis
IV, UV, UA preferred. May give IM.
Gentamicin:

	<1 week of age	>1 week of age
Preterm		
<1000 gm	2.5 mg/kg q24 hr	2 mg/kg q12 hr
>1000 gm	2 mg/kg q12 hr	2 mg/kg q12 hr
Term		
>37 wks	2 mg/kg q12 hr	2.5 mg/kg q8 hr

Using a two-syringe method, dilute with 1 cc of sterile water. Give over at least 20 minutes, IV, UV, or UA

Paper Work

The following items must be sent with the transport team:
Xeroxed copies of the infant's and mother's chart
Infant's X-Rays (these will be returned)
10 cc of cord blood in a clot tube
10 cc of mother's blood in a clot tube

Parents

Please remind parents that they are welcome to call and visit the nursery at any time of the day or night. If the mother is planning to breastfeed, provide her with breastfeeding information and encourage her to pump her breasts.
All breast milk should be collected in a sterile container (you can use Gerber bags and then double bag for the freezer).
Label all containers with the name, date and time collected.
The milk should be frozen immediately.

Report

When the transport team arrives, you will need to report on the infant's history and condition since birth, and your assistance with stabilization for transport. If the shift changes before the transport team arrives, please give a complete report to your relief nurse.

Special Circumstances

For *all* infants, closely monitor temperature and dextrostix.

Asphyxia

Monitor blood gases if in oxygen.
Fluid restrict to 50 cc/kg/day.
Do baseline neuro and head exam.
Observe closely for seizure activity.
Keep a high index of suspicion for Persistence of Fetal Circulation.

Persistence of Fetal Circulation (PFC or Pulmonary Hypertension)

Suspect PFC in any infant who has suffered asphyxia and whose oxygenation fluctuates greatly with small changes in FIO_2, whose hypoxemia seems to be out of proportion to the degree of lung disease, and who shows marked improvement with 100% oxygen.
Goal of therapy: vasodilate pulmonary arterioles, maintain BP, and prevent hypoxia and acidosis.
Monitor blood gases.
May obtain simultaneous gases: UA & Rt Radial to determine presence of a Right to Left shunt through PDA.
Keep well oxygenated: pO_2 100–150 in term, pO_2 80–90 in preterm.
Keep pCO_2 20–30.
Keep alkalotic: pH 7.55–7.60.
Wean *very* gradually (1 to 2% at a time), and with caution.
Maintain systemic blood pressure.
Minimize stresses to baby to prevent hypoxia and vasoconstriction of pulmonary vessels.

Seizures

Suction stomach contents ASAP.
Phenobarbitol 5–10 mg/kg. May repeat up to a loading dose of 20 mg/kg/per day. Maintenance dose = 3–7 mg/kg/day.
Phenobarbitol doses must be double checked.
Phenobarbitol may cause respiratory depression or hypotension.
Watch respiratory effort–Have bag and mask ready.
Monitor blood pressure closely–Have Albumin available.
Monitor Dextrostix!

Tracheo-esophageal Fistula (TEF)

Elevate HOB.
Keep NPO. Maintain IV.
#8 or #10 feeding tube to blind pouch on low intermittent suction.
Keep infant from crying to prevent distension.
Frequent oral-pharyngeal suctioning.
Use positive pressure ventilation only if absolutely necessary to avoid forcing air through the fistula into the GI tract where it can not be vented.

Omphalocele/Gastroschisis

Cover the defect with warm, sterile, normal saline moistened lap pads and wrap with Saran wrap. Support defect so that there is no torque, kinking, or drying of the bowel.
If possible place baby in a plastic bag to neck or nipple line.
Keep NPO
IV–Keep well hydrated: D5 1/3 NS 150 cc/kg/day.
N/G tube to low intermittent suction for G.I. decompression.
Maintain temperature!

G.I. Obstruction/Abdominal Distension

Keep NPO.
Maintain IV
N/G tube to low intermittent suction.
Elevate HOB.

Diaphragmatic Hernia

Do *not* mask bag if possible.
If assisted ventilation is required, intubate immediately and ventilate rapidly and gently to prevent pneumothorax.
Be sure the ETT is not below the carina.
N/G tube to low intermittent suction for G.I. decompression.

Myelomeningocele

Cover defect with warm, sterile normal saline soak and wrap in Saran wrap, chux or diaper.
If possible, place baby in a plastic bag to include area above defect.
Keep infant on stomach.
Maintain temperature!

Cardiac

Administer oxygen as needed.
Monitor blood gases.
Prevent crying for maximum pulmonary blood flow.
Assess pulses, perfusion, BP, HR, murmur, precordial activity.
Minimize stresses that will lead to hypoxia.

Pulmonary Air Leak

Assess for equal breath sounds, chest excursion, PMI.
Chest X-Ray as soon as possible.
Have pneumo kit for needling chest (alcohol wipe, #20 gelco, T connector, stopcock, 20cc syringe).
If chest needled, continue to evacuate air until chest tube is placed.
Chest tube placement: Have chest tray, #8, #10, #12, or #14 feeding tube with water seal and suction setup.

Copyright 1988. Children's Hospital, Oakland.

Index

A

Abdellah, Faye G., 41
Abdomen
  assessment of, 323–328, 559
    postpartum, 487–488
  exercises for, 468–469, 475–476, 478–480
  length of gestation and, 323–326
  lie, presentation, and fetal position and, 326–328
  muscle tone following cesarean section, 481
Abdominal touch picture, 327
Abdominal wall check, 479
Abdominal wall exercises, 472–473
Abduction contracture, congenital, 563
Abnormal presentation, 682
  cesarean section for, 697
ABO antigens, 429
Abortion
  bleeding with, 660
  as contraceptive method, 72–73
  danger signs in, 73
  ethical issue of, 138–139
  funding of, 134
  genetic, 793–795
  history of, 318
  issue of, 46
  liberalized laws on, 101
  loss with, 793
  maternal mortality from, 43
  in pregnant adolescents, 829
  psychological aspects of, 73, 794–795
  therapeutic, 657
Abruptio placentae
  bleeding with, 660–662
  complications of, 664–665
  etiology of, 705
  treatment of, 664, 707
Abstinence, 71–72
  periodic, 70–71
Accommodation, 630
Accountability, 941–942
Acetylcholinesterase level testing, 276–277
Acidosis, newborn, 409

Acini, 439
Acquired immunodeficiency syndrome (AIDS), 46, 102
  children with, 908t
  comfort for victims of, 907t
  fear of, 909
  HIV virus and, 906–909
  legal controversy of, 153
  in pregnancy, 907–908
  sex education and, 824
  testing for, 321
Acrocyanosis, 552
Acrosome reaction, 167
Acupuncture, 396
Acyclovir, 902
Adaptation
  to death, 792
  strategies, 785
Adenosine, respiratory depression with, 887
Admission nursery, 590
Adolescent
  follow-up needs of, 836–838
  as high-risk patient, 836–838
  in hospital, 836
  needs of, 831–832
  pregnancy of 46, 93–94, 100, 821–842
    in antepartum period, 828–834
    early intervention in, 828–830
    issues of increase in, 823–826
    during labor and delivery, 834–835
    new approaches and programs for, 841–842
    physical characteristics and medical risks in, 827–828
    postpartum period of, 836–838
    preventions of, 841
    psychologic characteristics and risk factors in, 826–827
    resources and referrals for, 838–841
    stage of adolescence and, 826
    statistics on, 823
Adolescent Pregnancy Programs, Office of, 46
Adoption, 101–102

Adrenal glands, during pregnancy, 209
Adrenal hormones, after delivery, 428
Advanced registered nurse practitioners (ARNP), 24
Advocacy, 942–944
Affection, 83
Affectional bond, 625
Affiliation, 83
Afterpains, 430, 488
Agnodice the Athenian, 26
AIB scale, 633
Ainsworth, Mary Salter, 40
Air ambulance, 762, 778
Alba lochia, 425
Alcohol
  abuse of, 882–884
  avoidance of, 265
  during breastfeeding, 461
  consumption, 261
  fetal effects of, 875, 882–883
  widespread use of, 46
Aldous's family development stages, 92
Alert but agitated state, 574
Alert state, 574
Allergy, special formulas for, 620–621
Alpha-fetoprotein level, 276
Alternate leg flexion/extension, 470
Alternative birth centers, 917. *See also* birthing centers
  advantages of, 924–925
  disadvantages of, 925
  legal basis for practice in, 924
  response to demands for, 920
Alveoli, 439
Ambulant labor, 931
Ambulation
  after delivery, 430–431
  postpartum assessment of, 491
Amenorrhea, 195
American College of Nurse-Midwives, 149
American Journal of Nursing, on ethical issues, 131
American Nurses' Association of Nurse Researchers, 952

American Nursing Association (ANA)
  educational requirements of, 148
  first article of, 131
  Standards of Maternal-Child Health Nursing Practice of, 147
American Red Cross, 33, 37
American Society for Psychoprophylaxis in Obstetrics, 40, 305
Amides, 394
Aminophylline, 674
Amnesia effect, 836
Amnesia-producing drugs, 390
Amnioblasts, 174
Amniocentesis
  consent for, 138
  definition of, 271
  in fetal maturity assessment, 278
  genetic disorders detected by, 272–274t
  indications for, 271–278
  nursing role in, 279–282
  procedure and interpretation of, 278–279
  in sex preselection, 107
  side-effects of, 279
Amniotic fluid, 174
  cytologic analysis of cells of, 278
  evaporation of, 407
  increase in, 191
  meconium-stained, 192, 279
  testosterone levels of, 107
Amniotic fluid embolus (AFE), 675
Amniotomy, 691, 692
  complications for, 694–695
Anabolic protein metabolism, 429
Analgesia, 387, 390
  decreased use of, 41
  inhalation, 395–396
Android pelvis, 349
Anemia
  nutritional, 255–256
  with spinal cord injury, 855–856
Anesthesia, 387
  decreased use of, 41
  first used in childbirth, 29, 913
  general, 395–396
  inhalation, 395–396
  local, 394–395
  infiltration, 390–391
  toxic effects on fetus of, 394–395
  regional, 390–395
  use of for delivery, 39
Ankle circles, 469
Ankle exercises, postcesarean, 483
Ankle flexion/extension, 469
Anorectal canal, development of, 191
Antepartum fetal death, 793
Anthropoid pelvis, 349
Anthropometric assessment, 256
Anthropometric measures, 605
Antibacterial agents, use of in newborns, 410–412
Antibiotics, for postpartum infections, 659–660
Antibodies, during pregnancy, 210
Antibody titers, 909
Anticipatory guidance, 334
Anticoagulation therapy, 670
  risk of, 674
Antimicrobial agents, fetal effects of, 876–877t
Antiplatelet agents, 675

Antiseptic techniques, 31
Anus, assessment of, 562
Anxieties
  of physically disabled parent, 865–866
  in pregnant adolescent, 832–833
Apgar, Virginia, 38, 402
Apgar scores, 376
  assignment of, 743–744
  fetal biophysical profile and, 293
  low, 695, 702
  resuscitation by, 744t, 755
Apgar scoring system, 38, 402–405
  1-minute, 744, 745
Apnea, 717–718
Aquamephyton, side-effects of, 412
Arab-Americans
  attitude toward pregnancy in, 116, 118
  postpartal practices of, 120–121
Arantius, 28
Areola, 439
Artificial feeding, dangers of, 437
Artificial insemination, 103–104
Artificial insemination donor (AID), 103
Artificial insemination homologous (AIH), 103
Artificial insemination husband donor (AIHD), 103
Ascorbic acid, 604
  iron absorption and, 248
Asphyxia, 400–401
  causes of, 400
  chemical changes with transient, 535–536
  prevention of, 400, 719
  risk of, 537
  in SGA infants, 728, 730
Assessment
  of adolescent mother, 836–838
  and diagnosis phase, 9–13
  equipment for, 551
  of normal newborn, 546–576
  procedure for, 551–576
  purpose of, 547
  skills, 362–365
  tools of, 547
Assimilation, 630
Asymmetry, 551
Attachment, 624. See also Bonding; Maternal-infant attachment
  behaviors of, 627–629
  of father, 811–814
  in premature infant, 629–630
  process of, 625–627
Audiologic testing, 850
Audiovisual materials, 519–520
Auditory assessment, 575–576
Auditory stimulation, 632–633
Auscultation, 362
Autonomy, 136–137
  issues of, 137–140
Autopsies, 800
Autosuggestion, conscious, 478
Awake and Aware, 305
Ayer's spatula, 329

B

Babinski reflex, 570
Baby foods, commercial, 614

"Baby M" case, 106
Backache
  postpartum assessment of, 490
  with pregnancy, 206
Ballottement, 196
Barbiturates, 388–390
Barlow test, 562
Barton, Clara, 32–33
Basal body temperature method, 70
Baseline data, determining and documenting of, 547
Baseline tonus, 375
Bassinets, 590–591, 593
Behavior,
  purposiveness of, 506
  reinforcement of, 507
Behavioral assessment, 571–576
Behaviorism, 503–504
Behavioristic learning theories, 503–505
Belief system, 115
Bending, postpartum, 474–475
Beneficence, 140, 142–143
Bertheau, Caroline, 30
Beta-mimetic drugs, 649
Bilirubin
  in amniotic fluid, 277–278
  indirect and direct, 714
  levels of, 542
Billings method, 70
Biochemical abnormalities, detection of, 272
Biochemical tests, 255–256
Bioethics
  nursing and, 131–134
  principles and rules in, 134–143
Biologic pregnancy tests, 197
Biparietal diameter, 269
Birth canal
  fetus descent through, 344–347
  trauma to, 432
Birth control, 825–826
  dissemination of information on, 33–34
  history of, 85
Birth control pill. See Oral contraceptives
Birth Control Review, 34
Birth defects, in in vitro fertilization, 105
Birthing beds, 4
Birthing centers, 4, 45. See also Alternative birth centers
  in-hospital, 925–928
  out-of-hospital, 924–925
  philosophy of, 924
  preparation for use of, 928–929
Birthing chairs, 4, 916
Birthing customs, 415
Birthing methods
  alternative, 915–932
  comparative advantages and disadvantages of, 929t
Birthing room, 4, 926–927
  delivery
    contraindications for, 927t
    transfer from to regular delivery room, 926–927
  objective of, 927
Birth intervals, 356
Birth rate, 42–45
Birth registration, 418

INDEX

Birth weight, 547
  maternal nutrition and, 245
Black Americans, postpartal practices of, 121
Blackwell, Elizabeth, 30
Bladder
  distended, 434
  infections of with spinal cord injury, 856
  postpartum assessment of, 488–489
  trauma to, 434
Blanching, 552
Blastocyst, 168
  implanted, *172*
Blastomere, 168
Blind parent, 851–852
  care and treatment issues for, 853–854
  childbearing process for, 852–853
  parenting strategies of, 868
  techniques to enrich obstetric care for, 854–855
Blood glucose levels
  in premature infant, 715
  stabilization of, 650
Blood group incompatibility, 428–429
Blood pressure
  changes in with pregnancy, 203, 427
  after delivery, 427
  in general health assessment, 320–321
Blood replacement therapy, 707
Blood typing, 429
Blood vessels
  changes in with pregnancy, 207
  development of, 175–176
  fetal, 185
Blood volume, after delivery, 426
Bloody show, 350, 352
Body fluids, assessment of, 321
Bonding, 624. *See also* Attachment; Maternal-infant attachment
  cultural differences in, 415, 418
  with father, 811
Bourgeois, Louise, 28
Bowel obstruction, with cesarean section, 690
Bowel sound, 487
Bowlby, John, 40
Bradley, Robert, 304, 305
Bradley method, 306–308, 313, 913
  disadvantages of, 307–308
Branchial arches, 176
Braun von Fernwald's sign, 196
Braxton Hicks contractions, 200, 342, 350
  with spinal cord injury, 858
Braxton Hicks sign, 196
Brazelton, T. Berry, 39–40
  on working parents, 88
Brazelton Neonatal Behavioral Assessment Scale (BNBAS), 571–572, 633
  infant's state in, 572–574
  usefulness of, 574, 636
Breastfeeding, 436–462
  adequate milk supply in, 450
  for adolescents, 836
  of adopted infants, 460
  afterpains and, 430
  assessment tool for, *442*
  avoiding supplemental feeding with, 445–446
  baby with cleft lip or palate, 459–460
  benefits of, 436
    emotional, 448
    to mother and newborn, 447–448
    psychosocial, 609–610
  breast assessment and, 322–323
  breast care and diet with, 448–450
  with cesarean births, 460
  colic with, 453
  contraception during, 71
  cultural attitudes toward, 121–122
    changing, 437–438
  decline in, 438
  on demand, 445
  drugs administered to mother during, 461–462
  early initiation of, 441
  education on, 312
  encouragement of, 40
  failure in, 447
  historical perspective on, 437
  with HIV virus, 908
  infant difficulty in attaching to breast, 452–453
  infant needs and feeding behavior with, 450
  information sources on, 450–451
  menstrual cycle and, 426
  while mother and infant are separated, 454–459
  mother's knowledge about, 447–448
  nursing assessment for, 438–441
  nursing management of, 441
  nutrient supplements with, 609–610
  positioning infant for, 441–445
  for premature or ill infant, 458–459
  problems with, 452–454
  psychologic support for, 446–447
  to release oxytocin, 356
  of SGA infants, 616
  slow weight gain with, 453
  with spinal cord injury, 857–858
  after stopping, 460, 461
  support for, 441–445
  timing of, 445
  twins, 459
  for working mother, 457–458
Breastfeeding support groups, 447
Breast milk
  low phenylalanine levels of, 620
  nutrients in, 609
Breast pumps, 454–456, 458
Breasts
  assessment of, 322–323, 440–441
  care of during breastfeeding, 448–450
  changes in with pregnancy, 195, 202–203
  engorgement of, 451–452
  fat and connective tissue of, 439
  glandular tissue of, 439
  innervation and blood supply to, 439
  mastitis of, 453–454
  postpartum, 426, 440–441, 487
  during pregnancy, 440
  skin of, 439
Breath, first, 533–536
Breathing, periodic, 717
Breathing pattern control, 309–310
Breckinridge, Mary, 35–36
Breech presentation, 326, *697*
  cesarean section with, 682

Brown, Louise, 104
Brown fat metabolism, 407
  fatty acid release with, 409
  in thermogenesis, 539
Brow presentation, *697*
Buccopharyngeal membrane, 189
Bulk flow, 182
Butanol-extractable iodine, 209
Buttocks lift, 475
Byrne, Ethel, 33

C

Caffeine
  during breastfeeding, 461
  fetal effects of, 886–887
Calcium, 603
  deficiency of, 209, 264–265
  extrauterine adaptation of, 541
  release of during labor, 342
  requirements, 248
  supplementation of, 250
Calcium gluconate, 647
Calipers, 323–324
Calorie needs, 247
Campbell, Dame Kate, 38
Candida albicans infections, 652
Capacitation, 167
Capillary hemangiomas, 554–555
Caput succedaneum, 536, 555, *556*
Carbohydrates, 602
  complex, 265
  intake of with diabetes, 650–652
  metabolism of
    after delivery, 429
    during pregnancy, 207–208
Carbon monoxide, 887
Cardiac compression, closed chest, 752–753
Cardiac loop, formation of, *185*
Cardiac output, during pregnancy, 203
Cardiff method, 328
Cardiopulmonary resuscitation, *405*
  in newborn, 404
Cardiorespiratory monitoring, 764
Cardiovascular system
  changes in during labor, 344
  changes in with pregnancy, 203
  immature, 718–719
Care
  family-centered, 593–594
  for normal newborn, 579–597
  recommended daily routine for, 594–597
Career counseling, 840–841
Caring
  advocacy and, 942–944
  as human sensitivity, 939–940
  and nursing education, 936
  in perinatal nursing, 935–944
  technology and, 938–939
Case studies, 519, 949
  application of, 950
Cataracts, 557
Catecholamines, increased circulating levels of, 887
Caudal anesthesia, 391–393
Cell membranes, breaks in, 182
Cellular immune response, 210
Central nervous system immaturity, 721

Central venous pressure monitoring, 707
Cephalhematoma, 537, 555–556
Cephalic presentation, 326
Cephalopelvic disproportion (CPD), 681, 695–696
Cerebrospinal fluid assessment, 895
Cerebrum, maturation of, 184
Ceremonial system, 115
Cervical cap, 57–58
Cervical mucosal changes, 162–163
Cervical range of motion exercise, 476
Cervix
  changes in during labor, 342, 350
  changes in with pregnancy, 200–201
  after delivery, 425
  dilation of, 352
  trauma to, 432
Cesarean birth classes, 306
Cesarean section
  abdominal assessment following, 488
  by abdominal incision, 684
  in adolescent patients, 834, 835
  anesthesia for, 395–396
  breastfeeding and, 460
  case presentation for, 686
  early ambulation after, 430–431, 481–482
  exercise program following, 480–485
  extraperitoneal, 684–690
  with fetal distress, 704
  gastrointestinal tract after, 428, 690
  increased rate of, 466, 683–684
  indications for, 681–684
  morphine injection during, 432
  need for family involvement in, 919
  psychosocial considerations in, 690–691
  pulmonary disturbances with, 690
  rates of use of, 39
  in Renaissance, 28
  repeat, 682
  risk of infection with, 685–690
  by uterine incision, 684
  vaginal birth after, 930–931
Chabon, Irwin, 305
Chadwick's sign, 195, 201
Chamberlen, Peter, 28–29
Chamberlen, William, 28–29
Change, 19–20. *See also* Emotional change; Physiologic change; Psychological change
  adoption and internalization of, 17–18
  cultural and social barriers to, 13
  definition of, 3–7
  by drift, 6
  economic barriers to, 13
  elements of, *8*
  failure to, 18
  in family, 18–19, 79–96
  identifying barriers to, 12–13
  implementation of, 15–16, 17
  levels of, 5
  participants in, 6
  physical barriers to, 13
  planned, 5–6, 7, 13–15
  process of, 7–9
  psychologic barriers to, 13
  research for, 946–954
  resistance to, 12–13
  in society, 98–108
  strategies for, 14, 15

stress and, 12
successful, 17–18
theories of, 7–9
victim versus agent of, 4
Change agent
  definition of, 6–7
  in recent past, 42
Change theorists, 7–9
Charting tips, 151*t*
Chastity girdles, 27
Chemical stressors, 537
Chemical teratogenesis, 875
Chest assessment, 559
  postpartum, 487
Chest expansion, upper, 482
Chest positioning, 494
Childbearing, 24. *See also* Childbirth
  cultural and socioeconomic influences on, 99–100
  cultural aspects of, 110–126
  education surrounding, 502–503
  effect of blindness on, 852–853
  historical overview of, 916–917
  phases of, 89–90
Childbearing centers, 925. *See also* Birthing centers
Childbirth. *See also* Natural childbirth
  alternative concepts of, 415, 915–932
  in ancient civilizations, 24–26
  in ancient Greece, 26–27
  Bradley method of, 306–308
  changes to prevent puerperal sepsis in, 30
  changing trends in education for, 303
  Christianity and, 27
  consumer movement and, 39–41
  cultural attitudes toward, 119–120
  in eighteenth century, 29
  father's experience of, 806
  historic view on pain of, 381–382
  Lamaze method of, 308–310
  methods of preparation for, 303–314
  in Middle Ages, 27
  in nineteenth century, 29–33
  prenatal education for, 303–314
  recent changes in, 36–42
  in Renaissance, 27–29
  into twentieth century, 33–36
Childbirth classes, 240–241
  encouragement to attend, 333
  European roots of, 304
  types of, 311
Childbirth coach, 918–919
Childbirth Without Fear, 305
Child care and the growth of love, 40
Childcare services, 87, 839–840
Childrearing
  changing practices of, 437–438
  cultural factors in, 814–815
  father's role in, 811
Children
  changing attitudes toward, 84
  cultural attitudes toward, 122–123
  response of to mother's pregnancy, 237–238
Children's Bureau, 37
  movement for, 34–35
Child spacing practices, 114
Chilling, postpartum, 431
China
  attitude toward pregnancy in, 116
  postpartal practices of, 120

Chlamydia conjunctivis, 897
Chlamydia infection, 329, 892, 896, 910
  epidemiology and transmission of, 896
  issues of, 896–897
  prevention of, 893
  screening for, 897
Chlamydiazyme test, 897
Chloasma, 430
Chloasma gravidarum, 195
Chloroform, use of in childbirth, 29
Choanal atresia, 557
  assessment for, 412–413
Cholecalciferol, 604
Chorioamnionitis, 893
Chorion, 170
Chorion frondosum, 170
Chorionic villi, 170
  sampling, 298–299
Chromosomes, 163
Cigarette smoking, fetal effects of, 887–888
Ciotti, G. B., 28
Circulatory system
  extrauterine adaptation of, 538–539
  fetal, 184–187, *188*
  intrauterine, 533, *534*
Circumcision
  on girls, 26
  hospital procedures for, 596–597
Claiming process, 627
Cleft lip/palate
  assessment for, 412
  breastfeeding with, 459–460
Clement, Jules, 29
Client interview, 251
Clinical nurse specialists, 148–149
Cloacal membrane, 189
Cloning, 108
Closure, crisis of, 99
Coagulation mechanism, alterations in during pregnancy, 670–671
Coagulation system, after delivery, 426–427
Coagulopathy, with severe hemorrhage, 666–669
Cobalamin, 603
Cocaine, fetal effects of, 885–886
Cognitive development stages, 630–631
Cognitive feedback, 507
Cognitive learning theory, 505–506
  principles of, 507
Cohorting system, 582
Coitus interruptus, 72
Cold application, in pain control, 396
Cold stress, 409
  problems associated with, 712–713
Cole, Eunice, 47
Colic, 619
  with breastfeeding infant, 453
Colobomas, 557
Color assessment, 551–552, 594
Colorado Intrauterine Growth Curve, 547–548
Colostrum, 202, 440
Comfort
  management of during labor and delivery, 379–398
  readiness for postpartal education and, 513–515
Common law, 146
Communal family, 81

Communication
  with deaf parents, 849–850
  with high-risk family, 786–787
  between nurse and couple, 936
Community health nurses, 316
Community hospital, 767
Community organizations, 10
Community practices, 146–147
Compensatory justice, 135–136
Complement system, 210
Computerized axial tomographic (CAT) scanning, 270
Comstock Law, 33
Conception age, 198
Conditioning
  without reinforcement, 503–504
  through reinforcement, 505
Condom, 58–59
  in disease prevention, 59
  female, 58
  foam with, 61
Conductive heat loss, 407, 540
Condyloma acumata, 898, 899
Condylomata, 654
Confidentiality issues, 139–140
Congenital anomalies
  assessment for, 412–413, 414t
  screening for, 413
  in SGA infants, 730–734
Congenital hip dislocation, 562
Congenital malformations
  assessment for, 412
  of eye, 557
Connective tissue, 207
Connecting stalk, 174
Connectionism, 503
Consent, 137, 138
  disputes over, 151
  to human research, 139
  patient rights and, 150–151, 152
Constipation, 619
  nutrition management of, 264
Consumer movement, 39–41
Contemporaneity principle, 506
Continuity, 5
Continuity hypothesis, 505
Continuous positive airway pressure, 763
Contraception, 76–77. See also Birth control; *specific methods of*
  with abstinence, 71–72
  access to, 839, 841
  adolescent and, 825–826
  barrier methods of, 55–67
  during breastfeeding, 461
  with coitus interruptus, 72
  considerations in choosing method of, 54–55
  contraindications for, 55
  dissemination of information on, 33–34
  effectiveness of, 54
  factors influencing use of, 52–54
  failure rates of various methods, 54t
  by fertility awareness methods, 70–71
  future trends in, 74
  historical perspective on, 51–52
  increased use of, 101
  issues of, 50–77
  lack of knowledge of, 52
  with lactation, 71
  nursing process and, 74–76

postcoital methods of, 72–73
  resistance to, 52
  safety and risks of, 54–55
  with sterilization, 67–69
Contraceptive sponge, 61–63
Contraction stress test (CST), 284–289
Contracts, patient-nurse, 941
Control
  locus of in family, 88
  social, 83
Convective heat loss, 408, 540
Coombs' test, 429
Copper T 380A, 65
Corona radiata, 167
Corpus albicans, 162
Corpus luteum, 160–162
  decline of, 340
Cortisol, circulating, 209
Cost-benefit analysis, 142
Cotyledons, 174
Counseling, of high-risk family, 788–789
Couples
  dual-career, 94–96
  establishment phase of, 85–87
  older, first pregnancy of, 94
  parenthood phase of, 87
Couvade ritual, 806
Couvade syndrome, 234, 806
Couvelaire uterus, 664
Cow's milk, 613
  allergy to, 620–621
Craniosynostosis, 555
Creatinine clearance, 205
Credibility, 10
Crimean War, nursing during, 32
Crisis, support through, 787–789
Crying, 574
  response to, 636
Cultural systems, 13, 111–112
  birthing and bonding customs and, 415
  childbearing behavior and, 112–113
  components of, 115
  defining characteristics of, 111
  diversity of, 943–944
  father's role and, 814–815
  individual experience of, 112
  Kay-Galen framework in evaluating influence, 115–122
  Newton framework in evaluating influence, 122–123
  nutrition and, 262–264
  role of in childbearing, 112–124
Cumulus oophorus, 161
Cyclopropane, 395
Cytogenetic abnormalities, 275–277
Cytomegalic inclusion disease, 654
Cytomegalovirus, 897
  epidemiology and transmission of, 898
  maternal and newborn issues of, 898
Cytotrophoblast, 170
Cytotrophoblastic layer, 174

D

Daily food guide, 254–255
Dalkon Shield, 825
Data collection tools, 547
da Vinci, Leonardo, 28

Day-care, problems of, 87
Deafness
  postlingual, 847–848
  prelingual or congenital, 847
Deaf parent, 846–847
  guidelines for communicating with, 849t
  heterogeneity of culture of, 847–848
  parenting strategies of, 868
  planning for, 848–850
  risk of deafness of child, 850
Death announcements, 800
Decidua, 170. See Endometrium
  maturing, *171*
Decidua basalis, 170
Decidua capsularis, 170
Decidual reaction, 170
Decidua parietalis, 170
Deep sleep state, 572–573
Deep vein thrombosis, 670
Deinstitutionalization, 845
DeLee catheter, 401, 402
Delivery
  adolescent patient during, 834–835
  for blind mother, 854
  comfort management during, 379–398
  cultural attitudes toward, 119–120
  father's role in, 818
  maternal position in, 931–932
  with spinal cord injury, 859
  support during, 367
  use of medication for, 114
Demand feeding, 445
Demerol (meperidine), 390
Demonstrations, 518–519
Dependence, 13
Depression, with cesarean section, 690
Descriptive methods, 948–950
  application of to research, 950–951
Desquamation, 553
Developmental crisis
  concept of, 219–220
  pregnancy as, 220–222
Developmental tasks, 608
Dewees, William P., 28
Dextrostix, 208
Dextrostix test, 409, 715
Diabetes mellitus, 649–650
  case presentation of, 651
  cesarean section with, 683
  classification system of for pregnancy, 650t
  management of, 650–652
  treat to mother and fetus with, 650
Diagnostic tests, 267–268
Diaphoresis, postpartum, 431, 491
Diaphragm, 56–57
  descent of after delivery, 429–430
Diaphragmatic breathing, 468, 471, 474
  postcesarean, 482
Diaphragms, foam with, 60–61
Diarrhea, nutritional care for, 619
Diastasis, abdominal exercise for, 479
Diastasis recti, 428, 559
Diastolic pressure, 320
DIC. See Disseminated intravascular coagulation
Dickens, Charles, 31–32
Dick-Read, Grantly, 304–305
Dick-Read method, 913
Diet, See also Nutrition
  for breastfeeding mother, 450

Diet (continued).
  requirement of during pregnancy, 208
  for spinal cord injury, 855
Dietary Guidelines for Americans, 265
Dietary intake form, 254
Diet for a Small Planet, 263
Diethylstilbestrol, 104
Differentiation, 506
Diffusion, 181
  facilitated, 181–182
Digestive system, 206
  immaturity of, 719–721
Digoxin, 674
Dilation, 342, 352
Disabled, problems facing, 845–846
Disabled movement, 845
Disabled parents, 844–869
  issues for, 865–868
  parenting strategies for, 867–868
  planning of, 866–867
Discharge, preparation for, 789
Disease Prevention and Health Promotion, Office of, 37
Disequilibrium, 630
Dispatch centers, 760
Disseminated intravascular coagulation
  intrapartal, 707
  risk factors for, 667–669
  with severe hemorrhage, 666–669
  treatment of, 664–665
Distributive justice, 134–135
Diuresis, postpartum, 431, 491
Divorce, increasing rate of, 99
Dizziness, postpartum, 431
DNA synthesis, 249
Documentation, 150
  of postpartal teaching, 524–527
Dole, Elizabeth, 41
Double effect, principle of, 140
Double leg sliding, 479–480
Douching, as contraceptive method, 73
Driving forces, 17
Drowsy state, 573–574
Drug abuse, 872–873
  incidence of, 874
  during pregnancy, 874
Drug abusers, characteristics of, 873–874
Drug dependence, 873
Drug use, 261, 873
Drugs
  during breastfeeding, 461–462
  considerations in use of during labor and delivery, 388
  dissociative or amnesia-producing, 390
  fetal effects of, 388, 878–881t
  for infant resuscitation, 406t, 754t, 755
  neonatal depression with, 390
  in pain control, 387–398
  for spinal cord injury, 855
  systemic, commonly used during childbirth, 389t
  transfer of across placenta, 388
  widespread use of, 46
Dual-career families, 94, 96
Dubowitz gestational age assessment, 550, 563
  scoring of, 567
Ductus deferens, 165
Ductus venosus, closure of, 538

Dunant, Henri, 32
Dysreflexia, 858–859
Dystocia, 681–682, 695
  case presentation of, 698–699
  danger of, 695–696
  fetal factors in, 695, 696–700
  pelvic, 695, 701
  shoulder, 700
  uterine, 695, 696

E

Early postpartum discharge, factors contributing to trend toward, 593
Early pregnancy classes, 332
Ears
  assessment of, 557
  of full-term and premature infants, 558
Eating behavior
  cultural influences on, 262–264
  ethnic influences on, 261–262
Eclampsia, 644
  risks of, 644
  treatment of, 645–647
Ectoderm, 174
Ectopic pregnancies
  bleeding with, 660
  treatment of, 662, 664
Edema
  dependent, during pregnancy, 203
  in newborn, 553
  pitting, during pregnancy, 208
Education
  of nurses, 148
  or parents, 501–527
  in pregnant adolescents, 830–831
  prenatal, 303–314
  value placed on, 88
Education, Department of, 37
Education Amendment, Title IX of, 830
Edwards-Steptoe conception method, 38
Effacement, 342
Effect, law of, 503
Effleurage, 308, 396
Egg donation, 106
Egnell electric breast pump, 455, 456
Elbow circles, 476–477
Electronic fetal monitoring, 363–364
  during acute fetal distress, 374
  application of, 365
  benefits of, 374
  impact of, 373–374
  nursing concerns with, 374
  procedure for, 375–376
  types of, 364–365
Embolectomy, pulmonary, 675
Embryo
  at 22–23 days, *176*
  at 24–25 days, *177*
  at 28 days, *177*
  at 6 weeks, *298*
  with amnion removed, *183*
  development of, 174–177, 192
  folding of, *175*
  gastrointestinal tract in, *191*
Embryoblast, 168
  embedding of, 170
Emergencies
  intrapartum risk for, 742

  postpartum risk for, 742
  preparing for, 741–742
  prepartum risk for, 742
Emotional assessment, 329–330
Emotional change, during pregnancy, 218–242
Emotional roles, 84
Emotional support, by father, 808–809
Empathic understanding, 939–940
Empathy, 939
Empirical-rational view, 940
Endocrine system
  changes in with pregnancy, 208–209
  after delivery, 427–428
  extrauterine adaptation of, 540–541
Endocrine tests, for pregnancy, 197
Endoderm, 174, 175
Endometrial cycle, 160
  changes in cervical mucosa with, 162–163
Endometritis, 658
  with *Chlamydia* infection, 897
  prevention of, 690
Endometrium, changes in during labor, 342
Endotracheal entubation, 749–752
Endotracheal tube suctioning, 764
Energy requirements, 247, 601–602
En face position, 494
  bonding and, 624, 629
Enfamil Premature Formula, 616
Engagement, 347, 353
Engrossment, 812–814
  indications of, 813
Entrainment, 625–627, 632
Enzyme defects, detection of, 271–272
Epidemics, among hospitalized infants, 590
Epididymis, 165
Epinephrine, 394
  in resuscitation, 747
Episiotomies, 354
  incisions of, 432
  lacerations with, 432–433
  pudendal anesthesia with, 391
  routine use of, 39
  timing of, 432
Equilibrium, 630
  definition of, 4
Ergesterol, 604
Ergonovine (Ergotrate), 430
Erikson, Erik, 608
Erythema toxicum, 553
Erythrocin ointment, 556
Erythromycin
  in neonates' eyes, 139
  prophylactic, 411
Esophagus
  changes in during pregnancy, 206
  development of, 189–190
Esters, 394
Estriol
  monitoring levels of, 292–294
  from placenta, 292
  plasma levels of, 295
  24-hour urinary chart of, 295
Estriole, 199
Estrogen
  breasts and, 440
  effects of, 199
  in endometrial cycle, 162–163

pituitary gland enlargement with, 208
production of, 160
Ethnic background, nutrition and, 261–262
Ethics. *See also* Bioethics
 basic concepts of, 130–131
 defective newborn rights and, 153
 issues of, 129–130
 law and, 130–131
 normative, 130
 in perinatal nursing, 129–143
Ethnographic research, 949–950
 application of, 951
Eugenics, 139
Evacuation apron, *581*
Evaluation, 16
 guidelines for, 16
Evaporated milk formulas, 613
Evaporative heat loss, 540
Evil eye, 121
Exercise, law of, 503
Exercise
 abdominal and pelvic tightening, 468–469
 function of, 468
 for pelvic realignment and muscle rebalance, 466–468
 postpartum, 465–485
  with cesarean births, 466
  goals of, 466
  in supine position, 469–470
Expected date of confinement (EDC), 225–226
Experience of Childbirth, The, 305
Experimental methods, 948
 applicability of to perinatal nursing research, 950
Expressive roles, 84
Extended family, 81
Extinction, 504
Extrauterine life
 adaptation to, 531–545
 circulatory system in, 538–539
 endocrine system in, 540–541
 establishing rhythmic respirations in, 537–538
 first breath in, 533–536
 gastrointestinal system in, 541–542
 hepatic system in, 542
 metabolic changes in, 541
 negative stressors of, 536–537
 periods of reactivity in, 542–544
 pulmonary system in, 533–538
 thermoregulation in, 539, 540
 transitional period of, 544–545
Extremities, malformations of, 561
Extrinsic factors, 12
Eyes
 assessment of, 556–557
 infections of with herpes virus, 901
Eye-to-eye contact, 627

F

Face presentation, *697*, *698*
Facies assessment, 556
Facilitative strategies, 15
Facilities, inadequate, 13
Failure, fear of, 13
Failure-to-thrive infants, nutritional care for, 618–619

Fainting spells, postpartum, 431
Family
 acceptance of coming child by, 231
 adolescent pregnancy and, 93, 827, 829–933
 adult, 93
 aging, 92
 allocation of power and decision making in, 88
 alternative lifestyles of, 100–102
 change in, 18–19
 changing roles in, 79–96
  problems with, 93–96
 chaotic, 92–93
 childhood, 93
 communal, 81
 criteria in determining strengths of, 82
 decreasing size of, 99
 definition and function of, 79–81
 developmental levels and tasks in, 89–92
 dual-career, 94–96
 dysfunctional, 830
 effects of change on, 80–81
 effects of pregnancy on, 241
 evolution of, 84
 expectant, 89
 extended, 81
 factors influencing roles in, 88–89
 forces in, 19
 forms of, 81, 82*t*
 function of in society, 81, 83–84
 high-risk, 782–785
  care of, 781–790
  needs of, 785–787
 historical stages of, 86*t*
 involvement of in birthing centers, 921
 as launching center, 91
 levels of functioning of, 92–93
 locus of control in, 88
 meetings with, 786–787
 members of, balancing needs of, 80
 in middle years, 91
 nuclear, 81, 84
 nursing assessments, interventions, and strategies in, 92–93
 of origin, 81
 with preschooler, 91
 psychologic and emotional changes with pregnancy, 218–219
 reconstituted or blended, 81
 reworking of relationships with pregnancy, 230
 with school-age child, 91
 single-parent, 81, 92, 100–101
 social trends affecting, 99
 socioeconomic status of, 89
 support for, 787–789
 with teenager, 91
 time orientation in, 88–89
 traditional roles in, 84
 universals of, 82
 value of education in, 8
Family-centered maternity care
 current practices, 917–918
 in hospitals, 920
 improvements in, 918–919
 nurse-midwife in, 920
Family establishment phase, 89
Family planning, society's expectations about, 113–114

Fantasy, 228
Fat, 602
 metabolism of during pregnancy, 208
Father
 in adolescent pregnancy, 833–834
 assessment of expectations of, 815–816
 binding-in of, 236
 dealing with illness and death of newborn, 814
 emotional support by, 808–809
 emotional symptoms of, 234
 experience of birth by, 805–806
 experience of during pregnancy, 233–237
 financial concerns of, 235
 gatekeeper function of, 809
 guidelines for participation of, 817–818
 interaction of with infants, 812
 meaning of pregnancy for, 806–807
 needs of in prenatal education, 313
 in pain control, 809–810
 participation in labor and birth by, 365–366, 807–808
  benefits of to father, 810–811
  benefits of to infant, 811–814
  benefits of to mother, 808–810
 paternal tasks of, 235–237
 phases of involvement in pregnancy by, 313
 predisposition to couvade in, 806
 preparation of, 814–817
 psychological adjustment of, 234–235
 reaction of to loss, 792
 response of to change in mother, 235
 role of, 805–819
 in role-playing about coming infant, 230–231
 types of, 236
Fatherhood, stages of, 236–237
Fatigue, with pregnancy, 196
Feedback, 16
Feeding. *See also* Breastfeeding; Infant formulas
 daily routine of, 595–596
 of SGA infants, 616–617
 support of, 608–609
 techniques of, 613
Feeding intolerances, 719–720
Feeling, 627
Fein v. *Permanente Medical Group*, 148
Ferning, 163
Ferraro, Geraldine, 41
Fertile period
 calculation of, 70
 risk-taking during, 71
Fertility awareness contraceptive methods, 70–71
Fertility rate, reduction in, 113
Fertilization, 165–169, 192
 stages of, *169*
Fetal abnormalities, sonographic detection of, 269
Fetal acceleration determination (FAD), 282
Fetal acid-base assessment, 702
Fetal alcohol syndrome, 882–833
Fetal biophysical profile, 291–292
 Apgar scores and, *293*

Fetal biophysical profile, (continued).
  fetal distress in labor and, 293
  perinatal death and, 294
Fetal blood pH, 376–378
  monitoring of, 701–702
Fetal blood transfusions, 300
Fetal breathing movements (FBMs), estimation of, 269
Fetal circulation, 533, 534
Fetal death
  antepartum, 793
  estriol levels and, 294
  spontaneous, 45
Fetal depression, with general anesthesia, 396
Fetal distress, 683, 701–702
  case presentation of, 702–703
  monitoring during, 374
  risk to infant with, 702–704
  treatment for, 704
Fetal glucose level, 409
Fetal head position, 358–359
Fetal heart rate (FHR), 198, 282, 284
  acceleration of, 282–284
  assessment of, 373
  beat-to-beat variability in, 374, 375
  deceleration, 289
    early, 375–376
    late, 376
  falling, 287
  monitoring of, 362–363, 375–376
    placement of equipment for, 283
  periodic accelerations of, 375
  periodic decelerations of, 375
  transient decelerations in, 376
  variable decelerations of, 376, 377
Fetal heart tones (FHTs), 282
  auscultation for, 328
Fetal hypoxia, 287, 289
Fetal malrotations, 698
Fetal-maternal response, assessment of, 363
Fetal monitoring, 4
  with contraction stress test/oxytocin challenge test, 284–289
  definition and indications for, 282
  direct, 365
  indirect, 364, 365
  introduction of, 38
  with nonstress test, 282–284
  nursing roles in, 289–291
  procedure and interpretation of, 282
Fetal monitors, 362
Fetal movement, 198
  monitoring of, 291–292
  pattern of, 328
  perception of by father, 234
Fetal "right to life" amendment, 152
Fetal scalp blood sampling, 376–378, 701
Fetal scalp kit, 377
Fetal skeletal problems, radiographic diagnosis of, 271
Fetopelvic disproportion, 24, 356–358
Fetoscope, 362
Fetoscopy, 268
  definition and indications for, 295–296
  nursing roles in, 297
  procedure and interpretation of, 296–297
Fetus
  adolescent mother and, 833
  amniocentesis in assessing maturity of, 278
  changes in during labor, 344–350
  circulatory system development in, 184–187
  descent of, 344–345, 353
  development of, 177
    at 9–12 weeks, 177–178
    at 13–16 weeks, 178
    at 17–20 weeks, 178–179
    at 21–24 weeks, 179
    at 25–28 weeks, 179–180
    at 29–32 weeks, 180
    at 33–36 weeks, 180
    at 37–40 weeks, 180–181
  effects of maternal substance abuse on, 875–889
  endocrine function in, 182
  expulsion of, 353
  extension of, 353
  factors affecting uterine nutritive function in, 182
  flexion of head, 353
  gastrointestinal system development in, 189–192
  high-risk factors for, 268t
  importance of maternal nutrition for, 244–245
  internal rotation of, 353
  lie of, 345, 346
  mechanical injuries to, 536–537
  nervous system development in, 182–184
  nursing assessment of, 373
  nutrient transfer in, 181–182
  organ system development in, 181–192
  outlining of, 196
  passing through pelvis, 347–350
  physiologic changes in, 159–192
  prenatal diagnosis and well-being of, 267–300
  presentation of, 345–347
  renal system development in, 187–188
  restitution and external rotation of, 353
  risk of radiation to, 271
  skull of, 345–347, 348
  stations of, 345, 347
  transition of from intra- to extrauterine life, 340
Fiber, requirement for, 265
Fibrinogen, during pregnancy, 426–427
Fibrinolytic agents, 675
Fibrinolytic system, after delivery, 426–427
Fibrosis, 538
First-come, first-served principle, 136
Fleidner, Fridereike, 30
Fleidner, Pastor Theodor, 30
Flowsheets, 524
Fluid therapy, 776
Fluorescence cell sorting, 107
Fluoride, supplementation of, 610
Flying exercise, 477
Foam test, 278
Folacin, 249
Folic acid, 603–604
  deficiency of, 617
Follicle-stimulating hormone (FSH), 160
  after delivery, 427
  pituitary gland and, 208
  release of, 165
Follicular atresia, 165
Follicular development, 160–161
Follow-up, for adolescent mothers, 839
Fontanelles, 555–556
  assessment of, 412
Food. See also Diet; Nutrition
  allergies to, special infant formulas for, 620–621
  hot-cold theory of, 117, 263t
  nutrients in, 244
Food diary record, 254
Food frequency list, 254
Food groups, protein in, 246
Foot, dorsiflexion of, 569
Footprinting procedure, 415–416
Foramen ovale, 185
Foramen primum, 184
Foramen secundum, 184
Forceps, 28–29, 704
  application, 698–700
  introduction of in childbirth, 916
Foregut, 189
  septation of, 190
Formula feeding, 610
  parental support during, 614
Fractional-antedating response, 505
Fractures, assessment for, 412
Fray, Margery, 40
Frontier Nursing Service, 36
FTA-ABS test, 895
Functioning, levels of, 92–93
Fundal height, 323
  estimated gestation and, 326t
  measurement of, 323–324
Funding, inadequate, 13
Funerals, 800
Furazolidone (Tricofuron), 654

G

Galactosemia, special infant formulas for, 620
Galen, 27, 30, 115
Gametogenesis, 163–165, 192
  normal, 166
Gamp, Sairey, 32
Gastric aspiration, 413
Gastrointestinal enzymes, 191
Gastrointestinal system
  changes in during labor, 344
  after delivery, 428
  development of, 177
  extrauterine adaptation of, 541–542
  fetal, 189–192
  nutritional care for problems of, 619
Gate control theory, 380, 381
  and alternative pain control approaches, 396
  cultural background and, 382
  effects of, 381
Gatekeeper function, 809
Gavage feeding tube insertion, 720–721
Generalization, 504
  cognitive, 506
Gene therapy, 108
Genetic abortion, 793
  psychology of, 794–795

Genetic counseling
  with amniocentesis, 279–282
  amniocentesis and, 271
Genetic disease
  detected by amniocentesis, 272–274t
  detection of by CVS, 299
  special infant formulas for, 619–620
Genetic engineering, 107–108
Genitals
  assessment of, 560
  female, 561
Genotype, 163
Gentian violet, 654
Germ theory, 31
Gestational age
  assessment for, 548, 563–570
    in postnatal examination, 549
  duration of labor and, 358
  estimation of, 198–199, 323–326
    methods for, 548–551
    sonographic, 269
  indexes of, 547
Gestational edema, 644
Gestational proteinuria, 644
Getting into bed procedure, 471
Getting out of bed procedures, 470
Glaucoma, 557
  effects on childbearing of, 852–853
Glomerular filtration rate
  augmented, 209
  after delivery, 428
  during pregnancy, 205
Glucose
  levels of
    extrauterine adaptation of, 541
    fetal, 409
  metabolism of during pregnancy, 209
Glucose tolerance test, 256
Glucosuria, during pregnancy, 205, 207–208
Gluteal fold asymmetry, 562
Gluteal tightening exercises, 469
Glycogen storage, 209
Goal-gradient hypothesis, 505
Goals, negotiating of, 13–14
Going-home phase, 493–494
Gonadotropin-releasing hormone, 160
Gonorrhea, 652, 910
  epidemiology and incidence of, 892–893
  maternal and newborn issues with, 893
  treatment of, 654–657
Goodell's sign, 196
Governmental agencies, 36–38
Graafian follicle, 161
  development of, 165
Grandparents
  psychological adjustment of, 239
  in psychological preparation for newborn, 241
  response of to pregnancy, 239–240
Granny midwives, 36
Granulosa cells, 162
Gravida, 318
Grief work, 495
  with perinatal loss, 799–800
  with pregnancy, 229
Ground ambulance, 762, 778
Group discussion, 518
Growth assessment, 600–601
Growth rate, 608

Growth spurts, 450
G/TPAL, 318
Gurney, 762
Gustatory assessment, 576
Gynecoid pelvis, 349

H

Habit, as restraining force, 13
Habit-family hierarchy, 505
Habituation, 575
Hair
  assessment of, 556
  growth of during pregnancy, 207
Halothane (Fluohane), 395
Handicapped infant care, 46
Handwashing techniques, 410
  with immune system immaturity, 716
  in newborn nurseries, 581, 582
Harvey, William, 28
HBsAg screening, 904
Head
  assessment of, 555–558
  circumference, 601
Head lift, 476
  modified, 483
Health, Education, and Welfare, Department, founding of, 37
Health and Human Services, Department of, 37
Health assessment, 319–322
Health care. *See also* Case
  change in, 4
  holistic, 943
  maintenance and promotion of during pregnancy, 330–334
Health care team, in nutritional assessment, 250
Health clinics, 841
Health habits, 322
Health history, 317
  content of, 317–319
  sample form for, 318
  taking of, 319
Healthy Mothers/Health Babies' public information program, 37
Hearing communication devices, 846, 848
Heart
  auscultation of, 321–322
  chambers, separation of, 184
  changes in with pregnancy, 203
  fetal, 184–186
Heartburn, 264
Heart failure, 718–719
Heart murmurs, during pregnancy, 203
Heart sounds, during pregnancy, 203
Heat application, in pain control, 396
Heat conservation mechanisms, 539–540
Heat loss
  conductive, 407
  convective, 408
  mechanisms of, 540
  radiative, 408–409
  through evaporation, 407
Heckler, Margaret, 41
Hegar's sign, 196
Helicopter, 778–779
Hemagglutination, 197

Hemangiomas, capillary, 554–555
Hematocrit, after birth, 409
Hematologic adaptations, 665–666
  during pregnancy, 203, 204t
Hematomas, 433
Hemoglobin, after birth, 409
Hemoglobinopathies, detection of, 295–296
Hemorrhage
  case presentation of, 705–706
  causes of, 660–666
  factors predisposing to, 665t
  with incomplete placenta delivery, 666–669
  intrapartal, 704–707
  intraventricular, 719
  management of, 662–666
  maternal mortality with, 662, 665
  postpartal, 665t, 667–669
    management of, 666–669
  risk of, 707
  treatment of, 707
Hemorrhoids, 433
  postpartum, 489
  treatment of, 433
Henderson, Victoria, 42
Heparin, 674
  cautions for use of, 674–675
Hepatic system, extrauterine adaptation of, 542
Hepatitis B Immune Globulin (HBIG) vaccine, 904, 905, 906
Hepatitis B virus, 892, 903
  CDC guidelines for, 905t
  epidemiology and transmission of, 904
  maternal issues of, 904
  newborn issues of, 905
  postexposure recommendations for, 906t
  prevention of, 905–906
Hepatitis vaccination, 904
Heroin, fetal effects of, 885
Herpes, genital, 654
Herpes simplex virus, 892, 900
  epidemiology and transmission of, 900
  maternal issues of, 900, 902–903
  newborn issues of, 901–902, 903
  nursing issues of, 903
  parent information on, 902t
  treatment and prevention of, 902
Heteronomy, 136–137
High-risk family, 782–785
  care of, 781–790
  case presentations of, 783–785
  needs of, 785–787
  nursing approaches to, 783–784
  preparation of for discharge, 789
High-risk newborn, 710–739
  resuscitation of, 740–755
Hindgut, 190
Hip hiking, 475
Hippocrates, 30
Hips, assessment of, 562
Hispanics
  attitudes toward pregnancy of, 116–118
  postpartal practices of, 120
Histogenesis, 184
Historical research method, 949
  application of, 951
HIV antibody screening, 907

HIV testing, 153
Hmongs, postpartal practices of, 121
Holistic assessment, 11
Holistic health care, 943
Holmes, Oliver Wendell, 30–31
Homans' sign, 490
Home birth, 45, 916, 920
  advantages of, 920–922
  back-up system for, 923
  disadvantages of, 922–923
  equipment and drugs for, 923t
  nurse-midwife in, 923–924
Homeostatic change, 5
Homeothermic control, 405–407
Home pregnancy tests, 198
Homosexuality
  AMA House of Delegates recommendations on, 102
  public expression of, 99
Homosexual parents, 102–103
Hospital births, 916
Hospitality, 943
Hospitals
  alternatives to, 45
  family-centered maternity care in, 917
Hot-cold food theory, 263t
HTLV-III virus testing, 321
Huffing, 482
Human chorionic gonadotropin (HCG), 104, 664
  corpus luteum hyperplasia and, 162
  detection of in pregnancy test, 197
  effects of, 199
  secretion of, 182
Human chorionic somatomammotropin (HCS), 182
Human history, transitions in, 99
Human immunodeficiency virus (HIV), 46, 906
  epidemiology and transmission of, 906–907
  maternal issues of, 907–908
  newborn issues of, 908–909
  nursing issues of, 909
  risk factors for, 911
Human papilloma virus (HPV), 898
  epidemiology and transmission of, 899
  issues of, 899–900
Human placental lactogen (HPL), 182, 292
  analysis of, 295
  effects of, 199
Hunter, John, 103
Husband-Coached Childbirth, 305
Husband-coached natural childbirth, 305
Hutchinson, Anne, 29
Hydatidiform mole
  bleeding with, 660
  treatment of, 664
Hydrocephalus, 695
  assessment for, 412
  diagnosis of, 270
Hydroxyzine (Atarax, Vistaril), 390
Hyperbilirubinemia, 714
  treatment of, 715
Hypercarbia, 409
  nursing actions for, 410
Hyperglycemia, 652
Hypermastia, 439
Hyperpigmentation, 207

Hyperreflexia, with spinal cord injury, 858–859
Hypertension
  gestational, 644
  during pregnancy, 644
  recognition of signs and symptoms of, 645
  risks of, 644–645
  treatment of, 645–647
  uterine blood flow and, 182
Hyperthermia, risk of, 755
Hypertonic contractions, 695
Hyperventilation, during labor, 344
Hypervitaminosis, 604
Hypnosis, 306, 396
Hypocalcemia, 209, 541, 715
Hypoglycemia, 541
  with diabetes, 650
  gastric suctioning and, 413
  in newborn, 409
  nursing actions for, 410
Hypoparathyroidism, 209
Hypospadias, 560
Hypotension
  nursing actions for, 410
  during pregnancy, 203
Hypothermia
  prevention of in newborn, 410
  risk of, 755
Hypotonia, 563–564
Hypovolemia
  with postpartal hemorrhage, 666
  postpartum, 431
Hypovolemic shock, 427–428
Hypoxia, 409
  chronic intrauterine, 730
  fetal adaptation to, 187
  fetal distress and, 702
  oxygen therapy for, 704
Hysterectomy, 68

I

Icteric skin, 542
Identification bands, 581
Identification process, 493–494
Identity, 83
Identity crisis, 942
IgA, 210
IgG, 210
IgM, 210
Immune globulin, 429
Immune system
  changes in with pregnancy, 209–210
  after delivery, 428–429
  immaturity of, 716–717
Immunoglobulins, 210
Implantation, 170
Incubator air temperatures, 713t, 714t
Incurvation reflex, 569
Independent living skills, 856
India, postpartal practices of, 120
Indwelling catheter, avoidance of, 434
Infant(s). *See also* Newborn
  appearance of, 634
  assessment of before discharge, 499
  attachment and stimulation of, 623–638
  benefits of father's participation to, 811–814
  born outside hospital environment, 582, 590

  characteristics of effecting relationships, 634–636
  choosing sex of, 106–107
  concern about performance of, 495
  crying of, 636
  effects of maternal stimulation on, 632–634
  factors in responses of, 549–551
  feeding of, 450, *451*, 605–608
  growth and development needs of, 600–601
  growth assessment of, 600–601
  gustatory responses of, 634–635
  mental and psychosocial growth of, 601
  nutritional needs of, 599–621
  nutritional therapy needs of, 617–621
  olfactory abilities of, 634
  physical growth of, 600
  physiologic state and responsiveness of, 635
  physiological considerations of, 608
  psychosocial needs of, 608–614
  responsiveness of, 636–637
  sensorimotor intelligence of, 630–632
  small, underdeveloped
    feeding of, 615–617
    nutrient supplements for, 617
    physical characteristics of, 614–615
    type of milk for, 615–616
  smiling of, 635–636
  of spinal-cord-injured mother, 859–862
  stool patterns of, 450
  visual responses of, 634
Infant baptism beliefs, 415
Infant formulas, 610–611
  comparison of, 611t
  conditions requiring special, 619–621
  cow's milk, 613
  evaporated milk, 613
  nutrients in, 612t
  osmolality of, 611–613
  stability of, 613
  in Third World countries, 40
Infant mortality rates, 44–46, 828
Infant teaching and discharge checklist, *525*
Infanticide, 153
Informed consent, 137, 150–151
Inhalation analgesia, 395
In-hospital birthing centers, 925
  advantages of, 925–927
  disadvantages of, 927
  preparation for use of, 928–929
Instrumental roles, 84
Insulin products, 652, 653t
Insulin resistance, 652
Integrating process, 494–495
Intercultural conflict, 93
Intergenerational conflict, 93
Intermittent positive pressure breathing (IPPB), 405
Intermittent positive pressure ventilation, 763
International Childbirth Education Association, 40, 305
Intestine
  changes in during pregnancy, 206
  development of, 190

Intimacy, 808
Intrapartum period
 nurse's role during, 361–378
 predisposition to stressors in, 742
 problems during, 679–708
 society's expectations about, 114–115
Intrauterine devices (IUDs), 65–66, 825
 contraindications for, 55
 risk of infection with, 55
 safety and effectiveness of, 66
 sexual effects of, 67
 side-effects of, 66–67
Intrauterine growth curves, 547–548
Intrauterine growth retardation (IUGR), 182, 722, 730
 causes of, 728
 with CMV infection, 898
 environmental factors in, 728
 estriol levels and, 294
 fetal factors in, 728–729
 placental factors in, 728
Intrauterine life
 fetal circulation in, 533
 pulmonary function in, 532–533
Intrauterine malnutrition, chronic, 729–730
Intrauterine surgery, 4
Intravascular clot formation, 671
Intravenous fluid administration, 753–754
Intravenous therapy, 764
Intrinsic factors, 12
Introjection-projection-rejection/acceptance (IPR/A), 228–229
Investigative research methods, 948–950
 applicability of to perinatal nursing research, 950–951
In vitro fertilization, 4, 38, 104–105
 cloning and, 108
Involution, 424, 430
Iodine, protein-bound, 209
Iodine requirements, 249
Iron, 603
 supplementation of, 250, 609
Iron deficiency anemia, 255–256
Iron requirements, 248
Isolation guidelines, 583–589t
Isolation nursery, 590
Isolette
 thermoregulation in, *713*
 transport, 762

J

Jaundice, 552
 in newborn, 542, 543t
 pathologic, 594
 physiologic, 594
Jewish culture, attitudes toward pregnancy of, 118
Justice, 134–136
 compensatory, 135–136
 distributive, 134–135

K

Kanamycin, 461
Karotype, determination of, 298–299
Kay, Margarita, 115

Kay-Galenic framework, 115–116
 in assessing Mexican-American mother, 125
 in assessing Vietnamese mother, 126
 during birth, 119–120
 extrinsic factors in, 115, 116–118
 in intrapartal period, 118–119
 in newborn period, 121–122
 in postpartal period, 120–121
 in prenatal period, 116–118
Kegel exercises, 466–468, 470
Kernicterus, 542
Kidneys
 palpation of, 559
 of premature infant, 715–716
Kinship system, 115
Kitzinger, Sheila, 305–306
Kleihauer Betke blood test, 429
Knee-to-chest stretches, 480
Knowledge system, 115
Knowles, Malcolm, 510

L

Labeling, criteria for, 142
Labia majora, 560
Labia minora, 560
Labor
 adolescent patient during, 834–835
 artificial induction of, 691–692
 augmentation of, 691
 biophysical changes in mother during, 340–350
 for blind mother, 854
 case presentation of, 692
 characteristics of, 351t
 comfort management during, 379–398
 complications with, 694–695
 in home births, 922
 rate of, 680–681
 in darkened setting, 932
 duration of, 356–359
 factors involved in initiation of, 341t
 false, 351
 father's participation in, 807–819
 fear of, 119
 fetus during, 344–350
 first stage of
  active phase, 352
  latent phase, 351, 352
  pain in, 384
  transitional phase, 352–353
 fourth stage of, 356
 hypertonic, 375
 hypotonic, 375
 impact of and coping during, 368–372t
 interference with process of, 680
 maternal position in, 931
 mechanism of, 344–345, 353, 357
 mother/fetus changes in, 339–359
 physiologic effects of pain in, 384–385
 premature, 647–649
  predisposition to, 225
 premonitory signs of, 350–356
 process of, 340
 second stage of, 353
  pain in, 384
 stages of, 351
 as stressor, 362

 support during
  active phase, 367
  fourth stage, 367–368
  latent phase, 367
  second stage, 367
  third stage, 367
  transitional phase, 367
 theories of onset of, 340
 third stage of, 353–355
 use of medication for, 114
Labor and delivery postpartum recovery rooms, 4
Laboring couple, nurse as support to, 365–368
Lact-Aid Nursing Trainer System, 460–461
Lactated Ringer's solution, 666
Lactation
 beginning of, 426, 440
 as contraceptive, 71
 drugs to stimulate, 460–461
 induced, 460, 461
 iron needs during, 248
 nutritional support for, 245, 609
 RDAs during, 246
 weight control during, 259–261
Lactation Consultant, Certified, 447
Lactiferous ducts, 439
Lactiferous sinuses, 439
Lacto-ovovegetarians, 262
Lactose excretion, 208
Lactose intolerance, 262
La Leche League, 40, 447, 450, 500
Lamaze, Fernand, 304, 305
Lamaze childbirth classes, 4, 914
Lamaze method, 305, 313, 913
 breathing patterns in, 309–310
Laminaria tents, 694
Landau reflex, 569
Lange caliper, 601
Lanugo, 178, 553
 shedding of, 180
Laparoscopy, in oocyte donation, 106
Laryngotracheal diverticulum, 189
Last menstrual period (LMP), 198, 548
La Valliere, Mlle., 29
Law
 ethics and, 130–131
 historical background and framework of, 146–147
 issues of in perinatal nursing, 145–154
 nursing practice and, 147–148
LcCommare O Reccoglitrice, 28
Learning
 definitions of, 501–502, 506
 environmental and organizational factors in, 509–510
 principles of, 507–508
 psychologic conditions for, 508–509
Learning theories
 behavioristic, 503–505
 cognitive-field, 505–508
LeBoyer techniques, 396, 926–927
Lecithin to sphingomyelin (L/S) ratio, 278
Lectures, 518
Leg cramps, nutrition management of, 264–265
Leg length inequality, 562
Legislative changes, 47
Length measurement, 601
Leopold's maneuvers, *326–327, 327, 328, 373*

Let-down reflex, 440
  enhancement of, 446
Leukocyte production, 204
Leukorrhea, 201
Lewin, Kurt, 7, 8–9
Lidocaine hydrochloride (Xylocaine), 390–391, 394
Life space, 505
Lifestyles
  alternative, 100–103
  lack of support for, 93–94
  radical changes in, 98–99
Lightening, 350
Light sleep state, 573
Limb differentiation, 176
Linea nigra, 195
Linoleic acid, 602
Lipids, plasma levels of during pregnancy, 208
Lister, Sir Joseph, 31
Lithotomy position, 931–932
Liver
  changes in during pregnancy, 206
  in extrauterine adaptation, 542
  fetal, 191–192
  immature, 714–715
  palpation of, 559
Lobenstein, Ralph Waldo, 36
Lobenstein Midwifery School, 36
Lochia, 425
  assessment of discharge of, 489
Lofenalac formula, 620
Lordosis, with pregnancy, 206
Loss, coping with, 791–792. *See also* Perinatal loss
Low-back discomfort exercises, 480–481
Low-birth-weight infants
  classification of, 711
  nutritional care for, 618
Lower extremities
  assessment of, 561–562
  of reflexes, 569–570
  asymmetry of, 562
  postcesarean exercises for, 483
  postpartum assessment of, 490
Low ovum transfer, 105
Low rib expansion, postcesarean, 482
Lubic, Ruth Watson, 45
Lumbar epidural anesthesia, 391–394
  contraindications and side-effects of, 394
Lumbo-pelvic realignment exercise, 469
Lung maturity, 38
  amniocentesis in calculating, 278
Lungs
  auscultation of, 321–322
  fetal, 185
Luteinization, 160
Luteinizing hormone (LH), 160
  breastfeeding and, 426
  effects of, 208
  release of, 165

M

Macrodantin, 654
Magnesium
  deficiency of, 264–265
  requirements, 248–249
Magnesium sulfate, 645–647, 649

Mainstreaming, 845
Maladaptation, 785
Male contraception, future trends in, 74
Maleficence, 140
Male midwives, 23, 28
Male role, traditional, 807
Mammary papilla, 439
Management functions, 15
Manipulation, 948
Marijuana
  abuse of, 873
  during breastfeeding, 461
  fetal effects of, 884–885
Marmet technique, 454
Marriage
  approval of, 220
  declining rates of, 99
Martin, Darrel, 42
Martin Chuzzlewit, 31–32
Maslow's hierarchy of needs, 11
Massage, after delivery, 472
Mastitis, 453–454, 659
Maternal attachment, 624
Maternal behavior
  in animals, 624–625
  effects of, 632–634
  in humans, 625–630
Maternal binding-in, 232–233
Maternal-fetal blood group incompatibility, 428–429
Maternal-fetal relationship
  during eighth month, 225
  during last weeks of pregnancy, 226–227
Maternal-fetal welfare issues, 137–138
Maternal history, 548–549
Maternal identity, development of, 227–228
Maternal-infant attachment. *See also* Attachment
  behaviors of, 627–629
  development of, 625–627
  research on, 40
Maternal mortality rate, 43, 828
  improvement in, 114
  racial differences in, 46
Maternal nutrition, 243–244
  historical perspectives on, 244
  importance of, 244–245
Maternal Nutrition and the Course of Pregnancy, 256
Maternal position
  duration of labor and, 359
  in labor and delivery, 931–932
Maternal role. *See also* Mother; Mothering behaviors
  binding-in to unknown baby in, 232–233
  learning to give of self in, 231–232
  securing acceptance in, 230–231
  seeking safe passage for self and baby in, 229–230
Maternal role taking process, 228–229
Maternal tasks, 229–233
Maternal transport, 758–759
  early identification of high-risk mother and, 760–761
  equipment and supplies for, 763
  indications for, 759
Maternicity, 493
  measures of, 493–494

Maternity care
  in ancient Egypt, 26
  change in, 4
  early efforts to improve, 34–36
  family-centered, 41, 917–920
  need to lower costs of, 46
Maternity Center Association (MCA), 35–36, 45, 304
  Childbearing Center of, 924, 925
  teaching aids developed by, 304
Maternity centers, 241
Maternity leave, 87
Maternity nursing
  beginning courses in, 24
  definitions of, 23–24
  effecting change in future of, 45–47
  historical developments in, 22–47
  recent changes in, 36–42
Maternity teaching checklist, 526
Maturity indexes, 547
Mauriceau, Francois, 28
McCormick, R. A., 141–142
McGill Pain Questionnaire, 383–384
Meal plan, sample, 255
Mean Corpuscular Volume (MCV) test, 256
Mechanical stressors, 536–537
Meconium, 192, 401
  aspiration of, 402
  production of, 178
Meconium staining, 553
Medela breast pump, 455
Median episiotomy, 432
Medicaid, 37
Medical ethics, 131
  versus nursing ethics, 131–133, 134
Medical records, patient rights and, 150
Medical standards, 148
Medical treatment
  allocation of, 134–135
  right to refuse, 137
Medicare, 37
Medications, *See also* Drugs
  duration of labor and, 358
  fetal effects of, 888
Mediolateral episiotomy, 432
Medullary respiratory centers, 184
Meiotic division, 163
Melasma gravidarum, 195
Menadione, 604
Menarche, 163
Menopause, 165
Menstrual age, 198
Menstrual cycle
  history of, 318
  midcycle bleeding in, 161
  physiology of, 51, 52–53
  return of, 426
Menstrual dates, calculation of, 548–549
Menstrual extraction, 72
Menstrual physiology, 53
Menstruation, 163
Mental growth, 601
Meperidine, 390
Mercurio, Scipione, 28
Mesoderm, 174
Mesonephrons, 187
Metabolic acidosis, in cold-stressed newborns, 409
Metabolic end product, fetal biotransformation of, 192

Metabolic immaturity, 715
Metabolism
  changes in with pregnancy, 207–208
  extrauterine adaptation of, 541
Metaethics, 130
Metanephrons, 187
Methadone maintenance programs, 885, 886
Methoxyflurane (Penthrane), 395
Methylergonovine maleate (Methergine), 430
Metronidazole (Flagyl), 654
Mexican-Americans
  attitudes toward pregnancy of, 116–119
  childbearing case study of, 125
  newborns, care of by, 121–122
  postpartal practices of, 120
Microallocation, 134–136
Midarm circumference, 601
Midgut, 190
Midwifery, Association for the Promotion and Standardization of, 36
Midwives. *See also* Nurse-midwives
  in ancient Greece, 26
  definition of, 23
  in early twentieth century U.S., 34–36
  in eighteenth century, 29
  importance of, 26
Milia, 553–554
Miliaria, 554
Milk
  expression of, 454–456, 458
  for SGA infants, 615–616
  storage of, 456–457
Milk line, 439
Mill, John Stuart, 137
Mimicry, 228
Mindell, Fania, 33
Minerals, 602–603
  metabolism of during pregnancy, 208
Miscarriage, 792–793
Mittelschmerz, 161
Molding, 347
Mongolian spots, 554
Monilial infections, risks of, 654
Montgomery's glands, 195, 202, 439
Montrice, 918–919
Moral character, 131
Morals, 130
"Morning after" pill, 73
Morning sickness, 195–196
Moro reflex, 567
Morphine
  during cesarean, 432
  fetal effects of, 885
Morula, 168
Mother. *See also* Maternal role
  biophysical changes in during labor, 340–350
  emotional and psychological considerations during labor, 366–367
  immediate postpartal feelings of, 496–497
  physiologic adaptations of in postpartal period, 423–434
  physiologic changes in system of, 194–217
  psychological development of, 227–228
  psychosocial concerns of, 366–367
  reaction of to loss, 792
  surrogate, 99, 105–106
    legal controversy over, 153–154
  unmarried, 94
Mother and Baby Care and Family Health, 304
Mother-child relationship
  acceptance of child by others and, 231
  family influence on, 234
Motherhood. *See also* Maternal role
  changing behavior of, 87
  traditional role of, 87
  transition to, 496–497
    first 3 months of, 497
    long-term adjustments in, 497
    nursing support in, 497–500
    role modeling for, 498
    support systems for, 497–500
Mother-infant bond
  establishment of, 493
  father's influence on, 810
  in first hours after birth, 413–415
  fostering of, 493–494
  tasks of, 494–496
Mothering behaviors, 491. *See also* Maternal role
  focus of, 493
  human, 627–629
  postpartum assessment of, 491–494
  species-specific, 624–625, 626t
  stimuli contributing to ineffective, 491–492
  three phases of, 492–494
Mothering skills, 495–496
Motivation, 11–12
  principles of, 507–508
Mouth
  assessment of, 558
  changes in during pregnancy, 206
Movement assessment, 563–567
Moving, 8
Moving phase, 13–16
Mucous plug, 200
Multiple births, special instruction for, 521
Multiple sclerosis
  communicating information about, 863
  genetic issue of, 862
  planning pregnancy with, 863–864
  pregnancy research and, 862–863
  social and emotional considerations in, 864
Muscle tone
  assessment of, 567
  exercises to restore, 428
  in premature infant, 712
Muscular activity, in thermoregulation, 407, 539
Musculoskeletal system
  changes in during labor, 344
  changes in with pregnancy, 206
  after delivery, 428
Myelination process, 181, 184
Myoepithelial cells, 439
Myometrium
  changes in during labor, 340–342
  function of, 340
Myrtiform caruncles, 425–426

N

Naloxon hydrochloride (Narcan), 390
  in resuscitation, 747
Narcotics, 390
  fetal effects of, 885–886
National Association of Childbearing Centers, 45
National Birth Control League, 34, 85
National Board of the Young Men's Christian Association, 37
National Center for Nursing Research, 953
National Coalition of Hispanic Mental Health and Human Services Organization, 37
National Committee on Federal Legislation for Birth Control, 34
National Federation for Specialty Nursing Organizations (NFSNO), 47
National Health Promotion Network, 37
National League for Nursing Education, accreditation by, 30
National Research Council's Committee on Maternal Nutrition report, 244
National Urban League, 37
Natural chance principle, 136
Natural childbirth, 40, 305, 396
  growing demand for, 916–917
  methods of, 929–930
Nausea, 264
Neck
  assessment of, 558
  exercises, 476–477
  of newborn, *559*
Necrotizing enterocolitis, 721
Needlescope, 296, 297
Needs, hierarchy of, 11
Neisseria gonorrhoeae, 652, 892
Neonatal intensive care centers, 4
  transport systems and, 758–759, 779
Neonatal nurse, 93
Neonatal transport, 757–758
  checklist for, *773*
  equipment and supplies for, 763–764, 765t
  indications for, 758
  notes form for, *775*
  preparation for, 768–772t
Nephrogenic cord development, *189*
Nervous system, fetal, 182–184
Neural groove, 182
Neural plate, 175, 182
Neural tube, 182
  closure of, 184
Neural tube defects
  detection of, 276–277
  epidemiologic observations about, 276t
Neurologic assessment, 563
  scoring system for, *564*
  techniques of, *565*
Neuromuscular-controlled relaxation, 308
Neuromuscular development, 176–177
Neurulation, 182
Newborn. *See also* Infant(s)
  adaptation of to extrauterine life, 531–545
  assessment of, 546–576

Newborn (continued).
  audiologic testing of, 850
  banding of, 416
  bathing of, 410
  care of, 579–597
    cultural attitudes toward, 121–122
    society's expectations about, 115
  characteristics of, 741
  death of, 794, 814
  defective, rights of, 152–153
  with drug withdrawal symptoms, 885–886
  establishing clear airway in, 400
  footprinting procedures for, 415–416
  high-risk, 710–739
    resuscitation of, 740–755
  hypercarbia in, 409, 410
  hypoglycemic, 409, 410
  hypotension in, 410
  hypoxia in, 409
  identification of, 416, 581
  illness of, 814
  initial assessment of, 402–405
  initial attachment to parents, 413–415
  initial breathing in, 400–402
  nursing assessment of, 399–418
  prevention of hypothermia in, 410
  prevention of infection in, 410
  reactions of with mothers and fathers, 812
  recording care plan for, 416–418
  registration of, 418
  resuscitation of, 401–402, 404–405
    drugs used in, 406t
  temperature control in, 405–409
  threats to, 400–402
  unique physical and physiological characteristics of, 754
  vitamin K for, 412
  vulnerability of, 400
Newborn nurseries
  antiseptic practices in, 581–582
  central, concept of, 590–591, 592
  cohorting baby system in, 582
  contagious diseases in, 582
  diarrhea in, 581
  equipment in, 580
  infectious agents in, 581
  isolation guidelines for, 583–589t
  persons entering, 582
  physical design of, 580–582
  special, 590
Newton, Niles, 122
Newton framework, 122–123
Niacin, 250, 603
Nicotine, 887
Nightingale, Florence, 30–33, 935
Nightingale Pledge, 140, 142
Nipple confusion, 446
Nipples, 439
  care of during breastfeeding, 448–450
  inverted, 449–450
  sore, 452
Nipple shields, 453
Nipple stimulation contraction stress test, 287
  nursing guidelines for, 288t
Nitrous oxide, 395
Noncontraceptor, chronic, 76
Nonmaleficence, 140–142

Nonstress test (NST), 282–284, 364
  actions based on, 286
  nonreactive, 287
  reactive and nonreactive, 285, 286
Norepinephrine release, 540
Normative ethics, 130
Normative-reeducative assumption, 940
Norms, 131
Norplant System, 74
Norton v. Argonaut Insurance Company, 147
Nose, assessment of, 557
Notes on hospitals, 32
Notes on nursing, 32
Notochord, 182
Nuclear family, 81
  roles of members in, 84
Nufer, Jacob, 28
Nurse
  accountability of, 941–942
  as advocate, 942–944
  anticipatory guidance by, 334
  in assessing parent readiness for postpartal education, 513–516
  assessment and management of pain during labor, 385–387
  assessments by, 362–363
  attitudes of toward father's participation, 815–817
  caring of, 936
  change model for, 9–17
  collaboration of with other health care providers, 47
  development of relationship with pregnant patient, 332–334
  diagnosis of postpartal educational needs, 516–517
  effects of change on, 4
  ethical codes of, 131–133
  expanded roles of, 148–150
  in family functioning, 93
  in fetal monitoring, 363–365
  guide for care during labor and birth, 368–372t
  in infant attachment and stimulation, 636–638
  in intrapartal period, 361–378
  licensure of, 147–148
  male, 42
  need for unity of, 46–47
  neonatal care record of, 596
  in newborn assessment, 549–551
  obligation triad of, 131–132
  in postpartal education, 502–503, 510
  in postpartum period, 486–500
  preconceptual counseling by, 316–317
  in prenatal period, 315–334
  in relieving family stress, 782–783
  role of in dealing with psychological needs of pregnancy, 240–241
  role of with alcoholic mother, 883
  with single-parent families, 101
  specialization of, 937–938
  support of laboring couple, 365–368
  view of patient by, 940
Nurse-midwifery, 34
Nurse-midwives, 149–150, 932
  in birthing centers, 925
  in first rural health center, 35–36

  in home births, 923–924
  role of, 920
    expanded, 917
  support for employment of, 42
Nurse practice acts, 147–148
Nurse practitioners, 149
Nurses' Association of the American College of Obstetricians and Gynecologists (NAA-COG), 46–47
  Standards for Obstetric, Gynecologic, and Neonatal Nursing, 147
Nurses' Coalition for Action in Politics (NCAP), 41
Nursing. *See also* Maternity nursing; Perinatal nursing
  advances in knowledge and techniques of, 38
  beginning of modern, 31–33
  bioethics and, 131–134
  cultural differences of patients and, 111–112
  cultural guidelines for, 115
  in holistic care of different cultural groups, 123–124
  legislative changes in, 41
  in Middle Ages, 27
  obstetric, 23
  professional, 148
  standard of care in, 147
Nursing assessment
  contraception and, 74–75
  of pregnant patient, 317–329
Nursing bra, 473
Nursing change model
  level III of, 16–17
  level II of, 13–16
  level I of, 9–13
Nursing diagnosis
  contraception and, 75
  use of in family change, 19
Nursing education
  caring and, 936
  changes in, 38–39
  in 19th-century U.S., 30
  paternalistic focus of, 936–937
Nursing interventions, in pain control, 387
Nursing research, 952–953
  organizations for, 952–953
  topics of, 954t
Nursing Research, 953
Nursing Service of the Joint Commission for the Accreditation of Hospitals, Standards for, 147
Nutrients, 600
  deficiencies of, 263–264
  essential, 246
  insufficient, 734–735
  sources of, 244
  supplementation of, 250
  for SGA infants, 617
Nutrition
  before conception, 245
  importance of during pregnancy, 244–245
  for infant, 599–621
  in pregnant adolescent, 832
  risk factors, 250–251, 260–261
Nutritional assessment, 250–261, 605

postpartum, 491
significant clinical signs in, 257t
tools for, 254
Nutritional care
for adolescent, 839
for failure-to-thrive infants, 618–619
with gastrointestinal problems, 619
for low birth weight infants, 618
planning of, 618
Nutritional history, 251–254
Nutritional needs, 246–250, 601–608
Nutritional status, 605
clinical signs of, 606–607t
duration of labor and, 358
Nutritional therapy needs, 617–621
Nutrition questionnaire, 254
prenatal, 252–253
Nystagmus, 557
effects on childbearing of, 853
Nystatin (Mycostatin), 654

O

Obesity, 261, 601
Obligations, 131
Observation nursery, 590
Obstetric examination, 549
Obstetricians, 23
Obstetric nurses, 23
Obstetrics, 23
O'Connor, Sandra Day, 41
Olfactory assessment, 576
Oligodendrocytes, 184
Oligospermia, 103
On-call system, 766
Oocyte
donation, 106
primary, 161
Oogenesis, 164–165
Oogonia, 164–165
Oophrectomy, 664
Operant conditioning, 505
Ophthalmia neonatorum, 410
prophylaxis against, 410–412
Ophthalmic ointment, 411
Oral contraceptives, 825
choice of, 55
effectiveness of, 64
introduction of, 51
prescribing of, 63–64
sexual effects of, 65
side-effects and safety of, 64–65
types of, 63
Organogensis, 174
Orque's cross-cultural tool, 123, 124
Orthostatic proteinuria, 205–206
Ortolani test, 562
Outcome objectives, establishing, 14
Outreach programs, 767
Ovarian cycle, 160–162
Over-the-counter medications, fetal effects of, 888
Ovulation, 160–161
method, 70
Ovum, fertilized, 168
Oxygenation, 776
Oxygen supply, insufficient, 735–739
Oxygen therapy, 674
with fetal distress, 704
for hemorrhaging, 707
Oxytocin, 282, 287

afterpains and, 430
as calcium releasers, 342
complications with, 694
discontinuance of, 376, 704
to induce labor, 691–692, 693t
overresponse to, 288, 289
protocol for administration of, 694
release of with breastfeeding, 356
secretion of, 209
sensory receptors for, 441
stimulation of milk production by, 440
Oxytocin challenge test (OCT), 282, 284–289, 364
nonnegative, 290

P

Paiget's cognitive development stages, 630–631
Pain
assessment and management of, 385–387
early theories of, 380–381
father in control of, 809–810
in labor, 384–387
measurement of, 382–384
nursing intervention in, 387
past experience with, 382
pathway of, 381
perception of, 381–382
as personal experience, 380
pharmacologic agents for, 387–396
physiologic effects of in labor, 384–385
psychologic factors in, 382
psychological approaches to, 396–398
sensory modulation of, 396
unrelieved, 384–385
variations in perception of, 381
Painless Childbirth, 305
Pain Rating Index (PRI), 384
Paired stimulus comparisons, 812
Palmar grasp reflex, 569
Pancreas, change in during pregnancy, 209
Papanicolaou (Pap) test, 654
for herpes testing, 900, 903
Paracervical block, 391
Parachute reflex, 569
Paradigm shifts, 952
Paralysis, 19–20
Paraplegic parents, 868
Parathyroid gland, change in during pregnancy, 209
Pare, Ambroise, 28
Parent education, 501–527
contracting for, 509
in infant attachment and stimulation, 636–637
Parent groups, 500
Parent-infant bonding, 627–629. See also Maternal-infant attachment
with home birth, 921–922
Parent-infant reciprocity, 631–632
Parent-infant services, evaluation of, 96
Parenting
alternative forms of, 103–108
changing attitudes toward, 84

changing behaviors of, 87–88
commitment with, 221
demands of, 85
encouragement for, 498
evolution of, 84–88
joys and frustrations of, 87
preparation for, 499
resources for, 500, 839
stages of, 87
strategies of for disabled parents, 867–868
Parents
adoptive, 101–102
blind, 851–855
deaf, 846–850
homosexual, 102–103
issues of for disabled, 865–868
with multiple sclerosis, 862–864
with physical disability, 844–869
with spinal cord injury, 855–862
Parity, 318
duration of labor and, 356
Pasteur, Louis, 31
Patent ductus arteriosus, 718
Paternalism, 142, 143
Paternal tasks, 235–237
Patient
communication about, 150
compliance to medical regimen of, 941
nurse's view of, 940
responsibility for self-care of, 940–941
teaching, 502
"Patient's Bill of Rights," 150
Patient records, 150
Patient rights, 150–152
Pediatrician, early securing of, 499
Peer pressure, 826
Pelvic alignment, while holding infant, 475
Pelvic cellulitis, 658
Pelvic examination, 328–329
Pelvic floor
assessment of, 475
comfort of, 473
muscle exercise, 469, 473
Pelvic inflammatory disease
with Chlamydia infection, 897
with gonorrhea, 892
with IUD use, 67
with salpingitis, 892
Pelvic inlet, 348–349
Pelvic joint, changes in with pregnancy, 206
Pelvic outlet, 349
Pelvic realignment exercises, 468–470
Pelvic thrombophlebitis, 658, 659
Pelvis
bones of, 348
false and true, 348
neuroanatomy of, 384
fetus passing through, 347–350
types of, 349–350
Penicillin, 654–657, 895
Pentothal, 395
Percutaneous umbilical blood sampling, 299–300
Perfection, 19
Performance roles, 84
Perinatal care, levels of, 757
Perinatal care team, 761

Perinatal care team (*continued*).
    composition of, 766
    principles of operation, 766–767
Perinatal crisis, mobilizing families during, 781–790
Perinatal infections, sexually transmitted disease and, 891–911
Perinatal loss, 45, 791, 801
    case presentation for, 796–799
    coping with, 792
    in first trimester, 792–793, 794
    grief response to, 799–800
    health care team and, 796
    information on, 796
    need to reduce, 46
    nursing interventions for, 796
    physiology or, 792–794
    practical information about, 800
    psychology of, 794–800
    in second trimester, 794
    self-help organizations for, 796–800
    subsequent pregnancies and, 795
    in third trimester, 794
Perinatal nursing
    AIDS and, 153
    as art and science, 938–939
    caring and, 935–944
    ethics and, 129–143
    expanded roles in, 148–150
    legal controversies in, 152–153
    legal issues in, 145–154
    patient rights in, 150–152
    research in, 952–953, 954t
    and research process, 947–951
    science and technology in, 937–938
    surrogacy and, 153–154
Perinatal research journals, 953
Perinatal screening, 364
Perineal care, teaching, 490
Perineal heat lamp, 490
Perineum
    changes in with pregnancy, 203
    postpartum assessment of, 489–490
Peritonitis, 658–659
Personal interview, 950
Personal relationship building, 9–11
Persuasive strategies, 15
Petechiae, 555
Phenothiazines, 460
Phenotype, 163
Phenylalanine, 620
Phenylketonuria, special infant formulas for, 620
Phoebe, 27
Phosphatidylglycerol levels, 278
Phosphorus requirements, 248
Photocardiography, 282
Phototherapy, 38
Phototherapy lights, 715
Physical assessment, postpartum, 487–491
Physical disability
    deinstitutionalization and, 845
    lack of information on, 844–845
    parents with, 844–869
    stigma associated with, 845
Physical growth, 600
    assessment of, 600–601
Physician liability insurance, 914
Physicians, role of in childbirth, 23
Physiologic change
    in fetus, 159–192

in maternal system, 194–217
Pica, 261
Pinocytosis, 182
Piskacek's sign, 196
Pituitary gland
    change in with pregnancy, 208–209
    failure of, 427–428
PKU testing, 139
Placenta
    delivery of, 354
        incomplete, 666
        support during, 367
    development of, 170–174
    in fetal circulatory system, 187
    full-term, 172
    function of, 181
    hormones and enzymes, levels of, 292–295
    meaning attached to, 120
    nutrient transfer across, 192
    separation of, 358, 427
    villa in, 173
Placenta accreta, 707
    etiology of, 705
Placental abnormalities, sonographic detection of, 269
Placental grading, 297–298
Placental hormones, 199
Placenta percreta, 705
Placenta previa
    bleeding with, 662
    case presentation of, 662–663
    treatment of, 664, 707
Planned Parenthood Federation, International, 85
Planned Parenthood Federation of America, 34
    study of, 825
Plantar grasp reflex, 569
Platypelloid pelvis, 349
Poke and tuck exercise, 476
Polar bodies, 165
Policies, 147
Polyamines, synthesis of, 200
Polycythemia, 730
Polydactyly, 561
Position, 326
Positive affirmations, 472
Postmature infants, 734
    case presentation of, 735–738
    physical characteristics of, 734
    physiological characteristics of, 734–739
Postpartal curriculum, 510–511
    determining entering behaviors in, 513
    objectives for, 511–512
    task analysis for, 512–513
Postpartal education
    assessment for, 513–516
    capability for, 516
    diagnosis for readiness for, 516–517
    documentation of, 524–527
    evaluation of, 521–524
    evaluation planning guide for, 522–523t
    individualizing of, 510–521
    instruction material for, 518–521
    motivation for, 515–516
    setting goals for, 517–518
    strategy for, 510–513
Postpartal infection, 657–658
    case presentation for, 660–661

extragenital, 659
    genital, 657–659
    predisposing risk factors to, 658t
    therapy for, 659–660
Postpartum period
    for adolescent, 836–838
    for blind mother, 854–855
    cultural attitudes toward, 120–121
    exercises for, 465–485
        recommended regime, 483–485
        safe activities for, 485
    maternal physiologic adaptations during, 423–434
    nurse's role in, 486–500
    predisposition to stressors in, 742
    society's expectations about, 115
    special problems of, 431–434
Postpartum support, 367–368
Postremity, 504
Posture assessment, in prone position, 568
Posture tone assessment, 563–567
Poverty, 261
Power-coercive assumption, 940
Power strategies, 15
Preconceptual counseling, 316–317
Preeclampsia, 644
    case presentation of, 646
    treatment of, 645–647
Pregnancy
    in adolescents, 46, 821–842
    bleeding in first half of, 660–666
    cost analysis of, 223
    cultural attitudes toward, 116–119
    ad developmental crisis, 220–222
    development of nurse-mother relationship during, 332–334
    Dietary guidelines and, 265
    drug abuse during, 874
    effects of on family, 241
    ethical issues of, 137–138
    excessive blood loss during, 665
    father's experience of, 233–237
    first, 220–221
    grandparents' experience of, 239–240
    health care and outcome of, 315–316, 330–334
    importance of nutrition in, 244–245
    increased vulnerability with, 224–225
    mask of, 195
    meaning of for fathers, 806–807
    minor discomforts of, 210, 211–217t
    need for emotional support during, 333–334
    nightmares during, 226
    nurse's role in, 240–241
    nursing assessment in, 317–329
    nutritional assessment during, 250–261
    nutrition management of discomforts in, 264–265
    nutritional needs during, 246–250
    in older couple, 94
    organ system changes with, 200–210
    patterns of interest in sex during, 331
    physiologic changes with, 194–217
    positive signs of, 198
    predisposition to stressors in, 742
    problems during, 643–676

psychologic and emotional changes of, 218–242
assessment in, 329–330
during first trimester, 222–223
during second trimester, 223–224
during third trimester, 224–227
second, 221–222
siblings' experience of, 237–238
signs and symptoms of, 195–199
society's expectations for behavior and, 113–123
spacing of, 261
taboos surrounding, 117
in teenagers, 100
tests for, 197–198
vulnerability during, 232–233
weight control during 256–259, 261
Pregnancy counseling, 842
Pregnancy-induced hypertension, 644
risks of, 644–645
"Pregnant Patient's Bill of Rights and Responsibilities," 150
Premature infant
anticipatory grief for, 630
attachment of, 629–630
breastfeeding of, 458–459
cardiovascular immaturity in, 718–719
case presentation of, 723–728
central nervous system immaturity in, 721
digestive immaturity in, 719–721
immune system immaturity in, 716–717
incidence of, 711
liver immaturity in, 714–715
metabolic immaturity in, 715
neurologic characteristics of, 712
parental reactions to, 629–630
physical characteristics of, 711–712
preparing family for, 785–786
reflexes and muscle tone in, 712
renal immaturity in, 715–716
respiratory immaturity in, 717–718
skin immaturity in, 721–722
small, 615
stimulation of, 633–634
temperature regulation in, 712–714
Premature labor, 647
case presentation of, 648
risks of, 649
with spinal cord injury, 858
treatment of, 649
Prenatal care
for blind mother, 854
in pregnant adolescents, 831–833
Prenatal childbirth classes, 240–241
Prenatal diagnosis, 267–300
by amniocentesis, 271–282
with CAT scan, 270
fetal biophysical profile and, 291–292
by fetal monitoring, 282–291
fetoscopic, 295–297
radiographic, 270–271
sonographic, 268–270
through chorionic villus sampling, 298–299
through percutaneous umbilical blood sampling, 299–300
through placental enzymes and hormones, 292–295
through placental grading, 297–298

Prenatal education, 314
assessment of learning needs in, 311–312
changing trends in, 303–304
childbirth classes in, 306–310
content of, 312–313
continuing, 332
economics of, 311
father's needs in, 313
history of, 304–306
key elements of, 310–313
structure of, 310–311
target of, 310
teaching strategies in, 312
timing and location of, 310
types of classes for, 311
Prenatal period
nurse's role during, 315–334
society's expectations about, 114
Prenatal screening techniques, 268. *See also specific techniques*
Preschoolers, 91
Presentation, determination of, 326–327
Present pain intensity (PPI), 384
Pressure transducers, 364
Prevention 82, 37
Prig, Betsy, 32
Primitive streak, 174
Primordial follicle, *167*
Problem-solving change model, 9
Procedures, 147
Procrastination, 19
Procreative imperative, 113
Professional organizations, 10
Progestasert-T, 65
Progesterone
effects of, 199
in endometrial cycle, 163
influence on uterine activity of, 342
secretion of, 160
withdrawal of to induce labor, 340
Progestogen, 63
Progressive relaxation, 472
Progress reports, 524–527
Prolactin, 208
breastfeeding stimulation of, 426
breasts and, 440
concentrations of during pregnancy, 209
sensory receptors for, 441
Pronephrons, 187
Prostaglandins
as calcium releasers, 342
complications for, 695
to induce labor, 692–694
synthesis of, 342
Protein, 602
complementary, 263
metabolism of during pregnancy, 207
requirements, 247
Proteinuria, 644
during pregnancy, 205–206
Psychologic change, during pregnancy, 218–242
Psychologic function, 506
Psychoprophylaxis, 396
Psychosocial assessment, 329–330
Psychosocial growth, 601
Psychosocial needs, 608–614
Puberty, miniature, 540
Public Health Services (PHS), 37

Pudendal block, 391
transvaginal technique for, *393*
Puerperal fever
contagiousness of, 31
discovery of cause of, 30–31
Puerperal sepsis
changes in childbirth practices to prevent, 31
during Middle Ages, 27
prevention of, 30
Puerperium. *See* Postpartal period
Pulmonary edema, 718–719
Pulmonary embolism, 669–670
alternative therapies for, 675
assessment for, 671–674
case presentation for, 672
causes of, 670–671
with cesarean section, 690
incidence of, 670
sources of, 675
therapy for, 674
Pulmonary system
adaptation to extrauterine life, 533–538
intrauterine function of, 532–533
Pyelonephritis, 659
Pyridoxine, 250, 604
Pyrimethamine, 657

Q

Quadriceps exercises, 469–470
Quality of life principle (QLP), 140–141, 142
Quasi-experimental method, 948
applicability of to perinatal nursing research, 950
Questionnaires, application of, 950–951
Quickening, 178, 196, 198
father's experience of, 234
psychologic effects of, 223

R

Radiant heat loss, 540
Radiant warmer, 407, 408, 774
Radiation
heat loss by, 408–409
risk of to fetus, 271
Radiography, 270–271
Radioimmunoassay, for pregnancy, 197
Radiopharmaceutical drugs, 461
Ramsey, P., 141–142
Randomization, 948
Rapid plasma reagin (RPR) test, 895
Rapport, establishing, 9
Raynalde, Thomas, 28
Reaching, 493
Reactive change, 5
Reactive inhibition, 505
Reactivity periods
first, 542–544
second, 544
Readiness, law of, 503
Reasonable man concept, 146–147
Receiving hospital, 767–772
Reciprocity, 631–632

Recommended Dietary Allowances (RDAs), 246, 604–605
  for nonpregnant women, 247t
  for pregnant and lactating women, 246t
Rectal examination, intrapartal, 373
Rectum
  assessment of, 562
  temperature of, 462
Red Cross, International, 32–33
Red reflex, 556
Reeducative strategies, 15
Referral calls, 767
Referral hospital, 758, 772–773
Referral patterns, 760
Referrals
  for long-term support, 789
  for pregnant adolescents, 838–841
Reflexes. See also specific reflexes
  assessment of, 567–570
  in premature infant, 712
Refractometer, 716
Refreezing phase, 8, 16–17
Regionalization system, 757
  concept of, 38
  handling of crises in, 782
  transport programs and, 759
Registered nurses (RNs), 148
Regulations, 146
Reinforcement, conditioning through, 505
Relactation, 460, 461
Relativism of interactions principle, 505–506
Relaxation
  in pain control, 387
  postpartum, 478
  techniques, 308–309, 396
    after delivery, 471–472
    postcesarean, 483
Religious affiliation, 415
Religious values, 13
Renal plasma flow, 205
Renal system
  changes in with pregnancy, 205–206
  after delivery, 428
  fetal, 187
  immature, 715–716
Reproductive system
  changes in with pregnancy, 99, 200–203
  female, 51
Research, 946–954
  applicability of to perinatal nursing, 950–951
  change and, 951–952
  process of, 947–951
  selecting method of, 951
  types of, 947–950
Research councils, 950
Resistance, 12–13
  overcoming, 15
Resources
  allocation of, 134–136
  analysis of, 14–15
  for pregnant adolescents, 838–841
Respiration
  establishment of rhythmic, 537–538
  factors influencing in fetus and newborn, 535t
Respiratory alkalosis, of pregnancy, 429–430
Respiratory center, factors influencing in fetus and newborn, 535t

Respiratory depression, 432
Respiratory exercises, postcesarean, 482
Respiratory failure, 717
Respiratory system
  changes in during labor, 344
  changes in with pregnancy, 203–205
  immature, 717–718
  with spinal cord injury, 857
Respondent superior doctrine, 151, 766
Responsibilities, resuming of, 496
Rest assessment, postpartum, 491
Restraining forces, 17
Restructurization, cognitive, 506
Resuscitation
  assessment in, 745, 748
  basic steps in, 745
  definition of, 741
  determining need for, 743–745
  drugs for, 754t, 755
  environment during, 747–748
  equipment for, 743, 750
    in newborn nursery, 580
  guidelines for, 749–750
  heart rate during, 746–747
  of high-risk newborns, 740–755
  objectives of, 745
  preparation for, 742–743
  procedure for, 750–752
  purpose of, 749
  ventilation in, 745–746
Resuscitation bag, 745–746
Retinal detachment, 852
Retinol, 603
Retinopathy of prematurity, 719
Retrolental fibroplasia, 719
Return transports, 779
Rewards, external, 16
Rh analysis, 277–278
Rh antibody formation, 278
Rh factor incompatibilities, 428–429
Rh negative infant, 410
Rho Gam, 38
RH type, 38
  determining of by PUBS, 299–300
Rhythm method, 70
Ribble, Margaret, 150
Rib expansion, 482
Riboflavin, 250, 603
Rights of Infants, The, 150
Rites of passage, 220
Ritodrine, 649
Ritual system, 115
Roesslin, Eucharius, 28
Rogers, Carl, 936
Role ambivalence, 112
Role behaviors, 219
  learning of, 220
Role modeling, 498, 519
Role play, 228, 519
Roles
  assignment of, 14
  definition of, 84
  redefining of, 496
Rooming-in, 591–594
  criteria for, 593
  early discharge and, 593
Roosevelt, Theodore, 34
Rooting reflex, 608
  assessment of, 567
Rosegarden of pregnant women and midwives, 28

Routine care, 579–580
Rubella, 654, 657
  vaccine, 38, 429
Rubra lochia, 425
Rupture of membranes (ROM), 350–351
  artificially, 351
  premature (PROM), 351, 909–910
  spontaneously, 351

S

Saddle block, 391
Sanctity of life principle (SLP), 140–141, 142
Sanger, Margaret, 33–34
Scalp assessment, 556
Scanzoni maneuver, 698
Scapular retraction/protraction, 477
Scapular rotation, 476
Schwann cells, 184
Scientific advances, in parenting, 103–108
Scrotum, size of, 560
Seconal, 388
Security, of family, 83
Sedatives, 388–390
Self-care responsibilities, 940–941
Self-determination. See Autonomy
Self-giving, 231–232
Self-understanding, 940
Seminiferous tubules, 165
Semmelweis, Ignaz Phillip, 31
Sensitivity, 939–940
Sensorimotor intelligence, 630–631
Sensory assessment, 575–576
Sensory modulation methods, 396
Sensory stressors, 537
Serosa lochia, 425
Servocontrol mechanism, 713–714
Seton, Elizabeth Bayley, 30
Sex
  patterns of interest in during pregnancy, 331
  selection of, 106–107
Sex chromosomes, 163
Sex education, 823–824, 841, 842
Sex hygiene, ancient attitudes toward, 26
Sexuality, disability and, 845
Sexually transmitted disease (STD), 46, 652–654, 891–892
  contraceptives in preventing, 55
  counseling and support with, 910–911
  fetal effects of, 910
  impact of on perinatal infections, 891–911
  nursing role in, 910–911
Sexual orientation, recognition of, 102–103
Sheehan's syndrome, 427–428
Sheppard-Towner Act, 35, 37
Shettles sex selection technique, 106–107
Shippen, William, 29
Shivering, 407, 539
Show, Dr. John, 29
Shunts, closing of, 538–539
Siblings, reaction of to loss, 792
Significant others, support of during labor, 366

Sign language, 846
Silver nitrate drops, 411
  in neonates' eyes, 139
Silver sulfadiazine cream, 410
Simpson, Sir James Y., 29
Single-parent families, 81, 100–101
  development stages of, 92
Sitting up in bed position, 473
Sitting in chair position, 473–475, 474
Sitz baths, 490
Six Practical Lessons for an Easier Childbirth, 305
Sizemore, Susan, 42
Skin
  changes in with pregnancy, 206–207
  daily care of, 594–595
    with spinal cord injury, 857
  immaturity of, 721–722
  integrity, 552–553
  lesions of in newborn, 553–555
  observation of, 594
  pigmentation of with pregnancy, 195, 430
Skin diseases, hereditary, 296
Skinfold thickness, 601
Sleep
  after labor, 430–431
  following reactivity period, 544
  postpartum assessment of, 491
Sleep hunger, 492
Sleep/wake cycle, 574–575
Small-for-gestational-age infants, 729
  case presentation for, 731–733
  chronic intrauterine hypoxia in, 730
  chronic intrauterine malnutrition in, 729–730
  congenital anomalies in, 730–734
  definition of, 722–728
  feeding methods for, 616–617
  food for and feeding of, 615
  nutrient supplements for, 617
  physical characteristics of, 614–615, 729
  type of milk for, 615–616
Smellie, William, 29
Smiling, 635–636
Smoking, 261
Social interaction model, 8–9
Socialization, 81, 83
  incongruence in, 112
Social psychology, principles of, 507–508
Social Security Act, 37
  amendments of, 37
  Title XX, 37
Social trends, 99
Social worth, 135–136
Society
  changing roles and expectations in, 98–108
  expectations of childbearing behavior of, 113–123
  history of, 99–100
Socioeconomic status, 89
Sodium bicarbonate therapy, 747
Solid food additions, 613–614
Somatomammotropin, 208
Somites, 185
Sonography, 198
  definition of, 268
  indications for, 268
  nursing roles in, 269–270
  in placental grading, 297–298
  procedure and interpretation of, 268–269
  real-time, 269
Soranus, 26–27
Southeast Asians, postpartal practices of, 120–121
Soybean formulas, 620–621
Spence, tail of, 439
Sperm
  in fertilization, 167
  mature, *165*
Spermatids, 174
Spermatocytes, 164
Spermatogenesis, 163–164
Spermatogonia, 164
Sperm donors, 103–104
Spermicides, 59–61
Spermiogenesis, 164
Spina bifida, 412–413
Spinal anesthesia, 391
Spinal canal puncture, 431–432
Spinal cord injury, 855
  autonomic dysreflexia or hyperreflexia with, 858–859
  delivery with, 859
  maternal and infant well-being with, 855–858
  nursing care plan for, 860–861*t*
  pregnancy outcome with, 859–862
  premature labor with, 858
Spinal headache, 431–432
Spine, assessment of, 562
Spousal consent, 139
Stabilization, 17
Standing pelvic realignment, 483
  exercise for, 478–479
Standing procedure, 470–471
State, assessment of, 572–575
Status quo
  assessing, 11
  threat to upset, 9
Statutes, 146
Steady state, 4
Sterilization, 67
  effectiveness of, 67
  factors in considering, 55
  female, 68
  male, 68–69
Stern vs. Whitehead, 106
Stillbirth, 793–794
Stimulation
  auditory, 632–633
  implementing program of, 637–638
  importance of, 630–632
  of premature infant, 633–634
  responsive, 811
  tactile, 632
Stimulus-response bond, 503
Stimulus-response patterns, 505–506, 631
Stimulus-response theories, principles of, 507
Stomach
  changes in during pregnancy, 206
  development of, 190
Stomedeum, 189
Strabismus, 557
Strategies, 14
  determination of, 15
Stress, change and, 12
Stressors, identification and mediation of, 362
Striae, 323, 324, 430
  with pregnancy, 207
Stromal cells, 161
Substance abuse, 872–889. *See also* Drug abuse
  fetal effects of, 875–889
Succinyl choline (Anectine), 395
Sucking calluses, 558
Sucking fat pad, 558
Sucking reflex, assessment of, 567–569
Suckling, 440
Suction machines, portable, 762
Sulfa drugs, 461
Sulfisoxazole (Gantrisin), 654
Sulfonamide, 657
Supine bicycle exercise, 475
Supplementation feedings, 445–446
Support
  for high-risk family, 787–789
  long-term, 789
Supported forward bending stretch, 480, *481*
Support groups
  parent-to-parent, 789
  for perinatal loss, 796
Support systems
  in single-parent families, 100
  for transition to motherhood, 497, 497–500
Surrogacy
  contracts, legality of, 106
  legal controversy of, 153–154
Surrogate mothers, 105–106
Survey method, 946
Sutures, 555
Symmetry, 551
Syncytium, 170
Syncytotrophoblast, 170
Syndactyly, 561
Synectics theory, 952
Syphilis, 652, 654
  congenital, *896*
  epidemiology and incidence of, 893
  maternal issues of, 893–895
  newborn issues of, 895
  nursing issues of, 895–896
  tertiary, 894
  testing for, 895
  treatment of, 654–657, 895
Systolic pressure, 320

T

Tactile assessment, 576
Tactile stimulation, 632
  of premature infant, 633
Taking-hold phase, 492–493
Taking-in phase, 492
Tar, 887
Target system, 7
  assessment of, 11
  characteristics of static and future-oriented, 12*t*
  determining what will motivate, 11–12
  getting cooperation of, 16
  goals of, 13–14
Task analysis, 512–513
Teaching
  barriers to, 521
  definitions of, 502
Teaching-learning transaction, 510
Technologic advances, 937–938
  caring and, 938–939

Technologic advances (continued).
  fear of, 13
  in parenting, 103–108
Teenagers, 91. See also Adolescent
  pregnant, 46, 93, 100, 821–842
  cultural attitudes toward, 116
  response of to mother's pregnancy, 238
  as unmarried parents, 94
  weight gain during lactation and postpartum, 261
Teeth, 206
Telephone consultation, 759
  with high-risk family, 787
Temperature
  monitoring of, 595
  regulation of in premature infant, 712–714
Teratogenesis, 875
Teratogenic drugs
  fetal effects of, 878t
  widespread use of, 46
Terbutaline, 649
Tertiary care centers, 757, 759
Test-tube babies, 38, 99, 104. See also In vitro fertilization
Tetany, 209
Tetracycline, 895
  during breastfeeding, 461
  prophylactic, 411
Tetracyclines, 654
Thank You, Dr. Lamaze, 305
THC, fetal effects of, 884–885
Theca externa, 161
Theca interna, 161
Theophylline, 460
Therapeutic relationship, building, 9–11
Therapeutic touch, 373
Thermal environment, neutral, 540, 713
  chart for, 776t
Thermal insulation, 407, 539
Thermogenesis, nonshivering, 539–540
Thermoregulation
  adaptation to extrauterine life of, 539–540
  mechanisms for, 405–407
  in premature infant, 714–715
  during resuscitation, 755
  standard interventions for, 774–776
Theutt of Hamburg, Dr., 27–28
Thiamin, 250, 603
Thiopental sodium (Pentothal), 395
Thorax, assessment of, 559
Thromboembolic disease, 669–674
  treatment for, 674
Thrombophlebitis, 490
  with spinal cord injury, 856–857
Thyroid gland, 209
Thyroid hormone, synthesis of, 249
Thyrotropin, 182
Thyroxin, 209
Time orientation, 88–89
Timing, 15
Tocodynamometers, 364
Tonic neck reflex, 570
TORCH complex, 654, 657
Torticollis, 558
Total parenteral nutrition, 720–721
Touch, 627
  therapeutic, 373
Touch-release techniques, 472

Toxemia, 64
  maternal mortality from, 43
Toxic shock syndrome, 62
Toxoplasmosis, 654
TPR assessment (temperature, pulse, respirations), 373
  postpartum, 487
Tradition, 13
Tranquilizers, 390
Transcutaneous electric nerve stimulation (TENS), 396
Transcutaneous oxygen monitoring, 764
Transcutaneous oxygen monitors, 762–763
Transitional nursery, 590
Transitional period, 544
Transport, active, 182
Transport center
  assessment in, 773–774
  data collection in, 764–766
  equipment for, 761–763, 765t
  estimate time of arrival for, 777–778
  factors in selecting, 778
  financial solvency of, 766
  fluid therapy in, 776
  in hospital, 595
  oxygenation/ventilation in, 776
  parental contact in, 777
  patient monitoring in, 777
  quality assurance for, 764
  safety in, 776
  team in, 776
  temperature regulation in, 774–776
Transport equipment, 761–762
  maternal, 763
  neonatal, 763–764
Transport programs, 759–760. See also Maternal transport; Neonatal transport; Transport center
  community hospital and, 767
  dispatch center for, 760
  establishing effective, 767
  liability risk of, 767
  receiving hospital and, 767–772
  referral hospital and, 772–773
  referral patterns of, 760
  in regionalized health care system, 757–758
  two-way, 757
  unique aspects of, 766–767
Transport vehicles, 758, 778–779
  cost of, 766
Transverse presentation, 697
Treponema pallidum, 654, 893
Triceps skinfold, 601
Trichloroethylene (Trilene), 395
Trichomonas infections, 654
Trichomonas vaginalis, 652
Triiodothyronine, 209
Trisomy, in SGA infants, 730
Trophoblast, 168
  cell layers in, 170
Truncus arteriosus, 185
Trust building, 10
Trust/distrust task, 413, 608
Tubal occlusion, 74
Tubal sterilization, 68
Twins
  breastfeeding of, 459
  loss of, 800
  position for nursing of, 474

U

Ultrasound. See Sonography
Ultrasound transducers, 364
Umbilical cord, 174
  clamping of, 353–354, 410, 538
  compression, 704
  cross-section of, 560
  inspection of, 559
  topical medications for, 410
Underwater birthing, 932
Underweight, 258
Unfreezing, 7–8, 9–13
Upper extremities, assessment of, 561
Ureters, dilatation of, 428
Urethra, trauma to, 434
Urinalysis, 256
Urinary frequency, 196, 205
Urinary tract infections, 652
  case presentation of, 656
  effects of during pregnancy, 665t
  risks of, 654
Urination problems, 489
Urine specimen, 321
Uterine blood flow, 192
Uterine blood perfusion, increased, 704
Uterine contractions
  assessment of, 363, 373
  decreased blood flow with, 287
  duration of, 363
  fetal heart rate and, 376
  frequency of, 363
  hypertonic, 695, 696
  hypotonic, 695, 696
  intensity of, 342, 363
  during labor, 342–344
  mechanical pressure of, 536
  monitoring procedures for, 375
  with oxytocin stress test, 287–288
  phases of, 344
  in second stage of labor, 353
  in third stage of labor, 354
Uterine dystocia, 696
Uterine nutritive function, factors affecting, 182
Uteroplacental insufficiency, 376
Uterotonic agents, 691–692
Uterus
  changes in during labor, 340
  changes in with pregnancy, 200
  couvelaire, 664
  endometrial lining of after delivery, 425
  evolution of spontaneous activity of, 343
  fundus
    after delivery, 424–425
    palpation of, 488
  involution of, 424, 430
  position of, 325
  postpartum changes in, 424–426
  progressive development of segments of, 343

V

Vacuum extraction, 700, 704
Vagina
  changes in with pregnancy, 201–202
  discoloration of mucosa of, 195

infections, 329, 652
  postpartum assessment of, 489–490
Vaginal birth, after cesarean birth, 930–931
Vaginal examination, intrapartal, 373
Vaginal suppository, insertion of, 60
Vagisec, 654
Valium, 390
Value system, 13, 115
  conflict of, 133–134
Vascular damage, 433
Vasectomy, 68–69
Vasomotor control, 405–407, 539
Vasopressin, 209
Vasospasm, 645
VDRL test, 895
Vegans, 262, 263
  lunch sample for, 264t
Vegetarians, 262–263, 264
Vena cava, relief of obstruction of, 426
Ventilation, 745–746, 776
  procedure and purpose of, 748
Ventilators, 762
Vernix caseosa, 178, 552–553
Vertex presentation molding, 536
Viability, definition of, 152
Vietnamese
  attitudes toward pregnancy of, 116–119
  childbearing case study of, 126
  newborns, care of by, 122
  postpartal practices of, 120–121
Visual assessment, 576
Visualization technique, 477–478
Visually disabled, 851–855
Vitalism, 140
Vital sign monitoring, for neonatal transport, 764
Vital Statistics, Bureau of, 418
Vitamin A, 603
  toxicity, 604
Vitamin A needs, 249
Vitamin B complex, 249–250, 603–604
Vitamin C, 604
Vitamin D, 604
  requirement of, 209, 249

supplementation of, 609
  toxicity, 604
Vitamin E, 604
  needs, 249
  for SGA infants, 617
Vitamin K, 412, 604
  administration of to newborns, 418, 541
  inefficient production of, 719
  supplementation of, 609
Vitamins, 603–604
  deficiencies of, 263–264
  fat-soluble, 249
  recommended dietary allowances of, 604–605
  supplementation, 250
  water-soluble, 249–250
Vitelline duct, 190
Voluntary agencies, 36–38
Vomiting
  functional, 619
  nutrition management of, 264
Vulva, trauma to, 433–434

W

Wage gap, 85t
Wald, Lillian, 34–35
Walking procedure, 471
Warming blankets, 407–408
Water metabolism, 208
Water needs, 602
Weight, desirable, 258t
Weight control, 256–259
  during lactation and postpartum, 259–261
  during pregnancy, 261
Weight gain
  assessment of, 256–259
  during pregnancy, 207, 226
Weight loss, after delivery, 430
Weight measurement, 601
  daily, 595
Wet nurses, 40
Wharton's jelly, 174

White House Conference on Food, Nutrition, and Health report, 244
Wide neighborhoods, 35
Women
  changing role of in society, 113–114
  health issues of, 50–77
  improved status of, 99
  reproductive anatomy and physiology of, 51
  roles of in society, 24
  in workforce, 99
Women, Infants, and Children (WIC), 37, 839
  nutritious foods offered by, 245, 247
Women's movement, 41
Women Rebel, 34
World Health Organization, origin of, 37

X

X-rays. *See* Radiography

Y

Yoga, 306
Yolk sac, 174

Z

Zakrzewska, Marie, 30
Zero population growth, 113
Zinc
  depletion, 619
  requirements for, 249
  supplementation of, 250
Zona pellucida, 165
  loss of, 168
  sperm penetration of, 167
Zona reaction, 167–168
Zygote, 168

Credits

These pages constitute an extension of the copyright page.

p. 6, Table 1–1: Adapted from Strategies and Techniques for the Nurse Change Agent, by E. Olson, *Nursing Clinics of North America*, 1979, 14(2), p. 325. Reprinted by permission of W. B. Saunders Company.

p. 7, Figure 1–1: Adapted from Green, C. P. 1983. Teaching strategies for the process of planned change. *J. Cont. Ed. Nursing.* 14(6), p. 17.

p. 9, Figure 1–2: Green, C. P. 1983. Teaching strategies for the process of planned change. *J. Cont. Ed. Nursing.* 14(6) p. 21.

p. 12, Table 1–4: Reprinted with permission from *Hospital Progress*, June 1973. Copyright 1973, Catholic Hospital Association.

p. 18, Figure 1–6: Welter, P. *Connecting with a Friend*. Wheaton, IL: Tyndale, pp. 68, 72, 1985.

p. 19, Figure 1–8: From Planning Change in the Family, by W. G. Dyer. In A. M. Reinhardt and M. D. Quinn, eds., *Family-Centered Community Nursing*, pp. 152–157. Copyright 1973, by the C. V. Mosby Company. Reprinted by permission.

p. 25. Figures 2–1, 2–2, 2–3, and 2–4, p. 28, Figure 2–5, and p. 29, Figure 2–6: From *A Pictorial History of Medicine*, by O. L. Bettmann. Springfield, IL: Charles Thomas Publisher, 1956.

p. 35, Figure 2–7: Mary Breckinridge, 1952. *Wide Neighborhoods*. New York: Harper and Row. Reproduced with permission from the Frontier Nursing Service, Hyden, Kentucky.

p. 43, Figure 2–8: From Prevention 82. Department of Health and Human Services (PHS) Publication No. 82-50157.

p. 43, Figure 2–9: From Prevention 82. Department of Health and Human Services (PHS) Publication No. 82-50157.

p. 43, Table 2–1: Adapted from Federal Security Agency, 1952. Vital Statistics, and Pratt, M. W. 1982. The demography of maternal and child health. *In Maternal and Child Health Practices: Problems, Resources, and Methods of Delivery*, eds. H. M. Wallace, E. M. Gold, and A. C. Oglesby. New York: John Wiley & Sons.

p. 43. Table 2–2: Health United States, 1984. DHHS Publication No. (PHS) 85-1232. Hyattsville, MD: Public Health Service.

p. 44, Figure 2–10: Federal Security Agency, 1952. Vital Statistics 26(17).

p. 44, Figure 2–11: National Center for Health Statistics (1968a).

p. 45, Figure 2–12: National Center for Health Statistics (1987b).

p. 51, Figure 3–1, and p. 52, Figure 3–2: From *Sexuality Today*, by G. D. Nass, and M. P. Fisher. Boston, MA: Jones and Bartlett, 1988.

p. 53, Figure 3–3, p. 54, Table 3–1, p. 55, Table 3–2 and p. 64, Table 3–4: From *Contraceptive Technology*, 1984–1985, by R. A. Hatcher, F. Guest, F. Stewart, G. K. Stewart, J. Trussell, S. Cerel, and W. Cates, 12th ed. New York: Irvington. 1984.

p. 56, Figure 3–4, p. 59, Figure 3–6, p. 60, Figure 3–7, p. 66, Figure 3–10, p. 68, Figure 3–11, and p. 69, Figure 3–12: *Sexual Choices: An Introduction to Human Sexuality*. 2nd ed., 1987. Boston: Jones and Bartlett. G. D. Nass, R. W. Libby and M. P. Fisher.

p. 57, Figure 3–5: From *Contraceptive Technology*, 1986–1987. 13th ed., by R. A. Hatcher, F. Guest, F. Stewart, G. K. Stewart, J. Trussell, S. Cerel, and W. Cates, eds. New York: Irvington, 1986.

p. 60, Figure 3–8: From *Information on Contraceptive Vaginal Suppositories*. Planned Parenthood/Alameda-San Francisco. 1983. San Francisco: Planned Parenthood.

p. 62, Figure 3–9: From *Human Sexuality*, by W. H. Masters, V. E. Johnson, and R. C. Kolodny. 3rd ed. Glenview, IL: Scott, Foresman and Company, 1988.

p. 63, Table 3–3: From *Nutrition and Family Planning: Oral Contraceptives*. Reno, NV: Washoe County Health Department.

p. 82, Table 4–1: Adapted from Sussman, M. B., 1973. Family Systems in the 1970's: Analysis, Policies, and Programs. In *Family Health Care*, D. P. Hymovich and M. U. Barnard, eds. New York: McGraw-Hill.

p. 86, Table 4–3: From *Family-Centered Care of Children and Adolescents*, by J. M. Tackett and M. Hunsberger. Copyright 1981 by W. B. Saunders Company. Reprinted by permission. Stage IV, reprinted by permission from Megatrends, copyright 1982, by John Naisbitt. Published by Warner Books, Inc.

p. 90, Figure 4–4: From E. M. Duvall, *Family Development*, 4th ed. Philadelphia: J. B. Lippincott, 1971. In *Community Health Nursing: Concepts and Practice*, by B. W. Spradley, 2nd ed. Boston: Little, Brown and Company, 1985. Reprinted by permission.

p. 94, Table 4-4: By J. A. Tapia, Fractionalization of the Family Unit. In *The Process of Human Development*, eds, C. S. Schuster and S. S. Ashburn. Boston: Little, Brown and Company, 1986.

p. 95, Figure 4-5: The Nursing Process in Family Health, by J. A. Tapia. 1972. *Nurs. Outlook.* 20(4):267-270.

p. 123, Figure 6-1: Adapted from *Social Work in Health Care*, by A. Brownlee, 1978. 4(2):179-198.

p. 124, Figure 6-2: M. Orque, 1981. Cultural components. In *Maternity Care: The Nurse and the Family*, ed, Jensen R. C.

p. 161, Figure 9-1, and p. 162, Figure 9-2: From *Williams' Obstetrics*. 17th ed., 1985. By J. A. Pritchard, P. D. MacDonald, and M. F. Gant. New York: Appleton-Century-Crofts.

p. 166, Figure 9-5, p. 171, Figure 9-9, p. 172, Figure 9-11: From *The Developing Human*, 2nd ed., by K. Moore. Philadelphia: W. B. Saunders Co., 1977.

p. 167, Figure 9-6, p. 168, Figure 9-7, p. 172, Figure 9-10, p. 183, Figure 9-22, and p. 185, Figure 9-23: From *Medical Embryology*, 4th ed., by J. Langman. Baltimore: Williams & Wilkins, 1981.

p. 169, Figure 9-8, p. 186, Figure 9-24, p. 188, Figure 9-25, p. 190, Figure 9-27: From *Clinical Embryology for Medical Students*, by R. S. Snell, 3rd ed. Boston: Little, Brown and Company, 1983.

p. 173, Figure 9-12, and p. 175, Figure 9-13: From *Illustrated Human Embryology:* Volume I Embryogenesis, by H. Tuchman-Duplessis, G. David, and P. Haegel. New York: Springer-Verlag, 1980.

p. 189, Figure 9-26, and p. 191, Figure 9-28: From *Illustrated Human Embryology*, Volume II: Organogenesis. New York: Springer-Verlag, 1974.

p. 197, Table 10-1: From Diagnosis of pregnancy, by B. A. Eskin. In L. Iffy and H. A. Kaminetzky eds., *Principles and Practice of Obstetrics and Perinatology.* Copyright 1981 by John Wiley & Sons, Inc. Reprinted by permission.

p. 197, Table 10-2: From *An Introduction to Midwifery*, by M. A. Hickman. Boston: Blackwell Scientific Publications, Inc., 1978; and *Williams' Obstetrics*, 17th ed., by J. A. Pritchard, P. C. MacDonald, and N. F. Gant. Norwalk, CT: Appleton-Century-Crofts, 1985.

p. 204, Table 10-3: From *Williams' Obstetrics*, 17th ed., by J. A. Pritchard, P. C. MacDonald, and N. F. Gant, Norwalk, CT: Appleton-Century-Crofts, 1985; and *Laboratory Tests—Implications for Nurses and Allied Health Professionals*, by C. J. Byrne, D. F. Saxton, P. K. Pelikan, and P. M. Nugent. Menlo Park, CA: Addison-Wesley, 1981.

p. 233, Table 11-2: Adapted from Maternal tasks in pregnancy, by R. Rubin. *Maternal-Child Nursing Journal*, 1975, 4(3), 143-153. Reprinted by permission.

p. 246, Table 12-1, and p. 247, Table 12-2: Food and Nutrition Board, Committee on Dietary Allowances, National Research Council, 1980. Recommended dietary allowances, 9th rev. Washington, DC: National Academy of Sciences.

p. 248, Table 12-4, p. 250, Table 12-5, p. 254, Table 12-6, p. 257, Table 12-10, and p. 258, Table 12-11: California Department of Health Services, Maternal and Child Health Branch. 1987. *Nutrition during pregnancy and the postpartum period: A manual for health care professionals.* (Review Draft.)

p. 255, Tables 12-7, and 12-8: March of Dimes Birth Defects Foundation. 1986. Recipes for healthy babies.

p. 256, Table 12-9: San Francisco Department of Health. 1987. Perinatal nutrition protocols. San Francisco perinatal forum nutrition committee.

p. 262, Table 12-12: Adapted from *Nutrition: Principles and Application in Health Promotion*, by C. M. Suitor and M. F. Hunter. Copyright 1984, J. B. Lippincott Company, Philadelphia. Reprinted by permission.

p. 263, Table 12-13: Nutrition Education Committee for Maternal and Child Nutrition Publications. 1986. *Cross-cultural counseling: A guide for nutrition and health counselors.* United States Department of Agriculture. Department of Health and Human Services.

p. 264, Table 12-15: Coalition for the Medical Rights of Women. 1987. *Natural remedies for pregnancy discomforts.* California Department of Health Services, Education Program Assoc., Inc.

p. 268, Table 13-1: From Fetal and Maternal Monitoring Antepartal Fetal Assessment, Part I, by M. S. Cranley. *American Journal of Nursing*, 78:2098-2102.

pp. 272-274, Table 13-2, and p. 296, Figure 13-18: From The Current Scope of Antenatal Diagnosis, by M. B. Golbus, *Hospital Practices*, 17(4):179-186. 1982. Reprinted by permission.

p. 275, Table 13-3, and p. 281, Figure 13-3: From Recurrence Risks of Malformations, by G. N. Wilson, *Journal of Reproductive Medicine*, 1982, 27(a):607-612. Reprinted by permission.

p. 276, Table 13-4, and p. 277, Table 13-5: From Neutral Tube Defects: Epidemiology, Detection, and Prevention, by F. L. Cohen. 1987. *J. Obstet. Gynecol. Neonatal Nurs.* 16(2):112.

p. 283, Figure 13-4, and p. 285, Figures 13-6 and 13-7: From Nonstress Antepartal Monitoring, by M. T. Lieber. Copyright 1980, American Journal of Nursing Company. Reproduced with permission from *Maternal/Child Nursing*, 5:335-339.

p. 286, Figures 13-8, and 13-9, and p. 287, Figure 13-10: From Fetal and Maternal Monitoring: Nonstress Test, (pictorial) by R. Kopf. Part VI. Copyright 1978. *Am. J. Nurs.* 78:2115-2117. Reproduced with permission.

p. 288, Table 13-6: From The Nipple Stimulation Contraction Stress Test, by C. Marshall. 1986. *J. Obstet. Gynecol. Neonatal Nurs.* 15(6):459-462.

p. 289, Figure 13-11: From Intrapartal Fetal Monitoring, by R. M. Lojek and M. J. Yunek. Copyright 1978, *Am. J. Nurs.* 78:2102-2109. Reprinted by permission.

p. 289, Figure 13-12, and p. 290, Figure 13-13: From Fetal and Maternal Monitoring Oxytocin Challenge Test, (pictorial) Part V, by S. Sethi. Copyright 1978. Reproduced with permission from the *Am. J. Nurs.* 78:2112-2115.

p. 292, Table 13-7, p. 293, Figures 13-14, and 13-15, and p. 294, Figure 13-16: From Antepartum Fetal Evaluation: Development of a Fetal Biophysical Profile, by F. A. Manning, L. D. Platt, and L. Sipos. Am. J. Obstet. Gynecol. 1980. 136:787-795. Reprinted by permission of C. V. Mosby Co.

p. 295, Figure 13-17: From Serial Estriol Determinations in High-Risk Pregnancies: Implications for Primary Care Nursing, by P. Burosh, 1976. J. Gynecol. Nurs. 5:34-40. Reprinted by permission.

p. 299, Figure 13-20: From Chorionic Villus Sampling, by J. S. Hogge, et al. 1986. *J. Obstet. Gynecol. Neonatal Nurs.* 15(1):25.

p. 331, Figures 15-11 and 15-12: From *Making Love During Pregnancy*, by Elizabeth Bing and Libby Coleman. New York: Bantam Books, 1977.

p. 343, Figure 16-1: From Oxytocin and Contractility of the Pregnant Human Uterus, by R. Caldeyro-Barcia and J. A. Serino, *Annals of New York Academy of Sciences*, Vol. 79, 1959, p. 814.

p. 343, Figure 16–2, p. 347, Figure 16–8, and p. 350, Figure 16–12: From *Williams' Obstetrics*, 17th ed., by J. A. Pritchard, P. C. MacDonald, and N. F. Gant. Norwalk, CT: Appleton-Century-Crofts, 1985.

p. 346, Figure 16–5, p. 348, Figure 16–9, and p. 349, Figure 16–10: From *Human Labor and Birth*, 4th ed., by H. Oxorn and W. E. Foote. Copyright 1980. New York: Appleton-Century-Crofts.

p. 349, Figure 16–11: From *Human Anatomy and Physiology*, by A. P. Spence and E. B. Mason, p. 150. Copyright 1979 by Benjamin/Cummings Publishing Company. Reprinted by permission.

p. 352, Figure 16–13: From Primigravid Labor: A Graphico-Statistical Analysis, by E. A. Friedman, *Obstet. Gynecol.*, 6:570. Reprinted by permission by Appleton-Century-Crofts. Copyright 1955.

p. 372, Table 17–1: From *Childbearing: A Nursing Perspective*, by A. L. Clark and D. D. Affonso. Philadelphia: F. A. Davis, 1979.

p. 375, Figure 17–5, p. 376, Figures 17–6 and 17–7, and p. 377, Figure 17–8: From *Fetal Monitoring and Fetal Assessment in High-Risk Pregnancy*, by S. M. Tucker. C. V. Mosby Company, 1978.

p. 380, Figure 18–1: Adapted from *The Challenge of Pain*, by R. Melzack and P. D. Wall. Reprinted by permission of Basic Books, Inc., 1983.

p. 383, Figure 18–3: From "Labor Is Still Painful After Prepared Childbirth Training," by R. Melzack et al., *Canadian Medical Association Journal*. 1981. 125:357–363. Reprinted by permission.

p. 385, Figure 18–5: Adapted from "Neutral Blockade for Obstetrics and Gynecology," by P. R. Brownridge, G. Taylor, and D. H. Ralston. In M. J. Cousins and P. O. Bridenbaugh, eds., *Neutral Blockade in Clinical Anesthesia and Management of Pain*. Philadelphia: J. B. Lippincott Company, 1980. Reprinted by permission.

p. 393, Figure 18–7: From *Williams' Obstetrics*, 17th ed., by J. A. Pritchard and P. C. MacDonald. East Norwalk, CT: Appleton-Century-Crofts, 1980.

p. 400, Figure 19–1: From *Childbearing: A Nursing Perspective*, by A. L. Clark, D. D. Affonso, and T. R. Harris. Philadelphia: F. A. Davis, 1979. Reprinted by permission.

p. 401, Table 19–1: Adapted from *Neonatology*, by B. Avery. Philadelphia: J. B. Lippincott, 1987.

p. 402, Table 19–2: Adapted from *Realities in Childbearing*, 2nd ed., by M. L. Moore. Philadelphia: W. B. Saunders Co., 1983.

p. 403, Table 19–3: Adapted from "Evaluation of the Newborn Infant-Second Report," by V. Apgar et al., *J. Am. Med. Assoc.* 168:1985–1988, 1958.

p. 405, Figure 19–3: Adapted from *Critical Care of the Newborn*, by W. Hodson, and W. Truog. Philadelphia: W. B. Saunders, 1983.

p. 414, Table 19–5: Adapted from Screening for Hidden Congenital Anomalies, by G. VanLeeuwen and L. Glenn, *Pediatrics*, 41, 147, 1968.

p. 416, Figure 19–8: From *Nursery Forms. Procedure Book.* 1983. Kearney, NB: Good Samaritan Hospital.

p. 424, Figure 20–1, and p. 432, Figure 20–2: Adapted from *Maternity Nursing*, 15th ed., by S. J. Reeder, L. Mastroianni, and L. Martin. Philadelphia: J. B. Lippincott. 1983.

p. 425, Table 20–1: From *Maternal-Newborn Nursing*, 2nd ed., by A. Pillitteri. Boston: Little, Brown and Company, 1981.

p. 427, Table 20–2: Adapted from *Perinatal Coagulation*, by W. E. Hathaway and J. Bonnar. Copyright 1978. San Diego: Grune and Stratton.

p. 437, Figures 21–1 and 21–2: Courtesy of the Maxwell Museum of Anthropology, University of New Mexico.

p. 449, Figures 21–12 and 21–15, and p. 455, Figure 21–21: Reproduced with permission of Happy Family Products, Inc.

p. 454, Figure 21–17: Reproduced with the permission of the Lactation Institute.

p. 455, Figure 21–20: Reproduced courtesy of Lopuco, Ltd.

p. 456, Figure 21–22: Reproduced with the permission of Egnel, Inc.

p. 458, Figure 21–25: Courtesy of Gerber Products Co.

p. 460, Figure 21–26: Courtesy of Lact-Aid International, Inc.

p. 504, Table 24–1: Adapted from *Learning Theories for Teachers*, 4th ed., by M. L. Bigge, Copyright 1981 Harper and Row Publishers, Inc. Reprinted by permission.

p. 511, Figure 24–1: Adapted from *Educational Psychology: The Science of Instruction and Learning*, by R. C. Anderson and G. W. Faust. New York: Dodd, Mead. 1973.

pp. 514–515, Figure 24–2: Women's Hospital of Texas, Houston.

pp. 522–523, Table 24–2: From *Practical Approaches to Patient Teaching*, by D. A. Bille. Boston: Little, Brown and Co., 1981.

p. 525, Figure 24–4, and p. 526, Figure 24–5: Alta Bates Hospital.

p. 532, Table 25–1 and p. 533, Figure 25–1: From *Assessment of the Newborn: A Guide for the Practitioner*, by M. Ziai, T. Clarke, and T. Merritt. Boston: Little, Brown. 1984.

p. 535, Table 25–2, and p. 536, Figure 25–3: Adapted from *Childbearing: A Nursing Perspective*, by A. Clark, D. Affonso, and T. Harris. 2nd ed. Philadelphia: F. A. Davis. 1979.

p. 536, Figure 25–4, and p. 537, Table 25–3: From *High-risk Newborn Infants: The Basis for Intensive Nursing Care*, by S. B. Korones. 3rd ed. St. Louis: C. V. Mosby. 1981.

p. 543, Figure 25–5: From Transition to Extrauterine Life, by H. W. Arnold, et al., Am. J. Nurs. 65(10):77–84.

p. 548, Figures 26–1 and 26–2: From A Practical Classification of Newborn Infants by Weight and Gestational Age, by F. C. Battaglia and L. O. Lubchenco, J. Pediatrics, 71(2):159–163. Reprinted by permission.

p. 550, Figure 26–3: From *The Neurological Assessment of the Preterm and Full-Term Newborn Infant*, by L. Dubowitz and V. Dubowitz. Philadelphia: J. B. Lippincott, 1981.

p. 554, Figure 26–6, p. 556, Figure 26–8, p. 557, Figure 26–9, p. 559, Figure 26–11, p. 562, Figure 26–16, and pp. 570–571, Figure 26–21: Courtesy of Mead Johnson Laboratories.

p. 560, Figure 26–13: Reprinted with the permission of Edward Wallenstein.

p. 563, Figure 26–17: From *Pediatrics*, 17th ed., by A. M. Rudolph and J. E. Hoffman. Copyright 1982. Norfolk, CT: Appleton-Century-Crofts, Reprinted by permission.

p. 564, Figure 26–18: From Clinical Assessment of Gestational Age in the Newborn Infant, by L. Dubowitz, V. Dubowitz, and C. Goldberg. 1970. J. Pediatrics. 77(1):1–10.

p. 568, Figure 26–19: From *Nelson Textbook of Pediatrics*, 12th ed., by R. Behrman and V. Vaughan. Philadelphia: W. B. Saunders, 1983. Reprinted by permission.

p. 569, Figures 26–10, 20, 14, 15: From *Assessment of the Newborn: A Guide for Practitioners* by M. Ziai, T. Clark, and T. Merritt. Boston: Little Brown & Co. 1984.

p. 572, Table 26–3, p. 573, Figure 26–22, and p. 574, Table 26–4: From *Neonatal Behavioral Assessment Scale*, by T. B. Brazelton. Philadelphia: J. B. Lippincott. 1973. Reprinted by permission.

p. 575, Table 26–5: From *Behrman's Neonatal-Perinatal Medicine: Diseases of the Fetus and Infant*, 3rd ed., by A. Fanaroff, and R. J. Martin. St. Louis: C. V. Mosby. 1983.

pp. 583–589, Table 27–1: From Isolation Guidelines For Obstetric Patients and Newborn Infants, by R. Weinstein, K. Boyer, and E. Linn. 1983. *Am. J. Obstet. Gynecol.* 146(4):353–360.

p. 592, Figure 27–4: Maternity Hospital, Western Reserve University Hospitals, Cleveland, Ohio.

p. 605, Table 28–1, p. 606, Table 28–2, p. 611, Table 28–4, and p. 612, Table 28–5: From *Nutrition and Diet Therapy*, 5th ed., by S. R. Williams. C. V. Mosby Company. 1985. Reprinted by permission.

p. 626, Table 29–1: From Maternal Behavior in Mammals, by M. A. Trause, M. H. Klaus, and J. H. Kennell, In M. H. Klaus and J. H. Kennell, (Eds.), *Parent-Infant Bonding*, 2nd ed. St. Louis: C. V. Mosby. 1982.

p. 631, Table 29–2: From *Human Development: A Life-Span Approach*, 2nd ed., by K. L. Freiberg. Copyright 1983 by Wadsworth, Inc. Reprinted by permission of the publisher, Wadsworth Health Sciences Division, Monterey, California.

p. 635, Figure 29–5: From Infancy and the Optimal Level of Stimulation, by D. J. Greenberg and W. J. O'Donnell. *Child Development*, 1972, 43, pp. 639–645. Reprinted by permission of The Society for Research in Child Development, Inc.

p. 650, Table 30–2: From Pregnancy and Diabetes: Medical Aspects, by P. White. 1965. *Med. N. Am.* 49:1016.

p. 653, Table 30–3: From *Medical Letter on Drugs and Therapeutics* (1981).

p. 657, Figure 30–1: From Postpartum Infection, by D. Charles, and T. A. Kelin. In *Obstetrical and Perinatal Infections*, eds. D. Charles and M. Finland. Philadelphia: Lea & Febiger. 1973.

p. 657, Figure 30–2, and p. 658, Table 30–5: From Puerpural Infections, by D. Eschenbach and G. Wager. *Clinical Obstetrics and Gynecology*, 1980, 23, 1003–1037: and Disorders of Immuno-Haematology in Pregnancy, by M. R. MacKenzie, *Clin. in Haematology*, 1978, 2, 515–523.

p. 659, Table 30–6, and p. 665, Table 30–8: From *Williams' Obstetrics*. 17th ed. New York: Appleton-Century-Crofts.

p. 670, Table 30–9: By permission of Mary M. Wagner, Clinical Nursing Specialist, University of Iowa Hospitals and Clinics. In Shock: Emergency Nursing Implications, by J. Royce. 1973. *Nurs. Clin. N. Amer.* 8:380.

p. 671, Tables 30–10, and 30–11, and p. 674, Table 30–12: Adapted from Thromboembolism and Pregnancy, by R. K. Laros and L. S. Alger. *Clin. Obstet. Gynecol.*, 1979, 22, 871–888.

p. 683, Figure 31–2: Based on Trends in Cesarean Section Rates for the United States, by P. Placek and S. Taffel, *Public Health Reports*, 1980, 95(6), 540–548. Reprinted by permission.

p. 685, Figure 31–4 and p. 684, Figure 31–3: From *Synopsis of Obstetrics*, 10th ed., by E. Sandberg. St. Louis: C. V. Mosby Company, 1978.

p. 700, Figure 31–7: Courtesty of Appleton-Century-Crofts.

p. 700, Figure 31–8, and p. 701, Figure 31–9: Courtesy of J. L. Waeltz.

p. 712, Figure 32–1: Courtesy of The National Foundation/March of Dimes (1976). Clinical Education Aids. The National Foundation-March of Dimes, White Plains, N.Y. 1976.

p. 713, Table 32–1, and p. 714, Table 32–2: Courtesy of The American Academy of Pediatrics. 1977. From *Standards and Recommendations for Hospital Care of New Infants*, 6th ed.

p. 746, Figure 33–1: From *Atlas of Procedures in Neonatology*, by M. Fletcher, and M. MacDonald, eds. Philadelphia: J. B. Lippincott. 1983.

p. 746, Figure 33–3 and p. 747, Figure 33–4: From Standards for CPR and ECC Part IV: Neonatal Advanced Life Support. *JAMA* 255(21):2969–2973. 1986.

p. 749, Figure 33–5: Adapted from Schreiner, R. L., *Neonatology for the Pediatrician Medical Education Resources Program*, Indiana University School of Medicine, 1978, p. 187.

p. 750, Figure 33–6: From Orotracheal Intubation in the Newborn Infant: A Method for Determining Depth of Tube Insertion, by M. Tochen. 1979. *J. Pediatrics*. 95:6.

p. 751, Figure 33–7: From *Care of the High-Risk Neonate*, by M. Klaus, and A. Fanaroff, 3rd ed. Philadelphia: W. B. Saunders. 1979.

p. 753, Figure 33–11: From Starting IVs in Neonates (slide/tape presentation) by H. Bean, T. Harris, and J. Cornett. *University of Arizona Biomedical Communications*, Tucson, Arizona. 1978.

p. 754, Table 33–3: From Standards for CPR and ECC Part IV: Neonatal Advanced Life Support. 1986. *JAMA* 255(21): 2969–2973; and Emergency Drug Doses for Infants and Children, *Pediatrics* 81:3. 1988. American Academy of Pediatrics, Committee on Drugs.

p. 763, Table 34–1: From Maternal Transport, by H. Giles. 1979. *Clin. Obstet. Gynecol.* 6:206–207.

p. 765, Table 34–2: Used with permission of The Children's Hospital, Oakland.

pp. 768–772, Table 34–3, p. 773, Figure 34–3, and p. 775, Figure 34–4: Used with the permission of The Children's Hospital, Oakland.

p. 797, Figure 36–1: Courtesy of Obstetrics Department, Alta Bates Hospital, Berkeley, California.

p. 813, Figure 37–4: Jeff Weisman, Courtesy of Alta Bates Hospital.

p. 816, Table 37–1: From Nursing Care for the Emerging Family: Promoting Paternal Behavior, by W. Kunst-Wilson and L. Cronenwett. 1981. *Res. Nurs. Health.* 4:208.

p. 817, Figure 37–5: From Assessing Early Father-Infant Attachment, by M. Wieser, and P. Castiglia. 1984. *MCN*. 9:105.

p. 822, Figure 38–1: Courtesy of Ken Wittenberg.

p. 824, Figure 38–2: Courtesy of Sybil Shelton/Peter Arnold, Inc.

p. 832, Figure 38–3: Courtesy of Erika Stone/Photo Researchers, Inc.

p. 835, Figure 38–4, p. 837, Figure 38–5, and p. 838, Figure 38–6: Courtesy of Mary Ellen Mark.

p. 849, Table 39–1: From Dos and Don'ts of Deaf-Patient Care, by L. Sabatino, *National Magazine for Nurses*, 1976, Vol. 39, No. 6, pp. 64–68. Copyright 1976. Medical Economics Company, Inc., Oradell, NJ. Reprinted by permission.

p. 867, Figure 39–3: Courtesy of Andre.

p. 876–877, Table 40–1: Courtesy of *The Medical Letter*, 1987.

p. 878, Table 40–2: Adapted from Drug Use During Pregnancy, by W. F. Rayburn and F. P. Zuspan, *Perinatal Press*, 4(134)115–117. 1980. Reprinted by permission.

p. 878–881, Table 40–3: From *Drugs Used with Neonates and During Pregnancy*, 2nd ed., by I. L. Stile, T. Hegyi, and I. M. Hiatt. Copyright 1984. Oradell, NJ: Medical Economics Books.

p. 883, Table 40–4: From The Fetal Alcohol Syndrome, by S. K. Clarren and D. W. Smith, N. Eng. J. Med., 1978, 298, pp. 1063–1067; and Fetal Alcohol Syndrome and Other Related Birth Defects, by P. A. McCarthy, *Nurse Practitioner*, 1983, pp. 33–37.

pp. 894–896, Figures 41–1, 41–2, 41–3, 41–4: From *High Risk Pregnancy: A Team Approach* by R. A. Knuppel and J. Drukkee, Philadelphia: W. B. Saunders Co. 1986.

p. 899, Figure 41–5, p. 901, Figure 41–6 and p. 903, Figure 41–7: From Herpes Facts and Fallacies by E. J. Bertoli. AJN. 82:924, 1982.

p. 902, Table 41–1: From Parent Information: Herpes Simplex, by Trish Barrett, 1988. Alta Bates Hospital, *Infection Control Manual*, Berkeley, CA.

p. 908, Tables 41–5 and 41–6, and p. 909, Table 41–7: Courtesy of R. Farnher.

p. 920, Table 42–1: From *Birth and The Family Journal*, by M. Estes, 5:155–157. 1978.

p. 923, Figure 42–4: From Adapting the Birth Center Concept to a Traditional Hospital Setting, by S. S. Averitt, *J. Obstet. Gynecol. Neonatal Nursing*, 1980, 9(2), 105–106. Reprinted by permission.

p. 924, Table 42–2 and p. 926, Table 42–4: From Childbirth in the 1980's: What Are The Options? by S. A. Gillespie, *Issues in Health Care of Women*, 1981, 3:101–108. Reprinted by permission from Hemisphere Publishing Corporation, New York and Washington, D.C.

Chapter 1, Figure 1–4; Chapter 4, Figure 4–2; Chapter 11, Figure 11–3; Chapter 12, Figure 12–4; Chapter 13, Figure 13–1, 2b; Chapter 14, Figure 14–3; Chapter 15, Figure 15–3; Chapter 16, Figures 13–a through l; Chapter 17, Figure 17–10; Chapter 21, Figures 21–19b, 22, 24; Chapter 23, Figure 23–3; Chapter 24, Figure 24–3, 6; Chapter 27, Figure 27–1, 27–4b, 27–5, 27–6; Chapter 28, Figures 28–2, 3, 4; Chapter 29, Figure 29–1, 2, 3, 6, 7, 8, 9; Chapter 30, Figure 30–2; Chapter 31, Figure 31–1; Chapter 32, Figure 32–4; Chapter 33, Figure 33–2, 8, 9, 10, 12; Chapter 34, Figure 34–1, 2, 5; Chapter 37, Figure 37–2, 3; Chapter 43, Figure 43–4, 5, 6; Chapter 44, Figure 44–1: photos supplied by Jeff Weissman, Oakland, CA

Appendix B: Reprinted with permission of the American Nurses' Association.

Appendix C: Reprinted with permission of the American Nurses' Association.

Appendix D: Reprinted with permission of the American Hospital Association, copyright 1972.

Appendix E: "The Pregnant Patient's Bill of Rights/The Pregnant Patient's Responsibilities," written by Doris Haire and members of ICEA, published by International Childbirth Education Association, P. O. Box 20048, Minneapolis, Minnesota 55420.

Appendix H: From "The Development of Family-Centered Maternity/Newborn Care in Hospitals," *Journal of Obstetric, Gynecologic and Neonatal Nursing*, 1978, 7(5), 55–58. Reprinted by permission.

Appendix K: Adapted with permission from *Contraceptive Technology, 1984–1985*.

Appendix M: Reprinted with permission from JOGNN; March/April 1985, pp. 125–126.

Appendix N: Reprinted with permission from Alta Bates Hospital.

Appendix P: Copyright 1988. Children's Hospital, Oakland, CA. Reprinted with permission.